Ivosic

Medical Microbiology

An Introduction to Infectious Diseases

Medical Microbiology

An Introduction to Infectious Diseases

John C. Sherris, *Editor*
Professor, Department of Microbiology and Immunology
School of Medicine
University of Washington
Seattle, Washington

Kenneth J. Ryan
Professor and Chief, Clinical Microbiology
Departments of Pathology and of Microbiology and Immunology
College of Medicine
University of Arizona
Tucson, Arizona

C. George Ray
Professor and Chief, Clinical Virology-Serology Section
Department of Pathology
Professor and Chief, Section of Infectious Diseases
Department of Pediatrics
College of Medicine
University of Arizona
Tucson, Arizona

James J. Plorde
Professor, Departments of Laboratory Medicine and Medicine
University of Washington
Chief, Clinical Microbiology Section
Chief, Infectious Disease Section
Veterans Administration Medical Center
Seattle, Washington

Lawrence Corey
Professor and Head, Clinical Virology Division
Departments of Laboratory Medicine and Microbiology and Immunology
School of Medicine
University of Washington
Seattle, Washington

John Spizizen
Professor and Head, Department of Microbiology and Immunology
College of Medicine
University of Arizona
Tucson, Arizona

Chapter 56, Dental and Periodontal Infections, contributed by
Murray R. Robinovitch
Professor and Chairman, Department of Oral Biology
School of Dentistry
University of Washington
Seattle, Washington

Elsevier
New York • Amsterdam • Oxford

Elsevier Science Publishing Co., Inc.
52 Vanderbilt Avenue, New York, New York 10017

Sole distributors outside the United States and Canada:

Elsevier Science Publishers B.V.
P.O. Box 211, 1000 AE Amsterdam, The Netherlands

Library of Congress Cataloging in Publication Data

Main entry under title:

Medical microbiology.

Bibliography: p.
Includes index.
1. Medical microbiology. 2. Communicable diseases. I. Sherris, John C. II. Ryan, Kenneth J. [DNLM: 1. Communicable Diseases. 2. Microbiology. WC 100 M489]
QR46.M473 1984 616'.01 84-10183
ISBN 0-444-00854-3

Current printing (last digit)
10 9 8 7 6 5 4 3 2

Manufactured in the United States of America

This book is dedicated to
the late John D. Lawrence,
Director of Medical Publications of Elsevier,
whose enthusiasm, guidance, confidence, and support led to its completion.
He was a good friend and a strong supporter of medical microbiology
and will be sorely missed.

Contents

Preface xi
Acknowledgments xiii

1 **Overview** 1
John C. Sherris

2 **Bacterial Structure, Physiology, and Growth** 9
John Spizizen

3 **Nature of Viruses** 23
John Spizizen

4 **Microbial Death: Sterilization, Pasteurization, Disinfection, and Sanitization** 33
John C. Sherris

5 **Bacterial Variation and Genetics** 41
John Spizizen

6 **Normal Microbial Flora** 50
John C. Sherris

7 **Pathogenesis of Infection: Initial Defenses, Infectivity, Virulence, and Immune Response** 59
John C. Sherris and C. George Ray

8 **Epidemiology of Infectious Diseases** 76
Lawrence Corey

9 **Laboratory Diagnosis of Infectious Diseases** 88
Kenneth J. Ryan and C. George Ray

10 **Antimicrobics and Chemotherapy** 123
John C. Sherris

11 **Staphylococci** 150
John C. Sherris

12 **Streptococci** 162
Kenneth J. Ryan

13 **Corynebacteria and Other Non-Spore-Forming Gram-Positive Rods** 182
Kenneth J. Ryan

14 **Bacillus** 188
Kenneth J. Ryan

15 **Clostridia, Gram-Negative Anaerobes, and Anaerobic Cocci** 193
John C. Sherris

16 *Neisseria* 205
Kenneth J. Ryan

17 *Haemophilus, Bordetella,* and *Gardnerella* 216
Kenneth J. Ryan

18 *Mycoplasma* and *Ureaplasma* 228
Lawrence Corey

19 *Legionella* 233
Kenneth J. Ryan

20 Enterobacteriaceae 238
Kenneth J. Ryan

21 *Vibrio* and *Campylobacter* 258
Kenneth J. Ryan

22 *Pseudomonas* and Other Opportunistic Gram-Negative Bacilli 264
Kenneth J. Ryan

23 Some Bacteria Causing Zoonotic Diseases 271
Kenneth J. Ryan

24 Spirochetes 280
John C. Sherris

25 Mycobacteria 291
John C. Sherris

26 *Actinomyces* and *Nocardia* 305
Kenneth J. Ryan

27 Rickettsiae and Rickettsial Diseases 310
Lawrence Corey

28 *Chlamydia* 318
Lawrence Corey

29 Characteristics of Fungi 326
Kenneth J. Ryan

30 Superficial Fungi and Mycoses 334
Kenneth J. Ryan

31 *Candida* and Other Opportunistic Fungi 339
Kenneth J. Ryan

32 Systemic Fungal Pathogens 347
Kenneth J. Ryan

33 Subcutaneous Fungi and Disease 358
Kenneth J. Ryan

34 Respiratory Viruses 361
C. George Ray

35 Viruses of Mumps and Childhood Exanthems 378
C. George Ray

36 Poxviruses 390
C. George Ray

37 Enteroviruses 394
C. George Ray

38 Hepatitis Virus 403
Lawrence Corey

39 Herpesviruses 413
Lawrence Corey

40 Viruses of Diarrhea 427
C. George Ray

41 Arthropod-Borne and Other Zoonotic Viruses 434
C. George Ray

42 Rabies 446
Lawrence Corey

43 Slow Viruses and Tumor Viruses 451
Lawrence Corey

44 **Introduction to Pathogenic Parasites** 460
James J. Plorde

45 **Sporozoan Infections** 469
James J. Plorde

46 **Rhizopod Infections** 484
James J. Plorde

47 **Flagellate Infections** 491
James J. Plorde

48 ***Pneumocystis carinii*** **Infections** 509
James J. Plorde

49 **Intestinal Nematodes** 513
James J. Plorde

50 **Tissue Nematodes** 526
James J. Plorde

51 **Cestode Infections** 535
James J. Plorde

52 **Trematode Infections** 545
James J. Plorde

53 **Skin and Wound Infections** 555
John C. Sherris

54 **Bone and Joint Infections** 562
C. George Ray

55 **Eye, Ear, and Sinus Infections** 567
C. George Ray

56 **Dental and Periodontal Infections** 574
Murray R. Robinovitch

57 **Upper Respiratory Tract Infections and Stomatitis** 580
C. George Ray

58 **Middle and Lower Respiratory Tract Infections** 584
C. George Ray and Kenneth J. Ryan

59 **Enteric Infections and Food Poisoning** 592
Kenneth J. Ryan

60 **Urinary Tract Infections** 601
James J. Plorde

61 **Central Nervous System Infections** 608
C. George Ray

62 **Intravascular Infections, Bacteremia, and Endotoxemia** 616
C. George Ray and Kenneth J. Ryan

63 **Infections of the Fetus and Newborn** 629
C. George Ray

64 **Sexually Transmitted Diseases** 637
Lawrence Corey

65 **Infections in the Immunocompromised Patient** 649
Lawrence Corey

66 **Nosocomial Infections and Infection Control** 655
Kenneth J. Ryan

New Developments in Medical Microbiology 665

Glossary 669

Index 677

Preface

Half a century ago, it was reasonable to expect medical and other health sciences students to acquire a rather comprehensive knowledge of all the scientific disciplines bearing on medicine. Over the intervening years, this objective has become increasingly impracticable because of the additions to knowledge of basic biologic mechanisms, the emergence of important new diseases, and the development of new biomedical procedures that have had to find their place in curricula. Thus, it has become increasingly important for the educator to be selective, and for education in medical microbiology to relate to the student's career objectives. In this book we have tried to illustrate basic biologic principles with medically applicable examples wherever possible and to develop the subject with a view to its application to clinical work.

We have focused on those aspects of microbiology that we believe to be essential to understanding the pathogenesis, epidemiology, laboratory diagnosis, prevention, and therapy of major infectious disease processes and have omitted details of microbiology that do not illustrate important principles or tend to be rapidly forgotten by those not specializing in the subject. We have not attempted to cover all microbial and parasitic diseases because we wished to avoid being excessively synoptic. Rather, we have covered particular diseases in some depth to give a better basis for understanding the processes involved. Tables and appendices have been used to illustrate the greater breadth of the subject, but, in general, should be considered illustrative and as sources of information and not to be committed to memory.

We have concentrated primarily on infections that occur in developed countries, but have also covered some of the major parasitic diseases of critical importance elsewhere. Throughout, the text is intended to serve as a basis for further study, and this is especially important for those who will work in areas where major tropical or parasitologic infections persist. A few references to monographs, reviews, and papers that we consider to be especially useful have been cited at the end of most of the microbiology chapters. Comprehensive bibliographies were beyond the scope of the book, and we consider that further readings to illustrate the processes of scientific thought and advance are best selected by course instructors.

We elected not to include a section on immunology because this subject has long outgrown its microbiologic origins. It is increasingly taught as an independent discipline, and there are several excellent immunology texts specifically designed for the medical and health sciences student. Chapter 7 on the pathogenesis of infectious diseases does, however, review some basic immunologic concepts that find application in subsequent chapters. Throughout the book we have assumed some prior knowledge of biochemistry, cell biology, anatomy, and histology, but we have included a glossary of terms, especially clinical and technical terms, that may be unfamiliar to some students.

The introductory chapter is an overview of the whole topic of the book and is intended to help place subsequent chapters within a broad perspective. It may merit rereading at a later stage. Chapters 1 through 10 are concerned with those general aspects of microbiology and infection that apply to most of the organisms and diseases considered elsewhere. Chapters 11 through 52 cover specific organisms and their relation to human health and disease. The final chapters are devoted to important disease syndromes or classes of infections as encountered in clinical or epidemiologic work. This approach involved some repetition and overlap, but we believe it is important to integrate the microbiologic material into the clinical context.

Marginal notations are used throughout to highlight key points and to serve as a rapid guide for review. Marginal illustrations of microbial morphology and arrangement are also used in many chapters. In these we have shown Gram-positivity of bacteria by shading within the organisms and Gram-negativity by drawing them in outline. Students may find the unused sections of the margins helpful for their own supplementary notes.

The study of medicine involves a continuous process of learning and updating, and it is unrealistic to expect a health sciences student to master, in a single course, all the material that may ultimately be needed and still retain a capacity for originality and scholarship. Thus, we have aimed to provide students with a book on which to build and to do it in as readable form as possible. We will have succeeded if it helps catch their interest and enthusiasm while developing a firm understanding of the principles of medical microbiology and infectious diseases.

John C. Sherris
Editor

Acknowledgments

The authors wish to acknowledge and thank many people who have helped us in preparation of the book: Doctors Joseph Davie, Charles Evans, Stanley Falkow, Hjordis Foy, Neal Groman, Mary Jane Hicks, George Kenny, Barbara Kirby, William Kirby, Frederick Neidhardt, Peter Perine, Howard Raff, Fritz Schoenknecht, and Peter Sherris reviewed sections of the manuscript. In particular Davise Larone reviewed the whole Mycology section. The final result is, of course, the sole responsibility of the authors.

The mycology and parasitology drawings and all but two of the marginal drawings were the work of Sam C. Eng, Clinical Technologist of the Clinical Microbiology Laboratories of the University of Washington. Sam C. Eng and Dr. Fritz Schoenknecht provided several of the color plates and figures.

Philip Schafer of Elsevier steered the book into production with skill and good humor, and Loretta Linser was responsible for the excellent copy editing.

Ellen Meyer and Elizabeth Sherris typed most of the various drafts of the manuscript, and Elizabeth Sherris devoted very many hours to the organization of the book (and of the editor) as it developed.

Medical Microbiology

An Introduction to Infectious Diseases

A. Staphylococcal pus (Gram)

B. Colonies of *S. aureus (top)* and *S. epidermidis (bottom)*

C. Streptococcal pus (Gram)

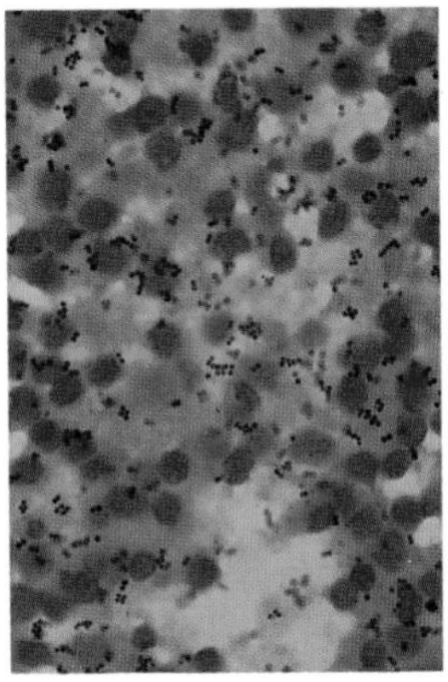
A

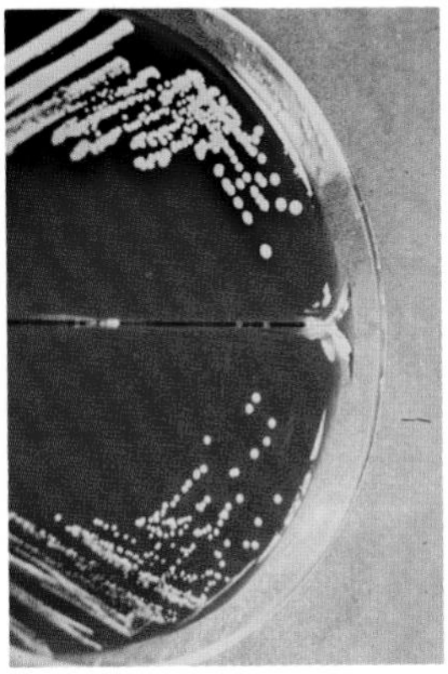
B

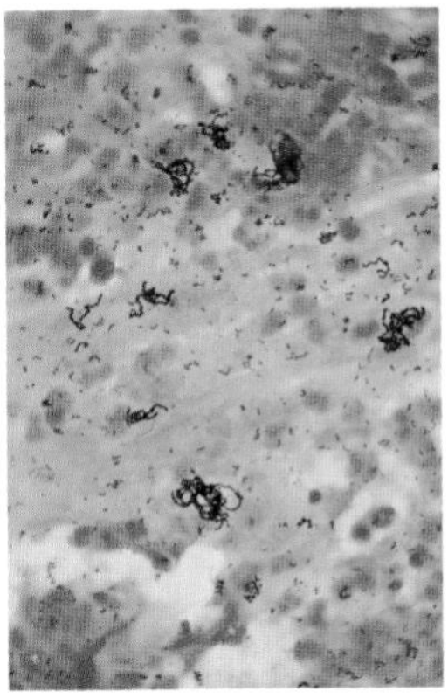
C

D. Pneumococci in CSF (Gram) of a case of fulminant meningitis

E. Fluorescence antibody staining of *S. pyogenes (Kindly provided by C.Evans Roberts)*

F. β hemolysis of *S. pyogenes*

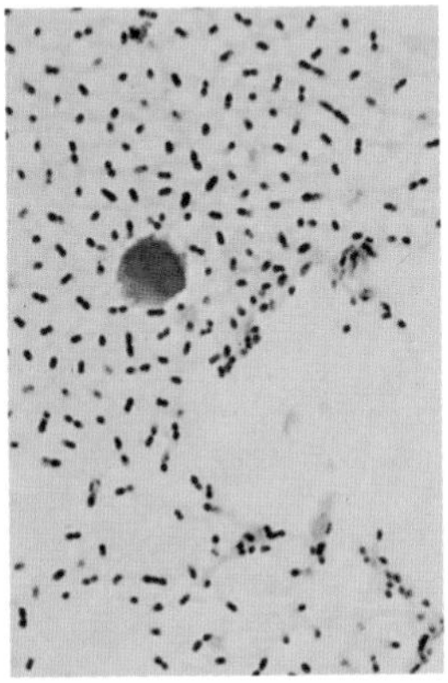
D

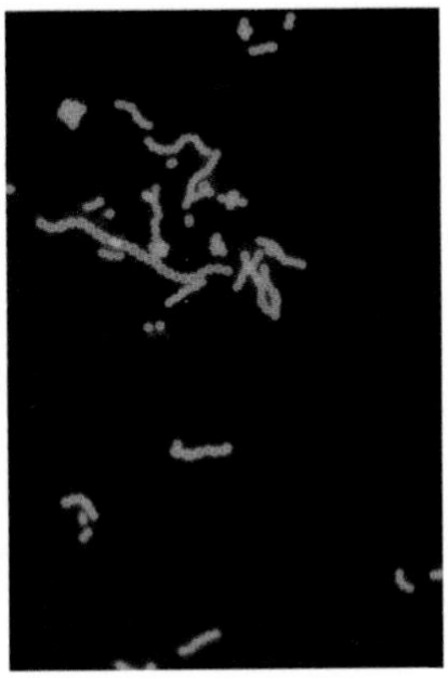
E

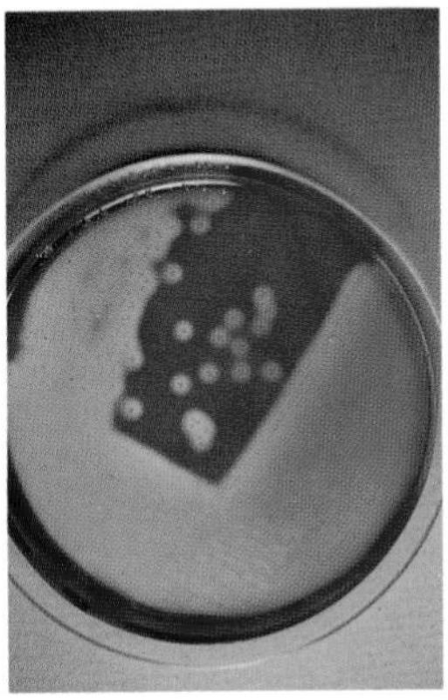
F

G. α hemolysis of *S. pneumoniae*

H. Listeria monocytogenes in CSF (Gram)

I. Low power of smear from clostridial myositis (Gram)

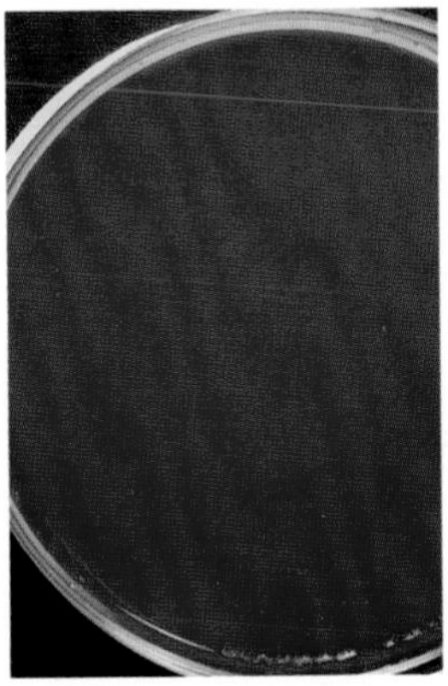
G

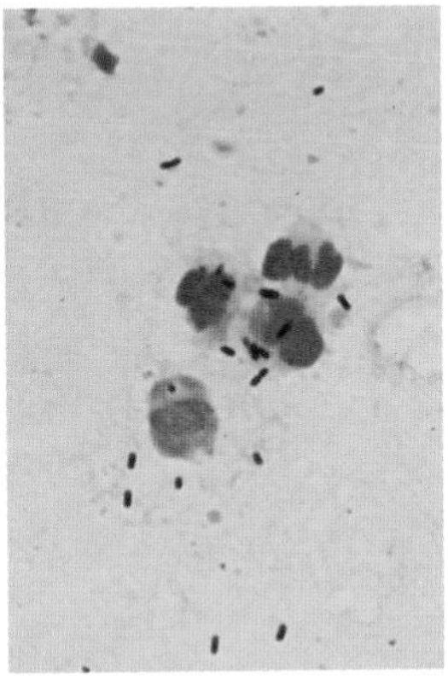
H

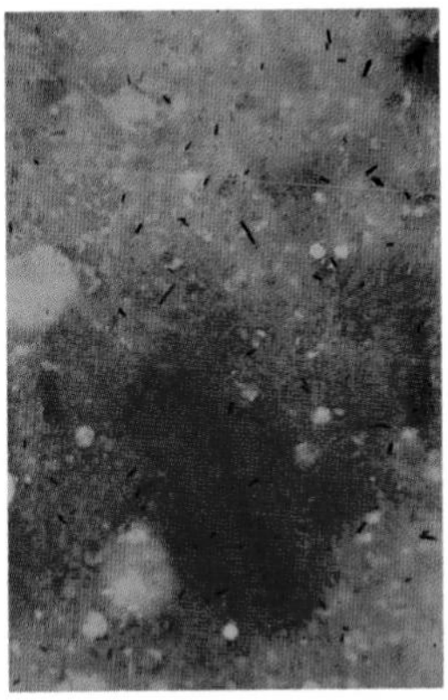
I

J. *C. perfringens* colonies on blood agar medium

K. Nagler test for *C. perfringens* α toxin (antitoxin incorporated at bottom)

L. Pus from subphrenic abscess due to mixed anaerobes (Gram)

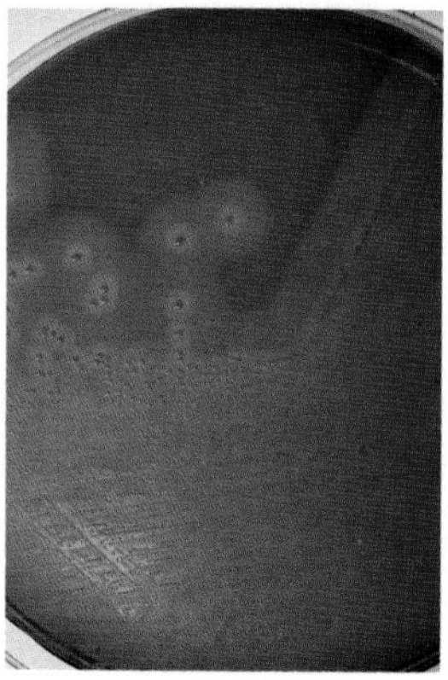

J

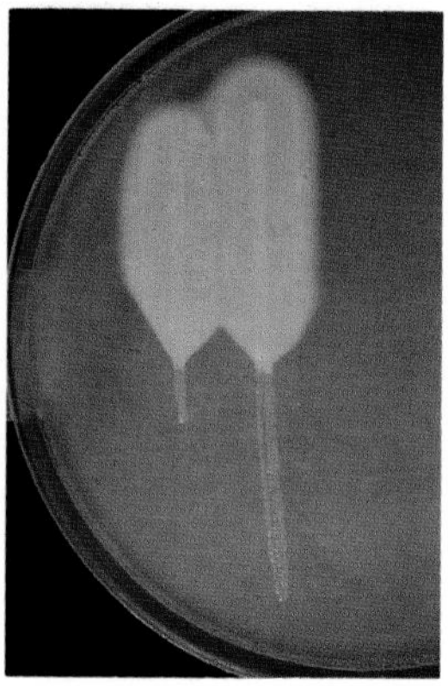

K

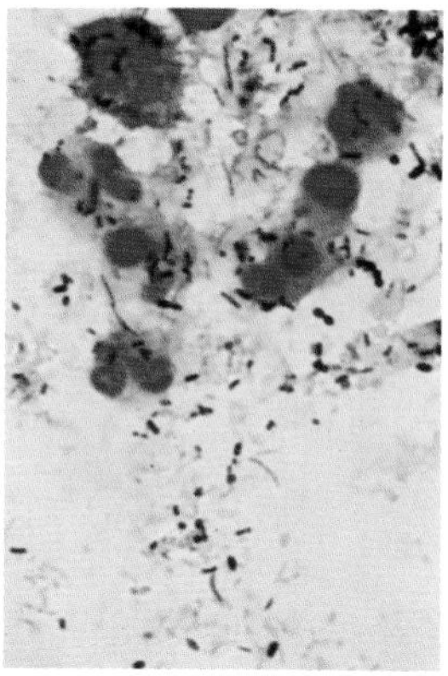

L

M. *N. gonorrhoeae* in urethral pus (Gram)

N. Oxidase reaction of gonococcal colonies on chocolate agar

O. *H. influenzae* in sputum of patient with pneumonia (Gram)

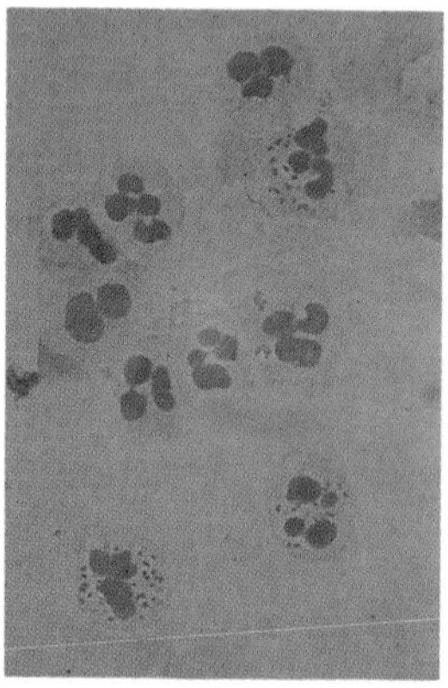

M

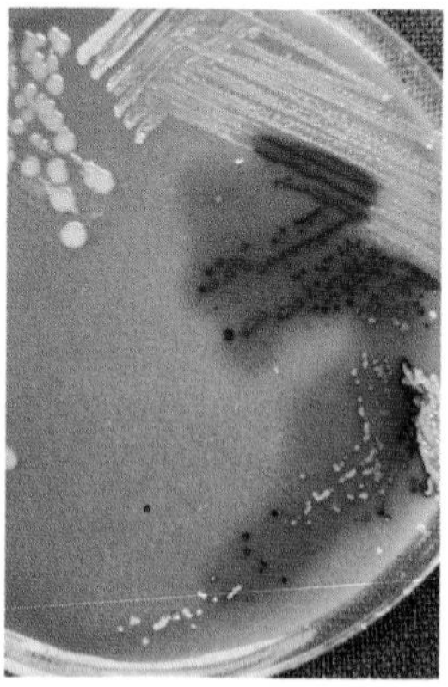

N

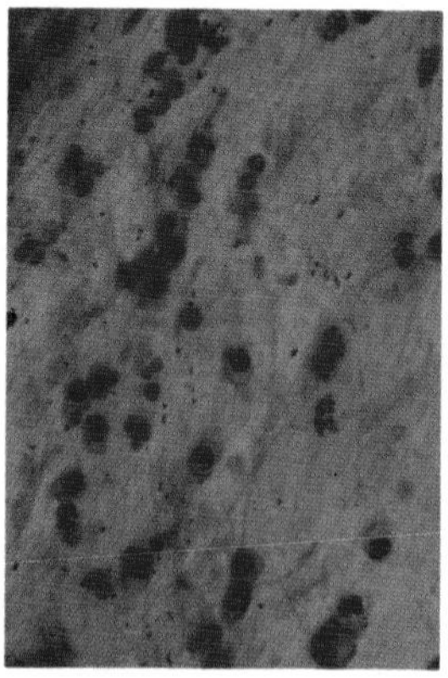

O

P. Direct Gram stain of *E. coli*-infected urine

Q. Colonies of lactose-fermenting *(red)* and nonfermenting species on MacConkey's agar

R. Colonies of *Mycoplasma* X200 *(kindly provided by G.E. Kenny)*

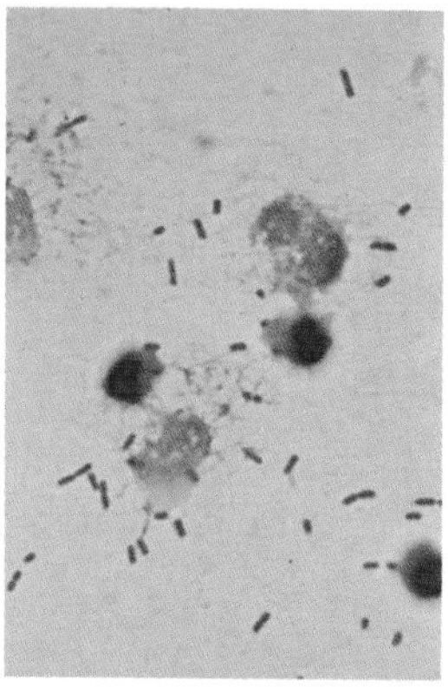

P

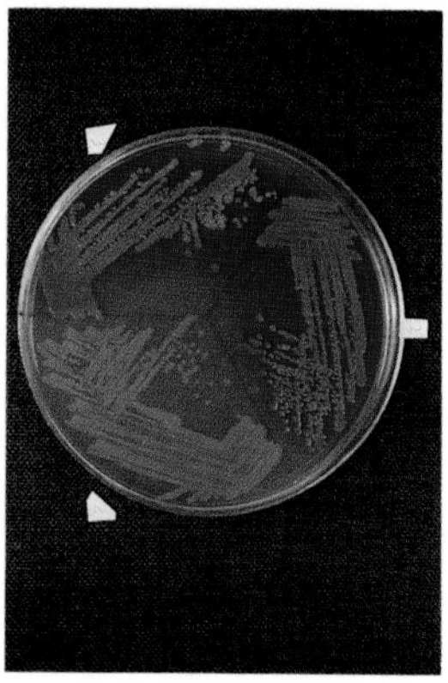

Q

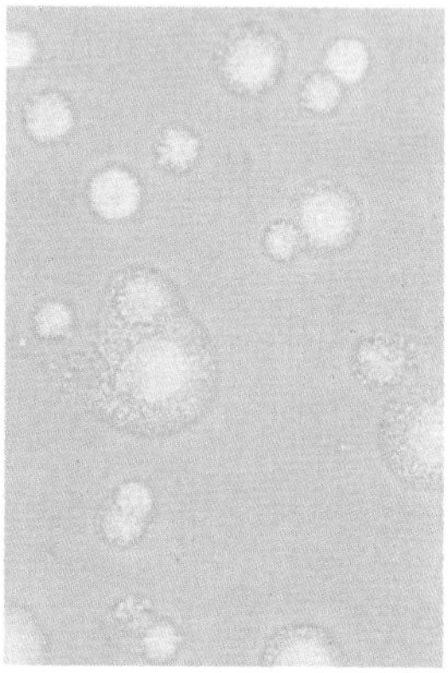

R

S. Overnight growth of *P. aeruginosa* on nutrient agar showing pigment

T. Acid-fast stain of sputum from a patient with tuberculosis

U. Acid-fast stain of smear of skin from patient with lepromatous leprosy *(from Armed Forces Institute of Pathology)*

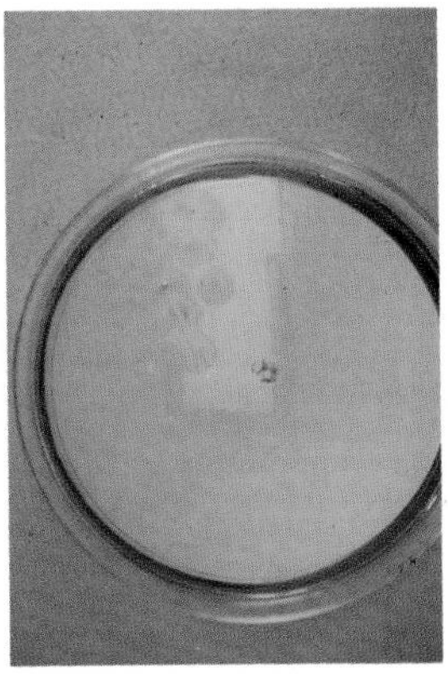

S

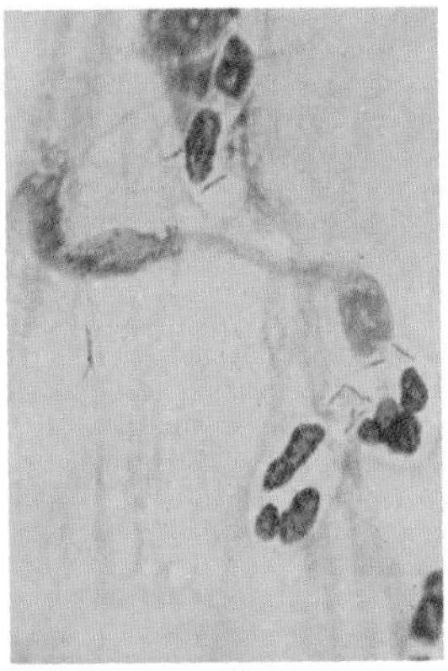

T

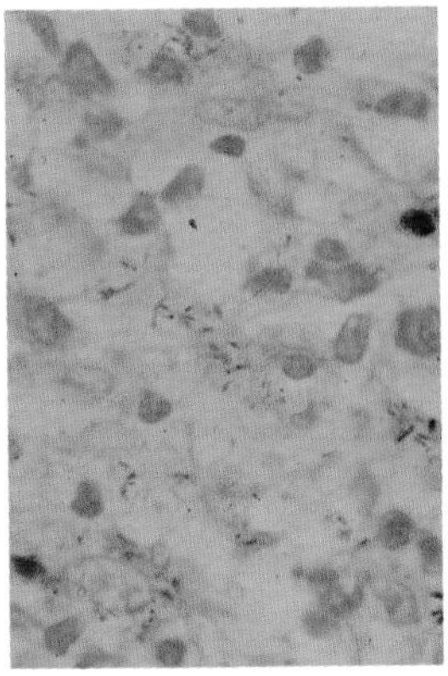

U

V. Crushed small sulfur granule from patient with actinomycosis X100

W. Macular rash in rubella

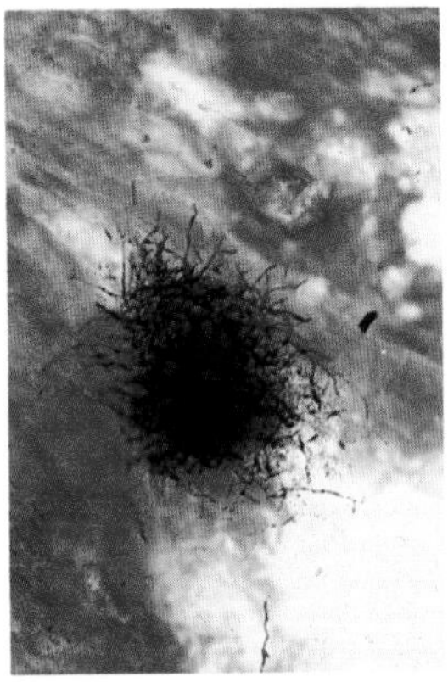

V

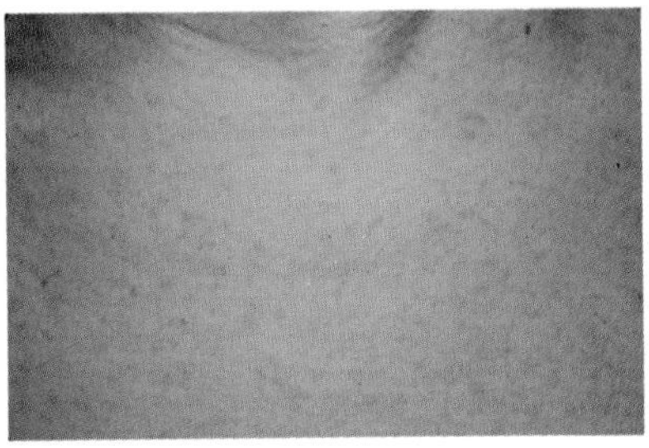

W

X. Maculopapular rash in measles

Y. Vesicles in a herpes simplex finger infection

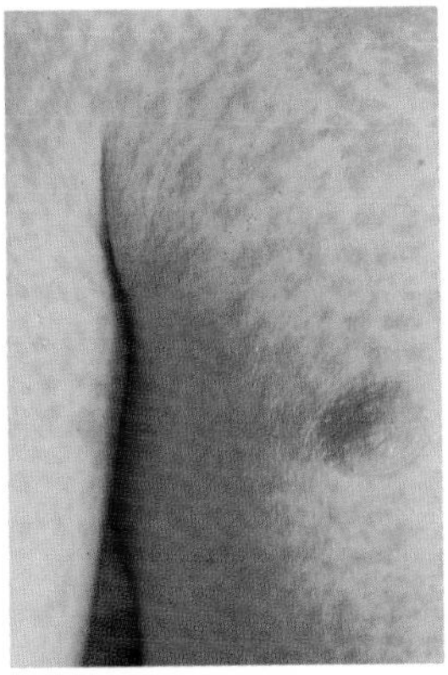

X

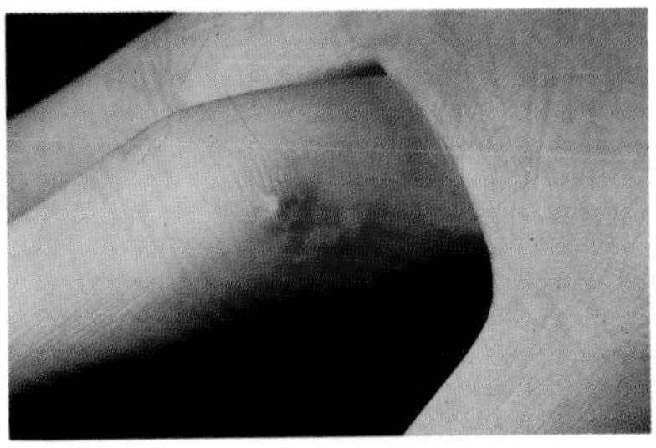

Y

Z. Varicella infection in an immunosuppressed child with leukemia

AA. Chromoblastomycosis tissue section *(reproduced with permission from Dr. E.S. Beneke and the Upjohn Company; Scope Publications, Human Mycoses).*

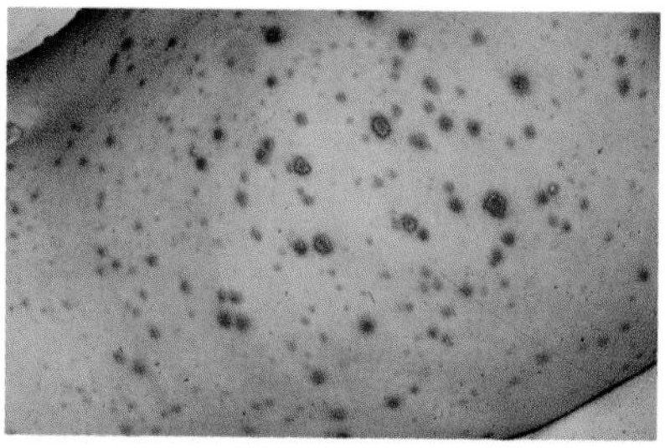

Z

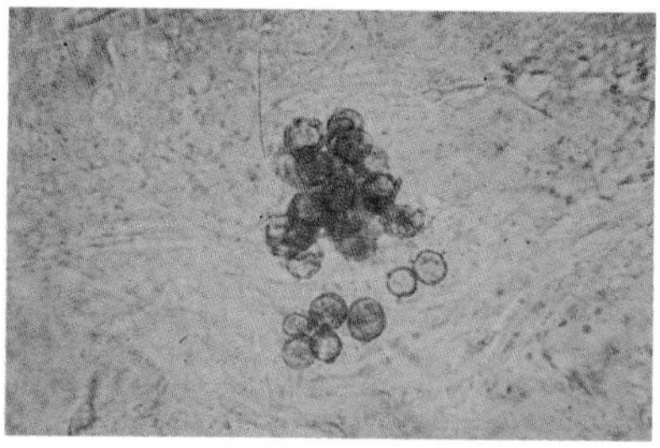

AA

BB. Zygomycosis nonseptate hyphae in tissue *(reproduced with permission from Dr. E.S. Beneke and the Upjohn Company; Scope Publications, Human Mycoses).*

CC. *Cryptococcus neoformans* in tissue *(reproduced with permission from Dr. E.S. Beneke and the Upjohn Company; Scope Publications, Human Mycoses).*

DD. Molds in culture *(reproduced with permission from Dr. E.S. Beneke and the Upjohn Company; Scope Publications, Human Mycoses).*

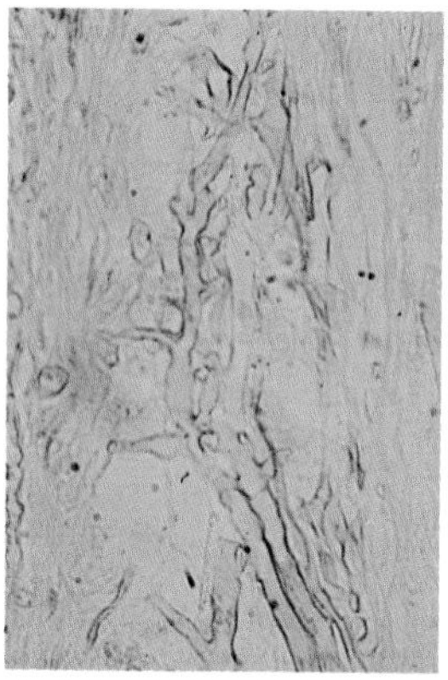

BB

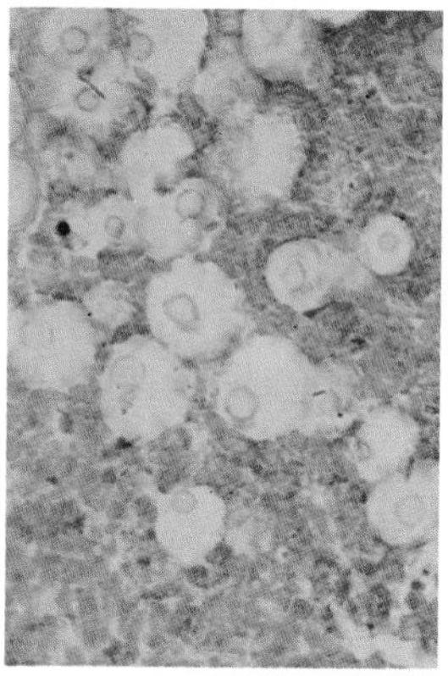

CC

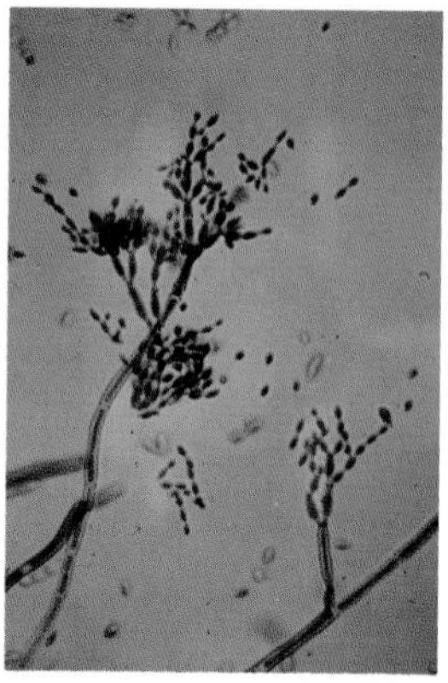

DD

Examples of Erythrocytic Stages of Malarial Parasites

	Trophozoite Ring Form	Late Trophozoite	Merozoite	Male Gametocyte
Plasmodium vivax	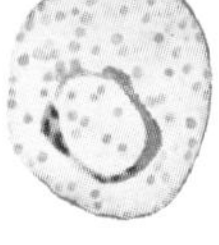	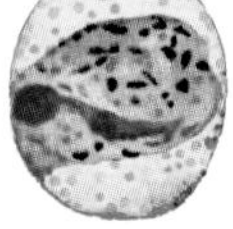	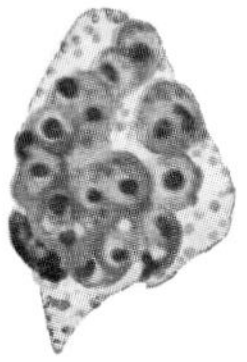	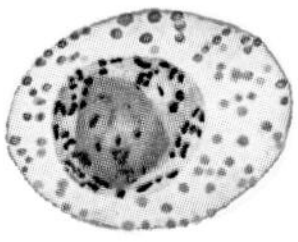
Plasmodium malariae	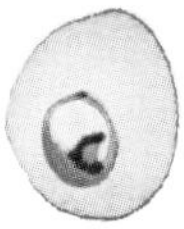	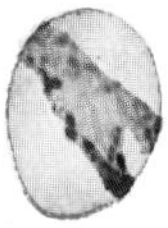	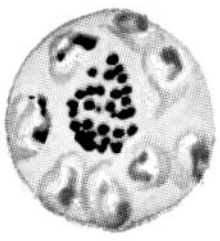	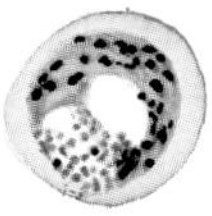
Plasmodium falciparum	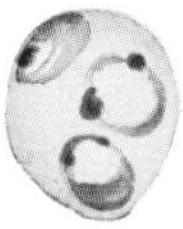	Not usually seen in blood. Occur in visceral capillaries		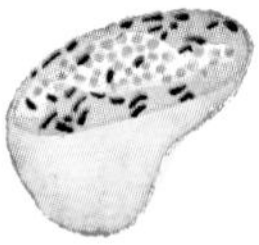

Source: Reproduced with permission from illustrations of a complete series of erythrocytic states in Brown, H.W. and Neva, F.A., *Basic Clinical Parasitology,* 5th ed., Appleton-Century-Crofts, East Norwalk, Connecticut. Copyright 1983 by Appleton-Century-Crofts.

John C. Sherris

Overview

1

Nine months of microbial innocence

During its development in the uterus, the fetus exists in a homeostatic environment, protected from contact with other living things by the cellular and humoral defenses of the mother and by the filtering capacity of the placenta. Thus, in most cases the fetal tissues are sterile, although occasionally microorganisms infecting the mother can transgress the placenta and invade the fetus. Congenital rubella and congenital syphilis, for example, can cause permanent damage to the developing fetus. Normally, however, the infant first encounters microorganisms immediately after the fetal membranes rupture; these microorganisms are usually derived from the normal inhabitants of the mother's uterine cervix and vagina.

Entry into microbial world

At birth, the infant enters an enormously complex microbial ecosystem. Some inhabitants of this microbial world have adapted to colonize the external, alimentary, upper respiratory, and vaginal surfaces of humans (and other creatures) in vast numbers—generally to their mutual benefit. A few have the capacity to cause disease by invading the tissues, producing toxic substances, or both. Most, however, are free living and nonparasitic to other organisms, and many play a central part in shaping the environment of our planet. Without these microbes other life forms as we know them could not exist.

Roles of microorganisms in nature

Microorganisms, which are by definition invisible to the unaided eye, are responsible for much of the breakdown and natural recycling of organic material in the environment. Some can fix atmospheric nitrogen to synthesize nitrogen-containing inorganic and organic compounds and thus contribute to the nutrition of living things that lack this ability. Some can use atmospheric carbon dioxide as a source of carbon for organic compounds; others (the oceanic algae) are instrumental in the production of atmospheric oxygen through their use of atmospheric CO_2 for photosynthesis. Thus, microorganisms play central roles in the nitrogen and carbon cycles and in maintaining the atmospheric oxygen level.

Microbial diversity

Very few areas on the surface of the planet do not support microbial life, because microorganisms have an astounding range of metabolic and energy-yielding abilities, and many can exist under conditions that are lethal to other life forms. For example, some bacteria can oxidize inorganic compounds such as sulfur or ammonium ions to generate energy, and some can survive and multiply in hot springs at temperatures over 75°C. Iron-oxidizing bacteria can cause serious damage to water pipes when the water contains other required nutrients at an optimum pH. Many microorganisms can only metabolize fermentatively, using substances other than oxygen as terminal hydrogen acceptors, and thus live under conditions of extreme reduction. Some of these are cellulolytic and can multiply rapidly in masses of decaying vegetation in the absence of oxygen. To many, oxygen is rapidly lethal.

Human exploitation of microbial world

The metabolic heterogeneity and diverse synthetic abilities of microorganisms have led to their application to human purposes. These uses include alcoholic fermentation in the production of wines, beers, and spirits, composting techniques, and the mass production of complex organic compounds such as vitamin B_{12} and various antibiotics or their precursors. In many cases, because microorganisms multiply rapidly and have a relatively simple genome, mutants that improve quality and yield have been readily selected in the laboratory. Recently, through the use of recombinant DNA techniques, genes coding for the synthesis of hormones such as human insulin have been added to the genetic makeup of bacteria, which may then produce the desired complex product in culture. Because of this relatively simple and manipulable genetic structure, the science of molecular biology developed from studies on microbial genetics and, in turn, led to practical application of this knowledge in areas such as recombinant DNA technology.

Symbiosis

Some microbial species have adapted to symbiotic relationships with higher forms of life. For example, bacteria that can fix atmospheric nitrogen colonize the root systems of legumes and of a few trees such as alders and provide the plant with its nitrogen requirements. When the plant dies or is plowed under, the fertility of the soil is enhanced by nitrogenous compounds originally derived from the bacterial metabolism. Ruminants can use grasses as their prime source of nutrition because the abundant flora of anaerobic bacteria in the rumen breaks down cellulose and other plant compounds into usable carbohydrates and amino acids and synthesizes essential nutrients, including some amino acids and vitamins. These few examples illustrate the protean nature of microbial life and their essential place in our ecosystem.

Classes of microorganisms that interact with humans

It is because these organisms are essential to the existence of life that the study of general microbiology and of the role of microorganisms in nature is of great interest. This book, however, has a narrower anthropocentric focus: it is concerned with those microorganisms directly involved in the maintenance of health or causation of disease in humans. Within this context, we will consider four broad classes of microorganisms that interact with humans: bacteria, fungi, viruses, and protozoa. We have extended our definition of microbiology to include some disease-producing multicellular parasites—the helminths and flukes—that are macroscopic at some stages of their life cycles; indeed, intestinal tapeworms can measure many feet in length and become discomfortingly obvious.

Fungi and protozoa

Among the microorganisms that infect or coexist with humans, the fungi and protozoa have many of the cellular characteristics found in mammalian or plant cells: nuclear membranes, diploid chromosomal arrangements, mitotic apparatus, mitochondria, sterol-containing cell membranes, and, in many cases, the ability to reproduce sexually. These microorganisms are termed *eukaryotes* because of their "true" nuclear structure. Their size is quite variable; although width or diameter rarely exceeds 10 μm (0.01 mm), length may be much greater. Most fungi and some protozoa can be grown in culture on artificial media.

Bacteria

The bacteria are generally smaller, simpler, and probably more primitive than the fungi and protozoa. Their nuclear material comprises a single, double-stranded, but very large DNA molecule without a structural nuclear membrane. They are thus described as *prokaryotic*; they are haploid with no true sexual mode of reproduction. Many possess autonomous self-replicating smaller circular DNA molecules, termed plasmids, which are transmissible between bacteria and code for properties that facilitate their survival. Bacteria have no mitochondria, their cytoplasmic membranes generally contain no sterols, and they have a unique and usually very rigid cell wall structure. Most divide by binary fission and can be grown in artificial culture, often with extraordinary rapidity. For example, many bacteria have a doubling time under ideal conditions of about 20 min; thus, under optimal growth conditions, a single organism can yield a population of more than 10^9 after only 8 hr. Such growth rates are rarely, if ever, achieved in the human body; severe bacterial disease, nevertheless, can develop very rapidly. The major differences between prokaryotic and eukaryotic cells are listed in Table 1.1.

Viruses

The viruses, a totally distinct group of infecting agents, are strict intracellular parasites of other living cells—not only of mammalian and plant cells but also of simple unicellular organisms, including bacteria (the bacteriophages). The viruses are simple forms of replicating, biologically active particles that carry genetic information in either DNA or RNA molecules, but never both. Most mature viruses have a protein coat over their nucleic acid and sometimes a lipid surface membrane derived from the cell that they infect. They lack the protein-synthesizing enzymes and structural apparatus for their own replication; they bear essentially no resemblance to a true eukaryotic or prokaryotic cell. Viruses replicate by using their genetically active nucleic acids to subvert the metabolic activities of the cell that they infect to bring about the synthesis and reassembly of their component parts. A cell infected with a single viral particle may thus yield many hundreds of viral particles, which can be assembled almost simultaneously under the

Table 1.1 Distinctive Features of Prokaryotic and Eukaryotic Cells

Cell Component	Prokaryotes	Eukaryotes
Nucleus	No membrane, single circular chromosome	Membrane-bounded, a number of individual chromosomes
Extrachromosomal DNA	May be present in form of plasmid (s)	In organelles
Organelles in cytoplasm	None	Mitochondria (and chloroplasts in photosynthetic organisms)
Cytoplasmic membrane	Contains enzymes of respiration. Active secretion of enzymes. Site of phospholipid and DNA synthesis	Semipermeable layer not possessing functions of prokaryotic membrane
Cell wall	Rigid layer of peptidoglycan (absent in *Mycoplasma*)	No peptidoglycan (in some cases cellulose present)
Sterols	Absent (except in *Mycoplasma*)	Usually present
Ribosomes	70S in cytoplasm	80S in cytoplasmic reticulum

direction of the viral nucleic acid. Cell death and infection of other cells by the newly formed viruses usually result. Sometimes, viral and cell reproduction proceed simultaneously without cell death.

The origin of viruses is obscure; they share characteristics with genes, with plasmids, and with certain simple, obligately intracellular bacteria. Indeed, different groups of viruses show such disparate characteristics that some could conceivably have originated from each of these sources.

viral integration

The close association of the virus with the cell sometimes results in the integration of viral nucleic acid into the functional nucleic acid of the cell, producing a latent infection that can be transmitted intact to the progeny of the cell. Integration may be facilitated by mutational changes in the host or viral nucleic acid. The integrated viral genome can be silent, producing no detectable metabolic effect, or it may encode the production of a new or altered protein. The production of diphtheria toxin, for example, is encoded by a bacteriophage integrated into the chromosome of the diphtheria bacillus.

latent viral infections

Carriage of viral nucleic acid may be passed longitudinally through successive generations of inbred animals; some of these latent viral infections are associated with a high incidence of specific tumors in animals. An excision of integrated viral nucleic acid sometimes leads to production of complete viral particles and death of the host cell. Other types of viral latency will be described in more detail in Chapter 3. Suffice it to say that in some cases, such as herpes simplex infections, latency between clinical attacks of disease may not be consequent to viral integration, but probably to a balance between the virus and the immunologic response of the host: when host immunity declines, relapse occurs.

Normal bacterial flora

Although certain viruses can coexist with humans without causing disease, most of the known normal microbial inhabitants of man are bacteria. The skin and the alimentary, upper respiratory, and vaginal tracts all play host to numerous bacteria that are amazingly well adapted to survive under the physiologic and nutritional conditions found in these sites. These organisms often maintain themselves by adhering specifically to epithelial cells and multiplying on their surfaces. In some cases, organisms of the normal flora are directly beneficial to the host: they prime the immune system or synthesize nutritionally useful products, such as vitamin K. The normal flora also benefits the host indirectly by providing formidable competition to colonization and infection by pathogenic bacteria. Elimination of this competition by removal of normal floral organisms with antibiotic treatment increases susceptibility to many bacterial infections.

Endogenous infections

Many members of the normal flora are not devoid of pathogenic potential: if sufficient numbers reach normally sterile areas of the body (for example, tissues, peritoneal cavity, bladder, or lower respiratory tract), they may cause severe or even fatal infections. These infections can result from mechanical causes, such as a ruptured intestine, or from a congenital or acquired failure of some critical component of the immune system that normally helps to prevent organisms from transgressing body surfaces or removes them when the day-to-day minor accidents of life deposit them in the tissues. This process is largely effected by the phagocytic cell system and enhanced by the early inflammatory response.

Exogenous infections

Infection by extraneous organisms (those not part of the body's indigenous flora) may be secondary to structural or functional damage to surface structures that normally exclude them (for example, a third-degree burn of the skin or damage to the bronchial ciliated epithelium from smoking) or result from invasion through intact epithelia. Organisms that can invade an individual with intact cellular and humoral immune mechanisms have specific determinants of virulence that allow them to multiply in the host and avoid eradication by the body's first line of phagocytic cell defenses. Determinants of virulence are multiple and differ for various species. Most virulent organisms can attach to and penetrate epithelial cell barriers and thus initiate infection. Some are resistant to phagocytosis, some produce substances that kill phagocytes or inhibit their migration, and some are resistant to destruction after phagocytosis. Intracellular existence and multiplication protect viruses and some bacteria, fungi, and protozoa from humoral immune mechanisms as long as they remain within the cell. Some bacteria produce enzymes that destroy immunoglobulin A. In most cases, the ability to circumvent the body's defenses is relative, and organisms must be numerous to initiate infection that may progress with simultaneous destruction and multiplication of the infecting agent.

Determinants of virulence

Mechanisms of damage to host

The mere presence of microorganisms multiplying in the tissues does not necessarily produce disease; however, many produce toxic substances, some highly potent and pharmacologically specific, that facilitate spread of the infection or damage remote organ systems. Damage also results from the body's response to infection through inflammation, through immediate or delayed hypersensitivity to microbial antigens, or through local or remote tissue responses to immune complexes. Some organisms can cause disease without penetrating mucous membranes through the effects of their highly potent toxins. Such toxins are often produced in the intestinal tract or, in some cases, in food before ingestion.

Immune responses of host

During the course of an infection, the body's adaptive immune mechanisms, both specific and nonspecific, come into play. The local inflammatory reaction mobilizes phagocytes and serum antimicrobial factors. Polymorphonuclear leukocytosis often develops in bacterial infections and increases the number of phagocytic cells; fever may slow down multiplication of some infecting agents and increase the effectiveness of specific antimicrobial processes in the body. Antigen, often processed by macrophages, primes and leads to multiplication of specific immunologically active lymphoid cells of both the T and B series. Antibody with specific attachment sites for the infecting agent and for phagocytic cells increases the efficiency of phagocytosis or abrogates the effectiveness of antiphagocytic surface components of some bacteria, a process in which complement collaborates. In some cases, direct killing of the pathogen results from the action of complement on antibody-coated cells; in others, antibody blocks attachment sites on the surface of strict intracellular parasites such as viruses, thus halting the cycle of spread from cell to cell. Cell-mediated immune mechanisms serve to increase the activity of macrophages and of other mechanisms directed against intracellular pathogens. Interferon production, which plays a major role in blocking the intracellular replication of viruses, also appears to interact with natural killer cells to increase their efficiency in destroying virus-infected cells. These processes are but a few of the diverse and often interacting defense mechanisms that the body mounts against infecting agents.

Outcome of infection

The outcome of an infection is determined by the size of the infecting dose, the site of infection, the virulence of the organism, and the speed and effectiveness of the immune response. Most infections transmitted between humans would ultimately be controlled by the body's defenses without therapeutic intervention, because selective pressures over the course of human history have been toward a balanced state of parasitism that ensures survival of both host and parasite. Organisms that are pathogenic to humans but for which the primary reservoirs are nonhuman may, however, show extraordinary virulence (for example, rabies virus), because they are not subject to pressure toward balanced parasitism in our species. Genetic recombination between human and nonhuman organisms may also produce strains of unusual virulence, which may account for the 1918–1919 influenza pandemic that took more lives than World War I.

Epidemic spread

Many infections, other than those caused by members of the normal flora, may spread epidemically. Epidemics range from those in small, closed communities or hospitals to those with massive, worldwide spread. The factors determining the occurrence, spread, and resolution of epidemics are complex, but can often be influenced by medical and public health intervention. To produce a transmissible epidemic, an organism must have a sufficient degree of infectivity and conditions must exist that permit spread. These conditions may include direct contact (impetigo), aerial transmission (influenza), contaminated food or water (typhoid), or the presence of essential insect vectors (malaria). The degree of innate and acquired immunity in the population must be sufficiently low for the rate of infection to be amplified as the disease spreads. Epidemic spread and disease are facilitated by malnutrition, poor socioeconomic conditions, natural disasters, and hygienic inadequacy. In previous centuries epidemics often caused high morbidity and mortality and massive dislocation of society because of the pervasive fear and helplessness they produced. Some of these epidemics were certainly caused by the introduction of "new" organisms of unusual virulence into the population affected. The possibility of recurrence of old pandemic infections, especially pandemic influenza, remains of concern. Our understanding of the epidemiology and immunology of individual diseases facilitates their control, however, and led to one of medicine's greatest successes: the eradication of smallpox. As the focus of medicine moves increasingly toward prevention, it becomes even more important for all health care workers to understand the principles and control of epidemic spread.

Chemotherapy

Over the past 40 years, therapeutic tools of remarkable potency and specificity have become available for the treatment of infections. These agents include all of the antibiotics and an array of synthetic chemicals with action against infecting organism, but minimal or acceptable toxicity for the host. Most are antibacterial and exploit the structural and metabolic differences between bacterial and eukaryotic cells to provide the selectivity necessary for good antimicrobial therapy. Penicillin, for example, interferes with the synthesis of the bacterial cell wall, a structure that has no analog in human cells. There are fewer antifungal and antiprotozoal agents, because of closer metabolic and structural similarities between the eukaryotic cells of the host and those of the parasite. Nevertheless, there are a series of significant differences, and effective therapeutic agents have been discovered or developed to exploit them.

Specific therapeutic attack on viral disease has posed more complex problems, because of the intimate involvement of viral replication with the metabolic and replicative activities of the cell. Thus, most substances that inhibit viral replication have unacceptable toxicity to host cells. Some successful antiviral agents have been developed, however; these include agents that interfere with the liberation of viral nucleic acid from its protective coat or are incorporated as base analogs into the viral nucleic acid and prevent its replication. Some experimental antiviral agents act indirectly by stimulating interferon production by the host target cells; others that prevent penetration of virus into the target cell have great promise.

After Fleming's discovery of penicillin, the earlier effective antibiotics were discovered by screening many fungi and bacteria for their possible production of antimicrobial agents. This approach yielded a rich harvest that included, among many others, such agents as streptomycin, chloramphenicol, the tetracyclines, and erythromycin. More recently, research and development have focused on molecular modification of naturally occurring agents to improve their ranges of activity, to enhance their pharmacologic characteristics, or to make them insusceptible to the resistance mechanisms that some bacteria have developed against the action of earlier agents. With increasing understanding of the molecular biology of viral replication, it seems certain that synthetic compounds targeted to interfere with essential aspects of attachment, replication, or assembly will be developed using computer modeling, and that similar approaches will increase the number of chemotherapeutic agents available for use against eukaryotic parasites.

Microbial resistance to chemotherapy

The response of bacteria, and to a lesser extent of protozoa and fungi, to the widespread use of specific antimicrobial agents in therapy and prophylaxis reflects their extraordinary genetic plasticity. Resistant strains have appeared among many species that were previously fully susceptible to a particular agent. This resistance has resulted from mutation in the microbial genome and, in the case of bacteria, from the acquisition of genetic determinants of resistance on extrachromosomal, self-replicating portions of DNA (plasmids). Some individual genetic sequences can move from plasmid to plasmid or to chromosomal DNA (transposons). Some plasmids carry multiple resistance determinants against several antibiotics and can be transferred within or between bacterial species. Thus, the selective pressure of a single antimicrobial agent can lead to the predominance of multiple resistance in a previously fully susceptible strain. These developments have had major implications for successful prevention and treatment of many bacterial infections, and the selective factors that have contributed to the spread of resistance must be understood and acted on if some of the benefits of the antibiotic revolution are not to be lost through excessive or inappropriate use.

Prevention by immunization

As indicated previously, new developments and understanding in medicine are increasing the emphasis on prevention of disease, and nowhere is prevention more important than in infectious diseases. Specific immunization by parenteral injection of nonliving purified or complex antigens has long been shown effective in preventing tetanus, pertussis, poliomyelitis, and influenza infections if immunization schedules are rigorously applied and maintained with appropriate boosters. Live vaccines using organisms of reduced virulence (attenuated) that undergo limited multiplication in the body have also been used for many decades in the prevention of smallpox, rabies, poliomyelitis, and tuberculosis. Such vaccines provide prolonged immunologic stimulus and thus obviate repeated immunization. This principle, extended more recently to measles, rubella, and mumps, has effected dramatic changes in the overall occurrence of infection in children and its toll of poor health, school absences, serious complications, and even death.

Many infectious diseases have not yet been controlled by boosting the body's defenses, either because effective immunizing antigens have not been discovered or because the parenteral routes of immunization are ineffective. New work has extended the range of useful immunizing agents available and has demonstrated the value of stimulating local immune mechanisms at the site of some infections, such as dysentery. It seems certain that selective application of new methods of immunization to populations or age groups at particular risk will reduce the overall impact of infections still further. Examples include immunization of children against *Haemophilus influenzae* type b, which can cause severe meningitis in this age group; immunization of the elderly and others at particular risk of developing pneumococcal pneumonia; and immunization of burn victims against certain organisms, associated with high mortality, that often infect their lesions.

Other prophylactic approaches

Other methods of prevention have been or will be exploited. Chemoprophylaxis with specific antibiotics for brief periods has extended the range of surgical procedures that can be performed safely; for example, patients with implanted heart valves or artificial hips can be protected from infection by organisms that gain access during surgery and may lead to loss of the prosthesis. Identification of the chemical nature of specific receptors for bacterial toxins may allow them to be used therapeutically on nonabsorbable particles to remove enteric toxins before they can attack living cells. Perhaps most importantly, there is increasing emphasis on stimulation of the body's nonspecific phagocytic immune system and on the physiologic and nutritional factors that influence resistance to infection. For example, it has been shown recently that a key factor in preventing the severely burned patient from succumbing to infection is the maintenance of general nutritional balance by parenteral feeding with essential nutrients. Those who have read George Bernard Shaw's *The Doctor's Dilemma* will deduce that we are coming full circle, and that "stimulation of the phagocytes," a major focus of research in the 1920s, is highly relevant today.

Diagnostic microbiology

All of the facts and concepts discussed herein have been developed from basic microbiologic and immunologic research, and their application to the specific diagnosis of infectious diseases likewise depends on laboratory work. Detection and identification of microorganisms or their products in clinical material are undertaken in clinical or public health microbiology laboratories. Most bacteria and fungi can be grown in artificial culture, studied for a variety of key taxonomic characteristics, and speciated rapidly. Once grown, they can be tested for their susceptibility to antimicrobial agents in the test tube, and the results used in the rational selection of therapy. Most viruses can be grown in cultures of eukaryotic cells derived from human or mammalian tissues, then speciated by appropriate techniques, such as reactivity with specific antibodies.

Interpretation of diagnostic tests

The isolation of a potentially pathogenic organism from clinical material, particularly from a site with a normal flora, often does not provide sufficient evidence of etiology. Knowledge of potential sources of contamination, the constituents of the normal flora, and the probability of a particular pathogen's association with the clinical manifestation must all be considered in deducing a probable or confirmed diagnosis. Thus, informed judgment plays a role in presumptive laboratory diagnosis of many specific infectious diseases. Many laboratory methods that measure the immunologic response of the host to a particular organism can be diagnostic (as in the case of syphilis) or provide confirmatory evidence of a suspected diagnosis, either in the individual case or during the course of an epidemic. It is essential that the student grasp the principles, methods, and pitfalls of the approaches used if the potentialities of the laboratory are to be applied correctly, and errors and misinterpretations avoided.

It is hoped that this overview will help the reader to understand how the different topics in this book relate to one another, and the reasons why the authors believe that the material presented is essential for students who will practice in any branch of medicine. There is much specific information in the book that must be learned, as well as principles that must be understood. We offer no apologies for the fact that some rote memorization is essential. One cannot deduce a staphylococcus or the manifestations of a staphylococcal infection. This knowledge must be learned and remembered, and memory continually reinforced and extended. Memorization without understanding, however, is no basis for the application of a discipline to the diagnosis, care, and treatment of disease: it is essential that the underlying principles be firmly grasped.

John Spizizen

Bacterial Structure, Physiology, and Growth

2

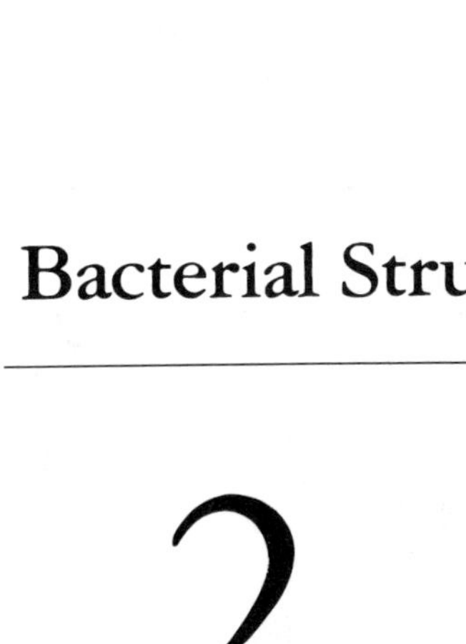
Diplococci
Streptococci
Staphylococci
Bacilli
Vibrio
Spirochete

Bacterial cells have a wide range of sizes and shapes. They generally measure 0.2–1.5 μm in diameter and 1–6 μm in length. A few bacterial species have longer cells, sometimes dependent on growth conditions. Bacterial cells can be seen with the ordinary light microscope, but often with some difficulty because the refractive index of the organisms is similar to that of the suspending liquid. Phase-contrast microscopy, which depends on changes of phase rather than amplitude of light waves, shows the general morphology of bacteria more clearly. Bacteria are most easily seen after staining with dyes.

There are four basic shapes of bacteria: spherical, rod-shaped, curved, and spiral. These shapes are illustrated in the marginal figures, where black indicates Gram positive and white Gram negative (Details of the Gram stain are discussed here and in Chapter 9). Spherical or oval cells, called *cocci,* generally appear in characteristic groups of two or more. Pairs are known as *diplococci,* chains as *streptococci,* and clusters are characteristic of *staphylococci.* Rods, termed *bacilli,* are found singly or in chains of varying lengths, depending on growth conditions. Short rods are known as *coccobacilli.* Some rods are uniform, but others are unusually shaped. For example, members of the genus *Corynebacterium* are often club-shaped at one end, whereas fusiform bacteria are tapered at each end. Short curved rods are characteristic of the vibrios. There are also spiral bacteria: Those with rigid cell walls are classified as *spirilla*; more undulating types are known as *spirochetes.* Bacterial cells may develop altered shapes under certain conditions, such as starvation or contact with antibiotics.

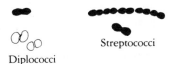

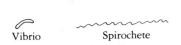

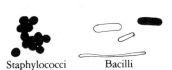

Cell Surface Structures

Cell surfaces comprise a complex, rigid cell *wall* surrounding a thin cell (cytoplasmic) *membrane.* Many bacterial cells have a capsular layer, which is often slimy and covers the wall. Some bacteria have appendages extending beyond the cell surface, including long flagella responsible for motility and short pili. These structures, shown schematically in Figure 2.1, are described in more detail below.

Capsule

Visualization

The outermost layer is usually known as a *capsule* when it is present as a distinct structure, and as *slime* when it forms a loose association with the wall. Capsules are often not visible by direct microscopy of living bacteria,

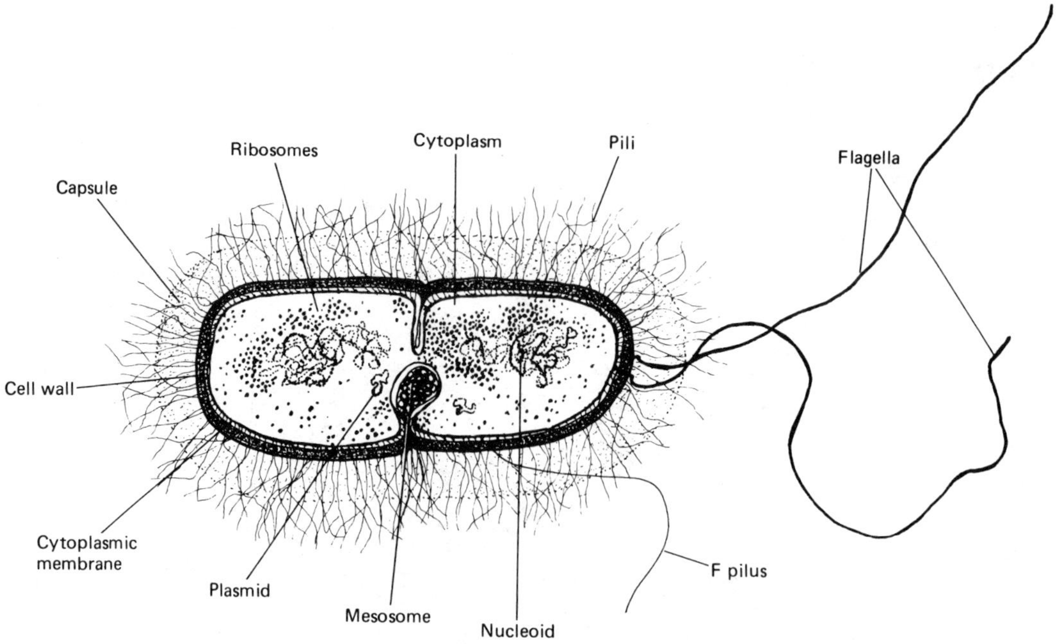

2.1 Schematic of structures of a dividing bacterium.

but can be observed by special stains or as a halo around the cell when it is suspended in a dark colloidal substance such as India ink. They also become visible and swollen in the presence of specific antibody that reacts with them.

capsule swelling reaction

This quellung or capsule swelling reaction can be used to identify different capsular antigenic types among some species of bacteria; for example, it can distinguish more than 80 serotypes of *Streptococcus pneumoniae.*

association with virulence

Capsules often have a protective function; their presence is frequently important in determining the pathogenicity of an organism by making it more resistant to ingestion by phagocytic leukocytes, and thus to destruction by the host. Mutants of many pathogenic bacteria that have lost the ability to synthesize capsules are no longer virulent. It must be realized, however, that many encapsulated bacterial species are not pathogenic. In nature, as opposed to culture, bacteria are often surrounded by an extensive hydrophilic polysaccharide matrix that they secrete, which apparently plays a role in attaching them to surfaces.

Capsule synthesis is greatly influenced by growth conditions. For example, *Streptococcus mutans,* an organism that causes dental caries, synthesizes a capsule consisting of a levan carbohydrate polymer derived from sucrose; the amount of capsular material produced is dependent on the concentration of sucrose. The capsule allows the bacterium to attach to tooth enamel and initiate the carious process.

most capsules are polysaccharide, some polypeptide

Most bacterial capsules are composed of polysaccharides of single or multiple sugar residues, but some consist entirely of polypeptides. Thus, the capsule of *Bacillus anthracis,* the causative agent of anthrax, consists of a polymer of D-glutamic acid (the unnatural form of the amino acid). This polypeptide serves to protect the capsule from the degrading effects of host proteolytic enzymes, which generally recognize only the natural forms of amino acids.

Cell Wall

Structure and function

The cell wall is a rigid layer that determines the shape of bacteria and protects their hypertonic internal contents from the environment. Thus, when the cell wall is removed or weakened (for example, by the action of enzymes such as lysozyme), the cell ruptures unless it is maintained in a medium of the same osmotic pressure as the cytoplasm. It can then exist in a spherical form termed a *protoplast* or *spheroplast,* derived from Gram-positive and -negative cells, respectively. Spheroplasts have some residual cell wall components and, in contrast to protoplasts, can multiply in media under high osmotic pressure. Cell-wall-deficient mutants of highly variable shape, called *L forms,* may also be selected in vitro or in vivo and can grow slowly in special media. A group of cell-wall-deficient bacteria, classified as *Mycoplasma,* that occur in nature include some species that cause disease in humans and animals. There is no evidence that they are derived from bacteria with complete cell walls.

Cell-wall-deficient organisms

Bacterial cell walls are unique structures with no analogs in mammalian cells. Their synthesis is thus a site of attack of antibiotics that kill bacteria but have little if any toxicity to the host (for example, penicillin).

Gram stain

The structure of the cell wall differs between two classes of bacteria, which can be differentiated by the Gram stain. In this procedure, bacteria are treated with a purple dye, crystal violet, followed by an iodine solution. When the organisms are washed with alcohol (or acetone), the dye–iodine complex is retained by some species and lost by others. The final step is counterstaining with a red dye such as safranine. Bacteria that retain the crystal violet are stained purple and are termed *Gram positive.* Those decolorized by the alcohol, stain with the red counterstain and are termed *Gram negative.* These differences in staining are shown in Plates A and P. They are of great taxonomic and diagnostic value, because they reflect major differences in cell wall structure. The Gram stain procedure is considered in more detail in Chapter 9.

Cell wall of Gram-positive organisms

The Gram-positive cell wall (Figure 2.2) is a thick layer, sometimes constituting as much as 15% of the dry weight of the cell. It is composed of a polymer known as *peptidoglycan* or *mucopeptide.* The peptidoglycan consists

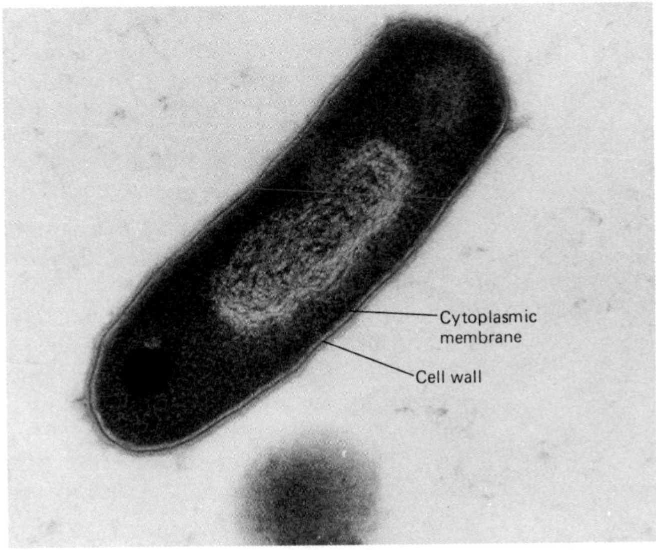

2.2 Electron micrograph of Gram-positive bacterium. Note cell wall and cytoplasmic membrane. (*Kindly provided by Dr. E.S. Boatman.*)

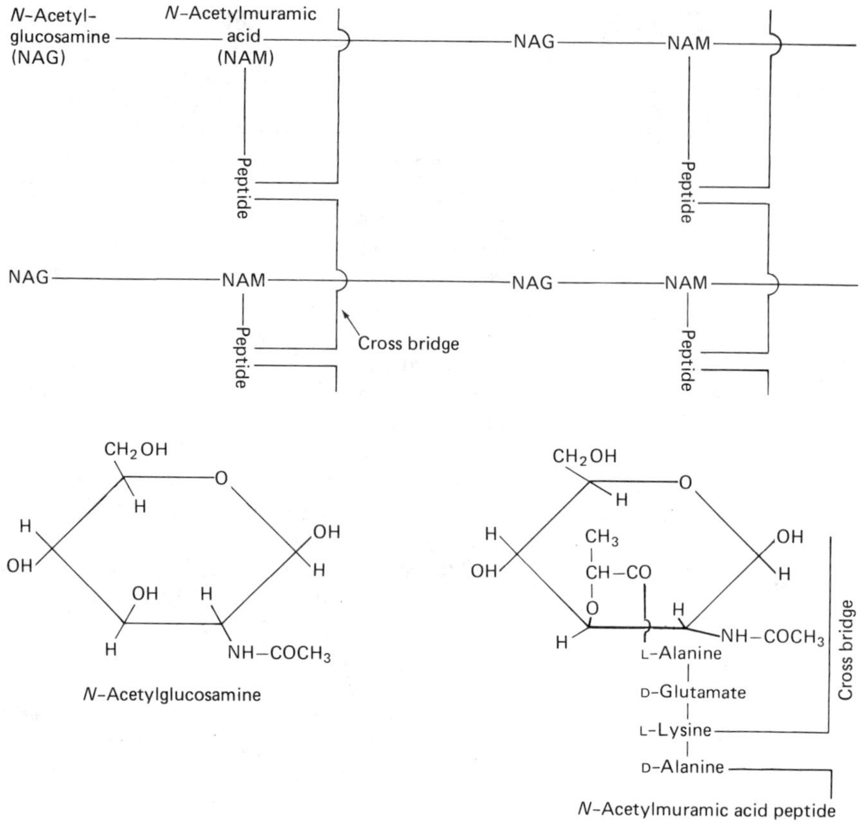

2.3 Schematic of mucopeptide (peptidoglycan).

structure of peptidoglycan

of a linear chain of two alternating sugars, *N*-acetylglucosamine and *N*-acetylmuramic acid, in 1:4 linkages. A tetrapeptide of alternating L- and D-amino acids is attached to the muramic acid sugar at its *O*-lactyl group (Figure 2.3). Adjacent chains are cross-linked by peptide linkage between the third amino acid and the terminal D-alanine on the other polymer chain. This cross-linking creates an interlocking network of mucopeptide. The network undergoes modification by autolytic enzymes during growth, which permits separation of the wall during cell division.

teichoic acid

Another component of the Gram-positive cell wall is a polymer of glycerol phosphate or ribitol phosphate known as *teichoic acid.* Sugars and D-alanine may occur as substituents in teichoic acid. The teichoic acid polymer is often linked to the mucopeptide chains by covalent linkage to the muramic acid. Teichoic acids are major cell wall surface antigens of Gram-positive bacteria.

outer antigenic layers

In certain Gram-positive organisms, notably the streptococci, other antigenic layers around the wall often allow serologic subtyping within a species and sometimes contribute to virulence. These layers may be carbohydrate or protein. The serologic specificity of these substances is useful for differentiating strains of medical importance.

Cell wall of Gram-negative organisms

The wall of Gram-negative bacteria is more complex (Figure 2.4). A thin peptidoglycan layer is present on the inner surface next to the cytoplasmic membrane. It is less cross-linked than that of the Gram-positive organisms, and teichoic acid is absent. Outside the peptidoglycan is a complex structure called the outer membrane, because it shares many features with the cyto-

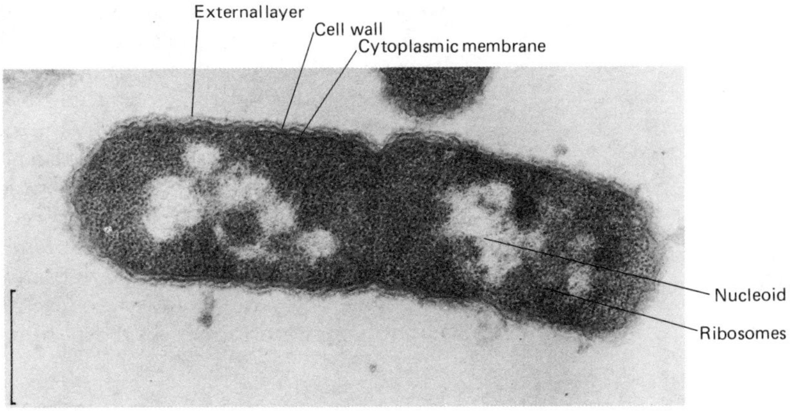

2.4 Electron micrograph of Gram-negative bacteria. (*Kindly provided by Dr. E.S. Boatman.*)

inner peptidoglycan layer and outer membrane

plasmic or cell membrane. It consists of a bilayer of phospholipids in which lipopolysaccharide (on the outer surface), lipoprotein, and specific proteins are embedded. Some of the proteins are part of transport systems for small molecules. Others function in protecting enzymes present between the wall and cell membrane. The lipoprotein may constitute as much as 40% of the dry weight of the wall. The lipopolysaccharide has been extensively investigated. Its basic structure (Figure 2.5) is composed of lipid A, which varies in structure in different species, and polysaccharide. The polysaccharide has a core component common to all Gram-negative bacteria and one or more components that vary in structure and are often specific for individual species. These carbohydrates are antigenic, and the variable components are termed *O* or *somatic* (body) *antigens.* Each *Salmonella* species, for example, has characteristic *O* antigens that provide valuable diagnostic criteria for identification. Antibodies directed against outer membrane proteins may be of special importance in immunity to some Gram-negative bacteria.

structure of lipopolysaccharide

O and outer membrane protein antigens

The lipopolysaccharide is also termed endotoxin and is responsible for the fever, shock, vascular collapse, and hemorrhage that may develop in severe Gram-negative bacterial infections. The lipid A moiety appears to be the principal component involved in toxicity, although the polysaccharide is also required for activity. Lipopolysaccharide may also help to protect the bacterial cell from phagocytosis in the host. The endotoxin is thus an important element in the pathogenicity of Gram-negative bacteria, and it is discussed in greater detail in Chapter 7. It is not destroyed by temperatures as high as 120°C, and its effects can be exhibited after injection of contaminated solutions, even when autoclaved.

endotoxic properties of lipopolysaccharide

heat stability of endotoxin

Cytoplasmic Membrane

Structure and enzymatic activities

The cytoplasmic membrane consists of a phospholipid bilayer in which various proteins are interspersed. These proteins constitute 60–70% of the

2.5 Unit of lipopolysaccharide (LPS).

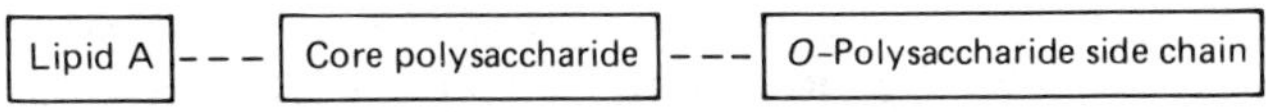

weight of the membrane, and many are enzymes. The cytoplasmic membrane is an active, selective permeability barrier, allowing only certain molecules to enter the cytoplasm. It contains the enzymes for oxidative phosphorylation and electron transport in aerobic bacteria, and thus has some of the functions of eukaryotic mitochondria. It is the site at which enzymes synthesize cell wall polymers and capsules, and it also plays an important role in the secretion of extracellular enzymes, some of which have significant functions in the pathogenicity of certain bacterial species.

enzymatic activities in periplasmic space

Between the cytoplasmic membrane and the cell wall is the periplasmic space, which contains some enzymes involved in active transport of nutrients and metabolites. Some antibiotic-inactivating enzymes that confer resistance to antibiotics are located in the periplasmic space.

Cytoplasm

The cytoplasm contained within the cell membrane is the main body of the cell and includes most of its proteins and enzymes. It also contains several defined structures that are discussed below and illustrated in Figure 2.1.

mesosomes

The mesosomes are complex invaginations of the cytoplasmic membrane that may be involved in cell division by associating with the chromosome. They are found mainly in Gram-positive bacteria.

Nucleoid: single, highly folded DNA molecule

Plasmids: smaller, circular DNA molecules

genetic contributions of plasmids

The nucleoid carries the primary genetic information of the cell. It consists of a single chromosome, but lacks the nuclear membrane characteristic of the analogous structure, the nucleus, in eukaryotic cells. The bacterial chromosome is a highly folded, double-stranded, circular DNA molecule with a molecular weight of approximately 3×10^9. Associated with the chromosomal DNA are polyamines and basic proteins, which neutralize the negative charges of the DNA. In addition to chromosomal DNA, many, but not all, bacteria contain small, circular, covalently closed, double-stranded DNA molecules called *plasmids*. Single or multiple copies of a plasmid or more than one type of plasmid may be present. Plasmids often contain genetic information for functions that protect the cell from adverse conditions or contribute to its virulence. For example, genes coding for antibiotic-inactivating enzymes or for production of certain toxins are often plasmid-borne. Plasmids may also carry genes coding for resistance to metal ions, for degradative enzymes, and for the fertility factor needed in some instances of bacterial conjugation. Genes for essential cellular functions, however, are chromosomal.

Functions of 70S bacterial ribosomes

Ribosomes exist throughout the cytoplasm of bacterial cells. They are granules 15–20 nm in diameter that consist of RNA and protein and are the centers of bacterial protein synthesis. Their number, which is influenced by nutritional conditions, is greatest in actively growing cells. Bacterial ribosomes are 70S and are composed of 50S and 30S subunits; in contrast, the larger 80S eukaryotic ribosomes are composed of 60S and 40S subunits. The distinctions between bacterial and mammalian ribosomes are exploited by antibiotics that interfere with protein synthesis by bacterial ribosomes, but have little if any effect on eukaryotic ribosomes. For example, the antibiotic erythromycin attaches to a small part of the 50S subunit of bacterial ribosomes and stops protein synthesis. Strains resistant to erythromycin can often methylate the RNA and prevent this attachment. The effect of antibiotics is considered in greater detail in Chapter 10.

inhibition of protein synthesis by antibiotics that attach to ribosomes

Cytoplasmic inclusion bodies are characteristically found in certain species of bacteria. Some are present as reserve material in the form of polymers.

Storage granules

Polymers of glucose in the form of glycogen and starch may be present. Some bacteria store polyhydroxybutyrate in visible granules. Such polymers disappear under restricted nutritional conditions. Others, notably *Corynebacterium diphtheriae,* produce visible structures of an inorganic phosphate polymer known as *volutin granules.* These structures, which are prominent as red particles when the cells are stained with methylene blue, are hence often termed *metachromatic granules.*

Appendages

Flagellar proteins and structure

H antigens of flagella

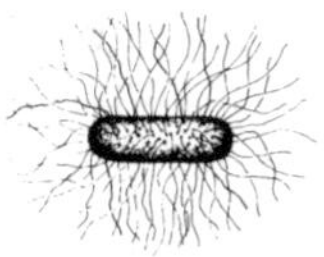

Motility is a characteristic of some bacteria. It results from the presence of locomotor organs, the flagella, which are long, thin, hollow structures. Flagella are helical in shape and are attached to the cell wall and membrane by a basal body through an intermediate structure, the hook. The basal body is composed of rings that appear to be able to rotate the entire flagellum and to provide the driving force for movement. Flagella consist of aggregates of proteins of a class termed *flagellins.* The amino acid composition of the flagellins differs among different bacterial species and can elicit the production of specific antibodies. They are designated as H or flagellar antigens, and antisera prepared against them can differentiate certain bacterial species (for example, within the genus *Salmonella*). In some bacterial families or genera, such as the Enterobacteriaceae, flagella appear around the entire cell surface. In others (for example, *Pseudomonas* and *Vibrio*), a single flagellum or a tuft of flagella is present at one or both ends of the cell.

specialized flagella in spirochetes

In spirochetes, structures called *axial filaments* are responsible for locomotion. They are morphologically similar to flagella, but are enclosed in a sheath wound around the long axis of the cell and located inside the cell membrane (Chapter 24). Rotation of the fibers leads to motility.

Pili

sex pili

role of attachment pili in virulence

Pili or fimbriae are filamentous protein appendages shorter than flagella that are numerous on the surface of some Gram-negative bacteria in nature. They are often lost after one or two subcultures. They are not organs of motility. One special type of pilus found in "male" strains of *Escherichia coli* (Chapter 5) is involved in conjugation or mating, with the transfer of DNA from donor to recipient probably accomplished through its core. Other types of pili are involved in the initiation of infection. For example, they mediate the attachment of *Neisseria gonorrhoeae* to the urethral epithelium and allow the colonization of the intestinal wall by some pathogenic enteric bacteria. Thus, loss of pili often results in loss of virulence.

Spores

resistance of spores

spore structure

Spores may be formed by a limited number of bacterial genera, the cells of which develop into these structures under conditions of starvation. Spores are dormant forms of the organism that are resistant to high temperatures, radiation, drying, and chemicals. Resistance is due to the specialized structure of spores, which have a very low water content and a high concentration of a unique compound, dipicolinic acid, in complex with calcium. When spores germinate under favorable conditions, the calcium dipicolinate diffuses out, which coincides with restoration of heat sensitivity. The wall consists of normal cell wall components, outside of which is a thick cortex of peptidoglycan differing in structure from normal cell wall peptidoglycan. Surrounding the cortex are layers of an insoluble structural protein responsible for protecting the spore from toxic chemicals. This spore coat, in turn, is surrounded by a lipoprotein and carbohydrate layer termed the *exosporium.*

The transition of a bacterial cell to the spore state involves several distinct stages, which are part of a differentiation process. The biochemical changes development of spores

and resultant structures are uniquely different from those of the original vegetative cell. It is of interest that a crystalline protein formed during sporulation of several species of *Bacillus* is toxic to certain insects. One of these proteins, produced by *Bacillus thuringiensis,* is used for the control of certain moth (Lepidoptera) larvae that consume important agricultural crops such as lettuce and cabbage.

Bacterial Metabolism

Origins of subunits for macromolecular synthesis

Energy generation

Synthetic processes

The bacterial cell exists and grows as a result of enzyme-catalyzed chemical reactions that provide energy for the synthesis of its components. The subunits required for the synthesis of macromolecules are synthesized by the cell from simpler compounds, obtained intact from the medium, or derived from the breakdown of more complex compounds. Cellular reactions involving degradation of compounds are known as *catabolic*; those in which synthesis occurs are termed *anabolic.* The catabolic reactions not only produce essential subunits, but provide the energy for synthetic processes. In some of these processes, primarily oxidation, energy is released in the form of high-energy phosphate, which is stored as adenosine triphosphate (ATP). The latter is then used to activate compounds for biosynthetic reactions. In this way, cell walls, proteins, nucleic acids, and other (for example, storage) compounds are produced for the growth of bacterial cells. Many of the biochemical reactions involved are similar to those in most other living cells. Some, however, are unique to certain bacterial species, particularly those in which compounds from the environment are used.

Aerobic respiration

Anaerobic fermentation by Embden–Meyerhof pathway

end products of fermentation

detection by gas chromotography

Many bacteria grow in the presence of oxygen and are thus termed *aerobic.* Aerobic bacteria are of two classes: obligate aerobes, which require oxygen for growth; and *facultative anaerobes*, which can also grow in the absence of oxygen. Obligate aerobes and most facultative species metabolize glucose and other sugars in the presence of oxygen by the process of respiration to generate 38 molecules of ATP for each molecule of glucose metabolized to carbon dioxide and water. Electrons are transported during this process to oxygen as a terminal acceptor. Some bacteria are *obligate anaerobes.* In the absence of oxygen obligate anaerobic and facultative species use the glycolytic or Embden–Meyerhof pathway, in which an organic compound is the electron acceptor for glucose oxidation. In this oxidation, for each molecule of glucose, two molecules of pyruvate, two molecules of ATP, and two molecules of reduced nicotinamide adenine dinucleotide are produced. The latter must be reoxidized to nicotinamide adenine dinucleotide, the oxidized form of pyridine nucleotide, by reduction of pyruvate. Direct reduction of pyruvate leads to the formation of lactic acid, a characteristic end product of the fermentation of carbohydrates by streptococci and certain lactobacilli. This process is called *homofermentation.* In other bacteria, pyruvate is metabolized further before reduction. Figure 2.6 depicts some of these unique fermentation patterns, which can yield products such as carbon dioxide, ethyl alcohol, formic acid, acetic acid, succinic acid, acetoin, and 2,3-butene glycol. These substances are detectable by gas chromatography, and their formation by certain species is so characteristic that it is useful for taxonomic and diagnostic purposes.

Extracellular enzymes

Certain bacteria have the unique ability to degrade compounds of high molecular weight in the environment by secreting enzymes into their surroundings. Thus, they may hydrolyze starch (amylases), proteins (proteolytic enzymes or proteases), lecithin (lecithinases), collagen (collagenases), lipid (lipases), or nucleic acids (nucleases). Some of these enzymes contribute to virulence, and the production of specific extracellular enzymes is often used for diagnostic characterization of the bacterial species or strain.

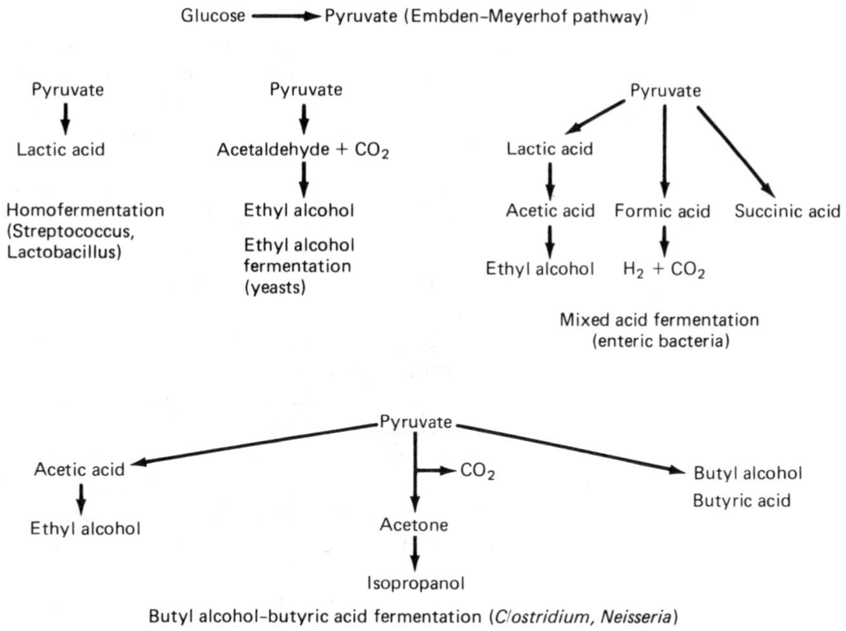

2.6 Some fermentation patterns in bacteria.

Bacterial Growth

Requirements

Culture media

Bacteria multiply in a variety of media and environments. In the laboratory, they are usually grown initially on complex media, which often contain many components of their natural environments (Chapter 9). The proper pH, temperature, salt concentration, and oxygen or other gaseous requirements must be provided to permit propagation of any given species.

essential requirements for growth

The essential requirements for multiplication are those that permit the biosynthesis of cellular components. They include a carbon source, which is often a source of energy as well, and sources of nitrogen, sulfur, and phosphorus. In addition, trace quantities of certain mineral elements are usually required.

hydrogen acceptors in respiration and fermentation

Oxidizable compounds such as glucose and other sugars can serve as sources of energy for growth. For biologic oxidation to proceed, a hydrogen acceptor is needed; oxygen acts as the ultimate acceptor in aerobic bacteria. In anaerobes, the hydrogen acceptors are certain organic compounds that are intermediates in fermentation. In some instances, inorganic compounds, such as sulfates, nitrates, or carbonates, can replace oxygen as the terminal hydrogen acceptors in a process termed *anaerobic respiration.*

heterotrophic organisms require organic sources of carbon

photosynthetic and lithotropic organisms use CO_2 as sole carbon source

The nutritional requirement for carbon is usually provided by a sugar, which may also be the energy source. Organisms with this requirement are termed *heterotrophs,* because exogenous organic compounds are needed. Certain bacteria, notably those that are photosynthetic (deriving energy from light sources) or lithotropic (obtaining energy from inorganic compounds), use CO_2 as their only source of carbon. These organisms are found in various natural environments and are not human parasites. Many heterotrophs also require CO_2 because it is a precursor in many important biosynthetic pathways, including those of purines and pyrimidines, as well as of organic intermediates in metabolic reactions. However, it is usually produced in sufficient amounts by the organism during the catabolism of carbohydrates.

Certain other bacteria, notably *N. gonorrhoeae,* require higher concentrations of CO_2 to initiate and maintain growth even on complex media, and the atmosphere in which cultures are grown must be supplemented with CO_2.

nitrogen requirements and sources of NH_3

The requirement for nitrogen is usually satisfied by ammonia. Amino acids are deaminated enzymatically to yield NH_3, or the amino groups are transaminated to keto acids. Ammonia is incorporated either directly or by transamination of α-ketoglutaric acid into the amino group of glutamic acid, which is a key amino acid in protein synthesis. Certain bacteria fix atmospheric nitrogen and metabolize it to NH_3.

mineral requirements

Of the minerals required, phosphorus is essential because it is a structural element of nucleic acids, ATP, and coenzymes. It is thus required in significant quantities in the form of inorganic phosphate. Sulfur, a constituent of proteins and other cell compounds, must also be provided. Other minerals, such as magnesium and potassium, are required for ribosome activity as well as for enzymatic activities. Calcium is a constituent of the cell walls of Gram-positive organisms as well as of spores. Iron, a constituent of cytochromes, is required for the expression of virulence mechanisms in some organisms, notably *C. diphtheriae.* The importance of iron in bacterial metabolism is indicated by the production of compounds called *siderophores* in response to iron deficiency. The siderophores form complexes with iron in the environment, making it available to the bacterial cell. As iron is oxidized in aerobic environments to the insoluble ferric form, this process of chelation is a mechanism developed by aerobic bacteria for assimilation of iron. Other minerals are also required in trace amounts to provide essential elements that are usually needed as cofactors for specific enzymes and in some cases as constituents of coenzymes.

sequestration of iron by siderophores

growth factor and vitamin requirements

Many bacteria require additional growth factors, which include coenzymes and their precursors (vitamins) as well as constituents of proteins, nucleic acids, lipids, and other essential cell substances. The requirement for growth factors results from the absence of or defects in biosynthetic pathways. Certain pathogenic bacteria such as *N. gonorrhoeae* need one or several specific amino acids for growth. *Haemophilus influenzae* requires hemin or hematin (X factor) and either the coenzyme nicotinamide adenine dinucleotide or nicotinamide adenine dinucleotide phosphate (V factor). Other *Haemophilus* species may require only one of these factors; for example, *Haemophilus parainfluenzae* requires V factor but not X factor. Certain organisms, such as lactobacilli, require an unusually large number of growth factors, including vitamins, purines, and pyrimidines.

Kinetics

cell growth before division

binary fission and cell cleavage

Bacterial growth leads to cell reproduction, which occurs by binary fission. Before division, all cell constituents, including surface structures and cytoplasmic components, increase in quantity; in addition, DNA is synthesized, leading to a doubling of the chromosome. At division, two daughter cells of equal size are produced, each containing a complete chromosome. Cleavage of the cell wall is the final stage of cell division; however, incomplete cleavage with failure of the cells to separate may occur under certain environmental conditions, or it may be a feature of a particular genus (for example, the streptococci, which produce chains of cells).

range of generation times

The generation time, which is the time required for a cell to divide, varies with nutritional status and with species. Thus, many bacterial species have generation time of 20–60 min under optimal conditions; others, such as *Mycobacterium tuberculosis,* divide only after 15 hr in culture and even more slowly in the body.

procedures
for measuring growth

The rate and extent of bacterial growth in a liquid medium can be measured directly by colony counting techniques. Dilutions of a growing culture are made at intervals and seeded onto the surface of a solid nutrient agar medium in petri dishes. These plates are incubated to allow visible growth to develop. Certain dilutions will permit isolated macroscopic colonies of bacteria to develop from a single bacterium or small clumps, which can then be counted. These counts provide an estimate of the numbers of viable bacteria at different times and thus their growth in the liquid culture can be followed. Growth can also be measured turbidimetrically and extrapolated to viable units.

Growth
in liquid medium

lag phase

When bacteria are inoculated into a liquid medium, there is an initial *lag period* during which they do not multiply, but undergo an adjustment to the new conditions. This interval is usually associated with a gradual increase in cell constituents. The duration of the lag period varies according to the previous history of the inoculated cells. It will, for example, be longer if the cells have not recently multiplied or if they have been grown in a different medium.

exponential phase

After the lag period the cells enter a phase of maximal growth rate, called the *logarithmic* or *exponential phase* of growth, in which numbers double with each generation time. Thus, a single cell of a species with a generation time of 20 min will yield 8 cells after 1 hr of log phase growth, 512 cells after 3 hr, and more than 1 million cells after 7 hr.

stationary phase

death phase

Eventually, use of essential nutrients during log phase growth results in their depletion and the accumulation of toxic products, which leads to a decrease and finally a cessation of growth. The cell population is then in a *stationary phase*, during most of which some cells die while others continue to divide slowly. This phase is followed by a *death phase*, during which most of the cells are dying. These phases are represented in Figure 2.7. It should be noted that the growth phases have different time spans, depending on the environment. In natural environments such as soil, water, or the human body, growth is much slower than in optimal media. In addition, the presence of other organisms will influence the rate and extent of growth of any particular strain.

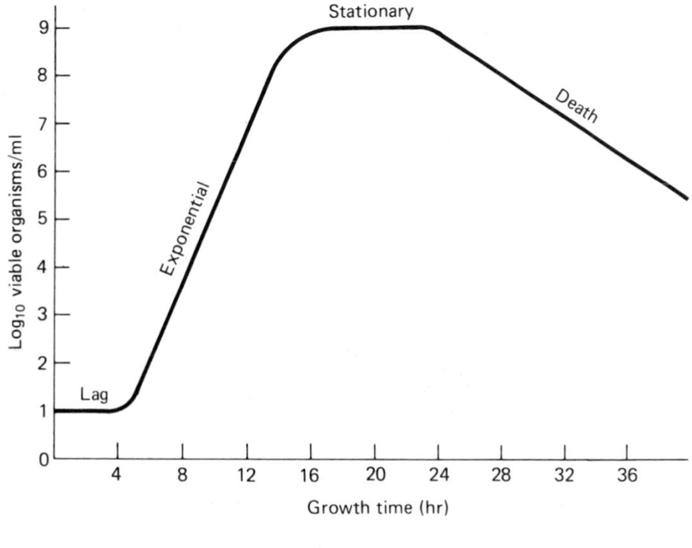

2.7 Phases of bacterial growth: example *E. coli.*

Bacteria that grow slowly or not at all in artificial culture

Some bacteria are grown with great difficulty on laboratory media and some, like the spirochete of syphilis, have not been grown in continuous culture. Cell-wall-deficient bacteria such as *Mycoplasma* and L forms show small colonies only after 3–6 days of incubation on specially supplemented or hyperosmotic nutrient agar media. Protoplasts cannot be grown at all.

Certain genera (for example, *Chlamydia* and *Rickettsia*) can only grow inside host cells. These obligate intracellular parasites resemble free-living bacteria in that they divide by binary fission, possess cell walls containing peptidoglycans, contain some of the enzymes of intermediary metabolism found in bacterial and higher cells, and can be inhibited by a number of antibacterial antibiotics. However, they lack the complete enzymatic machinery needed for independent growth in artificial media, which makes them obligate parasites.

Bacterial Classification

Binomial classification

Bacteria are classified into genera and species according to a binomial Linnean scheme similar to that used for higher organisms. For example, in the case of *Staphylococcus aureus, Staphylococcus* is the generic name and *aureus* the species designation. Some genera with common characteristics are further grouped into families. Bacterial taxonomy, however, has posed special problems because phylogenetic relationships, fossil records, and cross-breeding experiments that are important determinants for taxonomy of higher organisms are generally not available for bacteria, which are haploid and usually divide asexually by binary fission. Thus, bacterial taxonomy was developed pragmatically by determining multiple characteristics and weighting them according to which seemed most important: for example, shape, spore formation, Gram reaction, aerobic or anaerobic growth, and temperature of growth were given special weighting in defining genera. Properties such as ability to ferment particular carbohydrates, production of specific enzymes or toxins, and antigenic composition of cell surface structures were often of major value in defining species. The detection of these properties continues to be of central importance in identification of unknown isolates.

pragmatic weightings of classic bacterial taxonomy

Numeric taxonomy

In recent years, methods based on sounder principles have become available for detecting relationships between microorganisms. The computer has allowed the use of a statistical approach, which gives equal weighting to a large range of independent characteristics and allocates bacteria to groups according to the proportion of shared characteristics. This method is known as *Adansonian* or *numeric taxonomy.* More sophisticated taxonomic criteria are now employed based on chemical analysis of chromosomal DNA. This approach is valuable as all traits observed are gene products. The base composition of DNA, usually expressed as the moles percent of guanine (G) plus cytosine (C) to total bases, can be analyzed. Organisms with differences of G+C of more than 10% are considered unrelated; however, similar percentages do not necessarily imply relatedness. Closer similarities of the genome can be detected by determination of base sequence homology. This determination is made by a method known as *DNA–DNA hybridization,* in which single strands of DNA from one organism are allowed to anneal with single strands from another. One of the strands is labeled with a radioactive isotope. The extent of hybridization as determined by double-strand formation (detected by the radioactive label in one of the strands) is taken as a measure of base sequence homology and hence of relatedness. The data obtained allow the quantitation of the relationship of organisms with some similar morphologic and physiologic characteristics. Thus, it is

determinations of DNA base ratio can prove unrelatedness but not relatedness

hybridization techniques for determining degree of base sequence homology revealed that *E. coli* and *Shigella sonnei* are more closely related to each other than to *Salmonella typhi.* These new taxonomic tools have generally validated the results of the pragmatic methods used previously; however, some important and unexpected relationships have been uncovered, and in the future determination of both DNA and RNA sequences will provide a sounder basis for classification.

Details of the procedures commonly used in practice for identification of bacteria are given in Chapter 9. Common genera and species of medical importance, as well as some of the diseases that they cause, are listed in Table 2.1.

Table 2.1 Classification of Bacteria of Major Pathogenic Significance

Diagnostic Characteristic	Genus	Common Species (Disease)
Gram-positive bacteria		
Cocci	*Staphylococcus*	*S. aureus* (furunculosis)
	Streptococcus	*S. pneumoniae* (lobar pneumonia)
Bacilli		
Aerobic	*Bacillus*	*B. anthracis* (anthrax)
	Mycobacterium	*M. tuberculosis* (tuberculosis)
	Nocardia	*N. asteroides* (nocardiosis)
Anaerobic	*Clostridium*	*C. tetani* (tetanus)
	Actinomyces	*A. israelii* (actinomycosis)
Facultative anaerobic	*Listeria*	*L. monocytogenes* (listeriosis)
	Erysipelothrix	*E. rhusiopathiae* (swine erysipelas)
	Corynebacterium	*C. diphtheriae* (diphtheria)
Gram-negative bacteria		
Cocci	*Neisseria*	*N. meningitidis* (meningitis)
Bacilli		
Aerobic	*Pseudomonas*	*P. aeruginosa* (wound and burn infections)
	Streptobacillus	*S. moniliformis* (rat-bite fever)
	Brucella	*B. abortus* (brucellosis)
	Bordetella	*B. pertussis* (whooping cough)
Anaerobic	*Bacteroides*	*B. fragilis* (anaerobic infections)
	Fusobacterium	*F. nucleatum* (fusospirochetal disease)
Facultative anaerobic	*Escherichia*	*E. coli* (enteritis)
	Salmonella	*S. typhi* (typhoid fever)
	Shigella	*S. flexneri* (dysentery)
	Klebsiella	*K. pneumoniae* (pneumonia)
	Yersinia	*Y. pestis* (plague)
	Vibrio	*V. cholerae* (cholera)
	Campylobacter	*C. fetus* (enteritis)
	Haemophilus	*H. influenzae* (meningitis)
Spiral	*Treponema*	*T. pallidum* (syphilis)
	Borrelia	*B. recurrentis* (relapsing fever)
	Leptospira	*L. icterohaemorrhagiae* (Weil's disease)
Other bacteria		
Wall deficient	*Mycoplasma*	*M. pneumoniae* (primary atypical or mycoplasmal pneumonia)
Obligate intracellular parasites	*Rickettsia*	*R. prowazekii* (louse-borne typhus)
	Coxiella	*C. burnetii* (Q fever)
	Chlamydia	*C. trachomatis* (trachoma)

Additional Reading and References

Mandel, M. 1969. New approaches to bacterial taxonomy: Perspective and prospects. *Annu. Rev. Microbiol.* 23:239–274.

Mandelstam, J., and McQuillen, K., Eds. 1973. *The Biochemistry of Bacterial Growth.* 2nd ed. New York: Wiley. Excellent description of microbial metabolism.

Osborn, M.J., and Wu, H.C.P. 1980. Proteins of the outer membrane of Gram-negative bacteria. *Annu. Rev. Microbiol.* 34:369. This gives detailed consideration of the structure of the Gram-negative cell surface.

Smith, H. 1977. Microbial surfaces in relation to pathogenicity. *Bacteriol. Rev.* 41:475–500.

John Spizizen

Nature of Viruses

3

host specificity

obligate intracellular parasites

Viruses are characteristically submicroscopic particles that infect living cells. The discovery of viruses involved their recognition as *filterable* infectious agents; that is, they could pass through filters that retained bacteria. This observation was first made in 1892 by Iwanowski, who was working with a virus infecting tobacco plants, and showed that infected fluids filtered through bacteria-retaining filters retained the ability to cause infection. Viruses range in size from 20 to 300 nm. Different viruses infect bacteria, plants, animals, and humans. They are highly specific for hosts, requiring specific attachment sites on host cells; after attachment, they can penetrate the cell surface. Viruses multiply within susceptible living cells, and thus cannot infect or replicate in their absence. In other words, in contrast to most other infectious agents, they are *obligate intracellular parasites.* Some bacteria, including members of the genera *Chlamydia* and *Rickettsia,* are also intracellular; however, they differ markedly from viruses in possessing cell walls containing peptidoglycans and other components found in bacterial cells and in their modes of reproduction.

Structure

contain either RNA or DNA, never both

capsids and envelopes

viroids are viruses lacking capsids

prions

double- and single-stranded DNA viruses

most RNA viruses are single stranded

Viruses have much simpler chemical compositions than bacteria. They lack the structural and enzymatic components of bacterial cells, such as walls, membranes, ribosomes, and the like. They contain a single type of nucleic acid, either RNA or DNA, and a protein shell known as a *capsid.* Some viruses may have, in addition, an external lipoprotein coat or envelope. An intact, infectious viral particle is termed a *virion.* A number of tiny viruses, called *viroids,* that cause certain diseases in plants (for example, potato spindle tuber disease) consist entirely of RNA in the form of linear or circular molecules. Other agents, which are probably causes of some degenerative neurologic diseases, consist only of small, self-replicating proteins, termed *prions,* with no associated nucleic acid. It is not known how they replicate. The causative agent of Creutzfeldt–Jakob syndrome is thought to be a prion.

In the true viruses affecting humans, the amount of nucleic acid present is relatively small, constituting a few percent or less of the particles. Viruses may have both double-stranded and single-stranded DNA. Viruses containing RNA are most frequently single stranded. The RNA may be present as a single or as several molecules. Basic proteins or polyamines are often associated with the nucleic acids, effectively neutralizing their acidic groups.

Table 3.1 Composition of Some Viruses

Virus	Size (nm)	Nucleic Acid	Capsid Symmetry
Parvovirus	20	DNA, single strand	Icosahedral
Papovavirus	45–55	DNA, double strand, supercoiled	Icosahedral
Adenovirus	60–90	DNA, double strand	Icosahedral
Bacteriophage, T-even	95 × 65 (100 × 25 with tail)	DNA, double strand	Complex
Herpesvirus	150 × 200	DNA, double strand	Icosahedral
Vaccinia virus	250 × 300	DNA, double strand	Complex
Picornavirus	28	RNA, single strand	Icosahedral
Reovirus	75	RNA, double strand, segmented	Icosahedral
Influenza virus	80–120	RNA, single strand, segmented	Helical
Paramyxovirus	150	RNA, single strand	Helical
Tobacco mosaic virus	300 × 17.5	RNA, single strand	Helical

protective role of viral protein capsids

capsomers and viral surface structure

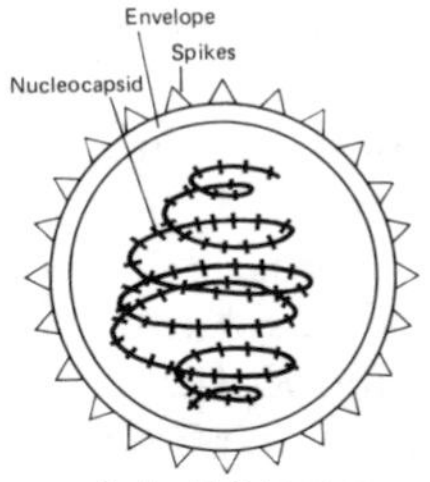

Enveloped helical structure

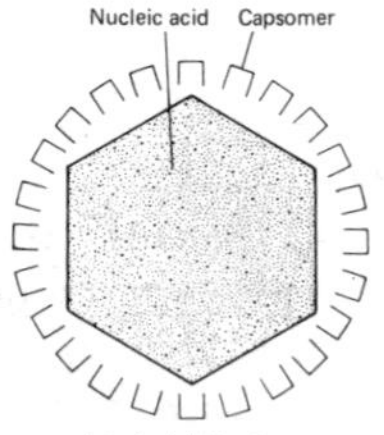

Icosahedral structure

The capsid proteins constitute the bulk of the viral structure. They surround the nucleic acid portion and serve to protect the nucleic acid from degradative enzymes. The protein consists of one or several kinds of subunits, termed *capsomers,* that are combined in a characteristic manner for each viral type. As a result, electron microscopy employing negative staining reveals the characteristic structure determined by the subunits. X-ray diffraction studies have revealed most viral structures to have either *helical* or *icosahedral* symmetry. With helical symmetry, the nucleic acid molecule is surrounded by protein molecules, the *nucleocapsid,* arranged helically to yield a structure with a single rotational axis. With icosahedral symmetry, the nucleocapsid is arranged into a uniform shape possessing 12 vertices, 20 triangular faces, and 30 edges. More complex structures are found in the large viruses and in bacteriophages (Table 3.1; Figures 3.1 and 3.2). Some viruses have a bilayer lipoprotein or phospholipid protein envelope surrounding the capsid. In the influenza virus, the phospholipid is derived from the cytoplasmic membrane of the host cell as a result of budding and applied when the virus is released from the cell in the final stages of its formation. Budding through the nuclear membrane of the cell also occurs with viruses such as herpes simplex, in which the viral phospholipid envelope has the composition of the inner nuclear membrane.

In addition to structural proteins, which constitute the bulk of the viral particle, functional proteins may be present. They include the proteins that mediate specific attachment to cells, as in influenza viruses. In many bacterial viruses, or bacteriophages, lysozyme is also present. This enzyme may func-

3.1 Sizes and shapes of selected viruses compared to bacteria. Length of average bacillus 4 μm.

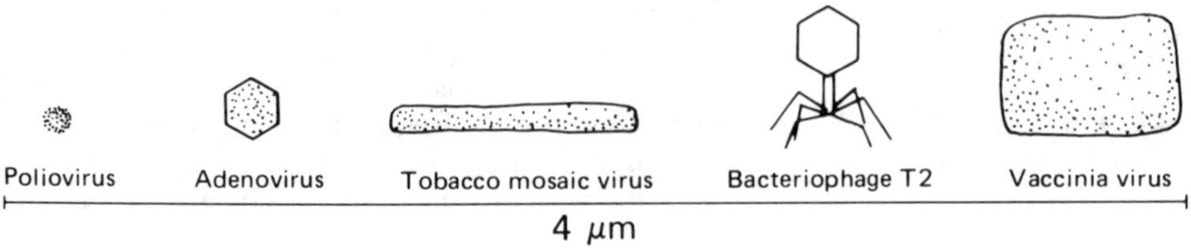

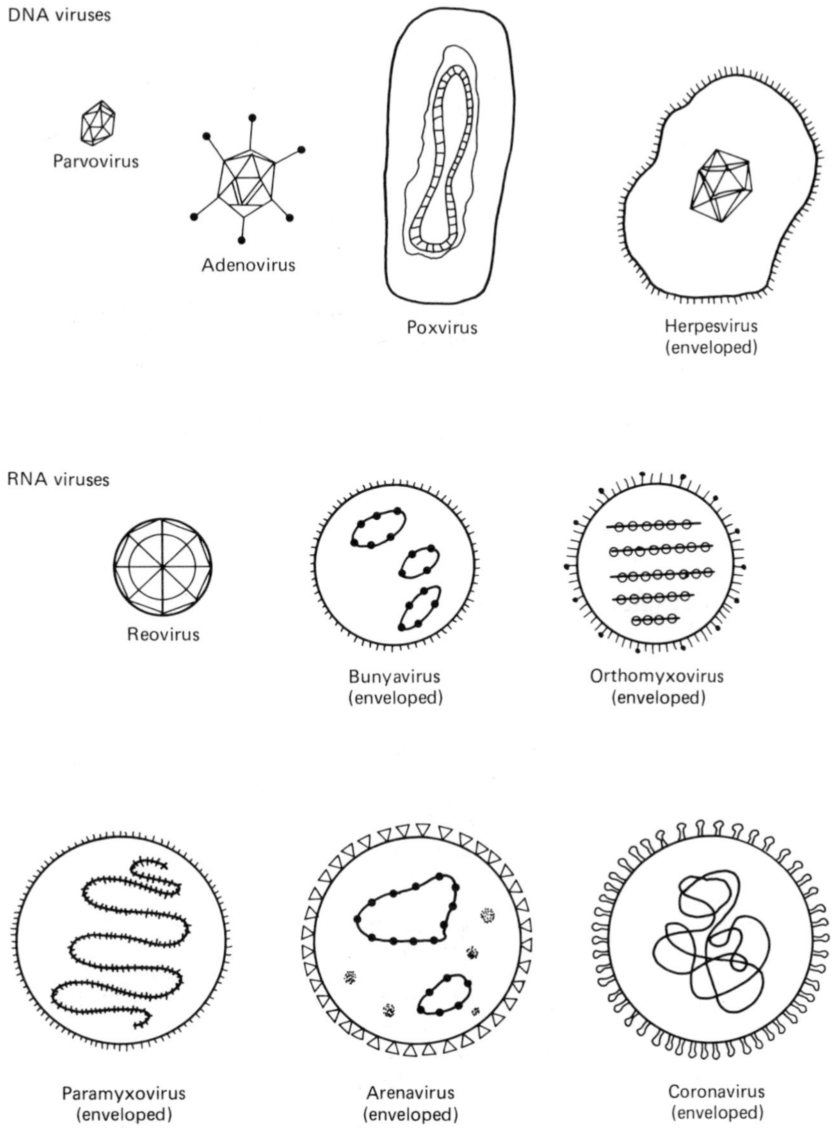

3.2 Comparative sizing and differing structural appearances of some viruses that affect humans.

functional and attachment viral proteins

reverse transcriptase of some RNA viruses

use of existing host cell enzymes for replication

tion in the entry and release of viral particles. Some viruses have enzymes that synthesize nucleic acids. For example, influenza virus contains an RNA polymerase that requires an RNA primer for activity. The RNA tumor viruses contain reverse transcriptase, a DNA polymerase that uses RNA as a primer. Except for these few cases in which enzymes are present in mature particles, viruses require additional enzymes for replication in the cell. In some instances, as with certain bacteriophages infecting *Escherichia coli* or with herpesviruses, host cell production of enzymes is induced or encoded by the DNA genes of the virus. Some of these enzymes are needed for the initiation of viral DNA replication. Most viruses use the existing enzymes of the host cell for replication, including protein and nucleic acid synthesis. This process is the basis of obligate intracellular parasitism.

Summary of viral structure

In summary, viruses are infective nucleoproteins containing either DNA or RNA, never both, and the nucleic acid may be single or double stranded. The bulk of the virus is the protein, which is mainly structural but may contain receptors for attachment to host cells. In addition, some viruses contain enzymes, such as lysozyme in bacteriophages, or polymerases for RNA or DNA synthesis. Lipoproteins derived from host cell membranes may also be present. Electron microscopy combined with X-ray diffraction has revealed the arrangement of capsid protein subunits in the form of helical or icosahedral structures. These forms are characteristic of most viruses; however, more complex structures are found in large viruses and some bacteriophages.

Classification

The large array of viruses has made classification difficult. Initially, viruses were categorized on the basis of diseases caused and host specificity. Thus, for viruses causing human diseases, categories were as follows:

1. *neurotropic viruses* (that is, viruses infecting the nervous system), including poliomyelitis, rabies, and equine encephalomyelitis;

Table 3.2 Classification of Animal and Human Viruses

Family	Representative Viruses	Size (nm)	Characteristics
	DNA Viruses		
Parvoviridae	Parvoviruses of rodents; adenovirus-associated satellite viruses (defective)	20	Replicate in nucleus of cell
Papovaviridae	Papilloma viruses; polyoma virus of mice; vacuolating, agent of monkeys (SV40)	45–55	Replicate in nucleus; latent; oncogenic
Adenoviridae	Respiratory disease viruses (39 types in human infection)	60–90	Many latent; produce tumors in newborn hamsters
Herpesviridae	Herpes simplex virus, types 1 and 2; varicella-zoster virus; cytomegalovirus; Epstein–Barr virus	100–200	Many latent; may cause recurrent infection, some associated with tumors (herpes type 2, Epstein–Barr virus)
Poxviridae	Smallpox; molluscum contagiosum; fibroma and myxoma of rabbits	230 × 400	Replicate in cytoplasm; DNA-primed RNA polymerase and other enzymes
	RNA Viruses		
Picornaviridae	Human enteroviruses, including poliovirus, Coxsackie virus, and echovirus; rhinoviruses; foot-and-mouth virus of cattle; hepatitis A	20–30	Replicate in cytoplasm
Reoviridae	Reoviruses (latent respiratory and enteric infections): orbiviruses, including Colorado tick fever and African horse sickness viruses; rotaviruses causing infantile gastroenteritis	60–80	Double-stranded RNA

2. *respiratory viruses* (that is, viruses infecting the respiratory tract), including influenza and the common cold;
3. *skin viruses,* including herpes and warts;
4. *liver viruses,* including serum hepatitis, infectious hepatitis, and yellow fever;
5. *salivary gland viruses,* including mumps and cytomegalovirus; and
6. *gastrointestinal viruses,* including rotavirus.

Families of DNA and RNA viruses

Our current knowledge of the chemical and physical structure of viruses has led to a classification scheme for those infectious to vertebrate animals and humans. The composition of the viral genome (that is, DNA or RNA) permits division of these viruses into two main groups. There are 5 families of DNA viruses and 10 families of RNA viruses (Table 3.2). It should be noted that within many families or genera of viruses are antigenic subtypes, which are differentiated primarily by serologic reactions using specific antibodies.

antigenic subtypes

Table 3.2 *(continued)*

Family	Representative Viruses	Size (nm)	Characteristics
	RNA Viruses		
Togaviridae	Alphaviruses, including Sindbis virus; flaviviruses, including yellow fever virus; rubiviruses, including rubella virus; pestiviruses, including mucosal diarrhea virus	40–70	Lipid envelope; arthropod-borne varieties replicate in arthropods and humans
Arenaviridae	Lassa virus; lymphocytic choriomeningitis virus of mice	50–300	Granules of RNA inside virion, some ribosomes from host cell
Coronaviridae	Respiratory viruses of man; infectious bronchitis virus of birds; calf diarrhea virus; swine enteric virus	80–30	Petal-shaped projections resembling solar corona
Retroviridae	RNA tumor viruses of mice, birds, and cats; visnavirus of sheep	100	Contain enzyme reverse transcriptase, which uses viral RNA to synthesize DNA transcript
Bunyaviridae	Rift Valley fever virus; Bunyamwera virus	90–100	Arthropod-borne, multiplying in arthropods; bud through cytoplasmic membrane
Orthomyxoviridae	Influenza viruses (types A, B, and C) of humans, swine, and horses	80–120	Segmented, single-stranded RNA; phospholipids, RNA-dependent RNA polymerase and neuraminidase
Paramyxoviridae	Mumps; measles; Newcastle disease viruses; canine distemper virus	150–300	Non-segmented, single-stranded RNA; RNA-primed RNA polymerase and neuraminidase
Rhabdoviridae	Rabies virus; bovine vesicular stomatitis virus	70–175	Helical, single-stranded RNA; bud through cytoplasmic membrane

Replication

use of host biosynthetic pathways for replication

viral integration

distinction between viral replication and bacterial multiplication

specificity of viral adsorption to host cells

passage of virus into cell and uncoating

Viruses infect living cells only, as they require the enzymes and the biosynthetic pathways of the host to replicate. Some viruses redirect cellular metabolic systems almost entirely to synthesize viral components. In some viral infections, however, cell metabolism is not significantly altered, although viral synthesis may occur. In the extreme case of certain latent viral infections, the virus does not replicate autonomously, but maintains its nucleic acid component by insertion into the host chromosome.

Unlike the mode of replication of bacterial cells, in which binary fission occurs, viral progeny are produced from the assembly of viral components, mainly protein and nucleic acids. These components are synthesized as a result of genetic control of the host cell by the nucleic acid of the infecting virus. A large number, often hundreds, of mature viral particles are formed from a single infecting virus.

Viruses gain entrance to host cells in several ways. In the case of bacteriophages and animal viruses, attachment sites on the cell surface are recognized by specific proteins in the viral coat. This process, known as *adsorption,* must then be followed by other processes that bring the nucleic acid inside the cell. Bacterial cell walls are pierced by bacteriophage lysozyme, and the nucleic acid is forced into the cell. In the case of animal viruses, the whole virus is often engulfed by the cell membrane and the protein coat digested away from the nucleic acid inside the cell, a process known as *uncoating.* Plant viruses enter at cell sites opened by surface abrasion or insect inoculation. In animal cells, viral replication differs with the type of infecting virus. More is known about the process of viral infection of bacterial cells, which will also be discussed.

Replication of Animal Viruses

RNA virus replication

positive and negative strand RNA viruses

Replication of poliomyelitis virus

To express viral genetic information, messenger mRNA must be made by transcription of viral nucleic acid. This process is accomplished in several ways, depending on the virus type. Thus, orthomyxoviruses contain RNA polymerases that transcribe viral RNA to mRNA inside the host cell. The mRNA is described as a *positive* strand, the single-stranded viral RNA as a *negative* strand. All orthomyxoviruses are negative-strand viruses, as are rhabdoviruses. In contrast, picornaviruses and togaviruses have a viral RNA that serves as its own mRNA; they are thus positive-strand viruses. In positive-strand viruses, the viral RNA or mRNA is immediately translated in the cell to produce RNA polymerase (Figure 3.3). This RNA polymerase synthesizes replicative intermediates, first a partially double-stranded RNA, then a complete double strand consisting of positive and negative RNA. In poliovirus, for example, the RNA (positive strand) directs the formation of early translational products, RNA polymerase and inhibitors of host cell synthetic processes. The newly synthesized RNA polymerase produces a replicative intermediate, a double-stranded RNA. Viral RNA in the form of single positive strands is then synthesized (Figure 3.3). These strands are translated into viral structural proteins, which then surround the viral RNA to produce viral particles. All of these events occur in the cytoplasm of the infected cells. Completed viruses are liberated after disintegration of the host cell.

unique structure of viral mRNAs

Most viral mRNAs have a unique structure, with polyadenylic acid at the 3′ end and methylated bases at the 5′ end. The methylated portion is an unusual structure called a *cap.* The cap facilitates initiation of translation of the RNA.

DNA virus replication

In general, DNA viruses replicate their DNA in the nucleus. The Poxviridae are an exception: they replicate their DNA, synthesize viral protein, and assemble their components in the cytoplasm. Viruses of the families Papovaviridae, Adenoviridae, and Herpesviridae uncoat their DNA after

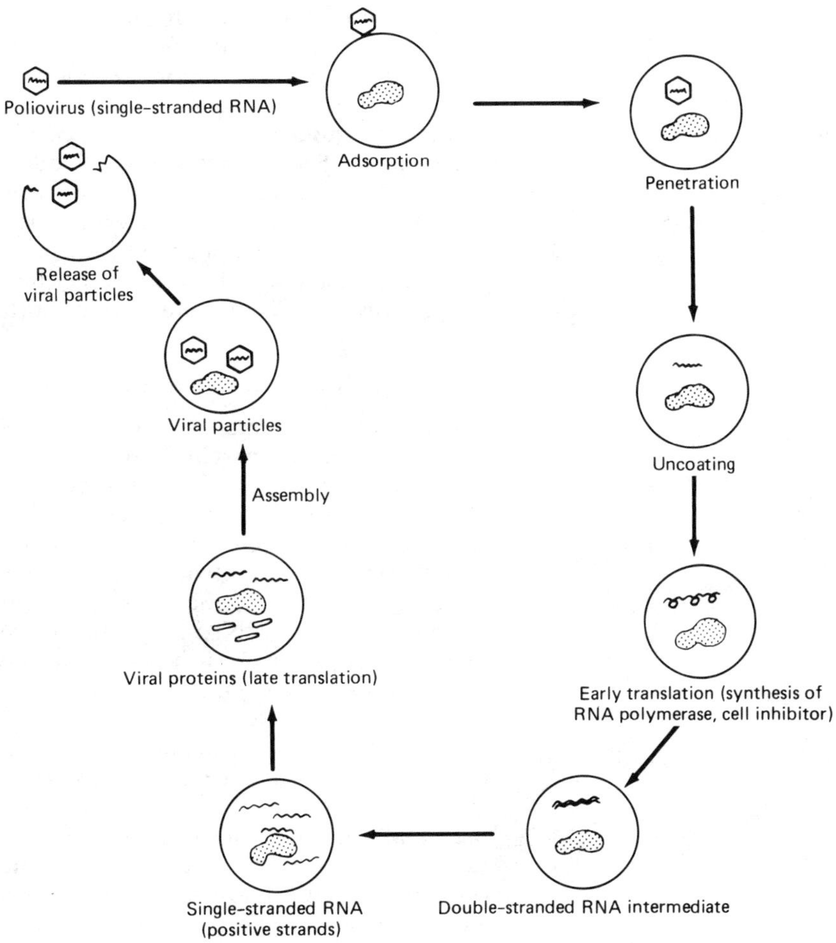

3.3 Poliovirus replication (positive-strand RNA).

cellular uptake, and the DNA enters the nucleus of the cell in some unknown fashion. The mRNA transcribed by the viral DNA is first translated to produce early virus-specific proteins, including enzymes for viral DNA replication. The mRNA is then transported to the cytoplasm for translation of viral structural proteins. The newly synthesized viral proteins are carried to the nucleus, where mature viral particles are assembled. Infective viral particles consisting of DNA and capsid proteins are released when host cells are disintegrated.

Persistent and Latent Infection

maintenance of viral infection with little or no cell destruction

Cell destruction after viral invasion and replication does not occur in all virus types. Some viruses cause *persistent* infections, in which viruses are replicating and released but the infected cells appear normal. Avian and mouse leukemia viruses, for example, cause persistent infections without affecting cell functions. Viral persistence may also occur as a result of the normal infection cycle in a small proportion of cells in a population at any time; in this case the infected cells are destroyed, but new susceptible cells continue to be formed to sustain viral replication. Some investigators believe that the production of *defective interfering particles* may be critical in the es-

defective interfering particles

tablishment of persistent infections. Such particles possess all the structural proteins of the parent virus but lack portions of the genome. These replicate only with the help of fully intact virions and impair normal replication of infectious viruses.

viral latency

Certain viruses may also cause infections in which no disease symptoms are apparent. Such inapparent, or "hidden," infections are called *latent* infections. For example, herpes simplex virus can produce an inapparent infection in which the virus resides in a sensory ganglion. Episodes of skin blisters recur at a site supplied by a nerve originating from the latently infected ganglion, and the virus can be cultured from the lesions. The nature of the virus in its latent state remains unclear.

Transformation and Endogenous Genes

Properties of cells transformed by oncogenic viruses

Viruses that cause tumors in animals, the so-called *oncogenic* viruses, produce an unusual type of persistent infection that results in cell *transformation.* When cells in culture are transformed, they behave differently from normal cultured cells. They can grow in semisolid media, require less serum for growth, and, unlike normal cells, are not inhibited by crowding. Furthermore, transformed cells can be grown through numerous passages in culture. In the DNA-containing oncogenic viruses, a specific protein is responsible for transformation, and the DNA is integrated into the genome of the cells. With other viruses, however, such as the human papilloma viruses, the DNA does not integrate; it exists in a free state and replicates as an extrachromosomal DNA package, or *episome.*

DNA tumor viruses

RNA tumor viruses and reverse transcriptase

The RNA viruses of the family Retroviridae contain the enzyme reverse transcriptase (RNA-dependent DNA polymerase), which produces a DNA copy of the RNA of the virus. Another enzyme, ribonuclease H, converts the DNA thus made to a double-stranded form. After integration of this DNA into the chromosome, viral RNA and mRNA are produced. In some cells, the mRNA is translated into viral proteins, and complete viral particles are subsequently produced. In other cells, however, the integrated viral genome, called the *provirus,* is present without viral replication. These proviral genes, which replicate with the chromosome as if they were normal chromosomal genes, are termed *endogenous* genes. Expression of these endogenous genes to produce viral proteins may occur, but it is regulated by other normal genes. Under certain conditions, these endogenous viral genes can be induced to produce infective viral particles. Endogenous viral genes have been found in many vertebrates, including humans, and are detected by DNA hybridization with known viral-specific DNA.

provirus

Replication of Bacteriophages

determinants of bacteriophage specificity

Viruses that infect bacteria are known as *bacteriophages* or *phages.* The extensive knowledge of certain bacteriophages and their mode of replication has provided a general model for viral replication. There is a great variety of phages, most of which are highly specific for bacterial hosts. The specificity of a given phage is partly attributable to its ability to attach to specific receptors on the bacterial surface, a process known as *adsorption.* The most thoroughly studied phages are a group of seven T phages that infect *E. coli* strain B. Although they infect the same host, they use different receptors on the cell surface as sites of attachment. Phages T2 and T6 adsorb to receptors in the lipoprotein layer, and phages T3, T4, and T7 attach to receptors in the lipopolysaccharide layer of the cell wall. There are numerous receptors for each phage on a cell. Alterations in receptors caused by mutations in host cells lead to resistance to infection.

receptors

Morphology of T phages

Studies of the structure of the T phages reveal the presence of a head and a tail. The head consists of a capsid protein with DNA in a tightly coiled form. The tail in the large T-even (that is, T2, T4, and T6) phages is composed of a contractile body with an inner channel and a base plate at the end. Fibers on the base plate are used in the attachment of the phages to cell wall receptors. After contact with the receptor, the tail contracts, thus transporting the DNA in the head through the tail and into the cell. This process involves a break in the cell membrane, which is subsequently sealed. The capsid and tail proteins, which do not penetrate the cell membrane, are left behind on the cell surface; however, small proteins closely associated with the phage DNA enter the cell with the injected nucleic acid. Smaller phages, which do not possess this contractile apparatus, depend on the cell to provide the energy needed for injection of DNA.

mechanism of insertion of phage DNA

early proteins and DNA synthesis

Once inside the cell, phage DNA directs the synthesis of a number of new enzymes, known as *early proteins.* These enzymes are required for phage DNA synthesis. They include a phage DNA polymerase and kinases for synthesis of the nucleotide triphosphates, the immediate precursors of DNA. In the T-even phages; the DNA of which contains hydroxymethylcytosine in place of cytosine, enzymes for synthesis of this unique base are also synthesized. Phage DNA replication is accomplished through the activity of these and other new enzymes. Substrates for synthesis are derived from medium components as well as from the degradation of host DNA. At later stages of DNA replication, phage structural proteins, termed *late proteins,* are synthesized. They include capsid tail proteins and lysozyme. The capsid (protein) subunit and the tail proteins assemble in an orderly fashion, and the DNA is incorporated to produce a mature phage particle. Each cell produces as many as 200 phage units, which are released after lysis of the cell wall. The lytic cycle of bacteriophage replication is shown in Figure 3.4A. Lysis of the bacterium is induced by the phage lysozyme. Some phages are released through the wall without lysis or death of the host cell.

late proteins and phage assembly

Bacterial lysis

Temperate Bacteriophages

Living in close association with many bacteria are phages that do not kill. These *temperate phages,* unlike the virulent T phages, usually infect without overtly affecting the host cell. When free, they can adsorb and inject their DNA in the same manner as T phages. The DNA of the temperate phages, however, integrates into the host chromosome at specific sites (Figure 3.4B). There it exists as a *prophage,* which replicates as a component of the host chromosome. One temperate phage, Mu, integrates randomly into the chromosome; when it integrates within a gene, it causes a mutation. Another phage, P1, does not integrate, but instead circularizes and replicates synchronously with the host chromosome without producing phage proteins. Thus, temperate phages provide models for some mammalian virus latencies.

nonlytic prophage infection

Bacteria that contain prophage are termed *lysogenic,* as a few cells may lyse because of phage replication and lead to eventual release of the temperate phage. The number of cells that become susceptible to phage replication and lysis varies with the strain and with cultural conditions. All cells containing prophage, however, can be induced by certain agents to produce mature phage. These agents include ultraviolet radiation, mitomycin C, and other DNA-damaging compounds. Induction has been shown to result from the proteolytic cleavage of repressor proteins. Repressors produced by temperate phages prevent the replication of phage by inhibiting excision of the prophage from the host chromosome. The presence of phage repressor proteins prevents infection of the lysogenic cell by other phages of the same or a similar type. This phenomenon, called *immunity,* should be distinguished

induction of lysogenic phage

repressor proteins and resistance to reinfection

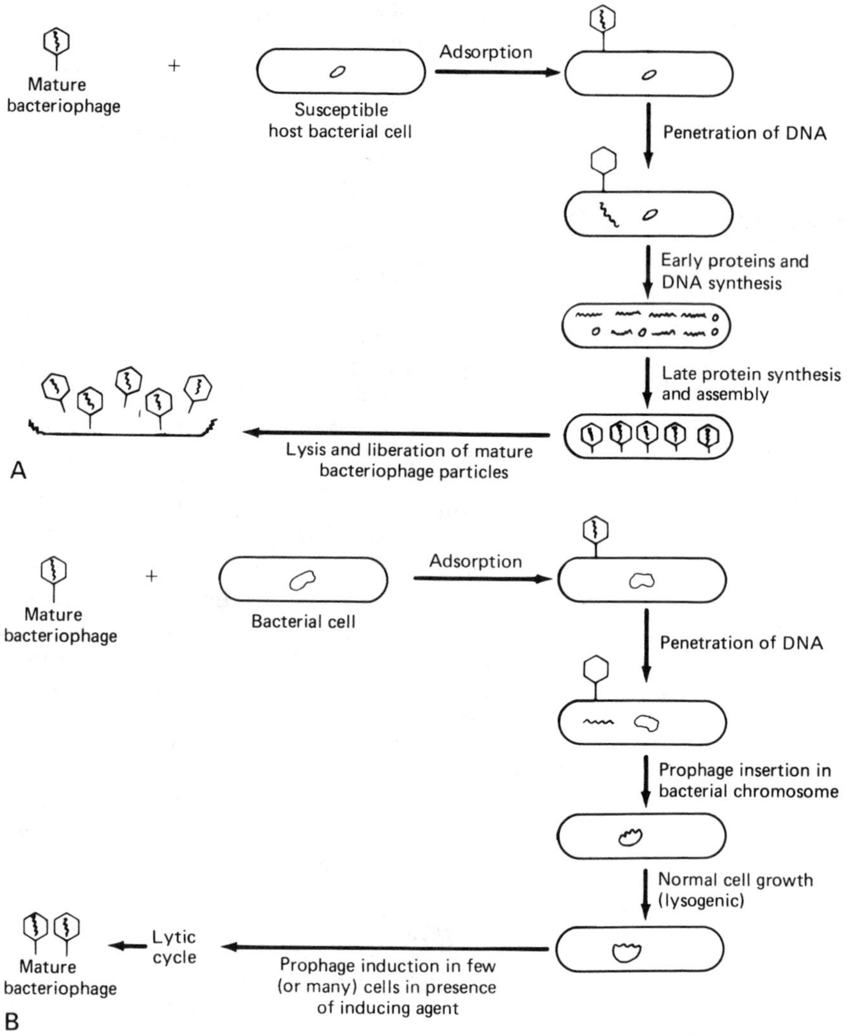

3.4 Bacteriophage replication. (**A**) Lytic (virulent) cycle. (**B**) Temperate cycle.

from resistance to virulent phage infection. In the latter case, it is the inability of the phage to adsorb to receptors that prevents infection.

Lysogenic conversion by temperate phages

Temperate phages may produce genetic changes in the host, an effect termed *lysogenic conversion.* Thus, in *Salmonella,* the presence of certain prophages alters the antigenic structure of the cell wall, producing new somatic or O antigens. In *Corynebacterium diphtheriae,* the presence of a specific temperate phage genome leads to the production of diphtheria toxin by all of the cells. The absence of the prophage results in an avirulent strain of *C. diphtheriae.*

Certain temperate phages have the ability to transfer pieces of chromosomes. This process, known as *transduction,* is discussed in Chapter 5.

Additional Reading and References

Joklik, W.K., Ed. 1980. *Principles of Animal Virology.* Norwalk, Conn.: Appleton-Century-Crofts. pp. 1–219. Excellent description of present knowledge of basic virology.

John C. Sherris

Microbial Death:
Sterilization, Pasteurization, Disinfection, and Sanitization

4

Definitions

Death, as it relates to microbial organisms, can be defined as a loss of ability to multiply under any known conditions. The complexity of the definition reflects the fact that organisms that appear to be irreversibly inactivated may sometimes recover when appropriately treated. For example, bacteria that have been inhibited by certain mercurial compounds such as merthiolate will fail to multiply because of inactivation of critical microbial —SH groups by free mercury ions. If they are placed in a medium containing compounds with free —SH groups, such as thioglycolate, the process can be reversed and viability restored. Similarly, ultraviolet (UV) irradiation of bacteria can result in the formation of thymine dimers in the DNA with loss of ability to replicate or of fidelity in replication. A period of exposure to visible light may then activate an enzyme that breaks the dimers and restores viability by a process known as *photoreactivation.* Mechanisms also exist for repair of the damage without light. Such considerations are of great significance in the preparation of safe vaccines from inactivated virulent organisms.

Sterilization involves complete killing, or removal of all living organisms from a particular location or material. It can be accomplished by incineration, nondestructive heat treatment, certain gases, exposure to ionizing radiation, some liquid chemicals, and filtration.

Disinfection involves the destruction of harmful microorganisms by liquid chemical agents known as *disinfectants.* These agents usually have some degree of selectivity, and bacterial spores, or organisms with waxy coats (for example, mycobacteria), show considerable resistance to most disinfectants. *Antiseptics* are disinfectant agents that can be used on body surfaces, such as the skin or vaginal tract, to reduce the numbers of the normal flora and of pathogenic contaminants. They have lower toxicity than disinfectants used environmentally, but are usually less active in killing vegetative organisms.

Sanitization is similar in principle to disinfection, but only involves providing an acceptable level of microbial cleanliness on inanimate objects such as surfaces used in food preparation.

Pasteurization is the use of heat at a temperature sufficient to inactivate certain harmful organisms in a liquid such as milk, but below that needed to ensure sterilization. For example, heating milk at a temperature of 74°C for 3–5 sec or 62°C for 30 min kills most pathogenic bacteria that may be present without altering its quality. Obviously, spores are not killed at these temperatures.

Asepsis, which involves prevention of microorganisms from reaching a protected environment, is usually applied to procedures used in the operating room, in the preparation of therapeutic agents, and in technical manipulations in the microbiology laboratory. An essential component of aseptic techniques is the sterilization of all materials and equipment used.

Microbial Killing

Exponential kinetics of killing

Killing of bacteria by heat, radiation, or chemicals is usually exponential with time, that is, a fixed proportion of survivors is killed during each time increment. Thus, if 90% of a population of bacteria is killed during each 5 min of exposure to a weak solution of a disinfectant, a starting population of 10^6/ml will be reduced to 10^5/ml after 5 min, 10^3/ml after 15 min, and theoretically to 1 organism (10^0)/ml after 30 min. Exponential killing corresponds to a first-order reaction or a "single-hit" hypothesis, in which the lethal change involves a single target in the organism and the probability of this change is constant with time. Thus, plots of the logarithm of the number of survivors against time will be linear; however, the slope of the curve will vary with the effectiveness of the killing process, which is influenced by the nature of the organism, lethal agent, concentration (in the case of disinfectants), and temperature. In general, the rate of killing increases exponentially with arithmetic increases in temperature or in concentrations of disinfectant. The data for developing killing curves are obtained from colony counts (Chapters 2 and 9) made on samples removed at intervals from a microbial suspension subjected to the sterilization process.

Sterility as a probability

An important consequence of exponential killing with most sterilization processes is that sterility is not an absolute term, but must be expressed as a probability. Thus, to continue the example given previously, the chance of a single survivor in 1 ml is theoretically 10^{-1} after 35 min. If a chance of 10^{-9} were the maximum acceptable risk for a single surviving organism in a 1-ml sample (for example, of a therapeutic agent), the procedure would require continuation for a total of 75 min.

Exponential killing

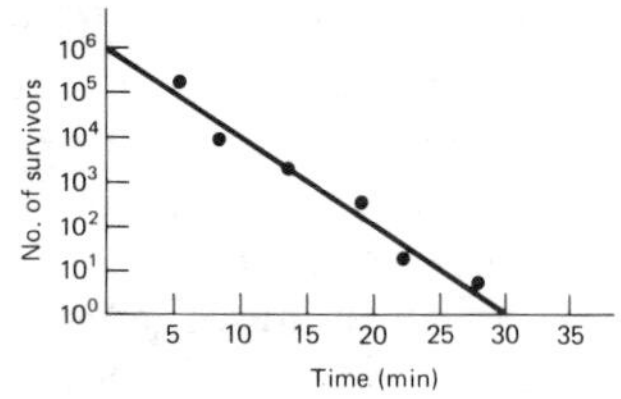

Deviation from exponential killing

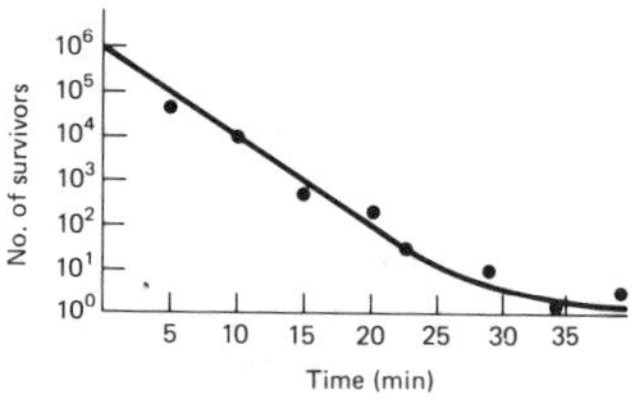

A simple single-hit curve often does not express the kinetics of killing adequately. If multiple targets are involved, the experimental curve will deviate from linearity. More significant, is the fact that microbial populations may include a small proportion of more resistant mutants or of organisms in a physiologic state that confers greater resistance to inactivation. In these cases, the later stages of the curve are flattened, and extrapolations from the exponential phase of killing may seriously underestimate the time needed for a high probability of achieving complete sterility. In practice, materials that will come into contact with tissues are sterilized under conditions that allow a very wide margin of safety, and the effectiveness of inactivation of organisms in vaccines is tested directly with large volumes and multiple samples before a product is made available for use.

Sterilization

The availability of reliable methods of sterilization has made possible the major developments in surgery and intrusive medical techniques that have helped to revolutionize medicine over the past century. Furthermore, sterilization procedures form the basis of many food preservation procedures, particularly in the canning industry.

Heat

Incineration

The simplest method of sterilization is to expose the surface to be sterilized to a naked flame. This technique is used in microbiology to sterilize the platinum or nickel chromium wire loop used to transfer cultures or spread inocula on solid media. It can be used equally effectively for emergency sterilization of a knife blade or a needle. Disposable material is, of course, rapidly and effectively decontaminated by incineration. Carbonization of organic material and destruction of microorganisms, including spores, will occur after exposure to dry heat of 160°C for 2 hr in a sterilizing oven. This method is applicable to metals, glassware, and some heat-resistant oils and waxes that are immiscible in water and cannot, therefore, be sterilized in the autoclave. A major use of the dry heat sterilizing oven is in preparation of laboratory glassware.

dry heat:
160°C for 2 hr

Moist heat

greater effectiveness than dry heat

boiling water fails to kill bacterial spores

Moist heat in the form of water or steam is far more rapid and effective in sterilization than dry heat, because reactive water molecules denature protein irreversibly by disrupting H bonds between peptide groups at relatively low temperatures. Most vegetative bacteria of importance in human disease are killed within a few minutes at 70°C or less, although many bacterial spores (Chapter 2) can resist boiling for prolonged periods. In the past, boiling water was widely used for sterilizing instruments; its effectiveness was often increased by adding sodium carbonate, which raised the temperature of boiling and the speed of killing and also helped to inhibit rusting. Currently, however, the use of boiling water has been replaced by the autoclave, which when properly used will ensure sterility by killing all forms of microorganisms.

autoclave effective because of increased temperature of steam generated under pressure

The *autoclave* is, in effect, a sophisticated pressure cooker (Figure 4.1). In its simplest form, it comprises a chamber in which the air can be replaced with pure saturated steam under pressure. Air is removed either by evacuating the chamber before filling with steam or by displacement through a valve at the bottom of the autoclave, which remains open until all air has drained out. The latter, which is termed a downward displacement autoclave, capitalizes on the heaviness of air compared to saturated steam. When the air has been removed, the temperature in the chamber is proportional to the pressure of the steam; autoclaves are usually operated at 121°C, which is achieved with a pressure of 15 psi. Under these conditions, spores directly exposed will be killed in less than 5 min, although the normal sterilization

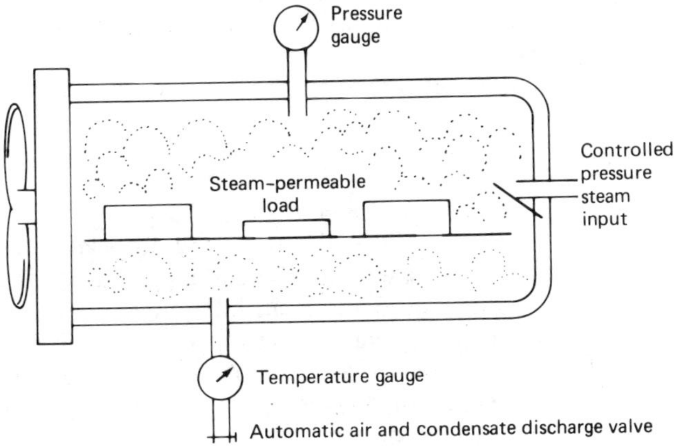

4.1 Simple form of downward displacement autoclave

killing rate increases logarithmically with arithmetic increase in temperature

role of condensation and latent heat in effectiveness of autoclave

Uses of autoclave

time is 10–15 min to account for variation in the ability of steam to penetrate different materials and to allow a wide margin of safety. As the volocity of killing increases logarithmically with arithmetic increases in temperature, a steam temperature of 121°C is vastly more effective than 100°C. For example, the spores of *Clostridium botulinum*, the cause of botulism, may survive 5 hr of boiling, but can be killed by 4 min at 121°C in the autoclave. The use of saturated steam in the autoclave has other advantages. Latent heat equivalent to 539 cal/g of condensed steam is immediately liberated upon condensation on the cooler surfaces of the load to be sterilized. The temperature of the load is thus raised very rapidly to that of the steam. Condensation also permits rapid steam penetration of porous materials such as surgical drapes by producing a relative negative pressure at the surface, which allows more steam to enter immediately. Autoclaves can thus be used for sterilizing any materials that are not damaged by heat and moisture, such as heat-stable liquids, swabs, most instruments, culture media, rubber gloves, and many others.

need for access of pure saturated steam

Causes of sterilization failures

It is essential that those who use autoclaves understand the principles involved. Their effectiveness depends on absence of air, pure saturated steam, and access of steam to the material to be sterilized. Pressure per se plays no role in sterilization other than to ensure the raised temperature of the steam. A temperature of less than 121°C at the bottom of the chamber with a pressure of 15 psi indicates that air is still present. A temperature of more than 121°C at this pressure indicates that the steam is superheated and no longer at the phase boundary with water. Superheated steam behaves as a gas and is no more effective in sterilization than air at the same temperature. Failure can also result from attempting to sterilize the interior of materials that are impermeable to steam or the contents of sealed containers. Under these conditions, a dry heat temperature of 121°C is obtained, which may be insufficient to kill even vegetative organisms. Large volumes of liquids require longer sterilization times than normal loads, because their temperature must reach 121°C before timing begins. Thermocouples may be needed to measure the internal temperature of such containers. When sealed containers of liquids are sterilized, it is essential that the autoclave cool without being opened or evacuated; otherwise, the containers may explode as the external pressure falls in relation to that within.

Flash autoclave

"Flash" autoclaves, which are widely used in operating rooms, often use saturated steam at a temperature of 134°C for 3 min. Air and steam are removed mechanically before and after the sterilization cycle so that metal instruments may be available rapidly.

Quality control of autoclaves depends primarily on ensuring that the appropriate temperature for the pressure used is achieved and that packing and timing are correct. Biologic and chemical indicators of the correct conditions are available and are inserted from time to time in the loads.

Gas

A number of articles, particularly certain plastics and lensed instruments that are damaged or destroyed by autoclaving, can be sterilized with ethylene oxide. Occasionally formaldehyde gas is used to decontaminate larger areas.

Ethylene oxide sterilization of heat-labile materials

Ethylene oxide is an inflammable and potentially explosive gas. It is an alkylating agent that inactivates microorganisms by replacing labile hydrogen atoms on hydroxyl, carboxy, or sulfhydryl groups. Ethylene oxide sterilizers resemble autoclaves and expose the load to 10% ethylene oxide in Freon or carbon dioxide at 50–60°C under controlled conditions of humidity. Exposure times are usually about 4–6 hr and must be followed by a pro-

need for aeration after ethylene oxide sterilization

longed period of aeration to allow the gas to diffuse out of substances that have absorbed it. Aeration is essential, because absorbed gas can cause damage to tissues or skin. Ethylene oxide is a mutagen, and special precautions are now taken to ensure that it is properly vented outside of working spaces. Used under properly controlled conditions, ethylene oxide is an effective sterilizing agent for heat-labile devices such as artificial heart valves that cannot be treated at the temperature of the autoclave.

Ultraviolet Light and Ionizing Radiation

UV light causes direct damage to DNA

Uses and limitations of UV light

Ultraviolet light in the wavelength of 240–280 nm is absorbed by nucleic acids and causes genetic damage, including the formation of the thymine dimers discussed previously. The practical value of UV sterilization is limited by its poor ability to penetrate. Apart from its use experimentally as a mutagen, its main application has been irradiation of air in the vicinity of critical surgical sites and aiding in the decontamination of laboratory facilities used for handling particularly hazardous organisms. In these situations, single exposed organisms are rapidly inactivated. It must be remembered that UV light can cause skin and eye damage, and workers exposed to it must be appropriately protected.

Effects of ionizing radiation

Ionizing radiation carries far greater energy than UV light. It, too, causes direct damage to DNA and produces toxic free radicals and hydrogen peroxide from water within the microbial cells. Cathode rays and gamma rays from cobalt-60 are widely used in industrial processes, including the sterilization of many disposable surgical supplies such as gloves, plastic syringes, and the like, because they can be packaged before exposure to the penetrating radiation.

Filtration

Membrane filters

Both live and dead microorganisms can be removed from liquids by positive- or negative-pressure filtration. Membrane filters, usually composed of cellulose esters (for example, cellulose acetate), are available commercially with pore sizes of 0.005–1 μm. For removal of bacteria, a pore size of 0.2 μm is effective because filters act not only mechanically but by electrostatic adsorption of particles to their surface.

Filtration is used for sterilization of large volumes of fluid, especially those containing heat-labile components such as serum.

Pasteurization and Tyndallization

Pasteurization involves exposure of liquids to temperature in the range of 55–75°C to remove all vegetative bacteria of significance in human disease. Spores are unaffected by the pasteurization process.

Pasteurization of milk, wine, and equipment for respiratory therapy

Pasteurization is used commercially to render milk safe and extend its storage quality. To the dismay of some of his compatriots, Pasteur proposed application of the process to winemaking to prevent microbial spoilage and vinegarization. This method was quickly adopted by the upstart California wine industry, and controlled experiments—anathema to the finest palates—indicated no effect on the quality or bouquet of wine when the process was undertaken properly. Most wines currently available have been filter sterilized. Pasteurization in water at 70°C for 30 min has also been used for rendering respiratory equipment free of organisms that may otherwise multiply in mucus and humidifying water and cause respiratory infections.

Tyndallization: limitations of use

Tyndallization is an ingenious procedure developed by John Tyndall in 1887 for killing both vegetative and spore-forming bacteria at temperatures of 100°C or below in nutrient materials such as certain culture media. The material is heated to kill vegetative organisms, held at room temperature for several hours to allow any spores present to germinate, and then reheated to kill the vegetative progeny of the spores. The process is usually repeated three times. Filtration has rendered this approach obsolete, but it is mentioned because its application to nonnutrient heat-sensitive materials has been reported occasionally. Obviously, it will be ineffective in sterilizing spore-forming organisms under these conditions, because the spores will not germinate.

Disinfection, Antisepsis, and Sanitization

general protoplasmic poisons

inactivation of disinfectants by organic material

Given access and sufficient time, disinfectants cause the death of pathogenic vegetative bacteria. Most are general protoplasmic poisons and are not currently used in the treatment of infections other than very superficial lesions, having been replaced by antimicrobics (see Chapter 10). Some, such as the quaternary ammonium compounds, alcohol, and the iodophors reduce the superficial flora and can eliminate contaminating pathogenic bacteria from the skin surface. Others, such as the phenolics, are valuable only for treatment of inanimate surfaces or for rendering contaminated materials safe. All are bound and inactivated to varying degrees by protein and dirt and lose considerable activity when applied to other than clean surfaces. Their activity increases exponentially with increases in temperature, but the relationship of increases in concentration to killing effectiveness is more complex and varies for each compound. Optimal in-use concentrations have been established for all available disinfectants. The major groups of compounds currently used are briefly discussed as follows.

Alcohols

alcohols require some water for antibacterial effectiveness

uses of ethanol and isopropyl alcohol

The alcohols are protein denaturants that rapidly kill vegetative bacteria when applied as aqueous solutions in the range of 70–95% alcohol. They are inactive against bacterial spores and many viruses. Solutions of 100% alcohol dehydrate organisms rapidly and fail to kill, because the lethal process requires water molecules. Ethanol (70–90%) and isopropyl alcohol (90–95%) are widely used as skin decontaminants before simple invasive procedures such as venipuncture. Their effect is not instantaneous, and the traditional alcohol wipe, particularly when followed by a vein-probing finger, is more symbolic than effective, because insufficient time is given for significant killing.

Isopropyl alcohol has largely replaced ethanol in hospital use because it is somewhat more active and is not subject to diversion to house staff parties.

Halogens

Effectiveness of tincture of iodine

allergenicity

Iodine is an effective disinfectant that acts by iodinating or oxidizing essential components of the microbial cell. It is commonly used as a tincture of 2% iodine in 50% alcohol. It kills more rapidly and effectively than alcohol alone, but has the disadvantage of sometimes causing hypersensitivity reactions and of staining materials with which it comes in contact. It is an excellent preparation for use on skin before drawing a blood culture, a procedure in which contamination must be excluded as much as possible. Tincture of iodine is applied and allowed to dry, and the iodine then removed with alcohol swabs. This procedure ensures an application time sufficient for adequate skin disinfection. Other preparations are available in which iodine is combined with organic compounds such as detergents in

Iodophors

dissociable complexes. These agents, termed *iodophors,* cause less skin staining and dehydration than tinctures and are widely used in preparation of skin before surgery. As they, too, are allergenic, iodophors should not be used on patients with a history of iodine sensitivity.

Chlorination of water and swimming pools

Chlorine is a highly effective oxidizing agent, which accounts for its lethality to microbes. It exists as hypochlorous acid in aqueous solutions that dissociate to yield free chlorine over a wide pH range, particularly under slightly acidic conditions. In concentrations of less than one part per million, chlorine is lethal within seconds to most vegetative bacteria, and it inactivates most viruses; this efficacy accounts for its use in rendering supplies of drinking water safe and in chlorination of water in swimming pools. Chlorine reacts rapidly with protein and many other organic compounds, and its activity is lost quickly in the presence of organic material. This property, combined with its toxicity, renders it ineffective on body surfaces; however, it is the agent of choice for decontaminating surfaces and glassware that have been contaminated with viruses or spores of pathogenic bacteria. For these purposes it is usually applied as a 5% solution of sodium hypochlorite.

use of NaOCl as a decontaminating agent

Surface-Active Compounds

Hydrophobic and hydrophilic groups of surfactants

effects on bacterial cell membrane

Surfactants are compounds with hydrophobic and hydrophilic groups that attach to and solubilize various compounds or alter their properties. Anionic detergents such as soaps are highly effective cleansers but have little direct antibacterial effect, probably because their charge is similar to that of most microorganisms. Cationic detergents, particularly the quaternary ammonium compounds ("quats") such as benzalkonium chloride, are highly bactericidal in the absence of contaminating organic matter. Their hydrophobic and lipophilic groups react with the lipid of the cell membrane of the bacteria, alter its surface properties and its permeability, and lead to loss of essential cell components and death. These compounds have little toxicity to skin and mucous membranes, and thus have been used widely in concentrations of 0.1% for their antibacterial effects. They are inactive against spores and most viruses.

problems with contamination of "quats"

The greatest care is needed in the use of "quats" because they will adsorb to most surfaces with which they come in contact, such as cotton, cork, and even dust. As a result, their concentration may be lowered to a point at which certain bacteria, particularly *Pseudomonas aeruginosa,* can grow in the solutions and then cause serious infections. Many instances have been recorded of severe infections resulting from contamination of ophthalmic preparations or of solutions used for treating skin before transcutaneous procedures. These compounds should be stored in small containers and never reused. Unless contraindicated, they are better used in tincture form because the alcohol avoids the risk of contamination. It should also be remembered that cationic detergents are totally neutralized by anionic compounds. Thus, the antibacterial effect of quaternary ammonium compounds is inactivated by soap.

neutralization of cationic detergents by soaps

Quats in much higher concentrations than those used in medicine (for example, 5–10%) are highly effective for sanitizing surfaces.

Phenolics

Environmental decontamination with phenols and cresols

Phenol, one of the first effective disinfectants, was the primary agent employed by Lister in his antiseptic surgical procedure, which preceded the development of aseptic surgery. It is a potent protein denaturant and bactericidal agent. Substitutions in the ring structure of phenol have substantially improved activity, and a range of phenols and cresols that are effective environmental decontaminants are now widely used in hospital hygiene. They are less deviated by protein than are most other disinfectants, have a detergentlike effect on the cell membrane, and are often formulated with soaps to increase their cleansing property. They are too toxic to skin and tissues to be used as antiseptics.

Skin decontamination with hexachlorophene and chlorhexidine

toxicity of hexachlorophene

Two diphenyl compounds, hexachlorophene and chlorhexidine, have been extensively used as skin disinfectants. Hexachlorophene is primarily bacteriostatic. Incorporated in a soap, it builds up on the surface of skin epithelial cells over 1–2 days of use to produce a steady inhibitory effect on skin flora and Gram-positive contaminants, as long as its use is continued. It was a major factor in controlling outbreaks of severe staphylococcal infections in nurseries during the 1950s and 1960s, but was then found to produce neurotoxic effects in some premature babies and, when applied in excessive concentrations, in older children. It is now a prescription drug. Hexachlorophene has been replaced by chlorhexidine solutions or tincture of chlorhexidine as a routine hand and skin disinfectant. Chlorhexidine is rapidly bactericidal and has very low toxicity.

Glutaraldehyde and Formaldehyde

Use of glutaraldehyde in decontamination of equipment

Glutaraldehyde and formaldehyde are alkylating agents highly lethal to essentially all microorganisms. Formaldehyde gas is irritative, allergenic, and unpleasant, properties that limit its use as a solution or gas. Glutaraldehyde is an effective sterilizing agent for apparatus that cannot be heat treated, such as some lensed instruments and equipment for respiratory therapy. Formaldehyde vapor, an effective environmental decontaminant under conditions of high humidity, is sometimes used to decontaminate laboratory rooms that have been accidentally and extensively contaminated with pathogenic bacteria, including those, such as the anthrax bacillus, that form resistant spores. Such rooms are sealed for processing and thoroughly aired before reoccupancy.

There are numerous other disinfectant compounds, but those discussed herein remain the most important.

Additional Reading and References

Favero, M.S. 1980. Sterilization, disinfection and antisepsis in the hospital. In *Manual of Clinical Microbiology.* 3rd ed. Lennette, E.H., Balows, A., Hausler, W.J., and Truant, J.P., Eds. Washington, D.C.: American Society for Microbiology. A good account of the practical use of disinfectants.

Perkins, J.J. 1982. *Principles and Methods of Sterilization in Health Sciences.* 2nd ed. Springfield, Ill.: Charles C Thomas. An excellent standard text and source of reference.

John Spizizen

Bacterial Variation and Genetics

5

Despite the differences in cellular organization of DNA between bacteria and higher life forms, the processes of DNA replication and of gene expression and control are essentially identical. This was extensively exploited in developing the new science of molecular biology because of the rapidity of bacterial growth, the ability to detect genetic alterations in single cells, and the ease with which large volumes of identical cells could be obtained for biochemical studies.

Like all other forms of life, heredity in bacteria is determined by genes, which specify the polypeptides of enzymes and other proteins. The individual traits that constitute the specific characteristics of a microbial cell make up the cell's *phenotype*, which is directed by the genes. The individuality of the genetic components of a cell is its *genotype*. In the case of bacteria, the genes are located in the single chromosome that constitutes the nucleoid, although two to four nucleoids may be present under certain conditions. The chromosome consists of a large, double-stranded molecule of DNA, which is circular and covalently closed. Chromosomal DNA is extensively coiled in the cell. If opened and extended, the chromosome of *Escherichia coli* would measure about 1 mm; in its native supercoiled state, however, it appears as a rounded discrete body, the nucleoid. Unlike the nucleus of eukaryotic cells (Chapter 1), the bacterial (prokaryotic) nucleoid has no nuclear membrane and the DNA is not associated with basic proteins or histones.

chromosome comprises covalently closed, double-stranded DNA

physical state of chromosomal DNA

In addition to the chromosome, many bacterial cells have extrachromosomal DNA in the form of plasmids. Plasmids are also covalently closed, circular molecules of double-stranded DNA, but they are considerably smaller than chromosomal DNA. The molecular weight of plasmids varies from 10^6 to 10^8. In contrast, the molecular weight of the chromosome of *E. coli* is about 3×10^9 and consists of 4.6×10^6 base pairs. Plasmids may exist as single or multiple copies in each cell. More than one type of plasmid may coexist.

plasmids are smaller, covalently closed, double-stranded DNA molecules

Still other forms of DNA may be present in microbial cells. The DNA of infecting bacteriophages may be inserted into the chromosome or its replicative intermediates may be present in the cytoplasm of the cell. Insertion sequences (the so-called IS elements) are present in different locations in the chromosome and plasmids of bacteria such as *E. coli.* These elements, which consist of double-stranded DNA segments, can move to new positions

Bacteriophage DNA

Transposable elements

on the chromosome or plasmids. They do not encode any detectable traits, but may have an influence on adjacent genes. Transposable elements that contain a gene for antibiotic resistance or other detectable phenotypes are known as *transposons.* Transposons usually consist of IS elements bounding a segment of DNA that encodes antibiotic resistance or other traits. The IS elements and transposons have inverted repeat nucleotide sequences at each end of the segments.

inverted repeat sequences of transposable elements

Thus, the bacterial cell contains genetic information mainly in its single chromosome, but accessory information may also exist in gene segments capable of movement within and without the chromosome. Some of these elements encode cellular traits; others do not. Some segments may contain bacteriophage genes. In addition, self-replicating extrachromosomal DNA may be present in the cell in the form of plasmids, which may or may not encode phenotypic traits.

Gene Expression

Genetic control of protein synthesis

The DNA in the chromosome or in plasmids consists of regions that have the necessary information for specifying the synthesis of proteins. The amino acids synthesized are determined by triplets of nucleotides. The sequence of nucleotide triplets in these regions determines the order in which the amino acids are placed in the synthesis of specific polypeptides. The chromosomal sections containing the specific nucleotide sequences are the genes, which direct the synthesis of polypeptides or larger protein subunits that aggregate with other subunits to form proteins, including enzymes. Although most proteins produced are structural and enzymatic, some have regulatory functions. These regulatory proteins bind to specific sites in the chromosome and thus can control the synthesis of other proteins specified by adjacent regions. In this way, the process of protein synthesis is regulated in microbial cells.

Regulatory proteins

Operons

One of the unique features of bacterial cells is the control of gene expression by means of an *operator* gene. This gene is often adjacent to a number of genes encoding enzymes of a metabolic pathway. Such a gene cluster under the control of a single operator is called an *operon. Repressor* proteins produced by the cell under certain conditions specifically bind to the operator gene and prevent the formation of the mRNA of the adjacent genes in the operon.

There are approximately 5000 genes in the chromosome of a bacterial cell such as *E. coli.* Their expression results in the synthesis of the complex enzymatic machinery of the cell, which may vary under different environmental conditions because of the influence of these conditions on regulatory processes. Other genes specify the synthesis of the structural proteins of membranes, cell walls, and other cellular components.

Mutation

Types of mutations

The ability of the microbial cell to maintain its identity after reproduction is due to the information content determined by the sequence of bases of the DNA. Because triplets of bases determine the specific amino acids formed, alteration in a single base will result in formation of a different amino acid and thus in a significant change in the protein for which the gene codes. If the protein is an enzyme, such a change usually results in complete loss of activity. Whole segments of DNA are sometimes lost or translocated to other portions of the chromosome, which also results in changes in the proteins synthesized. Such alterations in base sequence are called *mutations. Point mutations* refer to single base changes, *deletions* to removal of sections of bases, and *frame-shift mutations* to additions or losses of single bases that alter the reading frame during the translation leading to protein synthesis.

Spontaneous mutation and mutagenesis

Mutations occur spontaneously and are the basis of many microbial variations. The cell containing the mutation, the so-called mutant, is generally not evident in a population of bacteria because any one mutation occurs infrequently and only comes to predominate in the presence of some specific selective factor favoring it over the "wild" type from which it was derived. Spontaneous mutation frequencies may be as low as 1 in 10^{10} or as high as 1 in 10^5 cells of population; however, frequencies can be increased markedly by a number of agents, collectively known as *mutagens*. Substances that react with DNA, for example, can produce alterations leading to base changes after DNA replication. Ethyl methane sulfonate and *N*-methyl-*N*-nitro-*N*-nitrosoguanidine are highly active in this regard, and ultraviolet light and ionizing radiation are also effective mutagens. Insertion sequences and transposons, when inserted into the chromosome, also act as mutagens by altering the sequence of bases. Bacteria have been used as indicators for testing the mutagenicity of substances that may pose problems for humans, because the rapid growth rate of bacteria allows genetic changes to be detected easily. Screening of large numbers of compounds is thus permitted.

use of bacteria as indicators for mutagenic compounds

Mutant selection

Methods for selecting mutants from a population of microbial cells are generally required for detection. Thus, mutants that confer antibiotic resistance can be detected readily by culturing in the presence of antibiotic concentrations that will inhibit or kill the sensitive cells, but allow the resistant mutant to grow. This process may also occur in vivo during antibiotic therapy (Chapter 10). Mutations that obviate a cell's requirement for a growth factor such as a vitamin or an amino acid are also readily selected by their ability to grow on media lacking the factor. Cells that require the growth factor are called *auxotrophs*; those that do not are known as *prototrophs*.

Auxotrophic mutants

Auxotrophic mutations are the result of a defect in an enzyme of a biosynthetic pathway, thus preventing the synthesis of a compound required for growth. The reverse mutation to prototrophy restores the enzymatic activity, so that the growth factor is no longer required.

Thus, microbial variation can result from mutation and subsequent selection. Selective forces such as antibiotics allow the mutants to predominate. Other mutants may grow better than the wild type under special environmental conditions (such as artificial culture), resulting in eventual replacement of the original wild-type population.

Gene (DNA) Transfer

Transformation, transduction, and conjugation

The transfer of genetic elements between bacterial cells also leads to variation. Chromosomal, plasmid, and bacteriophage DNA can all be transferred by several methods. These processes include DNA transformation, bacteriophage transduction, and cell conjugation. In transformation, free DNA from another bacterium crosses the cell wall barrier of the recipient strain. If it is homologous to the chromosomal DNA of the recipient, it can pair with the resident chromosome, leading to recombination. If it is extrachromosomal, it may be able to replicate autonomously in the new cell. In transduction, bacteriophage particles carry over chromosomal or extrachromosomal DNA to the cell that they infect. In cell conjugation or mating, chromosomal or extrachromosomal DNA is transferred when "male" and "female" cells are brought into contact (Figure 5.1).

transformation of pneumococcal capsules and virulence

Transformation by DNA was first demonstrated with pneumococci in classic experiments that identified DNA as the carrier of genetic information. In these studies, purified DNA from a virulent encapsulated pneumococcus of capsular type III was added to a culture of an avirulent nonencapsulated

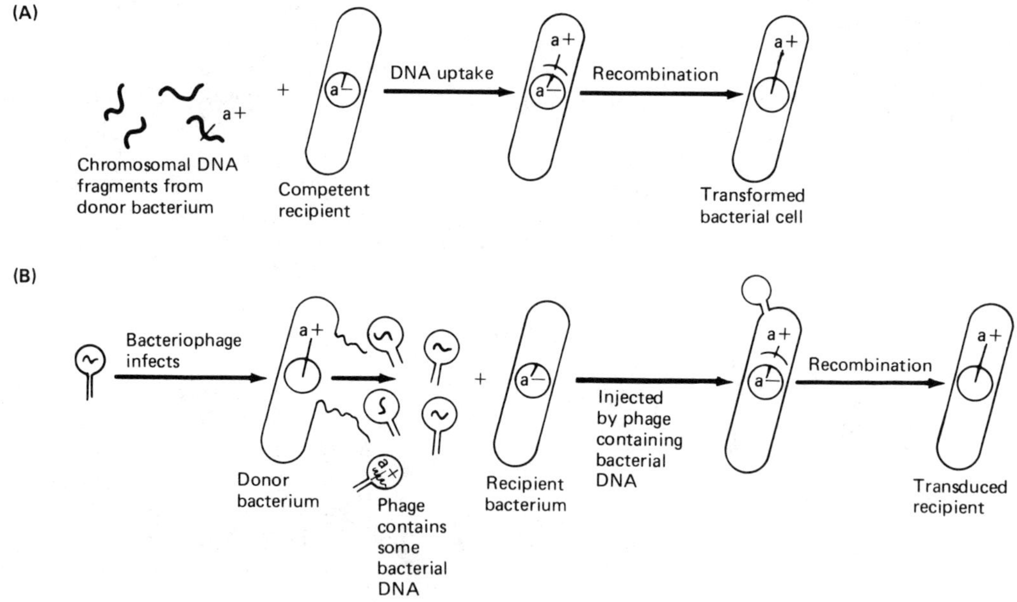

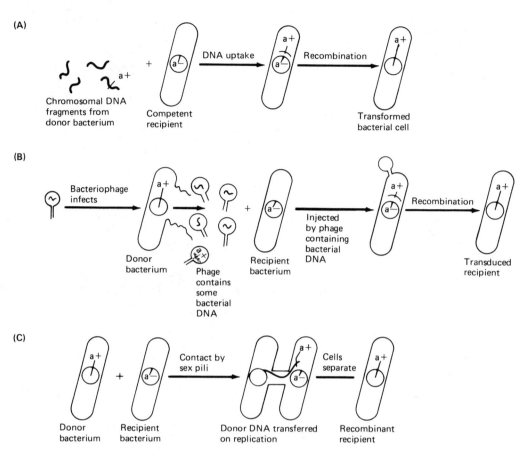

5.1 Chromosomal gene transfer mechanisms in bacteria. (**A**) Transformation. (**B**) Transduction. (**C**) Conjugation.

strain originally derived from one of capsular type II. The DNA contained the information for synthesis of the type III capsular polysaccharide and was incorporated into the genome of the capsule-defective strain by recombination. In this way, some cells of the avirulent nonencapsulated strain were transformed into virulent encapsulated cells of the capsular serotype of the DNA donor (type III) and could be selected by their ability to cause lethal infections in mice. Subsequently, numerous other traits have been shown to be transferable by transformation within several bacterial species.

Competence

transformation within few species only

The transforming DNA attaches and penetrates the recipient cells only if they are in the "competent" stage of growth. Competence is usually found near the end of the logarithmic phase of growth. Only a few microbial species can become competent for DNA transformation when intact cells are used. In some other species, however, transformation can be achieved with spheroplasts, cells from which the walls have been partially removed by enzyme treatment. The intact cell wall thus appears to be a barrier to DNA penetration.

Characteristics of DNA required for transformation

Transforming DNA containing chromosomal genes is taken up most actively by competent cells when it exists as double-stranded linear fragments larger than 0.5 megadaltons. Single-stranded DNA may transform under special conditions that protect it from degradation by extracellular nucleases.

chromosomal transformation requires DNA homology; plasmid or phage DNA transformation does not

An essential requirement for activity of transforming chromosomal DNA is homology of its base sequence with that of the recipient DNA. Thus, chromosomal DNA transformation is restricted to closely related species. Transformation by plasmid or bacteriophage DNA, however, does not require sequence homology, and such DNA can cross species lines more readily. It is not clear whether transformation occurs in nature to any significant extent.

Transduction by bacteriophage possible in all bacterial species

occasional incorporation of host DNA into phage coat

incorporation of transduced DNA into recipient cell

Transduction of chromosomal gene fragments and of plasmid DNA appears to be universal among bacteria. Bacteriophage (phage) particles containing chromosomal or plasmid DNA from the host cell are formed during their replication cycle, when host DNA fragments are incorporated within the phage coat instead of bacteriophage DNA. This phenomenon occurs in only a small fraction of the phage population. The host DNA fragments must be of proper size to be encoated, and nucleases formed as a result of bacteriophage activity fragment the chromosomal DNA during bacteriophage replication. The DNA incorporated into the transducing phage particles is double stranded and linear and, as in the case of transformation, can be incorporated into the resident genome by genetic recombination only if homology exists. As with transformation, however, transduction of plasmid DNA is not confined to homologous species.

requirements for phage receptors and nonlethality in transduction

Transduction thus requires the ability of the bacteriophage to attach to specific receptors on the cell and inject its DNA. As the infected cell must not be killed by the bacteriophage, a temperate bacteriophage is more likely to perform transduction than a virulent type. Transduction has many similarities to transformation, but differs in that the DNA of the transducing bacteriophage is protected by the protein coat from the action of the enzyme deoxyribonuclease, whereas transforming DNA is readily inactivated by the enzyme.

Conjugation

sex pili and cell-to-cell contact

most transfers by conjugation involve plasmids and plasmid DNA

Conjugative and nonconjugative plasmids

In conjugation or bacterial mating, DNA transfer is mediated by thin protein structures, called *sex pili,* produced by the donor cell. Several sex pili are formed by the donor, and contact is made to specific receptor sites on a recipient cell; this process is followed by retraction, which allows cell contact. The DNA may actually be transferred through the core of the pilus. Most transfers by conjugation among bacteria involve plasmid DNA. Many plasmids, the so-called conjugative plasmids, contain genes known as *tra* (transfer) *genes,* which are responsible for the production of sex pili and other functions required for the conjugative process. A single-stranded copy of the plasmid DNA is transferred to a recipient cell, where a complementary strand is made and replication occurs. Some cells contain both a self-transmissible and a nontransmissible plasmid.

chromosomal material may be transferred with integrated conjugative plasmid

F and Hfr

F′ plasmid

Portions of the chromosome, or sometimes the entire chromosome, may be transferred through the sex pili as a consequence of integration into the chromosome of a conjugative plasmid. Thus, in the case of the F or fertility plasmid of *E. coli* K12, recombination of the plasmid into the chromosome results in the production of Hfr (high frequency of recombination) cells. Conjugation is then promoted by the *tra* genes of the integrated F plasmid, and chromosomal fragments are transmitted to cells lacking F plasmid, the so-called F^- cells. All Hfr cells can transfer chromosomal material. Unlike free plasmid DNA, transferred fragments of chromosomal DNA cannot self-replicate and must recombine with the resident chromosome to survive. Occasionally the F genome, along with a small fragment of the chromosome, will detach from the chromosome in an Hfr cell, converting it to a plasmid termed *F′*. Subsequent reintegration of the F′ plasmid into the chromosome occurs at high frequency.

plasmid transfer by conjugation can cross species lines

Transfer of plasmid DNA by conjugation generally occurs more frequently than transfer of chromosomal DNA. The frequencies of transfers of plasmid DNA are greatest among closely related strains; unlike chromosomal transfer, however, plasmid transfer can occur with distantly related species and genera, because plasmids are self-replicating and do not require homology with the resident chromosome.

Plasmid Phenotypes

Nonessential plasmid genes

Plasmid gene conferring antibiotic resistance or virulence

Plasmid-coded metabolic properties

plasmids and bacteriocins

Plasmids may contain genes responsible for traits that are not essential characteristics of a microbial species, but which allow the survival of bacteria under particular environmental conditions or in some cases determine their pathogenicity. Examples of some plasmid-coded traits are shown in Table 5.1. Some plasmids are cryptic, that is, they have no discernible phenotypic effect or function. The occurrence of plasmid-carried genes for antibiotic resistance, and their selection and spread as a result of extensive use of antibiotics, is of paramount significance in infectious diseases and is discussed in greater detail in Chapter 10. Some plasmid genes encode toxin production or other determinants of virulence such as pilus production (Table 5.2). In other cases, plasmids provide the cell with genes that permit the utilization of compounds not normally metabolized by the species. For example, enteric pathogens of the genus *Salmonella* characteristically do not utilize lactose; this feature is useful in differentiation of *Salmonella* from *E. coli*, which ferments lactose. Occasionally *Salmonella* will acquire a plasmid containing the gene coding for lactose utilization, which removes this important differential trait. Plasmids can also carry genes coding for the production of a protein termed *bacteriocin*, which is lethal to some bacterial strains other than those that produce it. In *E. coli*, the bacteriocins are termed *colicins*. Various colicins are produced that are active against different strains of *E. coli* and can be used to subtype this species. The function of bacteriocins may be to eliminate competing strains and to help establish the producing strain in a particular ecologic niche. Many other plasmid-coded traits are known (Table 5.1) that provide bacteria with increased versatility.

movement of transposable genes between plasmids and chromosomes

mutations produced by chromosomal insertion of transposons

In some bacteria, genes commonly found on plasmids may also occur on the chromosomes. For example, some genes that confer resistance to antibiotics or code for toxins may be present in either site, perhaps because they are situated on transposons. For example, the *ent* gene of *E. coli* (Table 5.2) is part of a transposon, as is the lactose-utilizing gene; these transposons can insert themselves into a number of sites on the chromosome, as well as into other plasmids. Insertion of a transposon into the chromosome usually results in mutation. In a recent experiment, insertion of a tetracycline-resistant transposon into the chromosome of a virulent strain of *Salmonella typhimurium* resulted in a mutation in the aromatic biosynthetic pathway, which produced a requirement for aromatic amino acids for growth with

Table 5.1 Plasmid-Coded Traits

Conjugation (sex factor)	Colonization antigens
Chromosome mobilization	Nitrogen fixation
Bacteriocins (e.g., colicins)	Plant tumors (crown gall)
Antibiotic resistance	Hydrocarbon degradation
Heavy metal resistance	Carbohydrate fermentation
Toxins	

Table 5.2 Examples of Some Virulence Factors Produced by Plasmid and Bacteriophage Genes

Plasmid or Phage	Bacterial Strain	Virulence Factor	Disease Produced
ent plasmid	*Escherichia coli*	Enterotoxin	Diarrhea
Surface antigen plasmid	*Escherichia coli*	Colonization antigens	Diarrhea
Colicin V plasmid	*Escherichia coli*	Invasive properties	
Exfoliative plasmid	*Staphylococcus aureus*	Exfoliative toxin	Scalded skin syndrome
Corynebacterium phage β	*Corynebacterium diphtheriae*	Diphtherial toxin	Diphtheria

inability to multiply in laboratory mice. The mutant strain, however, produced immunity in mice and was able to protect them against the virulent parent organism. This example illustrates how the use of transposon mutation techniques may be useful in developing vaccines.

Recombinant DNA Techniques

Insertion of extraneous DNA

Recent advances in knowledge of microbial genetics and of the chemistry of nucleic acids have allowed the insertion into DNA molecules of specific exogenous genes that will replicate when they are inserted into microbial cells. This new technology has facilitated study of the molecular nature of heredity and allowed production of some complex mammalian biologic products in quantity by bacteria or yeasts. Recombinant DNA techniques developed from the discovery of specific enzymes derived from bacteria that break DNA molecules at defined sites. These enzymes are called *restriction endonucleases* or *restriction enzymes*, because they recognize foreign DNA (for example, viral DNA) and degrade it unless it has been modified by another enzyme that inserts methyl groups on certain bases. Restriction enzymes attach to and subsequently cleave a defined oligonucleotide sequence in double-stranded DNA, with production of discrete fragments of DNA. Some of the enzymes make breaks in both strands of the DNA; however, these breaks are several nucleotides apart from each other on the two strands. The result is the production of single-stranded ends that are termed *sticky* or *cohesive*, because they can easily associate with complementary single-stranded ends of other DNA molecules by base pairing (for example, adenine associates with thymine and guanine with cytosine by hydrogen bonding). The fragments may also circularize by the same mechanism. Other restriction enzymes produce flush-ended fragments, which cut DNA at the recognition site on directly opposite sides of the double-stranded molecules.

Restriction endonucleases

Sites of enzyme cuts

Plasmids with single cleavage sites for specific restriction enzymes are found to be useful as vehicles for gene cloning. When DNA from another source is cut with the same enzyme, the fragments can then associate with the cleaved plasmid. Thus, in Figure 5.2, DNA molecule P represents a singly cut plasmid and molecule C a fragment of enzyme-cleaved DNA from another source. The cohesive single-stranded ends will associate to circularize the molecule. After association, the enzyme DNA ligase is added to seal the nicks in the hybrid molecule. Such recombinant DNA molecules can be transformed into bacteria such as *E. coli*. If the plasmid contains a marker gene for antibiotic resistance, the transformed cell can be isolated on media

Plasmid vectors in gene cloning

Selection of cells transformed with recombinant plasmid

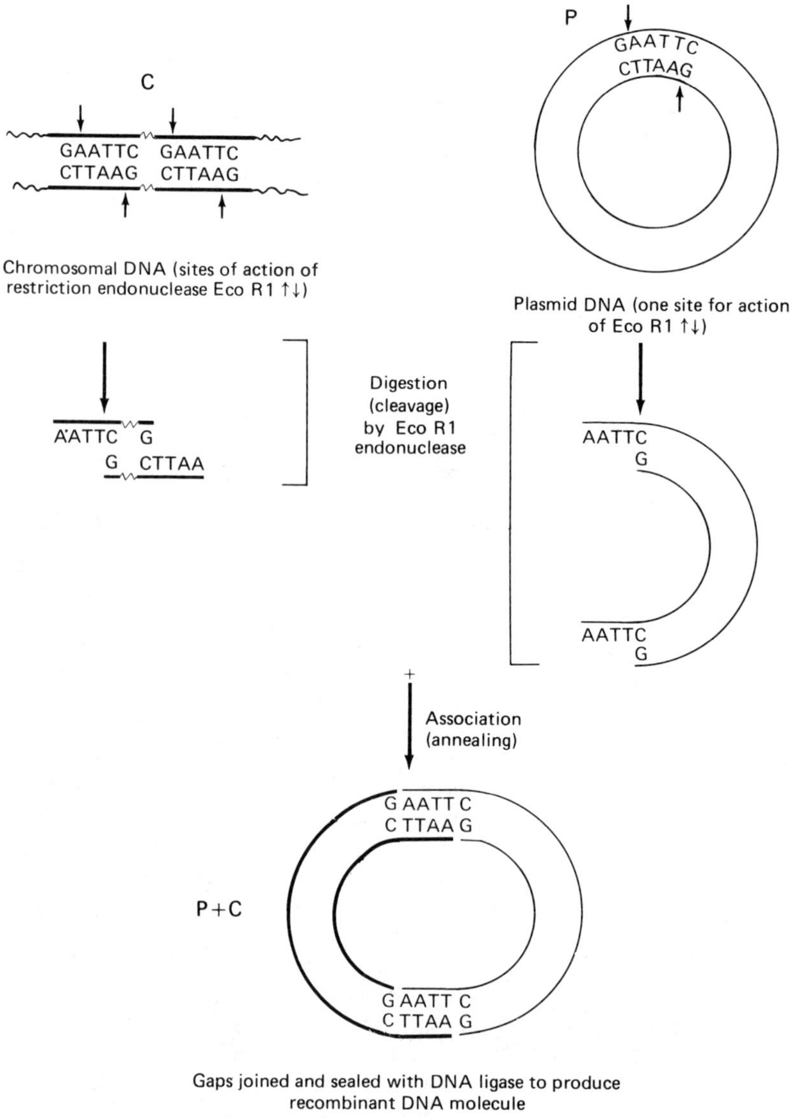

5.2 Construction of a recombinant DNA molecule. C represents chromosomal fragments. P represents plasmid.

containing the relevant antibiotic. The recombinant molecule then replicates as a plasmid in the recipient bacteria, and the gene insert is maintained and replicated. In principle, any gene can thus be replicated in *E. coli* or other recipient bacteria, a process called *gene cloning*. A plasmid used for gene cloning is called a *cloning vector*. Bacteriophages are also used as cloning vectors.

Bacteriophage vectors

Theoretic and practical implications of gene cloning

Gene expression in *E. coli* has been demonstrated for many gene inserts from a variety of microbes and higher organisms. Recombinant DNA technology thus has far-reaching importance in increasing our ability to investigate gene function, including viral genes. It is of great practical importance in that it makes possible large-scale production of biologic compounds such as insulin and growth hormones, which could only be obtained previously with great difficulty and at great expense from mammalian tissues. These compounds can now be produced in bacteria, which can be readily propagated in large amounts.

Additional Reading and References

Avery, O.T., MacLeod, C.M., and McCarty, M. 1944. Studies on the chemical nature of the substance inducing transformation of pneumococcal types. *J. Exp. Med.* 79:137–158. The first demonstration that DNA transforms bacterial cells and thus contains genetic information.

Cohen, S.N., and Shapiro, J.A. 1980. Transposable genetic elements. *Sci. Am.* 242:40–49. Mobile genes and their role in bacterial variation.

Drake, J.W., and Baltz, R.H. 1976. The biochemistry of mutagenesis. *Annu. Rev. Biochem.* 45:11–37. The mechanisms of mutation and DNA damage.

Elwell, L.P., and Shipley, P.L. 1980. Plasmid-mediated factors associated with virulence of bacteria to animals. *Annu. Rev. Microbiol.* 34:465–496. Genes present in plasmids which code for virulence factors.

Old, R.W., and Primrose, S.B. 1981. *Principles of Gene Manipulation. An Introduction to Genetic Engineering.* 2nd ed. University of California Press. Recombinant DNA and its cloning genes from various living cells.

John C. Sherris

Normal Microbial Flora

6

The term *normal* or *indigenous flora* is used to describe microorganisms that are frequently found in particular sites in normal, healthy individuals. The constituents and numbers of the flora vary in different areas of the body, and sometimes at different ages. They comprise microorganisms whose morphologic, physiologic, and genetic properties allow them to colonize and multiply under the conditions that exist in particular sites, to coexist with other colonizing organisms, and to inhibit competing intruders. Thus, each accessible area of the body presents a particular ecological niche, colonization of which requires a particular set of properties of the invading microbe.

Organisms of the normal flora can be classified as *parasites,** which live at the expense of the host; *symbionts,* which benefit the host; and *commensals,* which have a neutral relationship to the host. In many instances, however, not enough is known about the organism's interactions with the host to make such distinctions. They can also be categorized as *residents,* which are present invariably or for many weeks or months in a particular site, and *transients,* which may establish themselves briefly for colonization or infection without disease, but tend to be excluded by competition from residents or by the host's innate or immune defense mechanisms. The distinction between the transient and the *carrier state* is blurred when potentially pathogenic organisms are involved. For example, *Streptococcus pneumoniae* (the pneumococcus), isolated from the upper respiratory tract of many healthy people during the winter months, is often considered part of the transient normal flora. In contrast, the presence of *Neisseria meningitidis* (the meningococcus) in the nasopharynx of healthy individuals during epidemics of meningococcal meningitis is usually regarded as carriage.

Residents and transients

normal flora and the carrier state

It is important for students of medical microbiology and infectious disease to have a good grasp of the role of the normal flora, because of its significance both as a defense mechanism against infection and as a source of potentially pathogenic organisms. It is also important to know its sites and composition to avoid confusion between members of the normal flora and specific organisms of disease when interpreting laboratory results.

*The term *parasite* is also used to describe members of the animal kingdom that infect humans or animals. These organisms are discussed in Chapters 44–48.

Origin of the Normal Flora

fetus is sterile

The healthy fetus is sterile until the birth membranes rupture. During and after birth, the infant is exposed to the flora of the mother's genital tract, to the skin and respiratory flora of those handling it, and to organisms in the environment. During the infant's first few days of life, the nature of the flora often reflects chance exposure to organisms that can grow on particular sites in the absence of competitors. Subsequently, as the infant is exposed to the full range of human floral organisms, those best adapted to colonize particular sites become predominant. Thereafter, the flora generally resembles that of other individuals in the same age group and cultural milieu.

Factors Determining the Nature of the Normal Flora

Physiologic conditions

Bacterial adherence

Bacterial interactions

Local physiologic and ecologic conditions determine the nature of the flora. They are sometimes highly complex, differing from site to site, and sometimes vary with age. These conditions include the amounts and types of nutrients available, pH, oxidation–reduction potentials, and resistance to local antibacterial substances such as bile or lysozyme. Many bacteria have a remarkable affinity for specific types of epithelial cells to which they attach and on which they multiply. This adherence, which is mediated by pili or other surface components, permits the bacteria to multiply while they avoid removal by the flushing effects of surface fluids and peristalsis. Various microbial interactions also determine their relative prevalence in the flora. These interactions include competition for nutrients, inhibition by the metabolic products of another organism (for example, by hydrogen peroxide), and production of antibiotics and bactericiocins.

With a complex flora, it is not possible to determine the relative importance of these factors, but the importance of interbacterial interactions is, however, clear and is illustrated by the dramatic distortions that can result from antibiotic therapy.

Normal Flora of Different Sites

The total normal flora of the body probably contains more than 100 distinct species of microorganisms. In this chapter the major members known to be important in preventing or causing disease will be considered, as well as those that may be confused with etiologic agents of local infections. These organisms are summarized in Table 6.1, and most will be described in greater detail in subsequent chapters. The student should not attempt to memorize unfamiliar names at this point.

Blood, Body Fluids, and Tissues

Sterile in health

transient bacteremia

In health, the blood, body fluids, and tissues are normally sterile. Occasional organisms may transgress epithelial barriers as a result of trauma (including physiologic trauma such as the act of heavy chewing or during childbirth); they may be briefly recoverable from the bloodstream before they are filtered out in the pulmonary capillaries or removed by cells of the reticuloendothelial system. Such transient bacteremia may be the source of infection of damaged or abnormal heart valves that leads to subacute bacterial endocarditis (Chapter 62).

Skin

Propionibacteria

The skin plays host to an abundant flora that varies somewhat according to the number and activity of sebaceous and sweat glands; variation between individuals may be substantial and consistent. Aerobic *diphtheroids* (corynebacteria) are abundant on normally moist skin areas (axillae, between

Table 6.1 Predominant and Important Flora of Various Body Sites in Health

Body Site	Flora
Blood	Sterile; occasional transient low-level bacteremia from physiologic trauma (e.g., viridans streptococci)
Tissues; cerebrospinal fluid; urinary bladder; uterus and Fallopian tubes; middle ear; paranasal sinuses	Sterile
Skin; distal urethra; external ear	*Propionibacterium acnes*; *Staphylococcus epidermidis*; diphtheroids
Mouth	
Tongue and buccal mucosa	Viridans streptococci; *Neisseria* spp.; *Branhamella*; occasional *Candida albicans*
Gingival crevices and tonsillar crypts	*Bacteroides* spp.; *Fusobacterium* spp.; *Peptostreptococcus* spp.; *Actinomyces*; other anaerobes
Nasopharynx	Oral organisms—transient carriage of *Streptococcus pneumoniae, Haemophilus* spp., and *Neisseria meningitidis*; oral anaerobes
Esophagus	Transient mouth flora
Stomach	Rapidly becomes sterile after meals
Small intestine	Scanty, variable, and ill-defined
Colon	
After weaning	*Bacteroides* spp.; *Fusobacterium* spp.; *Clostridium* spp.; *Peptostreptococcus* spp.; *Escherichia coli*; *Proteus* spp.; other Enterobacteriaceae; *Pseudomonas aeruginosa*; numerous other bacteria and yeasts
During breast-feeding	*Bifidobacterium*; lactobacilli; aciduric streptococci
Vagina	
Prepubertal and postmenopausal stages	Skin and some colonic organisms
Childbearing years	Lactobacilli; aciduric streptococci and yeasts

toes). *Staphylococcus epidermidis* and members of the genus *Propionibacterium* occur all over the skin. Propionibacteria are slim, anaerobic, Gram-positive rods that grow in subsurface sebum and break down skin lipids to fatty acids. They are thus most numerous in the ducts of hair follicles and of the sebaceous glands that drain into them (pilosebaceous units). They cannot be removed from skin sites bearing pilosebaceous units even by the most vigorous washing or application of antiseptics, and small numbers are often isolated from biopsy materials because of contamination from the skin during the operative procedure. Propionibacteria and *S. epidermidis* are nonpathogenic, except in certain situations in which general or local host defenses are compromised. Organisms of the skin flora are resistant to the bactericidal effects of skin lipids and fatty acids, which inhibit or kill many extraneous bacteria.

Stability of skin flora

Conjunctival Sac

In health, the conjunctivae have a very scanty flora of nonpathogenic corynebacteria and *S. epidermidis*. The low bacterial count is maintained by lysozyme and the flushing effect of tears.

Intestinal Tract

Mouth and pharynx

The mouth and pharynx contain large numbers of facultative and strict anaerobes. Many species of facultative streptococci are encountered, most of which are α-hemolytic or nonhemolytic (see Chapter 12). Different streptococci predominate on the buccal and tongue mucosa because of different adherence characteristics; one species, *Streptococcus mutans,* shows specific adherence to teeth and plays an etiologic role in caries. Gram-negative diplococci of the genera *Neisseria* and *Branhamella* make up the balance of the facultative organisms most commonly isolated. Strict anaerobes and microaerophilic organisms of the oral cavity have their niches in the depths of the gingival crevices surrounding the teeth and in sites such as tonsillar crypts, where anaerobic conditions can develop readily. Anaerobic members of the normal flora are major contributors to the etiology of periodontal disease.

Although it varies from site to site, the total number of organisms in the oral cavity is very high. Saliva usually contains a mixed flora of about 10^8 organisms per milliliter, derived mostly from the various epithelial colonization sites.

Stomach

The stomach contains few, if any, resident organisms in health because of the lethal action of gastric hydrogen chloride and peptic enzymes on bacteria.

Small intestine

The resident flora of the small intestine is scanty, except in the lower ileum, where it begins to resemble that of the colon. Many animal species have bacteria very closely associated with the epithelium, which have been grown in artificial culture with difficulty or not at all. The extent to which analogous situations may exist in humans is still unclear. These mucosa-associated organisms probably evolved as symbionts with the host species.

Colon

The adult colon carries the most prolific flora in the body (Figure 6.1). Feces are 25% or more bacteria by weight (about 10^{10} organisms per gram).

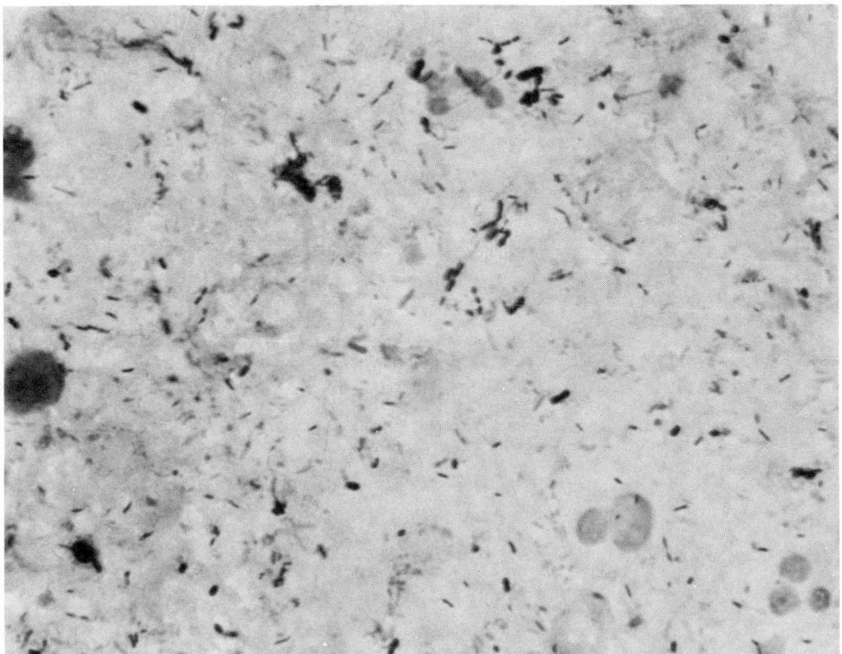

6.1. Gram-stained smear of feces, showing great diversity of microorganisms.

6.2. Gram-stained smear of stool of breast-fed infant. Note homogeneous flora of Gram-positive rods.

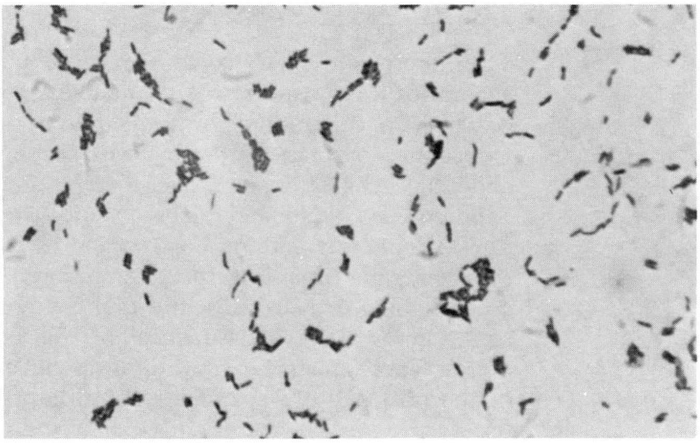

predominant anaerobic flora

More than 90% are anaerobes, predominantly members of the genera *Bacteroides* and *Fusobacterium,* although *Clostridium perfringens,* a major etiologic agent of gas gangrene, is invariably present. The remainder is composed of facultative organisms such as *Escherichia coli,* fecal streptococci (enterococci), yeasts, and numerous other species. There are considerable differences in adult flora depending on the diet of the host. Those whose diets include substantial amounts of meat have more *Bacteroides* and other anaerobic Gram-negative rods in their stools than those on a predominantly vegetable or fish diet.

colonic flora of breast-fed infants

bifidobacteria

effect of artificial feeding

The fecal flora of breast-fed infants differs from that of adults; up to 99% comprises anaerobic Gram-positive rods of the genus *Bifidobacterium* (Figure 6.2). Human milk is high in lactose and low in protein and phosphate, and its buffering capacity is poor compared to that of cow's milk. These conditions select the bifidobacteria, which ferment lactose to yield acetic acid and grow optimally under the acidic conditions (pH 5–5.5) that they produce in the stool. Infants fed cow's milk, which has a greater buffering capacity, tend to have less acidic stools and a flora more similar to that found in the colon of the weaned infant or of the adult. These findings also apply to infants fed some artificial formulas.

Respiratory Tract

Anterior nares

S. aureus carriage

The external 1 cm of the anterior nares is lined with squamous epithelium and has a flora similar to that of the skin except that it is the predominant site of carriage of a pathogen, *Staphylococcus aureus.* About 25–30% of healthy people in the community carry this organism at any given time, 15% permanently and 15% transiently. The organism may spread to other skin sites or colonize the perineum; it can be disseminated by hand-to-nose contact, by desquamation of the epithelium, or by droplet spread during upper respiratory infection.

Nasopharynx

The nasopharynx has a flora similar to that of the mouth; however, it is often the site of carriage of potentially pathogenic organisms such as pneumococci, meningococci, and *Haemophilus* species.

Lower respiratory tract

The respiratory tract below the level of the larynx is protected in health by the action of the epithelial cilia and by the movement of the *mucociliary blanket* (Chapter 7); thus, only transient inhaled organisms are encountered in the trachea and larger bronchi. The accessory sinuses are normally sterile and are protected in a similar fashion, as is the middle ear by the epithelium of the eustachian tubes.

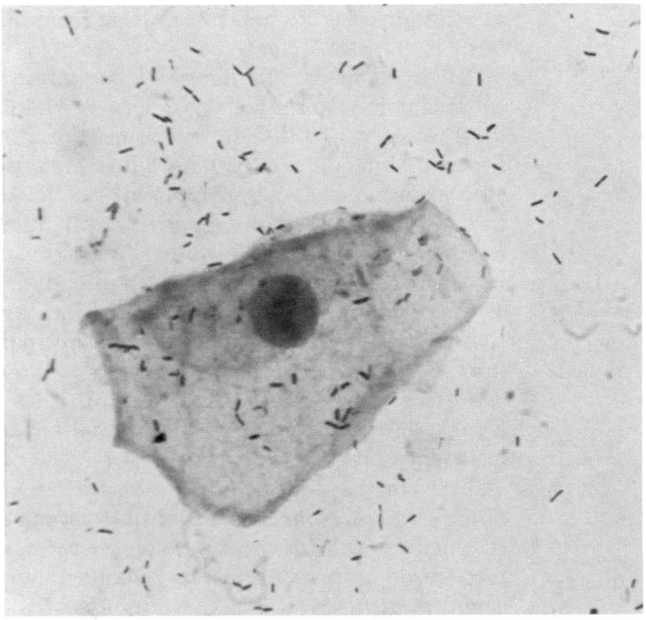

6.3. Gram-stained smear of normal adult vagina, showing lactobacillary flora and squamous epithelial cells.

Genitourinary Tract

Urinary tract

The male genitourinary tract and the female urinary tract are sterile in health; the distal 1 cm of the urethra, however, has a scanty flora derived from the perineum. Thus, in health the urine within and above the bladder is sterile.

Vagina

Hormonal effects on vaginal flora

utilization of glycogen by lactobacilli

The flora of the vagina varies according to hormonal influences at different ages. Before puberty and after menopause, it is mixed, nonspecific, relatively scanty, and contains organisms derived from the flora of the skin and colon. During the childbearing years, it is composed predominantly of anaerobic and microaerophilic members of the genus *Lactobacillus,* with smaller numbers of anaerobic Gram-negative rods, Gram-positive cocci, and yeasts that can survive under the acidic conditions produced by the lactobacilli. These conditions develop because glycogen is deposited in vaginal epithelial cells under the influence of estrogenic hormones and metabolized to lactic acid by lactobacilli. This process results in a vaginal pH of 4–5, which is optimal for growth and survival of the lactobacilli, but inhibits many other organisms. The consistency of the lactobacilliary adult flora is seen in Gram-stained preparations of vaginal smears (Figure 6.3).

Role of the Normal Flora in Disease

Urinary tract and abdominal infections

Subacute bacterial endocarditis

Many species among the normal flora are opportunists; they can cause infection if they reach protected areas of the body in sufficient numbers or if local or general host defense mechanisms are compromised. For example, *E. coli* can reach the urinary bladder by ascending the urethra (Chapter 60) and cause acute urinary tract infection, usually in sexually active women. Perforation of the colon from a ruptured diverticulum or a penetrating abdominal wound will release feces into the peritoneal cavity; this fecal contamination may be followed by peritonitis, primarily caused by facultative members of the flora, and by intraabdominal abscesses, primarily caused by Gram-negative anaerobes. Viridans streptococci from the oral cavity may reach the bloodstream as a result of physiologic trauma or injury (for example, tooth extraction) and colonize a previously damaged heart valve, initiating bacterial endocarditis (Chapter 62). These and other diseases, such as actinomycosis (Chapter 26), result from displacement of normal flora into body cavities or tissues.

Opportunistic infections in the immunocompromised

Vincent's angina

Reduced specific immunologic responses, defects in phagocytic activity, or weakening of epithelial barriers by vitamin deficiencies can all result in local invasion and disease by normal floral organisms. This source accounts for many infections in patients whose defenses are compromised by disease (for example, diabetes, lymphoma, or leukemia) or by cytotoxic chemotherapy for cancer. One specific local infection of this type is Vincent's angina of the oral mucosa, a local invasion and ulceration apparently caused by the combined action of oral spirochetes and members of the genus *Fusobacterium.* Death after lethal radiation exposure usually results from massive invasion by normal floral organisms, particularly those of the intestinal tract.

Caries and periodontal disease

Caries and periodontal disease are both caused by organisms that may be considered members of the normal flora. They are considered in detail in Chapter 56.

Nonspecific adverse effects

Early in the 20th century, it was widely believed that the normal flora of the large intestine was responsible for many "toxic conditions," including rheumatoid arthritis, degenerative diseases, and a range of conditions now recognized as psychosomatic. Ritualistic purging and colonic lavage flourished, particularly at expensive mineral spas, and some patients were even subjected to colectomy as the ultimate cure. The concept was given respectability by Metchnikoff, who suggested that the longevity of Georgian peasants in Russia was attributable to their heavy consumption of yogurt, resulting in replacement of their colonic flora with lactobacilli to the general benefit of their health. These concepts fell into disrepute as the etiology of the "toxic" diseases was clarified, and when it was found that lactobacillary replacement of flora of the adult colon did not occur under the conditions used.

Blind-loop syndrome

More recently, however, attention has again been focused on the less specific contributions of the normal flora to health and disease. In patients with large or multiple blind-ended diverticula in the small intestine, heavy colonization by the anaerobic intestinal flora may occur. This colonization results in bacterial breakdown of bile acids needed for absorption of fat and fat-soluble vitamins and in competition for vitamin B_{12}. Similar situations sometimes occur in the elderly when the small intestine is invaded by colonic flora. If the primary cause (for example, Meckel's diverticulum) cannot be eliminated surgically, these conditions can be ameliorated with antibiotic therapy and fat-soluble vitamin supplements. An analogous situation occurs in tropical sprue, in which secondary colonization of the jejunum by facultative Gram-negative enteric bacteria leads to fat malabsorption and vitamin B_{12} and folic acid deficiencies.

Tropical sprue

Ammonia and hepatic encephalopathy

Under certain conditions, a "toxemia" can result from the action of the normal colonic flora. In severe hepatic cirrhosis, the portal circulation may be partially diverted to the systemic circulation. The detoxification by the liver of ammonia produced by bacterial action on protein residues is bypassed, and severe dysfunctions of the central nervous system (hepatic encephalopathy) can result. This problem can be ameliorated with a strict low-protein diet.

Intensive husbandry and antibiotic feeds

There is considerable evidence that cattle and poultry maintained under conditions of intensive husbandry may have slower growth rates than those kept under more stringent hygienic conditions, and that this disparity is caused by differences in their normal flora. Addition of antibiotics to feed may improve growth; the development of antibiotic-resistant flora, however, poses important ecologic problems.

Beneficial Effects of the Normal Flora

Priming of Immune System

Sterile animals

Organisms of the normal flora play an important role in the development of immunologic competence. Animals delivered and raised under completely aseptic conditions ("sterile" or gnotobiotic animals) have a poorly developed reticuloendothelial system, low serum levels of immunoglobulins, and no antibodies to normal floral antigens, which often cross-react with those of pathogenic organisms and confer a degree of protection against them. Many bacteria that are nonpathogenic to normal hosts can be lethal to gnotobiotic animals, presumably because immunologic priming has not occurred under the protection of maternally derived antibody.

Exclusionary Effect

beneficial effect of breast-feeding

The normal flora produces conditions that tend to block the establishment of extraneous pathogens and their ability to infect the host. The bifidobacteria in the colon of the breast-fed infant produce an environment inimical to colonization by enteric pathogens; this protective effect is aided by ingested maternal immunoglobulin A. Breast-feeding has clearly been shown to help protect the infant from enteric bacterial infection.

effect of normal vaginal flora

The normal vaginal flora has a similar protective effect. Before the introduction of antibiotic therapy, it was found that institutional outbreaks of fomite-transmitted gonococcal vulvovaginitis in prepubertal girls were controlled by synthetic estrogen therapy. This treatment led to glycogen deposition in the vaginal epithelium and establishment of a protective lactobacillary flora. The possible hazard of such therapy in this age group was not then recognized.

Superinfection secondary to antibiotic therapy

Candidiasis

Staphylococcal enterocolitis

Antibiotic therapy, particularly with broad-spectrum agents, may so alter the normal flora of the gastrointestinal tract that antibiotic-resistant organisms multiply in the relative ecologic vacuum produced, sometimes causing significant infections. The pathogenic yeast *Candida albicans*, a minor constituent of the normal flora, may multiply dramatically and cause diarrhea and superficial fungal infections in the mouth, vagina, or anal area. Certain resistant strains of *S. aureus* may largely replace the facultative flora of the colon during antibiotic therapy, particularly after gastrointestinal surgery, and produce a severe necrotizing enterocolitis that is often fatal. Fortunately, although the reasons are not clear, this disease is now rare. More recently, a nonstaphylococcal pseudomembranous colitis associated with antibiotic therapy was shown to result from proliferation of a toxin-producing anaerobe, *Clostridium difficile*, which can be a minor constituent of the flora or acquired from an external source. It may be resistant to several antibiotics, particularly lincomycin and clindamycin, and can multiply and elaborate its toxin during and after therapy. The toxin is responsible for the damage to the colonic epithelium.

C. difficile pseudomembranous enterocolitis

Superinfections in the immunocompromised

Many other such superinfections could be cited; for example, antibiotic-resistant organisms that replace some of the oral and intestinal flora during therapy may cause respiratory, urinary, and other severe systemic infections in immunocompromised patients.

The exclusionary effect of the flora in health has been demonstrated in numerous experiments on gnotobiotic and antibiotic-treated animals. For example, *C. albicans* attaches to oral epithelial cells of germ-free rats; however, prior colonization with certain viridans streptococci that attach to similar epithelial cells prevents establishment of *C. albicans*. In another experiment, the infecting oral dose for mice of streptomycin-resistant *Salmonella typhimurium* was shown to be approximately 10^5 organisms in untreated animals. Oral streptomycin treatment, which inhibits many members of the normal flora, reduced the infecting dose by approximately 1000-fold.

Production of Essential Nutrients

Vitamin production

In ruminants, the action of the extensive anaerobic flora in the rumen is essential to the nutrition of the animal. The flora digests cellulose to usable form and provides many vitamins, including 70% of the animal's vitamin B requirements. In humans, members of the vitamin B group and vitamin K are produced by the normal flora; except for vitamin K, however, the amounts available or absorbed are small compared to those in a well-balanced diet. Bacterial vitamin production is reduced during broad-spectrum antibiotic therapy, and supplementation with vitamin B is indicated in malnourished individuals.

Manipulation of the Normal Flora

Attempts to manipulate the normal flora have usually been fruitless and have sometimes been dangerous. Manipulation has proved useful, however, in two situations. Patients whose immunologic defenses are massively compromised (for example, during whole body irradiation and bone marrow transplantation in the treatment of leukemia) may have their normal flora greatly reduced by judicious use of combined chemotherapy, reduction or exclusion of extraneous organisms by sterilization of food and supplies, and by aseptic nursing procedures. These conditions substantially reduce the risk of infection during a highly vulnerable period.

It has also been shown that nursery outbreaks of *S. aureus* infections, a major problem in the 1950s and 1960s, may be controlled by deliberate colonization of the infant's nares with *S. aureus* 502A, a strain of low virulence that tends to exclude more virulent strains of *S. aureus*. Unfortunately, some infections have also occurred with the 502A strain. As greater understanding of the complex ecology of the normal flora is gained, it is probable that other techniques for its manipulation will be developed to augment protection from infection.

Additional Reading and References

Bitton, G., and Marshall, K.C., Eds. 1980. *Adsorption of Microorganisms to Surfaces.* New York: John Wiley and Sons. An up-to-date account of knowledge of bacterial adherence, including adherent members of the normal flora.

Gibbons, R.J., and Van Houte, J. 1975. Bacterial adherence in oral microbial ecology. *Annu. Rev. Microbiol.* 29:19–44. A pioneering review of the role of bacterial adherence in the oral cavity.

Noble, W.C. 1981. *Microbiology of Human Skin.* 2nd ed. London: Lloyd Luke.

Rosebury, T. 1970. *Life on Man.* New York: Berkeley Publishing Co. A delightful, wry, and instructive paperback. Highly recommended for recreational reading.

Skinner, F.A., and Carr, J.G., Eds. 1974 *The Normal Microbial Flora of Man.* The Society for Applied Bacteriology Symposium No 3. London: Academic Press. This and the Noble reference give excellent coverage of their topics and are good reference sources.

John C. Sherris and C. George Ray

Pathogenesis of Infection:
Initial Defenses, Infectivity, Virulence, and Immune Response

7

The factors that determine the initiation, development, and outcome of an infection involve a series of complex and shifting interactions between the parasite and the host, which can vary with different infecting organisms. They include the host's primary physical barriers against invasion and the ways in which they can be breached, the ability of an organism to evade destruction by host defenses, the manner in which an organism spreads and causes disease, and the body's adaptive immunologic ability to control and eliminate invading parasites.

Despite the complexity of interactions between different parasites and hosts, several components of pathogenetic processes and principles have broad application to infectious diseases and will be described in this chapter with appropriate examples. More details of individual organisms and diseases will be given in subsequent chapters. As indicated in the preface to the book, a general understanding of immunology from study of one of the several excellent modern texts that are available will be presupposed, and only those immunologic phenomena directly involved in the pathogenesis and control of infectious diseases will be considered.

Species immunity and susceptibility

In considering the present topics, it is essential to bear in mind that the ability of an organism to infect or cause disease depends on the susceptibility of the host and that there are remarkable species differences in host susceptibility for many infections. For example, dogs do not get measles, and people do not get distemper. Thus, the term *pathogenicity,* which is defined as the ability to cause disease, must be qualified according to the host species involved. In recent years, increasing numbers of infections have been caused by organisms previously considered nonpathogenic. These infections develop in patients whose immunologic or cellular defenses are compromised by genetic defects, disease, or therapy. Therefore, the concept of pathogenicity requires further qualification, and it is useful to consider organisms as *primary pathogens,* which may initiate disease in previously healthy individuals, and *opportunists,* which are frequent causes of disease in the immunocompromised host or when first-line defense barriers are breached. *Virulence,* as applied to infectious agents, is defined as the degree of pathogenicity. Thus, a pathogenic organism may be of high or low virulence for a particular host species, or particular strains of a pathogenic species of bacteria may have lost a critical determinant of virulence and be categorized as *avirulent.*

Primary and opportunistic pathogens

Virulence is degree of pathogenicity

First-Line Defenses Against Microbial Invasion

First-line defenses are those that block access of organisms to subepithelial tissues or prevent colonization of certain body surfaces. They are summarized in Table 7.1 and considered in more detail herein according to the structures and processes involved.

Epithelial Barrier

Skin

sites of penetration

chemical defenses of skin

Vaginal epithelium

conjunctiva

Respiratory epithelium

mucociliary escalator

A simple mechanical barrier to microbial invasion is provided by intact epithelia, the most effective of which is the multilayered stratified squamous epithelium of the skin with its superficial cornified anucleate layers. Organisms can only gain access to the underlying tissues by breaks or by way of hair follicles, sebaceous glands, and sweat glands, which traverse the stratified layers. The surface of the skin is inhibitory to the growth of most microorganisms because of low moisture and pH and the presence of inhibitory substances such as lactic acid from sweat glands and free fatty acids, waxes, and alcohols from the secretions of sebaceous glands or the metabolic activity of commensal organisms. Higher moisture (for example, beneath occlusive dressings) can increase the number of potential pathogens on the skin surface, and significant destruction of skin is invariably followed by infection, as in the case of severe burns. The vaginal epithelium, a modified squamous epithelium, is primarily protected during the childbearing years by the low pH and exclusionary effects produced by the normal flora discussed in Chapter 6. The conjunctiva is primarily protected by the flushing effects of the tears, aided by a high concentration of lysozyme.

The epithelium of the paranasal sinuses and of the respiratory tract from the level of the larynx to the alveoli is a less effective mechanical barrier but is protected by a mucus covering to which microorganisms adhere and by the epithelial cilia, which move the mucus away from the area at risk. In the respiratory tract, particles larger than 5 μm are trapped in this fashion, moved upward at a rate of about 1 cm/min to pass through the larynx, and are then swallowed and destroyed by the defenses of the alimentary tract. Interference with the action of cilia from toxic substances or from infections

Table 7.1 Nonspecific Defenses Against Colonization with Pathogens

Site	Mechanical Barrier	Ciliated Epithelium	Competition by Normal Flora	Mucus	Immunoglobulin A
Skin	+++	—	+	—	—
Conjunctiva	++	—	—	—	+
Oropharynx	+++	—	+++	—	+
Upper respiratory tract	++	+	+++	++	++
Middle ear and paranasal sinuses[a]	++	+++	—	++	?
Lower respiratory tract[a]	++	+++	—	++	++
Stomach	++	—	—	++	—
Intestinal tract	++	—	+++	+++	+++
Vagina	+++	—	+++	+	+
Urinary tract[a]	++	—	—	—	+

Abbreviations: +, ++, +++ = relative importance in defense at each site; — = unimportant.

[a] Sterile in health.

such as influenza or whooping cough can permit colonization and infection of the lower respiratory tract with pathogenic bacteria, leading to the development of bronchitis or pneumonia.

Gastrointestinal epithelia

chemical defenses

Like the epithelium of the respiratory tract, that of the intestinal tract below the esophagus is a less efficient mechanical barrier than the skin, but there are other effective defense mechanisms. The high level of hydrochloric acid and gastric enzymes in the normal stomach kill many ingested bacteria, and others are susceptible to pancreatic digestive enzymes or to the detergent effect of bile salts. Again like the respiratory tract, the intestinal epithelium (or mucous membrane) is coated with a film of mucus that traps many organisms directly or, as discussed later, by reaction with immunoglobulin (Ig)A secreted into it. The mucus and attached particles are continuously passed along and out of the alimentary tract by contractile peristaltic waves. Inhibition of these processes decreases the infecting dose of various pathogens or permits colonization of areas, such as the small intestine, that usually have a limited normal flora. The net result is an increased risk of infection. For example, the infecting dose of the cholera vibrio is lowered by several orders of magnitude in patients who have achlorhydria (absence of gastric hydrochloric acid) because of disease or malnutrition. Stagnation of intestinal contents from several causes is also associated with abnormal bacterial overgrowth (Chapter 6).

effect of mucus

removal by peristalsis

Urinary tract

urine as culture medium

protective effects of flushing and low pH

infection with stasis

The transitional epithelium of the urinary tract is multilayered and resistant to invasion, especially in the undistended state. Urine is a good culture medium for many bacteria, however, and if they reach the normally sterile bladder, they can multiply to very large numbers (for example, more than 10^5/ml), particularly if there is urinary stasis. Primary mechanisms of defense are the flushing effect of urine and its relatively low pH, which tend to inhibit microbial growth. Urinary tract infections are much more common in young women than young men because the shortness of the urethra allows easier passage of organisms to the bladder, and, as a result, infections are often associated with sexual intercourse. Infections are also common in any situation that produces urinary stasis, such as partial obstruction by an

Table 7.1 *(continued)*

Lymphoid Follicles	Low pH	Flushing Effects of Contents	Peristalsis	Special Factors
—	++	—	—	Fatty acids from action of normal flora on sebum
—	—	+++	—	Lysozyme
yes	—	++	—	
yes	—	+	—	Turbinate baffles
—	—	+	—	
yes	+++	—	—	Mucociliary escalator; alveolar macrophages; cough reflex
—	+++	+	+	Production of hydrochloric acid
yes	—	+	+++	Bile; digestive enzymes
—	+++	—	—	Lactobacillary flora ferments epithelial glycogen
—	+	+++	—	

enlarged prostate, or when passage of bacteria into the bladder is facilitated by the use of catheters.

Secreted Antimicrobial Products

Lysozyme and lactoferrin

In addition to some antimicrobial substances mentioned previously, most mucosal secretions and those of adjacent glands produce other nonspecific inhibitory substances, including lysozyme (Chapter 2), which disrupts the peptidoglycan of Gram-positive cell walls, and lactoferrin, which competes for the iron essential to microbial multiplication.

Secretory IgA

origin of sIgA

Secretory IgA (sIgA) and, to a lesser extent, secretory IgM antibodies can traverse epithelial cells of the respiratory, intestinal, and upper urinary tracts and are also found in saliva and milk. Secretory IgA is produced in subepithelial tissues by plasma cells derived from antigenically stimulated lymphoid tissues, which are associated with hollow viscera; IgA-producing cells can migrate to mucosal surfaces remote from the site of the original antigenic stimulus. The sIgA antibodies can attach specifically to microorganisms possessing the antigens that elicited them or to cross-reacting antigens. This occurs at the epithelial surface or in its covering mucus and prevents attachment of the microorganisms to epithelial cells and thus colonization of the epithelial surface, which is often the first step in cell or tissue invasion. It also agglutinates bacteria and partially inhibits their multiplication and neutralizes viruses by blocking their attachment to cell receptors. However, sIgA does not opsonize or mediate complement fixation and complement-dependent bacterial killing. Secretory IgA in mucus can also prevent absorption of soluble antigens, such as certain toxins against which it is directed. It is resistant to the action of proteolytic enzymes and is thus well adapted to functioning near the intestinal epithelial surface. It is not essential to immunity, because many patients with genetically determined absence of this class of antibody can nonetheless mount effective IgG and IgM responses to invading organisms; however, it has been shown to be an important primary immune mechanism for preventing a variety of infections, such as cholera and giardiasis, and some respiratory virus diseases that depend on initial attachment to mucosal surface receptors. Secretory IgA in human milk plays an important role in protecting the infant from intestinal infections.

blocking of microbial adhesion

viral neutralization

sIgA prevents initiation of some infections, but is not essential to immunity

significance of sIgA in human milk

Secreted antimicrobial substances can probably act cooperatively, and it has been shown that sIgA can increase the speed of bacterial inactivation by lysozyme.

Normal Microbial Flora

The role of the normal microbial flora in protection against infection has been considered in Chapter 6. It is therefore sufficient to stress its great significance in competing with pathogenic intruders for particular ecologic niches and in priming the immune system.

Alveolar and Other Surface Macrophages

ingest particles that reach alveoli

Macrophages, which are found free in the alveoli of the lungs play a very important role in ingesting and destroying organisms that are inhaled in very small droplet nuclei (less than 5 μm) and escape the mucociliary defenses of the trachea and bronchial tree. Similarly, a few macrophages reach the surface of other mucous membranes, but are less significant in defense. The mechanisms of killing by phagocytes are discussed in the next section.

Second-Line Defenses Against Invasion

Once a microorganism has breached the surface epithelial barrier, it is subject to a series of nonspecific processes designed to remove, inhibit, or destroy it. These defenses are complex, dynamic, and interacting, but will be considered under the general headings of the initial environment, the inflammatory response, phagocytic activity, and other clearance mechanisms.

Initial Environment

Lysozyme in tissues

Effects of iron-binding proteins

Tissue histiocytes

Lymph flow

Microorganisms that reach the subepithelial tissues are immediately exposed to the intercellular tissue fluids, which have some defined properties that act to inhibit multiplication of many bacteria. For example, most tissues contain lysozyme in sufficient concentrations to disrupt the cell wall of some Gram-positive bacteria, and other less well-defined inhibitors from leukocytes and platelets have been described. Tissue fluid itself is a suboptimal growth medium for most bacteria and deficient in free iron. Iron is essential for bacterial growth, but it is sequestered by the body's iron-binding proteins such as transferrin and lactoferrin and is thus inaccessible to organisms that do not themselves produce iron chelators. Tissue histiocytes, which are phagocytic cells derived from the monocytic series, can phagocytose and destroy many infectious agents even when they are not activated by lymphokines or when the organisms are not specifically opsonized. Furthermore, the turnover of tissue fluids from the blood capillary circulation to the lymphatic drainage system serves to move the occasional invading organism to a lymph node, in which fixed phagocytic cells can remove and destroy it. Pathogenic bacteria, almost by definition, can overcome these initial defenses, and, as they multiply, secondary nonspecific defenses come into play that enhance those described previously.

Inflammatory Response and Its Effects

vasodilatation and fluid extravasation

polymorphonuclear inflammation

Mediators of inflammation

Local defensive role of inflammation

Immune stimuli

Mobilization of polymorphonuclear leukocytes from bone marrow, and leukocytosis

When bacteria multiply in the tissues, the usual result is an inflammatory response. The blood-carrying capillaries dilate, which leads to local extravasation of fluid containing high levels of protein, immunoglobulins, and complement components. Polymorphonuclear leukocytes are attracted to the infected site and reach the tissue fluids by passing between the capillary endothelial cells. The inflammatory response is mediated and activated by substances such as histamine, serotonin, lysosomal enzymes, and small peptide kinins liberated when leukocytes or tissue cells are destroyed by bacterial products. Complement components produced by activation of either direct or alternate complement pathways also contribute to inflammation. The end results are the classic inflammatory manifestations of swelling (tumor), vasodilatation of surface vessels with redness (rubor) and increased skin temperature (calor), pain from increased pressure and tissue damage (dolor), and loss of function because of reflex nerve inhibition or the pain caused by movement. The inflammatory response has several immediate defensive effects. It first increases tissue fluid flow from the bloodstream to the lymphatic circulation and brings phagocytes, complement, and any existing antibody to the site of infection. Later, the deposition of fibrin may contribute to the walling off of the lesion before the healing process begins. A major effect of the increased lymphatic drainage serves to bring microbes or their antigens into contact with the cells in the local lymph nodes that mediate the development of specific immune response.

A local inflammatory response can also produce important systemic effects. Polymorphonuclear leukocytes are mobilized from the bone marrow pool to increase the numbers of those present at the infected site and to replace those destroyed or at the end of their life span. Thus, polymorphonuclear leukocytosis, primarily involving neutrophils, is a common feature of most bacterial infections and serves to increase the immediately available phagocytic defenses. Fever, a common concomitant of inflammation, is mediated by the peptide endogenous pyrogen, which is released by phagocytic cells (for example, on exposure to bacterial endotoxin). Endogenous pyrogen acts on the hypothalamus to increase the "setting" of the body's thermostatic mechanisms. The value of fever is not completely clear; however, it increases the effectiveness of several processes involved in phagocytosis and microbial killing and frequently reduces the multiplication or replication rate of bacteria or viruses below that maintained at 37°C.

Fever and endogenous pyrogen

Phagocytic Defenses

Polymorphonuclear and mononuclear phagocytes

Phagocytic cells include polymorphonuclear leukocytes (particularly neutrophils), blood monocytes, macrophages, tissue histiocytes, and the fixed phagocytic cells of the reticuloendothelial system. All are derived from the same stem cells, and blood monocytes that reach the tissues assume the characteristics of macrophages when they reach inflammatory sites. Despite the differences between them, all of these cells share certain common mechanisms for ingesting and attempting to destroy invading microorganisms.

Neutrophil chemotaxis

Phagocytosis

metabolic burst

myeloperoxidase–halide system

lysosomal enzymes in phagolysosome

The neutrophil leukocyte is short-lived (circulating half-life, 7 hr), metabolically active, and demonstrates marked chemotaxis to some bacterial products, derivatives of the C3 and C5 components of complement, and to other products of the inflammatory process. These factors attract leukocytes to the sites of microbial invasion. Particles, including bacteria, that attach to the surface of polymorphonuclear leukocytes are ingested in a vacuole called the *phagosome,* which is bounded by the portion of the cytoplasmic membrane involved in their uptake. Once within the cell, there is a burst of metabolic activity with increased oxygen uptake and production of superoxide, hydrogen peroxide, and free oxygen radicals, all of which are active against many bacteria and viruses. Oxidation of chloride and iodide ions is brought about by myeloperoxidase in the presence of H_2O_2 to generate substances with marked bactericidal properties. Lysosomal granules of the cell then fuse with the phagocytic vacuole to produce a *phagolysosome,* in which surviving ingested organisms are exposed to its range of enzymes and in most cases destroyed. The pH of the phagolysosome is approximately 3.0–4.0 and its enzymes include peroxidase, acid and alkaline phosphatases, nucleases, lysozyme and several others that make the environment highly hostile to most organisms. The various responses of phagocytes are summarized in Table 7.2. Lysosomal enzymes are also substantially damaging to the tissues when released in large amounts on death of neutrophils; they thus contribute to the formation of pus and to the breakdown of tissue cells and collagen that leads to abscess formation.

effects of lysosomal enzymes on tissue

Macrophages

macrophage cooperation with immunoresponsive cells

The macrophage, which is longer lived than the neutrophil, can resynthesize its lysosomal enzymes and granules and attack successively phagocytosed microorganisms or debris from the infective process. It thus plays a more stable and continuing role in control of an infection. Macrophages are seen in greatly increased numbers during resolution of an acute infection and in chronic infections such as tuberculosis and many fungal diseases. They cooperate with cells of the lymphoid immune system by "processing" antigen to increase its effectiveness as an immunologic stimulus. This process is accomplished by breaking down structures such as bacterial cell walls to

Table 7.2 Microbicidal Responses of Phagocytes

A. Degranulation: phagosome formation
   1. Cationic proteins
   2. Proteases
   3. Lactoferrin
   4. Lysozyme
   5. Acid hydrolases
   6. Myeloperoxidase

B. Oxidative respiratory burst
   1. Myeloperoxidase-associated
      a. Hydrogen peroxide, myeloperoxidase, halide
      b. Iodination
      c. Chemiluminescence via luminol
   2. Superoxide, singlet oxygen, and other reactive oxygen radicals

Reproduced with permission from Quie, P.G. 1983. *J. Infect. Dis.* 148:189–193, copyright 1983 by University of Chicago, publisher.

release antigenic components or by associating antigens with immunoresponse sites on the surface of the macrophage and presenting them to the appropriate lymphocytes. In turn, lymphokines produced by cells of the lymphatic system can enhance the number and effectiveness of the macrophages in an infectious lesion. For example, macrophage inhibition factor inhibits macrophage motility and retains them within the area in which they are immediately needed. Other lymphokines derived from antigenically stimulated lymphocytes "activate" macrophages to higher metabolic levels and increase their capacity to destroy microorganisms. The stimulus for activation is immunologically specific, but the effect is nonspecific; for example, a macrophage in which activation has resulted from a tuberculous infection will have enhanced activity against any microorganism.

effects of lymphokines on macrophages

activation of macrophages

The phagocytic cells of the reticuloendothelial system are present in the lymph node sinuses and along small blood vessels and vascular sinuses of the liver, spleen, and bone marrow. Microorganisms that escape from a local lesion into the lymphatic circulation or bloodstream are rapidly cleared by reticuloendothelial cells or arrested in the small pulmonary capillaries and then ingested by phagocytic cells. This process is so efficient that when a million organisms are injected into a vein of a rabbit few if any will usually be recoverable in cultures of blood taken 15 min after injection, although the ultimate result of such clearance may not be a cure.

clearing effects of reticuloendothelial cells

The processes of phagocytosis are enhanced greatly by the presence of any IgG and IgM antibodies directed against the infecting organism, as well as by the presence of complement. Phagocytic cells have surface receptors for the Fc fractions of IgA and for the C3b derivative of complement. Thus, bacteria and viruses with attached antibody are brought to the surface of phagocytic cells to facilitate ingestion, and this process is enhanced by activation of the complement cascade. Even in the absence of specific antibody, many bacterial products (particularly endotoxin) and viruses activate the alternate pathway of complement, which also improves the efficiency of phagocytosis. These processes are known as *opsonization* (preparation for eating), and the antibody or complement components that enhance phagocytosis are termed *opsonins.*

Opsonization by antibody and complement

activation of alternate complement pathway

It must be remembered that phagocytosis and the mechanisms for intracellular killing are not always effective, because organisms have evolved that resist ingestion, that are insusceptible to lysosomal enzymes, or that interfere with fusion of the lysosome with the phagosome.

Microbial Infectivity

Ability to multiply on epithelial surfaces

temperature requirements

resistance to local antibacterial conditions

To invade the tissues, an organism must be able to overcome the initial epithelial barriers. This process sometimes involves direct spread through wounds, human or animal bites, or bites of insect vectors. Often, however, a primary pathogen establishes itself locally by colonizing the epithelial surface, then enters the tissues through the epithelium. Thus, a requirement for infectivity by many primary pathogens is an ability to survive and, if necessary, multiply under the conditions that obtain on a surface epithelium or in a tissue into which they are deposited. The ability to grow at a body temperature of 37°C is an obvious essential requirement for organisms that infect any area except the skin or nasal mucosal surfaces, which have a lower temperature. Some pathogenic organisms, such as the rhinoviruses of the common cold and the fungi that cause ringworm of the skin, grow poorly if at all at 37°C and thus cannot invade deeper tissues. Other examples of ability to survive local conditions are the lysozyme insusceptibility of bacteria that cause conjunctivitis and the resistance of pathogens of the lower intestinal tract to the antibacterial effects of bile and the digestive enzymes.

adherence to epithelial cells

viral receptors

bacterial adhesins

colonization of epithelium

effects of toxins

mucolytic enzymes

A general prerequisite for infection is the capacity to adhere to the surface of epithelial cells. Most viruses have specific attachment sites to target cells. For example, the influenza viruses attach specifically to neuraminic-acid-containing glycoprotein receptors on the surface of respiratory epithelial cells before penetrating to the interior of the cell. With some bacteria, the attachment is highly specific and mediated by an affinity of chemical groups on the microbial surface, termed *adhesins,* for receptors on the epithelial surface. In bacteria, the adhesins are frequently on pili, which are surface appendages. For example, certain strains of *Escherichia coli* that cause gastroenteritis in piglets produce a surface antigen, K88, encoded by plasmid genes. This antigen has a specific affinity for mannose-containing surface components on the small intestinal epithelium. Adhesion by this mechanism is essential for infectivity. Adherence thus facilitates colonization and penetration of epithelia, because it brings the organism into intimate contact with its target and prevents its removal by the flushing effects of visceral contents or secretions or, in the respiratory tract, by the action of cilia. Also, the activity of bacterial toxins on epithelial cells is enormously enhanced by this juxtaposition; certain organisms, such as *Bordetella pertussis,* directly inhibit ciliary action. In some bacteria and viruses, mucolytic enzymes assist in penetration to the epithelial surfaces; in others, the penetration of mucus appears to require active motility to penetrate mucus and possibly a chemoattractant response.

IgA Protease

resistance to aveolar macrophage ingestion and killing

Microorganisms that reach mucosal surfaces will often encounter secretory IgA antibody, which can react with them and inhibit their adherence to epithelia and growth. Some species, such as the gonococcus, the meningococcus, and *Haemophilus influenzae* produce an IgA protease, which presumably facilitates colonization and penetration of the epithelial barrier. In the pulmonary alveoli, an organism immediately encounters phagocytic alveolar macrophages; however, many successful pulmonary pathogens, such as the pneumococcus and *Klebsiella pneumoniae,* possess capsules that inhibit their ingestion. Others, particularly the tubercle bacillus, are taken up by alveolar macrophages, but can multiply within them and be carried to sites such as regional lymph nodes. These processes, which are of great importance in the pathogenesis of disease itself, will be considered in greater detail in the next section.

Mechanisms of Virulence of Invasive Organisms

Bacterial mechanisms for obtaining iron

Microorganisms that can invade and cause disease possess a variety of mechanisms to avoid or subvert the defenses of the host and a range of methods for producing pathologic lesions and systemic illness. First, however, they must have the ability to obtain the iron they require in an environment in which free iron is highly restricted by the host's iron-binding proteins. This requirement is satisfied by their production of iron-chelating compounds, such as enterochelin from pathogenic Enterobacteriaceae, or by their ability to utilize iron-containing compounds derived from hemoglobin. It is of interest that many nonspecific and immune defensive mechanisms will themselves reduce even further the amount of free iron in plasma and tissue fluids. Conversely, injection of iron compounds into infection sites will considerably increase the severity of disease.

Avoidance of Host Defense Mechanisms

Antiphagocytic effects of capsules

Leukocidins

Several important pathogenic bacteria are rapidly destroyed when phagocytosed, and to multiply and cause disease they must avoid this situation. Several, such as *Streptococcus pneumoniae* and *H. influenzae,* produce polysaccharide capsules that protect the unopsonized organism from phagocytosis in tissue fluids and reduce phagocytic effectiveness on epithelial surfaces. Consequently, extracellular multiplication proceeds relatively unimpeded until an effective opsonizing antibody response is mounted against the invader. Other organisms, such as *Staphylococcus aureus* and *Clostridium perfringens,* produce extracellular toxic products that are lethal to polymorphonuclear leukocytes (and other cells, in the case of *C. perfringens*) and thus directly attack the host defense system.

Intraphagocytic survival and multiplication

In some cases already discussed briefly, microorganisms can survive the phagocytic process, and migration of the macrophage may contribute to their spread. *Coxiella burnetii* (a species of *Rickettsia*), for example, can multiply under the seemingly hostile conditions that exist in the phagolysosome. Others, such as *Mycobacterium tuberculosis,* are ingested, but then inhibit lysosomal fusion by a mechanism that remains unclear. Some of the mechanisms employed by various agents to subvert the action of the phagocyte are summarized in Table 7.3.

Deviation of opsonizing antibody by free antigen

In addition to the production of enzymes that destroy secretory IgA, various mechanisms are available for avoiding or delaying the effects of the

Table 7.3 Microbial Pertubations of Intraphagocytic Microbicidal Mechanisms

A. Inhibition of lysosome-phagosome fusion
   1. *Mycobacterium tuberculosis*[a]
   2. *Toxoplasma gondii*
   3. *Chlamydia psittaci*
   4. *Histoplasma capsulatum*
   5. *Neisseria gonorrheae*

B. Resistance to lysosomal enzymes
   1. *Mycobacterium lepraemurium*
   2. *Leishmania mexicana*
   3. *Salmonella typhimurium*

C. Exotoxin-induced cytotoxicity
   1. *Pseudomonas aeruginosa*
   2. *Staphylococcus aureus*

D. Inhibition of phagocyte oxidative response
   1. *Legionella pneumophila*[b]
   2. *Listeria monocytogenes*
   3. *Salmonella typhi*

E. Inhibition of phagocyte function by bacterial adenylate cyclase
   1. *Bordetella pertussis*

F. Inhibition of lysosome-phagosome fusion and phagocyte oxidative response
   1. Influenza A virus

Reproduced with permission from Quie, P.G. 1983. *J. Infect. Dis.* 148:189–193, copyright 1983 by University of Chicago, publisher.

[a]By bacterial sulfatide. [b]By toxin.

immune response. In some cases, protective antibody is neutralized by bacterial products before it can reach the organism. The antiphagocytic capsular polysaccharide of a pneumococcus, for example, is soluble, and it may be found in considerable amounts in body fluids during a pneumococcal infection. It can react with anticapsular antibody, thus protecting the organism itself. Only when sufficient antibody is produced to neutralize the free carbohydrate can the organism be effectively opsonized. In fact, the outcome of an untreated pneumococcal infection is a race between production of capsular polysaccharide and of anticapsular antibody. The spirochete that causes relapsing fever, *Borrelia recurrentis,* has a unique method of circumventing host humoral immune mechanisms. Mutations producing alteration of a major virulence-determining surface antigen occur at high frequency, and the mutated form does not react with the protective antibody that has developed against the previous antigen. Thus, the organism changes the rules of the game, and the infection may relapse two or three times with successive mutations. Many strains of *S. aureus* have a unique defense against opsonizing antibody. Their surface contains protein A, which reacts with the Fc portion of IgG and thus prevents its attachment to Fc receptors on phagocytes.

Mutations of surface antigens in *B. recurrentis*

Protein A of *S. aureus*

Diseases caused by organisms that can multiply within phagocytes are little affected by circulating antibody; these infections are controlled by the cellular immune defense systems described in the next section. Likewise, obligate intracellular parasites, especially the viruses, rickettsiae, and chlamydiae, are protected in their host cells from antibody, and they only become directly accessible to immunologic attack when they are released into the humoral environment or express their antigens on the surface of the infected cell. Some viruses, such as herpes simplex, can pass from cell to cell by intercellular bridges and are often inaccessible to humoral defenses. This inaccessibility accounts, in part, for their latency and stability as parasites.

Intracellular protection from antibody

Microbial Determinants of Disease

The damage to the host's cells and tissues that constitutes disease can be brought about in a variety of ways. In many viral infections, lysis and necrosis are the direct result of interference with the cell's metabolic and synthetic processes by viral action. Both discharge of intracellular contents and antigen–antibody reactions involving released virus components can initiate chronic inflammatory reactions, which are superimposed on the cell necrosis. Similar damage is produced by the obligate intracellular rickettsiae and chlamydiae, but in this case specific toxins may also be involved.

Direct damage by intracellular parasites

Infections with the pneumococcus are always extracellular and associated with little cytologic damage to the infected tissues; however, a dramatic acute inflammatory response develops that is itself responsible for disease manifestations. Thus, in pneumococcal pneumonia, the lung alveoli become filled with exudate and polymorphonuclear leukocytes from the pulmonary capillaries, resulting in failure of respiratory exchange, fever, and leukocytosis. If the patient survives, resolution of the disease is rapid and recovery of the normal structure and function of the lung is complete, because significant tissue death did not occur.

Disease resulting from inflammation

In many infections caused by Gram-negative organisms, the lipopolysaccharide endotoxin (Chapter 2) of the cell wall is believed to be a significant component of the disease process. The major characteristics of endotoxin (Chapter 20) are contrasted with those of exotoxins in Table 7.4. Endotoxin in nanogram amounts causes fever in humans by release of endogenous pyrogen from phagocytic cells. In larger amounts, whether on intact Gram-

Endotoxin of Gram-negative bacteria

effects of endotoxin

Table 7.4 Differential Characteristics of Endotoxins and Exotoxins

Characteristic	Endotoxins	Exotoxins
Chemical nature	Lipopolysaccharide (lipid A component)	Protein
Part of Gram-negative cell wall	Yes	No
Most from Gram-positive bacteria	No	Yes
Extracellular	No	Yes
Phage or plasmid coded	No	Many
Antigenic	WR	Yes
Can be converted to toxoid	No	Many
Neutralized by antibody	WR	Yes
Differing pharmacologic specificities	No	Yes
Stable to boiling[a]	Yes	No

Abbreviation: WR = weak reaction.

[a]Enterotoxin of *Staphylococcus aureus* withstands boiling.

negative organisms or cell wall fragments, it produces dramatic physiologic effects. These include hypotension, lowered polymorphonuclear leukocyte and platelet counts from increased margination of these cells to the walls of the small vessels, hemorrhage, and sometimes disseminated intravascular coagulation from activation of clotting factors. Rapid and irreversible shock may follow passage of endotoxin into the bloodstream. This syndrome is seen when materials that have become heavily contaminated are injected intravenously, or when a severe local infection leads to massive bacteremia. The role of endotoxin in more chronic disease processes is less clear, but some manifestations of typhoid fever and meningococcal septicemia, for example, are fully compatible with the known effects of endotoxin in humans. It should be noted that endotoxins are considerably less active than many exotoxins, incompletely neutralized by antibody against their carbohydrate component, and stable even to autoclaving. The latter characteristic is important, because materials for intravenous administration that have become contaminated with Gram-negative organisms are not detoxified by sterilization.

endotoxic shock

heat stability of endotoxins

In contrast to endotoxins, exotoxins (Table 7.4) are strikingly diverse proteins of very high toxicity with different specific activities against a wide variety of cellular structures and functions. For example, tetanus toxin acts on the nervous system by interfering with normal activity of neuromotor synapses and cholera toxin on the transport of fluids and electrolytes across the epithelial cells of the small intestine Exotoxins are excreted into the surrounding fluid by the organisms that produce them or liberated on bacterial lysis. They are antigenic and neutralized by the specific antibodies that they elicit; several, by treatment in vitro with formaldehyde, can be converted to toxoids, which retain the antigenicity of the toxin but lose its toxicity. Toxoids are highly valuable as immunizing agents against diphtheria and tetanus, in which the toxin is the major determinant of virulence and of the disease process. In some bacteria, production of exotoxin is determined by genes carried on temperate phages (diphtheria, scarlet fever, and botulism toxins) or on plasmids (*E. coli* enterotoxins). In these cases, toxigenicity can be transferred from toxigenic to nontoxigenic strains. At present, there is

exotoxins: toxicity and specificity

antigenicity of exotoxins and toxoids

phage- and plasmid-coded exotoxins

no satisfactory explanation for the high frequency of association of exotoxin genes with such transmissible elements.

remote effects of exotoxins

Some exotoxins are the primary determinants of disease caused by organisms that multiply on an epithelial surface (for example, diphtheria) or in a restricted local site in the tissues (for example, tetanus). In these cases the major effects of the toxins are in tissues remote from the infection, such as the heart muscle in diphtheria and the spinal cord and medulla in tetanus.

exotoxins contributing to invasion

Other exotoxins contribute to the capacity of an organism to invade and spread; the lecithinase α-toxin of *C. perfringens,* for example, disrupts the cell membranes of a wide variety of host cells, including the leukocytes that might otherwise impede the organism, and produces the necrotic anaerobic environment in which it can spread.

exotoxins produced outside of body

Still other exotoxins are produced outside the body in contaminated foods and cause disease when they are eaten. For example, the spores of *Clostridium botulinum* can survive inadequate food preservation processes and germinate under appropriate anaerobic conditions. Toxin synthesis follows as the vegetative cells grow. The toxins that cause such food poisoning are resistant to digestive enzymes. In the case of staphylococcal enterotoxins they are also resistant to boiling, so that disease may follow ingestion of contaminated foods in which the organism has already been killed.

enterotoxins: exotoxins affecting gastrointestinal tract

The term *enterotoxin* has been used widely for exotoxins that act directly or indirectly on the intestinal epithelium to produce diarrhea and vomiting. This terminology has caused some confusion; it is best to regard enterotoxins simply as exotoxins that have an effect on the intestinal tract.

nontoxic enzymes contributing to virulence

Many bacteria produce one or more enzymes that are nontoxic per se, but facilitate tissue invasion or help to protect the organism against the body's defense mechanisms. For example, various bacteria produce collagenases or hyaluronidases or convert serum plasminogen to plasmin, which has fibrinolytic activity. Although the evidence is not conclusive, it is reasonable to assume that these substances facilitate spread of infection. Hemolysins, some of which are highly cytotoxic, are produced by many bacteria and may liberate necessary growth factors for some of them. Deoxyribonucleases, elastases, and many other biologically active enzymes are also produced by some bacteria, but again their function in the disease process or in providing nutrients for the invaders is uncertain. All are proteins and have most of the characteristics of exotoxins, but do not produce specific toxicity.

In recent years, the molecular mechanisms of action of several exotoxins has been determined; these mechanisms will be considered in other chapters. In some cases, exotoxin genes have been cloned. In several instances, the toxins have been found to have a subunit that mediates attachment to the

protective effect of antitoxin

host cell, as well as a toxic subunit. Antibody to the former, produced in response to both toxins and toxoids, provides protection by preventing the toxic component from reaching its site of action. It is probable that genetically engineered toxoids will become available in the future for some exotoxins that are not toxoidable with formalin.

Tissue Damage from Immune Reactions

Tissue damage and the manifestations of disease may also result from interaction between the host's immune mechanisms and the invading organism or its products.

Immune complex diseases

Reactions between high concentrations of antibody, soluble microbial antigens, and complement can deposit immune complexes in tissues and cause acute inflammatory reactions and immune complex disease.

Antibody cross-reacting with host tissues

In poststreptococcal acute glomerulonephritis, for example, the complexes are sequestered in the glomeruli of the kidney, with serious interference in renal function from the resulting tissue reaction. Sometimes, antibody produced against microbial antigens can cross-react with certain host tissues and initiate an autoimmune process. Such cross-reaction is almost certainly the explanation for poststreptococcal rheumatic fever, and it may be involved in some of the lesions of tertiary syphilis.

Pathologic changes from delayed-type hypersensitivity reactions

In some other infections, the pathologic and clinical features are largely due to delayed-type hypersensitivity reactions to the organism or its products. Such reactions are particularly significant in tuberculosis and other mycobacterial infections. The mycobacteria possess no significant toxins and, in the absence of delayed hypersensitivity, their multiplication elicits little more than a mild inflammatory response. The development of delayed-type cell-mediated hypersensitivity to their major proteins leads to dramatic pathologic manifestations, which in tuberculosis are manifested as a chronic granulomatous response around infected foci with massive infiltration of macrophages and lymphocytes followed by central devascularization and necrosis. Rupture of a necrotic area into a bronchus leads to the typical pulmonary cavity of the disease, and rupture into a blood vessel can produce extensive dissemination or massive bleeding from the lung. Injection of tuberculoprotein into an animal with an established tuberculous lesion can lead to acute exacerbation and sometimes death. Thus, the body's defense mechanisms are themselves contributing to the severity of the disease process.

These examples illustrate processes that are probably involved to varying degrees in the pathology and course of most infections. As will be discussed in a subsequent section, the humoral or cell-mediated immune interactions, or both, are essential to the control of essentially all infectious diseases; they are potentially damaging to the host, however, particularly when large amounts of antigens are involved and the host response is unusually active.

Alterations in Virulence of Pathogenic Organisms

Attenuation

Virulence, which is usually determined by a number of properties of an organism, is not an immutable characteristic. Changes, usually toward lower virulence, may develop during prolonged epidemic or endemic associations of a pathogenic organism with a particular host species and contribute to a more balanced state of parasitism. Virulence may also be manipulated experimentally to yield *attenuated* organisms that retain the antigenic specificity of the wild type and the capacity to multiply in vivo, but lose the ability to cause serious disease. Many of the most successful "live" vaccines have been prepared in this way. Attenuation of many species for vaccine production was achieved pragmatically by passing the organism repeatedly through a host species that it normally does not infect or by growing it in vitro under suboptimal conditions, such as unphysiologic temperatures.

loss of virulence determining plasmids

temperature-sensitive mutants

defective interfering particles

The mechanisms involved in such attenuation are now understood more clearly. For example, Pasteur's classic attenuation of the anthrax bacillus to provide an effective vaccine for cattle is now known to have resulted from loss of a plasmid coding for anthrax toxin when the organism was grown at elevated temperature. Likewise, temperature-sensitive mutants that fail to produce the full complement of an essential metabolite or structure at body temperature can lose part or all of their virulence, as can defective interfering viral particles that have all of the structural proteins of the wild type, but lack an essential portion of the viral genome.

Adaptive Immune Responses of Host to Systemic Infection

The adaptive immune responses to infection comprise antibody synthesis by cells derived from the B-lymphocyte series, cell-mediated immunity determined by T lymphocytes, and the interferon systems. The first two are mainly antigen specific; the latter, however, can be activated by a variety of viral and other stimuli and can inhibit a wide range of virus species, irrespective of the initiating stimulus.

Antibody-Mediated Immunity

Natural antibody

Normal serum contains low concentrations of immunoglobulins, predominantly of the IgG class, with a variety of specificities. They are probably formed in response to absorption of antigens from the normal flora or in food or to antigenic stimuli from any infecting organisms that may have been encountered. These "natural" antibodies offer protection against some pathogenic species with cross-reacting antigens, although their specificities are unpredictable in the individual subject. Likewise, low concentrations of IgA are found on mucous membranes. Immunoglobulin A has already been considered as part of the first line of defense.

Antibody response to infection

anamnestic responses

longevity of IgG response

When an infection occurs, B cells programmed to react to specific microbial antigens proliferate and mature into plasma cells that produce IgM, IgG, or IgA antibodies. Effective amounts of antibody are rarely detectable before 5 days after first exposure to newly encountered antigen; however, an anamnestic response developed from memory cells occurs within a day or so of a subsequent stimulus and lasts much longer. In natural infections, these two responses tend to merge into each other. The presence of IgM antibody is of relatively short duration and usually indicates concurrent or recent infection. In contrast, specific IgG antibody may be detectable for years after control of an infection.

opsonization

complement-mediated bacterial killing

antitoxins

reduction of effectiveness in presence of increased iron

As discussed in previous sections, antibody plays many roles in defense against extracellular organisms and their toxic products. It opsonizes many bacteria, particularly those with antiphagocytic capsules, and the process is enhanced by binding and activation of complement. In the presence of complement, both IgG and IgM can initiate direct complement-mediated killing of many Gram-negative organisms, which may account in part for the failure of some organisms, such as the cholera vibrio, to invade the subepithelial tissues. Antibody is also produced against soluble bacterial carbohydrates and proteins, including toxins and extracellular enzymes, and will neutralize them directly or lead to their engulfment and destruction by macrophages. Thus, the protective power of antibody is great, and it is widely exploited in use of vaccines and toxoids for the prevention of many specific infections. It is interesting that most of the protective effects of humoral immunity are reduced if the iron concentration increases. This phenomenon is well illustrated by the increased susceptibility to some bacterial infections of patients with chronic hemolytic anemia, in whom serum iron concentrations tend to be elevated.

role of antibody in intracellular infections

The role of antibody in the prevention and control of intracellular organisms such as viruses is more complex. None of the immunoglobulins can penetrate the infected cell, but specific antibody will combine with free virus and prevent its attachment or entry into uninfected host cells. Cytotoxic T lymphocytes and nonspecific natural killer cells can act alone or in concert with antibody and the alternate complement pathway to destroy infected cells that have virus-coded surface antigens, and the released extracellular virus is then neutralized by antibody to prevent further spread of the infection. These processes are not always effective in controlling intracellular infections. For example, latent virus is inaccessible to antibody, and agents such as herpes simplex virus that can pass from cell to cell by intercellular bridges may not be reached by antibody once the infection is established. Furthermore, if viral antigens are not expressed at the cell surface, immune lysis of infected cells may not occur.

In many facultative or obligate intracellular bacterial infections, direct killing or neutralization of free organisms by antibody and complement does not occur, and opsonizing antibody does not eliminate infection because of the organism's capacity to survive or grow within phagocytic cells.

Cell-Mediated Immunity

Interactions of immune T cells with other cells

activation of T cells

macrophage processing of antigen

T-cell-mediated immunity is more complex, in that it involves, at the effector stage, a series of interactions with macrophages, other lymphocytes, and in some cases tissue cells. Some of these interactions are mediated by specific compounds termed interleukins. Most T cells have a surface receptor for a particular antigen, and, when that antigen is recognized, the cell is activated and differentiates to produce one of the functions described herein. The clones of cells with activity against the particular antigen multiply rapidly and become disseminated widely throughout the body. The initial step of antigenic stimulus often requires the collaboration of macrophages that "process" and present the antigen to the T cell in juxtaposition to a product of an immunoresponse gene so that it is recognized as foreign. As multiplication proceeds, the cells differentiate to yield some that have direct cytotoxic effects on host cells that they recognize, some whose major function is to produce various soluble lymphokines that carry messages to other cells, some that modulate both T- and B-cell immune response activity, and some that serve as memory cells for subsequent anamnestic responses.

Helper T cells

Helper T cells are primarily involved in signaling to B cells the need to differentiate into plasma cells and secrete immunoglobulin specific for the antigen to which they have been exposed. These T cells also enhance overall T-cell maturation when stimulated by specific or nonspecific factors.

Suppressor T cells

The suppressor T cells modulate both antibody production and the processes of cell-mediated immunity, and their function appears to be to ensure immune responses sufficient to achieve control of an infection, but below levels that are excessively damaging to the host.

T killer cells

Action of lymphokines

effect on macrophages

chemotactic effects

Two other types of effector T lymphocytes are produced upon specific stimulation. T killer cells can lyse infected or "foreign" cells independent of antibody. The second effector cells produce lymphokines, which have a wide variety of activities. One of these, macrophage migration inhibition factor, retards movements of macrophages and thus retains them where they are needed in the infected focus. Another activates macrophages to greater metabolic activity and killing effectiveness. One class of lymphokines is chemotactic and attracts neutrophils, monocytes, and other lymphocytes to an infected area. Thus, a hallmark of these T cells is collaboration with other cells in producing conditions that control infection.

Delayed-type hypersensitivity

chronic inflammatory response and lesions

relationship of cell-mediated immunity to delayed-type hypersensitivity

A major phenomenon associated with T-cell-mediated immune activities produced by the effector cells mentioned above is delayed-type hypersensitivity, which is a concomitant of many bacterial, viral, fungal, and parasitic infections. Lymphokines produced by T cells in response to protein antigens mobilize and activate macrophages and other lymphocytes at the site of infection and produce a chronic inflammatory response. This reaction serves to wall off and control many infections, but also produces pathologic lesions (for example, those of tuberculosis). There is no clear dissociation between delayed-type hypersensitivity and cell-mediated immunity, because each is a manifestation of the same basic processes. Demonstration of delayed-type hypersensitivity by intradermal inoculation of antigen (for example, in purified protein derivative skin test for tuberculosis) is used to determine previous or present infection with the pathogen from which the antigen was derived.

Null cells

Lymphocytes that lack typical T or B receptors (null cells) but have Fc receptors can recognize antibodies on infected cells and lyse them. This mechanism is known as *antibody-dependent cell-mediated cytotoxicity.* Another type is the natural killer cell, which can lyse infected cells without specific antigenic stimulation. This latter activity is enhanced by interferons.

Interferons

interferons are glycoproteins

viruses and other stimuli initiate interferon synthesis

immune interferon production

Interferons are carbohydrate-containing proteins (glycoproteins) produced by several cell types, including fibroblasts and many epithelial cells, but particularly lymphocytes and cells of the mononuclear phagocyte series. They are synthesized when the cell is exposed to a number of stimuli. Viral infections in particular lead to interferon production, as do endotoxin, some other bacterial products, and double-stranded natural or synthetic RNA. Production by lymphocytes can be stimulated by reaction of the cells with the specific antigen to which they are responsive or by mitogens. Their production is blocked by inhibitors of protein and RNA synthesis.

inhibition of viral protein synthesis

passage to uninfected cells

Interferons inhibit viral replication. They do not affect absorption, but act by inducing synthesis of a structural protein within the cell that inhibits synthesis of viral protein. In addition to their activity within the infected cell, they protect uninfected cells that may have taken up viruses. The phenomenon of viral interference (inability of another virus to superinfect during a primary viral infection) is largely due to interferon production in response to the first infecting virus. Some interferons also act as lymphokines to activate natural killer cells, which can destroy viral infected cells and some normal or cancerous cells in the absence of specific immune responses. The role of natural killer cells in the control of infections is not yet clear.

role in control of viral infections

host species specific but not virus specific

The interferons clearly play a critical role in the early control of many acute viral infections pending the development of humoral and cellular immune mechanisms that will supplement their action. On the other hand, there are some instances in which interferons may excessively enhance the inflammatory process by activating natural killer and cytotoxic T cells. They are generally specific for each animal species, and thus interferon for human therapeutic studies was originally obtained with great cost and effort from human blood leukocytes. Several interferon genes have now been cloned in bacteria and yeasts, and their products have been expressed in these organisms. Consequently, more complete studies are now under way on the application of interferon to the prophylaxis and treatment of viral diseases.

Conclusion

Host–parasite interactions are enormously complex and have evolved in a manner that has tended to produce a more balanced state of parasitism between well-established species and the microorganisms with which they frequently come into contact. In this chapter the components of these interactions have been discussed separately, but it is important to recognize the dynamic and shifting nature of their role in determining the course and outcome of an infection. Overlying the specific determinants of virulence and immunity discussed here are broader determinants such as the general health, nutrition, and quite probably the psychologic status of the host. There is increasing evidence that hormonal and diurnal controls of various aspects of the immune processes may be important. Study of these factors offers considerable hope for the possibility of manipulating general host resistance mechanisms more effectively in the future.

Additional Reading and References

Beachey, E.H. 1981. Bacterial adherence: Adhesin–receptor interactions mediating the attachment of bacteria to mucosal surfaces. *J. Infect. Dis.* 143:325–345.

Bullen, J.J. 1981. The significance of iron in infection. *Rev. Infect. Dis.* 3:1127–1138. A thorough review of a developing area of interest and importance.

Fields, B.N., and Greene, M.I. 1982. Genetic and molecular mechanisms of viral pathogenesis: Implications for prevention and treatment. *Nature* 300:19–23. Using a reovirus model, the authors illustrate nicely the specialized role of certain outer capsid proteins and suggest ways to control viral infections at the molecular level.

McNabb, P.C., and Tomasi, T.B. 1981. Host defenses at mucosal surfaces. *Annu. Rev. Microbiol.* 35:477–496. An excellent account, particularly of the activity of immunoglobulin A.

Mims, C.A. 1982. *The Pathogenesis of Infectious Disease.* 2nd ed. London: Academic Press. A very readable, up-to-date, and balanced account of the pathogenesis of infection.

Peterson, P.K., and Quie, P.G. 1981. Bacterial surface components and the pathogenesis of infectious diseases. *Annu. Rev. Med.* 32:29–43.

Quie, P.G. 1983. Perturbations of the normal mechanisms of intraleukocytic killing of bacteria. *J. Infect. Dis.* 148:189–193. A succinct discussion of organism–phagocyte interactions.

Smith, H., Skehel, J.J., and Turner, M.J., Eds. 1980. *The Molecular Basis of Microbial Pathogenicity.* Berlin: Verlag Chemie. A series of papers on the molecular rather than the phenomenologic aspects of host–parasite interactions.

Swanson, J., Sparling, P.F., and Puziss, M., Eds. 1983. Bacterial virulence and pathogenicity. *Rev. Infect. Dis.* S.5:633–S.832. The proceedings of a recent conference covering many of the topics considered in this chapter.

Lawrence Corey

Epidemiology of Infectious Diseases

8

Epidemiology, the study of the distribution of determinants of disease and injury in human populations, is a discipline that includes both infectious and noninfectious diseases. Most epidemiologic studies of infectious diseases have concentrated on the factors that influence acquisition and spread, because this knowledge is essential for developing methods of prevention and control. Historically, epidemiologic studies, and the application of the knowledge gained from them, have been central to the control of great epidemic diseases such as cholera, plague, smallpox, yellow fever, and typhus, which were major threats to human life and health throughout the world until the mid-20th century, and some of which remain so.

epidemiological responsibilities of medical attendants

An understanding of the principles of epidemiology and the spread of disease is essential to all medical personnel, even though their work may be with the individual patient rather than the community. Most infections must be evaluated in their epidemiologic setting; for example, what is the risk to the patient's family, schoolmates, and work or social contacts? Has the patient recently traveled to an area of special disease prevalence? Is there a possibility of nosocomial infection from recent hospitalization? Is the patient suffering from a reportable disease? The physician must never hesitate to enlist the help of public health authorities, who have the knowledge, organization, and responsibility to undertake the epidemiologic studies and control measures needed to protect the community.

Sources and Communicability

Infectious diseases of humans may be caused by exclusively human pathogens such as the measles virus, by environmental organisms such as *Legionella pneumophila,* or by organisms that have their primary reservoir in animals, such as the plague bacillus. They can generally be classified as noncommunicable or communicable.

noncommunicable infections

Noncommunicable diseases include 1) those caused by the patient's normal flora, such as peritonitis after rupture of the appendix; 2) those caused by the ingestion of preformed toxins, such as botulism and staphylococcal food poisoning; 3) infections caused by certain organisms common in nature, such as gas gangrene and Legionnaires' disease contracted from the environment. Many zoonotic infections (diseases transmitted from animals to humans), such as rabies and brucellosis, are rarely, if ever, transmitted between humans under natural conditions, although readily communicable within their animal reservoir.

single-source epidemics from noncommunicable diseases

These diseases may occur as epidemics that involve a common source of infection. For example, ingestion of a chicken salad heavily contaminated with an enterotoxin-producing *Staphylococcus aureus* can produce acute food poisoning within an hour or two in those who ate it, but the disease is not transmissible to others. Likewise, extensive dissemination of *Legionella* through an air-conditioning system may lead to many cases of pulmonary infection, particularly in immunocompromised hosts, but without secondary spread.

endemic, epidemic, and pandemic spread of communicable diseases

Infectious diseases communicable from person to person can be *endemic*, which implies that the disease may be present at a low but fairly constant level, or *epidemic*, which involves a level of infection above that usually found in a community or population. They may be widespread in a region and sometimes worldwide with high attack rates, in which case they are termed *pandemic*. A communicable infection requires that an organism be able to multiply in or on the body and to leave the body in a form directly infectious to others or indirectly infectious after development in an animate vector or in a suitable environment. An example of direct communicability is the respiratory spread of the influenza virus. In contrast, the malarial parasite requires a developmental cycle in a biting mosquito before another human can be infected.

Infection and Disease

distinction between infection and disease

subclinical infection and the carrier state

An important consideration in the study of the epidemiology of communicable organisms is the distinction between infection and disease. Infection involves multiplication of the organism in or on the host. Disease represents a clinically apparent response of the host to infection. With many communicable microorganisms, infection is much more common than disease, and apparently healthy infected individuals play an important role in disease propagation. Inapparent infections are termed *subclinical*, and the individual is sometimes referred to as a *carrier*. The latter term is also applied to situations in which an infectious agent establishes itself as part of a patient's flora or causes low-grade chronic disease after an acute infection. For example, the clinically inapparent presence of *S. aureus* in the anterior nares is termed *carriage*, as is a chronic gallbladder infection with *Salmonella typhi* which can follow an attack of typhoid fever and result in fecal excretion of the organism for years. With some infectious diseases, such as smallpox or measles, infection is invariably accompanied by clinical manifestations of the disease itself. These manifestations facilitate epidemiologic control, because the existence and extent of infection in a community is readily apparent.

some diseases have no carrier state

infectivity and virulence

The inherent infectivity and virulence of a microorganism are properties discussed in Chapter 7. They are important determinants of attack rates of disease in a community because, in general, organisms of high infectivity spread more easily and those of greater virulence are more likely to cause disease than subclinical infection. Some infectious agents, such as the chickenpox (varicella) virus, are of high infectivity but low virulence, and the disease they cause is quite mild; others, such as the leprosy bacillus, are of low infectivity but high virulence in established infections. The infective dose of an organism also influences the chance of infection and development of disease. A large dose of an organism of low virulence is more likely to cause disease than a small dose. Host factors such as age, race, genetic predisposition, and immune status can dramatically influence the manifestations of an infectious disease and are largely responsible, with differences in infecting dose, for the wide spectrum of disease manifestations that may be seen during an epidemic. For example, in an epidemic of measles in an isolated population in 1846, the attack rate for all ages averaged 75%; however, mortality was 90 times higher in children less than 1 year of age

role of infecting dose

Host factors influencing manifestations of disease

age

(28%) than in those 1–40 years of age (0.3%). Conversely, in one outbreak of poliomyelitis, the attack rate of paralytic polio was 4% in children 0–4 years of age and 20–40% in those 5–50 years of age. Likewise, infections caused by Epstein–Barr virus are asymptomatic when acquired in childhood, but will frequently result in infectious mononucleosis when primary infection occurs in early adulthood. Racial differences markedly influence the progression of the fungal disease coccidioidomycosis, which is contracted from the soil of some Sonoran and other southwestern desert areas: clinical disease and dissemination to organs such as bone and brain are more common in Filipino, black, and Asian subjects than in white subjects. Sex may also be a factor in disease acquisition; for example, for male subjects the likelihood of becoming a chronic carrier of hepatitis B is twice that for females.

race

sex

Routes of Transmission

direct and indirect spread

vector spread

congenital transmission of infection

Various transmissible infections may be acquired from others by direct contact, by aerosol transmission of infectious secretions, or indirectly through contaminated inanimate objects or materials. Some, such as malaria, involve an animate insect vector. The major horizontal routes of transmission of infectious diseases are summarized in Table 8.1 and discussed herein. Certain diseases can spread from the mother to the fetus through the placental barrier. This mode of transmission involves organisms that can be present in the blood and may occur at different stages of pregnancy with different organisms. Examples of transplacental spread include congenital rubella infection, congenital syphilis, and congenital toxoplasmosis.

respiratory spread

respiratory aerosol and droplet spread

Many infections are transmitted by the respiratory route, often by aerosolization of respiratory secretions with subsequent inhalation by others. The efficiency of this process depends in part on the extent and method of propulsion of discharges from the mouth and nose, the size of the aerosol droplets, and the resistance of the infectious agent to desiccation and inactivation by ultraviolet light. In still air, a particle 100 μm in diameter requires only seconds to fall the height of a room; a 10-μm particle will remain airborne for about 20 min, smaller particles even longer. When inhaled, particles with a diameter of 6 μm or more are usually trapped by the mucosa of the nasal turbinates, whereas particles of 0.6–6.0 μm will attach to mucus sites at various levels along the upper and lower respiratory tract and may initiate infection. Respiratory secretions are often transferred on hands or inanimate objects (fomites) and may reach the respiratory tract of others in this way. For example, spread of the common cold often involves transfer of infectious secretions from nose to hand by the infected individual with transfer to others by hand to hand contact, and then from hand to nose by the unsuspecting victim. Nose rubbing as a form of greeting, although little practiced in the West, would seem likely to improve the efficiency of rhinovirus transmission.

manual and fomite spread of respiratory infections

salivary spread

Some infections, such as herpes simplex and infectious mononucleosis, can be transferred directly by contact with infectious saliva through kissing or through bites. Salivary transmission of infectious secretions among children in day-care centers through shared toys and utensils often accounts for the rapid dissemination of agents such as respiratory syncytial virus, *Haemophilus influenzae* type b, and the meningococcus.

fecal–oral spread

direct and indirect contamination of food and water

Fecal–oral spread is an important means of transmission of a variety of bacterial, viral, and parasitic diseases. It is a route associated with poor hygiene and may involve direct or finger-to-mouth spread, the use of night soil as a fertilizer, or fecal contamination of food or water. Food handlers who are infected with an organism transmissible by this route constitute a special hazard. Some viruses disseminated by the fecal–oral route infect and

Table 8.1 Common Routes of Transmission[a]

Route of Exit	Route of Transmission	Example
Respiratory	Aerosol droplet inhalation	Influenza virus; tuberculosis
	Nose or mouth → hand or object → nose	Common cold (rhinovirus)
Salivary	Direct salivary transfer (e.g., kissing)	Oral–labial herpes; infectious mononucleosis
	Animal bite	Rabies
Gastrointestinal	Stool → hand → mouth and/or stool → object → mouth	Enterovirus infection; hepatitis A
	Stool → water or food → mouth	Salmonellosis; shigellosis
Skin	Skin discharge → air → respiratory tract	Poxvirus infection; varicella
	Skin to skin	Infectious warts; syphilis
Blood	Transfusion or needle prick	Hepatitis B; cytomegalovirus infection; malaria
	Insect bite	Malaria; relapsing fever
Genital secretions	Urethral or cervical secretions	Gonorrhea; herpes simplex
	Semen	Cytomegalovirus infection
Urine	Urine → hand → catheter	Hospital-acquired urinary tract infection
	Urine → aerosol (rare)	Tuberculosis
Eye	Conjunctival	Adenovirus
Zoonotic	Animal bite	Rabies
	Contact with carcasses	Tularemia
	Arthropod	Plague; Rocky Mountain spotted fever

[a] The examples cited are incomplete, and in some cases more than one route of transmission exists.

properties of intestinal pathogens

multiply in cells of the oropharynx, then disseminate to other body sites to cause infection. Commonly, however, organisms that are spread in this way multiply in the intestinal tract and may cause intestinal infections. They must, therefore, be able to resist the acid in the stomach, the bile, and the gastric and small-intestinal enzymes. Many bacteria and enveloped viruses are rapidly killed by these conditions, but Enterobacteriaceae and unenveloped viral intestinal pathogens are more likely to survive. Even with these organisms, the infecting dose in patients with reduced or absent gastric hydrochloric acid is often much smaller than in those with normal stomach acidity, which accounts in part for the greater attack rates in malnourished hosts. The carrier of enteric pathogens poses a particular hazard to others, especially when involved in food preparation and when personal hygienic practices are inadequate (for example, failure to wash hands after defecation).

greater risk of infection in achlorhydric host

hazards posed by intestinal carriers

skin-to-skin transfer

Skin-to-skin transfer occurs with a variety of infections in which the skin is the portal of exit. Examples are the spirochete of syphilis (*Treponema pallidum*), strains of group A streptococci that can cause impetigo, and the dermatophyte fungi that cause ringworm and athlete's foot. In the case of direct and fomite spread

syphilis, transfer is by direct contact because the rapid death of the spirochete outside the body precludes spread by fomites. Other diseases may be spread through fomites such as shared towels or inadequately cleansed shower and bath floors. Skin-to-skin transfer usually occurs through abrasions of the epidermis, which may be unnoticed.

blood-borne transmission

insect vectors

direct transmission with infected blood

Blood-borne transmission through insect vectors is an essential feature of some protozoal, bacterial, and viral diseases. In some instances the infectious agent requires a period of multiplication or alteration within an insect vector before it can infect another human host; such is the case with the yellow fever virus in the *Aedes aegypti* mosquito and with the malarial parasite. Direct transmission through blood has become increasingly important in modern medicine because of the use of blood transfusions and blood products and the increased use of self-administered illicit drugs by intravenous or subcutaneous routes, using shared unsterile equipment. Hepatitis B virus in particular has been frequently transmitted in this way.

genital tract transmission

significance of chronic, asymptomatic and recurrent infection

Disease transmission through the genital tract has emerged as one of the most common infectious problems in the latter half of the 20th century and reflects changing social and sexual mores. Spread can be between sexual partners or to the infant at birth. A major factor in these infections has been the persistence of organisms such as *Chlamydia trachomatis* and cytomegalovirus in genital tract secretions for periods of months, the high rate of asymptomatic gonococcal carriage in women, and the chronicity and recurrence of genital herpes infections.

urinary tract nosocomial transmission

Numerous organisms can infect the urinary tract and be excreted in the urine. Spread by person-to-person contact, although possible, is only a significant problem in the hospitalized patient. Transmission between patients with indwelling urethral catheters, which is particularly important, has been shown to occur by way of the inadequately washed hands of medical attendants and staff members.

eye-to-eye transmission

Infections of the conjunctiva may occur in epidemic or endemic form. Epidemics of *Haemophilus* conjunctivitis may occur in institutions and are highly contagious. The major endemic disease is trachoma, caused by *Chlamydia*, which remains a frequent cause of blindness in developing countries. These diseases may be spread by direct contact or by secretions passed manually or through fomites such as towels.

zoonotic transmission

blind-ended infections

transmission of zoonotic infection between humans

Some infections are spread from animals, where they have their natural reservoir, to humans. These infections are termed *zoonotic diseases*. Some zoonotic infections, such as rabies contracted from the bite of a rabid animal, are blind-ended in humans in that infection is rarely, if ever, transferred from person to person. Others may be transferred between humans once the disease is established in a population. Plague, for example, has a natural reservoir in rodents. Human infections contracted from the bites of rodent fleas may produce pneumonia, which may then spread to others by the respiratory droplet route.

Incubation Period and Communicability

determinants of short and long incubation periods

The incubation period is the time between exposure to the organism and the appearance of the first symptoms of disease. Generally, organisms that multiply rapidly and produce local infections, such as gonorrhea and influenza, are associated with short incubation periods (for example, 2–4 days). Diseases such as typhoid fever, which depend on hematogenous spread and multiplication of the organism in distant target organs to produce symptoms, often have longer incubation periods (for example, 10 days to 3 weeks). Some diseases have even more prolonged incubation periods because of slow passage of the infecting organism to the target organ, as in rabies, or slow growth of the organism, as in tuberculosis. Incubation periods may

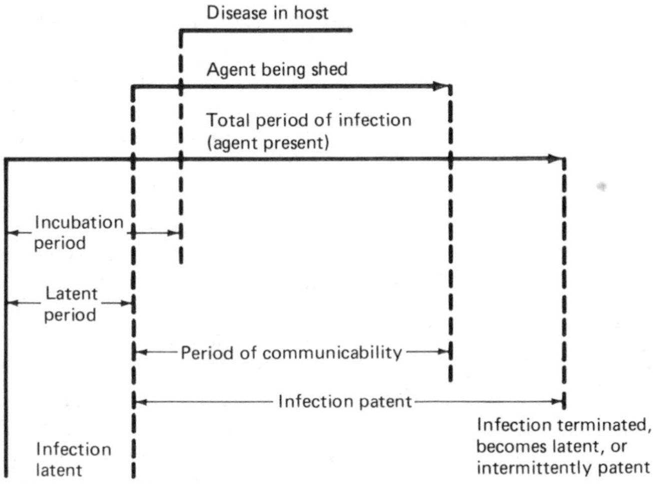

8.1 Schematic of stages of infection. (*Reprinted with permission from Fox, J.P., Hall, C.E., and Elveback, L.R. 1970. Epidemiology, Man and Disease. New York: Macmillan, copyright 1970 Macmillan Publishing Co., Inc.*)

also vary widely depending upon route of acquisition and infecting dose; for example, the incubation period of hepatitis B infection may vary from 7 to more than 200 days.

duration of shedding and communicability

The rapidity with which a disease is spread is also related to how soon the agent is shed from the host and the duration of communicability. These factors are not necessarily related to the development or duration of disease. For example, asymptomatic carriers of *Chlamydia* or gonococci in the uterine cervix can shed the agent for a longer time and be more infectious to others than those who are symptomatic and come to medical attention. Conversely, some agents, such as *S. aureus,* are more contagious from symptomatic infection than from asymptomatic carriers. The stages of infection in the host are illustrated schematically in Figure 8.1.

Epidemics

definitions and quantitation

infectivity

pathogenicity

virulence

incidence

rate

prevalence

The characterization of epidemics and their recognition in a community involve several quantitative measures and some specific epidemiologic definitions. Infectivity, in epidemiologic terms, equates with attack rate and is measured by the frequency with which an infection is transmitted when there is contact between the agent and a susceptible individual. Pathogenicity can be expressed as the number of persons who develop the disease divided by the total number infected, and virulence by the number of fatal or severe cases over the total number of cases. Incidence, the number of new cases of a disease within a specified period, is most often described as a rate in which the number of cases is the numerator and that in the population under surveillance is the denominator. Prevalence, which can also be described as a rate, is the total number of cases existing in a population at risk at a point in time or during a defined period.

Epidemics can be a common source or propagated by spread from person to person. An example of the former would be an outbreak of *Salmonella* food poisoning in which a number of people consume a food heavily contaminated with *Salmonella enteritidis.* An example of a propagated epidemic would be an outbreak of influenza.

common-source epidemics

Common-source epidemics from preformed toxin in food, such as that causing botulism, are not associated with secondary spread. A secondary wave of propagated infections, however, may result from common-source outbreaks caused by transmissible organisms.

propagated epidemics

The prerequisites for a propagated epidemic are a sufficient degree of infectivity to allow the organism to spread, sufficient virulence for an increased incidence of disease to become apparent, and a sufficient level of susceptibility in the host population to permit transmission and amplification of the infecting organism. Thus, the extent of an epidemic and its degree of severity are determined by complex interactions between parasite and host.

factors influencing susceptibility of a population

innate immunity and its origin

The degree of susceptibility of a population to a potentially epidemic disease depends on genetic factors and on the level of acquired immunity. Prolonged and extensive exposure to a pathogen during previous generations will select for a higher degree of innate immunity in a population. For example, extensive exposure of Western urbanized populations to tuberculosis during the 18th and 19th centuries conferred a degree of resistance greater than that among the progeny of rural or geographically isolated populations. The disease spread rapidly and in severe form, for example, when it was first encountered by the North American Indian. An even more dramatic example concerns the resistance to the most serious form of malaria that is conferred on peoples of West African descent by the sickle-celled trait (Chapter 45). These instances are clear cases of natural selection, a process that accounts for many differences in racial immunity.

acquired immunity

impact of degree of immunity on epidemic frequency

Acquired immunity and its level in a population are often the major determinants of the frequency and duration of epidemics. For example, measles is highly infectious and attacks most susceptible members of an exposed population. Infection, however, gives solid lifelong immunity. Thus, in populations in which the disease was maintained in endemic form, epidemics occurred at about 3-year intervals when a sufficient number of nonimmune hosts had been born to permit rapid transmission between them. When a sufficient immune population was reestablished, epidemic spread was blocked and the disease again became endemic. When immunity is short-lived or incomplete, epidemics can continue for decades if the mode of transmission is unchecked, thus accounting for the prolonged urban epidemic of tuberculosis during the last two centuries and the present epidemic of gonorrhea.

pandemics of infection to which immunity is low or absent

Occasionally, an epidemic arises from an organism against which immunity is essentially absent in a population and that is either of enhanced virulence or appears to be of enhanced virulence because of the lack of immunity. When such an organism is highly infectious, the disease it causes may become pandemic and worldwide. The most recent incidents have been with major antigenic variants of influenza A virus, against which there was little if any cross-immunity from recent epidemics with other strains. The 1918–1919 pandemic of influenza, for example, was responsible for more deaths (about 20 million) than World War I. Subsequent but less serious pandemics have occurred at intervals because of the development of strains of influenza virus with major antigenic shifts (Chapter 34). Some diseases of extraordinary severity and mortality, such as the sweating sickness of the 13th century, have appeared suddenly and disappeared equally suddenly, and their cause remains unknown. Possibly they involved a mutational or recombinational event that produced such enhanced virulence in a previously common pathogen that the variant was unable to maintain itself because of the death of so many of its victims.

epidemics associated with unusual virulence

social determinants of epidemic diseases

A major feature of serious epidemic diseases is their frequent association with poverty, malnutrition, disaster, and war. The association is multifactorial and includes overcrowding, contaminated food and water, an increase in arthropods that parasitize humans and can carry some epidemic diseases, and the reduced immunity that can accompany severe malnutrition or certain types of chronic stress.

In recent years in developed countries, increasing attention has been nosocomial epidemics

opportunistic infections

given to hospital (nosocomial) epidemics of infection. The hospital is not immune to the epidemic diseases that occur in the community; however, most nosocomial infections involve opportunistic organisms and result from the close association of infected patients with those who are unusually susceptible because of chronic disease, immunosuppressive therapy, or the use of bladder, intratracheal, or intravascular catheters and tubes. Control depends on the techniques of medical personnel, hospital hygiene, and effective surveillance. This topic is considered in greater detail in Chapter 66.

Control of Epidemics

surveillance and recognition

The first principle of control is to recognize the existence of an epidemic. This recognition is sometimes immediate because of the high incidence of disease, but often the evidence is obtained from ongoing surveillance activities, such as routine disease reports to health departments and records of school and work absenteeism.

cause and route of spread

The causative agent must be identified as soon as possible and characterized antigenically if more than one serotype exists. Studies to determine route of transmission (for example, in outbreaks of food poisoning) must be initiated immediately unless it is known from the organism's identity.

methods of control

Measures must then be adopted to control the spread and development of further infection. These methods include 1) blocking the route of transmission if possible (for example, improved food hygiene or arthropod control); 2) identifying, treating, and if necessary, isolating infected individuals and carriers if they are important contributors to maintenance of the epidemic; 3) raising the level of immunity in the uninfected population by immunization, where effective; 4) selective use of chemoprophylaxis for subjects or populations at particular risk of infection, as in epidemics of meningococcal infection; and 5) correcting conditions such as overcrowding or contaminated water supplies that have led to the epidemic or facilitated transfer.

General Principles of Immunization

active immunization

Artificial immunization, the most effective method of specific individual and community protection against many epidemic diseases, is becoming applicable to a broader range of infections as greater sophistication is attained in identifying and purifying specific immunizing antigens and in preparing and purifying specific antibodies for passive protection. Immunization can be active, with stimulation of the body's immune mechanisms through administration of a vaccine, or passive, through administration of plasma or globulin containing preformed antibody to the agent desired. Active immunization with living attenuated organisms generally results in a subclinical or mild illness that duplicates to a limited extent the disease to be prevented. These *live vaccines* generally provide both local and durable humoral immunity. Killed or inactivated vaccines such as influenza, rabies, or typhoid vaccines or diphtheria or tetanus toxoids provide immunogenicity without infectivity. They generally involve a larger amount of antigen than live vaccines and must be administered parenterally with two or more spaced injections to give a satisfactory secondary response. Immunity usually develops more rapidly with live vaccines, but serious overt disease from the vaccine itself can result in patients with immunodeficiency syndromes or in those whose immune responses have been suppressed. Live attenuated virus vaccines are generally contraindicated in pregnancy because of the risk of infection and damage to developing fetus. Current vaccines and their uses are listed in Appendices 8.1 and 8.2.

advantages and disadvantages of live attenuated vaccines

passive immunization

Prophylaxis or therapy of some infections can be accomplished or aided by passive immunization. This procedure involves administration of pre-

advantages of human antibody preparations

use of specific hyperimmune globulins

formed antibody obtained from humans, derived from animals actively immunized to the agent, or produced by hybridoma techniques. Animal antisera induce immune responses to their globulins that result in clearance of the passively transferred antibody within about 10 days and carry the risk of hypersensitivity reactions such as serum sickness and anaphylaxis. Thus, human antibodies are preferable and are detectable in the circulation for several weeks. Two types of human antibody preparations are generally available. Immune serum globulin (gamma globulin) is the immunoglobulin G fraction of plasma, pooled from a large group of donors that contains

Appendix 8.1 Vaccines

Disease	Type of Vaccine	Administration and Frequency	Comments
		Routine Vaccination of Children and Adults	
Diphtheria, tetanus	Adsorbed toxoid	Childhood series followed by IM at least every 10 yr[a]	
Pertussis	Inactivated bacilli	Childhood series IM[a] combined with DT	
Poliomyelitis	Live attenuated	Oral polio vaccine[a]	Preferred for routine use and during epidemics
	Formalin inactivated	Inactivated polio vaccine SC	Selective use in unimmunized adults
Rubella	Live attenuated	SC once[a]	Routine use in children and in adult women who are antibody (HI) negative if pregnancy can be prevented for 3 mo after vaccination
Rubeola	Live attenuated	SC once[a]	Administer after 13 mo of age
Mumps	Live attenuated	SC once[a]	Routine use in children and for prevention of orchitis in susceptible seronegative male patients
		High Risk of Acquisition of or Complications from Disease	
Influenza	Inactivated	SC yearly	Directed at reducing morbidity and mortality in those at risk of complications of influenza (i.e., those with chronic heart and pulmonary disease and those over 65 yr old)
Pneumococcal	Purified multivalent polysaccharide	SC once	Same population as for influenza vaccination; also, patients with functional or surgical asplenia, agammaglobulinemia, cirrhosis, multiple myeloma, or nephrotic syndrome
Hepatitis B	Inactivated subunit		Groups at high risk for acquisition of hepatitis B, including household contacts of hepatitis B patients, patients requiring large volumes of clotting factors, homosexual men, and selected medical and dental personnel
		Populations Exposed to Localized Outbreaks	
Meningococcal A, C, AC	Purified capsular polysaccharide	SC once	Control of localized epidemics and adjunct to chemoprophylaxis in household contacts
Rubeola	Live attenuated	SC once	Control of outbreaks, usually among adolescents and young adults

Abbreviations: IM = intramuscularly; SC = subcutaneously; HI = hemagglutination inhibition; BCG = bacillus Calmette–Guérin; PO = per oS.

[a]Recommended schedules are listed in Appendix 8.2.

antibody to many naturally occurring diseases. Hyperimmune globulins are purified antibody preparations from the blood of subjects with high titers of antibody to a specific disease that have resulted from natural exposure or hyperimmunization. Hepatitis B immune globulin, rabies immune globulin, and human tetanus immune globulin are examples of the latter. Details of the use of these globulins can be obtained from the chapters that discuss the diseases in question. Appendix 8.3 lists the diseases in which passive immunization has proved to be useful in preventing acquisition of disease. Passive antibody is most effective when given during the incubation period.

Appendix 8.1 *(continued)*

Disease	Type of Vaccine	Administration and Frequency	Comments
		Populations Exposed to Localized Outbreaks (continued)	
Tuberculosis	Live attenuated BCG	SC or intradermally once	Used in groups at excessive risk of new infection with tuberculosis or in individuals persistently exposed to sputum positive for tuberculosis
Adenovirus	Live attenuated bivalent (types 4 and 7)	PO once	Used only in military recruits
Typhoid	Inactivated bacilli	SC in two doses	Used for those with unusual exposure: e.g., household contacts of documented *Salmonella typhi* carriers
Rubella	Live attenuated	SC once	Control of outbreaks among adolescents and young adults (must screen post-pubertal female patients with HI test before vaccination)
		Travelers to Foreign Countries	
Smallpox	Live vaccinia virus	Intradermally every 3–5 yr	Not recommended except for those traveling to countries still requiring vaccination certificates
Yellow fever	Live attenuated	SC once every 10 yr	Administered at yellow fever vaccination centers
Cholera	Phenol-inactivated suspension of *Vibrio cholerae*	SC approximately every 6 mo	Only 50% effective and not effective in decreasing transmission of disease
Typhoid	Inactivated bacilli	SC in two 4 wk apart	Efficacy of 70–90% in "normal" exposure
Typhus	Formaldehyde-inactivated *Rickettsia prowazekii*	SC in two doses	Administered only to persons in close contact where disease is indigenous
Plague	Formaldehyde-inactivated *Yersinia pestis*	SC in three injections of 0.5 ml at least 1 wk apart, booster every 2 yr	Agricultural workers who reside in endemic areas
Poliomyelitis	Oral or inactivated polio	[See text]	Most adults already immune
Hepatitis A	Immune serum globulin	IM every 3 mo	[See section on passive immunization]

Appendix 8.2 Recommended Schedule for Active Immunization of Normal Infants and Children

Recommended Age	Vaccine	Comment
2 months	DTP, OPV	Can be initiated earlier in areas of high endemicity
4 months	DTP, OPV	Interval of 2 months desired for OPV to avoid interference
6 months	DTP (OPV)	OPV optional for areas where polio might be imported (e.g., some areas of southwestern United States)
12 months	Tuberculin test[a]	May be given simultaneously with MMR at 15 months
15 months	Measles, mumps, rubella (MMR)	MMR preferred
18 months	DTP, OPV	Consider as part of primary series; DTP essential
4–6 years[b]	DTP, OPV	
14–16 years	Td	Repeat every 10 years for lifetime

Reproduced with permission from Report of the Committee on Infectious Diseases, 19th ed., Table 1. Copyright 1982 by the American Academy of Pediatrics.

For all products used, consult manufacturer's brochure for instructions for storage, handling, and administration. Biologic agents prepared by different manufacturers may vary, and those of the same manufacturer may change from time to time. The package insert should be followed for a specific product.

Abbreviations: DTP = diphtheria and tetanus toxoids with pertussis vaccine; OPV = oral attenuated poliovirus vaccine containing poliovirus types 1, 2, and 3; MMR = live measles, mumps, and rubella viruses in a combined vaccine; Td = adult tetanus toxoid (full dose) and diphtheria toxoid (reduced dose) in combination.

[a]Mantoux test (intradermal purified protein derivative) preferred. Frequency of testing depends on local epidemiology. Annual or biennial testing is recommended unless local circumstances dictate less frequent or no testing.

[b]Recommended up to 7th birthday.

Appendix 8.3 Passive Immunization

Disease	Preparation	Route	Comment
Hepatitis A	Human immune serum globulin	IM	Used in household contacts
Hepatitis B	Human hepatitis B immune globulin Human immune serum globulin	IM IM	Prophylaxis of direct parenteral exposure (needle prick) or mucous membrane contact in susceptible hosts; both hepatitis B immune globulin and immune serum globulin containing anti-hepatitis B surface antigen antibody (anti-HBs) may be useful in preventing nonparenteral transmission
Herpes zoster	Human zoster immune globulin	IM	Prevention and amelioration of varicella in susceptible immunosuppressed hosts
Diphtheria	Equine diphtheria antitoxin	IM or IV	Dose dependent on extent of membrane and degree of toxicity; may also be used in unimmunized household contacts
Tetanus	Human tetanus immune globulin	IM	When given with tetanus toxoid, use different syringes and sites
Rabies	Human rabies immune globulin	Locally and IM	Used for postexposure prophylaxis
	Equine anti-rabies globulin	Locally and IM	Same as for human rabies immune globulin
Measles	Human immune serum globulin	IM	Used in susceptible household contacts, those less than 1 yr old, exposed susceptible pregnant women, and immunodeficient hosts
Rubella	Human immune serum globulin	IM	Used in exposed susceptible pregnant women who will not consider termination of pregnancy

Abbreviations: IM = intramuscularly; IV = intravenously.

Additional Reading and References

Benenson, A.S., Ed. 1981. *Control of Communicable Diseases in Man.* 13th ed. Washington, D.C.: American Public Health Association. This excellent and authoritative, inexpensive paperback provides the major features of infectious diseases and methods for their identification and control.

Committee on Infectious Diseases of the American Academy of Pediatrics. 1982. *Report of the Committee on Infectious Diseases.* 19th ed. Evanston, Ill.: American Academy of Pediatrics. This reference manual of the Expert Committee of the American Academy of Pediatrics provides short synopses of the most important infectious diseases in children.

Fox, J.P., Hall, C.E., and Elveback, L.R. 1970. *Epidemiology, Man and Disease.* New York: Macmillan. This reference book remains an excellent overview of the principles and concepts of infectious disease epidemiology.

McNeill, W.H. 1976. *Plagues and People.* Garden City, N.Y.: Anchor Press/Doubleday. This interesting book describes the impact of infectious diseases on the rise and fall of civilizations and how epidemics have influenced human affairs and history.

Kenneth J. Ryan and C. George Ray

Laboratory Diagnosis of Infectious Diseases

9

diagnosis of microbial infections

The diagnosis of a microbial infection begins with an assessment of clinical and epidemiologic features, leading to the formulation of a clinical hypothesis. Anatomic localization of the infection with the aid of physical and radiologic findings (for example, right lower lobe pneumonia, subphrenic abscess) is usually included. This clinical diagnosis suggests a number of possible etiologic agents based on knowledge of infectious syndromes and their courses (Chapters 53–66). The specific etiologic diagnosis is then established by the application of the methods described in this chapter. A combination of science and art on the part of both the clinician and the laboratory worker is required: The clinician must select the appropriate tests and specimens to be processed and, where appropriate, suggest the suspected etiologic agents to the laboratory. The laboratory worker must design a battery of methods that will demonstrate the probable agents and be prepared to explore other possibilities suggested by the clinical situation or the findings of the laboratory examinations. The best results are obtained when communication between the clinic and the laboratory is maximal.

The Specimen

General Considerations

critical nature of specimen

The prime interface between the clinic and the diagnostic laboratory is the specimen submitted for processing. If it is not appropriately chosen and/or collected, no degree of laboratory skill will rectify the error. Failure at the level of specimen collection is the most common reason for failure to establish an etiologic diagnosis, or worse, for suggesting a wrong diagnosis. The primary problem lies in distinguishing normal floral organisms and surface contaminants from those causing the infection. Specimens may be divided into three categories on the basis of probability of contamination with normal flora. Details for individual specimens are provided in Chapters 53–66.

Direct tissue or fluid samples. Direct specimens are collected from normally sterile tissues (lung, liver) and body fluids (cerebrospinal fluid, blood). The methods range from careful aspiration of a superficial pustule to surgical biopsy. In general, such collections require the direct involvement of a physician and may carry some risk for the patient. The results are always useful, because positive findings are diagnostic and negative findings exclude infection at the suspected site.

Indirect samples. Indirect samples are specimens of inflammatory exudates (expectorated sputum, voided urine) that have passed through sites known to be colonized with normal flora. The site of origin might be sterile in healthy persons; however, some assessment of the probability of contamination with normal flora is necessary before these specimens can be reliably interpreted. This assessment requires knowledge of the potential contaminating flora as well as the probable pathogens to be sought. Indirect samples are usually more convenient for both physician and patient, but carry a higher risk of misinterpretation.

importance of seeking specific pathogens in normal floral sites

Samples from sites with a normal flora. Frequently the primary site of infection is in an area known to be colonized with many organisms (pharynx, large and small intestine). In such instances, examinations are made only for organisms known to cause infection that are not normally found in the infected site. The laboratory workup is thus directed toward isolation and identification of a limited number of organisms. For example, *Salmonella, Shigella,* and *Campylobacter* may be sought in a stool specimen or group A β-hemolytic streptococci in a throat swab. It is neither practical nor relevant in these circumstances for the laboratory to describe the normal flora. Samples from sites with a normal flora are only useful for diagnosis or prediction of infections at remote sites when the organism sought is not encountered in health. For example, detection of *Streptococcus pneumoniae* in a throat swab is useless in the diagnosis of pneumonia, because the organism is often found in the throat in healthy persons. The specimen must have been taken from the lung to be useful. On the other hand, isolation of influenza virus from the throat is useful in the diagnosis of influenzal pneumonia, because the virus is not normally present in the respiratory tract.

Types of Specimens

limitation of swabs

best specimens from infected fluids or tissue

The sterile swab is the most convenient and most commonly used tool for specimen collection; however, it provides the poorest conditions for survival and can only collect a small volume. The worst possible specimen is a dried-out swab; the best involves collection, when possible, of 5–10 ml or more of the infected fluid or tissue, because infecting organisms present in small numbers may not be detected if too small a sample is taken. Furthermore, a sample of several milliliters will serve as its own transport medium. Swabs should be used only when fluid or tissue collection is not possible, and they should be processed quickly or placed in a suitable transport medium. In infections such as tuberculosis, in which the numbers of *Mycobacterium tuberculosis* are usually small, swabs are unacceptable for collecting specimens.

Specimen Transport

rapid loss of viability of some bacteria

problems of overgrowth by some species after specimen collection

Specimens should be transported to the laboratory as soon after collection as possible, because some microorganisms survive only briefly outside the body. For example, unless special transport media are used, isolation rates of the bacteria that cause whooping cough (*Bordetella pertussis*) and gonorrhea (*Neisseria gonorrhoeae*) are decreased when processing is delayed beyond a few minutes. Many respiratory viruses survive poorly outside the body. On the other hand, some bacteria survive well and may even multiply after the specimen is collected. The growth of enteric Gram-negative rods in specimens awaiting culture may in fact compromise specimen interpretation by altering the numbers and relative proportions of different organisms, and thus interfere with the isolation of more fastidious organisms. Significant changes are associated with delays of more than 3–4 hr.

transport media

Various transport media have been developed to minimize the effects of the delay between specimen collection and laboratory processing. In general, properly buffered fluid or semisolid media containing minimal potential nutrients will prevent drying, maintain a neutral pH, and minimize growth. Other features may be added to meet special requirements, such as an oxygen-free atmosphere for obligate anaerobes.

Diagnostic Methods

The general approaches to laboratory diagnosis vary with different microorganisms and infectious diseases. The types of methods, however, will usually be some combination of the following:

1. *Direct examination.* Of the infectious agents discussed in this book, only some of the parasites are large enough to be seen with the naked eye. Bacteria can be seen clearly with the light microscope when appropriate methods are used; individual viruses can be seen only with the electron microscope, although aggregates of viral particles in cells (viral inclusions) may be seen by light microscopy. Various stains are used to visualize and differentiate bacteria in smears and histologic sections. The sensitivity and specificity of microscopic examinations can be improved with the combined use of serologic reagents (specific antibodies), as in immunofluorescence.
2. *Culture.* Growth and identification of the infecting agent in vitro, usually the most sensitive and specific means of diagnosis, is thus the method most commonly used. Bacteria can be grown in a variety of artificial media, but human and animal viruses can be isolated only in cultures of living eukaryotic cells.
3. *Antibody detection (serologic diagnosis).* Detection and quantitation of specific antibodies formed by the host in response to an infection can provide evidence of present or previous infection with a particular infectious agent. Numerous methods are employed using antigens prepared from a wide range of infectious agents.
4. *Antigen detection.* Isolation and direct examination methods require living or morphologically intact organisms. In some cases, specific antigens of the infecting agent can be detected in the patient, particularly if they are released from the organism into body fluids or blood. Antigen detection procedures use antibodies of known specificity to test for the presence of suspected antigens, the reverse of serologic diagnosis.

In this chapter, we shall consider these principles in their application to the diagnosis of diseases caused by bacteria and viruses. Many of the methods to be described can also be applied, with certain variations, to the diagnosis of diseases caused by fungi, *Mycoplasma, Rickettsia, Chlamydia,* and parasites; however, because of the special features of each of these groups, the specific approaches to their isolation and identification will be discussed in subsequent chapters. As the serologic diagnosis of all infectious diseases utilizes common basic concepts, these concepts will be considered separately in the last section of this chapter.

Diagnosis of Bacterial Infections

Direct Examination

limits of resolution of microscope

Direct examination of stained or unstained preparations by light microscopy is particularly useful for detection of bacteria. Even the smallest bacteria (0.15 μm wide) can be visualized, although some require special lighting techniques. As the resolution limit of the light microscope is near 0.2 μm, the optics must be ideal if the organisms are to be seen clearly by direct transmission microscopy. These conditions may be achieved with a 100×

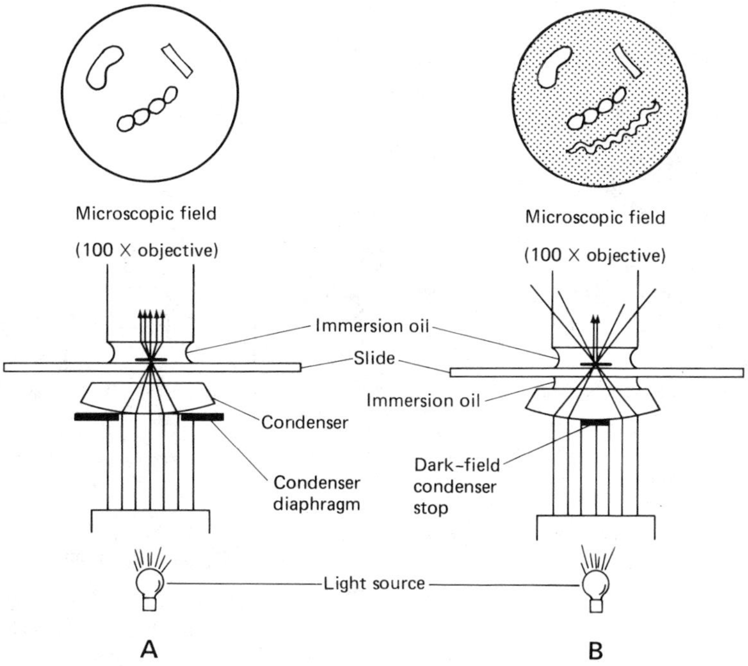

9.1 Bright- and dark-field illumination for light microscopy. (**A**) Bright-field illumination properly aligned. The purpose is to focus light directly on the preparation for optimal visualization against a bright background. (**B**) In dark-field illumination, a black background is created by blocking the central light. Peripheral light is focused so that it will be collected by the objective only when it is reflected from the surfaces of particles (for example, bacteria). The microscopic field shows bright halos around some bacteria and reveals a spirochete too thin to be seen with bright-field illumination.

oil immersion objective, a 5–10× eyepiece, and optimal lighting, as shown in Figure 9.1. Some bacteria, such as *Treponema pallidum,* the cause of syphilis, are too slim to be visualized with the usual bright-field illumination. They can be seen by use of the *dark-field* technique. With this method, a condenser that focuses only diagonal light on the specimen is used, and only light reflected from particulate matter such as bacteria reaches the eyepiece (Figure 9.1). The angles of incident and reflected light are such that the organisms are surrounded by a bright halo against a black background. This type of illumination is also used in other microscopic techniques, in which a high light contrast is desired, and for observation of fluorescence. Fluorescent compounds, when excited by light of one wavelength, emit light of a longer wavelength and thus a different color. Fluorescence microscopy involves the use of illumination sources that produce light in or near the ultraviolet range, combined with dark-field illumination. Barrier filters permit visualization of emitted light, but protect the observer from ultraviolet light. When the fluorescent compound is conjugated with an antibody as a probe for detection of specific antigen, the technique is called *immunofluorescence*, or fluorescent antibody microscopy(Plate E).

dark-field microscopy

fluorescence microscopy

Stains

Gram and acid-fast techniques assist bacterial classification

Bacteria may be stained by a wide variety of dyes, including methylene blue, crystal violet, carbol–fuchsin (red), and safranin (red). The two most important methods, the *Gram* and *acid-fast* techniques, employ staining, decolorization, and counterstaining in a manner that helps to classify as well as stain the organism.

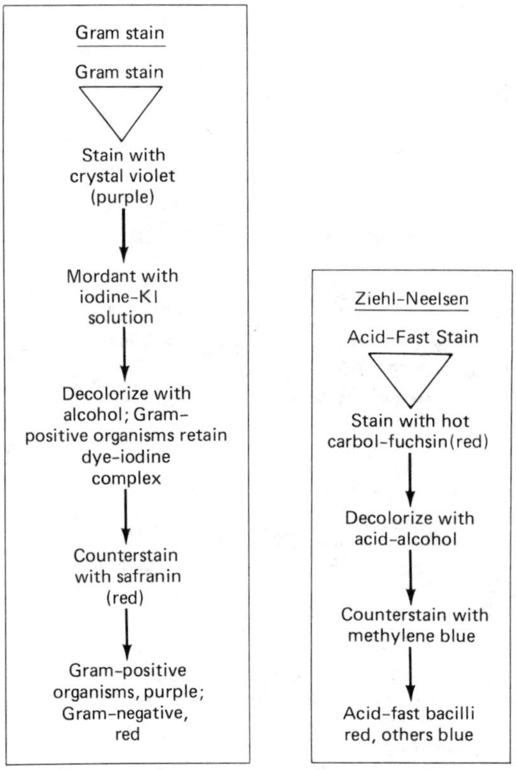

9.2 Gram stain and acid-fast stain for bacteria.

Gram stain. The differential staining procedure described in 1884 by the Danish physician Hans Christian Gram has proved one of the most useful in microbiology and medicine. The procedure (Figure 9.2) involves the addition of a solution of iodine in potassium iodide to cells previously stained with certain acridine dyes, such as crystal violet. This treatment produces a mordanting action in which purple insoluble complexes are formed with the cell's ribonucleic acid. The difference between Gram-positive and Gram-negative bacteria is in the permeability of the cell wall to these complexes upon treatment with alcohol or mixtures of acetone and alcohol. Gram-negative bacteria lose the purple iodine–dye complexes, whereas Gram-positive bacteria retain them. An intact cell wall is necessary for a positive reaction; Gram-positive bacteria may fail to retain the stain if the organisms are old, dead, or damaged by antimicrobial agents. No similar conditions cause a Gram-negative organism to appear Gram positive. The stain is completed by the addition of safranin, a red counterstain taken up by bacteria that have been decolorized. Thus, cells stained purple are Gram positive, and those stained red are Gram negative (Plates A and P). As indicated in Chapter 2, Gram positivity and negativity correspond to major structural differences in the cell wall.

When the Gram stain is applied to clinical specimens, the purple or red bacteria are seen against a Gram-negative (red) background of leukocytes, fluid, and debris. Retention of the purple dye in tissue or fluid elements, such as the nuclei of polymorphonuclear leukocytes, is an indication that the smear has been inadequately decolorized. In smears of uneven thickness, judgments on the Gram reaction can be made only in well-decolorized areas.

etiologic bacteria often seen in direct Gram smears of specimens

In many bacterial infections, the etiologic bacteria are readily seen on stained Gram smears of pus or fluids. This information, combined with the clinical findings, may guide the management of infection before culture results are available. Interpretation requires knowledge of the probable etiologic agents for the clinical syndrome, of their morphology and Gram reaction, and of any organisms normally present in health at the infected site. An accurate reading of the Gram smear requires considerable experience.

stain with difficulty, but resist decolorization once stained

Acid-fast stain. Acid fastness is a property of the mycobacteria (for example, the tubercle bacillus) and related organisms (for example, some species of *Nocardia*). Acid-fast organisms generally stain very poorly with dyes, including those used in the Gram stain. They can, however, be stained with prolonged application, more concentrated dyes, and heat treatment. Their unique feature is that once stained, acid-fast bacteria resist decolorization by concentrations of mineral acids and ethanol that remove dyes from other bacteria. This combination of weak initial staining and strong retention once stained is probably related to the high lipid content of the mycobacterial cell wall. Acid-fast stains are completed with a counterstain to provide a contrasting background for viewing the stained bacteria (Figure 9.2).

acid-fastness related to cell wall lipid content

Ziehl–Neelsen technique

The standard acid-fast procedure is the Ziehl–Neelsen stain in which the slide is flooded with carbol–fuchsin (red), heated, and then decolorized with a 3% solution of hydrochloric acid in alcohol. When counterstained with methylene blue, acid-fast organisms appear red against a blue background (Plate T). A variant of this method is the Ponder–Kinyoun (cold) acid-fast stain, in which a more concentrated fuchsin is used and heating is omitted. Another variant is the fluorochrome stain, which uses a fluorescent dye, auramine, or an auramine–rhodamine mixture followed by decolorization with acid–alcohol. Acid-fast organisms retain the fluorescent stain, which allows their visualization with fluorescence microscopy. Fluorescing organisms can be detected at lower magnification (×250), which increases the speed with which smears may be read. A comparison of the procedures used for Gram staining and for acid-fast staining by the Ziehl–Neelsen technique are shown in Figure 9.2.

fluorescent method

Culture

Almost all medically important bacteria can be cultivated outside the host in artificial culture media. Usually, a single bacterium placed in the proper culture medium and environment will multiply to numbers sufficient to cause macroscopic changes or be detectable by other means, such as microscopic examination. Beginning with those of Louis Pasteur and Robert Koch, growth medium formulations of increasing sophistication have been developed to match the growth requirements of pathogenic bacteria.

defined and undefined media

Media are of two basic types, defined and undefined. Defined media are prepared from chemically known ingredients. Undefined media are essentially recipes prepared from partial digests of animal or vegetable protein, often supplemented with substances such as yeast extract, serum, blood, or glucose, to meet the metabolic requirements of the organism. Their chemical composition is therefore complex, and their success depends on the similar nutritional requirements of most heterotrophic living things. Most diagnostic bacteriology utilizes undefined media because of their lower cost and ability to support growth of a broad range of pathogenic organisms. Defined media are useful for characterization of the biochemical activities of organisms and in research requiring tight control of all variables.

most diagnostic media are undefined

growth in broth medium

Growth media are initially prepared in the fluid state as broths to which bacteria or clinical specimens may be added directly. The presence of bacteria in broth medium will not be grossly apparent until they attain numbers sufficient to produce turbidity or macroscopic clumps. Turbidity results from reflection of transmitted light by the bacteria; depending on the size of the organism, a minimum of 10^7–10^8 bacteria per milliliter of broth is usually required. Some strictly aerobic bacteria may grow as a film on the surface; other bacteria grow as a sediment.

agar media

special properties of agar

The addition of a gelling agent to a broth medium allows its preparation in solid form: as plates when poured into petri dishes and as slants in tubes. The universal gelling agent for diagnostic bacteriology is *agar*, a polysaccharide extracted from certain types of seaweed. Agar has the convenient property of becoming liquid when boiled but not returning to the solid state as a gel until cooled to less than 50°C. At the temperatures used in the diagnostic laboratory (37°C or lower), agar–broth mixtures produce a smooth, solid, nutrient gel; its firmness depends on the agar concentration. This medium, usually termed "agar," may be qualified with a description of any supplement (for example, blood agar).

plate streaking for isolation

bacterial colonies

Separation of bacteria may be accomplished by spreading a small sample over the surface of an agar plate in a structured form with a sterile wire loop. This procedure is termed *plate streaking*. Bacteria well separated from others grow as isolated colonies. The time of appearance of macroscopic colonies, which contain billions of organisms, depends on the generation time of the organism. Well-streaked plates will yield isolated colonies regardless of the numbers in the specimen (Figure 9.3 and Plates F and Q).

use of plates in isolating pure cultures

differences in colonial morphology

Growth of bacteria on solid media has advantages over the use of broth cultures for diagnostic work. It allows isolation of bacteria in pure culture, because a colony well separated from others can be assumed to arise from a single organism or an organism cluster (colony-forming unit). Colonies from different species or genera vary greatly in size, shape, texture, color, and other features, but are consistent when developed from the same strain. Differences in colonial morphology are very useful for separating bacteria in mixtures and as clues to their identity. Experienced bacteriologists learn to recognize subtle differences in colonial morphology, including those seen with growth on different bacteriologic media.

other methods of detecting bacterial growth or growth products

New methods that do not depend on visual changes in the growth medium or colony formation may also be used to detect bacterial growth in culture. These techniques include release of radiolabeled products of bacterial metabolism, changes in the electric impedance of the medium, bioluminescence, and chromatographic detection of bacterial metabolic products in the medium. The extraordinary sensitivity of the latter method has also permitted detection of metabolic products in clinical specimens. The only one of these methods currently used in a significant number of clinical laboratories is a radioisotopic method that measures ^{14}C-labeled carbon dioxide released from labeled substrates in nutrient broth. This approach, which has been automated, can detect bacterial growth before the development of turbidity or colony formation. Once detected, bacteria are strained, subcultured, and identified in the usual way.

Bacteriologic Media

Over the past 100 years, countless media have been developed by bacteriologists to aid in the isolation and identification of medically important bacteria. Only a few have found their way into routine use in clinical laboratories. These media may be classified as nutrient, selective, or indicator.

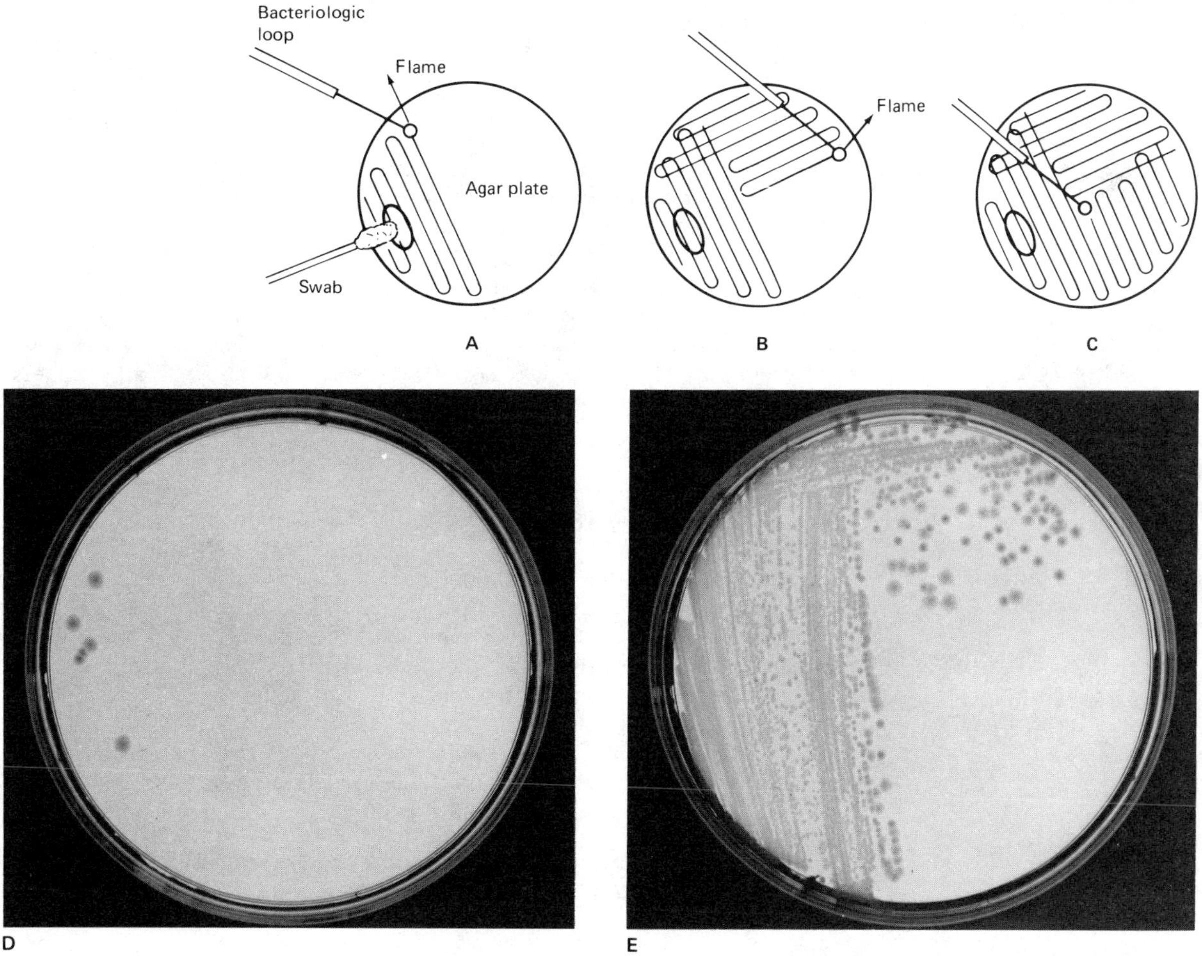

9.3 Bacteriologic plate streaking. Plate streaking is essentially a dilution procedure. The specimen is placed on the plate with a swab, loop, or pipette, and evenly spread over approximately one-fourth of the plate surface with a sterilized bacteriologic loop. (**A**) The loop is flamed to remove residual bacteria. (**B**) A secondary streak is made, overlapping the primary streak initially but finishing independently. (**C**) The process is repeated in a tertiary streak. (**D**) and (**E**) Two plates streaked in a similar manner. (**D**) Only a few bacteria grew. (**E**) A large number of bacteria grew. In each case, however, isolated colonies were produced for further study.

Most media now used in clinical laboratories are purchased commercially in dehydrated form.

Nutrient media. The nutrient component of a medium is designed to satisfy the growth requirements of the bacteria to permit growth and isolation. For medical purposes, the ideal isolation medium would allow rapid growth of all bacteria. No such medium has been and probably cannot be developed; however, several undefined media suffice for good growth of medically important bacteria. These media are prepared with enzymatic or acid digests of animal or plant products such as muscle, milk, or beans. The digest reduces the native protein to a mixture of polypeptides and amino acids termed *peptone*, which also includes trace metals, coenzymes, and various undefined growth factors. For example, tryptic or trypticase soy broth contains a pan-

bacteriologic peptones are enzymatic digests of protein

creatic digest of casein (milk curd) and a papaic digest of soybean meal. To this nutrient base, salts, vitamins, or body fluids such as serum may be added to provide obligate or opportunistic pathogens with the conditions needed for optimum growth.

used when specific pathogens are sought among normal flora

Selective media. Selective media are used when specific pathogenic organisms are sought in sites with an extensive normal flora (for example, *N. gonorrhoeae* in specimens from the uterine cervix or rectum). In these cases, other bacteria may overgrow the suspected species in simple nutrient media, either because the pathogen grows more slowly or because it is present in much smaller numbers. Selective media usually contain chemicals, dyes, or antibiotics inhibitory to contaminating flora, but not the suspected pathogen. Selective fluid media are called *enrichment broths* because they allow small numbers of pathogens to outgrow inhibited organisms before subculture on plates.

enrichment broths

detection of pH changes, hemolysis, etc.

Indicator media. Indicator media contain indicator systems designed to demonstrate features characteristic of specific pathogens or to separate the possible identities of the isolate into groups. The addition of one or more carbohydrates and a pH indicator is most common. Fermentation of the carbohydrates, which results in a color change in the colony, indicates the presence of acid products (Plate Q). Other indicator media may enhance the production of a pigment or stimulate other changes useful for early recognition of certain bacteria. The addition of red blood cells to plates allows the hemolysis produced by some organisms to be used as a differential feature (Plates F and G).

In practice, nutrient, selective, and indicator properties are often combined to various degrees in the same medium. It is possible to include an indicator system in a highly nutrient medium and also make it selective by adding appropriate antibiotics. Culture media commonly used are listed in Table 9.1, and more details of their constitution and use are provided in Appendix 9.1.

Cultural Conditions

incubation usually at 35–37°C

Once inoculated, cultures are placed in an incubator with temperature maintained at 35–37°C. Slightly higher or lower temperatures are used occasionally to selectively favor a certain organism or organism group. For example, *Yersinia enterocolitica* (Chapter 20) at 4°C and *Campylobacter fetus*, subspecies *jejuni* (Chapter 21), at 42°C will outgrow most competitors.

CO_2 required by some species, enhances growth of others

Most bacteria that are not obligate anaerobes will grow in air; however, CO_2 is required by some and enhances the growth of others. Incubators that maintain a concentration of CO_2 in the atmosphere of 2–5% are frequently used for primary isolation, because this level is not harmful to any bacteria and improves isolation of some. A less expensive method is the *candle jar*, in which a lighted candle is allowed to burn to extinction in a sealed jar containing plates. This method adds 1–2% CO_2 to the atmosphere.

candle jar for CO_2 production

growth of anaerobes in presence of reducing agents

Anaerobic incubation is a special case: strictly anaerobic bacteria will not grow under the conditions described previously, and many will die if exposed to atmospheric oxygen or high oxidation–reduction potentials. Most medically important anaerobes will grow in the depths of liquid or semisolid media containing any of a variety of reducing agents, such as cysteine, thioglycolate, ascorbic acid, or even iron filings. Growth is facilitated by boiling to remove dissolved oxygen. Plates of solid medium are incubated in anaerobic jars or large chambers from which all oxygen is removed or excluded. The latter can be achieved by replacing air with a gas mixture

anaerobic jars and chambers for plated media

Table 9.1 Media Used for Isolation of Bacterial Pathogens

Medium	Growth Characteristics
General purpose media	
Trypticase soy broth Brain–heart infusion broth Columbia broth	Most bacteria, particularly when used for blood culture
Thioglycolate broth	Anaerobes, facultative bacteria
Blood agar	Most bacteria (demonstrates hemolysis)
Chocolate agar	Most bacteria, including fastidious species (e.g., *Haemophilus*)
Selective media	
MacConkey agar Eosin–methylene blue agar	Gram-negative rods (nonfastidious)
Phenylethyl alcohol agar	Gram-positive bacteria only
Hektoen agar Xylose–lysine–deoxycholate agar *Salmonella–Shigella* agar	*Salmonella* and *Shigella*
Selenite F broth	*Salmonella* enrichment (less effective for *Shigella*)
Special purpose media	
Löwenstein–Jensen medium Middlebrook agar	*Mycobacterium tuberculosis* and other mycobacteria (selective)
Thayer–Martin medium	*Neisseria gonorrhoeae* and *Neisseria meningitidis* (selective)
Fletcher medium (semisolid)	*Leptospira* (nonselective)
Tinsdale agar	*Corynebacterium diphtheriae* (selective)
Charcoal agar Bordet–Gengou agar	*Bordetella pertussis* (selective)
Charcoal–yeast extract agar	*Legionella* species (nonselective)
Campylobacter (Skirrow) blood agar	*Campylobacter fetus* (selective)
Cysteine–glucose blood agar	*Francisella tularensis* (nonselective)
Cycloserine–cefoxitin–fructose agar	*Clostridium difficile* (selective)
Thiosulfate–citrate–bile–sucrose agar	*Vibrio cholerae* and *Vibrio parahemolyticus* (selective)

containing 10% hydrogen and 5% CO_2 in 85% nitrogen and allowing the hydrogen to react with residual oxygen on a palladium catalyst to form water. A convenient commercial system generates hydrogen and CO_2 from a packet to which water is added before the jar is sealed. Anaerobiosis takes longer to develop, but the system is adequate for medically important anaerobes, which are rarely exquisitely oxygen sensitive. Specimens suspected to contain significant anaerobes are transmitted to the laboratory and processed under conditions designed to minimize exposure to atmospheric oxygen at all stages.

need to maintain continuous anaerobiosis

Routine laboratory systems for processing specimens differ because no single medium or atmosphere is ideal for all bacteria, and selection of combinations depends on the nature of the specimens and the organisms sought. Routines for different types of specimens are organized as shown

supplements to routines

Table 9.2 Routine Use of Gram Smear and Isolation Systems for Selected Clinical Specimens[a]

Medium (Incubation)	Specimen							
	Blood	Cerebrospinal Fluid	Wound, Pus	Genital, Cervix	Throat	Sputum	Urine	Stool
Gram smear		X	X	X		X	X	
Trypticase soy broth (CO_2)	X	X	X					
Selenite F broth (air)								X
Blood agar (CO_2)		X	X	X		X	X	
Blood agar (anaerobic)			X		X[b]			
MacConkey agar (air)			X	X		X	X	X
Chocolate agar (CO_2)		X	X	X		X		
Thayer–Martin agar (CO_2)				X				
Hektoen agar (air)								X
Campylobacter agar (CO_2, 42°C)[c]								X

[a] The added sensitivity of a nutrient broth is used only when contamination by normal flora is unlikely. Exact media and isolation systems may vary between laboratories.
[b] Anaerobic incubation used to enhance hemolysis by β-hemolytic streptococci.
[c] Incubation in a reduced oxygen atmosphere.

responsibility of clinician

in Table 9.2. They include combinations of broth and solid plated media and aerobic, CO_2, and anaerobic incubation. Broths are most sensitive for detecting scanty numbers of bacteria because a larger volume of specimen can be added; plates, however, facilitate rapid isolation of pure cultures and early indications of identity. Established routines may vary between laboratories and, for practical reasons, specialized media for rare organisms are seldom included (for example, those for *Leptospira* or *Corynebacterium diphtheriae*). For detection of these organisms, the laboratory must be informed of the clinical possibility of their presence. To ascertain that appropriate media and procedures are employed, the physician should always indicate any suspicion of less common organisms in the request.

Bacterial Identification

need for a pure culture

Once growth is detected in any medium, the process of identification begins. Identification involves the use of methods to obtain pure cultures from single colonies, followed by tests designed to characterize and identify the isolate.

classes of identification tests

levels of identification in clinical practice

Positive broth cultures are Gram stained and subcultured to plated media. Representative colonies on these or on primarily seeded solid media are stained and subcultured for any additional cultural, biochemical, or serologic characterization that may be needed. The exact tests and their sequences vary with different groups of organisms, and the level of identification to be achieved varies according to the clinical usefulness of the information. Identification of genus, species, or occasionally subspecies or serotype level may be required. In other cases, only a general description or the exclusion of particular organisms is important in the management of a patient. For example, the report of "mixed oral flora" in a sputum specimen or "no *N. gonorrhoeae*" in a cervical specimen provides all of the information needed.

Cultural characteristics, an extension of basic observations of bacterial nature and pattern of growth in various types of culture media, can have nutritional requirements, growth characteristics, and sensitivity to inhibitors

great taxonomic significance. They include the demonstration of properties such as unique nutritional requirements, pigment production, and the ability to grow in the presence of certain potentially inhibitory substances (sodium chloride, bile) or on different media (MacConkey, nutrient agar). Demonstration of the ability to grow at a particular temperature or to affect certain natural substances such as milk, egg yolk, or meat is also useful. The nature and pattern of hemolysis can also be considered a cultural characteristic.

Biochemical characteristics, which include the ability to attack various substrates or to produce particular metabolic products, have the broadest application to the identification of bacteria. Most of these tests are carried out in a simple peptone-based medium, unless this substrate will not support growth of the organism. The most common properties examined are the following:

1. *Carbohydrate breakdown.* The ability to produce acidic metabolic products, fermentatively or oxidatively, from a range of carbohydrates (for example, glucose, sucrose, lactose) has been applied to the identification of most groups of bacteria. Such tests are crude and imperfect in defining mechanisms, but have proved useful for taxonomic purposes. More recently, gas chromatographic identification of specific short-chain fatty acids produced by fermentation of glucose has proved useful in classifying many anaerobic bacteria.
2. *Catalase production.* The enzyme catalase catalyzes the conversion of hydrogen peroxide to water and oxygen. When a colony is placed in hydrogen peroxide, liberation of oxygen as gas bubbles can be seen. The test is particularly useful in differentiation of staphylococci (positive) from streptococci (negative), but also has taxonomic application to Gram-negative bacteria.
3. *Citrate.* An agar medium that contains sodium citrate as the sole carbon source may be used to determine ability to utilize citrate. Bacteria that grow on this medium are termed *citrate positive.*
4. *Coagulase.* The enzyme coagulase acts with a plasma factor to convert fibrinogen to a fibrin clot. It is used to differentiate *Staphylococcus aureus* from other, less pathogenic staphylococci (Chapter 11).
5. *Decarboxylases and deaminases.* The decarboxylation or deamination of the amino acids lysine, ornithine, and arginine is detected by the effect of the amino products on the pH of the reaction mixture or by the formation of colored products. These tests are used primarily with Gram-negative rods.
6. *Hydrogen sulfide.* The ability of some bacteria to produce H_2S from amino acids or other sulfur-containing compounds is helpful in taxonomic classification. The black color of the sulfide salts formed with heavy metals such as iron is the usual means of detection.
7. *Indole.* The indole reaction tests the ability of the organism to produce indole, a benzopyrrole, from tryptophan. Indole is detected by the formation of a red dye after addition of a benzaldehyde reagent. A spot test can be done in seconds using isolated colonies.
8. *Nitrate reduction.* Bacteria may reduce nitrates by several mechanisms. This ability is demonstrated by detection of the nitrites and/or nitrogen gas formed in the process.
9. *O-Nitrophenyl-β-D-galactoside (ONPG) breakdown.* The ONPG test is related to lactose fermentation. Organisms that possess the β-galactoside necessary for lactose fermentation but lack a permease necessary for lactose to enter the cell are ONPG positive and lactose negative.

10. *Oxidase production.* The oxidase tests detect the *c* component of the cytochrome–oxidase complex. The reagents used change from clear to colored when converted from the reduced to the oxidized state. The oxidase reaction is commonly demonstrated in a spot test, which can be done quickly from isolated colonies.
11. *Proteinase production.* Proteolytic activity is detected by growing the organism in the presence of substrates such as gelatin or coagulated egg.
12. *Urease production.* Urease hydrolyzes urea to yield two molecules of ammonia and one of CO_2. This reaction can be detected by the increase in medium pH caused by ammonia production. Urease-positive species vary in the amount of enzyme produced; bacteria can thus be designated as positive, weakly positive, or negative.
13. *Voges–Proskauer test.* The Voges–Proskauer test detects acetylmethylcarbinol (acetoin), an intermediate product in the butene glycol pathway of glucose fermentation.

Biochemical and cultural tests for bacterial identification are analyzed with reference to tables that show the reaction patterns characteristic for individual species (Table 9.3). Such tables, which represent the sum of testing with many strains of each species, are published in books, pamphlets, and scientific papers and by institutions such as the Centers for Disease Control in Atlanta. As methods for performing many tests differ, it is important for laboratories to use procedures identical to those on which the table is based. Shortened versions are often used in routine practice. Given the phenotypic variation possible with bacterial species, the results with an unknown isolate may not match those in the table precisely; a final decision may therefore require further testing.

In recent years, instrumentation, automation, and computer analysis have been applied to speciation and identification of bacterial families such as the

Table 9.3 Biochemical Reactions for Differentiation of *Salmonella* Species

Test	*Salmonella* Species Reaction		
	S. choleraesuis	*S. typhi*	*S. enteritidis*
Indole	—	—	—
Citrate	(+)	—	+
Urease	—	—	—
Lysine decarboxylase	+	+	+
Ornithine decarboxylase	+	—	+
Fermentation			
Glucose	+	+	+
Gas from glucose	+	—	+
Lactose	—	—	—
Dulcitol	v	— or (+)	+
Inositol	—	—	v
Trehalose	—	+	+
Arabinose	—	—	+
Rhamnose	+	—	+
Hydrogen sulfide	v	+	+

Data published by the Centers for Disease Control, Atlanta, Georgia.
Abbreviations: — = less than 10% of strains positive; (+) = delayed reaction, requiring 3 or more days; + = more than 90% of strains positive; v = variable, 10–90% of strains positive.

automation and computer analysis in bacterial identification

Enterobacteriaceae, which show a great diversity of biochemical activity. These systems employ the same biochemical principles but use miniaturized reaction cuvettes, automatic readers, and a computerized data base to determine the most probable identification for the observed test pattern. Identification and taxonomic classifications from a range of phenotypic characteristics are satisfactory procedures, but increased use of more direct analyses of the bacterial genome can be expected in the future.

Demonstration of toxin production and pathogenicity is sometimes needed to confirm a clinical diagnosis. In laboratory animals, a localized or lethal infection with a characteristic pattern of lesions may develop after inoculation with some species. The organisms should be demonstrated in the lesions to confirm the diagnosis. In diseases caused by production of a specific bacterial toxin, the toxin may be detected in vivo in experimental animals or in vitro through cell cultures or immunologic methods. In either case, neutralization of the toxic effect with specific antitoxin should be demonstrated to confirm its nature.

Susceptibility or resistance to antimicrobics or chemical substances is sometimes helpful in the identification of bacteria, but involves properties that may be variable. Such tests are usually considered presumptive or ancillary to methods that determine the final identification.

Serologic identification. As discussed in Chapter 2, bacteria possess many structures that may be antigenic, such as capsular polysaccharides, flagellar proteins, and several cell wall components. Serology involves the demonstration of specific antigen–antibody interactions in vitro and, in bacterial identification, uses antibodies of known specificity to detect antigens present on whole bacteria or free in bacterial extracts (soluble antigens). Several methods are used for demonstrating antigen–antibody reactions.

optimum antigen–antibody ratios needed for precipitate formation

Precipitin tests. When soluble antigen and antibody combine in the proper proportions, a visible precipitate is formed (Figure 9.4A). Optimum antigen–antibody ratios are produced by allowing one (or both) to diffuse slowly into the other. This test may be done in capillary tubes, where the antigen and antibody solutions are placed in direct contact, or with immunodiffusion procedures, where they diffuse through agar. In capillary tubes the precipitate is formed at or near the interface. In immunodiffusion, one or more precipitin lines are formed between the antigen and antibody wells; the number of lines depends on the number of different antigen–antibody reactions occurring. Counterimmunoelectrophoresis (CIE) is immunodiffusion carried out in an electrophoretic field. The pH and other conditions are adjusted so that the negatively charged antigen migrates to the anode while the less charged antibody is swept toward the cathode with the flow of buffer ions. The net effect is that antigen and antibody are rapidly brought together in the space between the wells to form a precipitin line. Both the speed and the sensitivity of immunodiffusion are improved by CIE.

agglutination involves particulate antigens

bacterial agglutination, hemagglutination, and latex agglutination

Agglutination. The amount of antigen and antibody necessary to produce visible reaction can be reduced if either is on the surface of a relatively large particle. This condition, which may occur with whole bacterial cells, can be produced by coating soluble antigens or antibody onto the surface of red blood cells or microscopic latex particles (Figure 9.4B). The relative proportions of antigen and antibody thus become less critical, and antigen–antibody reactions are easily detectable by clumping when immune serum and particulate antigen are mixed in test tubes or on a slide. When bacteria

A

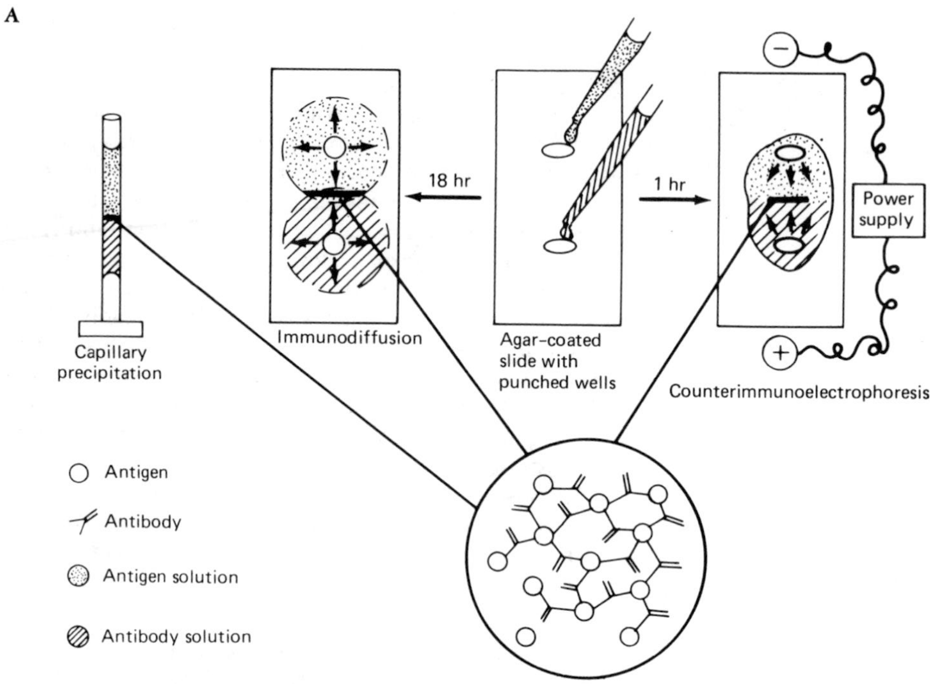

9.4 Precipitin formation and agglutination. (**A**) Three methods are shown for demonstrating antigen–antibody interaction with formation of a precipitate. In the capillary tube procedure, the antigen and antibody solutions are layered on each other. As they diffuse at the interface, an antigen–antibody complex is formed. In both immunodiffusion and counterimmunoelectrophoresis, the test is begun by adding the antigen and the antibody to separate wells cut in an agar gel; the precipitate forms as a line(s) where the antigen and antibody meet. In immunodiffusion, both antigen and antibody diffuse radially, with overlap between the wells; in counterimmunoelectrophoresis, the electrophoretic field concentrates both in the same area. The precipitate, composed of a lattice of antigen and antibody, is the same regardless of the method used. (**B**) Agglutination requires a particulate antigen small enough to produce smooth turbidity, but large enough to show visible aggregates when linked by specific antibody. The antigen may be 1) on the surface of the organism itself (simple agglutination); 2) coated on the surface of the red blood cell or latex particle (hemagglutination or latex agglutination); or 3) coagglutination, which is more complex, as the antibody is bound by its Fc receptor end to the protein A on the surface of a dead *Staphyloccus aureus.* Visible agglutination is produced when these particles combine with a soluble antigen or another particulate antigen as shown.

S. aureus as passive antibody carrier in coagglutination

serve as the antigen, the process is termed *bacterial agglutination.* When red cells or latex particles serve as antigen or antibody carriers, the test is termed *passive hemagglutination* or *latex agglutination.* A variant of this procedure, *coagglutination,* utilizes the unique ability of protein A on the surface of *S. aureus* to bind the Fc fragment of immunoglobulin G(IgG), leaving the Fab portions free to react with homologous antigen. Thus, *S. aureus* cells can become a diagnostic reagent when antibody with specificity to any of a variety of antigens is attached to their surface protein.

immunofluorescence procedures

RIA and ELISA procedures

Labeling methods. Detection of antigen–antibody interactions may be enhanced by attaching a label to one (usually the antibody) or both, then measuring the label after removal of unbound reagents. The most common method of this type in diagnostic microbiology is *immunofluorescence,* in which the antibody is labeled with a fluorescent dye, usually fluorescein isothiocyanate, that can then be detected by fluorescence microscopy. Fluorescence localizes the position of the antibody and thus of the antigen to which it is

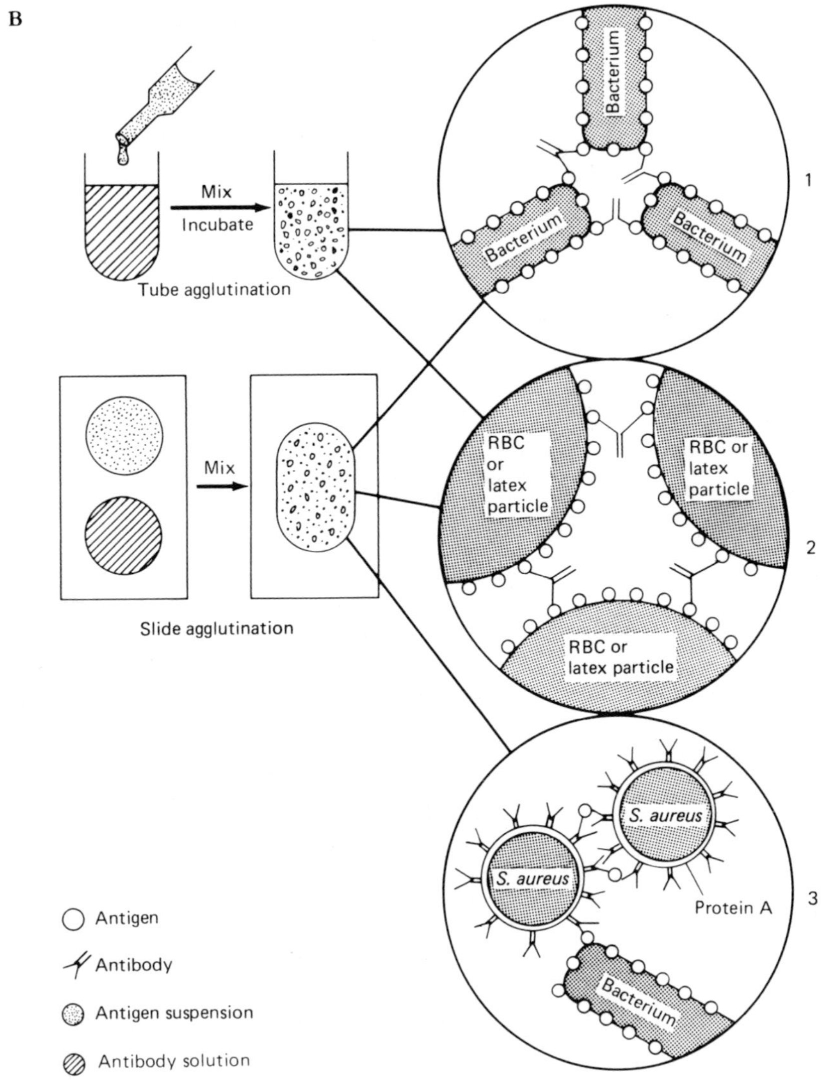

bound. Two newer methods, radioimmunoassay (RIA) and enzyme-linked immunosorbent assay (ELISA), are now being used increasingly. The principles of these techniques are described and illustrated later in the sections on serologic detection of viruses, although they are equally applicable to other microorganisms.

antigenic analysis

The application of these techniques to the development of systems for serologic identification of microorganisms is a complex process. It begins with selection of strains to be differentiated. Whole inactivated cells or antigens prepared from them by physical, chemical, or enzymatic treatment are injected repeatedly into animals (usually rabbits) to produce high antibody titers. After several weeks the animals are bled, the blood is allowed to clot, and the serum is separated. These immune sera (antisera) are cross-tested against homologous and heterologous strains using one of the antigen–antibody tests discussed previously, and the pattern of reactions is analyzed to determine the relatedness of the strains. An example of this process, taken from Dr. Rebecca Lancefield's work with streptococci, is shown in Table

immunization of laboratory animals and cross-testing with homologous and heterologous strains

Table 9.4 Lancefield Serologic Classification of β-Hemolytic Streptococci

Organism			Precipitin Formation when Reacted with Rabbit Antiserum Prepared with Extract of Strain:						Serologic Group Assignment
Strain	Source	Disease	C203	K96	K107	K126	K155	C6	
C203	Human	Scarlet fever	+	+	—	—	—	—	A
K96	Human	Pneumonia	+	+	—	—	—	—	A
K107	Cow	Mastitis	—	—	+	+	—	—	B
K126	Cow	None	—	—	+	+	—	—	B
K155	Horse	Pleuropneumonia	—	—	—	—	+	—	C
C6	Cheese	None	—	—	—	—	—	+	D

Data from one of Dr. Lancefield's studies (*J. Exp. Med.* 57:571–595, 1933) are presented as an example of the development of a serologic system. Note that extract from each strain produces a precipitin reaction with rabbit antiserum prepared with extract from the same strain, indicating that the product is antigenic. The two human strains (C203, K96), which react with each other but not with the nonhuman isolates, were assigned to group A. Strains K107 and K126, which also react with each other but not with the other strains, were assigned to group B. Strains K155 and C6 are serologically unique and were assigned the new groups C and D. New isolates may be classified in one of the existing groups or assigned a new one, depending on their reaction with known antisera. Continued application of these methods to streptococci has led to the recognition of groups A through T.

9.4. This method allowed recognition of many distinct Lancefield groups of streptococci of greatly differing significance in human and animal disease.

adsorption techniques for removing cross-reacting antibody

The development of serologic classification schemes to detect specific antigens is often greatly complicated by the presence of some common and cross-reacting antigens in related organisms. If the specific antigens cannot by purified for immunization of the experimental animal, the mixture must be used. The antisera that develop thus contain both specific and cross-reacting antibodies. The latter must be removed by adding the heterologous organism to the antiserum, allowing the cross-reacting antibody to adsorb to its surface, and removing both organism and unwanted antibody by centrifugation. The process is repeated until only the strain-specific antibody is left in the serum.

complexity of some serologic classifications

Serologic classifications become enormously complex when multiple antigens are present in species with numerous distinct but overlapping serotypes, such as *Salmonella enteritidis* (Chapter 20). Classification schemes of this complexity have been developed through the dedicated work of a few individual microbiologists, and thus their availability is uneven among the different bacterial groups.

In most cases, serotyping serves to subclassify organisms below the genus level. With some genera and species, the serologic detection of antigens allows fundamental taxonomic differentiation, as with the β-hemolytic streptococci (Chapter 12), or provides the most rapid means of diagnosis, as with *Legionella* (Chapter 19). With others, it is of primary value for epidemiologic and research purposes.

Other methods. Many other methods have demonstrated potential for use in the identification of bacteria and other microorganisms. They include determination of the chemical composition of cell components (capsule, cell wall, cell membranes), determination of nucleic acid:base ratios, and identification of DNA sequences by DNA homology techniques (Chapter 2). These methods are now being applied to the taxonomic study of many bacterial groups, but have not yet been adapted for use in clinical laboratories.

DNA base ratios and homology tests

Antigen detection. Theoretically, any of the methods described for detecting antigen–antibody interactions could be applied directly to clinical specimens to detect free antigen, thus offering the possibility of bypassing direct eximportance of free specific antigen

amination, culture, and biochemical identification tests to achieve a diagnosis. Success with this approach requires a highly specific antibody, a sensitive detection method, and the presence of the homologous antigen in an accessible body fluid. The latter is an important limitation, because not all organisms are known to release free antigen in the course of infection. Furthermore, the antigen should not cross-react serologically with antigens from other possible infecting organisms. At present, diagnosis by antigen detection is limited to bacteria with polysaccharide capsules, such as *Haemophilus influenzae,* and certain viruses and fungi. The techniques of CIE, latex agglutination, coagglutination, RIA, and ELISA can detect free antigen in serum, urine, cerebrospinal fluid, and joint fluid. As live bacteria are not required for antigen detection, these tests are useful when the causative organism has been eliminated by antimicrobial therapy. Antigen detection procedures have the advantage of speed: they can yield results within an hour or two, sometimes within a few minutes. They are less sensitive than cultures that can detect a single bacterium, however, and are thus considered ancillary tests.

antigen detection techniques

Diagnosis of Viral Infections

Specimen Selection and Transport

The selection of specimens for viral diagnosis is based primarily on the clinical history to determine which etiologic agents should be considered. Some selected situations are illustrated in Table 9.5. For example, it can be seen that mumps and enteroviruses are among the more common viruses involved in acute infection of the central nervous system. Specimens that

Table 9.5 Some Appropriate Specimens for Viral Isolation[a]

	Specimen					
Agent	Throat	Stool	Cerebrospinal Fluid	Urine	Vesicle Fluid	Other
Meningitis and encephalitis						
Mumps	++++	—	++	+	—	—
Enteroviruses	+++	++++	++	—	—	—
Herpes simplex	±	—	±	—	+	++++ (brain biopsy)
Arboviruses[b]	—	—	+	—	—	++ (brain) + (blood)
Respiratory diseases						
Influenza and parainfluenza viruses	++++	—	—	—	—	
Adenoviruses	++++	++++	—	—	—	
Exanthems						
Measles	++++	—	—	+	—	
Rubella[b]	++++	—	—	+	—	
Varicella	—	—	—	—	++++	
Herpes simplex	++	—	—	—	++++	
Cytomegalovirus	++	—	—	++++	—	+ (leukocytes)

Abbreviations: — = no yield; ± to ++++ = relative yield (low to high).

[a] In general, it should be remembered that virus shedding often diminishes rapidly after onset of acute illness; it is therefore important to attempt specimen collection as early as possible.

[b] Because it is frequently very difficult to isolate these agents from the disease in question, it is emphasized that serologic tests are particularly important to ensure a diagnosis.

might be expected to yield these agents on culture would include throat, stool (for enteroviruses), and cerebrospinal fluid. On the other hand, the diagnosis of herpes simplex encephalitis may require brain biopsy, and the arbovirus-caused illnesses often require serologic study for confirmation. Specimens for culture should be processed and inoculated as soon after collection as possible, because many viruses in the extracellular habitat are labile on prolonged exposure to temperatures above 4°C or on freezing.

Viral Isolation Methods

There are several common methods of viral isolation, including inoculation of cell culture (most frequently used), of embryonated hen's eggs, and of experimental animals.

Cell cultures from a variety of sources are used, each of which can support the replication of some viruses but not others. The preparation of cell culture monolayers is illustrated in Figure 9.5. The cells are derived from a tissue source by outgrowth of cells from a tissue fragment (explant) or by dispersal with chemical agents such as trypsin. They are allowed to grow in the presence of nutrient media on a glass or plastic surface until a confluent layer one cell thick (monolayer) is achieved. In some circumstances, a tissue fragment with a specialized function (for example, fetal trachea with ciliated epithelial cells) is cultivated in vitro and used for viral detection. This procedure is known as *organ culture.*

cell monolayers

organ culture

Three basic types of cell culture monolayers are used in diagnostic virology. The primary cell culture, in which all cells have a normal chro-

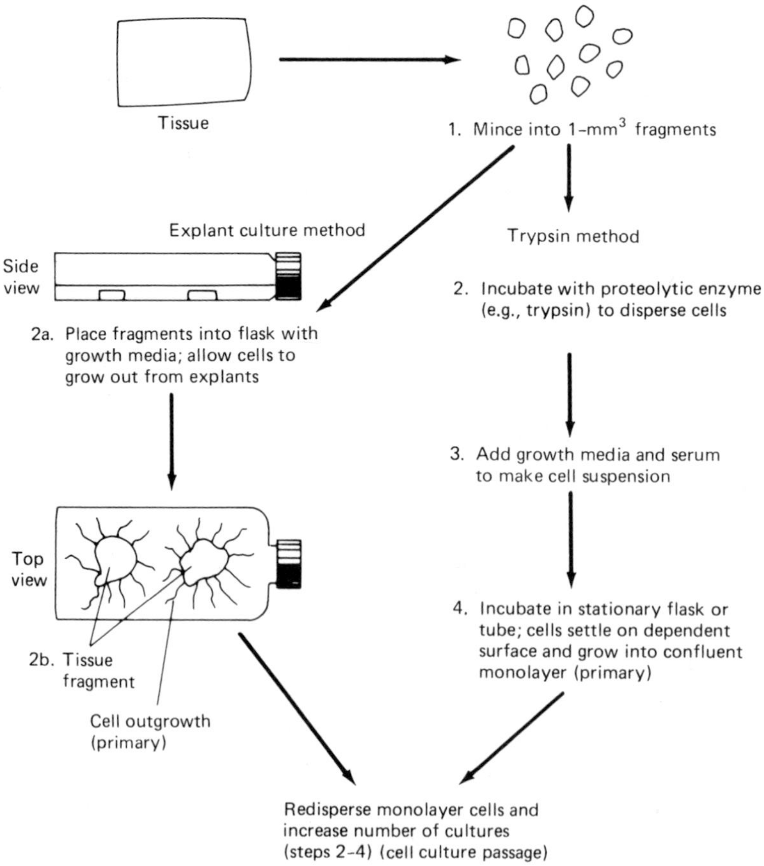

9.5 Preparation of cell culture monolayers.

primary and secondary cell cultures of limited viability

mosome count (diploid), is derived from the initial growth of cells from a tissue source. Redispersal and regrowth produces a secondary cell culture, which usually retains characteristics similar to those of the primary culture (diploid chromosome count and virus susceptibility). Examples of primary and secondary cultures commonly used are monkey and human embryonic kidney cell cultures.

transformed haploid or heteroploid lines may multiply indefinitely

Further dispersal and regrowth of secondary cell cultures usually leads to one of two outcomes: the cells eventually die, or they undergo spontaneous *transformation,* in which the growth characteristics change, the chromosome count varies (haploid or heteroploid), and the susceptibility to virus infection differs from that of the original. These cell cultures have characteristics of "immortality"; that is, they can be redispersed and regrown many times (serial cell culture passage). They can also be derived from cancerous tissue cells or produced by exposure to mutagenic agents in vitro. Such cultures are commonly called *cell lines.* A common cell line in diagnostic use is the Hep-2, derived from a human epithelial carcinoma.

diploid cell lines

A third type of culture is often termed a *cell strain.* This culture comprises diploid cells, commonly fibroblastic, that can be redispersed and regrown a finite number of times; usually 30–40 cell culture passages can be made before the strain dies out or spontaneously transforms. Human embryonic tonsil and lung fibroblasts are common cell strains in routine diagnostic use.

effect of viral growth on cells

cytopathic effect

Viral growth in susceptible cell cultures can be detected in several ways. The most common effect in seen with lytic or cytopathic viruses; as they replicate in cells, they produce alterations in cellular morphology (or cell death) that can be observed directly by light microscopy under low magnification (×30 or ×100). This *cytopathic effect* (CPE) varies with different viruses in different cell cultures. For example, enteroviruses often produce cell rounding, pleomorphism, and eventual cell death in various culture systems, whereas measles and respiratory syncytial viruses cause fusion of cells to produce multinucleated giant cells (syncytia). The microscopic appearance of some normal cell cultures and the CPE produced in them by different viruses are illustrated in Figures 9.6–9.12.

syncytia

hemadsorption and hemagglutination

Other viruses may be detected in cell culture by their ability to produce hemagglutinins. These hemagglutinins may be present on the infected cell membranes, as well as in the culture media as a result of release of free, hemagglutinating virions from the cells. Addition of erythrocytes to the infected cell culture, followed by a period of incubation under proper temperature conditions (which vary according to the virus sought), will result

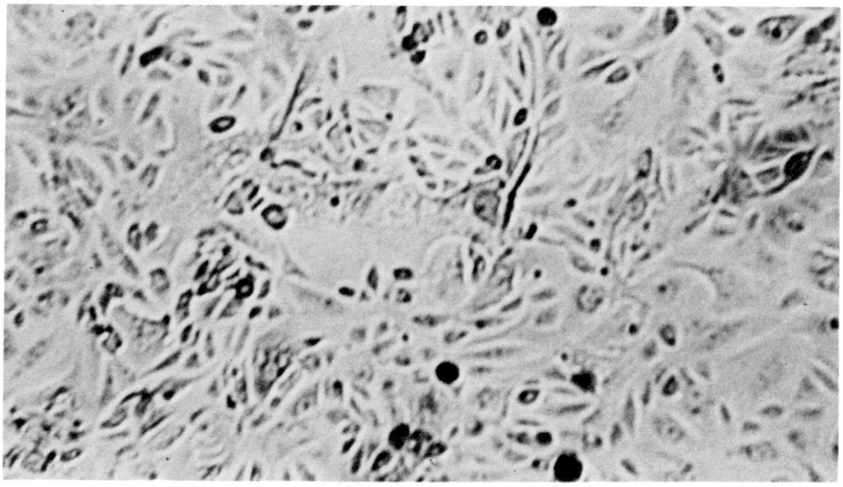

9.6 Normal monkey kidney cell culture monolayer (original magnification ×40).

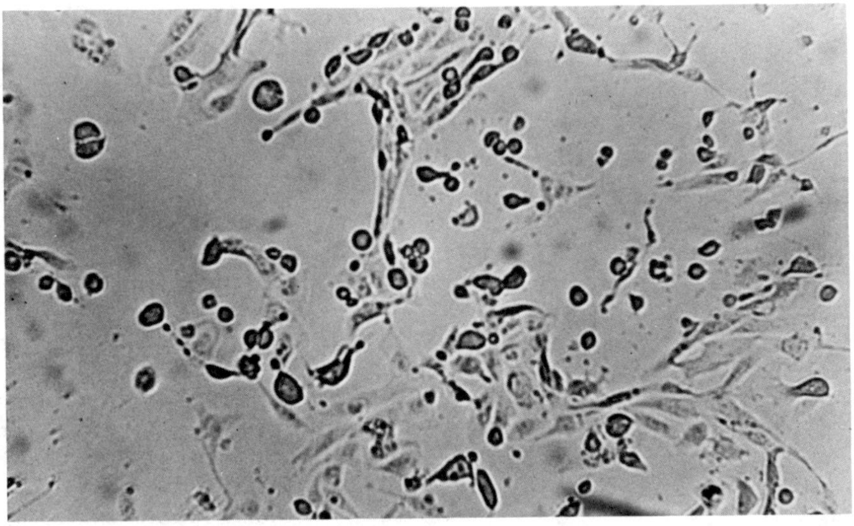

9.7 Enterovirus cytopathic effect in a monkey kidney cell monolayer (original magnification ×40).

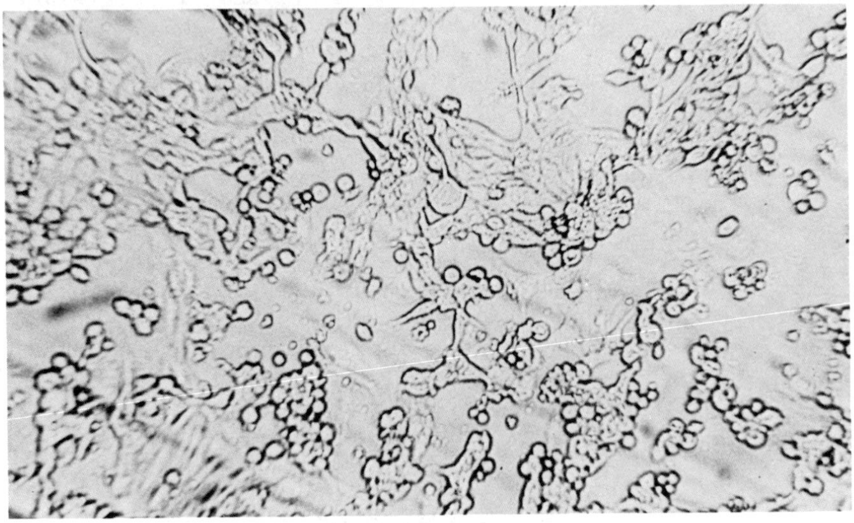

9.8 Adenovirus cytopathic effect in a monkey kidney cell monolayer (original magnification ×40).

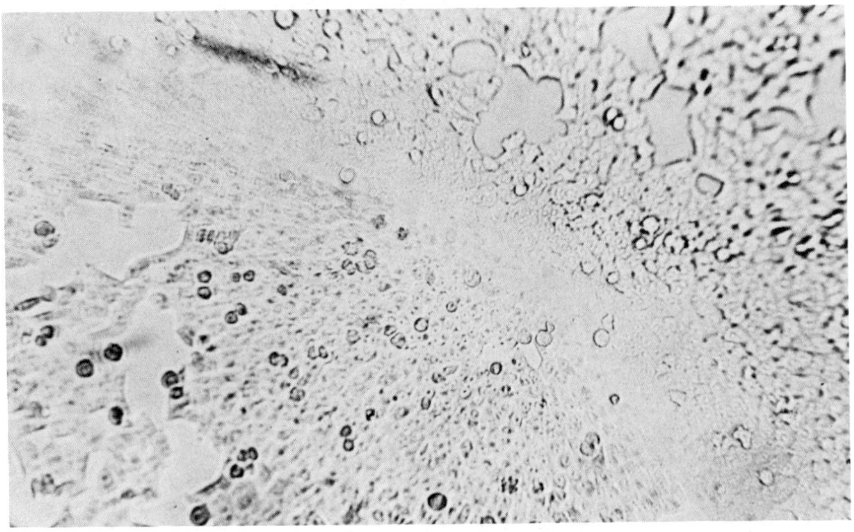

9.9 Normal heteroploid cell (Hep-2) monolayer (original magnification ×40).

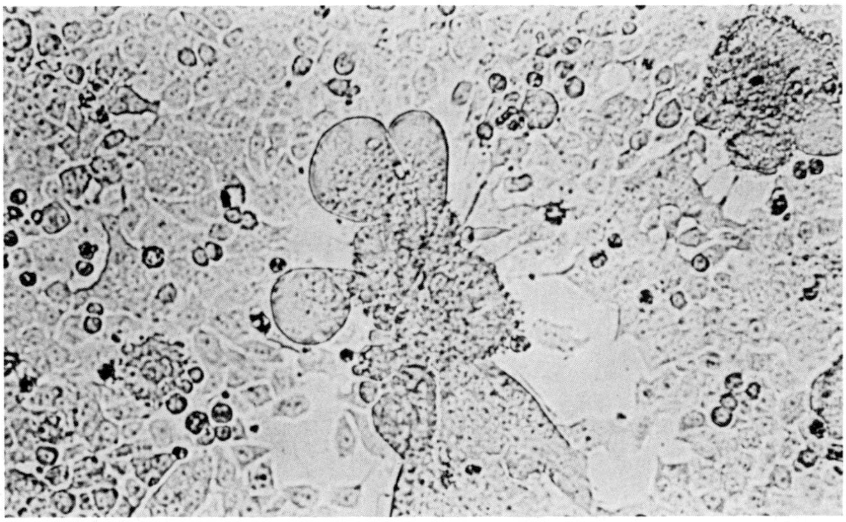

9.10 Respiratory syncytial virus cytopathic effect (giant, syncytial cell formation) in Hep-2 cell monolayer (original magnification ×40).

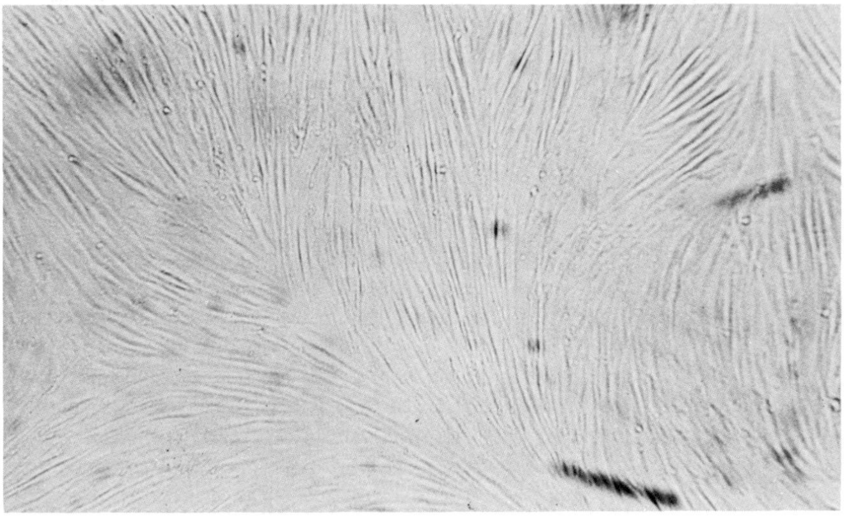

9.11 Normal human diploid fibroblast cell monolayer (original magnification ×40).

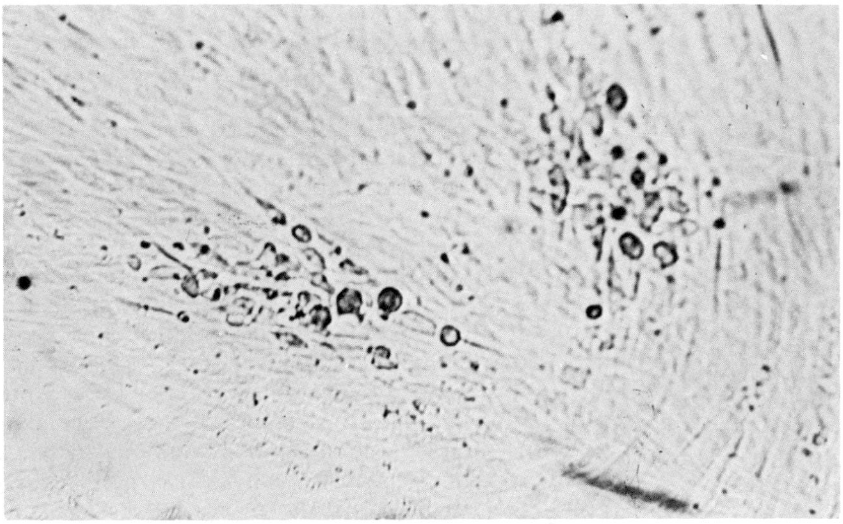

9.12 Cytomegalovirus cytopathic effect in human diploid cell monolayer (original magnification ×40).

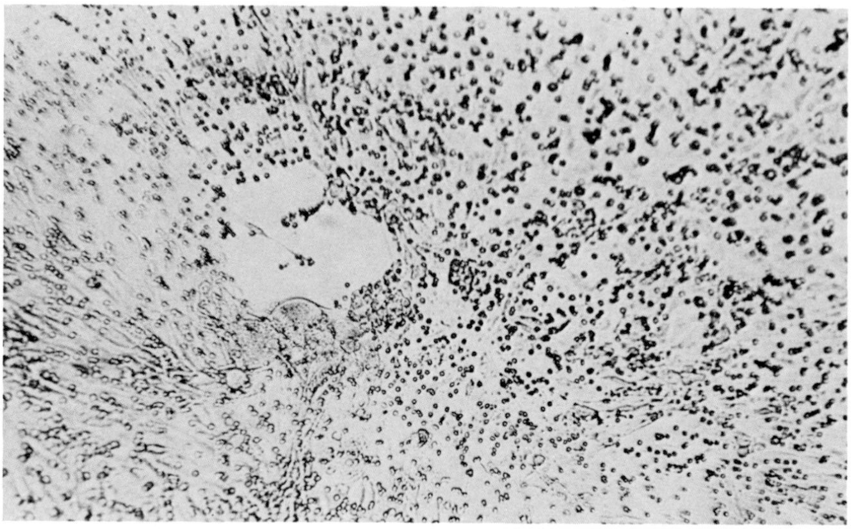

9.13 Parainfluenza virus in monkey kidney cell monolayer. Addition of guinea pig erythrocytes followed by incubation at 4°C for 30 min has resulted in hemadsorption (original magnification ×40).

in adherence of the erythrocytes to the cell surfaces, a phenomenon known as *hemadsorption* Figure 9.13). Influenza, parainfluenza, and mumps viruses are common examples of agents that can be detected in this fashion. If sufficient numbers of virions have been released into the fluid media of the culture, they may be detected by the presence of hemagglutination when erythrocytes are mixed with the fluid and incubated.

detection of virus by interference

A third method of viral detection in cell culture is by *interference.* In this situation, the virus that infects the susceptible cell culture produces no CPE or hemagglutinin, but can be detected by "challenging" the cell culture with a different virus that normally produces a characteristic CPE. The second, or *challenge,* virus fails to infect the cell culture because of interference by the first virus, which is thus detected. This method is obviously cumbersome, but has been applied to the detection of rubella virus in certain cell cultures, such as those derived from African green monkey kidney.

detection of incomplete virus by immunologic or nucleic acid probes

In other situations, only incomplete virus may replicate in cell cultures. Detection may therefore require immunologic *probes,* such as immunofluorescence for detection of intracellular viral antigen. Other methods of study may include much more sophisticated techniques, such as DNA or RNA hybridization, which will not be discussed here.

Some viruses do not readily infect cell culture monolayers; thus, in vivo methods for isolation may be required. These methods can include animal inoculation or the use of embryonated hen's eggs; each has special uses, which will be considered briefly.

growth of virus in embryonated hen's egg

The embryonated hen's egg (Figure 9.14) is still used by many laboratories for the initial isolation and propagation of influenza A virus. It is also required for isolation of influenza C virus, which grows poorly in cell cultures. Several routes of inoculation are available, depending upon the agent sought. Virus-containing material is inoculated on the appropriate membrane, and the egg is incubated to permit viral replication and recognition.

viral isolation in experimental animals: use of suckling mouse

Animal inoculation is used for some viruses. The usual animal host for viral isolation is the mouse; suckling mice in the first 48 hr of life are especially susceptible to many viruses. Intracerebral, subcutaneous, or intraperitoneal inoculation is used, depending upon the virus. Evidence for viral replication is based on the development of illness, manifested by such signs as paralysis, convulsions, poor feeding, or death. The nature of the infecting virus can be further elucidated by histologic and immunofluores-

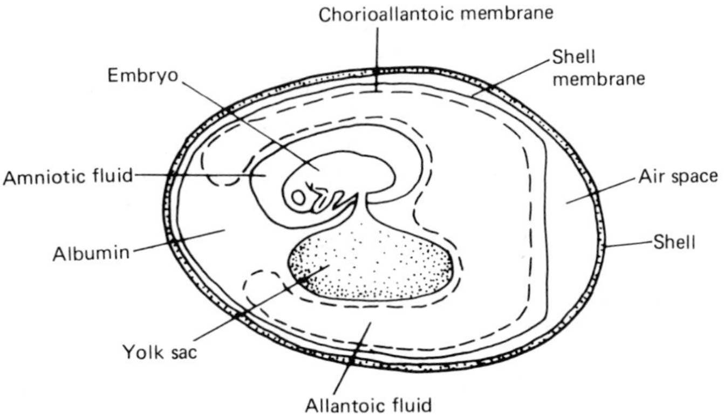

9.14 Inoculation of embryonated hen's egg for isolation of viruses, *Rickettsia*, or *Chlamydia*. Routes of inoculation include amniotic fluid (influenza virus); allantoic fluid (paramyxoviruses); chorioallantoic membrane (poxviruses, herpes simplex); and yolk sac (*Rickettsia*, *Chlamydia*).

cent examination of tissues or by detection of specific antibody responses. Many arboviruses, group A Coxsackie viruses, and rabies virus are best detected in this system.

With this background of viral isolation in mind, it is now possible to summarize the steps involved in this process. First, the viruses believed most likely to be involved in the illness are considered, and appropriate specimens are collected. Next, the specimens are processed; a schematic example is shown in Figure 9.15. Antibiotics and centrifugation or filtration are frequently required with respiratory or fecal specimens to remove organic

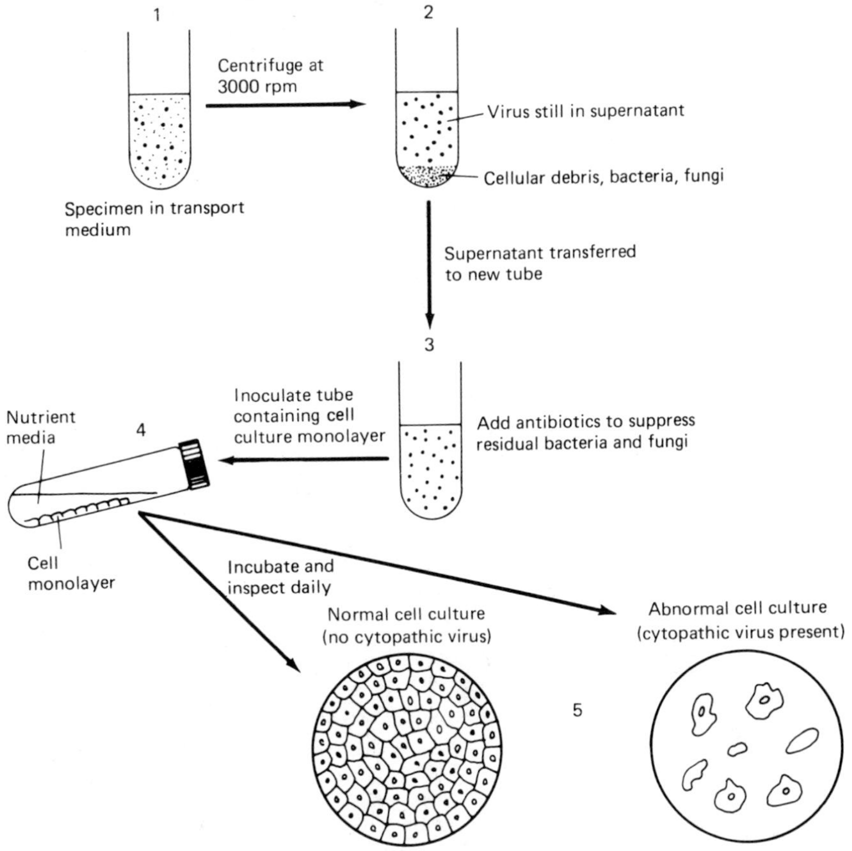

9.15 Preparation and inoculation of a specimen for isolation in cell culture (cytopathic virus).

matter, cellular debris, bacteria, and fungi, which can interfere with viral isolation. The specimens are then inoculated into the appropriate cell culture systems and observed. The time between inoculation and initial detection of viral effects varies; for most viruses, however, positive cultures are usually apparent within 5 days of collection. With proper collection methods and application of the diagnostic tools discussed subsequently, many infections can be detected within hours or a few days. On the other hand, some viruses may require culture for a month or more before they may be detected.

Viral Identification

viral passage

Effect on cell cultures. Upon isolation, a virus can usually be tentatively identified with regard to family or genus by its cultural characteristics (for example, type of CPE produced). Confirmation and further identification of the isolate may require enhancement of viral growth to produce adequate quantities for testing. This result may be achieved by inoculation of the original isolate into fresh culture systems (viral passage) to amplify replication of the virus, as well as improve its adaptation to growth in the in vitro system.

neutralization, immunofluorescence, and hemagglutination inhibition

Serologic detection. Of the several ways to identify the isolate, the most common is to neutralize its infectivity by mixing it with specific antibody to known viruses before inoculation into cultures. Figure 9.16 illustrates the use of this method for identification of a cytopathic virus. Other methods

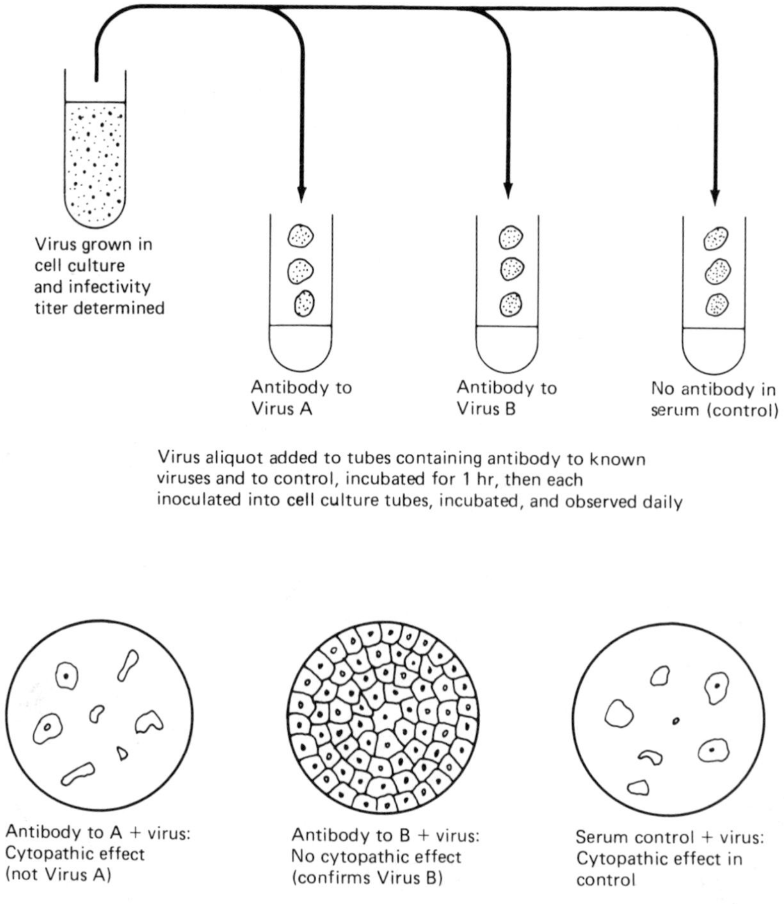
Virus grown in
cell culture
and infectivity
titer determined
Antibody to
Virus A
Antibody to
Virus B
No antibody in
serum (control)
Virus aliquot added to tubes containing antibody to known
viruses and to control, incubated for 1 hr, then each
inoculated into cell culture tubes, incubated, and observed daily
Antibody to A + virus:
Cytopathic effect
(not Virus A)
Antibody to B + virus:
No cytopathic effect
(confirms Virus B)
Serum control + virus:
Cytopathic effect in
control

9.16 Identification of a virus isolate (cytopathic virus) as "Virus B."

9.17 Detection of viral antigen in cells by direct immunofluorescence. (1) Acetone-fixed cells on slide. (2) Add fluorescein-conjugated antiserum and incubate. (3) Unattached antibody removed by washing. (4) Examine for fluorescence under UV illumination (the actual wavelength of light used is that which excites the fluorochrome; a dark-field condenser is used to provide indirect illumination). (A) Herpes simplex virus antigen in a neuron; bright areas of fluorescence show presence of antigen. (B) Respiratory syncytial virus antigen in cytoplasm of cells in culture.

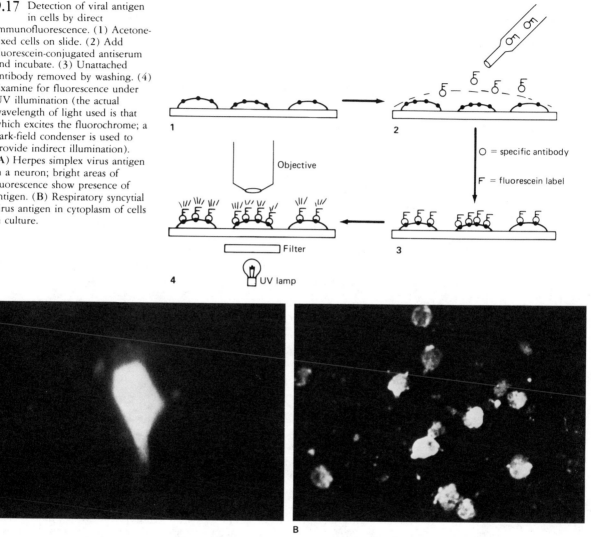

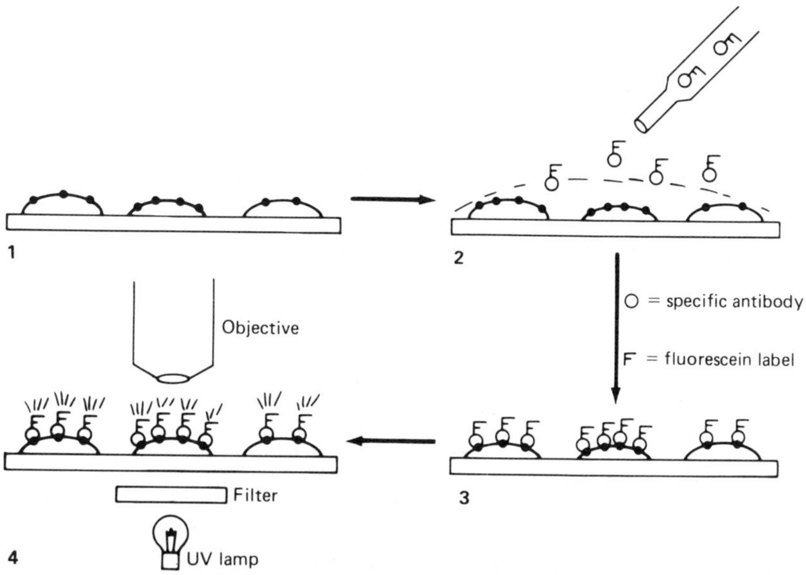

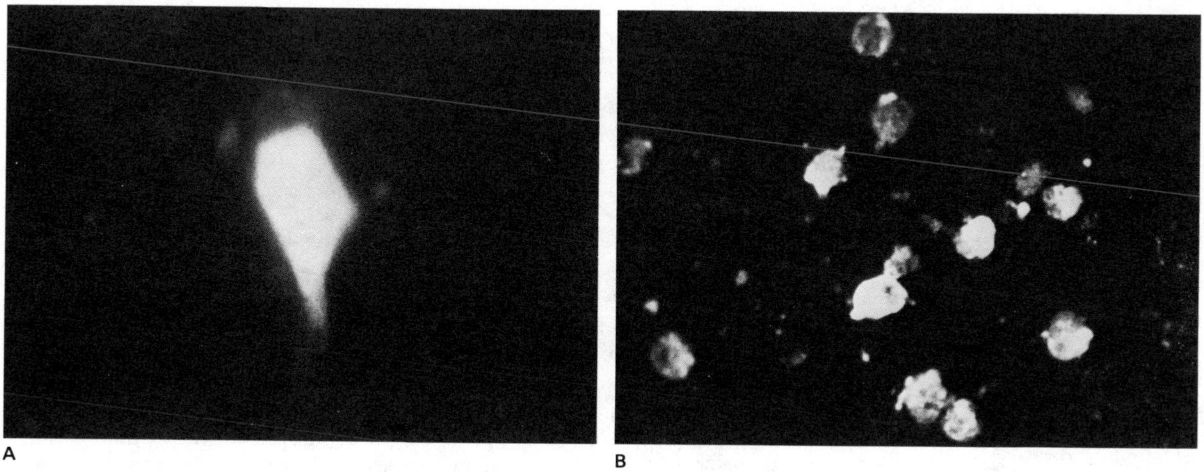

A

B

of identification include demonstration of specific attachment of fluorescein-labeled antiviral antibody to viral antigens in infected cells (Figure 9.17) and specific antibody inhibition of other viral properties such as hemagglutination (hemagglutination inhibition).

Other methods of viral detection. Some viruses (for example, human rotaviruses, hepatitis A and B viruses) grow poorly or not at all in the laboratory culture systems currently available. These viruses have been demonstrated in some instances by inoculation of susceptible human volunteers, and some will replicate and cause disease in subhuman primates such as chimpanzees. Obviously, such methods of cultivation cannot be used in routine diagnosis. Alternative methods for rapid detection of these and other viruses are summarized as follows.

direct examination

immune electron microscopy

Electron microscopy. Direct examination of fluids and tissues from affected body sites, using negative staining techniques, has sometimes enabled visualization of viral particles. When the virions are present in sufficient numbers, they may be further characterized antigenically by specific agglutination

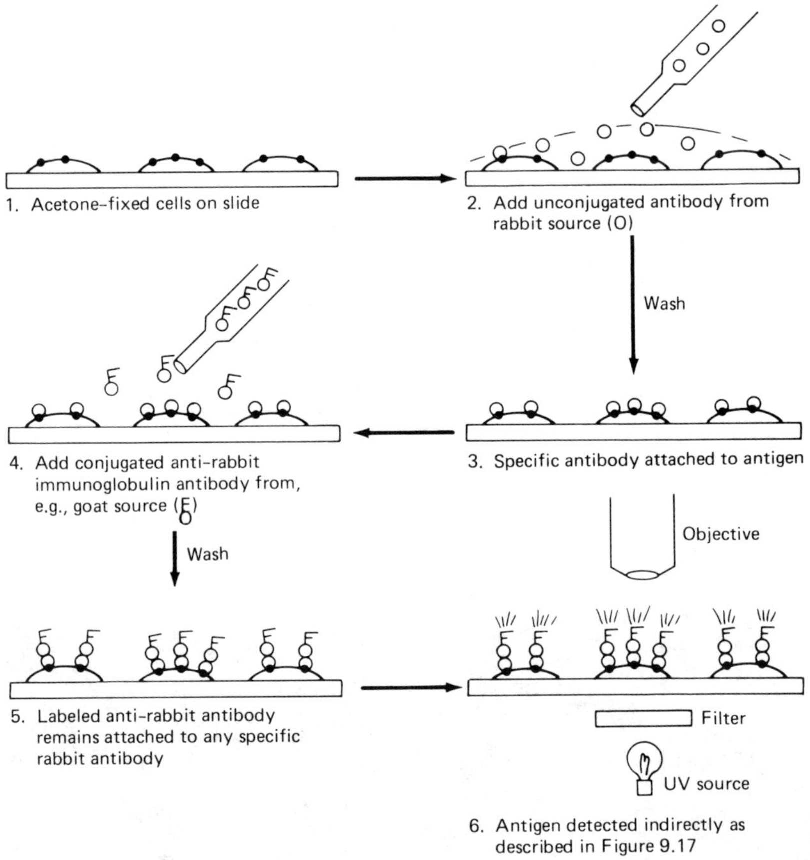
1. Acetone-fixed cells on slide
2. Add unconjugated antibody from rabbit source (O)
Wash
3. Specific antibody attached to antigen
4. Add conjugated anti-rabbit immunoglobulin antibody from, e.g., goat source
Wash
5. Labeled anti-rabbit antibody remains attached to any specific rabbit antibody
Objective
Filter
UV source
6. Antigen detected indirectly as described in Figure 9.17

9.18 Detection of viral antigen in cells by indirect immunofluorescence.

of viral particles upon mixture with type-specific antiserum. This technique, *immune electron microscopy,* can be used to identify viral antigens specifically or to detect antibody in serum using viral particles of known antigenicity.

direct and indirect immunofluorescence, RIA and ELISA techniques

Labeled antibody procedures. The principles of application of immunofluorescence, RIA, and ELISA to viral antigen detection are illustrated in Figures 9.17–9.19. Variations on direct immunofluorescence (Figure 9.17) include 1) *indirect methods,* whereby the antigen is first reacted with an unlabeled, specific antibody, which is then detected with a labeled antibody from a different species directed against the immunoglobulins that comprise the specific antibody (labeled anti-antibody) (Figure 9.18); and 2) *sandwich methods,* whereby the antigen adsorbs to a specific antibody, which has been attached to a surface. A second layer of labeled, specific antibody is used to detect the "trapped" antigen (Figure 9.19). These extremely sensitive techniques will be discussed further with regard to antibody detection.

Other methods of viral antigen detection include complement fixation, immunoprecipitation, thin-layer chromatography, and the like. Some are currently used primarily as research tools; details of others will be provided later in this chapter.

intranuclear and cytoplasmic inclusions

Cytology and histology. In some instances, viruses will produce specific cytologic changes in infected host tissues that aid in diagnosis. Examples include specific intranuclear inclusions, which can be seen in some herpesvirus and adenovirus infections (Figures 9.20 and 9.21); cytoplasmic inclu-

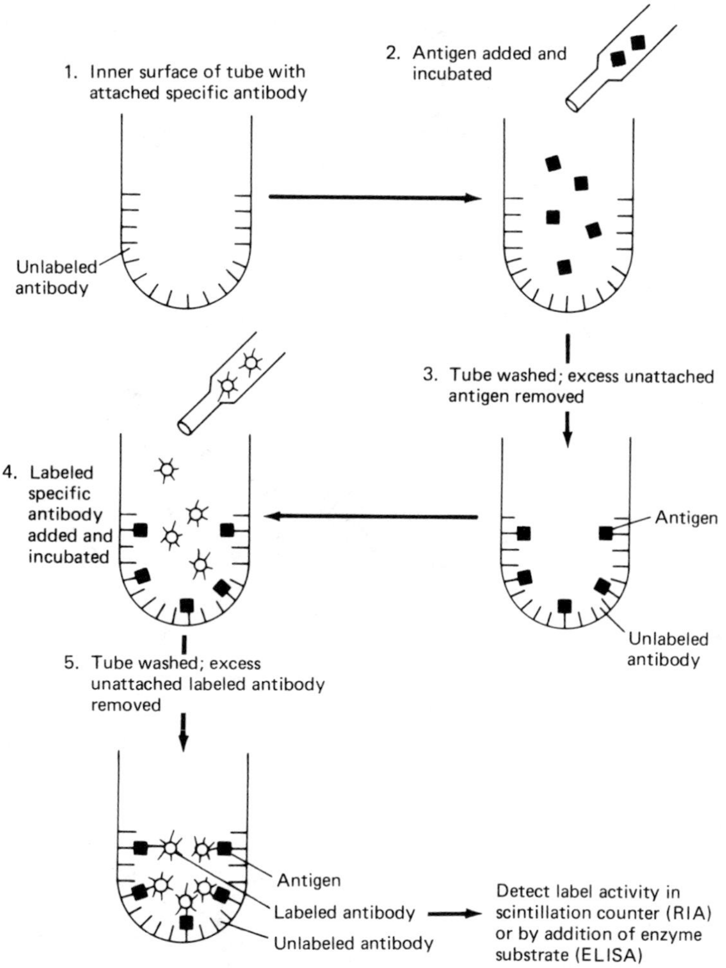
1. Inner surface of tube with attached specific antibody
Unlabeled antibody
2. Antigen added and incubated
3. Tube washed; excess unattached antigen removed
Antigen
Unlabeled antibody
4. Labeled specific antibody added and incubated
5. Tube washed; excess unattached labeled antibody removed
Antigen
Labeled antibody
Unlabeled antibody
Detect label activity in scintillation counter (RIA) or by addition of enzyme substrate (ELISA)

9.19 Detection of extracellular antigen by "sandwich" method.

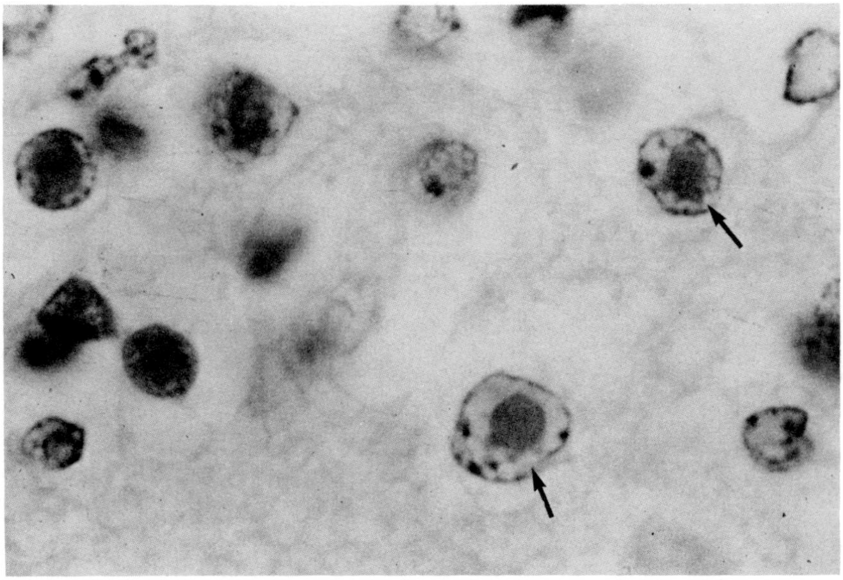

9.20 Brain biopsy from a patient with herpes simplex encephalitis. Arrows indicate typical intranuclear inclusions in infected neurons (hematoxylin–eosin stain; original magnification ×400).

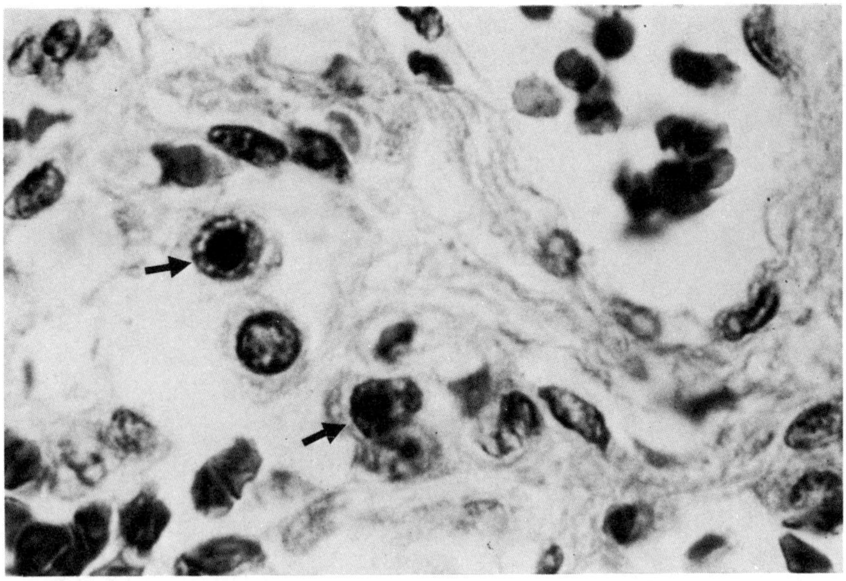

9.21 Lung tissue from a patient with adenovirus pneumonia. Arrows indicate "smudgy" intranuclear inclusions in alveolar epithelial cells (hematoxylin–eosin stain; original magnification ×400).

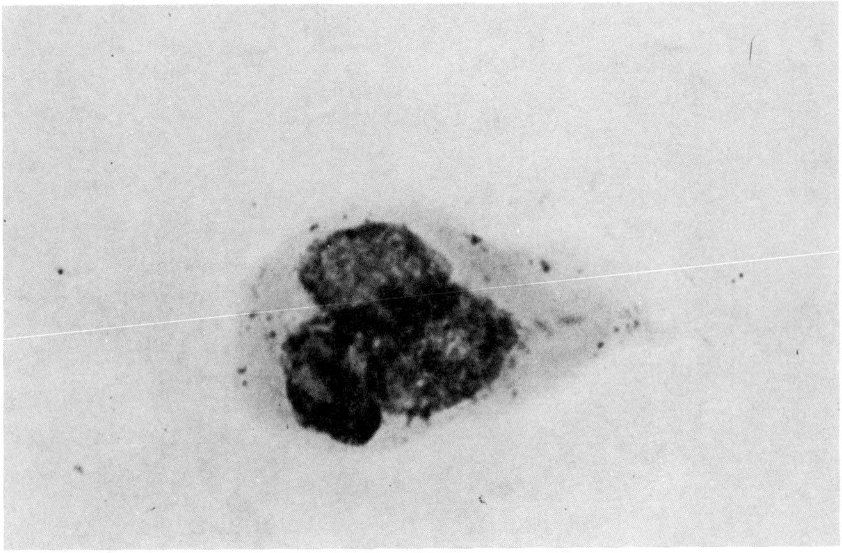

9.22 Multinucleated epithelial cells from a vesicle scraping of a patient with chickenpox. Cell fusion of this type can be seen with both varicella-zoster and herpes simplex infections (Wright's stain; original magnification ×400).

sions; and cell fusion, which results in multinucleated epithelial giant cells (Figure 9.22). Although such findings are useful when seen, their overall diagnostic sensitivity and specificity are usually considerably less than that of the other methods outlined herein.

Serologic Diagnosis of Infection

In infection, whether viral, bacterial, fungal, or parasitic, the host normally responds with the formation of antibodies, which can be detected by various methods. The temporal patterns of development and increase in quantities of specific antibodies in response to a typical viral infection are illustrated in Figure 9.23. These responses can be utilized to detect evidence of recent or past infection. Several basic principles must be emphasized:

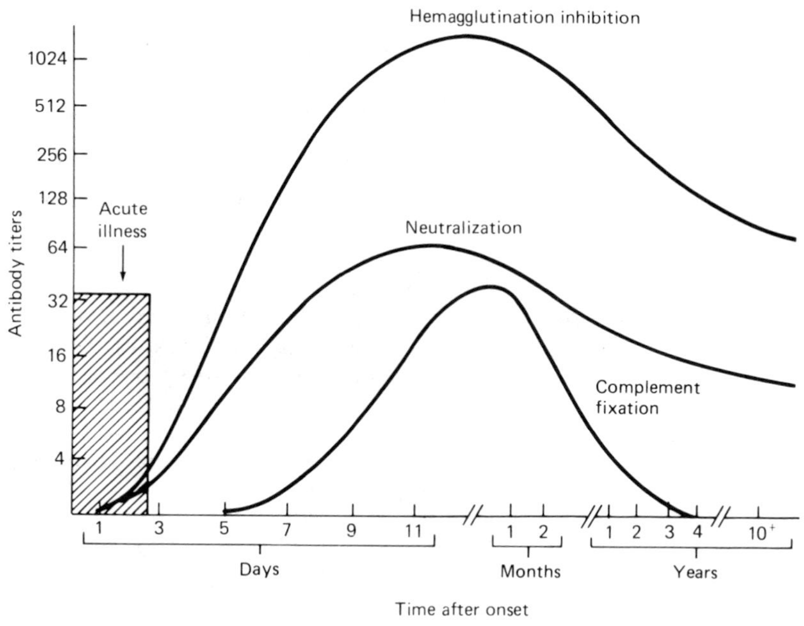

9.23 Patterns of antibody responses, measured by three different methods, to acute infection.

comparison of amount of antibody in acute and convalescent sera

1. In an acute infection, the antibodies usually appear early in the illness, then rise sharply over the next 10–21 days. Thus, a serum sample collected shortly after the onset of illness (acute serum) and another collected 2–3 weeks later (convalescent serum) can be compared quantitatively for changes in specific antibody content.
2. Antibodies can be quantitated by several means. The most common method is to dilute the serum serially in appropriate media and determine the maximal dilution that will still yield detectable antibody in the test system (for example, serum dilutions of 1:4, 1:8, 1:16, and so on). The reciprocal of the highest dilution that retains specific activity is called the *antibody titer.*

antibody titer

seroconversion and significant titer increases

3. The interpretation of significant antibody responses (evidence of specific, recent infection) is most reliable when definite evidence of *seroconversion* is demonstrated; that is, detectable specific antibody is absent from the acute serum (or preillness serum, if available) but present in the convalescent serum. Alternatively, a fourfold or greater increase in antibody titer supports a diagnosis of recent infection; for example, an acute serum titer of 4 and a convalescent serum titer of 16 or greater would be significant.

value of determining presence of specific IgM

4. In instances in which the average antibody titers of a population to a specific agent are known, a single convalescent antibody titer significantly greater than the expected mean may be used as supportive or presumptive evidence of recent infection. This finding, however, is considerably less valuable than those obtained by comparing responses of acute and convalescent serum samples. An alternative and somewhat more complex method of serodiagnosis is to determine which major immunoglobulin subclass constitutes the major proportion of the specific antibodies. In primary infections, the IgM-specific response is often dominant during the first days or weeks after onset, but is replaced progressively by IgG-specific antibodies; thus, by 1–6 months after infection, the predominant antibodies belong to the IgG subclass. Consequently, serum containing

a high titer of antibodies of the IgM subclass would suggest a recent, primary infection.

procedures used

The immunologic methods that can be used to identify a bacterial or viral agent have been discussed in relation to serologic identification of bacteria and viruses. Most of these methods can also be applied to serologic diagnosis by simply reversing the detection system: that is, using a known rather than an unknown antigen to detect the presence of an antibody. The methods of serologic diagnosis to be employed are selected on the basis of their convenience and applicability to the antigen in question. As shown in Figure 9.23, the temporal relationships of antibody response to infection vary according to the method used. Of the methods for measuring antigen–antibody interaction discussed previously, those now used most frequently for serologic diagnosis are agglutination, hemagglutination, RIA, and ELISA. In the remainder of this chapter, some of the additional tests and test modifications used primarily in serologic diagnosis (antibody detection) will be considered briefly.

Neutralization. Neutralization is commonly employed in serodiagnosis of viral infection. The principle is relatively simple in concept: some observable function of the agent (for example, cytopathic effect) is neutralized by first reacting the agent with antibody, then placing the antigen–antibody mixture into the test system. In viral neutralization, a single antibody molecule can bind to surface components of the extracellular virus and interfere with one of the initial events of the viral multiplication cycle, such as adsorption, penetration, or uncoating. Neutralizing antibodies often persist for the life span of the patient, and they correlate well with resistance to reinfection.

Agglutination. In the agglutination test, the known antigen may be a suspension of whole infectious particles, such as bacteria, or represent antigenic material adsorbed and fixed (for example, with glutaraldehyde) to the surface of a particulate carrier (for example, latex particles or erythrocytes). The presence of specific antibody results in immune aggregation of the particles, which can be read microscopically (or macroscopically in some systems) as agglutination (Figure 9.4).

Hemagglutination inhibition. Some antigens will react with naturally occurring receptors on cell membranes; for example, influenza viruses will agglutinate erythrocytes from certain animal and avian species. This phenomenon can be utilized in the hemagglutination inhibition test (Figure 9.24). First, the known antigen is reacted with serum; then the erythrocytes are added. If the antigen has reacted with adequate amounts of specific antibody, its ability to agglutinate the erythrocytes is abrogated (or "neutralized"), and agglutination is inhibited.

complement bound if antigen–antibody reactions occur in test system

unbound complement detected in sheep RBC: anti-sheep RBC indicator system

absence of hemolysis indicates positive test

Complement fixation. Complement fixation assays depend on two properties of complement. The first is the ability to cause hemolysis of sheep red blood cells (RBCs) coated with anti-sheep RBC antibody (sensitized RBCs). The second, under the proper conditions, is fixation (inactivation) of complement upon formation of antigen–antibody complexes. Complement fixation assays are performed in two stages: The *test system* reacts the antigen and antibody in the presence of complement; the *indicator system,* which contains the sensitized RBCs, detects residual complement. Hemolysis indicates that complement was present in the indicator system and therefore that antigen–antibody complexes were *not* formed in the test system. Primarily used to detect and quantitate antibody, complement fixation is gradually being re-

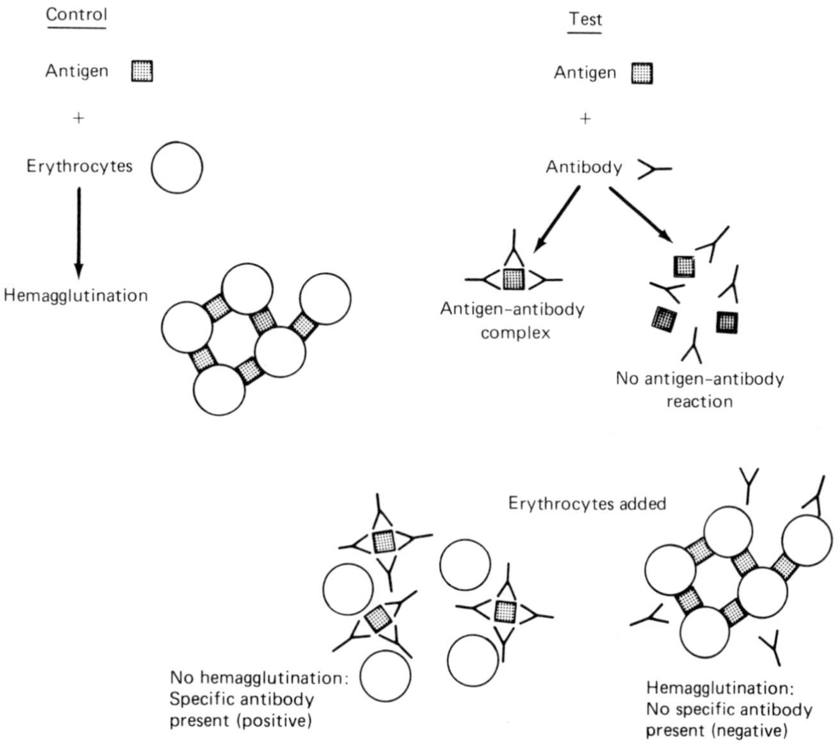

9.24 Hemagglutination inhibition for antibody detection (used when antigen agglutinates erythrocytes).

placed by simpler methods. The principles involved are shown in Figure 9.25.

Indirect immunofluorescence. Indirect immunofluorescence was detailed previously as one way to detect and identify antigens. In serodiagnosis, the known antigen is reacted with dilutions of the test serum, and the specific antibody that remains attached is detected by the addition of labeled antihuman immunoglobulin antibody.

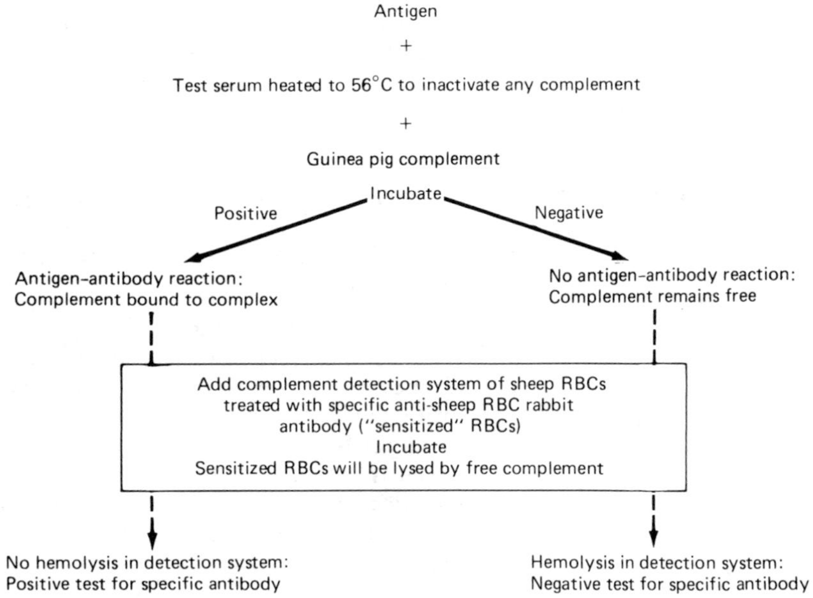

9.25 Complement fixation test.

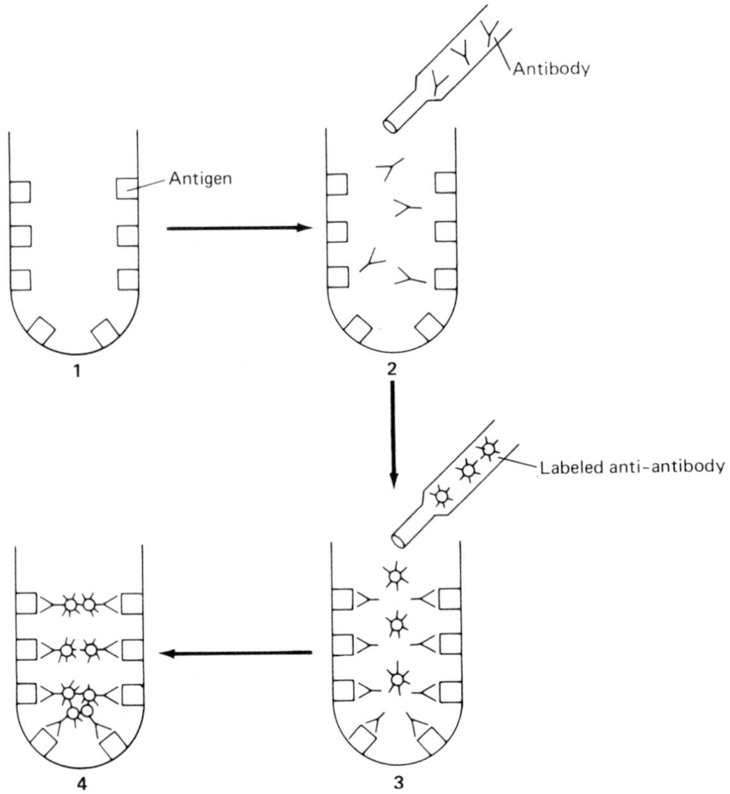

9.26 Solid-phase immunoassay for antibody detection. (1) Tube with known antigen attached to interior surface. (2) Add antibody-containing serum and incubate. (3) Specific antibody binds to antigen, wash and add labeled anti-antibody from different species, and incubate. (4) Wash off excess anti-antibody and measure activity of label.

Immunoassays. Figure 9.26 outlines the basic steps involved in antibody detection by solid-phase immunoassays. In essence, the known antigen is chemically fixed to the surface of a tube or latex bead (solid phase); succeeding steps involve reaction with the test serum, followed by incubation with specifically labeled antibody to human immunoglobulins. The result is measured by counting radioactivity (RIA) or by addition of a substrate for the enzyme label that will undergo a color change in the presence of specific binding (ELISA).

Appendix 9.1

1. *Nutrient broths.* Some form of nutrient broth is used for culture of all direct tissue or fluid samples from sites that are normally sterile to obtain the maximum culture sensitivity. Selective or indicator agents are omitted to prevent inhibition of more fastidious organisms.

2. *Blood agar.* The addition of defibrinated blood to a nutrient agar base enhances the growth of some bacteria, such as streptococci. It often yields distinctive colonies and provides an indicator system for hemolysis. Two major types of hemolysis are seen: a) β-hemolysis, a complete clearing of red cells from a zone surrounding the colony; and b) α-hemolysis, which is incomplete (that is, intact red cells are still present in the hemolytic zone) but shows a green color caused by hemoglobin breakdown products. The net effect is a hazy green zone extending 1–2 mm beyond the colony. A third type, α'-hemolysis, produces a hazy, incomplete

hemolytic zone similar to that caused by α-hemolysis, but without the green coloration.

3. *Chocolate agar.* If blood is added to molten nutrient agar at about 80°C and maintained at this temperature, the red cells are gently lysed, hemoglobin products are released, and the medium turns a chocolate brown color. The nutrients released permit the growth of some fastidious organisms, such as *Haemophilus influenzae,* that fail to grow on blood or nutrient agars. This quality is particularly pronounced when the medium is further enriched with vitamin supplements. Given the same incubation conditions, any organism that grows on blood agar will also grow on chocolate agar.

4. *Thayer–Martin medium.* A variant of chocolate agar, Thayer–Martin medium is a solid medium selective for the pathogenic *Neisseria* (*N. gonorrhoeae* and *N. meningitidis*). Growth of most other bacteria and fungi in the genital or respiratory flora is inhibited by the addition of antimicrobics. A current formulation includes vancomycin, colistin, trimethoprim, and anisomycin.

5. *MacConkey agar.* MacConkey agar is both a selective and an indicator medium for Gram-negative rods, particularly members of the family Enterobacteriaceae and the genus *Pseudomonas.* In addition to a peptone base, the medium contains bile salts, crystal violet, lactose, and neutral red as a pH indicator. The bile salts and crystal violet inhibit Gram-positive bacteria and the more fastidious Gram-negative organisms, such as *Neisseria* and *Pasteurella.* Gram-negative rods that grow and ferment lactose produce a red (acid) colony often with a distinctive colonial morphology.

6. *Hektoen enteric agar.* The Hektoen medium is one of many highly selective media developed for the isolation of *Salmonella* and *Shigella* species (Chapter 20) from stool specimens. It has both selective and indicator properties. The medium contains a mixture of bile, thiosulfate, and citrate salts that inhibits not only Gram-positive bacteria, but members of the Enterobacteriaceae other than *Salmonella* and *Shigella* that appear among the normal flora of the colon. The inhibition is not absolute; recovery of *Escherichia coli* is reduced 1000- to 10,000-fold relative to that on nonselective media, but there is little effect on growth of *Salmonella* and *Shigella.* Carbohydrates and a pH indicator are also included to help to differentiate colonies of *Salmonella* and *Shigella* from those of other enteric Gram-negative rods.

7. *Anaerobic media.* In addition to meeting atmospheric requirements, isolation of some strictly anaerobic bacteria (Chapter 15) on blood agar is enhanced by reducing agents such as L-cysteine and by vitamin enrichment. Sodium thioglycolate, another reducing agent, is often used in broth media. Plate media are made selective for anaerobes by the addition of aminoglycoside antibiotics, which are active against many aerobic and facultative organisms but not against anaerobic bacteria. The use of selective media is particularly important with anaerobes because they grow slowly and are commonly mixed with facultative bacteria in infections.

8. *Highly selective media.* Media specific to the isolation of almost every important pathogen have been developed. Many will allow only a single species to grow from specimens with a rich normal flora (for example, stool). The most common of these media are listed in Table 9.1; they are discussed in greater detail in following chapters.

Additional Reading and References

Cowan, S.T. 1974. *Cowan and Steel's Manual for the Identification of Medical Bacteria.* 2nd ed. New York: Cambridge University Press. This book is essentially a series of taxonomic tables linked by a scholarly (and sometimes entertaining) discussion of their application to bacterial identification. Media, reagents, and tests are also covered in greater detail than in the present chapter.

The CUMITECH Series. Washington, D.C.: American Society for Microbiology. Cumulative Techniques and Procedures in Clinical Microbiology (CUMITECH) is a series of 10- to 25-page pamphlets, each of which covers important topics related to diagnostic microbiology (blood cultures, urinary tract infections, antimicrobial susceptibility testing, and the like). Each pamphlet is jointly written by at least three authors representing the clinical as well as the laboratory viewpoint and includes clinical, specimen collection, isolation, and identification recommendations for all agents pertinent to the topic.

Lennette, E.H., Balows, A., Hausler, W.J., Jr., and Shadomy, J., Eds. 1985. *Manual of Clinical Microbiology*. 4th ed. Washington, D.C.: American Society for Microbiology. A widely used comprehensive text for clinical microbiology and virology.

John C. Sherris

Antimicrobics and Chemotherapy

10

One of the major revolutions in medicine has been the introduction of a large range of clinically effective antimicrobial agents over the past 50 years. Natural materials with some activity against microbes were used in folk medicine in earlier times, such as the bark of the cinchona tree (containing quinine) in the treatment of malaria; however, rational approaches to chemotherapy began with Ehrlich's development of arsenical compounds for the treatment of syphilis early in the century. Many years then elapsed before the next major development, which was the discovery of the therapeutic effectiveness of a sulfonamide (prontosil rubrum) by Domagk in 1935. Penicillin, which had been discovered in 1929 by Fleming, could not be purified at that time; however, it was later characterized and produced in sufficient quantities for therapeutic use by Florey and his colleagues in the early 1940s, when its clinical effectiveness was demonstrated. Since then, numerous new antimicrobial agents have been discovered or developed, and many have found their way into clinical practice. These agents have played an important role in the extraordinary decline in morbidity and mortality from bacterial diseases in developed countries.

selective toxicity

exploit differences between microbial and host cells

Clinically effective antimicrobial agents all exhibit selective toxicity toward the parasite rather than the host, a characteristic that differentiates them from the disinfectants (Chapter 4). In most cases, selective toxicity is explained by action on microbial processes or structures that differ from those of mammalian cells. For example, some agents inhibit synthesis of bacterial cell walls. Others act on functions of the 70S bacterial ribosome, but not the 80S eukaryotic ribosome. Some antimicrobial agents, such as penicillin, are essentially nontoxic to the host, unless hypersensitivity has developed. Others, such as the aminoglycosides, have a much lower therapeutic index, which is defined as the ratio of the dose toxic to the host to the effective therapeutic dose; as a result, control of dosage and blood levels must be much more precise.

therapeutic index

bactericidal and bacteriostatic activity

Some antimicrobial agents, such as those that inhibit cell wall synthesis (for example, the penicillins and cephalosporins) may be able to kill susceptible microorganisms without the intercession of humoral or cellular immune defenses. In the case of bacteria, this process is termed *bactericidal activity.* Others, such as the sulfonamides, simply inhibit essential metabolic processes, and metabolism can recommence when their level becomes subinhibitory. This process is termed *bacteriostatic activity,* and the ultimate destruction of an infecting organism depends on host defenses. Analogous terms for antifungal agents are *fungicidal* and *fungistatic activity,* respectively.

MIC and MLC or MBC

The basic measures of the in vitro activity of an antimicrobial agent against an organism are the minimum inhibitory concentration (MIC) and the minimum lethal concentration (MLC) or, in the case of bacteria, minimum bactericidal concentration (MBC). The MIC is the least amount that prevents growth of the organism under standardized conditions; the MLC is the least amount required to kill a predetermined portion of an inoculum (usually 99.9%) in a given time. The procedures for determining MICs and MLCs are considered in greater detail later in this chapter. For most clinically effective antimicrobial agents, the MICs for fully susceptible organisms range from 100 to 0.01 μg/ml or less, and successful therapy usually appears to require levels above the MIC at the site of the infection.

clinical pharmacology

The pharmacologic characteristics of antimicrobial agents are critical in deciding their use, their dosage, and the routes and frequency of administration. Among such characteristics are whether they are absorbed from the upper gastrointestinal tract, whether they are excreted and concentrated in active form in the urine, whether and how rapidly they are metabolized, and the duration of effective antimicrobial levels in blood and tissues. Most agents are bound to some extent to serum albumin, and the protein-bound form is usually unavailable for antimicrobial action. The amount of free to bound antibiotic can be described as an equilibrium constant that varies for different antibiotics. In general, high degrees of binding lead to more prolonged but lower serum levels of active antimicrobial agent after a single dose.

protein binding

sources and terminology

antibiotics

derived from other organisms

There are three sources of antimicrobial agents. The true antibiotics are of biologic origin and probably play an important part in microbial ecology in the natural environment. Penicillin, for example, is produced by several molds of the genus *Penicillium,* and the prototype cephalosporin antibiotics were derived from other molds. The largest source of naturally occurring antibiotics is members of the genus *Streptomyces,* which are Gram-positive, branching bacteria found in soils and freshwater sediments. Streptomycin, the tetracyclines, chloramphenicol, erythromycin, and many others were discovered by the screening of large numbers of *Streptomyces* isolates from different parts of the world. A few antibiotics, mostly with low therapeutic indices, are derived from soil bacteria of the genus *Bacillus,* but because of their toxicity are now limited mostly to local application rather than systemic use. Antibiotics are mass produced by techniques derived from the procedures of the fermentation industry.

chemotherapeutics

synthetic chemicals

The true chemotherapeutics are chemically synthesized antimicrobial agents. Most of the early chemotherapeutics were discovered among compounds synthesized for other purposes and tested for their therapeutic effectiveness in animals. The sulfonamides, for example, were discovered as a result of routine screening of aniline dyes. More recently, active compounds have been synthesized with structures tailored to be effective inhibitors or competitors of known metabolic pathways. Trimethoprim, which inhibits dihydrofolate reductase, is an excellent example.

molecular manipulations of antibiotics and chemotherapeutics

The third source of new antimicrobial agents is by molecular manipulation of previously discovered antibiotics or chemotherapeutics to broaden their range and/or degree of activity against microorganisms or improve their clinical pharmacologic characteristics. This approach has been the major thrust of developments over the past 20 years, particularly with the antibiotics. Examples include the development of the penicillinase-resistant and broad-spectrum penicillins, as well as a large range of aminoglycosides and cephalosporins of increasing activity, spectrum, and resistance to inactivating enzymes.

antimicrobics

The distinction between antibiotics and chemotherapeutics has become increasingly irrelevant, because some antibiotics, such as chloramphenicol, are now produced synthetically. The terms continue to be used, but the generic terms *antimicrobic* or *antimicrobial agent* to describe both classes of compounds are being used increasingly, and the term *chemotherapy* is used to describe treatment with antimicrobics or antitumor compounds.

spectra

narrow-spectrum agents

broad-spectrum agents

The range of activity of each antimicrobic is called its *spectrum,* a term used to describe the genera and species against which it has been shown to be active. Spectra overlap, but are usually characteristic for each broad class of antimicrobic. Some antibacterial antimicrobics are known as *narrow-spectrum agents;* for example, benzyl penicillin is highly active against many Gram-positive and Gram-negative cocci, but has little activity against enteric Gram-negative bacilli. Chloramphenicol and tetracycline, on the other hand, are broad-spectrum agents that inhibit a wide range of Gram-positive and Gram-negative bacteria, including some obligate intracellular organisms. Spectra relate to the general behavior of a genus or species at the time when the antimicrobic was introduced; resistant strains are frequently selected within many species, and thus the spectrum of an antimicrobic often does not indicate or predict the behavior of an individual strain. For example, the spectrum of benzyl penicillin is considered to include *Staphylococcus aureus,* although most strains now are penicillin resistant.

innate resistance to antimicrobics

acquired resistance

R plasmids

Bacterial resistance to antimicrobics may be innate to all members of a species, which thus fall outside the spectrum of activity of the agent. Innate resistance may be caused by absence of the specific target site of the antimicrobic, failure to permeate to the target site, ability of the organism to circumvent a blocked metabolic pathway, or production of an enzyme that inactivates the antimicrobic. Resistance may also be acquired by many organisms by the genetic mechanisms discussed in Chapter 5. It can result from mutation or by acquisition from another organism of resistance genes, which are sometimes grouped on plasmids that were previously termed *R factors* and that code for resistance to several different antibiotics. Resistant or multiresistant strains of many previously susceptible species are now encountered, sometimes as the predominant phenotype. Acquired resistance can involve all of the mechanisms responsible for innate resistance, but most frequently results from production of antimicrobic inactivating enzymes in the case of resistance determined by R plasmid genes.

effects of antimicrobic combinations

Different classes of antimicrobics acting together may be synergistic, additive, or antagonistic. *Synergy* means that the combined effect is greater than the sum of its parts. For example, penicillin and streptomycin kill enterococci far more effectively than either acting alone, because inhibition of cell wall synthesis by penicillin allows passage of the highly lethal streptomycin into the cell. An *additive effect* means that the effect of the combination is no greater than the sum of its parts. *Antagonism* means that one antimicrobic, usually that with the least important properties, partially prevents the second from expressing its activity. Antagonism occurs with certain combinations of bacteriostatic antimicrobics with the penicillins. Penicillin exerts its bacterial effect only on dividing cells, and inhibition of growth by a bacteriostatic antimicrobic may prevent the lethal activity of penicillin.

unpredictability of many combinations

Unfortunately, there are no firm rules for predicting the effects of new combinations. Laboratory tests to determine synergy or antagonism are helpful, but the ultimate test is clinical trial. Some clearly defined indications and contraindications for combined therapy have been established in this way and will be referred to elsewhere.

combinations in preventing resistance

One particular indication for combined therapy with different classes of antimicrobics is a large population of infecting organisms with a relatively high frequency of mutational resistance. If a lesion contains 10^9 organisms, and the frequency of resistant mutants to two antimicrobics, A and B, is 10^{-6} for each, the chance of relapse by selection of a resistant mutant is high with single therapy. The chance of a double mutant, however, is only 10^{-12}, and combined therapy will usually prevent this development. Pulmonary tuberculosis is an example, and established tuberculosis is always treated with two or more effective antimicrobics to reduce the risk of emergence of resistance.

double mutants extremely rare

These aspects of antimicrobics, chemotherapy, and resistance will now be considered in more detail, first under the headings of the major groups of antimicrobial agents. Major principles will be stressed using antimicrobics commonly employed. Details on specific antimicrobic use, dosage, and toxicity should be sought in one of the specialized texts or handbooks written for that purpose.

β-Lactam Antibiotics

origin from mold

6-aminopenicillanic acid nucleus

β-Lactamase (penicillinase)

Penicillins. The first penicillins were derived from cultures of molds of the genus *Penicillium.* All were derivatives of 6-aminopenicillanic acid, the basic structure of which is a β-lactam ring linked to a thiazolidine ring (Figure 10.1). Side chains of the β-lactam ring confer antibacterial activity and determine the pharmacologic properties and spectrum of the penicillin. The integrity of the β-lactam ring is essential for the activity of penicillins. It can be opened by enzymes termed *β-lactamases* (or penicillinases in the case of penicillin) produced by a wide range of bacteria. The action of these enzymes results in loss of all antibacterial activity.

benzyl penicillin and derivatives

The prototype penicillin is benzyl penicillin (penicillin G), from which earlier semisynthetic penicillins were derived. The action of an enzyme, amidase, breaks the bond between the β-lactam ring and the side chain, allowing other side chains to be added.

classification of penicillins

Examples of commonly used penicillins, their side chains, and their major properties are shown in Table 10.1. They can be classified conveniently as

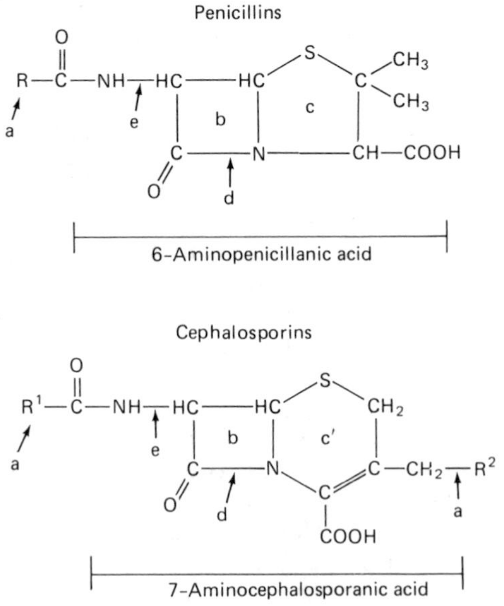

10.1 Basic structure of β-lactam antibiotics. (a) Different side chains determine degree of activity, pharmacologic properties, resistance to β-lactamases, and spectrum; (b) β-lactam ring; (c) thiazolidine ring; (c′) dihydrothiazine ring; (d) site of action of β-lactamases; (e) site of action of amidase.

Table 10.1 Some Representative Penicillins

Class	Compound	Side Chain	Route of Administration: Parenteral	Route of Administration: Oral	Long Activity	Resistance to Staphylococcal β-Lactamase	Activity Against Some Enterobacteriaceae	Activity Against Some Pseudomonas
Basic spectrum	Benzyl penicillin G	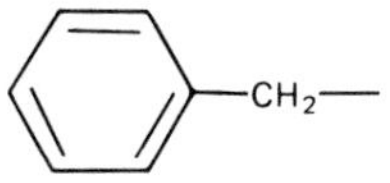	+	−	−	−	−	−
	Benzathine penicillin G[a]		+	−	+	−	−	−
	Penicillin V	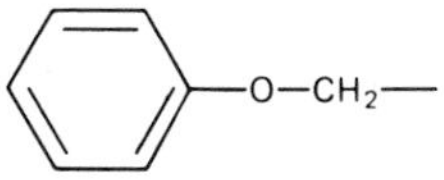	−	+	−	−	−	−
Penicillinase resistant	Methicillin	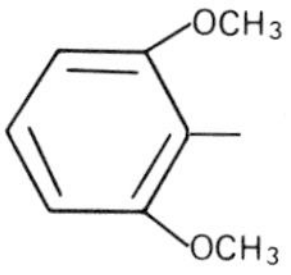	+	−	−	+	−	−
	Dicloxacillin	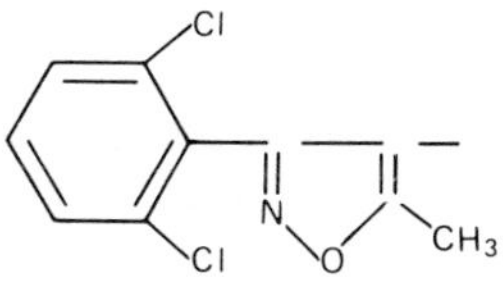	−	+	−	+	−	−
Extended spectrum	Ampicillin	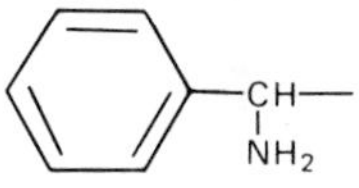	+	+	−	−	+	−
	Carbenicillin	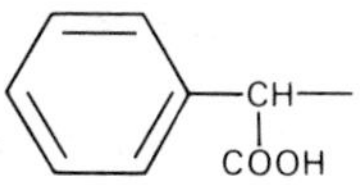	+	−	−	−	+	+

[a] Salt of combination of ammonium base and penicillin G (*N,N'*-dibenzylethylenediamine dipenicillin G).

narrow-spectrum penicillins, narrow-spectrum penicillins resistant to staphylococcal penicillinase, and broader-spectrum penicillins.

narrow-spectrum penicillins

failure to penetrate cell wall of Gram-negative bacteria

Acid instability of benzyl penicillin G

long-acting penicillins

The narrow-spectrum penicillins are active mainly against Gram-positive organisms and some Gram-negative cocci. They have little action against most Gram-negative bacilli, because the lipopolysaccharide–protein outer membrane of the Gram-negative cell wall prevents passage of these antibiotics to their sites of action on cell wall synthesis. Of the three narrow-spectrum penicillins shown in Table 10.1, penicillin G is the least toxic and least expensive; however, it is unstable in acid and, when given by mouth, may be largely destroyed by gastric hydrochloric acid. The modification of the molecule in penicillin V confers acid resistance, and this preparation is reliable when used orally. Benzathine penicillin is a combined form of penicillin from which active penicillin is slowly released into the bloodstream. Blood levels are low, but detectable for long periods. This agent can be used in the treatment of patients infected with highly susceptible organisms.

penicillinase-resistant penicillins

The penicillinase-resistant penicillins also have narrow spectra, but are active against penicillinase-producing *S. aureus.* They appear to owe their insusceptibility to the enzyme to steric hindrance resulting from the configuration of their side chain.

extended-spectrum penicillins

penicillins active against *Pseudomonas*

The extended-spectrum penicillins owe their expanded activity to the ability to traverse the outer membrane of some Gram-negative cell walls. Some, such as ampicillin, have excellent activity against a range of Gram-negative pathogens, but are ineffective against an important opportunistic pathogen, *Pseudomonas aeruginosa.* Others, such as carbenicillin and its derivatives, are active against many *Pseudomonas* strains when given in very high dosage, but are less active than ampicillin against some other Gram-negative organisms. It should be noted that broader-spectrum penicillins are all inactivated by staphylococcal penicillinase.

action of penicillins

penicillin-binding proteins

inhibitors of transpeptidation reaction

weakening of cell wall

role of autolytic enzymes

bactericidal action on growing cells

resistance of cell wall-deficient mutants and spheroplasts

tolerance

The penicillins are inhibitors of cell wall synthesis. They attach to several penicillin-binding proteins that are adjacent to the cytoplasmic membrane and variously represented in different susceptible species. Some penicillin-binding proteins have been identified as active in the steps leading to the development and structural strength of the cell wall. Penicillin acts by inhibiting cell wall synthesis, particularly in blocking the transpeptidation reaction that links the peptidoglycan molecules by pentapeptide bridges and provides structural strength to the wall. Inhibition of cell wall synthesis, when not accompanied by inhibition of other metabolic processes, leads to the development of weakened areas at the sites of active cell wall deposition. These areas are particularly susceptible to the activity of autolytic enzymes normally associated with cell wall turnover. The end result is bulging and rupture of the cytoplasmic membrane as water is drawn into the hypertonic cytoplasm of the cell. The effect of the penicillins on susceptible strains is thus exhibited on growing cells and is bactericidal if the external osmotic pressure is lower than that of the interior of the cell, and if autolytic enzymes are active. Nongrowing cells are inhibited, but not killed, by the antibiotic, and some cell-wall-deficient mutants, or osmotically stabilized spheroplasts, can grow in its presence. Recent work has indicated that different β-lactam antibiotics may have a predominant effect on different combinations of penicillin-binding protein enzymes involved in cell wall synthesis, and different morphologic effects may result. Furthermore, mutational loss of autolytic enzyme activity may abrogate the bactericidal effect of the antibiotic and produce a condition described as *tolerance*, in which sensitive bacteria are inhibited, but are much more slowly killed than the wild type.

explanation of selective toxicity

The selective toxicity of the penicillins results from the absence of a mammalian cell analog to the bacterial cell wall.

resistance

multistep mutational resistance

occurrence in gonococci and pneumococci

Acquired resistance to the penicillins can be mutational or by acquisition of plasmid genes. Significant degrees of mutational resistance require a number of separate mutational steps involving cell wall synthesis and often the loss of some determinants of virulence. Thus, in vivo mutational resistance is a rare event, but has occurred in certain species after many years of use of the antibiotic. Non-β-lactamase-producing gonococci of considerably increased resistance to penicillin are widely encountered and have been shown to result from a series of sequential mutations. Recent reports from various parts of the world of the isolation of pneumococci of increased resistance to penicillin appear to reflect a similar phenomenom. Mutational resistance may also be responsible for methicillin-resistant staphylococci. Occasionally, mutational resistance occurs in closed-lesion infections after prolonged low-dose treatment with one of the penicillins.

resistance from β-lactamase production

acquisition of β-lactamase by *H. influenzae* and *N. gonorrhoeae*

The major mechanism of acquired resistance to many penicillins is by production of β-lactamases. The genes coding for these enzymes are usually plasmid-borne. In some cases they are potentially transposable and may sometimes integrate into the chromosome. The β-lactamase of *S. aureus* causes resistance to all penicillins, except those that are specifically resistant to attack by the enzyme. Plasmid-determined β-lactamases found in some enteric organisms confer resistance to broader-spectrum penicillins. The transposal gene coding for one of them, the TEM β-lactamase, has recently been acquired by plasmids of *Haemophilus influenzae* and *Neisseria gonorrhoeae*, and strains of these species that are completely resistant to penicillin and ampicillin are being encountered with increasing frequency. The so-called penicillinase-resistant penicillins, which are resistant to hydrolysis by staphylococcal β-lactamase, are *not* resistant to the TEM β-lactamase. Fortunately, despite these developments many species that were originally susceptible to penicillin have retained their susceptibility over the four decades of use of the antibiotic.

toxicity of and hypersensitivity to penicillins

The penicillins are among the least toxic agents used in therapy. Very high concentrations may be associated with convulsions, but doses on the order of 50 g a day of benzyl penicillin or carbenicillin are usually well tolerated. Occasionally, hypersensitivity develops to the penicillins. This reaction may be manifested as an anaphylactic type of response (which may sometimes be very severe) or more commonly as a serum sickness.

origin and nomenclature

cefamycins

Cephalosporins. The first cephalosporin antimicrobics were derived from cultures of *Cephalosporium* molds. Some of the newer members of the group, obtained from cultures of a genus of branching bacteria related to the *Streptomyces*, have been termed the *cefamycins*. Their basic chemical structure is the same, however, and herein we will refer to all of them as cephalosporins.

structure

7-aminocephalosporanic acid

resistance to staphylococcal β-lactamase

The cephalosporins resemble the penicillins in possessing a β-lactam ring, the integrity of which is essential to their activity. They differ from the penicillins in that the five-membered thiazolidine ring is replaced by a six-membered dihydrothiazine ring. The nucleus of the cephalosporins, 7-aminocephalosporanic acid, like 6-aminopenicillanic acid, has little antibacterial action. Activity, pharmacologic properties, and spectra are conferred on the molecule by side chains in the positions indicated in Figure 10.1. The structure of the cephalosporins confers substantial or complete resistance to hydrolysis by staphylococcal penicillinase (β-lactamase), but the β-lactam ring of the earlier members of the group was opened by β-lactamases of effects of Gram-negative β-lactamases

many Gram-negative bacilli. The more recently introduced cephalosporins are much more resistant to β-lactamases of Gram-negative bacilli, which accounts in part for their wider spectrum.

mode of action similar to penicillins

The mode of action of the cephalosporins is essentially the same as that of the penicillins. They bind to and inactivate enzymes or compounds essential for cell synthesis, and they are usually lethal to susceptible growing cells.

range of cephalosporins

Many semisynthetically produced cephalosporins are now available with extended spectra and varying pharmacologic properties, and new compounds continue to be introduced while others decline in popularity. It would thus be quite unrewarding for the student to attempt to learn the specific details of those currently available. Even for the clinician, it is best to become familiar with two or three cephalosporins and learn to use them well. For these reasons, we will consider only a few representatives of the group, ranging from those with the narrowest to those with the broadest spectrum.

first-generation cephalosporins

Six cephalosporins are considered in Table 10.2. Those designated first-generation agents have a more restricted spectrum than those developed subsequently. Their spectrum against Gram-positive organisms resembles that of the penicillinase-resistant penicillins, but they are also active against some Gram-negative bacilli (Appendix 10.1). They continue to have therapeutic value because of their high activity against Gram-positive organisms and because a broader spectrum may be unnecessary and is more likely to predispose the patient to the problem of superinfection. Of the two first-generation cephalosporins listed in Table 10.2, cephalothin must be given parenterally, but the side chains of cephalexin confer acid stability and absorbability and make it an effective oral preparation.

Table 10.2 Cephalorsporins

		Route of Administration		
Class	Compound	Parenteral	Oral	Spectrum
First generation	Cephalothin	+	−	*Staphylococcus aureus* (penicillinase producing and nonproducing) Streptococci other than enterococci and peptostreptococci *Escherichia coli*; *Haemophilus influenzae*; *Klebsiella* species; *Proteus mirabilis*
	Cephalexin	−	+	
Second generation[a]	Cefamandole	+	−	First-generation spectrum expanded to indole-positive *Proteus* species; *Enterobacter*, and *Citrobacter*
	Cefoxitin	+	−	First-generation spectrum expanded to *Serratia*, indole-positive *Proteus*, and many Gram-negative anaerobes
Third generation[a]	Cefotaxime	+	−	Spectrum of cefamandole expanded to give high activity against *Haemophilus influenzae* and *Neisseria gonorrhoeae*, including β-lactamase-producing strains, and activity against *Pseudomonas aeruginosa* and many Gram-negative anaerobes
	Cefoperazone	+	−	

[a] Second- and third-generation cephalosporins have less activity than first-generation agents against Gram-positive organisms. Each agent has specific advantages in activity against particular organisms.

second-generation cephalosporins

Second-generation cephalosporins are resistant to chromosomally or plasmid-determined β-lactamases of some Gram-negative organisms that inactivate first-generation compounds. For example, cefoxitin is active against many strains of *Bacteroides fragilis* and *Serratia* species that are resistant to first-generation compounds and also resists breakdown by the TEM-type β-lactamase.

third-generation cephalosporins

Third-generation cephalosporins, such as cefotaxime, have an even wider spectrum and are active against Gram-negative organisms in extremely low concentrations. They are resistant to many β-lactamases. Both second- and third-generation cephalosporins are generally less active against Gram-positive cocci than those of the first generation or the penicillins.

resistance

cephalosporinase

β-lactamase

Resistance to cephalosporins may result from failure to permeate the cell membrane, absence of binding proteins, lack of cell wall, or plasmid or chromosomally determined β-lactamases. Many chromosomal β-lactamases of Gram-negative bacilli are cephalosporinases, which inactivate all first-generation compounds. The newer agents are progressively more resistant to such attack, as well as to enzymes that are plasmid coded. Mutational resistance to several cephalosporins occurs at relatively high frequency (10^{-6}–10^{-8}), particularly in *Enterobacter* species. Resistance is caused by markedly enhanced production of chromosomally determined cephalosporinase as a result of mutation in a repressor gene, the function of which is to control the amount of enzyme.

toxicity and hypersensitivity

The cephalosporins now in use are of low toxicity and can be given in large doses for complex infections. Hypersensitivity may develop, but cross-sensitivity to the penicillins is unusual.

agents of choice for susceptible infections

Clinical use. The β-lactam antibiotics are usually the drugs of choice for infections by susceptible organisms because of their very high therapeutic index and bactericidal action. They have also proved of great value in the prophylaxis of many infections. They are excreted by the kidney and achieve very high urinary levels. Penicillins reach the cerebrospinal fluid when the meninges are inflamed and are used in the treatment of meningitis due to susceptible organisms. First- and second-generation cephalosporins show poor penetration even with inflammation and are not appropriate for the treatment of meningitis. In contrast, the third-generation cephalosporins penetrate much better, and their marked activity makes them agents of choice in the treatment of meningitis caused by some Gram-negative organisms.

The β-lactam antibiotics often enhance permeability of the bacterial cell to the aminoglycosides, and synergistic combinations of these two classes of antimicrobics are indicated for a number of severe infections.

Aminoglycoside–Aminocyclitol Antibiotics

origin and structure

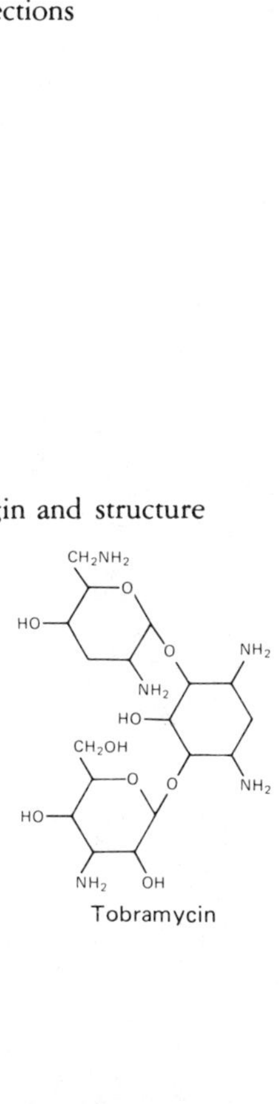

Tobramycin

The aminoglycoside–aminocyclitol antibiotics are a group of bactericidal agents characterized by combinations of six-membered aminocyclitol rings with varying side chains, which determine their spectra and degrees of resistance to inactivating enzymes. The structure of tobramycin is shown in the marginal figure. Streptomycin and other earlier members of the group were produced from species of *Streptomyces*. The newer members are semisynthetic derivatives.

The most important and commonly used members of the group are listed in Table 10.3, together with some key properties. Streptomycin is now rarely used, except for treatment of tuberculosis or in combination with penicillin for treatment of bacterial endocarditis, because high-level and stable resistant mutants are frequently selected during therapy. Kanamycin,

Table 10.3 Characteristics of Commonly Used Aminoglycosides

Compound	Single-Step High Mutational Resistance	Anti-Pseudomonas Activity	Susceptibility to Aminoglycoside-Inactivating Enzymes
Streptomycin	+	−	+++
Neomycin	+	−	+++
Kanamycin	±	−	++
Gentamicin	−	+	+
Tobramycin	−	+	±
Amikacin	−	+	±

Number of plus signs in the fourth column indicates the degree of susceptibility to enzymatic attack.

gentamicin, tobramycin, amikacin, netilmicin, etc.

in combination with a β-lactam antibiotic, is still used in the treatment of neonatal infections of uncertain etiology because of extensive experience with the drug. Otherwise, its use has declined in relationship to the newer agents. Neomycin, the most toxic aminoglycoside, is used as an oral preparation to reduce the facultative flora of the large intestine before certain types of intestinal surgery. It is very poorly absorbed, and most of its activity is expressed in the bowel. Gentamicin, tobramycin, amikacin and netilmicin have extended spectra that include activity against many strains of *P. aeruginosa*. Tobramycin has a wider spectrum of resistance to plasmid-coded aminoglycoside-inactivating enzymes than gentamicin. Amikacin is still more resistant to inactivation and may thus act on some gentamicin- and tobramycin-resistant strains.

mode of action

irreversible inhibition of protein synthesis

bactericidal effect

The aminoglycosides inhibit protein synthesis by combining with bacterial ribosomal proteins of the 30S ribosomal subunit. In the case of streptomycin, a ribosomal protein designated S12 appears to be involved exclusively. With the newer and more active aminoglycosides, other ribosomal binding sites are also involved, resulting in a broader spectrum of activity that includes many streptomycin-resistant strains. In sufficient concentrations, aminoglycosides bind to the ribosome irreversibly, block initiation complexes, and prevent elongation of polypeptide chains, resulting in a rapid bactericidal effect. Lower concentrations lead to distortion of the site of attachment of messenger (m)RNA, misreading of the message, and failure to produce the correct proteins with dramatic effects on growth and bacterial structure.

active transport into bacterial cells

inactivity under anaerobic conditions

The aminoglycosides are actively transported into the bacterial cell by a mechanism that involves oxidative phosphorylation. Thus, they have little or no activity against strict anaerobes or facultative organisms that only metabolize fermentatively (for example, streptococci). It appears highly probable that aminoglycoside activity against facultative organisms is similarly reduced in vivo when the oxidation–reduction potential is low.

Eukaryotic ribosomes are resistant to aminoglycosides, and the antimicrobics are not actively transported into eukaryotic cells. These properties account for their selective toxicity and also explain their ineffectiveness against intracellular bacteria such as *Rickettsia* and *Chlamydia*.

spectra

The newer aminoglycosides, gentamicin, tobramycin, amikacin and netilmicin have a broad spectrum of bactericidal action against many aerobic and facultative Gram-positive and Gram-negative rods, including *P. aeruginosa*. Their detailed spectrum is given in Appendix 10.1. It merits restressing that all anaerobes are resistant to their action and that they have little activity against streptococci, except when cell penetrability is increased by simultaneous action of a β-lactam antibiotic.

mutational resistance

High-level mutational resistance to streptomycin can occur in a single step because of its single target protein. With more than one molecular target, mutational resistance to the newer aminoglycosides is much less common and of lower level. When it does occur, it usually involves loss of the active transport mechanism across the cell wall, thus leading to increased resistance to all aminoglycosides.

plasmid-determined enzymatic resistance

newer compounds increasingly resistant to inactivation

The most common cause of bacterial resistance involves production of one of more of a range of enzymes that can acetylate, adenylate, or phosphorylate various critical groups on the aminoglycoside molecule. This mechanism abrogates or greatly reduces antibacterial activity. Production of these enzymes is determined by plasmid-borne genes. Aminoglycosides have been successively developed with few sites susceptible to such inactivation, and amikacin and netilmicin are currently among the most resistant. In the community and in many hospitals, plasmids coding for resistance to gentamicin and subsequently developed aminoglycosides are not widespread, and the antimicrobics have retained a broad activity and value.

toxicity

toxicity to eighth cranial nerve

need for blood level monitoring

All of the aminoglycoside antimicrobics are toxic to varying degrees to the vestibular and auditory branches of the eighth cranial nerve. Kanamycin and amikacin primarily affect hearing, whereas streptomycin and gentamicin are most toxic to vestibular function. The damage can lead to complete and irreversible loss of hearing and balance. These agents may also be toxic to the kidneys. Toxicity to the eighth cranial nerve greatly limits dosage, and even the most recent aminoglycosides have a very low therapeutic index for infections with *P. aeruginosa*. For example, the maximum safe blood level for gentamicin is approximately 9 μg/ml, whereas its MIC for many strains of *P. aeruginosa* is 2–4 μg/ml. Monitoring blood levels during therapy is often essential to ensure adequate, yet nontoxic dosage, especially when renal impairment diminishes excretion of the antimicrobic. The mechanism of toxicity appears to involve concentration in the inner ear fluids and destruction of the critical sensory cells mediating hearing and balance.

clinical uses

synergistic activity with β-lactam antimicrobics

The clinical value of the aminoglycosides resides in their rapid bactericidal effect, their broad spectrum, the slow development of resistance to the agents now most often used, and their action against *Pseudomonas* strains that resist many other antimicrobics. They cause fewer disturbances of the normal flora than other broad-spectrum antimicrobics, probably because of their lack of activity against the predominantly anaerobic flora of the bowel, and because they are only used parenterally for systemic infections. The β-lactam antibiotics often act synergistically with the aminoglycosides, probably because they facilitate aminoglycoside penetration into the bacterial cell. This effect has been exploited in treatment of bacterial endocarditis using combinations of penicillins and aminoglycosides, and of severe *P. aeruginosa* infections using carbenicillin and one of the aminoglycosides. Synergism is apparent in both in vitro bactericidal studies and in clinical trials. Unexpectedly, it has been found that carbenicillin can slowly inactivate gentamicin in solution. Therefore, these agents are never mixed in the same intravenous bottle.

The aminoglycosides are often used in combination with a β-lactam antibiotic in the initial treatment of life-threatening infections of unknown etiology until the results of cultures are available to allow more specific therapy.

Tetracyclines

general properties

The tetracyclines are a group of antimicrobics of which the prototype, chlortetracycline, was derived from a species of *Streptomyces*. The newest agents are produced semisynthetically. All are absorbed orally and have similar and broad spectra (Appendix 10.1), with relatively inconsequential differences

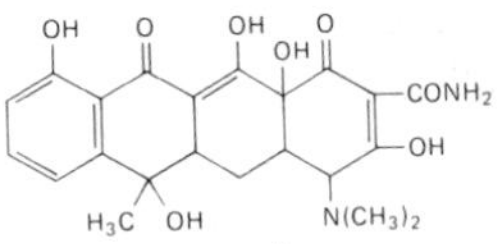
Tetracycline

in ranges of activity. Acquired resistance to one generally confers resistance to all. Chemically, the tetracyclines are polycyclic compounds that differ from each other in their side groups.

longer-acting tetracyclines

Two classes of compound are now in common use, tetracycline, which produces relatively short therapeutic levels after single doses and is about 65% protein bound, and longer-acting tetracyclines, which are more highly protein bound but are better absorbed and give higher and more prolonged blood levels. In general, they also have a slightly expanded spectrum. Minocycline and doxycycline are examples of longer-acting agents.

protein synthesis inhibitors

bacteriostatic activity

Like the aminoglycosides, the tetracyclines are inhibitors of protein synthesis. They are taken into the cell by an energy-dependent process, bind to the 30S subunit of the ribosome, and block attachment of amino-acyl transfer (t)RNA to the mRNA–ribosome complex. Unlike the aminoglycosides, their effect is reversed on dilution; thus, they are bacteriostatic rather than bactericidal agents.

spectrum of activity

broad-spectrum agents

The tetracyclines are broad-spectrum agents with a range of activity that encompasses most common pathogenic species, including Gram-positive and -negative rods and cocci and both aerobes and anaerobes. They are also active against cell-wall-deficient organisms such as *Mycoplasma* and L forms and against some obligate intracellular bacteria, including members of the genera *Rickettsia* and *Chlamydia*. There are a few minor differences in spectrum between members of the group. For example, doxycycline has some activity against tetracycline-resistant anaerobic Gram-negative rods of the genus *Bacteroides*, and minocycline has greater activity than tetracycline against meningococci and *Nocardia*.

resistance

Resistance to the tetracyclines, whether innate, mutational, or plasmid determined, appears to involve failure of the antimicrobics to permeate the cell. In contrast to most other groups of antimicrobics, inactivating enzymes do not appear to play a role. Resistant strains of most pathogenic species are now common and have been selected by the extensive use of these antimicrobics.

absorption and excretion

The tetracyclines are readily absorbed from the upper gastrointestinal tract, the usual route of administration, in the absence of divalent cations. They are chelated by Ca^{2+}, Mg^{2+}, and Al^{2+} and their absorption and activity are both reduced. Thus, tetracycline taken with dairy products or many antacid preparations may not be absorbed. Tetracyclines are excreted in the bile and urine in active form.

adverse effects

tooth discoloration

superinfection

The tetracyclines have a strong affinity for newly formed bone and for developing teeth, to which they give a yellowish color. There is a risk of staining of permanent teeth if the antibiotic is used in children up to 8 years of age in whom teeth are developing. A common complication of tetracycline therapy is gastrointestinal disturbance with nausea, vomiting, and diarrhea. This reaction is sometimes caused by direct irritation, but more often follows disturbance of the normal flora and superinfection with tetracycline-resistant bacteria or with an opportunistic yeast, *Candida albicans*. Vaginal or oral candidiasis (thrush) is a common complication of tetracycline therapy. Occasionally, severe hepatic damage can result from tetracycline therapy if blood levels are excessive.

clinical uses

Because of their broad spectrum, the tetracyclines have been used extensively in the treatment of polymicrobial infections or infections of unknown etiology derived from the respiratory or gastrointestinal tracts. They have been widely used in the treatment of otitis media and sinusitis, because the most common etiologic agents are usually susceptible. In many cases, however, they have been used in the treatment of viral infections, against which they are quite inactive.

Tetracyclines are agents of choice in the treatment of infections caused by the obligate intracellular parasites *Rickettsia* and *Chlamydia* and by *Mycoplasma*. They have been used as alternates to penicillin in the treatment of the spirochete of syphilis and of the gonococcus, although many strains of gonococci are now relatively resistant. They were used in the past as primary agents in the treatment of infections caused by intestinal anaerobes, but many are now resistant. Probably no group of antimicrobics has been more overprescribed, and thus has contributed significantly to the overall problem of resistance.

Chloramphenicol

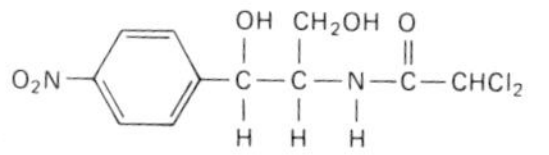

Chloramphenicol

Chloramphenicol is a broad-spectrum, orally adsorbed antimicrobic originally derived from a culture of *Streptomyces*. Its relatively simple structure allowed its complete synthesis, and it has since been produced commercially in this way.

bacteriostatic protein synthesis inhibitor

Chloramphenicol acts at the level of the 50S ribosomal subunit by inhibiting peptidyl transferase and thus prevents protein synthesis. Its action is usually reversed by dilution, and it is thus bacteriostatic. It has little effect on eukaryotic ribosomes, which explains its selective toxicity. Chloramphenicol is a broad-spectrum antibiotic that, like tetracycline, has a wide range of activity against both aerobic and anaerobic species (Appendix 10.1).

permeability into cells and across blood–brain barrier

It permeates readily into mammalian cells and is active against *Rickettsia* and *Chlamydia*. It also permeates the blood–brain barrier and attains excellent levels in the cerebrospinal fluid. Its use is restricted, however, by its occasional severe toxicity.

resistance

plasmid-determined acetylase

Acquired resistance to chloramphenicol is determined by plasmid genes coding for production of the enzyme chloramphenicol acetyl transferase. This enzyme acetylates and inactivates the antimicrobic. Resistance is most common among enteric Gram-negative rods and staphylococci, but occasionally occurs in other species, including *H. influenzae*. It is of interest that chloramphenicol resistance is much less common than tetracycline resistance, which probably reflects the less frequent use of chloramphenicol because of its toxicity.

absorption and metabolism

Chloramphenicol is readily adsorbed from the upper gastrointestinal tract. It is conjugated in the liver to the glucuronide form, which has no antimicrobial activity. Little of the dose is excreted in the urine or bile. Unlike those of most antimicrobics, urine levels of chloramphenicol are low, and it is not useful in urinary tract infections.

toxicity

bone marrow aplasia

aplastic anemia and agranulocytosis

High and prolonged doses of chloramphenicol result in some inhibition of blood-forming cells in the bone marrow (marrow hypoplasia). This inhibition is reversed on cessation of therapy and probably results from the action of the antimicrobic on mitochondrial 70S ribosomes. Occasionally, and probably by a different mechanism, progressive bone marrow aplasia with aplastic anemia and agranulocytosis develops even after low dosages and it is often fatal. The development of this complication in about 1 in 50,000 patients restricted the use of the antimicrobic to a limited number of highly specific indications. Chloramphenicol may also produce gray syndrome in the neonate, with abdominal, circulatory, and respiratory dysfunction. This syndrome, which can be fatal, results from excessive levels of active antibiotic because of failure of the infant liver to conjugate chloramphenicol to the glucuronide. Use of the drug is usually avoided in infants less than 1 month of age.

gray syndrome

clinical uses

The use of chloramphenicol is now largely restricted to treatment of severe infections for which its spectrum and diffusibility make it particularly valuable. These infections include typhoid fever, ampicillin-resistant *H. influenzae* meningitis, pyogenic coccal meningitis infections when penicillin is contraindicated, intraabdominal anaerobic Gram-negative infections, and some cases of cerebral abscess. It is also an alternative to tetracycline in the treatment of *Rickettsia* infections. Chloramphenicol is usually administered intravenously in such cases.

Erythromycin and Lincosamide Antibiotics

general properties

Erythromycin is the most commonly used of a group of antimicrobics termed the *macrolides*. The lincosamides, lincomycin and clindamycin (7-chlorolincomycin), are chemically unrelated to the macrolides but have similar modes of action and spectra, and are thus considered with them.

protein synthesis inhibitors

predominant bacteriostatic effect

spectra

Erythromycin and lincomycin are derived from different species of *Streptomyces*. Both act on protein synthesis at the ribosomal level by binding to the 50S subunit and blocking the translocation reaction. The effect on sensitive bacteria is primarily bacteriostatic, but a higher proportion of the population are killed than is the case with chloramphenicol. Erythromycin has a spectrum of activity that is close to that of benzyl penicillin, but also includes penicillinase-producing *S. aureus, Legionella pneumophila, Mycoplasma pneumoniae,* and *Chlamydia trachomatis*. Lincomycin has a generally similar spectrum. Clindamycin, a more active compound, is highly effective against many Gram-negative and Gram-positive anaerobic bacteria (Appendix 10.1).

mutational and plasmid-determined resistance

Mutational and plasmid-determined resistance occurs with both erythromycin and lincomycin. The former sometimes develops during therapy and may decrease permeability or affect the ribosomes so that the antimicrobics are not bound. Plasmid-determined resistance involves methylation of ribosomal RNA, which is induced by erythromycin and prevents its binding. Interestingly, induction with erythromycin leads to clindamycin resistance, although the reverse is unusual.

absorption and excretion

Oral and intravenous preparations of both erythromycin and the lincosamides are available. Both classes of antimicrobics are eliminated by the liver, in the bile, and, to a much lesser extent, through the kidney.

toxicity

pseudomembranous enterocolitis

Erythromycin in the estolate form can cause a reversible hepatitis, but is otherwise of low toxicity. Clindamycin can also be mildly hepatotoxic, but the most serious complication of treatment is pseudomembranous enterocolitis as a result of inhibition of most of the anaerobic flora of the bowel and overgrowth by the clindamycin-resistant *Clostridium difficile*, which elaborates an important enterotoxin. This enterotoxin is discussed in more detail in Chapter 15.

therapeutic uses

Erythromycin is the drug of choice in treating Legionnaires' disease and, in the event that they need treatment, *Campylobacter* intestinal infections. It is effective in some *Chlamydia* and *Mycoplasma* infections and can be used for many Gram-positive coccal infections when the penicillins are contraindicated.

Clindamycin has displaced lincomycin in therapy, and its major role is in treating serious infections caused by Gram-negative, or mixed, anaerobic organisms.

Sulfonamides

origin

structure

Shortly after Domagk's demonstration of the chemotherapeutic effectiveness of Prontosil rubrum in 1935, Trefouel in Paris showed that the active portion of the molecule was para-aminobenzene sulfonamide, which was termed

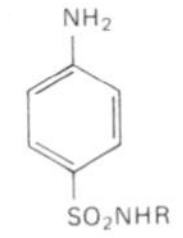

Sulfonamides

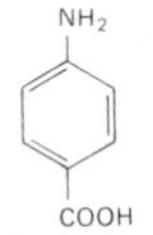

p-Aminobenzoic acid

sulfanilamide. Subsequently, numerous compounds were synthesized with substitutions of the amide group. These compounds provided increased activity and special pharmacologic properties, such as higher or more prolonged blood levels, greater solubility in urine, or failure to be absorbed from the intestinal tract.

competitive inhibition of PABA metabolism

effect on folate synthesis

explanation of selective toxicity

Sulfonamides are structural analogs of para-aminobenzoic acid (PABA), an essential metabolite involved in the pathway for folic acid synthesis for many bacteria. Sulfonamides compete for the enzyme handling PABA (dihydropterate synthetase) and block folic acid synthesis. Absence of folate inhibits a variety of metabolic processes in the cell, because the reduced form of folic acid is an essential coenzyme in the synthesis of some amino acids, purines, and thymidine, and thus indirectly of protein and DNA. Eukaryotic cells (and some bacteria) do not synthesize folate but derive folic acid from exogenous sources; they are thus unaffected by sulfonamides, which accounts for the selective toxicity of these agents. Differences in the activity of the various sulfonamides largely reflect their ability to compete with PABA for the enzyme system that handles it.

bacteriostatic

The effect of sulfonamides is exclusively bacteriostatic, and addition of PABA to a medium that contains them neutralizes the inhibitory effect and allows growth to resume. This quality is exploited in the clinical laboratory by adding PABA to blood cultures drawn from patients on sulfonamide therapy.

Spectrum

Originally, the more active sulfonamides had a very broad spectrum that included pathogenic streptococci, pneumococci, a number of enteric Gram-negative rods (especially *Escherichia coli*), the gonococcus and meningococcus, and *Chlamydia.* They also had some activity against pathogenic staphylococci and anaerobes. Unfortunately, resistance developed quickly, and their activity is now unpredictable without laboratory tests for measuring susceptibility.

Resistance

Both mutational and R-plasmid-mediated resistances are common in susceptible species. Resistance coded by R plasmids usually involves decreased permeability to sulfonamides. Mutational resistance can involve decreased affinity for sulfonamides of the enzyme handling PABA, decreased permeability, or occasionally enhanced PABA production.

Absorption and excretion

Sulfonamides are well absorbed by the oral route, except those specifically designed to act only within the intestinal tract. They penetrate readily into host cells and across the blood–brain barrier. They are excreted in the urine, predominantly in active form, and very high urine levels are achieved.

Toxicity

Most toxic effects of the sulfonamides are hypersensitivity phenomena. They include fever, rashes, and a serum-sickness-like syndrome. Occasionally, bone marrow depression occurs, which may progress to agranulocytosis or aplastic anemia. Deposition of sulfonamide crystals in the renal tubules was a problem with earlier, less soluble sulfonamides. It is now uncommon with the use of agents such as sulfisoxazole (Gantrisin).

Clinical uses

Sulfonamides are among the agents of choice for treatment of uncomplicated primary urinary tract infections, because most strains of *E. coli* encountered in the community have retained their sulfonamide susceptibility. They are also used in the treatment of some *Chlamydia* infections, in prophylaxis of meningococcal infections during epidemics caused by susceptible strains, and in the treatment of *Nocardia* infections (Chapter 26). Sulfonamides have little or no activity in abscesses or markedly purulent exudates, because disintegrating inflammatory cells provide many of the end products of folate activity that, like PABA, can neutralize the effects of sulfonamides. This neutralization accounts in part for their limited clinical usefulness compared to the more powerful antibiotics. The range of utility of sulfonamides is extended when combined with trimethoprim.

Trimethoprim

Origin

competitive inhibitor of dihydrofolate reductase

Trimethoprim is a synthetic structural analog of the pteridine portion of the folic acid molecule. It competitively inhibits the activity of bacterial dihydrofolate reductase, which catalyzes the conversion of folate to its reduced active coenzyme form. Trimethoprim has little activity against the mammalian enzyme. As would be expected, this effect is not neutralized by PABA, but can be reversed by end products of essential reactions for which tetrahydrofolate serves as a coenzyme, particularly by thymidine. Trimethoprim is primarily bacteriostatic. When combined with a sulfonamide, the sequential blockade of the pathway leading to production of tetrahydrofolate often results in synergistic bacteriostatic or bactericidal effects. This quality is exploited in therapeutic preparations combining both agents in concentrations designed to give optimum synergy in vivo.

Bacteriostatic

Synergism of mixtures with sulfonamides

Spectrum

Trimethoprim inhibits a considerable range of Gram-positive and Gram-negative facultative bacteria (Appendix 10.1), including those causing enteric and urinary tract infections. It is also active against some eukaryotic pathogens, including the malarial parasite and *Pneumocystis carinii* (Chapter 48).

Resistance

Acquired resistance can be mutational or plasmid mediated. The latter involves production of large amounts of a plasmid-coded tetrahydrofolate reductase for which trimethoprim has a lower affinity.

Absorption excretion, and toxicity

Trimethoprim is readily absorbed by mouth and is excreted in the urine, yielding very high levels. Combinations with sulfonamides have a range of toxicities similar to that of the sulfonamides themselves. The most important potential side effect of trimethoprim is folate deficiency. Despite its poor affinity for mammalian dihydrofolate reductase, those on the verge of folate deficiency may develop it during trimethoprim therapy. For this reason, trimethoprim is avoided in the newborn and during pregnancy.

Clinical uses

Trimethoprim is used alone in the treatment of many urinary tract infections caused by susceptible organisms. It has been found effective in combination with sulfonamides in the treatment of otitis media and sinusitis (partly because of its activity against *H. influenzae*), prostatitis, typhoid fever, and bacillary dysentry.

Polypeptide Antibiotics

A number of polypeptide antimicrobics are produced by bacteria of the genus *Bacillus,* which are aerobic, Gram-positive, spore-forming rods living primarily in soil. All of the polypeptide antibiotics are relatively toxic, and those with major activity against Gram-positive cocci, such as bacitracin, are only used topically because many better agents are available for systemic use. Polymyxin B, however, is occasionally used systemically because of its activity against *P. aeruginosa,* which is resistant to many other antimicrobics.

polymyxin activity against *P. aeruginosa*

Detergentlike effect on cell membrane

bactericidal activity

Toxicity

Polymyxin B has a cationic detergentlike effect. It combines with the cell membrane of susceptible organisms, alters its permeability, and leads to loss of essential cytoplasmic components and bacterial death. As it is not absorbed orally, it must be administered intravenously. Its reactivity with cell membranes extends to those of the host, resulting in nephrotoxicity and neurotoxicity. Polymyxin B is now essentially restricted to the treatment of serious *P. aeruginosa* infections caused by strains resistant to safer drugs such as carbenicillin and the aminoglycosides.

Vancomycin

Bactericidal activity

Gram-positive spectrum

Activity against methicillin- and cephalosporin-resistant staphylococci

Vancomycin is a bactericidal antibiotic that prevents cell wall synthesis by acting at an earlier stage of the synthetic process than the penicillins. It is active against certain Gram-positive organisms, particularly staphylococci. It must be given intravenously for systemic infections, because it is not absorbed from the gastrointestinal tract and is toxic to tissues on injection. It may cause thrombophlebitis of the vein into which it is injected. It also has some nephrotoxicity and may cause nerve deafness.

Vancomycin was displaced some years ago by the penicillinase-resistant penicillins and cephalosporins in the treatment of penicillin-resistant *S. aureus* infections, except in those patients with hypersensitivity to β-lactam antibiotics. The emergence of strains resistant to these antimicrobics, however, has led to increased use of vancomycin again. Its bactericidal effect is rapid, and it has sometimes successfully eradicated staphylococcal infections on implanted plastic devices without requiring their removal.

Table 10.4 Some Other Antibacterial Antimicrobics

Compound	Route of Administration		Mechanism	Major Spectrum	Clinical Usage	Special Properties
	Parenteral	Oral				
Nalidixic acid	–	+	DNA synthesis inhibition	Enteric Gram-negative rods	Urinary tract infections	Absent blood levels, high mutation rate to resistance
Nitrofurantoin	–	+	?	Enteric Gram-negative rods and enterococci	Urinary tract infections	Absent blood levels
Spectinomycin	+	–	Protein synthesis inhibition	Gonococcus	Penicillin-resistant gonorrhea	Unique aminoglycoside
Rifampin	–	+	Blocks initiation of translation	Gram-positive bacteria, Neisseria, and Mycobacteria	Tuberculosis meningococcal carriage	High mutation rate to resistance
p-Aminosalicyclic acid	–	+	PABA antagonist	Mycobacteria	Tuberculosis	Gastrointestinal disturbances
Isoniazid	–	+	? Inhibition of lipid synthesis	Mycobacteria	Tuberculosis	Neurotoxicity and nephrotoxicity
Ethambutol	–	+	?	Mycobacteria	Tuberculosis	Visual disturbances
Sulfones	–	+	PABA antagonists	*Mycobacterium leprae*	Leprosy	Anemia; hypersensitivity reactions
Metronidazole	–	+	Interference with anaerobic metabolism	Anaerobic Gram-negative rods; some protozoa	Anaerobic infections	? Teratogenic

Abbreviations: PABA = para-aminobenzoic acid. ? = mechanisms yet to be fully determined.

Other Clinically Valuable Antibacterial Agents

Several other effective antimicrobics are in use for special types of infections such as tuberculosis, urinary tract infections, and anaerobic infections. It is beyond the scope and intent of this book to provide comprehensive coverage of all available agents, if only because the field is rapidly changing. Table 10.4 lists a number of the commonly used agents that are not discussed herein, together with their more important properties and uses.

Laboratory Tests in Chemotherapy

Uses of laboratory tests

The discovery of the great majority of effective antimicrobics and the characterization of their spectra were based on in vitro tests in the laboratory, and similar tests have become increasingly important in clinical work. Susceptibility tests to determine the responsiveness of individual strains of a species are often needed when resistance has become common through widespread use of the antimicrobic. Tests to determine bactericidal activity of single or combined antimicrobics are used increasingly because infections in immunocompromised patients may only be controlled by agents or combinations that will kill the infecting strain in the absence of host defense factors. Measurements of levels of antimicrobics in blood or other fluids have become routine with those agents, such as the aminoglycosides, for which the toxic and therapeutic levels are relatively close. It is, therefore, important to understand the principle of these tests.

Antimicrobic susceptibility tests

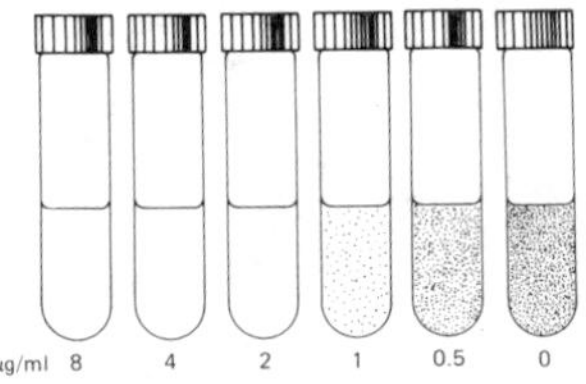

Dilution susceptibility test

Antimicrobic susceptibility tests, which are used to determine the inhibitory activity of an antimicrobic against a particular strain, are of two broad classes termed *dilution* and *diffusion tests.* Dilution susceptibility tests are the most direct. In a typical macrodilution test, twofold dilutions of the antimicrobic are prepared in 1-ml amounts of broth in test tubes to span a clinically significant range of concentrations. A control tube without antimicrobic is included. One-milliliter quantities of broth containing 10^5–10^6 bacteria to be tested are then added to each tube, thus diluting the original antimicrobic concentration in half. The tubes are incubated overnight and examined for turbidity from bacterial growth. The least amount of antimicrobic to prevent any visible growth is taken as the MIC of the organism.

Macrodilution tests such as that described are cumbersome, and mechanized, automated, and microdilution test procedures have been developed for routine use. Results of susceptibility test procedures are influenced by a variety of methodologic factors; however, reference procedures and standard control strains of defined performance have allowed the different routine procedures to give reasonably comparable results. In most clinical situations, successful treatment requires that the MIC of an antimicrobic for an organism should be substantially below the level achieved at the site of infection.

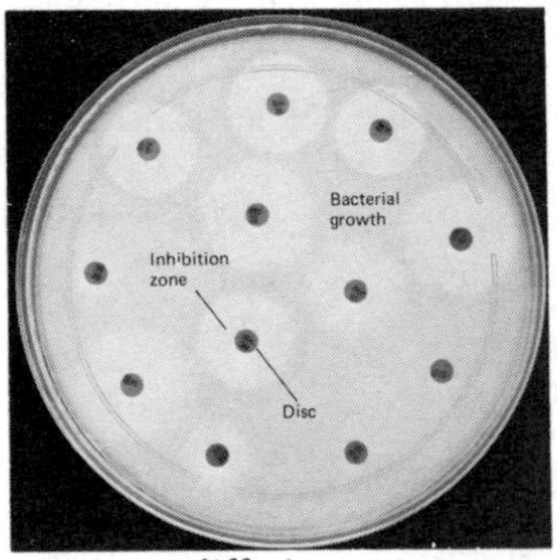

diffusion test

Diffusion susceptibility tests are less direct, but are simple, economic, and flexible for routine use. A standardized inoculum of the organism to be tested is seeded onto the surface of an agar plate, and filter paper discs containing defined amounts of antimicrobics are applied. The plates are then incubated overnight. The antimicrobic diffuses from each disc into the medium at a rate dependent on its chemical and physical characteristics. Zones of inhibition of growth of the organism develop, the diameter of which is determined by the susceptibility (MIC) of the organism, its growth rate, and the diffusibility of the antimicrobic. For common pathogenic bacteria such as the Enterobacteriaceae, *Pseudomonas,* staphylococci, and enterococci, differences in growth rate are relatively unimportant, and there is an inverse linear relationship between log MIC of such organisms and zone diameter. Thus, semiquantitative susceptibilities can be determined by a standardized procedure. The National Committee for Clinical Laboratory Standards (Kirby–Bauer) method used in the United States is such a standardized diffusion procedure. The diameters of the zones of inhibition obtained with the various antibiotics are measured and converted to "sensitive," "resistant," and "intermediate" categories by reference to a table. *Sensitive* implies that the organism is readily inhibited by the concentrations of antibiotic attainable in the blood (or urine, in the case of those agents only active in the urinary tract) with doses appropriate for treatment of uncomplicated systemic infections caused by the infecting organism. *Resistant* implies that the organism is not inhibited by normally attainable levels. Organisms in the *intermediate* range should be specially studied if therapy with that agent is to be used. The categories were developed by comparisons of zone diameter, MIC, and blood level data and from studies on the distribution of zone diameters (susceptibilities) of many species of known clinical responsiveness.

Interpretation of categories of susceptibility

Resistance and sensitivity are not always absolute. For example, relatively nontoxic antimicrobial agents, such as the penicillins or cephalosporins, can be administered in massive doses and may thereby inhibit some pathogens that would normally be considered resistant in vitro. Furthermore, in urinary infections, urine levels of some antimicrobics may be very high, and organisms that are seemingly resistant in vitro may be eliminated. When such therapy is considered, dilution tests are often needed for guidance. Diffusion tests with slow-growing organisms and with very poorly diffusing antimicrobics such as the polymyxins must be interpreted with caution. Resistance is significant, but sensitivity may need checking by a dilution test if systemic infections are to be treated. Obviously, diffusion tests do not measure bactericidal effects.

qualifications to resistance and sensitivity

Tests of Bactericidal Activity

Killing curves

Broth dilution tests can be adapted to determine the bactericidal or bacteriostatic effects of the antimicrobic on the organism tested. The number of viable organisms in the inoculum is measured, and samples are removed at intervals from tubes containing antimicrobic for viable counts (Chapter 2). Such counts can indicate the rate of killing if precautions are taken to ensure that the entire inoculum is exposed to antimicrobic and that antimicrobic carried over to the counting medium is either sufficiently diluted or neutralized to prevent any inhibition on the agar plate. A more commonly used procedure is simple measurement of the MBC, which is defined as the least amount of antimicrobic to kill 99.9% of an inoculum under standardized conditions after overnight incubation. Unfortunately, this measurement is subject to a series of technical problems that make it considerably less valuable than the more complex study of the rate of killing.

MBC tests

Limits of Sensitivity Tests

Other factors influencing selection of antimicrobic

In selecting therapy, the results of laboratory tests cannot be taken alone, but must be considered with information about the clinical pharmacology of the agent, the cause of the disease, the site of infection, and the pathology of the lesion. All of these factors will be taken into account in selecting the appropriate antimicrobic from those to which the organism has been reported as sensitive. Obviously, if the agent cannot reach the site of infection (for example, within an abscess), it will be ineffective. Furthermore, in some instances (for example, bacterial endocarditis or agranulocytosis), it is necessary to use an agent that is bactericidal, and an ordinary sensitivity test will not indicate this property. Previous clinical experience is also critical. In typhoid fever, for instance, chloramphenicol is effective and aminoglycosides are not, even though the typhoid bacillus may be sensitive to both in vitro. This finding appears to result from the failure of aminoglycosides to achieve adequate concentrations inside infected cells.

Antimicrobic Assays

Physical, chemical, and immunologic procedures

Levels of antimicrobic in blood and body fluids may be measured biologically or, in some cases, by techniques such as high-pressure liquid chromatography or radioimmunoassay. In the usual bioassay, a large agar plate is seeded with a stock strain of an organism (for example, *Sarcina lutea*) highly susceptible to the antimicrobic to be assayed. A series of spaced holes are then made in the plate by removing plugs of agar. Some are filled with different concentrations of a standard preparation of the antimicrobic, others with the material to be assayed. After overnight incubation the diameters of the zones of inhibition that develop around the holes are measured, and a curve is plotted from the standards to relate antimicrobic concentration to zone sizes. The concentration of antimicrobic in the material being assayed can then be determined by translating the zone diameter that it yields to its concentration using the standard curve. It is important for the laboratory to know whether more than one antimicrobic is being used to treat a patient, so that steps are taken to ensure that only the activity of the agent under consideration is being measured. For example, if gentamicin levels are to be measured in the presence of carbenicillin, a β-lactamase preparation can be added to inactivate the penicillin.

Bioassay

Other Tests

Tests of serum activity against infecting strain

Sometimes it is desirable to determine directly the effectiveness of antimicrobic levels in the patient's serum against the infecting organism. Dilutions of the patient's serum can be made in normal serum and equal amounts of broth added containing 10^5/ml of the infecting organism. After incubation, the inhibitory activity and, if desired, the lethal activity are measured as in MIC and MBC tests and expressed according to effective dilutions of the patients' serum. Tests of the activity of combinations of antimicrobial agents are sometimes important. These tests are made by inoculating the infecting organism into broth containing clinically relevant amounts of the antibiotics being studied, both alone and in combination. The tubes are incubated and quantitative counts made at intervals. This approach will indicate whether the effects of the combinations are synergistic, additive, or antagonistic.

Tests of antibiotic combinations

Antifungal Antimicrobics

Fungi are eukaryotic organisms with cell surface structures, cell membranes, and ribosomes different from those of the prokaryotic bacteria. Thus, antibacterial agents are usually ineffective against fungi. There are, however, several effective antifungal antimicrobics that depend on differences between fungal and mammalian cells.

The *polyene antifungal* antimicrobics are complex macrolide antifungal agents derived from species of *Streptomyces.* Several have been described, but only two, nystatin and amphotericin B, are commonly used to treat human infections. Their action depends on the presence of ergosterol in the fungal cell membrane, to which they attach. They then alter the permeability of the membrane, which leads to loss of vital cytoplasmic components and cell death. Bacterial cell membranes contain no sterols, and cholesterol,

activity of polyenes on cytoplasmic membrane

which predominates in mammalian cell membranes, has less affinity for polyenes.

nystatin

Nystatin is highly toxic when given parenterally, and its use is largely limited to topical application for the treatment of superficial yeast infections of the skin, vagina, or oral cavity.

amphotericin B

value and toxicity of amphotericin B in systemic fungal infections

Amphotericin B is administered intravenously in many severe systemic fungal infections (Chapters 31 and 32). It is sometimes given intrathecally in the treatment of fungal meningitis. It is effective against a wide range of fungi, but has considerable toxicity, particularly to the kidneys, because of some attachment to cholesterol of the host cell membranes. Thus, its therapeutic index is low, but it remains the antimicrobic of choice for most severe fungal infections because of its fungicidal properties.

fungistatic effects

The *imidazole antifungal* agents alter membrane permeability of susceptible yeasts and fungi, probably by inhibiting ergosterol synthesis. Buildup of hydrogen peroxide in the cells may also contribute to inhibition. Their major effects are fungistatic rather than fungicidal.

topical use of miconazole

ketaconazole in systemic infections

hepatotoxicity of ketaconazole

Two major imidazoles are now available. Miconazole is used primarily for topical application to superficial yeast and fungal infections. Ketaconazole, the most recently developed imidazole, is readily absorbed orally and has a wide spectrum of activity against yeasts and systemic and opportunistic fungi. Unfortunately, relapses are common on cessation of treatment, particularly in immunocompromised individuals, because of the purely fungistatic action of the drug. Furthermore, with increased experience, ketaconazole has been found to have considerable and sometimes serious toxicity to the liver. Nevertheless, it is considerably less toxic than amphotericin B and, whether used alone or in combination with amphotericin, its development constitutes a significant advance in the treatment of serious systemic infections.

buildup in keratin; activity against dermatophytes

duration of therapy

Griseofulvin is produced by a *Penicillium* mold. It is readily absorbed from the upper gastrointestinal tract and is taken up in high concentrations by newly formed keratin in the skin. It has inhibitory activity against a variety of fungi (dermatophytes) that cause superficial skin or nail infections. It takes a considerable time to act effectively, however, because synthesis of new keratin is required to bring it into contact with the fungus for effective action. Thus, it may be necessary to continue treatment of severe fungus infections of the nails for several months. Griseofulvin is believed to inhibit synthesis of fungal cell walls.

Effect against yeasts

Development of resistance

5-Fluorocytosine (flucytosine) was originally developed and tested for the treatment of cancer. It is a pyrimidine analog that inhibits DNA synthesis and has specific activity against certain yeasts. It is readily absorbed by the oral route to yield high levels in the blood. It is lethal to susceptible yeasts, but unfortunately also has some toxicity to the blood-forming cells in the bone marrow. Some strains of yeast are resistant to 5-fluorocytosine on first isolation, and resistant mutants are frequently selected during therapy.

Antiviral Agents

Sites of attack of antiviral agents

Because the method of replication of viruses is so intimately associated with the metabolism of the host cell (Chapter 3), there is less opportunity for the development of nontoxic agents that attack the processes of viral synthesis than for agents that inhibit bacterial or fungal growth. Nevertheless, viral attachment, penetration, and assembly are rather unique processes, and certain virus-specified enzymes required for replication offer sites of attack. These characteristics have been exploited with some clinically useful agents.

At present, antiviral agents have been most applicable to infections caused by the larger, more complex viruses and to those that become rapidly apparent because they affect body surfaces or the respiratory tract. The principal agents in current use are considered as follows.

Amantidine and rimantidine

prophylaxis of influenza infection

Amantidine and rimantidine are synthetic amines that specifically block the uncoating of influenza A viruses, but are inactive against influenza B virus. They are taken by mouth, have low toxicity, and have been used to provide temporary protection during acute epidemics to particularly susceptible subjects, such as nursing home residents. The agents have also been reported to reduce the severity of the disease if given within the first few hours of development of symptoms.

Idoxuridine

Trifluorothymidine

Idoxuridine, 5-iodo-2′-deoxyuridine (IUdR) is a halogenated pyrimidine that blocks nucleic acid synthesis through incorporation into DNA in place of thymidine to produce a nonfunctional molecule. Systemically it has considerable toxicity, but can be used locally as an effective treatment for herpetic infection of the cornea (keratitis). Trifluorothymidine is another pyrimidine analog effective in the treatment of herpetic infections of the cornea, including those caused by some strains that fail to respond to IUdR.

Adenine arabinoside

Adenine arabinoside (vidarabine) is a purine that inhibits DNA polymerase and has some selective action, in that herpes group viral polymerases are about 15–30 times more susceptible than the host cell enzyme. When given intravenously, adenine arabinoside reduces the mortality of herpes encephalitis, and it has been shown useful in the treatment of neonatal herpes simplex infection and herpes zoster in immunocompromised patients. It is used topically for treatment of herpetic infections of the eye, in which it has approximately the same effectiveness as IUdR. It is less toxic than IUdR, but can lead to destruction of blood-forming elements in the bone marrow with high dosages.

Acyclovir

mode of inhibition of herpes viral DNA polymerase

use in herpes virus infection

Acyclovir (acycloguanosine), a new and promising agent, serves as a substrate for virus-specified thymidine kinase produced by the herpes group of viruses, but not for host cell thymidine kinase. The triphosphate derivative produced by the enzyme inhibits viral DNA polymerase. Because of its mode of action, acyclovir has little toxicity to the host cell. This agent is effective in reducing the severity and duration of primary herpes simplex attacks and of disseminated varicella-zoster infections in immunocompromised patients.

ribavirin

Ribavirin is a synthetic nucleoside that is active in vitro and in vivo in experimental animals against a range of DNA and RNA viruses. It inhibits the synthesis of guanosine 5′-phosphate, which is required for synthesis of viral nucleic acid. It shows some promise for use as an aerosol in the prevention and treatment of some respiratory viral infections, especially influenza A and B, and respiratory syncytial viral infection.

Methisazone

Poxvirus inhibition

Methisazone (*N*-methylistan-β-thiosemicarbazone) is a specific inhibitor of poxvirus infections by blocking late viral protein synthesis. It thus leads to production of incomplete virus. It has been proved effective in the prophylaxis of poxvirus infections but, because of the elimination of smallpox from the world, it now is of historic interest only in human medicine.

Interferons

The interferons and their role in defense against viral infections have been considered in Chapter 7. Definition of their role in the therapy or prophylaxis of viral infections has been restricted because of their host specificity and the difficulty of obtaining sufficient leukocyte interferon for clinical trials. Most interferon inducers, such as synthetic double-stranded RNAs and endotoxin, produce too many side effects to be effectively employed.

production of interferon by recombinant DNA techniques

This situation is now changing rapidly, because the application of recombinant DNA techniques has allowed the relatively inexpensive production of human interferon by some bacteria and yeasts. Current results indicate a definite role of interferon in the treatment or prophylaxis of herpes zoster possible wide spectrum of clinical usefulness

and cytomegalovirus infections in immunocompromised patients and in the treatment of chronic active hepatitis B liver infection. Topical application under experimental conditions has been shown to have an effect in preventing colds caused by one type of rhinovirus, but it is unclear whether this approach will have practical clinical application. Unfortunately, the interferon preparations that have been tested clinically all show some toxicity in the doses used, and it remains to be determined whether other interferons will prove more effective and less toxic for therapy and prophylaxis.

Epidemiology of Antimicrobic Resistance

Development of Increased Resistance

Response predictable when antimicrobics first introduced

Development of resistance and multiresistance

When each antimicrobic was first introduced, its activity against individual isolates of a species was almost completely predictable from studies of its spectrum of activity. Some species were uniformly naturally resistant, and others were susceptible with few, if any, exceptions. With the use of most antimicrobics, resistant strains of many previously susceptible species became increasingly common—sometimes very rapidly—with serious clinical and epidemiologic consequences. For example, most strains of *S. aureus* were fully susceptible to penicillin when it was first introduced in 1944. By 1950, only about 30% of hospital isolates were susceptible; the current figure is about 15%, and many isolates are multiresistant to several previously active antimicrobics. Similarly, many enteric Gram-negative rods developed resistance to antimicrobics such as ampicillin, cephalosporins, tetracycline, chloramphenicol, and aminoglycosides, with many strains becoming multiresistant to as many as 15 agents. Fortunately, these developments have not been universal, and the spirochete of syphilis, the meningococcus, and the group A streptococcus, for example, have thus far retained their susceptibility to penicillin. Even this list may change, however, because 5 years ago it would have included the pneumococcus, but resistant strains of this organism have now been isolated in many countries.

Some species retain predictable susceptibility

Origin of Resistant Strains

Selection of preexisting resistant strains

Resistant mutants

Plasmid-determined resistance

Transposable elements

Resistant strains were occasionally found in a very small proportion of members of a species before introduction of an antimicrobic, and their proportion was greatly increased by its use. This situation was unusual, but partly explains the origin of penicillinase-producing *S. aureus*. In other cases, resistance involved the mutational or recombinational events discussed in Chapter 5. Most resistant mutants are genetically unstable in the absence of the selecting agent, but some, such as low-level penicillin-resistant gonococci and pneumococci and streptomycin-resistant mycobacteria, retain their virulence and can undergo epidemiologic spread. More important, plasmids carrying resistance markers have little, if any, adverse influence on the capacity of most organisms to survive, spread, and infect, and they frequently confer multiresistance. Transposable resistance genes introduce considerable genetic plasticity, and resistance determinants to new antimicrobics can be added to plasmids very quickly.

The origin of plasmid-carried determinants of resistance remains somewhat obscure. Some known to have preexisted the clinical use of the antimicrobic may have played a role in nature by protecting an organism against another that produced the agent. Some may have been derived from antibiotic-producing *Streptomyces*, in which they served to protect the cell from its own antibiotic. Some may have been chromosomal genes transposed to plasmids, and some may have been plasmid genes that mutated to provide altered specificity.

Enhancement and Spread of Resistance

Effect of antimicrobics on susceptibility to infection with resistant strains

ecologic vacuum

The central factors involved in increasing incidences of resistance are the selective effect of the use of antimicrobics, the spread of infection in human populations, and the ability of plasmids to cross species lines. Use of antimicrobics therapeutically or prophylactically, particularly agents with a broad spectrum of activity, produces a relative ecologic vacuum on surface lesions or in normal floral sites and allows resistant organisms to colonize or infect with less competition from others. In the case of multiresistance, treatment with a single antimicrobic may select for strains that are also resistant to many other agents. Thus, chemotherapy can both enhance the opportunity for acquiring resistant strains from other sources and increase their numbers in the body. The amplifying effect of antimicrobic therapy on resistance is also apparent with the transfer of resistance plasmids to previously susceptible strains. This effect occurs primarily in the lower intestinal tract, where the antimicrobic may reduce the flora resulting in an increased oxidation–reduction potential that favors plasmid transfer to the same or other species.

amplification of resistance with R plasmid transfer

example of acquisition and spread of plasmid-borne resistance determinants

As an example, consider a patient harboring as a very small part of his facultative intestinal flora a strain of *E. coli* carrying a plasmid coding for resistance to tetracycline, ampicillin, chloramphenicol, and the sulfonamides. He develops an infection with a *Shigella* dysentery bacillus susceptible to all of these antimicrobial agents and is treated with tetracycline. Most of the normal flora and the *Shigella* are inhibited, and the resistant *E. coli* becomes predominant because its multiplication is not impeded and competition is removed. Plasmid transfer occurs between the resistant *E. coli* and some surviving *Shigella*; the latter then multiply, causing a relapse of the disease with a strain that is now multiresistant. Any endemic or epidemic spread of dysentery from this patient to others will now be with the multiresistant *Shigella* strain, and its ability to infect will be enhanced if the recipient is on prophylaxis or therapy with any of the four antimicrobics to which it is resistant.

characterization and tracing of the spread of R plasmids

Such occurrences are commonplace and involve both virulent organisms and members of the normal flora, especially enteric Gram-negative rods. They account for the much higher incidence of resistance and multiresistance that characterizes hospital-acquired as opposed to community-acquired strains. Techniques have been developed for characterizing plasmids by molecular weight and "fingerprinting" them by demonstrating the pattern of fragments produced by restriction endonucleases. Thus, it has been possible to trace "epidemic" spread of plasmids through different species of organisms.

Major Selective Factors

Central role of hospital in antimicrobic resistance

community-acquired resistance

The hospital remains the major source and reservoir of resistant organisms that affect humans, although similar selection and spread occur in the community. Isolates of group A β-hemolytic streptococci and pneumococci are frequently resistant to tetracycline and reflect the widespread and often inappropriate community use of that agent. Most strains of gonococci now show substantially higher resistance to penicillin than was the case when the antibiotic was introduced.

environmental contamination and animal feed supplementation

There are selective factors other than use of antimicrobics in therapy and prophylaxis. Antimicrobic contamination of the hospital environment, as with antimicrobic from aerosols produced during administration or from high concentrations in urine, may be sufficient to inhibit the susceptible normal flora of the anterior nares of personnel and increase the carriage rate of resistant *S. aureus*. This contamination has been shown to occur in human and veterinary hospitals and in an antibiotic processing plant, and its significance requires further study. Much attention has been paid to the use of antimicrobics in animal feeds both prophylactically and for their growth-promoting effects, which are economically important but involve mechanisms not yet fully characterized. Cattle or poultry that consume feed supplemented with antimicrobics rapidly develop a resistant enteric flora that spreads throughout the herd. Resistance is largely plasmid determined and has been shown capable of spreading to the flora of farmers and of those living in close proximity to cattle-rearing farms. *Salmonella* species, which commonly infect intensively raised cattle and poultry, usually acquire the resistance plasmids, and zoonotic spread to humans can result in individual infections or epidemics caused by multiresistant *Salmonella*. Except for these specific examples, there is little clear evidence that antimicrobics in animal feeds are a major component of the resistance problem in humans; nonetheless, many countries have banned or controlled such use of antimicrobics that are useful for systemic therapy in humans. An important theoretic concern is that stabilization of plasmids may occur under such intensive pressure, and that they may then persist and spread in the absence of the selective effect of antimicrobics and acquire other undesirable genetic traits, such as enhanced virulence. The major problem in human medicine, however, remains the large-scale use of antimicrobics for treating actual or assumed infections and epidemiologic spread of resistant strains both in hospitals and in the community under the selective pressure of antimicrobic use.

concern of stabilization of R plasmids

Control of Resistance

loss of resistance on withdrawal of selective agent

In the past, numerous examples in the literature showed that the extent of resistance in a hospital directly reflects the extent of usage of an antimicrobic, and that withdrawal or control can lead to rapid reduction of the incidence of resistance. Obviously such measures will have little impact on the level of resistance in the community, and they can rarely be applied in practice. It is also possible that some resistance determinants have now become so stabilized that they are less likely to be lost in the absence of the selective agent. Experience and our understanding of the mechanisms and spread of resistance, however, indicate certain principles that can help to keep the problem under control, can sometimes reverse it, and are compatible with good therapeutic practice:

Principles for controlling resistance

1. Conservative and specific use of antimicrobics in therapy.
2. Adequate dosage and duration of therapy to eliminate the infecting organism and reduce the risk of selecting resistant variants.
3. Whenever possible, selection of antimicrobics according to the proved or anticipated known susceptibility of the infecting strain.
4. Use, when possible, of narrow rather than broad-spectrum antimicrobics when the specific etiology of an infection is known.
5. Use of antimicrobic combinations known to prevent emergence of resistant mutants in diseases like tuberculosis.
6. Prophylactic use of antimicrobics only in situations in which it has been proved valuable and for the shortest possible time to avoid selection of a resistant flora.
7. Avoidance of environmental contamination.
8. Application of careful, standard aseptic and hand-washing procedures to help to prevent spread of resistant organisms.

9. Use of containment isolation procedures for patients infected with resistant organisms that pose a threat to others and of protective precautions for those who are highly susceptible.
10. Epidemiologic monitoring for resistant organisms or determinants in an institution, and the application of enhanced control measures if a problem develops.
11. Restriction of the use of therapeutically valuable antimicrobics for nonmedical purposes.

Appendix 10.1 Usual Susceptibility Patterns of Common Bacteria to Some Commonly Used Bacteriostatic and Bactericidal Antimicrobics

Antimicrobic	Bactericidal	Bacteriostatic	*Staphylococcus aureus*	Enterococci	Other streptococci	*Neisseria*	*Haemophilus*	*Legionella*	*Mycoplasma*	*Escherichia coli*	*Proteus mirabilis*	Other *Proteus* spp.	*Klebsiella*	*Enterobacter*	*Serratia*	*Pseudomonas aeruginosa*	*Bacteroides fragilis*	Other Gram-ve anaerobes	*Clostridium*	*Rickettsia*	*Chlamydia*	
Benzyl penicillin	+		1 ◕	C ▨	1 ◔	1 ◔	▨◔	●	●	●	▨	●	●	●	●	●	●	1 ◔	1 ○	●	●	Narrow-spectrum agents
Penicillinase-resistant penicillins	+		1 ◔	●	2 ◔	●	●	●	●	●	●	●	●	●	●	●	●	●	●	●	●	Narrow-spectrum agents
Erythromycin	±	+	2 ◔	1 ○	2 ◔	◔	–	1 ○	1 ○	●	●	●	●	●	●	●	–	–	–	–	2 ○	Narrow-spectrum agents
Clindamycin	±	+	2 ◔	–	◔	●	●	–	–	●	●	●	●	●	●	●	1 ◔	1 ◔	–	–	–	Narrow-spectrum agents
Vancomycin	+		2 ○	1 ○	2 ○	●	●	●	●	●	●	●	●	●	●	●	–	–	1 ○	–	–	Narrow-spectrum agents
Ampicillin	+		2 ◕	1 ◔	2 ◔	1 ◔	1 ◔	●	●	1 ◔	1 ◔	●	●	●	●	●	●	–	1 ○	●	●	Broad-spectrum agents
Piperacillin	+		–	○	○	–	◔	●	●	–	1 ○	1 ◔	1 ◔	1 ◔	1 ◔	1 ◔	2 ◔	1 ○	–	●	●	Broad-spectrum agents
Cephalothin	+		2 ◔	●	2 ◔	–	●	●	●	◔	○	●	◔	●	●	●	●	◔	◔	●	●	Broad-spectrum agents
Cefoxitin	+		–	●	1 ○	1 ○	–	●	●	1 ○	1 ○	1 ○	1 ○	●	◔	◔	2 ◔	○	–	●	●	Broad-spectrum agents
Cefaperazone	+		–	–	–	–	○	●	●	1 ○	1 ○	1 ○	1 ○	2 ◔	2 ◔	◔	◔	–	–	●	●	Broad-spectrum agents
Gentamicin	+		◔	C ●	●	–	–	●	–	1 ◔	1 ○	1 ○	1 ◔	1 ◔	1 ◔	1 ◔	●	●	●	–	–	Broad-spectrum agents
Amikacin	+		◔	C ●	●	–	–	●	–	1 ◔	1 ○	1 ○	1 ◔	1 ◔	1 ◔	1 ◔	●	●	●	–	–	Broad-spectrum agents
Tetracycline		+	◔	●	◕	◔	○	2 ○	1 ○	◔	●	●	◔	◔	◕	●	◑	◔	◔	1 ○	1 ○	Broad-spectrum agents
Chloramphenicol		+	◔	◔	◔	◔	2 ◔	●	–	◔	◔	◔	◔	◔	○	●	1 ◔	2 ○	–	1 ○	–	Broad-spectrum agents
Sulfonamides		+	–	●	◔	◔	◔	●	–	1 ◔	●	●	–	◔	–	●	–	–	–	●	3 –	Broad-spectrum agents
Sulfamethoxazole + trimethoprim	±	+	–	–	–	–	1 ◔	–	–	1 ◔	◔	◔	◔	◔	◔	●	–	–	–	–	3 –	Broad-spectrum agents

Proportions of susceptible and resistant strains: ○ = 100% susceptible; ◔ = 25% resistant; ● = 100% resistant; ▨ = intermediate susceptibility.

Abbreviations: – = no present indication for therapy or insufficient data; 1 = antimicrobic of choice for susceptible strains; 2 = second-line agent; 3 = *C. trachomatis* sensitive, *C. psittaci* resistant; C = useful in combination of a β-lactam and an aminoglycoside.

These data reflect results in a single institution. Proportions of resistant strains may vary in different locations.

Behavioral aspects of problem of antimicrobic resistance

The problem of antimicrobic resistance and its spread has a considerable behavioral component. Needless and excessive therapy, failure to observe basic rules for preventing spread of infection to others, and lack of understanding of the process all serve to increase the problem. Conversely, intelligent, conservative, and specific use of chemotherapy with adequate precautions to prevent cross-infection provides the best chance of retaining the value of many of the agents we now possess.

Additional Reading and References

Falkow, S. 1975. *Infectious Multiple Drug Resistance.* New York: Academic Press. An excellent account of the genetics, molecular biology, ecology, and clinical significance of R factors.

Gilman, A.G., Goodman, L.S., and Gilman, A., Eds. 1980. *The Pharmacological Basis of Therapeutics*, 6th ed. New York: Macmillan. A standard reference text with excellent sections on antibiotics and chemotherapy.

Pratt, W.B. 1977. *Chemotherapy of Infection.* New York: Oxford University Press. An exceptionally informative and well-written account of basic chemotherapy and the characteristics of antibiotics.

Tompkins, L.S., Plorde, J.J., and Falkow, S. 1980. Molecular analysis of R factors from multi-resistant nosocomial isolates. *J. Infect. Dis.* 141:625–636. An excellent description of the use of newer methods to analyze the spread of R plasmids.

John C. Sherris

Staphylococci

11

Gram-positive cocci in clusters

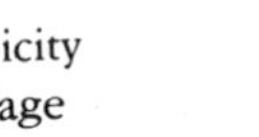

Staphylococcus

Members of the genus *Staphylococcus* (commonly called *staphylococci*) are round, Gram-positive cocci that can divide in any plane and tend to be arranged in grapelike clusters (from the Greek *staphyle,* bunch of grapes). Some single cells and pairs are also seen. Occasional short chains, which can occur as a chance feature of the organisms' mode of division, should not be confused with the regular occurrence of chains among the streptococci. Staphylococci have a typical Gram-positive cell wall structure. Like all medically important cocci, they are nonflagellate, nonmotile, and non-spore forming.

facultative

catalase production

Staphylococci grow best aerobically, but are facultatively anaerobic. They can oxidize or ferment various carbohydrates. Unenriched nutrient broth or nutrient agar supports their growth, and their doubling time (mean generation time) can be as short as 20 min. In contrast to streptococci, staphylococci produce catalase.

There are three medically important species of staphylococci: *Staphylococcus aureus, Staphylococcus epidermidis,* and *Staphylococcus saprophyticus.*

S. aureus

pathogenicity and carriage

coagulase positive

toxins

Staphylococcus aureus colonizes the anterior nares and sometimes other skin sites of about 30% of people in the community; more may be colonized in hospitals. The species is pathogenic and can cause a variety of infections in many otherwise healthy individuals. It can also colonize or infect some animal species. Its name (*aureus,* gold) was suggested by the golden color that develops in older colonies of many, but not all, strains grown on agar plates. The primary distinguishing characteristic of *S. aureus* is its production of the enzyme *coagulase,* which leads to coagulation of plasma. It also produces a number of toxins and extracellular enzymes known or believed to contribute to disease processes; however, many gaps remain in our understanding of the pathogenesis of staphylococcal infections.

S. epidermidis

coagulase negative

opportunistic infections

Staphylococcus epidermidis is a member of the normal skin (epidermal) flora of essentially all humans and many animals. Its colonies often show white pigmentation, and it does not produce coagulase. The organism causes disease only in those whose local or systemic defenses are compromised; such individuals constitute an increasing proportion of hospital populations, however, and more infections have been seen in the past few years.

S. saprophyticus

coagulase negative

Staphylococcus saprophyticus is free living in nature, but may also colonize the skin. Like *S. epidermidis,* it is coagulase negative and rarely causes infections in healthy individuals, although it can cause primary urinary tract urinary tract infections

infections in women. In contrast to *S. aureus* and *S. epidermidis,* it is resistant to the antibiotic novobiocin. Many diagnostic laboratories do not routinely differentiate the two coagulase-negative species; they report both as *S. epidermidis* or as coagulase-negative staphylococci.

Staphylococcus aureus

Morphology and Staining

In young cultures and untreated lesions, the cells of *S. aureus* are quite regular in size, with a diameter of approximately 1 μm. They fit together in their clusters with the precision of a collection of pool balls and are rather uniformly Gram positive. In older cultures, in resolving lesions, and in the presence of some antibiotics the cells often become more variable in size, and many lose the Gram positivity. The typical morphology of staphylococci in culture is shown in the marginal figure and in pus from a staphylococcal abscess in Plate A.

Cell Wall and Other Surface Structures

teichoic acid

protein A

The cell wall of *S. aureus* consists of a peptidoglycan, the backbone of which comprises alternating molecules of *N*-acetylglucosamine and *N*-acetylmuramic acid (Chapter 2). The peptidoglycan is interspersed with molecules of ribitol–teichoic acid, which is antigenic and relatively specific for *S. aureus.* In most strains, the peptidoglycan of the cell wall is overlaid with protein A; this unique protein has a strong affinity for the Fc portion of immunoglobulin G(IgG) molecules, which are firmly bound to the staphylococcal cell, leaving their Fab portions directed externally. The significance of this phenomenon in test systems for detecting free antigens is discussed in Chapter 9. It probably contributes to the virulence of *S. aureus* by interfering with opsonization. Rare strains of *S. aureus* have an external morphologic capsule with a marked antiphagocytic effect. These strains are virulent to mice and have been used extensively in experimental studies. Most infections in humans are caused by noncapsulate strains, and the mechanisms of virulence and immunity differ from those of the capsulate strains in experimental animals.

Cultural Characteristics

rapid growth

variable hemolysis

mannitol salt agar

Under aerobic conditions, *S. aureus* grows rapidly and diffusely in liquid medium. After overnight incubation on blood agar, it produces soft, regular, low, convex colonies approximately 2–3 mm in diameter. Most, but not all, strains show a rim of β-hemolysis surrounding the colony (Plate B). The buff-golden color of the colonies, when present, can be seen when they are drawn up into a small pile with a bacteriologic loop. Occasional strains require the addition of 2–10% carbon dioxide to the atmosphere for growth. In contrast to other staphylococci, *S. aureus* grows well on agar medium containing 7.5% sodium chloride and is able to ferment mannitol to yield organic acids and an acidic reaction. These characteristics have been exploited in a selective medium, mannitol salt agar, which incorporates a pH indicator (phenol red) to detect acid from mannitol fermentation; *S. aureus* forms colonies that turn the indicator yellow (pH < 6.8) against the pink background of the medium (pH 7.2). This medium is frequently used in environmental and public health studies when it is necessary to detect *S. aureus* among many contaminating organisms. Colonial characteristics on mannitol salt agar are not sufficiently specific for definitive identification.

Tests for Identification and Subtyping

Tube coagulase test

Mechanism of coagulase action

The single most important test used to distinguish *S. aureus* from other staphylococci (and micrococci) demonstrates production of coagulase. A loopful of staphylococcal growth from solid medium is inoculated into diluted rabbit or human plasma and incubated at 35–37°C. Coagulase production results in development of a fibrin clot, usually within 4 hr. Coagulase activates prothrombin or a prothrombin derivative that initiates the terminal clotting sequence: thrombin + fibrinogen → fibrin.

Slide clumping test

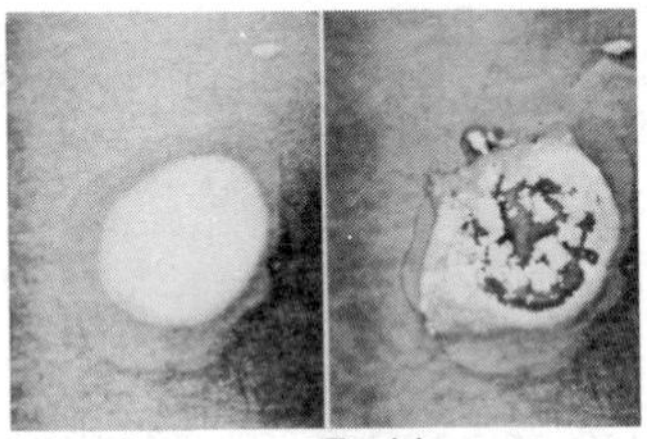

Negative Positive

A simple procedure, the slide coagulase or slide clumping test, is an excellent screening technique. A dense emulsion of staphylococcal colonies is made in a drop of water, mixed with undiluted plasma, and stirred with the loop. Immediate clumping enhanced by stirring denotes a positive test; the reaction can be readily distinguished from immune or nonspecific agglutination, which develops more slowly and is not enhanced by stirring. In this test, a cell-bound coagulase (or clumping factor) leads to deposition of fibrin on the surfaces of the staphylococci, which renders them "sticky" and results in clumping. The cell-bound coagulase differs from the free coagulase detected by the definitive tube test, but the two methods show about 95% correspondence. False-positive slide tests should not occur, but negative results may require verification with the tube test.

phage typing

Strains of *S. aureus* can be subdivided by bacteriophage typing and thus "fingerprinted" for epidemiologic purposes. The procedure depends on differing subjectivity to lysis of different strains by bacteriophages. It employs an international set of more than 20 bacteriophages derived originally from lysogenic strains of *S. aureus*. The bacteriophages are propagated on special strains of *S. aureus,* which also serve as controls for the specificity of the bacteriophages. The phages are dropped onto a plate seeded with the strain to be tested, using a template and an orientation marker. The pattern of lysis is read after overnight incubation (Figure 11.1). Most strains of *S. aureus* are lysed by more than one phage in the typing set. A phage type may be reported, for example, as 52/52A/80/81. Mutation or lysogenization during the course of an epidemic may occasionally change the reaction of a staphylococcus to particular phages. Thus, interpretation of phage typing results requires assistance from those familiar with the test. In general, typing patterns can be grouped together to reflect some common characteristics; four such groups (I, II, III, and IV) are recognized. Grouping is insufficiently precise to determine whether staphylococcal isolates have a common source;

variation in phage type

Phage groups

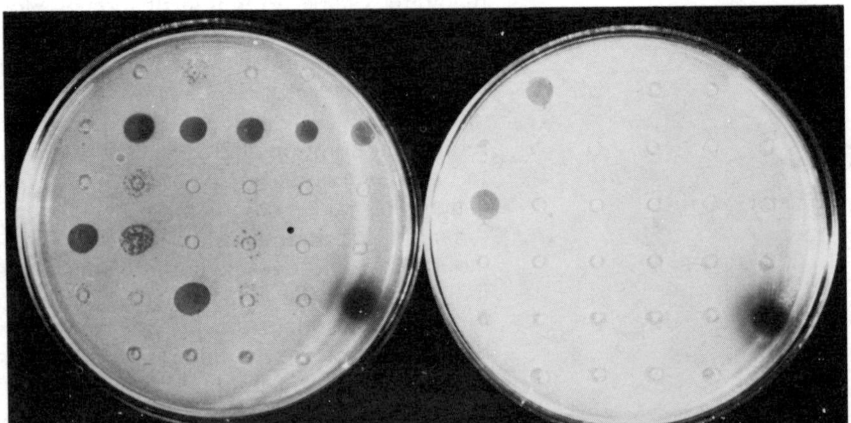

11.1. Bacteriophage typing of two strains of *Staphylococcus aureus*: results after overnight incubation. Lysis is indicated by absence of growth at the site of deposition of individual phages to which the strain is susceptible. The test shows that the two strains are not of common origin.

it has been helpful in pathogenic studies, however, because certain diseases are usually associated with a particular group (for example, bullous impetigo with phage group II strains). Normally, bacteriophage typing of an isolate from an individually infected patient has no diagnostic or therapeutic significance in contrast to its epidemiologic value.

Antigenic structure

Like all bacteria, *S. aureus* has many antigenically active components. Although strains can be subdivided serologically on the basis of surface protein and cell wall structural antigens, serotyping has not proved as valuable for epidemiologic studies as bacteriophage typing.

Toxins and Biologically Active Extracellular Enzymes

Strains of *S. aureus* produce a wide range of substances that contribute or possibly contribute to their virulence. The most important of these substances appear to be the following.

α-Hemolysin (α-toxin). α-Hemolysin is a low molecular weight, antigenic protein extotoxin that is lethal to many cells in low concentrations. It hemolyzes red cells, destroys platelets, kills leukocytes, causes necrosis of skin (dermonecrosis) when injected intradermally, and is lethal to experimental animals when sufficient amounts are injected intravenously. Although α-hemolysin can be converted to toxoid, neither toxoid nor anti-α-hemolysin has proved of significant value in the treatment or prevention of chronic staphylococcal infection.

Leukocidin. Leukocidin is an exotoxin, distinct from the α-hemolysin, that is lethal to polymorphonuclear leukocytes.

Resistance to boiling

Enterotoxins. Certain strains of *S. aureus* (particularly those of phage groups III and IV) produce one of several antigenically distinct exotoxins that cause acute gastrointestinal symptoms, usually within 2–5 hr of ingestion. These toxins are thus termed *enterotoxins.* They are low molecular weight proteins that retain activity after 30 min of boiling and are resistant to gastric and jejunal enzymes. Production of some has been shown to be coded by temperate bacteriophage. Ingestion of sufficient preformed toxin in food results in staphylococcal food poisoning. The toxin appears to act on neural receptors in the upper gastrointestinal tract, leading to stimulation of the vomiting center in the brain.

Exfoliatin. Certain strains of *S. aureus* belonging to phage group II produce exfoliatin, an exotoxin that leads to separation and loss of the most superficial layers of the epidermis. Production of the toxin is usually plasmid determined. Sufficient toxin may be produced at a local site of infection to cause marked epithelial desquamation at remote sites of the body (Ritter's disease, or scalded skin syndrome). The toxin is antigenic, and circulating antibody confers immunity to its effect.

Toxin associated with toxic shock syndrome. Evidence is growing that toxic shock syndrome is caused by a staphylococcal exotoxin distinct from all of those mentioned previously, but which may have enterotoxic properties. This toxin has not yet been fully characterized.

Coagulase. Although coagulase is not a toxin, it probably plays some role in the pathogenesis of staphylococcal infections and in determining their characteristics. Staphylococci coated with fibrin are resistant to phagocytosis, and fibrin deposition in the area of a staphylococcal infectious focus may help to localize the lesion.

Other extracellular products. Strains of *S. aureus* produce several other extracellular, biologically active substances, including hyaluronidase, nuclease, lipase, protease, and a plasminogen activator. Their roles in the pathogenesis of staphylococcal infection remain obscure.

Other Probable Contributors to Virulence

The morphologic capsule possessed by a few strains of *S. aureus* protects them from ingestion by phagocytes in experimental animals; it may play a similar role in human infections caused by such strains. Protein A, by binding the Fc portion of IgA molecules, may have an antiopsonic effect and help to protect the staphylococcus from phagocytosis. Once phagocytosed, *S. aureus* strains are much more resistant to lysosomal killing than are coagulase-negative staphylococci, and they may multiply within and kill the phagocyte. Furthermore, *S. aureus* can multiply in fresh human serum, whereas the growth of many coagulase-negative strains is partially or completely inhibited.

multifactorial nature of virulence

Thus, *S. aureus* has a variety of characteristics and products that may contribute to its virulence, although no single factor has been identified as the major contributor to its ability to multiply and cause lesions in tissues. Not all strains that cause infection possess all of the putative virulence factors discussed previously, and a single candidate for an effective immunizing vaccine appears unlikely.

Resistance

Resistance to drying

Like all medically important non-spore-forming bacteria, *S. aureus* is rapidly killed by temperatures above 60°C. It is also susceptible to all disinfectants and antiseptics commonly used. Unlike many pathogenic vegetative organisms, however, it can survive long periods of drying; for example, recurrent skin infections can result from use of uncleaned clothing contaminated with pus from a previous furuncle.

Antibiotic Susceptibility

Penicillinase production

When penicillin was first introduced, most strains of *S. aureus* were highly susceptible to it. Now, because of penicillinase β-lactamase production encoded by plasmid genes, most isolates from the community as well as from hospitals are penicillin resistant.

Methicillin-resistant strains

Most penicillin-resistant isolates are fully susceptible to the penicillinase-resistant penicillins and cephalosporins, although hospital epidemics caused by methicillin-resistant strains have occurred in most countries. This resistance is relative and mutational in origin. It appears to be associated with cell wall or penicillin-binding protein alterations, and is not due to β-lactamase production. As there are some technical problems in detecting this type of resistance, strains found resistant to methicillin or oxacillin should be considered of potentially increased resistance to all of the penicillinase-resistant penicillins and cephalosporins, even if routine susceptibility test reports indicate sensitivity.

multiresistance

Staphylococcus aureus may also be resistant to all other antimicrobics with antistaphylococcal action, except apparently vancomycin. Such multiresistance is usually plasmid determined. Multiresistant strains pose serious therapeutic problems. Plasmid-determined resistance is acquired by transduction, and multiple plasmids carrying different resistance markers may occur in single staphylococcal cells. It should also be noted that transduction is often associated with lysogenization by a new bacteriophage, which can lead to alteration in phage typing patterns. The extent of multiresistance in a population or hospital reflects the extent of antibiotic use and of cross-infection.

Susceptibility data from an American hospital are illustrated in Appendix 10.1; it must be realized, however, that very different, and often higher, proportions of resistant strains may be encountered in other institutions and populations.

Diseases

Pyogenic, suppurative lesion

Infections. Staphylococcal infections are characterized by intense suppuration, necrosis of local tissues, and a tendency for the infected area to become walled off with the formation of a pus-filled local abscess.

Furuncle

The prototypic, and most common, infection is the furuncle or boil, a superficial skin infection that develops in a hair follicle, sebaceous gland, or sweat gland. Blockage of the gland duct with inspissation of its contents causes predisposition to infection; thus, furunculosis is often a complication of acne vulgaris. Infection at the base of the eyelash gives rise to the common stye. The infected patient is often a carrier of the offending staphylococcus, usually in the anterior nares. The course of the infection is usually benign; no specific treatment is needed, and the infection resolves upon drainage of pus.

Stye

Chronic furunculosis

Some individuals are subject to chronic furunculosis, in which repeated attacks of boils are caused by the same phage type of *S. aureus*. There is little, if any, evidence of acquired immunity; indeed, delayed-type hypersensitivity to staphylococcal products appears responsible for much of the inflammation and necrosis that develops. Chronic staphylococcal disease may be associated with factors that depress host immunity; it is more common in patients with diabetes or congenital defects of polymorphonuclear leukocyte function (Chapter 65). In most instances, however, predisposing disease other than acne is not present.

defects in leukocyte function

Carbuncle

Infection may spread from a furuncle to the subcutaneous tissues, with the development of one or more abscesses extending to subcutaneous tissues known as *carbuncles*. These abscesses occur most often on the back of the neck, but may involve other skin sites. They are serious lesions that may result in bloodstream invasion (bacteremia).

Bullous impetigo

Certain strains of *S. aureus*, especially of phage type 71, can cause *bullous impetigo*, a highly communicable superficial skin infection characterized by large blisters containing many staphylococci in the superficial layers of the skin. Bullous impetigo is seen most often in infants and children under conditions in which direct spread can occur (for example, sharing of contaminated towels). The strains produce exfoliatin, and the disease can thus be considered a localized form of scalded skin syndrome. Another common *S. aureus* infection is paronychia, which involves the soft tissue around the nails. Paronychia may result from autoinfection or from an external source.

Paronychia

Deep lesions

Staphylococcus aureus can cause a wide variety of infections of deep tissues, by bacteremic spread from a skin lesion that may be unnoticed. These infections include osteomyelitis (usually of the metaphysis of the long bones in children); arthritis; cerebral, pulmonary, and renal abscesses; and breast abscesses in the nursing mother. Bacteremia and endocarditis can develop. All are serious infections that constitute acute medical emergencies. The organism can also cause bacterial pneumonia, which is always secondary to

osteomyelitis

abscesses

bacteremia and endocarditis

Staphylococcal pneumonia

some other insult to the lung or tracheobronchial tree, such as influenza, aspiration of gastric contents, or severe pulmonary edema. If untreated, multiple pulmonary abscesses develop. In all of these situations, diabetes, leukocyte defects, or general reduction of host defenses by alcoholism, malignancy, old age, or steroid or cytotoxic therapy can be a predisposing factor. Severe *S. aureus* infections, including endocarditis, are particularly common in drug abusers using injection methods. Occasionally a severe and life-threatening enterocolitis may develop when certain strains of *S. aureus* replace much of the normal colonic flora after a broad-spectrum antibiotic treatment to which the staphylococcus is resistant.

Staphylococcal enterocolitis

Wound infection

The organism is also a major cause of wound infection. The source may be the patient's own carrier state, other carriers (for example, physicians or nurses), or other infected patients. Cross-infection of the umbilical stump of the newborn infant can lead to extensive contamination of the infant and its environment. Spread to other infants and mothers in the hospital can result in a variety of staphylococcal infections, such as furuncles, conjunctivitis, breast abscess, and other deep infections. Surgical wound infections can be very severe, and infections at the site of intravenous lines can result in bacteremia and metastatic infection.

Scalded skin syndrome

Diseases caused by staphylococcal toxins. Scalded skin syndrome (Ritter's disease) results from the production of exfoliatin in a staphylococcal lesion, which can be quite minor (for example, conjunctivitis). The toxin is absorbed into the bloodstream, and erythema and intraepidermal desquamation may occur at remote sites from which *S. aureus* cannot be isolated (Figure 11.2). The disease is most common in neonates and in children less than 5 years old. The face, axilla, and groin tend to be affected first, but the erythema, bullous formation, and subsequent desquamation of epithelial sheets can spread to all parts of the body. The disease occasionally occurs in adults, particularly those who are immunocompromised.

Staphylococcal scarlet fever

Milder versions of what is probably the same disease are staphylococcal scarlet fever, in which erythema occurs without desquamation, and bullous impetigo, in which local desquamation occurs.

Toxic shock syndrome

Toxic shock syndrome is a serious, recently recognized disease associated with *S. aureus*. It is most common in young women during or immediately

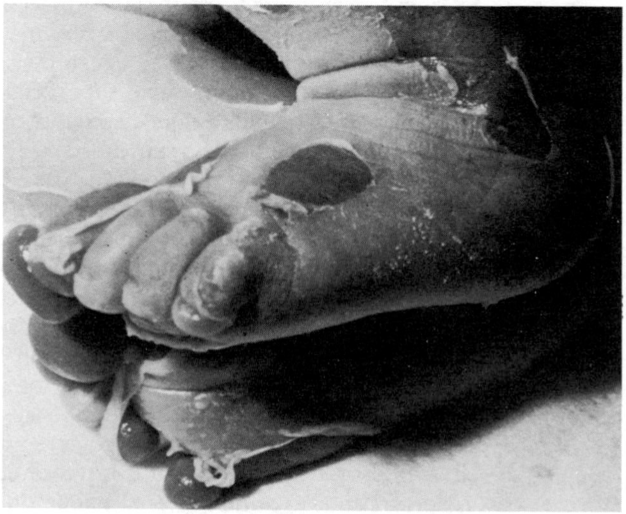

11.2 Staphylococcal scalded skin syndrome in a neonate. The staphylococcal infection was a breast abscess.

association with tampons

after menstruation and has been associated with the use of highly absorbent intravaginal tampons. The association was greatest with a particular brand that has since been withdrawn from the market; *S. aureus* grew in large numbers in and around the tampon with apparent absorption of an exotoxin. The disease is characterized by the development of high fever, vomiting, diarrhea, sore throat, and muscle pain. Within 48 hr, it may progress to severe shock with evidence of renal and hepatic damage. A skin rash may develop, followed by exfoliation at a deeper level than in scalded skin syndrome. Blood cultures are usually negative. The disease appears to be caused by an exotoxin that remains to be fully characterized.

Staphylococcal food poisoning

conditions for multiplication

resistance of toxin to boiling

Staphylococcal food poisoning results from production of staphylococcal enterotoxin in food before ingestion. It is an intoxication, not an infection. Characteristically, the food is moist and highly nutritious to *S. aureus*, as well as to people. Potato salads and creamy dishes are often involved. The food is contaminated by a carrier or, more often, by a preparer with a staphylococcal lesion. If the food is not refrigerated or refrigeration is inadequate, staphylococcal multiplication can result in 10^5 or more *S. aureus* per gram. If the strain produces enterotoxin, the food becomes toxic. Because of the heat resistance of the toxin, toxicity persists even if the food is subsequently heated to boiling.

short incubation

rapid recovery

Ingestion of the food results in acute vomiting and diarrhea within 1–5 hr. There is prostration, but usually no fever. Recovery is rapid, except sometimes in the elderly and in those with another disease. Staphylococcal food poisoning has been an unhappy and embarrassing sequel to innumerable group picnics and wedding parties in which gastronomic delicacies have been exposed to temperatures that allow bacterial multiplication.

Infectivity, Pathogenesis, and Immunity

variations in virulence

There is excellent epidemiologic evidence that strains of *S. aureus* differ considerably in infectivity and virulence, although the mechanisms involved are not understood. Multiresistant strains of phage type 80/81, prominent in the 1950s and 1960s, were associated with unusually serious outbreaks of staphylococcal disease in hospital patients. Many family outbreaks also occurred when carriers of the hospital strains returned home. Fortunately, this problem has diminished greatly (for reasons that are quite unclear), and present isolates of type 80/81 appear no more virulent than those of other phage types.

Influence of local conditions on infectivity

In general, strains of *S. aureus* are of quite low infectivity unless local conditions provide special opportunities for multiplication in the body. Experiments in medical student volunteers in the 1950s showed that intradermal injection of approximately 10^5–10^6 organisms was needed to initiate a small, local, infected lesion; in the presence of a suture, however, less than 10^2 organisms were required. Needless to say, these experiments were performed under conditions in which effective antibiotic therapy was immediately available to control complications, although none occurred. Similar situations, involving foreign material or local reduction in blood supply, play a role in many naturally occurring infections.

acute inflammatory response

survival in leukocytes

Once infection is initiated, the pathogenesis of staphylococcal disease becomes extremely complex and obscure. Some of the parameters have been discussed previously. There is an acute inflammatory response, initiated by microbial products and by tissue and leukocyte damage. The lesion tends to be localized, perhaps in part because of fibrin deposition through the action of staphylococcal coagulase. The organisms may multiply within and destroy leukocytes; in addition, various mechanisms, including production of protein A, serve to protect them from phagocytosis. Staphylococcal α-hemolysin and delayed hypersensitivity responses to staphylococcal proteins contribute to the necrosis of the lesions.

Resolution of infection

The resolution of staphylococcal infection in the absence of medical intervention usually results from an abscess "pointing" to the skin, with superficial necrosis followed by drainage of pus and healing by granulation and fibrosis. This process can occur with a small lesion, such as a furuncle, or with a large subcutaneous abscess. Immune mechanisms are undoubtedly involved; however, the relative roles of humoral and cellular immune mechanisms are again uncertain, and attempts to induce immunity artificially with various staphylococcal products have been disappointing at best. The natural history of staphylococcal infections indicates that immunity is of short duration and incomplete. Chronic furunculosis, for example, can recur over many years; staphylococcal osteomyelitis, if not effectively treated in its early stages, is notorious for its chronicity and is often associated with sinuses that drain the infected site to the skin surface for long periods. This chronicity, however, results in part from the poor vascularity of the affected bone.

uncertain role of immune mechanisms

multiple factors influencing pathogenesis and immunity

It seems likely that the imprecision of our understanding of staphylococcal infection and immunity reflects its multifactorial nature, in which different toxins, biologically active enzymes, antigens, and immune responses have a different constellation of roles in different cases.

Epidemiology

The basic habitat of *S. aureus* is the anterior nares. About 30% of individuals in the community carry the organism in this site at any given time. Nasal carrier rates among hospital personnel and patients may be much higher when staphylococcal infections both result from and contribute to the staphylococcal environmental load. Some individuals have extensive colonization of the perineum. They, and some nasal carriers, may disseminate the organism extensively with desquamated epithelial cells and thus constitute a source of infection to others.

Community infections

Most *S. aureus* infections acquired in the community are autoinfections with strains that the subject has been carrying in the anterior nares, on the skin, or both. Community outbreaks of bullous impetigo in children, mentioned previously, are usually associated with poor hygiene and fomite transmission from case to case.

Hospital infections

Routes of cross-infection

Hospital epidemics caused by a single phage type of *S. aureus* are a continuing and recurrent problem. Outbreaks are usually associated with nurseries or with patients who have undergone surgical or other invasive procedures. The initial source of the outbreak may be a patient with an overt or inapparent (for example, decubitus ulcer) staphylococcal infection; spread to other patients can occur through fomites, occasionally through air transmission, but is usually through the hands of personnel. A nasal or perineal carrier among medical, nursing, or other hospital staff may be the source of an outbreak, especially if carriage is heavy and numerous organisms are disseminated. A more serious source is the medical attendant with a staphylococcal lesion (for example, a furuncle on the wrist), whose hands may become heavily contaminated with *S. aureus* of proved pathogenicity.

Increased carriage rate

Hospital outbreaks of *S. aureus* infection can be self-perpetuating: infected patients and those who attend them frequently become carriers, and the total environmental load of the causative staphylococcus is increased. The principles of control of epidemics in general and of hospital outbreaks are described in Chapters 8 and 66.

In *S. aureus* outbreaks, it is critical to define the extent of infection with the responsible strain and to detect carriers who may have initiated or contributed to continuation of the outbreak. For these purposes, phage typing and determination of patterns of resistance to antimicrobics (antibiograms) are critical epidemiologic tools.

Laboratory Diagnosis

direct Gram smear

In general, laboratory procedures to assist in diagnosis are quite simple. Most staphylococcal lesions contain numerous polymorphonuclear leukocytes and large numbers of *S. aureus*. These findings are readily demonstrated by a direct Gram smear of pus (plate A) unless the patient has been treated with antibiotics. This method is also applicable to properly collected sputum samples from cases of staphylococcal pneumonia and to stool specimens from patients with staphylococcal enterocolitis.

culture

coagulase

susceptibility tests

The organism can usually be grown aerobically on blood agar, and typical colonies 2 mm or more in diameter develop overnight. A slide or tube coagulase test can be performed directly from these colonies. Antibiotic susceptibility tests are usually indicated because of the unpredictability of staphylococcal susceptibility patterns.

blood cultures

Blood cultures from untreated bacteremic patients are usually positive after overnight incubation. The organism produces colonies in the sedimented blood layer of unshaken blood culture bottles, probably because fibrin deposited on the surface by coagulase prevents separation and diffuse growth.

serodiagnostic procedures and limitations

Possible deep staphylococcal infection, such as osteomyelitis or perirenal abscess, poses special diagnostic problems when the lesion cannot be aspirated. Antibodies to staphylococcal hemolysin, nuclease, and cell wall ribitol–teichoic acid can be detected by a variety of immunologic techniques, including counterimmunoelectrophoresis and radioimmunoassay. Unfortunately, the sera of many individuals without deep staphylococcal infections may also contain such antibodies, and overlap is considerable in antibody titers of infected and uninfected subjects. Thus, these procedures are ancillary at best: their results must be interpreted with caution, and they are not generally available in clinical laboratories.

Prevention

Control of carriage and reinfection

In patients subject to recurrent infection, such as chronic furunculosis, preventive measures are aimed at controlling reinfection and, if possible, eliminating the carrier state. Clothes and bedding that may cause reinfection should be washed at a sufficiently high temperature to destroy staphylococci (70°C or higher) or dry-cleaned. In adults, the use of hexachlorophene soaps in showering and washing increases the bactericidal activity of the skin (see Chapter 4); however, their potential for neurotoxicity with prolonged use must be borne in mind. Anterior nasal carriage can be reduced and sometimes eliminated by nasal creams containing antimicrobics not used for systemic infections, such as neomycin and bacitracin. Similar measures may eliminate or reduce *S. aureus* dissemination from carriers proved to be a source of infection to others.

Hospital hygiene

In the hospital, control involves the application of the hygienic and epidemiologic approaches considered here and in Chapters 8 and 66. Careful hand washing by all medical attendants, the single most important factor, cannot be overstressed.

Chemoprophylaxis is mandatory in surgical procedures such as hip and cardiac valve replacements, in which infection with coagulase-positive or -negative staphylococci can have devastating consequences for the prosthesis and for the patient. It has been clearly shown that brief high-dose chemoprophylaxis around the time of surgery is highly protective, and the superinfections that often complicate longer periods of antibiotic administration are avoided.

Treatment

For superficial staphylococcal lesions, and usually for deeper chronic lesions as well, the most useful component of treatment is drainage.

Antimicrobic therapy

Acute, serious staphylococcal infections (for example, pneumonia or bacteremia) require immediate antibiotic therapy. A penicillinase-resistant penicillin or cephalosporin would normally be used pending the results of a susceptibility test. Infections proved to be caused by strains susceptible to benzyl-penicillin are thus best treated with that antibiotic. Severe infections caused by strains resistant to the penicillinase-resistant penicillins (methicillin-resistant staphylococci) may require vancomycin treatment.

Combined therapy

There is evidence of synergy between cell-wall-active antibiotics and the aminoglycosides when the staphylococcus is sensitive to both. Such combinations are often used in severe systemic infection, particularly in the compromised host, when effective and rapid bactericidal action is needed.

Some chronic infections, as well as recurrent infections in the compromised host, can be controlled by administration over months or years of an oral preparation of one of the penicillinase-resistant penicillins.

Coagulase-Negative Staphylococci

endocarditis

prosthetic device infections

prostatitis

Staphylococcus epidermidis is an almost universal inhabitant of the skin. It can cause infection, however, when local systemic defenses are compromised. The organism occasionally causes subacute bacterial endocarditis (Chapter 62), and it is the single most common cause of infection on or around prosthetic heart valves. It may infect peripheral vascular grafts and the sites of intravenous catheters. After *S. aureus*, *S. epidermidis* is the most common cause of infection following total hip joint replacement. It is also the organism most likely to cause infection of artificial cerebrospinal fluid shunts used in the treatment of hydrocephalus. Infection of the prostate and urinary tract in older men, especially after obstruction or instrumentation, also occurs.

S. saprophyticus urinary tract infections

Staphylococcus saprophyticus, which is widely dispersed in the environment, has a similar, but restricted ability to cause opportunistic infection in the compromised host. It is the etiologic agent in 10–20% of primary urinary tract infections in young women.

coagulase negative staphylococci in blood cultures

Coagulase-negative staphylococci are common contaminants of surface wounds and of specimens obtained by transcutaneous puncture or biopsy. Interpretation of a single blood culture that grows a coagulase-negative staphylococcus is a frequent diagnostic problem. In most cases, this finding is attributable to skin contamination; however, when the patient's defenses are compromised, it may be significant. The distinction can usually be made by observing several blood cultures and comparing the biochemical reactions and antibiotic susceptibilities of any coagulase-negative staphylococci isolated.

Resistance to antimicrobics

Most coagulase-negative staphylococci now encountered are resistant to penicillin, either because of penicillinase production or because of intrinsic resistance. Some are also resistant to the penicillinase-resistant penicillins (such as methicillin and cloxacillin), as well as to other antibiotics with spectra of activity that include many Gram-positive cocci. Strains resistant to the penicillinase-resistant penicillins often show varying degrees of resistance to the cephalosporins; this resistance may be detectable only with dilution tests. Treatment of coagulase-negative staphylococcal infections of prosthetic devices frequently requires removal of the device, as well as chemotherapy to prevent recurrence.

Micrococci

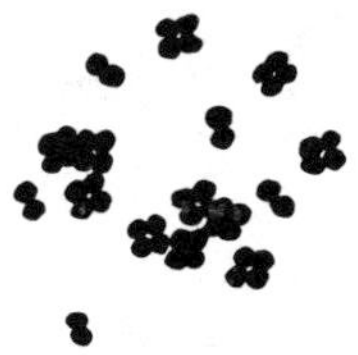

Micrococcus

A genus related to *Staphylococcus* is *Micrococcus*. The micrococci comprise commensal, free-living, Gram-positive cocci that are often larger than *S. aureus* and often arranged in regular packets of four or eight, depending on whether they divide in two or three planes before separation. They are coagulase negative and, like the staphylococci, produce catalase. In contrast to the staphylococci, micrococci metabolize oxidatively only and cannot grow anaerobically. Their pathogenic significance is similar to that of the coagulase-negative staphylococci.

Additional Reading and References

Cohen, J.O. Ed. 1972. *The Staphylococci*. New York: John Wiley and Sons. A good multiauthored review.

Elek, S.D., and Conan, P.E. 1957. The virulence of *Staphylococcus pyogenes* for man. A study of the problems of wound infections. *Br. J. Exp. Pathol.* 38:573–586. A classic study of the factors influencing the development of staphylococcal wound infections in humans.

Elias, P.M., Fritsch, P., and Epstein, E.H., Jr. 1977. Staphylococcal scalded skin syndrome. *Arch. Dermatol.* 113:207–219.

Larkin, S.M., et al. 1982. Toxic shock syndrome: clinical laboratory and pathologic findings in nine fatal cases. Ann. Intern. Med. 96:858–864. This and the Elias, Fritsch, and Epstein reference give excellent descriptions of two diseases related to staphylococcal exotoxins.

Musher, D.M., and McKenzie, S.O. 1977. Infections due to *Staphylococcus aureus. Medicine* (Baltimore) 56:383–409. A review of clinical experience with infections and of the factors that contributed to disease.

Kenneth J. Ryan

Streptococci

12

The genus *Streptococcus* comprises species of Gram-positive, spherical or oval cocci that tend to be arranged in chains. Most grow best in enriched bacteriologic media. Streptococci form a significant portion of the indigenous microflora of humans and animals; most of these species are found in the respiratory tract, but some inhabit the intestinal tract. Because of their complex growth requirements, they are not commonly found in the environment except as survivors from human and animal flora. Although most species rarely cause disease, the genus includes three of the most important pathogens of humans: *Streptococcus pyogenes,* the group A streptococcus, causes a variety of acute infections and can stimulate the poststreptococcal sequelae of rheumatic fever and acute glomerulonephritis. *Streptococcus agalactiae,* the group B streptococcus, is one of the most important causes of neonatal meningeal infection. *Streptococcus pneumoniae* is a major cause of both acute bacterial pneumonia and acute purulent meningitis.

Group Characteristics

Morphology

arrangement in chains

Gram positivity

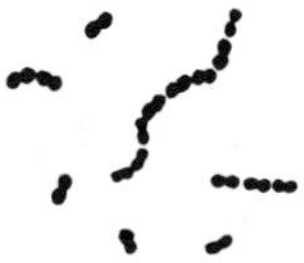

Streptococcus

non-spore forming and nonmotile

Streptococci stain readily with common dyes, demonstrating coccal cells 0.5–1 μm in diameter. In contrast to staphylococci, streptococcal cells are generally smaller and ovoid in shape. They are usually arranged in chains with oval cells touching end to end; however, length may vary from a single pair to continuous chains of over 30 cells, depending on the species and growth conditions. The Gram reaction is positive, although some cells in older cultures or purulent discharges may lose their ability to retain crystal violet and thus appear Gram negative. This finding is particularly likely if the organisms have been exposed to antimicrobics that inhibit cell wall synthesis, such as the penicillins and cephalosporins.

Medically important streptococci are not acid fast, do not form spores, and are nonmotile. Some members form capsules composed of polysaccharide complexes or hyaluronic acid.

Cultural and Biochemical Characteristics

Enriched media

blood agar

Streptococci grow best in media enriched with digests of animal tissues, serum, or defibrinated blood. The plating medium most commonly used is blood agar, which consists of a meat broth to which agar and animal blood are added. Sheep blood is preferred by most bacteriologists because of its catalase-negative facultative anaerobes

clear demonstration of streptococcal hemolytic patterns. Medically important species grow best at temperatures of 35–37°C. Streptococci are facultative anaerobes and can grow under atmospheric conditions ranging from aerobic to strictly anaerobic. They metabolize fermentatively and fail to produce catalase. Growth of many strains is enhanced by the presence of 2–10% carbon dioxide. Strictly anaerobic strains, previously called *anaerobic streptococci,* are now classified in the genus *Peptostreptococcus* (Chapter 16).

Growth characteristics

In broth cultures, streptococci that occur in pairs or very short chains (for example, pneumococcus) grow diffusely; those that form longer chains (group A streptococci, viridans streptococci) demonstrate a more granular appearance and frequently sediment to the bottom.

α- and β-hemolysis

nonhemolytic streptococci

After incubation for 18–24 hr on blood agar plates, small colonies ranging from pinpoint size to 0.5–2 mm in diameter are produced. A distinctive feature of streptococcal growth on blood agar is the production by many species of α (green) or β (clear) hemolysis of the erythrocytes suspended in the agar (Plates F and G)(Chapter 9). Hemolysis is dependent on several cultural features, including the incubation atmosphere and the species of blood used. Nonhemolytic variants of typically hemolytic species may be seen, and some species are inherently nonhemolytic. The term *γ-hemolytic,* sometimes used to describe the latter, is confusing and should be abandoned.

Lactic fermentation

Extracellular products

Streptococci are biochemically active, attacking a variety of carbohydrates, proteins, and amino acids. Glucose fermentation yields mostly lactic acid. Extracellular enzymes with substrates such as hyaluronic acid and DNA are produced by certain species and may contribute to virulence. Although potent exotoxins are not prominent among the streptococci, at least one, the erythrogenic toxin, is produced by some group A strains.

Classification

Lancefield antigenic groups

Hemolytic and biochemical characteristics

β-hemolytic streptococci assigned Lancefield groups; also some α-hemolytic and nonhemolytic strains

Understanding the classification of streptococci is complicated by the fact that an established taxonomy based primarily on hemolytic and biochemical reactions was dramatically changed by the work of Rebecca Lancefield. She demonstrated major and consistent antigenic differences in the cell wall carbohydrates of β-hemolytic streptococci with different biologic and pathogenic characteristics. This finding permitted allocation of these organisms to serologic groups. The presence of these group-specific antigens has been universally accepted as the primary taxonomic criterion for those species that have them. Hemolytic, cultural, and biochemical features, however, remain important for the taxonomy of other streptococci and for the initial detection and presumptive classification of all streptococci. β-Hemolysis indicates the strain has one of the Lancefield group antigens, but strains of some Lancefield groups may be α-hemolytic or nonhemolytic. The streptococci will be considered as follows: 1) pyogenic streptococci (Lancefield groups); 2) pneumococcus; 3) viridans streptococci; and 4) other, principally nonhemolytic, streptococci. This classification scheme is illustrated in Table 12.1.

comprise Lancefield groups A–T; most strains β-hemolytic

Pyogenic streptococci. The primary characteristic of pyogenic streptococci is the presence of one of the Lancefield cell wall polysaccharide or teichoic acid antigens, designated as *groups A–T.* The most common Lancefield groups of streptococci isolated from humans are A, B, C, D, F, and G. Many of these group designations correlate with species names previously assigned on the basis of cultural, biochemical, and pathogenic features, such as *S. pyogenes* (group A) and *S. agalactae* (group B). The importance of the serologic definition is emphasized by the common description of isolates according to their group (for example, Group A β-hemolytic streptococci)

Table 12.1 Classification of Streptococci by Hemolytic and Serologic Reactions

Group	Common Terms	Hemolysis
Pyogenic		
S. pyogenes	Group A streptococcus	β
S. agalactiae	Group B streptococcus	β, occasionally α or nonhemolytic
S. faecalis, *S. faecium*, *S. durans*	Enterococci	α or nonhemolytic (rarely β)
S. bovis, *S. equinus*	Nonenterococcal group D streptococci	α or nonhemolytic
Other species		β, occasionally α or nonhemolytic
Pneumococcus (*S. pneumoniae*)	Pneumococcus	α
Viridans and nonhemolytic		
S. sanguis, *S. salivarius*, *S. mitis*, *S. milleri*, *S. mutans*, Other species	Viridans streptococci or nonhemolytic streptococci (depending on hemolytic reaction)	α or nonhemolytic

rather than by the species name. Not all strains possessing Lancefield group antigens are β-hemolytic, especially in group D; however, all that are β-hemolytic are included among the pyogenic streptococci.

antigenic polysaccharide capsule, but no Lancefield group antigen; α-hemolytic

Pneumococcus. The pneumococcus group contains a single species, *S. pneumoniae.* Its distinctive feature is the presence of a polysaccharide capsule. Differences in the constitution and, thus, the antigenic specificity of the capsule of different pneumococci have allowed the identification of more than 80 immunotypes. Although the pneumococcal cell wall shares some common antigens with other streptococci, it does not possess any of the Lancefield group antigens. The pneumococcus is α-hemolytic.

α-hemolytic; several species among normal flora

Viridans streptococci. Viridans streptococci are α-hemolytic and lack both the group carbohydrate antigen of the pyogenic streptococci and the capsular antigens of the pneumococcus. The term encompasses several species, including *Streptococcus salivarius* and *Streptococcus mitis.* Viridans streptococci commonly appear among the normal respiratory flora of humans. They almost never demonstrate invasive qualities, although some species (*Streptococcus milleri*) have been associated with deep tissue abscesses and several with bacterial endocarditis.

Table 12.1 *(continued)*

Serologically Specific Antigens			
Lancefield Cell Wall	Surface Protein	Surface Polysaccharide	Disease Association
A	60+ M protein	—	Pyogenic, scarlet fever, rheumatic fever, glomerulonephritis
B	—	Ia, Ib, Ic, II, III	Pyogenic, neonatal sepsis, meningitis
D	—	—	Pyogenic, urinary infection
D	—	—	Low virulence, endocarditis
C, E–T	—	—	Pyogenic
—	—	80+	Pyogenic, pneumonia, meningitis
—	—	—	Low virulence, endocarditis, pyogenic; *S. mutans* associated with dental caries

Other streptococci (nonhemolytic). A variety of other streptococci may be encountered that lack the features of the pyogenic streptococci or pneumococci; they would be classified with the viridans group, except they are not α-hemolytic. Such strains are usually assigned descriptive terms such as *nonhemolytic streptococci* or *microaerophilic streptococci.* They have been less thoroughly studied, but generally have the same biologic behavior as the viridans streptococci.

Streptococcus pyogenes (Group A)

β-hemolysis by streptolysins S and O

Growth Characteristics

Group A β-hemolytic streptococci typically appear in purulent lesions or broth cultures as spherical or ovoid cells in chains of short to medium length (4–10 cells). On blood agar plates, colonies are compact, small, and surrounded by a 2- to 3-mm zone of β-hemolysis that is easily seen and sharply demarcated (Plate F). β-Hemolysis is caused by streptolysin S and the oxygen-labile streptolysin O, both of which are produced by most group A strains. Occasional strains lack streptolysins S, and β-hemolysis by streptolysin O occurs only under anaerobic conditions. This feature is of practical importance, because such strains would be missed if incubated under the usual aerobic conditions.

Structure

Cell wall Lancefield group A antigen

M protein type-specific antigens

fimbriae contain M protein and LTA antigens

variable hyaluronic acid capsule

The structure of group A streptococci is illustrated in Figure 12.1. The cell wall is built upon a peptidoglycan matrix that provides rigidity, as in other Gram-positive bacteria. Within this matrix lies the group-specific antigen, which is composed of rhamnose and *N*-acetylglucosamine. By definition all group A streptococci possess this antigen. The M protein is a surface component extending beyond the limits of the cell wall in association with hairlike fimbriae (Figure 12.2). Group A streptococci are divided into more than 60 serotypes based on antigenic differences in the M protein. A secondary typing system sometimes used in epidemiologic studies is based on another cell wall component, the T protein. There is no consistent relationship between the M and T proteins. A more recently studied structural component, lipoteichoic acid (LTA), appears on the fimbriae in a manner similar to that of the M protein. Some strains have an overlying nonantigenic hyaluronic acid capsule.

Toxins, Hemolysins, and Biologically Active Extracellular Products

Various exotoxins and hemolysins are produced, primarily by the group A streptococci. Some other pyogenic streptococci, however, may produce similar extracellular products.

Oxygen-labile antigenic hemolysin

Streptolysin O. One of two hemolysins responsible for hemolysis on blood agar plates is streptolysin O. It is an antigenic protein that is only active in

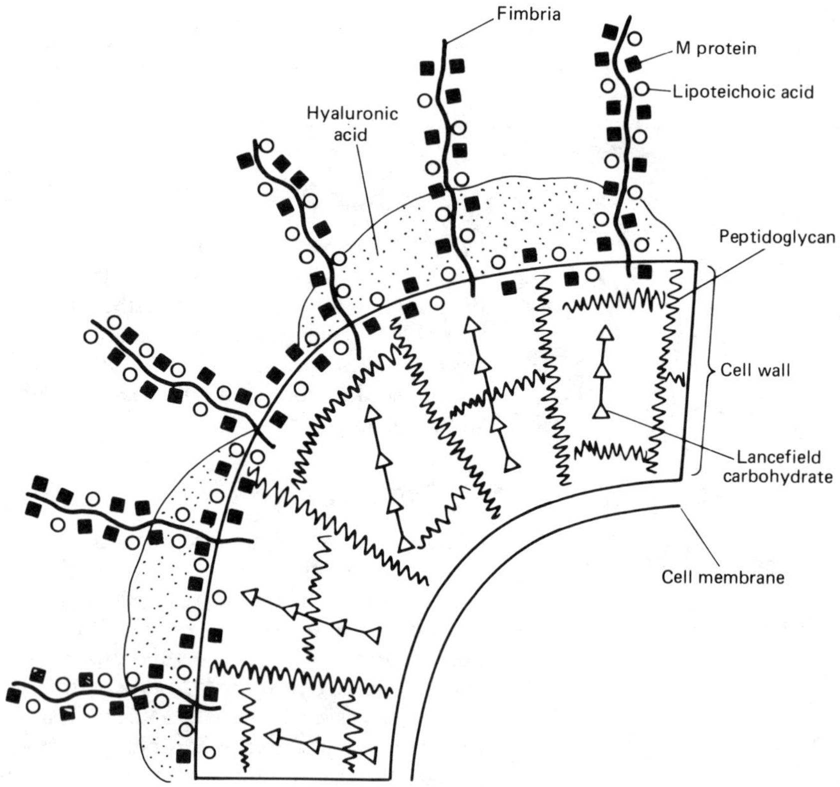

12.1 Antigenic structure of *Streptococcus pyogenes.* Diagram shows locations of peptidoglycan and Lancefield carbohydrate antigen in the cell wall. M protein and leipoteichoic acid are associated with the cell surface and fimbriae. A hyaluronic acid capsule may be the most external layer.

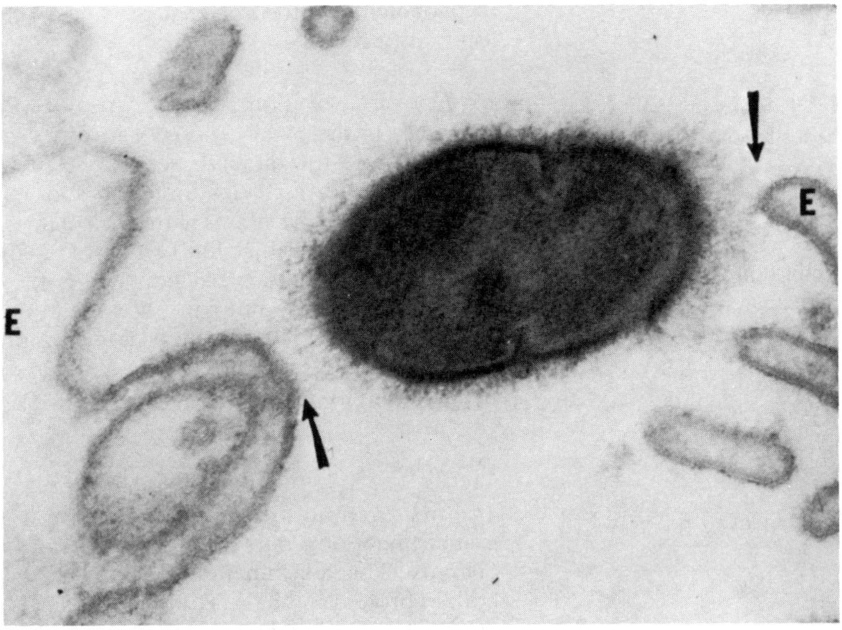

12.2 A group A β-hemolytic streptococcus is shown attaching to the cell membrane of a human oral epithelial cell (E). Note the hairlike fimbriae (*arrows*), which mediate the attachment. As in Figure 12.1, both M protein and lipoteichoic acid are associated with the fimbriae. (*Reproduced with permission from Beachey, E.H. and Ofek, I. 1976 J. Exp. Med. 143:764, Figure 2.*)

Cytotoxic activity

Antistreptolysin O

the reduced form, hence its designation O for oxygen lability. Streptolysin O is a general cytotoxin, lysing leukocytes, tissue cells, and platelets. The hydrolytic enzymes released into surrounding tissues from leukocytic granules probably contribute to cell death. Antibodies against streptolysin O are often formed as a result of *S. pyogenes* infection, and inhibition of hemolysis by these antibodies is the basis of the antistreptolysin O test.

Streptolysin S. Another hemolysin, streptolysin S, is oxygen stable but not antigenic. It is responsible for the hemolysis seen around colonies of group A streptococci on blood agar plates incubated aerobically.

fibrinolysis by activating serum plasminogen

Streptokinase. Filtrates of most strains of *S. pyogenes* cause lysis of fibrin clots through production of streptokinase. The action is not direct, but through conversion of plasminogen in normal plasma to a protease, plasmin. Streptokinase is antigenic, and antistreptokinase antibodies appear after group A streptococcal infection.

Deoxyribonuclease (DNA-ase). Various antigenic nucleases with activity against DNA and, to a lesser extent, RNA are formed by group A streptococci. Of the several immunologically distinct classes described, the most important is DNA-ase B. This enzyme is that produced most consistently in group A streptococcal infections.

spreading factor

Hyaluronidase. Because of its solubilizing action on the ground substance of mammalian connective tissues, hyaluronidase has been called the *spreading factor.* It is tempting to associate this enzyme with the diffuse, spreading lesions characteristic of streptococcal cellulitis, but its precise role in pathogenesis is not known. Many streptococci have hyaluronic acid capsules, including some that produce hyaluronidase; however, the two features usually do not coexist. Although hyaluronidase is produced by several groups of pyogenic streptococci, that produced by group A strains is immunologically distinct.

association with scarlet fever

Erythrogenic toxin. Some group A strains form erythrogenic toxin. It has no clear role in the pathogenesis of invasive streptococcal disease; however, it is responsible for the rash seen in scarlet fever. It is a protein exotoxin complexed with a carrier molecule and appears in three immunologically distinct forms. Only strains with particular temperate bacteriophages produce toxin. Intradermal injection of the toxin (the Dick test), which produces a localized erythematous reaction unless the subject has circulating specific antibody against it (antitoxin), was used in the past to measure susceptibility to scarlet fever. The rash of scarlet fever is probably caused by a combination of the direct effect of the erythrogenic toxin on the skin and delayed-type hypersensitivity to toxin.

production determined by temperate phages

Pathogenesis of Infection

Attachment by fimbriae

The first event in streptococcal infection in individuals with intact epithelia is attachment of group A streptococcal cells to epithelial cells, usually of the pharynx. This attachment is accomplished by the fimbriae, which contain both M protein and LTA. Although M protein-negative mutants fail to attach, the balance of current evidence favors LTA as the primary mediator of this process. Upon attachment, local epithelial damage occurs. In many *S. pyogenes* infections, however, invasion occurs through epithelial breaks.

M proteins protect against phagocytosis

type-specific immunity with opsonizing anti-M protein antibody

Possible effects of extracellular enzymes

After these initial events, any hyaluronic acid capsule may act to retard phagocytosis; however, the M protein plays the key role in allowing the streptococcal infection to become established. Strains containing M protein can resist phagocytosis by polymorphonuclear leukocytes, and they grow readily in tissue fluids and serum. Strains lacking M protein do not exhibit these features and are avirulent. Antibody directed against the M protein provides a type-specific immunity that lasts for many years, because opsonized *S. pyogenes* are rapidly killed when ingested by phagocytic cells. The precise role of other factors in the pathogenesis of infection is uncertain, but the combined effect of streptokinase, DNA-ase, and hyaluronidase may prevent effective localization of the infection while the streptolysins produce tissue injury. Antibodies against all of these components are formed in the course of streptococcal infection, although immunity is M type specific.

Antimicrobic Susceptibility

Penicillin susceptibility

Group A streptococci are highly susceptible to penicillin G. Concentrations as low as 0.01 μg/ml have a bactericidal effect, and penicillin resistance is so far unknown. Numerous other antimicrobics are also active, including other penicillins, cephalosporins, tetracyclines, chloramphenicol, and erythromycin, but not aminoglycosides. Tetracycline resistance has been found in 5–10% of strains, and erythromycin resistance also occurs when that agent is widely used.

Diseases

The group A streptococcus is unique in its ability to cause a variety of acute pyogenic infections and two nonsuppurative diseases that can follow streptococcal infection but do not involve the live organism. The latter diseases, acute rheumatic fever and glomerulonephritis, are known as *poststreptococcal sequelae,* or nonsuppurative complications of streptococcal infection.

A. Infections

most common
in childhood

Streptococcal pharyngitis. One of the most common bacterial infections is streptococcal pharyngitis. Although it may occur at any age, it is most frequent between 5 and 15 years. The illness is characterized by acute sore throat, malaise, fever (38.9–40°C), and headache. Infection typically involves the tonsillar pillars, uvula, and soft palate, which become red, swollen, and covered with a yellow-white exudate. The cervical lymph nodes that drain this area may also become swollen and tender. No single finding or combination of clinical features is sufficient to make or exclude a diagnosis of group A streptococcal pharyngitis in an isolated case, because the condition can be indistinguishable from viral pharyngitis. Streptococcal pharyngitis can only be diagnosed by demonstrating the presence of the organism with laboratory tests.

diagnosis requires culture

Suppurative complications

Group A streptococcal pharyngitis is usually self-limiting. Typically, the fever is gone by the third to fifth day, and other manifestations subside within a week. Occasionally the infection may spread beyond the pharynx to produce peritonsillar or retropharyngeal abscesses, otitis media, suppurative cervical adenitis, and acute sinusitis. Rarely, more extensive spread occurs, producing meningitis, pneumonia, or bacteremia with metastatic infection in distant organs. In the preantibiotic era, these suppurative complications were responsible for a mortality of 1–3% from acute streptococcal pharyngitis. Such complications are much less common now, and fatal infections are rare.

Impetigo. Group A streptococcal infection of healthy skin usually produces a localized skin disease known as *impetigo.* Invasion is through minor trauma, such as skin abrasions or insect bites. The primary lesion of streptococcal impetigo is a small (up to 1 cm) vesicle surrounded by an area of erythema. The vesicle enlarges over a period of days, becomes pustular, and eventually breaks to form a yellow crust. The lesions usually appear in 2- to 5-year-old children on exposed body surfaces, typically the face and lower extremities. Multiple lesions may coalesce to form deeper ulcerated areas. Streptococcal impetigo is often caused by nephritogenic strains, especially in the tropics. An early vesicle yields a pure culture of group A streptococci; an older, crusted lesion, however, may become secondarily colonized with *Staphylococcus aureus.* There is no evidence that staphylococci play any role in the natural history of streptococcal impetigo, although it should be recalled that *S. aureus* can produce its own clinically distinct form (bullous impetigo). The presence of staphylococci that produce penicillinase does not appear to compromise the effectiveness of penicillin therapy.

Skin infection, usually
in children

Secondary colonization
with *S. aureus*

Dermal infection
with spreading
erythema and edema

Erysipelas. Erysipelas is a distinct form of streptococcal infection of the skin and subcutaneous tissues, primarily affecting the dermis. It is characterized by a spreading area of erythema and edema with rapidly advancing, well-demarcated edges, pain, and systemic manifestations, including fever and lymphadenopathy. Infection usually occurs on the face, and a previous history of streptococcal sore throat is common. Erysipelas is a serious disease that requires immediate antimicrobic therapy, usually with penicillin.

Risk of cross-infection
Failure of skin grafts

Wound and burn infections. Although less common than in the past, group A streptococcal infections of wounds and burns can develop and spread rapidly to adjacent tissues, with the risk of sepsis and bacteremia. Burn infections are associated with failure of skin grafts. Burn and wound infections in hospitalized patients carry a substantial risk of cross-infection to other patients with similar conditions.

Life-threatening, contagious, postpartum infection

Puerperal infection. Infection of the endometrium at or near delivery is a life-threatening form of group A streptococcal infection. Fortunately, it is now relatively rare. Spread to other pelvic organs and the bloodstream via the lymphatic vessels produces a rapidly progressive infection, which can be fatal unless appropriate antimicrobic therapy is initiated early in its course. The disease is highly contagious, and special precautions are needed to prevent its spread to other hospitalized patients.

B. Disease Due to Erythrogenic Toxin

circumoral pallor

strawberry tongue and rash

Scarlet fever. Infection with strains that elaborate the erythrogenic toxin may superimpose the signs of scarlet fever on a streptococcal pharyngitis in subjects with no circulating antibody to the toxin. In scarlet fever, the buccal mucosa, temples, and cheeks are deep red, except for a pale area around the mouth and nose (circumoral pallor). Punctate hemorrhages appear on the hard and soft palates, and the tongue becomes covered with a yellow-white exudate through which the red papillae are prominent (strawberry tongue). A diffuse red rash appears on the second day of illness, spreading from the upper chest to the trunk and extremities. Close examination of the skin shows the rash to consist of multiple, discrete, red pinpoint elevations, which impart an irregular "sandpaper" feel to the skin. For unknown reasons, scarlet fever is both less frequent and less severe than earlier in the century. The disease can occur with any type of *S. pyogenes* infection caused by an organism that produces erythrogenic toxin.

C. Delayed Nonsuppurative Noninfectious Complications

complications of streptococcal pharyngitis

Rheumatic carditis

recurrence with subsequent *S. pyogenes* infections

Valvular damage

Rheumatic fever. Rheumatic fever is a nonsuppurative inflammatory disease characterized by fever and inflammation of the joints, heart, subcutaneous tissue, and central nervous system. The major clinical manifestations are carditis, subcutaneous nodules, chorea, and migratory polyarthritis. Attacks typically begin 3 weeks (range 1–5 weeks) after a group A streptococcal pharyngitis, and in the absence of antiinflammatory therapy last 2–3 months. During this period the clinical manifestations vary in severity at different times. The most serious manifestation of rheumatic fever and the only one with a major potential to produce long-range disability is carditis, which involves the connective tissue and the endocardium, particularly of the valves. Cardiac enlargement, valvular murmurs, and effusions are seen clinically and reflect endocardial, myocardial, and epicardial damage, which can lead to heart failure either acutely or through the production of chronic lesions. Acute rheumatic fever also has a marked predilection for recurrence with subsequent streptococcal infections. The first attack usually occurs between the ages of 5 and 15 years. The risk of recurrent attacks after subsequent group A streptococcal infections continues into adult life and then decreases. Repeated attacks lead to progressive damage to the endocardium and heart valves, with scarring and valvular stenosis or incompetence (rheumatic heart disease).

role of *S. pyogenes* in pathogenesis group rather than type-specific

prophylaxis

The association between group A streptococci and rheumatic fever is based on epidemiologic studies demonstrating prior episodes of streptococcal pharyngitis and marked immune responses to streptococcal products. Rheumatic fever does not follow nonrespiratory infections or infections with streptococci other than *S. pyogenes* (group A). Although some strains may be more likely to cause initial attacks, the events involved in recurrent rheumatic fever and the subsequent cardiac damage indicate that the pathogenesis of the disease is group rather than type-specific, because recurrences can be caused by many M protein types. Prophylactic penicillin therapy is used to prevent recurrent rheumatic fever by preventing subsequent streptococcal infections.

Possible pathogenetic mechanisms

Several theories have been advanced to explain the role of group A streptococci in rheumatic fever: 1) an autoimmune mechanism caused by similarities between streptococcal and human tissue antigens; 2) a serum sickness-like state mediated by antigen–antibody complexes; 3) residual toxicity of streptococcal products such as streptolysin S or O; and 4) persistence of the organisms in tissues (for example, as cell wall defective forms).

Probable autoimmune etiology

Of these theories, the first has the most experimental support. Patients with rheumatic fever have higher levels of various antistreptococcal antibodies than those with streptococcal infections who do not develop rheumatic fever. Some of these antibodies have been shown to react with both heart tissues and streptococcal antigens. For example, antibodies directed against streptococcal cell wall and cell membrane antigens cross-react with cardiac sarcolemmal sheaths, smooth muscle of vessel walls, and cells of the endocardium. There has been much debate over which of these cross-reactions is the most important. Recent evidence favors antibody evoked by a polypeptide fragment, which reacts with sarcolemmal membranes of human heart muscle. Cross-reactions between the group A polysaccharide and a glycoprotein isolated from heart valves have also been described. These observations correlate with the long-known heightened humoral immune response of patients with rheumatic fever to a variety of streptococcal products. Such patients also show greater cell-mediated immunity to streptococcal antigens. A cellular reaction pattern consisting of lymphocytes and macrophages aggregated around fibrinoid deposits is found in human hearts. This lesion called the Aschoff body is characteristic of rheumatic carditis.

Genetic and socioeconomic factors

Genetic factors are probably also important in rheumatic fever, because only a small proportion of individuals infected with group A streptococci develop the disease. Attack rates are highest among those of lower socioeconomic status and vary among those of different racial origins. The gene for an alloantigen, found on the surface of B-lymphocytes, appears among rheumatic fever patients at a frequency fourfold to fivefold greater than the general population. The localization of this gene in a region associated with immune response further suggests a genetic predisposition to hyperreactivity to streptococcal products. The incidence of rheumatic fever in the United States is much lower now than in the past.

Acute glomerulonephritis. The group A streptococcus is one of several microorganisms associated with glomerulonephritis. It is primarily a disease of childhood, characterized clinically by edema, hypertension, hematuria, and proteinuria and pathologically by diffuse proliferative lesions of the glomeruli. The clinical course is usually benign, with spontaneous healing over weeks to months. Occasionally a progressive course leads to renal failure and death. The frequency with which acute glomerulonephritis leads to chronic nephritis is not conclusively established, except that it is much more common in adults than children.

course usually benign

may follow respiratory or skin infection by specific M types (nephritogenic strains)

Poststreptococcal glomerulonephritis may follow either respiratory or cutaneous group A streptococcal infection. It involves only certain strains, known on epidemiologic grounds as *nephritogenic.* The average latent period between infection and glomerulonephritis is 10 days from a respiratory infection, but generally about 3 weeks from a skin infection. Nephritogenic strains are of a few M protein serotypes only, such as type 12 (respiratory) and type 49 (skin). Second attacks require infection with a nephritogenic strain of another M type; this event is rare, however, and recurrences are unusual.

immunologic etiology

As in rheumatic fever, the pathogenesis of acute glomerulonephritis appears to involve immunologic mechanisms. Immunoglobulins, complement components, and antigens that react with antibodies against group A streptococci have been identified in the diseased glomerulus. The renal injury may be caused by cross-reactions between renal tissue and antistreptococcal antibodies or simply by deposition in the glomerulus of preformed antigen–antibody complexes. Such complexes have been identified in the serum during acute disease and together with complement as discrete deposits in the glomerulus.

Epidemiology

Pharyngitis

direct or droplet spread

influence of crowding

Group A streptococcal pharyngitis is spread by respiratory secretions. Acquisition can be by direct contact with the mucosa or secretions, or through large droplets produced by coughing, sneezing, or even conversation. Droplet transmission is most efficient at short distances (2–5 feet). Spread is common in families and may be accentuated by crowding in institutions such as schools and military barracks. Food, although a less common vehicle of transmission, has been the source of many outbreaks. Environmental sources and fomites are not important means of spread, although group A streptococci survive for some time in dried secretions.

role of carriers

The acute case of streptococcal pharyngitis is the most important source of the organism. Without treatment, the organism is often present for 1–4 weeks after symptoms have disappeared. Asymptomatic carrier rates are usually very low; however, rates of more than 10% have sometimes been documented in children. Carriage may be both pharyngeal and nasal, and occasionally anal. The epidemiologic importance of asymptomatic and convalescent carriers is clearly less than that of acute cases. Nasal carriers have greater infectivity than those who carry *S. pyogenes* in the throat only.

"Ping-pong" infections

Recurrent infections are sometimes seen in families when prompt antimicrobial therapy has prevented the development of type-specific immunity. This situation allows reinfection from other infected or colonized siblings when antimicrobic treatment is stopped. Such "ping-pong" infection–reinfection cycles sometimes require simultaneous treatment of the entire family to prevent continued transmission.

Impetigo

prior skin colonization

transmission

Impetigo caused by *S. pyogenes* has an earlier peak age incidence (2–5 years) than streptococcal pharyngitis. Clinical impetigo is often preceded by skin colonization, which is favored by poor hygiene. Minor trauma of colonized skin (for example, insect bites) then leads to development of the lesions. Transmission involves direct contact or shared fomites such as towels. Certain flies have been shown to serve as vectors. Impetigo is most common among lower socioeconomic groups, in hot climates, and at times when insect bites are frequent. The M protein types of *S. pyogenes* associated with impetigo are different from those causing respiratory infection, and some are nephritogenic.

Nosocomial wound and puerperal infections

outbreaks associated with anal carriage of *S. pyogenes*

Group A streptococci were once a leading cause of nosocomial postoperative wound and puerperal infections (Chapter 66). The primary mode of transmission from patient to patient was by the hands of physicians or other medical attendants and through poor hygienic practices. The potential for hospital spread, however, is still present. Infections may be derived from staff or patients ill with pharyngitis or carrying the organism in the pharynx or nose. Contaminated particles or epithelial cells from nonrespiratory carriage sites can also be a source of infection. For example, two recent nosocomial outbreaks of group A streptococcal infections were traced to anal carriers who disseminated the organisms widely in operating rooms.

Treatment and Prevention

continued universal susceptibility to penicillin

Streptococcus pyogenes remains universally highly susceptible to penicillin G, the antimicrobic of choice. Patients allergic to penicillin are usually treated with erythromycin if the organisms are susceptible or with a cephalosporin if cross-allergy is absent. Adequate penicillin treatment of streptococcal pharyngitis within 10 days of onset will prevent rheumatic fever by removing the antigenic stimulus; it has a relatively minor effect on the duration of the pharyngitis, however, because of the short course of the natural infection. Penicillin does not prevent the development of acute glomerulonephritis.

prevention of rheumatic fever

prophylaxis for recurrences of rheumatic fever

Penicillin prophylaxis with long-acting preparations is used to prevent recurrences of rheumatic fever during the most susceptible ages (5–15 years). Patients with a history of rheumatic fever or known rheumatic heart disease usually receive antimicrobial prophylaxis while undergoing procedures known to cause transient bacteremia, such as dental extraction.

Laboratory Diagnosis

direct Gram smears unhelpful in diagnosis of pharyngitis

culture on blood agar

A typical clinical picture with demonstration of the organism in the infected site is the usual means by which active *S. pyogenes* infection is diagnosed. In pharyngitis, a swab of the posterior pharynx and tonsils is taken to include all inflamed areas. A direct Gram-stained smear is unhelpful because of the many other streptococci in the normal pharyngeal flora. Direct Gram smears from normally sterile sites will usually demonstrate streptococci (Plate C). Blood agar plates are seeded and incubated at 35–37°C. When *S. pyogenes* alone is sought (throat swabs), many laboratories use anaerobic incubation because of its favorable effect on the demonstration of β-hemolysis.

Presumptive differentiation of *S. pyogenes* from other β-hemolytic streptococci

After overnight incubation, β-hemolytic colonies are Gram stained to confirm that they are streptococci, then speciated according to group. Although definitive speciation is primarily through immunologic techniques, nonimmunologic methods can be used because of their good correlation with the definitive test. The *bacitracin test* is based on the exquisite susceptibility of group A strains to bacitracin and the relative resistance of strains of other groups. When a disc containing a small amount of bacitracin (0.02 U) is placed on a plate streaked from an isolated colony, more than 99% of group A strains show zone inhibition, whereas 90–95% of non-group A strains do not. The low rate of false-negative results has made this method a valuable presumptive test in hospital laboratories. Definitive identification of *S. pyogenes* requires demonstration of the group A specific antigen by precipitin, immunofluorescence, or agglutination procedures. Typing according to M or T antigens may be done for epidemiologic purposes; the procedure is serologic, using precipitin techniques with type-specific antisera.

Serologic detection of group A antigen

Epidemiologic subtyping

Serologic tests in rheumatic fever

Several serologic tests have been developed to aid in the diagnosis of poststreptococcal sequelae. They include the antistreptolysin O, anti-DNAase B, antistreptokinase, and antihyaluronidase tests. As characteristically high titers of antistreptolysin O are usually found in sera of patients with rheumatic fever, that test is used most widely.

Streptococcus agalactiae (Group B)

larger colonies than group A strains

β-hemolysis less distinct

In broth culture and in purulent lesions, group B streptococci produce short chains and occasional pairs of spherical or ovoid Gram-positive cells. In comparison with those of group A strains, the colonies produced on blood agar are larger and softer and may show yellow to orange pigments with anaerobic incubation. β-Hemolysis is less distinct and may be absent, particularly under aerobic conditions. In addition to their Lancefield antigen, group B streptococci possess polysaccharide capsular antigens. This characteristic forms the basis of a serologic typing system for strains within the group. The type antigens are designated Ia, Ib, Ic, II, and III. Sialic acid is the major immunodeterminant for types Ia, II, and III and is present in all five capsules. Although extracellular products and hemolysins have been identified in group B streptococci, their association with virulence has not been studied extensively.

penicillin susceptibility less than in group A

Group B streptococci are susceptible to the same antimicrobics as group A organisms; however, they are less susceptible to penicillin G (MIC, 0.2–1.0 μg/ml) and more frequently resistant to tetracycline.

Diseases

Neonatal pneumonia, sepsis, and meningitis

Group B streptococci are a leading cause of pneumonia, sepsis, and meningitis during the first 2 months of life. The incidence of group B infections in this age group has been estimated at 1–3 cases per 1000 births, and the mortality is between 30 and 60% of infected cases. Most cases, which develop in the immediate perinatal period, result from contamination of the infant with group B streptococci from the female genital tract. As group B streptococci are present in the vagina in one-third of all normal women, factors other than simple exposure must be involved in infection. The capsular sialic acid may be important as it has been associated with virulence and shown to prevent activation of the alternate complement pathway. For type III strains type-specific antibody has been shown to be protective; therefore, it is probable that only those infants who have not received specific transplacental immunoglobulin G(IgG) from their mothers are susceptible. A "late onset" syndrome may also occur 3–8 weeks after birth. These cases usually involve type III strains and have a lower mortality than those with early onset. Most cases with late onset have fever with no obvious primary site or meningitis. Some are examples of nosocomial cross-infection; others acquire the organisms after leaving the hospital.

probable protection by transplacental IgG

late onset syndrome in infants

Other group B streptococcal infections

Group B streptococci may also colonize the throat in children and adults, in whom they have been associated with a variety of pyogenic infections at nonrespiratory sites. Prominent examples are puerperal fevers and infections associated with gynecologic manipulations or surgery. As indicated by the species name *agalactae,* these organisms cause mastitis in cattle; however, pasteurization of milk has eliminated this source as an important link to human disease. Group B streptococci are not associated with rheumatic fever or acute glomerulonephritis.

Combination therapy

Because the organisms' susceptibility to penicillin is slightly less than that of many other streptococci, group B streptococcal infections are often treated with combinations of penicillin and an aminoglycoside.

Laboratory diagnosis

The laboratory diagnosis of group B infection is by culture on blood agar medium both aerobically and anaerobically, the latter to demonstrate hemolysis more clearly. Definitive identification involves serologic determination of the Lancefield group; however, presumptive identification tests with a high degree of correlation (for example, demonstration of ability to hydrolyze *hippurate*) are commonly used in clinical laboratories.

Group D and Other Pyogenic Streptococci

resistance of enterococci to bile salts and NaCl

The terms *group D streptococci* and *enterococci* are often used interchangeably, because the first demonstration of the group D antigen was in several species commonly found in the gastrointestinal tract. This usage is not correct, however, as the enterococci are a subset of species within group D (Table 12.1). Enterococci are found in the intestinal tract and have many biochemical and cultural features that reflect their habitat, such as the ability to grow in the presence of high concentrations of bile salts and sodium chloride. Morphologically, the enterococci are often oval and form diplococci or short chains. Several different species are biochemically distinct (see Table 12.1). Some are β-hemolytic, but most produce nonhemolytic or α-hemolytic colonies that are larger than those of other streptococci.

relative resistance to penicillin

The enterococci are the most resistant of the streptococci to antimicrobics. They require 4–16 μg/ml penicillin for inhibition and much higher concentrations for bactericidal effect. Enterococci are consistently resistant to aminoglycosides and sulfonamides, often resistant to tetracycline, and occasionally resistant to erythromycin and chloramphenicol. Ampicillin is the antimicrobial agent most consistently active. Despite their resistance to aminoglycosides, many strains of enterococci are inhibited and rapidly killed by combinations of low concentrations of penicillin and aminoglycosides. Under these conditions, the action of penicillin on the cell wall allows the aminoglycoside to enter the cell, reach its ribosomal receptor site, and kill the cell.

synergistic effects of penicillin and aminoglycosides on enterococci

Nonenterococcal group D streptococci

Since the original Lancefield classification was developed, the teichoic acid group D antigen has been found in some streptococcal species previously considered ungroupable. These organisms, termed *nonenterococcal group D streptococci,* resemble the viridans streptococci more than the enterococci in their cultural, biologic, and antimicrobic susceptibility features.

Pathogenicity of group C, G, and F streptococci

Streptococci of groups C, G, and F may be isolated from humans and other animals. These organisms can cause pyogenic infection, but do so much less frequently than those of groups A, B, or D. In general, their susceptibility to antimicrobial agents is similar to that of group A and B streptococci.

Diseases

Enterococcal infections

Enterococci cause opportunistic urinary tract infections, and occasionally wound and soft tissue infections, in much the same fashion as members of the Enterobacteriaceae. Infections are often associated with urinary tract manipulations, malignancies, biliary tract disease, and gastrointestinal disorders. There is often an associated bacteremia, which can result in the development of endocarditis on previously damaged cardiac valves.

Treatment of enterococcal infection depends on its site and severity. Ampicillin is effective in most urinary tract and minor soft tissue infections. More severe infections, particularly endocarditis, require treatment with combinations of a penicillin and an aminoglycoside.

Identification of enterococci in the laboratory depends on demonstration of their ability to grow in the presence of bile salts and high concentrations of NaCl (6.5%). Despite their Lancefield group D antigen, most strains of enterococci are not β-hemolytic.

Infections caused by pyogenic streptococci of other groups

The other pyogenic streptococci occasionally produce various respiratory, skin, wound, soft tissue, and genital infections, which may resemble those caused by group A and B streptococci. None has been clearly associated with poststreptococcal sequelae. The role of pyogenic streptococci other than those of group A in acute pharyngitis is unestablished. A few case reports of food-borne outbreaks have shown some strains of group C and G streptococci to cause pharyngitis, but the evidence is not yet strong enough to draw this conclusion in individual cases.

Streptococcus pneumoniae

Morphology

encapsulated, Gram-positive, lanceolate diplococci

In clinical material or culture, cells of *S. pneumoniae* appear as Gram-positive, oval diplococci with their axes end to end (Figure 12.3). They sometimes form short chains. The adjacent ends of a pair tend to be rounded, the distal ends more pointed, giving the individual cell a bullet or lancet shape. Older cells or those exposed to antimicrobial agents may appear Gram negative and show morphologic distortion. Virulent strains are encapsulated, but the capsules are not apparent in Gram-stained preparations.

Cultural Characteristics

Pneumoccoci are fastidious organisms, requiring a relatively complex medium for isolation. Rapid growth is frequently followed by autolysis. Initially turbid broth may clear on continued incubation; once formed, colonies begin to lyse in the center and even disappear. This behavior is caused by their susceptibility to autolytic enzymes and to peroxides produced during growth. Another growth-limiting feature is the lowered pH caused by lactic acid produced by fermentation or carbohydrates in the medium. Autolysis can be hastened with surfactants such as detergents and bile; this quality forms the basis of the bile solubility test.

autolysis and bile solubility

On blood agar, encapsulated pneumococci produce round, glistening colonies (0.5–2 mm in diameter after 18 hr) surrounded by a zone of α-hemolysis. Because of autolysis, the colonies often develop a dimpled, then a craterlike appearance. Pneumococcal colonies may be indistinguishable from those of viridans streptococci, particularly in young cultures.

α-hemolysis and colony autolysis

Virulence and the Pneumococcal Capsule

The structural features of pneumococci are similar to those of other streptococci; the important exception is their surface antigenic capsules, which are composed of complex polysaccharides forming hydrophilic gels. The recognition of more than 80 distinct serotypes of capsule (types 1,2, . . . , 24, and so on) forms the basis of a pneumococcal serotype classification system. The chemical structure of the polysaccharides has been determined for only a few types, but shows unique features for each. It is of interest that antibodies against capsules of certain serotypes are known to cross-react with polysaccharides produced by certain serotypes of other bacteria (*Haemophilus, Klebsiella*) and even with human blood group B isoantigen.

more than 80 antigenic types of pneumococcal polysaccharide capsules

The physical nature of the polysaccharide capsule of the pneumococcus inhibits its engulfment by phagocytes and is the major determinant of virulence. Unencapsulated mutants are avirulent in experimental infections. Specific anticapsular antibody, whether produced by active or passive immunization, opsonizes capsulate strains and confers type-specific immunity to infection. Capsule production, and thus virulence, can be conferred on noncapsulate strains by transformation with DNA extracted from a capsulate strain. Thus, an avirulent noncapsulate mutant of a type II pneumococcus can be transformed to a virulent capsulate type III strain with DNA from another type III strain.

antiphagocytic effect of capsule is major determinant of virulence

type-specific anticapsular antibody opsonizes organism and confers immunity

Transformation of capsule type

Toxins and Extracellular Enzymes

A pneumolysin, a neuraminidase, and a substance that causes purpura and dermal hemorrhage in experimental animals have been isolated from pneumococci. The pneumolysin has some properties similar to those of streptolysin O, including toxicity in experimental animals, and the neuraminidase may contribute to invasiveness by splitting membrane glycoproteins and glycolipids. There is no convincing evidence, however, that these substances play an important role in pneumococcal infection. Virulence is largely attributable to the antiphagocytic properties of the capsule, and disease to the acute inflammatory response to infection; however, these findings do not fully explain some of the clinical features of infection with *S. pneumoniae,* such as the abrupt onset, the toxicity, and the fulminant course and disseminated intravascular coagulation seen in some cases. For these reasons, interest in toxins continues, but their role is presently inconclusive.

Pathogenicity

The pneumococcus is pathogenic for humans and many animals. Under experimental conditions mice and rabbits are highly susceptible, and murine inoculation of clinical material was used in the past for primary isolation of the organism. The virulence of different serotypes varies for both humans and animals.

Antimicrobial Susceptibility

usually susceptible to penicillin

recent development of penicillin resistance

Pneumococci generally follow the pattern of group A streptococci in their susceptibility to antimicrobics. They are usually highly susceptible to penicillin and other β-lactam agents. Tetracycline resistance is common (3–30%), but resistance to erythromycin or chloramphenicol is rare. Aminoglycosides are not effective. Recently, pneumococci resistant to penicillin and other antimicrobics have been reported from South Africa. These strains require penicillin concentrations of 0.12–4.0 μg/ml for inhibition, whereas fully susceptible strains are inhibited by 0.01–0.05 μg/ml. Patients with pneumonia and meningitis caused by the more resistant strains respond poorly or not at all to penicillin therapy. The mechanism of resistance appears to be mutational and involves alterations of penicillin-binding proteins, rather than penicillinase production.

Although such strains are still rare in the United States, the development of penicillin-resistant pneumococci is very disturbing. For more than 30 years penicillin had been effective in the treatment of pneumococcal infections, and it appeared that mutational resistance was incompatible with virulence. We can no longer feel secure about the long-range stability of penicillin susceptibility in other species, such as *S. pyogenes.*

Diseases

predisposing factors

Pneumococcal pneumonia. Streptococcus pneumoniae is by far the most common cause of bacterial pneumonia. As with other bacterial pneumonias, viral respiratory infection and underlying chronic disease are important predisposing factors. Although infection may occur at any age, the incidence and mortality of pneumococcal pneumonia increase sharply after 50 years. Alcoholism, diabetes mellitus, chronic renal disease, and some malignancies are all associated with more frequent and serious pneumococcal pneumonias. In the preantibiotic era, the mortality in hospitalized patients was 20–30%; it has now been reduced to 5–10%. Although these mortality estimates are probably higher than those for cases in the community, the disease remains an important cause of death.

Normal host defenses and factors that impair them

Pneumococcal pneumonia begins with aspiration of respiratory secretions containing pneumococci. This event must be common, as 10–30% of normal people carry one or more serologic types of *S. pneumoniae* in the throat. Aspirated organisms are normally cleared rapidly by the defense mechanisms of the lower respiratory tract, including the cough and epiglottic reflexes, the mucociliary "blanket," and phagocytosis by alveolar macrophages. Events that impair the combined efficiency of these defenses can allow pneumococci to reach and multiply in the alveoli. They include the chronic illnesses mentioned previously, damage to bronchial epithelium from smoking or air pollution, and respiratory dysfunction from alcoholic intoxication, narcotics and other drugs, anesthesia, and trauma.

type-specific immunity and course of infection

In immune individuals with a sufficient level of circulating antibody against the capsular polysaccharide of organisms that reach the alveoli, the infection is controlled rapidly; in nonimmune individuals, however, alveolar multiplication is followed by a profuse outpouring of serous edema fluid, which facilitates growth and spread of pneumococci to adjacent alveoli and interferes with gas exchange. The fluid outpouring is quickly followed by an influx of polymorphonuclear leukocytes and erythrocytes, the latter as a result of capillary fragility. By the second or third day of illness, the lung segment has increased three- to fourfold in weight through accumulation of this cellular, hemorrhagic fluid. By the fourth or fifth day, neutrophils predominate in the consolidated alveoli, which usually affect a single lobe of the lung. Although some surface phagocytosis and destruction of pneumococci occurs in the absence of opsonizing antibody, it is outpaced by multiplication of the organism, and bacteremia is common. Even when formation of anticapsular antibody begins, it may be neutralized by free soluble capsular polysaccharide in the exudate and bloodstream. If antibody production is sufficient to overcome this neutralization, however, the pneumococci are readily phagocytosed and destroyed. When actively growing pneumococci are no longer present, macrophages replace the granulocytes and resolution of the lesion ensues. A remarkable feature of pneumococcal pneumonia is the lack of structural damage to the lung, which usually leads to complete resolution on recovery.

consolidation caused by inflammation: interference with gas exchange

lobar distribution

effect of free capsular polysaccharide

absence of structural damage

Clinical manifestations

Clinically, pneumococcal pneumonia begins abruptly with a shaking chill and high fever. Cough with production of sputum pink to rusty in color (indicating the presence of red blood cells) and pleuritic chest pain are common. Physical findings usually indicate pulmonary consolidation. Children and young adults typically demonstrate a lobar consolidation on chest radiography, whereas older patients may show a less localized bronchial distribution to the infiltrates. Without therapy, sustained fever, pleuritic pain, and productive cough continue until, in patients who recover, a "crisis" occurs 5–10 days after onset of the disease. The crisis involves a sudden decrease in temperature and of improvement in the patients condition. It is associated with effective levels of opsonizing antibody reaching the lesion.

crisis associated with effective levels of opsonizing antibody

Pneumococcal meningitis. With *Neisseria meningitidis* and *Haemophilus influenzae, S. pneumoniae* is one of the three leading causes of bacterial meningitis. The signs and symptoms are similar to those produced by other bacteria (Chapter 61). Acute purulent meningitis may follow pneumococcal infection at another site or appear with no apparent antecedent infection. It may also develop after trauma involving the skull. All ages are affected; in young children, however, meningitis caused by *H. influenzae* is more common. In later life, pneumococcal meningitis is the most common form of the disease. The mortality and frequency of sequelae are slightly higher with pneumococcal meningitis than with other forms of pyogenic meningitis.

age and predisposing factors

sinusitis and otitis media

Upper respiratory tract infections. Pneumococci are common causes of sinusitis and otitis media. The latter frequently occurs in children in association with viral infection. Chronic infection of the mastoid or respiratory sinus sometimes extends to the subarachnoid space to cause meningitis. Pneumococci do not cause pharyngitis or tonsillitis.

Other infections. Pneumococci may also cause endocarditis, arthritis, and peritonitis, usually in association with bacteremia. Patients with ascites caused by diseases such as cirrhosis and nephritis may develop spontaneous pneumococcal peritonitis.

Treatment and Prevention

penicillin therapy for susceptible strains

As the great majority of pneumococci are fully sensitive to it, penicillin is the antimicrobic of choice. Infections caused by the more resistant strains encountered recently may require treatment with erythromycin or chloramphenicol. The therapeutic response to treatment of pneumococcal pneumonia is often (but not always) dramatic. Reduction in fever, respiratory rate, and cough can occur in 12–24 hr, but may occur gradually over several days. Chest radiography may yield normal results only after several weeks.

Polyvalent capsular polysaccharide vaccine

A vaccine has been prepared from capsular polysaccharide extracted from the 14 types of *S. pneumoniae* most commonly encountered. This vaccine, which is protective against these 14 types, is recommended for patients particularly susceptible to pneumococcal infection because of age, underlying disease, or immune status.

Laboratory Diagnosis

direct Gram smears

need for adequate specimens

Gram smears of material from sites of pneumococcal infection usually show typical Gram-positive, lancet-shaped diplococci (Figure 12.3); in partially treated cases, however, many cells may be swollen and show a loss of Gram positivity. A properly collected sputum sample comprising inflammatory exudate from the affected lung segment will usually reveal the typical appearance. Sputum collection may be difficult, however, and specimens contaminated with respiratory flora are useless for diagnosis. Other types of lower respiratory specimens may be needed for diagnosis (Chapters 9 and 58).

Culture

Streptococcus pneumoniae grows well overnight on blood agar medium incubated aerobically. Supplementation with carbon dioxide often enhances

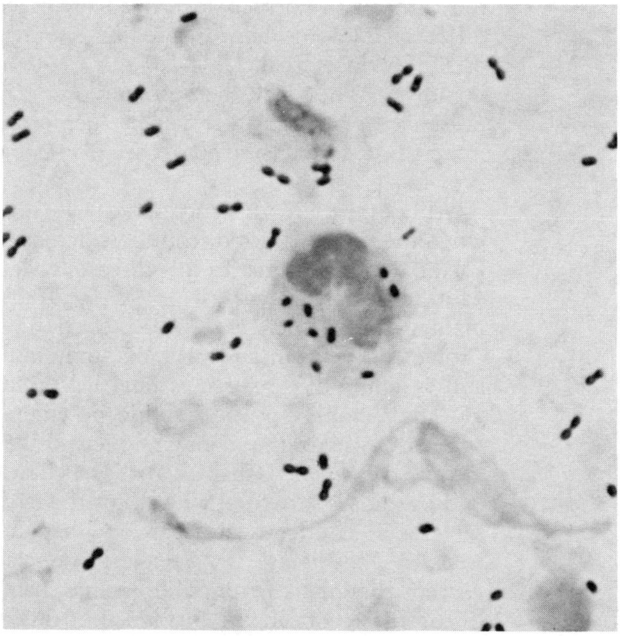

12.3 *Streptococcus pneumoniae* in sputum of patient with pneumonia. Note the marked tendency to form oval diplococci.

growth. Colonies are surrounded by a zone of α-hemolysis. The pneumococcal capsule, which is not visible in unstained preparations, can be demonstrated by special staining techniques or through the quellung (capsular swelling) reaction. When capsulate pneumococci are mixed with type-specific antisera, the opsonized capsule absorbs water, becomes increasingly refractile and visible under the light microscope, and appears swollen.

Quellung reaction

Distinguishing factors from viridans streptococci

The pneumococcus is distinguished from viridans streptococci by several tests, including:

1. Susceptibility to the synthetic chemical ethylhydrocupreine (Optochin), which can be demonstrated by a disc diffusion test; viridans streptococci are resistant.
2. Bile solubility; viridans streptococci are insoluble.
3. Presence of a capsule.
4. Virulence for mice.
5. Capsular swelling reaction with type-specific or pooled polyvalent sera against the pneumococcal capsule.

Blood culture

Bacteremia is common in pneumococcal pneumonia and meningitis, and blood cultures are valuable supplements to cultures of local fluids or exudates.

Detection of pneumococcal antigen in clinical material

If high-titer specific antisera are available, pneumococcal capsular material can frequently be demonstrated in body fluids, serum, and urine using counterimmunoelectrophoresis, latex agglutination, or coagglutination methods (Chapter 9). The quellung technique can also be applied directly to clinical specimens if organisms are visible.

Viridans Streptococci

α-hemolytic organisms

bile insoluble, optochin negative, noncapsulate

The viridans group comprises all α-hemolytic streptococci that remain after the criteria for defining pyogenic streptococci and pneumococci have been applied. Characteristically members of the normal flora of the oral and nasopharyngeal cavities, they have the basic bacteriologic features of streptococci, but lack the specific antigens, toxins, and virulence of the other groups. Although the viridans group includes several species (Table 12.1), they are usually not characterized in clinical practice because there is little difference among them in medical significance. Viridans streptococci generally produce small (0.5–1.0 mm) colonies surrounded by a zone of α-hemolysis. They lack the autolytic properties of pneumococci, even in the presence of surface-active agents such as bile salts. The procedures for distinguishing viridans streptococci from pneumococci have been described previously.

Subacute bacterial endocarditis

Although their virulence is very low, viridans strains can cause disease when they are protected from host defenses. The prime example is subacute bacterial endocarditis. In this disease, viridans streptococci reach previously damaged heart valves as a result of transient bacteremia associated with manipulations, such as tooth extraction, that disturb their usual habitat. Protected by fibrin and platelets, they multiply on the valve, causing local and systemic disease that is fatal if untreated. Extracellular production of glucans, complex polysaccharide polymers, may enhance their attachment to cardiac valves in a manner similar to the pathogenesis of dental caries by *Streptococcus mutans* (Chapter 56). The clinical course of viridans streptococcal endocarditis is subacute, with slow progression over weeks or months (Chapter 62). It is effectively treated with penicillin, but uniformly fatal if untreated. The disease is particularly associated with valves damaged by recurrent rheumatic fever. The decline in the occurrence of rheumatic heart disease has reduced the incidence of this particular type of endocarditis.

Additional Reading and References

Lancefield, R.C. 1933. A serological differentiation of human and other groups of hemolytic streptococci. *J. Exp. Med.* 57:571–595. The classic study that changed streptococcal classification.

Unny, S.K., and Middlebrooks, B.L. 1983. Streptococcal rheumatic carditis. *Microbiol. Rev.* 47:97–120. This current review covers all aspects of the pathogenesis of rheumatic myocarditis and valvulitis including the evidence for immunologic cross-reactions.

Wannamaker, L.W. 1970. Differences between streptococcal infections of the throat and of the skin. *N. Engl. J. Med.* 282:23–31. Some important clinical, epidemiologic, and immunologic features are summarized in greater detail than in the present chapter.

Wannamaker, L.W., and Matsen, J.M. Eds. 1972. *Streptococci and Streptococcal Diseases: Recognition, Understanding, and Management.* New York: Academic Press. This comprehensive monograph contains in-depth discussions on topics ranging from pathogenesis of sequelae to clinical aspects of streptococcal infections.

Kenneth J. Ryan

Corynebacteria and Other Non-Spore-Forming Gram-Positive Rods

13

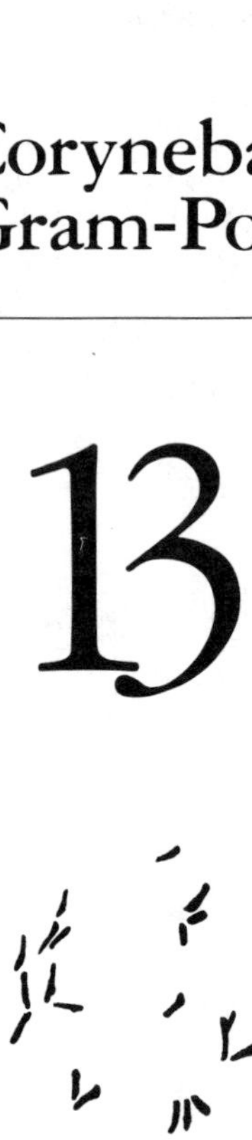

Corynebacterium diphtheriae

Corynebacteria are small, pleomorphic, Gram-positive rods, which in some species tend to have clubbed ends (from the Greek *koryne*, club). The cells often remain attached after division, forming "Chinese letter" or palisade arrangements. Spores are not formed. Some species contain polyphosphate granules that stain red-purple with methylene blue (metachromatic granules). Growth is generally best under aerobic conditions, but many strains will grow under microaerophilic or anaerobic conditions on media enriched with blood or other animal products.

Colonies on blood agar are usually small (1–2 mm); however, some strains of *Corynebacterium diphtheriae* may produce colonies 3 mm in diameter after incubation for 24 hr. Most are nonhemolytic. Catalase is produced, and many strains form acid (usually lactic acid) through carbohydrate fermentation. The species *C. diphtheriae* produces a powerful exotoxin, which is responsible for the disease diphtheria and which usually results from a pharyngeal infection. Some corynebacteria, which are primarily pathogenic to animals, produce other toxins. Others are nonpathogenic commensal inhabitants of the pharynx, nasopharynx, distal urethra, and skin; they are collectively designated as diphtheroids.

Corynebacterium diphtheriae

Loeffler's medium

metachromatic granules

Because it is clinically important to distinguish *C. diphtheriae* rapidly from members of the respiratory flora, several media and methods have been developed to demonstrate this organism. That used by Loeffler in 1887 in the discovery of *C. diphtheriae* is still used in clinical laboratories. It consists of 75% serum and 25% broth, which is coagulated by heat. *Corynebacterium diphtheriae* grows more rapidly on this medium than members of the normal oral flora, such as streptococci and *Neisseria* species, and the "Chinese letter" morphology and metachromatic granules typical of *C. diphtheriae* are particularly well developed. These morphologic features are not seen consistently in clinical specimens or in preparations from other common laboratory media.

Tellurite selective media

Selective media have been developed containing potassium tellurite, which inhibits many members of the normal oral flora. *Corynebacterium diphtheriae* also reduces the potassium tellurite to produce gray or black colonies, the morphology of which differs with each of three types of the organism: *gravis, mitis,* and *intermedius.* Differentiation of *C. diphtheriae* from other corynebacteria depends on several biochemical reactions, including carbo-

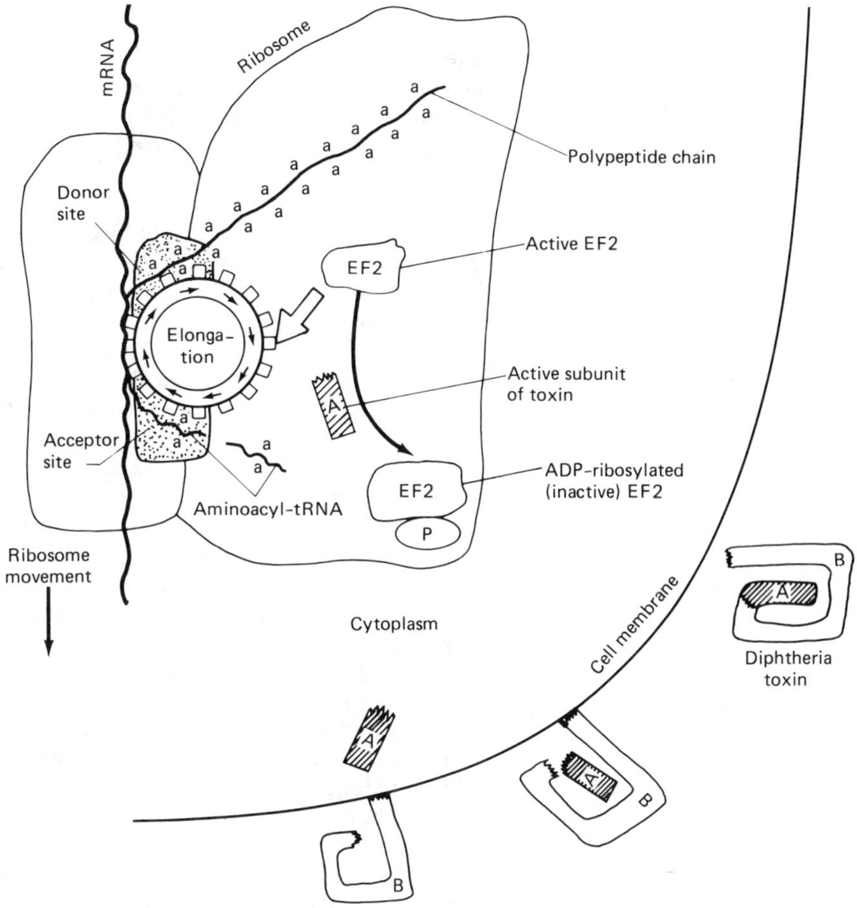

13.1 Action of diphtheria toxin. The toxin-binding (**B**) portion attaches to the cell membrane, allowing the active (**A**) portion to dissociate and enter the cell. In the cell, active toxin catalyzes a reaction that ADP-ribosylates and thus inactivates elongation factor 2 (EF2). This factor is essential for ribosomal reactions at the acceptor and donor sites, which transfer triplet code from messenger RNA (mRNA) to amino acid sequences via transfer RNA (tRNA). Inactivation of EF2 stops building of the polypeptide chain.

Diphtheria exotoxin

B fragment binds to cell receptor

A fragment is protein synthesis inhibitor

toxin coded by temperate phage

antitoxin and toxoid

Nontoxigenic strains

lysogenic conversion

hydrate fermentation tests. Virulence is determined by production of diphtheria exotoxin, a protein with potent cytotoxic features. It inhibits protein synthesis in cell-free extracts of virtually all eukaryotic cells, from protozoa and yeasts to higher plants and humans. However, it is only toxic to the intact cells of certain mammals. The toxin is composed of two fragments, A and B (Figure 13.1). The B fragment binds to a specific surface receptor on sensitive mammalian cells and mediates the transport of the A fragment, the active moiety, into the cell. Once in the cell, the A fragment inactivates the elongation factor required for transfer of polypeptidyl–transfer RNA from acceptor to donor site on the ribosome. The toxin acts on the EF-2 elongation factor found in eukaryotic cells but not that of bacteria. The toxin is highly potent. A single molecule has been shown to inhibit protein synthesis in a cell within a few hours. The structural gene for the diphtheria toxin molecule is contained in a bacteriophage (β phage), and strains of *C. diphtheriae,* which are lysogenic for this phage, produce toxin. The toxin is antigenic, stimulating the production of antitoxin antibodies during natural infection. Formalin treatment of toxin produces *toxoid,* which retains the antigenicity but not the toxicity of native toxin and is used in immunization against the disease. It is clear that this process functionally inactivates fragment B. Whether it also inactivates fragment A or prevents its ability to dissociate from fragment B is not known. Nontoxigenic strains of *C. diphtheriaea* can produce pharyngitis, but not the toxic manifestations of diphtheria. They can be converted to toxicity by lysogenization in vitro with β phage, and this process can probably occur in vivo.

Diphtheria

localized pharyngeal or upper respiratory infection

membrane

After an incubation period of 2–4 days, diphtheria acquired by the respiratory route usually presents as pharyngitis or tonsillitis; however, nasal diphtheria may resemble the common cold. Infection is localized and does not invade deep tissues or other organs. Typically, malaise, sore throat, and fever are present, and a patch of exudate or membrane develops on the tonsils, uvula, soft palate, or pharyngeal wall. The gray-white membrane is caused by the action of the diphtheria toxin on the epithelium at the site of infection. It is composed of a coagulum of fibrin, leukocytes, cellular debris, and bacteria, adheres to the mucous membrane, and may extend from the oropharyngeal area down to the larynx and into the trachea. Associated cervical adenitis is common, and in severe cases cervical adenitis and edema produce a "bullneck" appearance. In uncomplicated cases, the infection gradually resolves and the membrane is coughed up after 5–10 days.

cervical lymphadenitis

respiratory obstruction

The complications and mortality of diphtheria are caused by obstruction by the local infection or by the systemic effect of diphtheria toxin absorbed at the site of infection. Mechanical obstruction of the airway produced by membrane, edema, and hemorrhage can be sudden and complete and can lead to suffocation death, particularly if large sections of the membrane separate from the tracheal or laryngeal epithelial surface. Diphtheria toxin absorbed into the circulation causes damage to various organs, the most serious of which is to the heart. Diphtheritic myocarditis appears during the second or third week in severe cases of respiratory diphtheria. It is manifested by cardiac enlargement and weakness, arrhythmia, and congestive heart failure with dyspnea. Electrocardiographic abnormalities can be detected before evidence of heart failure. Paralyses caused by involvement of cranial and peripheral nerves later in the course of disease, most often involve the soft palate, oculomotor (eye) muscles, or motor paralysis of select muscle groups. Paralysis is reversible, and it is generally not serious unless respiratory muscles such as the diaphragm are involved.

remote effects of toxin on heart

neurologic manifestations

Cutaneous diphtheria

Corynebacterium diphtheriae may produce nonrespiratory infections, particularly of the skin. Cutaneous infection may occur with toxigenic or nontoxigenic strains alone or in association with *Staphylococcus aureus* or β-hemolytic streptococci. The characteristic lesion ranges from a simple pustule to a chronic, nonhealing ulcer and is most common in tropical and hot, arid regions. Cardiac and neurologic complications from these infections are infrequent, suggesting that the efficiency of toxin production or absorption is low compared to that in respiratory infections. Cases of cutaneous diphtheria can serve as an epidemiologic reservoir for spread of respiratory as well as nonrespiratory diphtheria.

little invasive capacity

It is important to remember that the manifestations of diphtheria are produced by multiplication of the organism and toxin production at the local site of infection. The organism has little invasive capacity, but the toxin causes tissue damage at both local and distant sites. Thus, *C. diphtheriae* is not isolated from the blood or from remote sites during the disease. The disease resolves with the formation of antitoxin antibody.

Epidemiology

droplet and fomitic spread

Carriers

Corynebacterium diphtheriae is transmitted by droplet spread, by direct contact with cutaneous carriers, and, to a lesser extent, by fomites. Some subjects become convalescent pharyngeal or nasal carriers and continue to harbor the organism for weeks to months or even for a lifetime. Other carriers have no history of the disease. Carriers represent the major reservoir for infection of nonimmune subjects. Diphtheria is currently rare in the United

States (100–300 cases per year) because of the routine practice of active immunization. Cases appear sporadically and as outbreaks in patients and populations who have not received adequate immunization, such as American Indians, migratory workers, and the transient and poor.

Treatment

Antitoxin therapy

adjunctive antimicrobic therapy

Treatment of diphtheria is directed at neutralization of the toxin with concurrent elimination of the organism. The former is accomplished by administering a diphtheria antitoxin produced in horses. This must be done as soon as possible because, whereas antitoxin neutralizes free toxin and that being produced, it has no effect on toxin already fixed to tissues. Hypersensitivity and serum sickness reactions can complicate this mode of therapy. *Corynebacterium diphtheriae* is susceptible to a variety of antimicrobics, including penicillins, cephalosporins, erythromycin, and tetracycline. Of these agents, penicillin and erythromycin have been used effectively as adjuncts to antitoxin therapy in acute disease. Erythromycin has been more effective than penicillin in eliminating the carrier state, but plasmid-determined erythromycin resistance is becoming common in some areas. The complications of diphtheria are managed primarily by supportive measures such as tracheostomy, cardiac monitoring and electric pacing, and drugs such as digitalis and antiarrhythmic agents.

Diagnosis

primary diagnosis is clinical

direct smears unreliable

Culture

Virulence tests

The initial diagnosis of diphtheria is entirely clinical. There are no laboratory tests of sufficient value to influence the decision regarding antitoxin administration. Direct smears of infected areas of the throat are not reliable diagnostic tools. Definitive diagnosis is accomplished by isolating and identifying *C. diphtheriae* from the infected site and demonstrating its toxigenicity. Isolation is usually achieved with Loeffler's medium and with a selective medium containing potassium tellurite. A recent formulation, Tinsdale agar, is highly selective; toxigenic strains produce a black colony with a brown halo. A toxigenicity (virulence) test is performed most easily by injecting two guinea pigs with the organism and protecting one with diphtheria antitoxin. Death of the test animal, with autopsy findings characteristic of the effects of diphtheria toxin, establishes the toxigenicity of the strain. Tissue culture and immunodiffusion methods for demonstrating toxigenicity are also available.

It should be acknowledged that while this diagnosis could be made and confirmed with great confidence in the past it is now more difficult because experience with the disease is rare. Most younger clinicians have never seen a case of diphtheria and many bacteriologists have never isolated the organism. As routine throat culture procedures will not isolate *C. diphtheriae,* the physician must advise the laboratory *in advance* of the suspicion of diphtheria. Laboratories without the appropriate media and experience must seek the assistance of reference facilities. Generally, 2 days are required to exclude *C. diphtheriae* (that is, they are not isolated on Tinsdale agar); however, more time is needed to complete identification and virulence testing of a positive culture.

Prevention

Toxoid immunization

The mainstay of diphtheria prevention is immunization. Three to four doses of diphtheria toxoid produce immunity by stimulating antitoxin production. The initial series is begun in the first year of life. Booster immunizations at

10-year intervals will maintain immunity. This vaccine is highly effective. Fully immunized individuals may become infected with *C. diphtheriae,* because the antibodies are directed only against the toxin, but the disease is mild. Serious infection and death occur only in unimmunized or incompletely immunized individuals. Susceptibility to diphtheria can be measured by the Schick test in which low concentrations of active and inactivated toxin are injected into the skin of opposite forearms. The inactivated toxin serves as a control. In subjects without circulating antitoxin, the action of the toxin causes redness and swelling in the test area within 24 hr. Presence of antitoxin results in a negative test. The Schick test is now used rarely, but it is of theoretic and epidemiologic importance.

Schick test

Other Corynebacteria

C. ulcerans and diphtheria toxin

Other diseases caused by corynebacteria

Corynebacteria other than *C. diphtheriae* are often called diphtheroids; some are commonly found in the normal flora of the skin and other body sites. The term actually encompasses several well-defined species, some of which have definite but unusual disease associations. Some species, such as *Corynebacterium ulcerans* may carry the β-phage and produce a small amount of diphtheria toxin and produce infections with mild toxic manifestations. Different toxins with dermonecrotic and/or hemolytic action may be produced also by *C. ulcerans, Corynebacterium hemolyticum,* and some other species, and many of them cause infection in animals that are occasionally the source of human disease. Clinical syndromes in humans include pharyngitis, pneumonia, granulomatous lymphadenitis, and skin infections. Corynebacteria may also produce disease in settings similar to those of *Staphylococcus epidermidis* (Chapter 13), the most common of which is endocarditis.

Group JK strains in immunosuppressed patients

One currently unnamed corynebacterium, group JK, has been increasingly associated with nosocomial infections in immunosuppressed patients. They include bacteremia, which is often associated with intravascular devices such as catheters and prosthetic heart valves. A striking feature of the JK corynebacterium is the extent of its antimicrobic resistance, which typically includes all common agents except vancomycin.

Other diphtheroids

Diphtheroids are not usually speciated in clinical laboratories, because the vast majority of isolates represent colonization or contamination rather than disease. When circumstances suggest that a diphtheroid isolate may be significant, further identification can be accomplished with several standard bacteriologic tests.

Listeria

Gram-positive rod

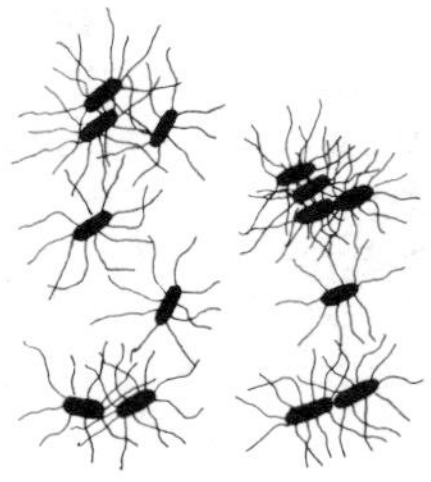

Listeria monocytogenes

Listeria monocytogenes is a Gram-positive rod with some bacteriologic features that resemble those of corynebacteria (Plate H). In stained smears of clinical and laboratory material, the organisms resemble diphtheroids. In culture, a small, smooth colony surrounded by a narrow rim of β-hemolysis is produced. *Listeria* species are catalase positive, which distinguishes them from streptococci, and produce a characteristic tumbling motility in fluid media that distinguishes them from corynebacteria.

Members of *Listeria* are widespread in nature. They can colonize or infect a wide variety of animals; human exposure usually involves transient colonization without disease. Resistance to infection involves T lymphocytes and mononuclear phagocytes as well as humoral mechanisms. Serious infections can occur and are seen most commonly in neonates and in immunocompromised individuals.

Meningitis and sepsis

The most common human infections are meningitis and sepsis. Neonatal and puerperal infections, associated with vaginal colonization by *Listeria,* appear in settings similar to those of infections with group B streptococci.

Intrauterine infections

Intrauterine infection results in the clinical syndrome of granulomatosis infantiseptica, in which the fetus is often stillborn with disseminated abscesses and/or granulomas. In most cases, an animal source cannot be found. Diagnosis of listeriosis is usually by culture of blood, cerebrospinal fluid, or focal lesions. *Listeria monocytogenes* is susceptible to penicillin G, ampicillin, erythromycin, and chloramphenicol, all of which have been used effectively.

Treatment

Erysipelothrix

Environmental and zoonotic sources

erythematous spreading lesion

Erysipelothrix rhusiopathiae is a Gram-positive rod with features similar to those of both corynebacteria and *Listeria*. This organism is widely distributed among animals and in decaying organic matter. Traumatic inoculation of *E. rhusiopathiae* into the skin produces *erysipeloid*, an occupational disease of fisherman, butchers, veterinarians, and others who handle animal products. Erysipeloid is a painful, slow-spreading, erythematous swelling of the skin. Penicillin is the treatment of choice, although the organism is also susceptible to erythromycin and tetracycline.

Lactobacilli

acidophilic Gram-positive non-spore forming rods

Lactobacilli are Gram-positive, non-spore forming rods. They are typically nonmotile and nonacid fast. The cells, which are usually long and slender with squared ends, are often arranged to form chains. They are aerobic and facultatively anaerobic and grow optimally at about pH 6. Lactobacilli actively ferment carbohydrates, forming lactic acid as the primary metabolic product. Numerous species have been described, of which the most commonly occurring in humans is *Lactobacillus acidophilus*.

member of the normal flora

Lactobacilli are important members of the normal human oral, gastrointestinal, and vaginal flora. Their reputation as beneficial members of the intestinal flora is responsible for the popularity of certain "natural" foods, such as yogurt, that contain lactobacilli and their fermentation products (Chapter 6). Lactobacilli are not pathogenic for humans or animals, although *L. acidophilus* has, from time-to-time been believed to play some role in the pathogenesis of dental caries.

Propionibacteria

The genus *Propionibacterium* resembles corynebacteria morphologically. Members are anaerobes or microaerophiles and are part of the normal skin flora (Chapter 6).

Additional Reading and References

Collier, R.J. 1975. Diphtheria toxin: Mode of action and structure. *Bacteriol. Rev.* 39:54–85. All aspects of diphtheria toxin are reviewed in detail, including the experimental evidence supporting current concepts of its biologic activity.

Koopman, J.S., and Campbell, J. 1975. The role of cutaneous diphtheria in a diphtheria epidemic. *J. Infect. Dis.* 131:239–244. This study shows that cutaneous diphtheria may be more contagious than respiratory infection.

McCloskey, R.V., Eller, J.J., Green, M., Mauney, C.U., and Richards, S.E.M. 1971. The 1970 epidemic of diphtheria in San Antonio. *Ann. Intern. Med.* 75:495–503. A clear and informative description of a modern diphtheria outbreak is provided. The clinical features are given in detail, including color photographs of diphtheritic membranes.

Kenneth J. Ryan

Bacillus

14

The genus *Bacillus* includes many species of aerobic or facultative, spore-forming, Gram-positive rods. With the exception of one species, *Bacillus anthracis,* they are low-virulence saprophytes widespread in air, soil, water, dust, and animal products. *Bacillus anthracis* causes the zoonosis *anthrax,* a disease of animals that is occasionally transmitted to humans.

Morphology and Staining

Gram-positive spore-forming rods

loss of Gram positivity

The genus comprises rod-shaped organisms approximately 0.7 μm wide and 3–10 μm long. The rods can thus vary from coccobacillary to rather long filaments, and they may be arranged in chains. The ends may be rounded or sharply truncated. Motile strains have peritrichous flagella. Formation of round or oval spores, which may be central, subterminal, or terminal depending on the species, is characteristic of the genus. Spores may be larger than the diameter of the bacillus, but usually are not. *Bacillus* species are Gram positive; however, positivity is often lost, depending on the species and the age of the culture. With some strains only very young (3–6 hr) cultures stain as Gram positive.

Growth and Resistance

aerobic growth

heat resistance of spores

Growth is obtained with ordinary media incubated in air and is reduced or absent under anaerobic conditions. Aerobic conditions are required for sporulation. The frequent development of a surface pellicle in broth cultures also reflects the aerobic preference. Colonies vary from 1 to 5 mm in diameter, and morphology ranges from mucoid to dry and pigmented. Some strains are β-hemolytic. The spores survive boiling for varying periods and are sufficiently resistant to heat that those of one species are used as a biologic indicator of autoclave efficiency.

Metabolism

Most species are metabolically active, producing acid but not gas from oxidation of glucose and various other sugars. They are catalase positive and produce proteolytic enzymes such as gelatinase. Many other biochemical reactions are variable among species and thus taxonomically useful.

Antigenic Structure

Multiple antigenic types have been described, primarily using agglutination reactions with antibody to cell wall or spore antigens. These procedures, however, are not used in routine diagnostic work.

Anthrax and Other Infections

Experiments of Koch and Pasteur on anthrax

The isolation of *B. anthracis,* the proof of its relationship to anthrax infection, and the demonstration of immunity to the disease are among the most important events in the history of science and medicine. Robert Koch rose to fame in 1877 by growing the organism in artificial culture using pure culture techniques. He defined the stringent criteria needed to prove that the organism caused anthrax (Koch's postulates), then met them experimentally. Louis Pasteur made a convincing field demonstration at Pouilly-le-Fort to show that vaccination of sheep, goats, and cows with an attenuated strain of *B. anthracis* prevented anthrax. He was cheered and carried on the shoulders of the grateful farmers of the district.

Bacillus anthracis

Morphological and cultural characteristics

In the clinical laboratory, *B. anthracis* is recognized by its tendency to form very long chains of rods with elliptic central spores. This appearance has sometimes been likened to that of bamboo rods (Figure 14.1). In infected tissues, chains are shorter and capsules are prominent, but spores do not develop. Colonies, which consist of parallel interlacing chains of bacilli, are characterized by a rough uneven surface with multiple curled extensions at the edge resembling a "Medusa head." *Bacillus anthracis* is nonmotile and nonhemolytic; these qualities, combined with other important bacteriologic features, help to differentiate the organism from other *Bacillus* species (Table 14.1).

Antiphagocytic effect of D-glutamic acid capsule

The anthrax bacillus differs from other *Bacillus* species in several important features. Of prime importance for virulence are its capsule and production of exotoxin. The capsule is a D-glutamic acid polypeptide of a single antigenic specificity. It has antiphagocytic properties and is required for virulence. As the "unnatural" isomer of glutamic acid, it is resistant to digestion by mammalian proteolytic enzymes. The exotoxin(s) produces extensive edema and death in a variety of animals. This activity has been separated into at least

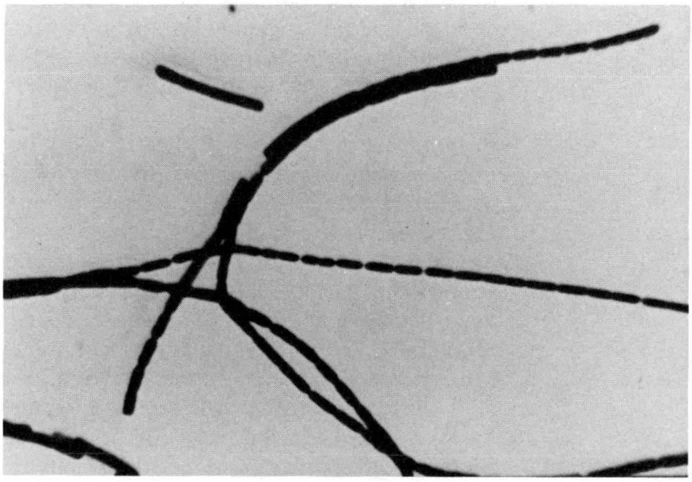

14.1 *Bacillus anthracis.* Large Gram-positive bacilli in chains are typical of this species. Other *Bacillus* species vary greatly in shape.

Table 14.1 Some Characteristics of *Bacillus* Species

Organism	Bacteriologic Features: Capsule	Hemolysis	Motility	Colony	Toxin Production	Distribution	Human Disease
B. anthracis	+	—	—	"Medusa head"	Exotoxin (EF, PA, LF)	Animals and contaminated soil where disease is enzootic	Anthrax
B. cereus	—	+	+	Granular, round	Enterotoxin; pyogenic toxin	Ubiquitous	Food poisoning; opportunistic infections (rare)
Other species	—	Variable	+	Variable	—	Ubiquitous	Opportunistic infections (rare)

Abbreviations: EF = edema factor; PA = protective antigen; LF = lethal factor.

three components: edema factor, protective antigen, and lethal factor. These factors are proteins or protein–carbohydrate complexes; their ability to produce pathologic lesions experimentally and stimulate immunity varies with the relative proportions of each. Strains repeatedly subcultured at 42°C become avirulent. This characteristic was the basis of Pasteur's attenuated vaccine, and has been shown to be due to loss of a virulence-determining plasmid.

attenuation of virulence

Anthrax

infection through small epithelial lesions

Spread of disease in herbivores and occasionally to humans

Anthrax is usually acquired through unrecognized breaks in skin or mucous membranes to which spores of *B. anthracis* gain access. The spores germinate to yield vegetative cells, which multiply and produce either localized or systemic infection depending on the animal species infected and the site inoculated. Herbivores such as horses, sheep, and cattle are most commonly affected and develop fatal septicemic disease. The disease is spread by spores in pastures contaminated with exudates of live or dead infected animals. Humans are usually infected by contact with infected animals or animal products. Because of the long survival of the spores, infection may result from contaminated hides, wool, bone, and even imported processed items such as fertilizers containing bone meal. The disease is now rare in developed countries, although animal anthrax persists in the southern United States. The incidence in humans in the United States has decreased from more than 100 cases annually in the 1920s to only a few reported cases each year. This dramatic reduction is associated with the control of animal anthrax through quarantine, sacrifice of infected herds, and immunization and with improved industrial hygiene. In the past, farmers, veterinarians, and meat handlers were infected most frequently; now, however, the rare case in the United States is usually related to contaminated imported materials.

Control of animal anthrax

Cutaneous anthrax

Cutaneous anthrax usually begins 2–5 days after inoculation of spores in an exposed part of the body, typically the forearm or hand. Scalp lesions have been associated with headgear contaminated with spores. The initial lesion is an erythematous papule, which may be mistaken for an insect bite. This papule usually progresses through vesicular and ulcerative stages over 7–10 days to form a black eschar surrounded by edema. This complex is known as the *malignant pustule,* although it is neither malignant nor a pustule. Associated systemic symptoms are usually mild, and the lesion typically heals after the eschar separates. Less commonly, the disease progresses with massive local edema, toxemia and bacteremia, and a fatal outcome if untreated.

Pulmonary anthrax

Pulmonary anthrax, contracted by inhalation of spores, can develop when contaminated hides, hair, wool, and the like are handled in a confined space. The infection was thus termed *woolsorter's disease,* as it was quite common among these workers at the turn of the century. Pulmonary anthrax has also developed following laboratory accidents. More ominous, it was once considered as a means of biologic warfare, which has now been outlawed by international treaty. After 1–5 days of nonspecific malaise, mild fever, and nonproductive cough, progressive respiratory distress and cyanosis ensue with massive edema of the neck, chest, and mediastinum. If untreated, progression to a fatal outcome is usually very rapid once edema has developed. Enormous numbers of organisms are found in the lungs, blood, and all organs. A gastrointestinal form of anthrax results from ingestion of raw or inadequately cooked meat containing *B. anthracis* spores. Infections at other sites, such as the meninges, may follow bacteremia in the course of cutaneous or pulmonary anthrax.

Other Bacillus Infections

Bacillus infections in immunocompromised hosts

As spores are widespread in the environment, isolation of one of the more than 20 *Bacillus* species other than *B. anthracis* from clinical material usually represents contamination of the specimen. Occasionally *Bacillus cereus, Bacillus subtilis,* and some other species produce genuine infections, including infections of the eye, soft tissues, and lung. Bacteremia and endocarditis may also result. Infection is usually associated with immunosuppression, trauma, an indwelling catheter, or contamination of complex equipment such as an artificial kidney. The relative resistance of *Bacillus* spores to disinfectants aids their survival in medical devices that cannot be heat sterilized.

Food poisoning from *B. cereus*

Bacillus cereus deserves special mention. It is the species most likely to cause opportunistic infection, which suggests a virulence intermediate between that of *B. anthracis* and the other species. A strain isolated from an abscess has been shown to produce a destructive pyogenic toxin. *Bacillus cereus* can also cause food poisoning by means of enterotoxins. One enterotoxin acts by stimulating adenyl cyclase production and fluid excretion in the same manner as toxigenic *Escherichia coli* and *Vibrio cholerae* (Chapters 20 and 21). One interesting strain has been shown to cause vomiting rather than diarrhea, but only with cultures grown on rice. It was isolated in association with an outbreak of nausea and vomiting that occurred 1–5 hr after consumption of cooked rice in a Chinese restaurant.

Diagnosis

Diagnosis of *Bacillus* infections follows the principles outlined in Chapter 9. The organisms are readily grown on a variety of media. *Bacillus anthracis* may be distinguished from other species by the characteristics listed in Table 14.1, by its virulence to experimental animals, and by other biochemical and cultural features. The appropriate tests may not be performed unless the suspicion of anthrax is communicated to the clinical laboratory. Isolates of other *Bacillus* species are usually contaminants; the rare situation in which they play a pathogenic role is suggested by multiple isolations, large numbers of organisms in fresh specimens, and the special circumstances of the case. Again, to ensure retention of the strain for further study, the laboratory must be advised that infection is suspected.

Treatment

Susceptibility of *B. anthracis* to penicillin

As *B. anthracis* is susceptible to penicillin, anthrax is treated with this agent. Antimicrobial therapy for other species must be guided by in vitro testing, because susceptibilities to penicillins, cephalosporins, aminoglycosides, tetracycline, and chloramphenicol are not predictable. Other modes of management of opportunistic *Bacillus* infections, such as removal of indwelling catheters, may be equally important.

Additional Reading and References

Melling, J., Capel, B.J., Turnbull, P.C.B., and Gilbert, R.J. 1976. Identification of a novel enterotoxigenic activity associated with *Bacillus cereus*. *J. Clin. Pathol.* 29:938–940.

Turnbull, P.C.B. 1976. Studies on the production of enterotoxins by *Bacillus cereus*. *J. Clin. Pathol.* 29:941–948. These two reports suggest some possible virulence mechanisms for intestinal and extraintestinal infections caused by *Bacillus cereus*.

John C. Sherris

Clostridia, Gram-Negative Anaerobes, and Anaerobic Cocci

15

All of the organisms discussed in this chapter are anaerobes, which can be considered as bacteria that fail to grow on the surface of solid medium when incubated in air and only metabolize fermentatively. They can be cultivated on enriched agar media when the plates are incubated in jars or chambers from which all oxygen is excluded. Oxygen can be removed by combination with hydrogen on palladium–asbestos or a similar catalyst. Anaerobes can also be grown in liquid media with a sufficiently low oxidation–reduction potential. The latter can be achieved by boiling, which removes dissolved oxygen, or by incorporating a reducing agent such as sodium thioglycolate, cysteine, meat fragments, or iron filings into the medium.

anaerobiosis

cultural techniques

oxygen sensitivity

Some anaerobes are killed so rapidly by exposure to oxygen that specimens taken for culture, media to be inoculated, and all transfer procedures must be maintained in its absence. Such exquisitely oxygen-sensitive organisms exist in highly anaerobic niches, such as the rumen of cattle and the depths of the gingival crevice of humans. They rarely contribute to disease, probably because they are inactivated by even the small amounts of oxygen dissolved in tissue fluids. It is the hardier aerotolerant anaerobes that usually play a pathogenic role in human infections. They are almost always derived from the patient's normal flora or, in the case of clostridia, from the environment. Case-to-case transfer is very rare.

explanations for anaerobiosis

Several explanations have been proposed for obligate anaerobiosis and oxygen toxicity. Anaerobes lack cytochromes and cannot use oxygen as a terminal hydrogen acceptor in energy-yielding reactions. Most, but not all, lack catalase and peroxidase enzymes, but possess flavoproteins; thus in the presence of oxygen they may produce hydrogen peroxide, which is toxic to many of them. Some anaerobes, which lack or produce low concentrations of the enzyme superoxide dismutase, may be inhibited or killed by other peroxides and toxic oxygen radicals. Certain critical enzymes (for example, fumarate reductase) of some anaerobes must be in the reduced state to be active; thus, aerobic conditions create a metabolic block. It therefore seems probable that no single characteristic is responsible for obligate anaerobic requirements or oxygen toxicity; some of those indicated previously, rather than being its cause, may have been selected *because* of the anaerobic nature of the organism.

resistance to aminoglycosides

Anaerobic organisms are resistant to the aminoglycoside antimicrobics, because active transport of these agents into the cell depends on oxidative phosphorylation reactions.

The major groups of medically significant anaerobes are as follows.

spore formers

Clostridia. The clostridia are Gram-positive, spore-forming motile or nonmotile bacilli. Some species are potentially highly pathogenic to humans or animals and produce potent exotoxins associated with particular disease syndromes. Others are nonpathogenic. Clostridia are found in soil (particularly soil fertilized with animal excreta) and in the lower intestinal tract of humans and animals. They are generally highly susceptible to penicillin.

Bacteroides. Members of the genus *Bacteroides* are Gram-negative, non-spore-forming rods. Some are markedly pleomorphic, but others are quite uniform. They are distinguished from *Fusobacterium* by the organic acids that constitute their metabolic end products. *Bacteroides* species appear among the normal flora of the oral cavity and colon in humans and animals.

Fusobacteria. Fusobacteria are also Gram-negative, non-spore-forming rods. Their morphology is fusiform with pointed ends, and they are distinguished from *Bacteroides* by metabolic end-product analysis. Their habitat is the same as that of *Bacteroides.*

Peptostreptococci. Peptostreptococci, also commonly known as *anaerobic streptococci,* are Gram-positive, nonmotile organisms that occur in chains. They are part of the normal flora of the upper alimentary and respiratory tracts and lower intestinal tract in humans and animals.

Peptococci. Peptococci resemble peptostreptococci, but form clusters rather than chains. They rarely play a pathogenic role.

Other genera and species of anaerobic organisms (for example, *Actinomyces israelii*) are considered elsewhere. Many others are not included in this chapter because they rarely cause disease, and because those discussed herein serve as satisfactory models for both specific and mixed anaerobic infections.

Clostridia

medically important clostridia

Many clostridia are of great significance as causes of disease in livestock and wildlife; however, these organisms are beyond the scope of this text. Discussion is limited to those that cause disease in humans, which may be categorized as follows:

1. The gas gangrene group, of which the most important is *Clostridium perfringens.* In addition to its role in gas gangrene, *C. perfringens* can cause anaerobic cellulitis, anaerobic puerperal sepsis, and a form of food poisoning.
2. *Clostridium tetani*, the cause of tetanus.
3. *Clostridium botulinum*, the cause of botulism.
4. *Clostridium difficile*, a recently recognized cause of toxic enterocolitis.

Clostridium perfringens

Subtypes based on toxin production

Importance of type A

Clostridium perfringens produces a remarkable number of exotoxins and extracellular enzymes with specific biologic activity. The species has been subdivided on the basis of these products (rather than serologically) into seven types (A–G), which have different pathogenic significance in different animal species. Type A is by far the most important in humans, and is found consistently in the colon and often in soil.

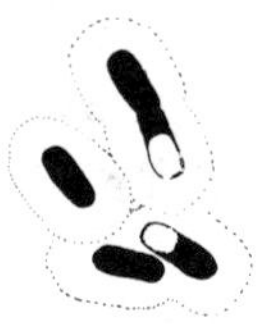

Clostridium perfringens

hemolytic toxins

gas production from carbohydrates

Morphologic, cultural, and metabolic characteristics. *Clostridium perfringens* is a large, Gram-positive, nonmotile encapsulated rod with squarish ends. Spores are rarely seen in culture or during infection, but develop in the natural habitat. The organism grows very rapidly overnight on blood agar medium or in broth under anaerobic conditions. Its mean generation time can be as short as 7 min. Incubation overnight on sheep or horse blood agar (usually used in diagnostic laboratories) produces round, smooth colonies about 2–3 mm in diameter; they are surrounded by a zone of complete hemolysis caused by θ-toxin and a wider zone of incomplete hemolysis caused by lecithinase α-toxin (Plate J). If the plate is refrigerated and rewarmed, the outer zone of hemolysis becomes complete. In broth containing fermentable carbohydrate, growth of *C. perfringens* is accompanied by the production of large amounts of hydrogen and carbon dioxide, which can result in markedly increased pressure in a sealed container. Much gas is also produced in vivo in necrotic tissues, hence the term *gas gangrene.*

heat-resistant spores of food poisoning strains

Resistance. Spores of *C. perfringens* are resistant to all disinfectants and to boiling for brief periods. The spores of some strains that cause food poisoning are often more heat resistant: they can withstand temperatures of 100°C for an hour or more, which accounts for their survival in cooked food. The vegetative cells are readily killed by disinfectants. They are susceptible to penicillin and many other antibiotics, except the aminoglycosides.

lecithinase activity

toxicity

Toxins and biologically active extracellular enzymes. *Clostridium perfringens* can produce several exotoxins and biologically active extracellular proteins that may contribute to virulence. The most important is α-toxin, a β-lecithinase that disrupts the cell membranes of various host cells, including erythrocytes, leukocytes, and muscle cells. Its production can be detected in vitro on a lecithin-containing agar medium, because it produces a precipitate of breakdown products of lecithin (phosphoryl choline and diglycerides) in the immediate vicinity of a streak of growth of *C. perfringens.* The reaction can be neutralized specifically by anti-α-toxin antibody (antitoxin), which provides a useful test for identifying the organism (Plate K). The median lethal dose (LD_{50}) of the toxin for experimental animals is approximately 5 μg/kg.

θ-toxin related to streptolysin O

θ-Toxin, a hemolytic substance with toxicity for heart muscle, is closely related to streptolysin O (Chapter 14). It is responsible for the complete β-hemolysis seen after overnight incubation on blood agar plates.

Enterotoxin

diarrhea production

Some strains of *C. perfringens* type A produce enterotoxin, an intracellular protein with toxicity for the intestinal tract. Enterotoxin is liberated from the bacterial cell in the upper gastrointestinal tract or on sporulation. It is heat labile and causes diarrhea by reversing the flow of water and electrolytes in the small intestine. The mechanism has not yet been defined.

Other biologically active extracellular products include a collagenase, a deoxyribonuclease, a hyaluronidase, and proteases. All may contribute to pathologic processes, but none share the central role of the α-toxin.

Diseases Caused by Clostridium perfringens

open wounds with muscle damage

other gas-gangrene-causing clostridia

Gas gangrene. Gas gangrene can develop in severe traumatic open lesions, such as compound fractures or bullet wounds, when there is muscle damage, contamination with dirt, clothing, or other foreign material, and if *C. perfringens* or, less commonly, one of the other gas-gangrene-causing clostridia (for example, *Clostridium novyi* or *Clostridium septicum*) is introduced. The disease is usually seen in war wounds, but is an occasional sequela of severe trauma in civilian life. It can develop within a few hours of wounding. As *C. perfringens* is sometimes present in bile in cholecystitis, gas gangrene of the abdominal muscles is an occasional complication of gallbladder or bile duct surgery, particularly when bile is spilled.

conditions for multiplication

If the oxidation–reduction potential in a wound is sufficiently low, *C. perfringens* spores can germinate and the organism can multiply very rapidly. Infections are always mixed; the presence of numerous facultative species contributes to the reduced Eh. *Clostridium perfringens* elaborates its α-toxin, which passes along the muscle bundles killing all cells, including inflammatory cells, and producing additional necrotic areas into which the organism can grow. Fermentation of muscle carbohydrate by *C. perfringens* produces gas in the subcutaneous tissues that can be felt when palpated (crepitation) and seen on radiography. As the disease progresses, α-toxin is absorbed into the bloodstream, producing marked systemic illness, and *C. perfringens* bacteremia develops. Untreated gas gangrene is always fatal.

α-toxin production

necrosis and gas production

constitutional signs and bacteremia

Role of α-toxin in pathogenesis

The critical role of anaerobiosis and of the α-toxin has been shown in animal experiments. *Clostridium perfringens* cells washed free of toxin and inoculated intramuscularly into guinea pigs cause no lesion. When substances causing muscle necrosis or actively metabolizing aerobic organisms are introduced, however, gas gangrene develops. Active immunization with α-toxin or passive immunization with anti-α-toxin antibody will prevent the disease.

Prevention of gas gangrene

Rapid and adequate surgical debridement with removal of dead tissue is the most important preventive measure. It is supplemented if possible with high doses of penicillin as soon after wounding as possible in an attempt to inhibit accessible clostridia and delay infection with other organisms that may promote clostridial disease. Antibiotic prophylaxis cannot replace surgical debridement, and the disease may develop in cases receiving such treatment because the antibiotics fail to reach the organism in devascularized tissues.

Treatment

Treatment must be initiated immediately. Excision of all devitalized tissue and massive doses of penicillin are most important. Frequently, amputation of a limb is required to prevent further spread. Placing the patient in a hyperbaric oxygen chamber has been shown to slow the spread of disease, probably by inhibiting bacterial growth and toxin production by increasing the tissue level of dissolved oxygen. This measure also appears to reduce the "toxicity" of the patient. In the past, gas gangrene polyvalent antitoxin was administered intravenously in large amounts to neutralize free toxin. It may help prevent hemolysis, but is of doubtful benefit in halting the gangrene.

Anaerobic cellulitis. Anaerobic cellulitis is a clostridial infection of wounds and surrounding subcutaneous tissue in which there is marked gas formation (more than that in gas gangrene), but in which the pain, swelling, and toxicity of gas gangrene are absent. It is much less serious than gas gangrene and can be controlled with less rigorous methods.

Clostridial endometritis. If *C. perfringens* gains access to necrotic products of conception retained in the uterus, it may multiply and infect the endometrium (Figure 15.1). Necrosis of uterine tissue and septicemia with massive intravascular hemolysis may then follow. Clostridial uterine infection was seen more commonly in the past, usually after incomplete illegal abortion with inadequately sterilized instruments. The disease is extremely serious and may require emergency hysterectomy and hemodialysis for renal shutdown resulting from hemoglobinemia.

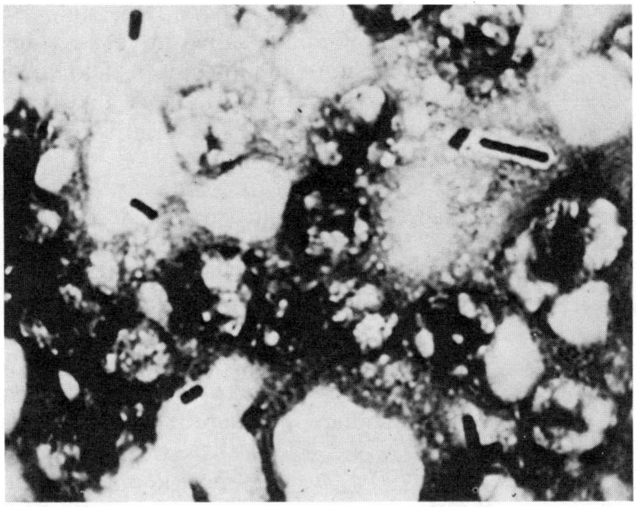

15.1. Gram smear of the uterus of a case of *Clostridium perfringens* endometritis. Note the absence of inflammatory cells.

incubation 8–24 hr
diarrhea without fever

Clostridial food poisoning. Clostridium perfringens can cause food poisoning if large numbers of an enterotoxin-producing strain are ingested. The incubation period of 8–24 hr is followed by nausea, abdominal pain, and diarrhea. There is no fever, and vomiting is rare. Recovery is usual within 24 hr. The disease is caused by the enterotoxin, which is liberated from the organism in the small intestine.

growth of *C. perfringens* in meat dishes

Outbreaks of the disease usually involve meat dishes such as stews, soups, or gravy. Heat-resistant spores of *C. perfringens* may survive the initial cooking and the organism multiplies rapidly if cooling and storage at room temperature are prolonged or if the food is rewarmed. Prevention involves good cooking hygiene and adequate refrigeration.

Diagnosis of Serious Clostridial Infections

diagnosis primarily clinical

Diagnosis is based ultimately on clinical observations. Bacteriologic studies are adjunctive. It is quite common, for example, to isolate *C. perfringens* from contaminated wounds without evidence of clostridial disease. The organism can also be isolated from the postpartum uterine cervix of healthy women or from those with only mild fever. Occasionally, *C. perfringens* is even isolated from blood cultures of patients who do not develop serious clostridial infection.

Direct Gram smears

absence of inflammatory cells

Gram smears from cases of gas gangrene show many clostridia and other organisms (for example, Enterobacteriaciae) that multiply in the necrotic tissue. Pieces of necrotic muscle may be seen, and the absence of inflammatory cells is noteworthy (Plate I). The appearance of smears from the endometrium in clostridial endometritis is similar, although in this case *C. perfringens* is usually the only organism present.

In clostridial food poisoning, isolation of more than 10^5 *C. perfringens* per gram of the ingested food in the absence of any other cause is usually sufficient to confirm the etiology of a characteristic food poisoning outbreak.

Clostridium tetani

Habitat

Clostridium tetani spores exist in many soils, especially if they are manured, and the organism is often present in the lower intestinal tract of humans and animals.

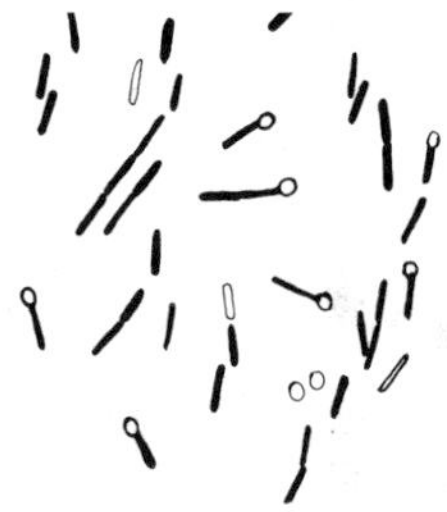

Clostridium tetani

Morphology. *Clostridium tetani* is a slim, Gram-positive rod; it may be predominantly Gram-negative in very young or old cultures. It forms spores readily in nature and in culture, yielding a typical round terminal spore that gives the organism a drumstick appearance before the residual vegetative cell disintegrates. The organism is flagellate and motile.

swarming growth on agar

Cultural characteristics. *Clostridium tetani* requires strict anaerobic conditions. Because of its motility, it spreads over the surface of anaerobic blood agar plates in a thin veil of growth. Its identity is suggested by cultural and biochemical characteristics, but definite identification depends on demonstration of its neurotoxic exotoxin.

heat-resistant spores

Resistance. *Clostridium tetani* spores remain viable in soil or culture for many years. They are resistant to most disinfectants and withstand boiling for several minutes. They are killed by autoclaving at 121°C for 15 min.

tetanospasmin exotoxin

conversion to toxoid

Toxin production. The most important product of *C. tetani* is its neurotoxic exotoxin, tetanospasmin, which is found extracellularly. It is a heat-labile antigenic protein readily neutralized by antitoxin and rapidly destroyed at 65°C and by intestinal proteases. Treatment with formaldehyde yields a nontoxic product, *toxoid,* that retains the antigenicity of toxin and thus stimulates production of antitoxin. The LD_{50} of the toxin for mice is on the order of 10^{-4} μg; less than 1 μg would probably be lethal to humans.

Tetanus

often small wounds

Predisposing conditions. Spores of *C. tetani* may be introduced into wounds with contaminated soil or foreign bodies. The predisposing wounds are often quite small, for example, a puncture wound containing a splinter. In contrast to those in gas gangrene, infected wounds often do not extend below the subcutaneous tissues. In some underdeveloped countries, contaminated salves applied to the umbilicus are a source of a frequently fatal infantile tetanus. Occasionally, the disease may follow severe burns; it has also occurred as a complication of chronic otitis media, probably when the organism gains access to the middle ear through a perforated eardrum.

low Eh from foreign bodies, necrosis, or other infections

The usual predisposing factor for tetanus is an area of very low oxidation–reduction potential in which tetanus spores can germinate. This can be provided by a large splinter, an area of necrosis from introduction of soil, or necrosis after injection of contaminated illicit drugs. Infection with facultative or other anaerobic organisms can contribute to the development of an appropriate anaerobic nidus for spore germination.

local multiplication only

action of toxin

Pathogenesis. Tetanus bacilli multiply locally and neither damage nor invade adjacent tissues. Tetanospasmin is elaborated at the site of infection and reaches the central nervous system mainly by ascending the motor nerves. In the spinal cord, it acts at the level of the anterior horn cells by blocking postsynaptic inhibition of spinal motor reflexes. Thus, an afferent stimulus produces spasmodic contractions of both protagonist and antagonist muscles, initially in the area of the causative lesion. In the more serious forms of the disease toxin extends up and down the spinal cord, and generalized spasms can result from minor stimuli such as a sound or a draft.

incubation period

Clinical presentation. The incubation period of the disease is from 4 days to several weeks. The shorter incubation period is usually associated with wounds in areas supplied by the cranial motor nerves, probably because of a shorter transmission route for the toxin to the central nervous system. In general, shorter incubation periods are associated with more severe disease.

local tetanus

effect of toxin on masseters

severe tetanus

spasms triggered by minor stimuli

mortality

Although tetanus may be localized to muscles in the region of the infection, it is usually more generalized. The masseter muscles are often the first to be affected, resulting in inability to open the mouth properly (trismus); this effect accounts for the use of the term *lockjaw* to describe the disease. As other muscles become affected, intermittent spasms can become generalized to include muscles of respiration and swallowing. In extreme cases, generalized convulsions produce opisthotonus, caused by massive contractions of the back muscles. Risus sardonicus (sardonic smile) is a late sign in which trismus combined with facial spasm leads to separation of the lips over clenched teeth. The untreated patient with tetanus retains consciousness and is aware of his plight, in which small stimuli can trigger massive contractions. In fatal cases, death results from exhaustion and respiratory failure. All of these results are attributable to very small amounts of tetanospasmin produced at the site of what is often a small, sometimes unrecognized local lesion. The amount of toxin is so small that unimmunized patients often do not have an antibody response. Untreated, the mortality caused by the generalized disease varies from 15 to more than 60%, according to the lesion, incubation period, and age of the patient. Mortality is highest in the neonate and in the elderly.

antitoxin

supportive measures

Treatment. Specific treatment of the disease involves neutralization of any unbound toxin with large doses of human tetanus immune globulin (TIG), which is derived from the blood of volunteers hyperimmunized with toxoid. In countries where TIG is unavailable, horse antitoxin is still used. Most important in treatment are nonspecific supportive measures, including maintenance of a quiet dark environment, sedation, and provision of an adequate airway. In severe cases, curarelike drugs are used to block nerve impulses at the neuromuscular junctions. These patients require artificial ventilation to maintain oxygenation despite respiratory paralysis. Such measures have resulted in a substantially reduced mortality.

active immunization with tetanus toxoid

Prevention. Routine active immunization with tetanus toxoid, combined with diphtheria toxoid and pertussis vaccine (DPT) for primary immunization in childhood, can completely prevent the disease. It has reduced the incidence of tetanus in the United States to less than 50 reported cases per year. Five doses of DPT are now recommended, to be given at the ages of 2, 4, 6, and 18 months, and once again between the ages of 4 and 6 years. Thereafter a booster of adult-type tetanus diptheria toxoid should be given every 10 years (see Chapter 8).

passive immunization

prophylactic booster dose of toxoid

Unimmunized subjects with tetanus-prone wounds should be given passive immunity with a prophylactic dose of TIG as soon as possible. This immunization provides immediate protection. Those who have had a full primary series of immunizations, and appropriate boosters, are given toxoid for tetanus-prone wounds if they have not been immunized within the previous 10 years in the case of clean minor wounds or 5 years for more contaminated wounds. If immunization is incomplete or the wound has been neglected and poses a serious risk of disease, TIG is also given.

Penicillin therapy is a prophylactic adjunct in serious or neglected wounds, but in no way alters the need for specific prophylaxis. All those who have not been actively immunized should be given a first dose of toxoid as soon as possible and followed up for a complete immunization series. If toxoid and TIG are given in opposite arms with different syringes there is no significant interference between them. Recommended immunization schedules change from time to time, and those responsible for their administration should be familiar with current recommendations.

Clostridium botulinum

Natural habitat

Spores of *C. botulinum* are found in soil, pond, and lake sediments in many parts of the world, including the United States. The major characteristic of medical importance is that strains of *C. botulinum* elaborate one of seven antigenically distinct neurotoxins of extraordinary toxicity: the estimated lethal dose for humans is less than 1 μg. Production of toxin is determined by carriage of lysogenic phage by the organism. *Clostridium botulinum* is classified into groups A–G based on the antigenic specificity of the toxin. Groups A, B, and E are most often associated with human disease.

neurotoxins

type differentiation

heat lability and mode of action of toxins

Clostridium botulinum neurotoxins are heat labile and destroyed rapidly at 100°C. They are resistant to the enzymes of the gastrointestinal tract and are readily absorbed by this route. They act on neuromuscular junctions by inhibiting release of acetylcholine, resulting in muscular paralysis. Both the voluntary and autonomic cholinergic nervous systems are affected.

spore survival at 100°C

germination and multiplication in food

Spores of *C. botulinum* resist boiling for long periods, but are rapidly destroyed by moist heat at a temperature of 121°C. Germination of spores and growth of *C. botulinum* can occur in a variety of alkaline or neutral foodstuffs when conditions are sufficiently anaerobic. Occasionally, under the same conditions, the organism can multiply in wounds or in the lower intestinal tract of infants.

toxin detection and typing

Clostridium botulinum is identified by its morphologic, cultural, and biochemical characteristics, particularly its toxin production. Toxin is detected by injecting culture supernatants into unprotected mice and into mice protected with antitoxins against the different serotypes of toxin. Unprotected mice and mice given heterologous antitoxin die of paralytic disease within 3 days. Mice protected against the specific serotype of toxin survive.

Botulism

Home canning of alkaline foods

Other sources

Botulism is usually associated with home-canned alkaline vegetables, such as green beans or mushrooms, that have not been heated at temperatures sufficient to kill *C. botulinum* spores. The organism multiplies on storage, often with no change in food taste or odor, and elaborates its toxin. If the food is ingested without cooking, botulism will result. Other sources include vacuum-packed freshwater fish and occasionally inadequately sterilized or faulty commercial canning. Acidic foods such as canned fruit do not support the growth of *C. botulinum.* The disease often occurs in small epidemics among those who have eaten the toxic food uncooked.

Symptoms and signs

effect on autonomic cholinergic nerve endings

After an incubation period of 18–96 hr, signs of paralysis develop, first involving the ocular, pharyngeal, laryngeal, and respiratory muscles. There may be extensive paralysis of voluntary muscles. Dry mouth, constipation, and urinary retention occur through the action of the toxin on the autonomic cholinergic nervous system. The mortality caused by the disease is over 20%, even with treatment.

antitoxin treatment

Treatment. Specific treatment involves the use of large doses of horse *C. botulinum* antitoxin to neutralize any free toxin. Supportive measures are designed to maintain respiration and a clear adequate airway.

adequate heating inactivates toxin

Prevention. Adequate pressure cooking or autoclaving in the canning process will kill spores. Heating food at 100°C for 10 min before eating will destroy the toxin. Food from damaged cans or those that present evidence of positive inside pressure should not even be tasted because of the extreme toxicity of the *C. botulinum* toxin.

Wound botulism. Very rarely, wounds infected with other organisms may allow *C. botulinum* to grow. Disease similar to that from food poisoning can develop.

Infant botulism. Recently, a syndrome associated with *C. botulinum* has been recognized in infants between the ages of 3 weeks and 8 months. The organism is apparently introduced with dietary supplements, especially honey, and multiplies in the infant's colon, with absorption of small amounts of toxin. The infant shows poor muscle tone, lethargy, and feeding problems, and may have ophthalmic and other paralyses similar to those in adult botulism. Infant botulism may contribute to the sudden infant death syndrome.

Laboratory diagnosis. Toxin can frequently be demonstrated in blood, intestinal contents, or remaining food, by inoculation into mice. Unprotected mice die, whereas those protected with specific antitoxin survive. *Clostridium botulinum* may also be isolated from stool or from foodstuffs apparently responsible for botulism.

Clostridium difficile

C. difficile enterotoxin

Recently, it has been shown that certain cases of antibiotic-induced pseudomembranous enterocolitis involving some colonic epithelial necrosis with bloody diarrhea are caused by a toxin of *C. difficile.* The organism shows unusual resistance to clindamycin and can multiply and elaborate its toxin in the relative ecologic vacuum produced in the colon by therapy with this antimicrobic. The disease has been reproduced in hamsters. *Clostridium difficile* is susceptible to vancomycin, and oral vancomycin has been helpful in treatment. Isolation of *C. difficile* from stool or detection of its toxin by its effect on cell cultures are helpful diagnostic procedures, when combined with clinical findings.

Anaerobic Gram-Negative Rods and Anaerobic Cocci

opportunists

Members of normal flora

Two large and important groups of organisms, anaerobic Gram-negative rods and anaerobic cocci, are considered together because they share many features in terms of habitat, diseases produced, and methods used in identification. They are more common causes of disease than the clostridia; those associated with human infections are opportunists, however, and their determinants of pathogenicity are more obscure. All are members of the normal flora of the upper alimentary and respiratory tracts, the female genital tract, or the colon.

Presumptive laboratory identification depends on morphologic and staining characteristics and on some biochemical tests; definitive speciation, however, increasingly involves the detection of characteristic organic acid metabolic end products by gas chromatography.

autoinfection

most infections mixed

Diseases caused by these organisms are almost invariably examples of autoinfection: the normal flora transgress epithelial barriers through trauma or pathologic conditions (for example, a ruptured appendix or colonic diverticulum) or because of compromised immune defenses. The result is usually abscess formation. The great majority of infections caused by the non-spore-forming anaerobes are mixed; that is, two or more anaerobes are isolated, often in combination with facultative bacteria such as *E. coli.* In some cases the components of these mixtures synergize each other's growth.

association with abscesses

Multiplication of these opportunistic pathogens in abscesses is facilitated by inhibition of leukocytic bactericidal function under the anaerobic conditions in the lesions. Many, but not all, anaerobic infections are associated with foul-smelling lesions, and thrombophlebitis is a common complication. The more aerotolerant anaerobes may occasionally cause endocarditis.

Bacteroides

B. fragilis

The most common opportunistic pathogen of the genus *Bacteroides* is *Bacteroides fragilis.* It is a slim, pale-staining, capsulate, Gram-negative rod that forms colonies overnight on blood agar medium and is relatively tolerant to atmospheric oxygen. The implication of fragility in its name is misleading, because it is actually among the hardier and more easily grown anaerobes.

minority member of colonic flora

It constitutes less than 10% of *Bacteroides* species in the normal colon, but predominates among Gram-negative infections in the abdominal cavity. Its polysaccharide capsule confers resistance to phagocytosis and stimulates abscess formation when injected into experimental animals. Its cell wall has minimum endotoxic activity. *Bacteroides fragilis* is almost always resistant to

penicillin resistance

penicillin, in part because of chromosomally determined β-lactamase production. Resistance to tetracycline is common, but most strains are susceptible to chloramphenicol, clindamycin, and metronidazole. Plasmids carrying resistance determinants have been demonstrated in *B. fragilis.*

B. melaninogenicus–asaccharolyticus group

The second most common cause of human infection in this genus is the *Bacteroides melaninogenicus–asaccharolyticus* group. *Bacteroides melaninogenicus* derives its name from the characteristic black colonies it forms as a result of production of a black pigment from hemoglobin derivatives. Organisms of this group are found in the oral cavity, upper alimentary and respiratory tracts, and colon. In contrast to that of *B. fragilis,* the cell wall has endotoxic properties, and the organisms are usually susceptible to penicillin. Infections

penicillin susceptibility

with *B. melaninogenicus* are usually derived from the oral flora; they include dental infections, pulmonary infections and abscesses, and infections of human bites. The latter tend to be serious and refractory unless treated ade-

derivation from oral flora

quately with debridement and antibiotics. This group of organisms is also encountered in abdominal and pelvic lesions.

Among several other designated species of *Bacteroides* are the predominant organisms in the adult colon. Their pathogenic potential is less than that of *B. fragilis* and of the *B. melaninogenicus–asaccharolyticus* group.

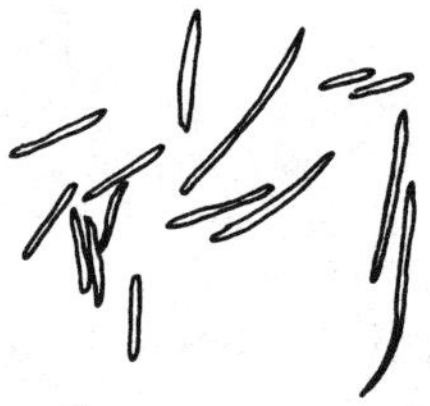

Fusobacterium nucleatum

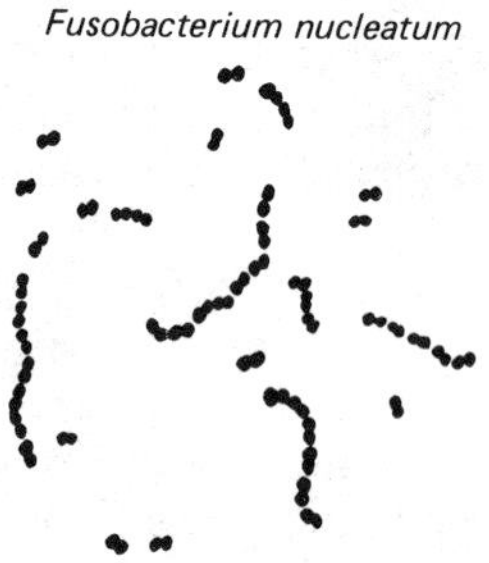

Peptostreptococcus

Fusobacterium

Fusobacterium nucleatum is the most common species of the genus in human infection. It is a spindle-shaped, slow-growing, Gram-negative, anaerobic rod that inhabits the oral cavity, the colon, and sometimes the female genital tract. It is less virulent than the two species of *Bacteroides* discussed previously and usually appears in mixed infections. It is sensitive to penicillin.

Other fusobacteria contribute to chronic ulcerative lesions of the gums, to abscesses deriving from the oral cavity and pharynx, and to a necrotic ulcerative lesion of the pharynx called *Vincent's angina* (Chapter 24).

Peptostreptococcus and *Microaerophilic Streptococci*

The taxonomy of this group of organisms has been shifting, and has thus been a source of considerable confusion. Some clinically important species, previously designated as peptostreptococci, although primarily anaerobic can grow slowly in reduced oxygen or increased CO_2 concentrations and have been reassigned to the genus *Streptococcus.* They have pathogenic potential similar to that of the peptostreptococci and will be considered here as microaerophilic streptococci.

abscesses

puerperal infections

thrombophlebitis

These organisms are usually small, Gram-positive cocci that tend to occur in long chains in clinical material and to lose their Gram positivity easily. They are members of the normal flora of the oral cavity, the colon, and the female genital tract. They are opportunists and are often found in lesions with other anaerobic and facultative organisms. Sometimes, anaerobic or microaerophilic streptococci are the sole etiologic agents in cerebral and other abscesses and in puerperal infections and pelvic peritonitis. They are often associated with septic thrombophlebitis, which may result in metastatic abscesses. Peptostreptococcal lesions tend to be foul smelling and to show gas production

subcutaneous tissue infections

These organisms can cause anaerobic cellulitis. Microaerophilic streptococci can also cause a form of spreading, synergistic, subcutaneous gangrene (Meleney's ulcer) in association with *Staphylococcus aureus,* usually after serious abdominal surgery. The infection arises in a suture line. Peptostreptococci and microaerophilic streptococci are sensitive to penicillin and usually to other antibiotics active against Gram-positive cocci, with the exception of the aminoglycosides.

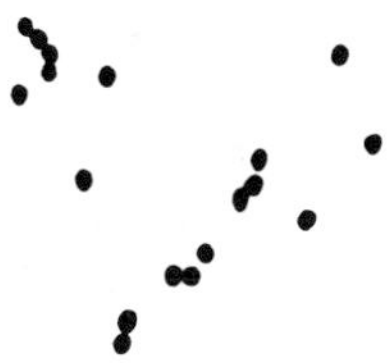

Peptococcus

Peptococcus

The peptococci are anaerobic organisms arranged in clusters; in contrast to the peptostreptococci, they are catalase positive. Their pathogenic significance is similar to that of the peptostreptococci, although their virulence is generally lower. *Peptococcus magnus* is the species most commonly associated with infection.

Other Nonclostridial Anaerobic Organisms

Many other anaerobic species of Gram-negative and non-spore-forming Gram-positive rods have been described. Their role in infection is usually only subsidiary, so they will not be discussed here. It is important to remember, however, that they probably play an important adjunctive role in lesions such as periodontal disease, the single major cause of tooth loss and oral sepsis. The genus *Veillonella,* which comprises small anaerobic Gram-negative cocci, merits special mention because it may be confused with *Neisseria* on Gram staining. It is often present in anaerobic lesions, but plays little role in infection.

Laboratory Diagnosis

Collection and transport

The key to detection and identification of anaerobes is a good specimen, preferably pus or fluid exudate from the infected site. It should be collected in special anaerobic transport tubes or in a syringe from which all air is excluded. These measures prevent loss of viability from contact with atmospheric oxygen. Specimens should, whenever possible, be taken to the microbiology laboratory immediately after collection for prompt placement in culture.

Direct Gram stain

discrepancy between Gram stain and aerobic culture

A direct Gram-stained smear of clinical material is often helpful. Numerous pale-staining Gram-negative rods are usually seen in anaerobic Gram-negative infections. They are often slim or fusiform and are frequently associated with some Gram-positive bacteria. Numerous polymorphonuclear leukocytes are usually seen (Plate L). These findings are highly suggestive of anaerobic Gram-negative infection, especially if little or no growth occurs on overnight aerobic culture.

Cultural identification requires special procedures. Media maintained under reduced or anaerobic conditions are used throughout, and exposure to atmospheric oxygen is kept to a minimum. Specific identification procedures, which vary according to species, include toxin detection among clostridia and end-product detection by gas chromatography among the Gram-negative rods and Gram-positive coccal species.

Clinical Manifestations and Treatment

As indicated previously, these normal floral organisms are opportunists, gaining access to tissues through trauma or other breakdown in normal host defenses. Those with the greatest virulence are selected out and multiply under conditions of sufficiently low Eh. Characteristically purulent and severe infections result, usually with abscess formation; anaerobic endocarditis occurs occasionally.

Surgical drainage and chemotherapy

In most cases, treatment requires detection of abscesses and drainage of the purulent material, in addition to appropriate chemotherapy. Frequently, chemotherapy alone is ineffective because of failure to penetrate the site of infection. Anaerobic organisms derived from the oral flora are usually susceptible to penicillin and are the most common cause of infection above the diaphragm. Fecal anaerobes, particularly *B. fragilis,* are usually resistant to penicillin and are the etiologic agents of most abdominal infections. They are most likely to respond to chloramphenicol, clindamycin, metronidazole, or an appropriate third-generation cephalosporin. It merits further emphasis, however, that surgical drainage is often essential to therapeutic success.

Additional Reading and References

Finegold, S.M. 1977. *Anaerobic Bacteria in Human Disease.* New York: Academic Press.

Smith, L.D-S. 1975. *The Pathogenic Anaerobic Bacteria.* 2nd ed. Publication 980. American Lecture Series. Springfield, Ill: Charles C. Thomas.

Willis, A.T. 1977. *Anaerobic Bacteriology. Clinical and Laboratory Practice.* 3rd ed. Butterworth and Co. These are three excellent texts. That of Finegold covers clinical syndromes in more depth.

Kenneth J. Ryan

Neisseria

16

Neisseria are Gram-negative diplococci. The genus contains two pathogenic and many commensal species, most of which are normal inhabitants of the upper respiratory and alimentary tracts. The pathogenic species are *Neisseria meningitidis* (meningococcus), a major cause of meningitis and bacteremia, and *Neisseria gonorrhoeae* (gonococcus), the cause of the venereal disease gonorrhea.

Morphology

Gram-negative bean-shaped diplococci

The organisms are Gram-negative cocci that typically appear in pairs with the opposing sides flattened. A "kidney bean" appearance, with the long axes of the cells parallel, is thus produced. This morphology is seen in cultured bacteria and in clinical specimens, although the typical features may not be demonstrable with every pair. Both gonococci and meningococci are readily phagocytosed by polymorphonuclear leukocytes (PMNs); cells containing 10 or more pairs of gonococci may be seen in Gram smears of pus (Plate M), although many organisms may be extracellular, particularly in the case of *N. meningitidis. Neisseria* are nonmotile, non-spore forming, and are non-acid fast. Their cell walls are typical of Gram-negative bacteria with a preptidoglycan backbone and endotoxic lipopolysaccharide complexed with protein in an outer membrane. Capsules and pili may be demonstrated by ultrastructure or by immunologic techniques.

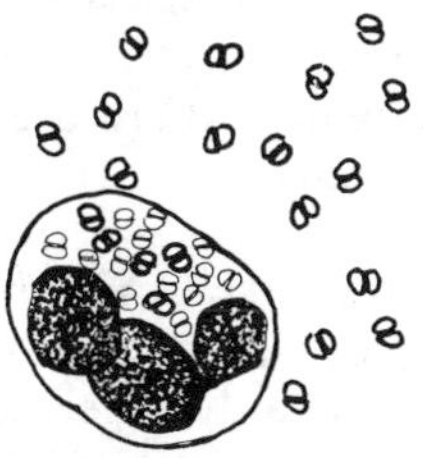

Neisseria gonorrhoeae in WBC

Cultural Characteristics

pathogenic species more fastidious than commensals

The gonococcus and the meningococcus require an aerobic atmosphere with added carbon dioxide and enriched media for optimal growth. The gonococcus grows more slowly and is more fastidious than the meningococcus, which can grow on routine blood agar. Both grow only at temperatures of 30–37°C. Other *Neisseria* are generally less fastidious and can grow at temperatures of 22–25°C.

Classification

oxidase-positive

Neisseria are oxidase-positive. Some of the bacteriologic and biochemical features used to distinguish the various species of *Neisseria* are illustrated in Table 16.1. Gonococci and meningococci may also be differentiated from

Table 16.1 Bacteriologic Features of *Neisseria* and *Branhamella*

	Growth			Acid Production from Sugars			
Organism	Blood Agar	Room Temperature	Special Medium[a]	Glucose	Sucrose	Maltose	Lactose
N. gonorrhoeae	–[b]	–	+	+	–	–	–
N. meningitidis	+	–	+	+	–	+	–
N. lactamica	+	v[c]	+	+	–	+	+
Other *Neisseria*	+	+	–	v	v	v	v
Branhamella	+	+	–	–	–	–	–

[a] Thayer–Martin or similar selective medium.
[b] Poor growth may occur with some strains.
[c] Reaction varies with different strains and species.

the other *Neisseria* by immunologic methods such as slide agglutination, coagglutination, and precipitin reactions.

Neisseria meningitidis

Growth and Structure

growth enhancement by CO_2

Meningococci grow on most nonselective routine laboratory media, and after overnight incubation on blood agar produce about 1.5-mm diameter colonies. Carbon dioxide enhances growth, but is not required. Most isolates produce a small capsule that is not detected by routine methods.

Antigenic Structure

serogroups on basis of capsular polysaccharide

Meningococci are divided into nine serogroups, largely on the basis of polysaccharide capsules. The most important serogroups are A, B, C, and Y. Not all strains can be grouped according to currently available antisera, and it is likely other antigens remain to be identified. The chemical structure of the group-specific polysaccharide has been identified for most serogroups. Purified groups A and C polysaccharides are immunogenic and are used as vaccines. In contrast, the polysaccharide of group B meningococci lacks the immunogenicity of those in groups A and C, although the reasons for this are not clear. In addition to the group antigens, several serotypes have been identified within group B and C meningococci. The group B serotypes are based on differences in outer membrane proteins. Further study is necessary to determine whether different serotypes within the serogroups are associated with predictable virulence or epidemiologic features.

Pathogenesis and Immunity

exclusively human parasite

Nasopharyngeal carriage

The meningococcus is an exclusively human parasite; like other pyogenic cocci (*Staphylococcus aureus, Streptococcus pneumoniae*), it can either exist as an apparently harmless member of the normal flora or produce acute disease. Carrier rates of meningococci in the upper respiratory tract are usually between 5 and 15% in healthy adults and children; higher colonization rates are found occasionally in closed populations such as military recruit camps and boarding schools. The carrier state is associated with the development of group specific antibodies and immunity, but before this develops, meningococci may sometimes spread from the nasopharynx to produce bacteremia, endotoxemia, and meningitis. The polysaccharide capsule is probably important in resisting phagocytosis, and the potent endotoxic activity of the

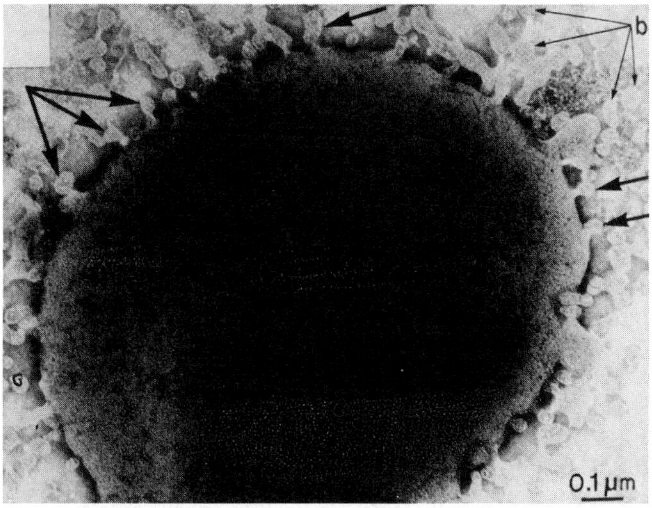

16.1 *Neisseria meningitidis.* Cell wall is shown shedding multiple "blebs" (*arrows*) containing LPS-endotoxin. Note the typical trilamellar Gram-negative cell wall structure in the wall and the blebs. *(Reproduced with permission from Devoe, I.W. and Gilcrist, J.E. 1973. J. Exp. Med. 138 (5):1160, Figure 3.)*

antiphagocytic effect of capsule and endotoxin activity

cell wall is responsible for some of the clinical manifestations. *Neisseria meningitidis* like gonococci have been shown to readily release endotoxin-containing blebs from the cell surface (Figure 16.1). The organism does not produce a significant exotoxin. It is unclear whether certain meningococcal strains are more virulent than others.

Mechanisms of immunity

Immunity to meningococcal infections is related to circulating group-specific opsonizing and bactericidal antibody, and antibody against endemic serogroups is present in many but not all adults. The peak incidence of serious infection is between 6 months and 2 years of age, which corresponds to the time between loss of transplacental antibody and the appearance of naturally acquired antibody (Figure 16.2). Infections later in life appear

16.2 Immunity to the meningococcus. The inverse relationship between bactericidal meningococcal antibody and meningococcal disease is demonstrated. The "blip" in the disease curve around age 20 is attributable in part to military and other closed population outbreaks. *(Adapted from Goldschneider et al. 1969.)*

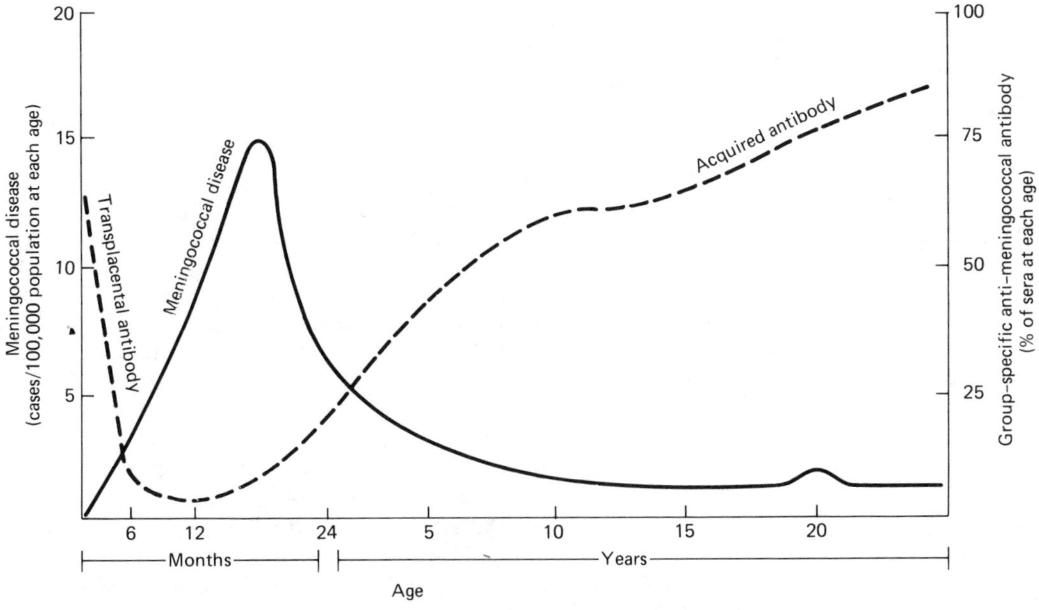

Populations at risk

when populations carrying virulent strains mix with susceptible individuals lacking specific antibody. Examples of this process include outbreaks of meningococcal disease among young adults in military recruit camps. In these outbreaks, *N. meningitidis* spreads among newly exposed recruits readily, but disease develops only in those lacking group-specific antibody.

acquisition of protective antibody

Protective antibody is usually acquired through subclinical or overt infection and through the carrier state, which produces immunity within a few weeks. However, natural immunization may not require infection or colonization with every serogroup or even with *N. meningitidis,* because antibody may be produced in response to cross-reacting antigens on other *Neisseria* species and even with other genera. For example, the K1 surface antigen of some *Escherichia coli* strains is chemically and immunologically identical to the group B meningococcal polysaccharide.

Epidemiology

Most endemic disease now due to groups B, C, or Y

Meningococcal infections must be reported by law in the United States, and usually more than 1000 cases per year are recorded. Most current cases are caused by group B, C, or Y strains in sporadic endemics or in small family or closed population outbreaks. Group A strains are more ominous and have the potential to cause widespread epidemics, which in the past have appeared in 8- to 12-year cycles. In the interim, group A meningococci curiously disappear, with only a few cases reported per year. It has been more than 30 years since such an epidemic has occurred in the United States, although serious group A epidemics have occurred in Brazil and South Africa in recent years.

epidemic potential of group A meningococci

Route and conditions for transmission

Transmission of meningococci is by respiratory droplets and requires both close contact and susceptibility (lack of antibody). This combination is most likely to occur in family members of an index case, particularly children. The attack rate of meningococcal infections among family members is 1000-fold higher than in the general population; prophylactic chemotherapy is indicated. Despite their contact with meningococcal infections, hospital employees have not shown an increased frequency of infection, probably because of the lack of prolonged close contact in a largely immune adult population.

Clinical Manifestations

Meningitis

The most frequent form of meningococcal infection is acute purulent meningitis with clinical and laboratory features similar to those of other causes of meningitis (Chapter 61). A distinguishing feature of meningococcal meningitis is the appearance of scattered skin petechiae, which may evolve into ecchymoses or a diffuse petechial rash. These features are manifestations of meningococcal bacteremia (meningococcemia) and thrombocytopenia, which develops with evolution of the disseminated intravascular coagulation (DIC) syndrome. Many of these features are similar to those of experimental endotoxic shock. Meningococcemia sometimes occurs without meningitis, and may progress to fulminant DIC and shock with bilateral hemorrhagic destruction of the adrenal glands (Waterhouse–Friderichsen syndrome). It is not always fulminant, however, and some patients have only low-grade fever, arthritis, and skin lesions that develop slowly over a period of days to weeks. The finding of *N. meningitidis* in the blood or even the cerebrospinal fluid (CSF) of patients with chronic meningococcemia is often unexpected from the clinical severity of the illness. Meningococci may also cause pneumonia, but this disease is uncommon and is not associated with the more common manifestations of meningococcal infection.

Meningococcemia and rash

Waterhouse–Friderichsen syndrome

Chronic meningococcal bacteremia

Diagnosis

direct smears

Culture and serogrouping

Direct Gram smears of CSF in meningitis may demonstrate the typical bean-shaped, Gram-negative diplococci. Definitive diagnosis is by culture of CSF, blood, or skin lesions. Although reputed to be somewhat fragile, the organism requires no special handling for isolation from presumptively sterile sites such as blood and CSF; *N. gonorrhoeae*, in contrast, is more fragile and fastidious. Good growth develops on blood or chocolate agar after 18 hr of incubation. If sufficient growth is present, confirmation and serogrouping may be done directly from the primary plates by slide agglutination methods. Speciation is based on carbohydrate fermentation patterns (Table 16.1).

Antigen detection in clinical material

For rapid diagnosis and in cases in which cultures are negative because of previous antimicrobic therapy, meningococcal polysaccharide antigen may be detected by methods such as counterimmunoelectrophoresis (Chapter 9). Meningococcal antigen has been detected in CSF, blood, and urine; false-negative results are common, however, particularly with group B strains.

Treatment

penicillin or chloramphenicol treatment

Penicillin is the treatment of choice for meningococcal infections because of its antimeningococcal activity and because it can penetrate inflamed meninges. Patients with penicillin hypersensitivity are treated with chloramphenicol. Although *N. meningitidis* is susceptible in vitro to a wide range of antimicrobics, relatively few are considered appropriate because of poor clinical results or lack of clinical experience. For example, cephalothin gives inconsistent clinical results despite good in vitro susceptibility. Some of the newer cephalosporins, however, may serve as alternatives to penicillin. Sulfonamides, although effective in the past, have been discarded in favor of penicillin and chloramphenicol. Resistance to penicillin or chloramphenicol has not been described, but sulfonamide-resistant meningococci are common.

Prevention

Chemoprophylaxis

sulfonamide-resistant strains

rifampin in chemoprophylaxis

indications for prophylaxis

In the past, the primary means of preventing secondary cases and further spread of meningococcal infection was chemoprophylaxis with sulfonamides. This approach was effective for populations ranging from individual family members to whole military camps. The development and spread of sulfonamide-resistant meningococci in the 1960s changed this situation. Currently, 40–50% of group C meningococci (one of the most common serogroups) are resistant to sulfonamides with lower incidences of resistance among group B and group Y strains. Sulfonamides are still the preferred prophylactic agents for susceptible strains, but in individual cases, sulfonamide susceptibility must be demonstrated before sulfonamides can be used. However, the time involved in susceptibility testing mandates initial selection of another agent. Rifampin is currently used for prophylaxis against sulfonamide-resistant meningococci or in situations in which the susceptibility is unknown. Penicillin is *not* effective as a prophylactic agent, probably because of inadequate penetration to the surface of the uninflamed nasopharyngeal mucosa. Selection of cases to receive prophylaxis is based on epidemiologic assessment of risk (see Epidemiology). Typically, family members are given prophylaxis but hospital employees are not, unless close contact such as mouth-to-mouth resuscitation has occurred. Culture findings play no role in these decisions, because they do not accurately predict risk of serious infection.

Meningococcal vaccines

Purified polysaccharide meningococcal vaccines have been shown to prevent group A and C disease in military and civilian populations. Unfortunately, their effectiveness in preventing disease in the major susceptible group is compromised by a poor antibody response to immunization in the first year of life. These vaccines are currently used in specialized populations such as military recruit camps and in the control of epidemics. The lack of an effective group B vaccine remains a problem.

Neisseria gonorrhoeae

Growth

fastidiousness of gonococci and CO_2 requirement

T1-4 colony types and association with virulence

different auxotypes

Neisseria gonorrhoeae grows well only on chocolate agar and on similar specialized media enriched to ensure its growth. It requires CO_2 supplementation. Small colonies appear after 18–24 hr of incubation and are well developed (2–4 mm) after 48 hr. The colonies are smooth and nonpigmented. Under specialized growth and illumination conditions four colony types have been recognized, designated T1 to T4. In general, T1 and T2 colonies are seen on primary isolation, are associated with virulence, and are able to produce experimental infections. Larger T3 and T4 colonies tend to appear on continued subculture and are avirulent. The ability to grow on defined media lacking specific nutrients has been used to develop an auxotyping scheme for gonococci. Over 30 types, some of which have been associated with particular clinical or epidemiologic features, can be separated with these procedures.

Structure

pili on T1 and T2 colony types

outer membrane proteins

In addition to the typical Gram-negative cell wall structure, gonococci possess numerous protein pili that extend through and beyond the peptidoglycan and outer membrane (Figure 16.3). In general, the T1 and T2 colony types typical of fresh virulent isolates have pili, but others do not. Gonococcal pili mediate attachment to mucosal surfaces and retard the rate of phagocytosis by neutrophils. The gonococcal outer membrane is composed of phospholipids, lipopolysaccharide, and several distinct proteins. The outer membrane proteins have been studied in a manner similar to that used for group B meningococci and have been found antigenically distinct. A serotyping scheme for *N. gonorrhoeae* has been developed on this basis. Gon-

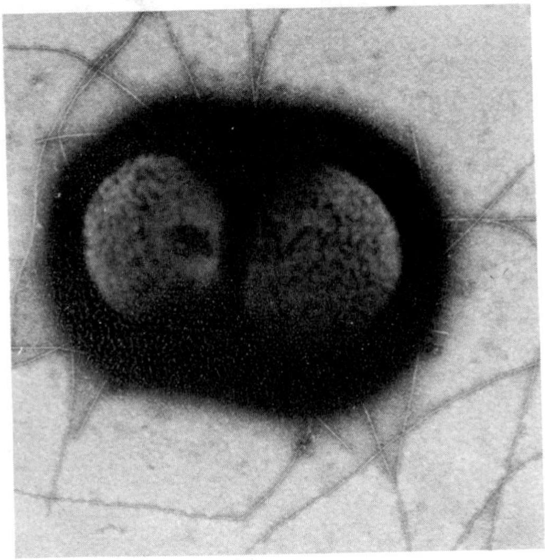

16.3 *Neisseria gonorrhoeae.* Surface pili are shown. These structures are associated with virulence and may mediate initial attachment to epithelial surfaces. *(Kindly provided by Dr. John Swanson.)*

ococcal strains have been shown to possess surface polysaccharide and capsules, but the pathogenic significance of these structures is not yet known.

Pathogenesis and Immunity

initial attachment mediated by pili

multiplication within epithelial cells

acute inflammatory response

direct extension to other sites

Gonococci are *not* normal inhabitants of the respiratory or genital flora. When introduced onto a mucosal surface by sexual contact with an infected individual, the organisms attach to mucosal epithelium, enter, and multiply within the epithelial cells. Attachment is probably mediated by the pili and is followed by endocytosis. Rapid intracellular multiplication leads to destruction of the epithelial cell and release of more gonococci. Spread to other cells eventually leads to an acute inflammatory response. Neutrophils readily phagocytose the gonococci, although this process is somewhat retarded by the pili and the inflammatory exudate tends to facilitate spread to other epithelial cells. Infection also extends to deeper structures by progressive infection of mucosal and glandular epithelial cells. These structures include the lining of the paracervical and paraurethral glands and of the fallopian tubes in women and the prostate and epididymis in men. Extension along the fallopian tubes from an initial cervical infection can lead to seeding of the pelvic cavity. In most cases the disease remains localized although bacteremia and hematogenous extension occur in a small proportion of cases. This is termed disseminated gonococcal infection (DGI). The strains involved in cases of DGI differ from other gonococci in possessing a greater resistance to the bactericidal effects of normal human serum and in commonly being of a single auxotype.

disseminated infection associated with one auxotype

immunity to reinfection weak

Immunity to gonococcal infection (or lack of immunity) remains poorly understood. Antibody directed against some components of the organism, such as the pili, has been demonstrated, but repeated gonorrhea infections are common. Whether these repeated infections result from failure of local immunity, "shielding" of gonococci in epithelial cells, or presence of multiple serotypes is still not known.

Epidemiology

recent epidemic of gonorrhea

difficulties in controlling the disease

Gonorrhea is a major worldwide public health problem. In the United States the number of reported cases has steadily increased since the 1950s. No truly effective means of control is yet in sight. Over one million cases have been reported annually in recent years; this figure does not reflect the true prevalence, however, as many cases, despite the legal requirement, go unreported. The reasons for our inability to control gonorrhea are complex and include changing sexual mores and practices, lack of an effective means to detect asymptomatic cases, decreased susceptibility of *N. gonorrhoeae* to penicillin (see Therapy), and, to some extent, lack of public appreciation of the importance of this disease. The latter is evidenced by failure of patients to seek medical care and of physicians to report cases to public health authorities to protect the privacy of their patients. In the minds of many, syphilis is dreaded and "unclean," whereas gonorrhea is only "the clap" (clap: archaic French clapoir, a rabbit warren; later, a brothel).

major reservoir is asymptomatic infections

The major reservoir for continued spread of gonorrhea is the asymptomatic patient. Screening programs and case contact studies have shown that almost 50% of infected women are asymptomatic or at least do not have symptoms usually associated with venereal infection. Most men (95%) have acute symptoms with infection. Many who are not treated become asymptomatic but remain infectious. Asymptomatic male and female patients can remain infectious for months. The attack rates for those engaging in genital intercourse with an infected patient are not known, but are estimated to be 20–50%. The organism may also be transmitted by oral–genital contact or by rectal intercourse. When all of these factors operate in a sexually promiscuous population, it is easy to explain the high prevalence of gonorrhea.

rarity of fomitic transfer

Although gonococci can survive for brief periods on the proverbial toilet seat, nonsexual transmission is extremely rare. Fomite transmission of a purulent vulvovaginitis in prepubescent girls has been reported, but currently most isolations of gonococci in children can be traced to sexual abuse by an infected adult.

Genital Gonorrhea

Urethritis and endocervicitis

In men, the primary site of infection is the urethra. Symptoms begin 2–7 days after infection and consist primarily of purulent urethral discharge and dysuria. Although uncommon, local extension can lead to epididymitis or prostatitis. The endocervix is the primary site in women, in whom symptoms include increased vaginal discharge, urinary frequency, dysuria, abdominal pain, and menstrual abnormalities. As mentioned previously, symptoms may be mild or absent in either sex, particularly in women.

Other Local Infections

Rectal infection

Pharyngeal infection

Rectal gonorrhea occurs after rectal intercourse or, in women, after contamination with infected vaginal secretions. This infection is generally asymptomatic but may cause tenesmus, discharge, and rectal bleeding. Pharyngeal gonorrhea is caused by orogenital sex and, again is usually asymptomatic. Sore throat and cervical adenitis may occur. Infection of other structures near primary infection sites, such as Bartholin's glands in women, may lead to abscess formation.

Conjunctivitis and ophthalmia neonatorum

Inoculation of gonococci into the conjunctiva produces a severe, acute, purulent conjunctivitis. Although this infection may occur at any age, the most common and serious form is gonococcal ophthalmia neonatorum acquired by an infant from an infected mother. This disease was formerly a common cause of blindness, and for this reason eye prophylaxis is used at birth. This disease had all but disappeared, but with the general increase in gonococcal infections it is now seen occasionally (Chapter 63).

Pelvic Inflammatory Disease

Salpingitis and pelvic peritonitis

The clinical syndrome of pelvic inflammatory disease (PID) includes fever, lower abdominal pain, adnexal tenderness, and leukocytosis with or without signs of local infection. These features are caused by spread of organisms along the fallopian tubes to produce salpingitis and into the pelvic cavity to produce pelvic peritonitis and abscesses. Although defined previously as a gonococcal disease, PID is now known to develop when other potential pathogens in the genital flora ascend by the same route. These organisms include anaerobes and *Chlamydia trachomatis,* which may appear alone or mixed with gonococci. The most serious complication of PID is infertility, which can result from a single attack and is common after multiple attacks, regardless of the microbial etiology.

Disseminated Gonococcal Infections

skin rash, arthralgia, and arthritis

Any of the local forms of gonorrhea or the local extensions such as PID may lead to bacteremia. In the bacteremic phase the primary features are fever, migratory polyarthralgia, and a petechial, maculopapular, or pustular rash. These features may be immunologically mediated, as gonococci are infrequently isolated from the skin or joints at this stage despite their presence in the blood. The bacteremia may lead to infections such as endocarditis or meningitis, but the most common is purulent arthritis. The arthritis typically follows the bacteremia and involves large joints such as elbows and knees. Gonococci are readily cultured from the pus.

Further consideration of gonorrhea is given in Chapter 64.

Diagnosis

Use and limitations of direct smear

Gram smear. The presence of multiple pairs of bean-shaped, Gram-negative diplococci within a neutrophil is highly characteristic of gonorrhea when the smear is from a genital site (Plate M). Unfortunately, other bacteria in the female genital flora may have a similar appearance. This finding, combined with the more acute exudate generally found in men has given the direct Gram smear a reputation for sensitivity and specificity in men, but insensitivity and nonspecificity in women; however, skilled microscopists, such as those in venereal disease clinics, who regularly see many cases can achieve a diagnostic accuracy in women that approaches that in men. The student or harried intern, however, cannot necessarily apply the same criteria with equal results despite published statistics, and cultural confirmation should be obtained. Cases in which the findings are unexpected or have particular social or medicolegal implications should always be confirmed by culture.

Selection of culture sites

Culture. Attention to detail is necessary for isolation of the gonococcus, as it is a fragile organism often mixed with hardier members of the normal flora. Success requires proper selection of culture sites, protection of specimens from environmental exposure, culture on appropriate media, and definitive laboratory identification. In men the best specimen is of urethral exudate or urethral scrapings (obtained with a loop or special swab). In women a cervical swabs yield most positive results: gonococci may also be isolated from the urethra and vagina, but the rate of positive results is significantly below that of cervical culture. The highest diagnostic yield in women is with the combination of a cervical and an anal canal culture, because some patients with rectal gonorrhea will have negative cervical cultures. Throat and rectal cultures in men are needed only if indicated by the patient's sexual practices.

immediate culture or use of transport media

Swabs may be streaked directly onto culture media or transmitted to the laboratory in a suitable transport medium (Stuart's) if the delay is not more than 4 hr. Laboratory requests must always specify the suspicion of gonorrhea, as specialized, selective media are required. These media satisfy the nutritional requirements of the gonococcus and inhibit competing normal flora, which may interfere with isolation. The most common is Thayer–Martin agar, an enriched selective chocolate-type agar. The exact formulation has changed over the years, but includes antimicrobics active against Gram-positive bacteria (vancomycin), Gram-negative bacteria (colistin, trimethoprim), and fungi (nystatin, anisomycin) at concentrations that do not inhibit *N. gonorrhoeae*. Other selective media with similar performance characteristics have been developed more recently. Self-contained kits shipped by mail have been successful in remote areas.

Thayer–Martin selective medium

Identification of Neisserial isolates

Colonies appear after 1–2 days of incubation in CO_2 at 35°C. They may be identified as *Neisseria* by demonstration of typical Gram-stain morphology and a positive oxidase test. Speciation is made by carbohydrate fermentation pattern (Table 16.1), immunofluorescence, or coagglutination. *Neisseria* other than *N. gonorrhoeae* are unusual in genital specimens, but speciation is the only way to be certain of the diagnosis.

Serology. Attempts to develop a serologic test for gonorrhea have not yet achieved the needed sensitivity and specificity. A test that would detect the disease in asymptomatic patients would be very useful in control of this disease.

Treatment

Penicillin

increasing mutational resistance

Penicillin was, for a long time, the primary treatment for gonorrhea, although two changes in the susceptibility of the organism have influenced its use. The first has been a slowly decreasing susceptibility of gonococci to penicillin, which has been noted since the 1950s. Older strains were uniformly inhibited by less than 0.1 μg/ml penicillin, whereas up to 25% of recent isolates in several U.S. cities require 0.5–2.0 μg/ml. This resistance is mutational; the strains do not produce penicillinase and can still be treated with a penicillin at high doses. Many of the more resistant isolates are also resistant to other antimicrobics.

plasmid-coded penicillinase production

In the late 1970s, penicillinase-producing *N. gonorrhoeae* (PPNG) appeared throughout the world, originating primarily in the Far East. These strains produced a plasmid-coded TEM-type β-lactamase identical to that of members of the Enterobacteriaceae and ampicillin-resistant *Haemophilus influenzae.* These gonococci are inhibited only by high concentrations of penicillin (4–64 μg/ml) and do not respond to penicillin therapy. Initially, most cases in the United States could be traced to the Far East through military or other contacts. There is now sustained disease transmission with PPNG in endemic foci in the United States, which has created further concern about the future of penicillin therapy for gonorrhea.

Spectinomycin

Erythromycin, tetracycline, spectinomycin and third-generation cephalosporins are alternate drugs for PPNG strains or for patients hypersensitive to penicillin. Of these, spectinomycin is preferred, unless the patient can be relied upon to complete a full course of oral medication. Present approaches to treatment are given in Chapter 64.

Prevention

Methods to block direct mucosal contact (condoms) or inhibit the gonococcus (vaginal foams, douches) have not been studied extensively, but it is likely that they provide protection against gonorrhea if used regularly. The classic public health methods of case-contact tracing and treatment have become more difficult with the increasing size of the primary reservoir. The availability of a good serologic test would greatly aid control, as it has for syphilis. The development of a gonococcal vaccine awaits further understanding of the immunology and epidemiology of gonorrhea.

Other *Neisseria*

Upper respiratory tract commensals

Many other *Neisseria* species exist primarily as normal inhabitants of the upper respiratory tract. Some have been shown to cause mild to serious infections, including meningitis, but only rarely. With the exception of *Neisseria lactamica,* these other *Neisseria* and *Branhamella* generally fail to grow on Thayer–Martin agar. They are distinguished from *N. gonorrhoeae* and *N. meningitidis* by biochemical and serologic tests. They can grow at 22–25°C and frequently produce dry, wrinkled, or pigmented colonies, which are readily distinguished from those of pathogenic species.

Branhamella

Organisms in the genus *Branhamella* were previously classified as *Neisseria* because, as oxidase-positive Gram-negative diplococci, they superficially resembled them. Studies of DNA homology have shown clear differences, however, and some clinical studies indicate that *Branhamella* may have a greater potential to produce respiratory tract infections than do true *Neisseria.*

Additional Reading and References

Goldschneider, I., Gotschlich, E.C., Liu, T.Y., and Artenstein, M.S. 1969. Human immunity to the meningococcus I–V. *J. Exp. Med.* 129:1307–1385. This series of five papers defines the basis of immunity to *Neisseria meningitidis* and the development of vaccines from the polysaccharide capsule.

Roberts, M., Elwell, L.P., and Falkow, S. 1977. Molecular characterization of two beta-lactamase-specifying plasmids isolated from *Neisseria gonorrhoeae. J. Bacteriol.* 131:557–562. This molecular study shows the mechanism of penicillinase production by gonococci and the relation of these plasmids to others, such as those found in *Haemophilus influenzae.*

Kenneth J. Ryan

Haemophilus, Bordetella, and *Gardnerella*

17

Haemophilus and *Bordetella* are small, Gram-negative rods that tend to assume a coccobacillary shape. They are nonmotile, non-spore forming, and require complex media for growth. Members of both genera cause respiratory infections, and *Haemophilus influenzae* is responsible for a variety of systemic infections, including purulent meningitis.

Haemophilus influenzae

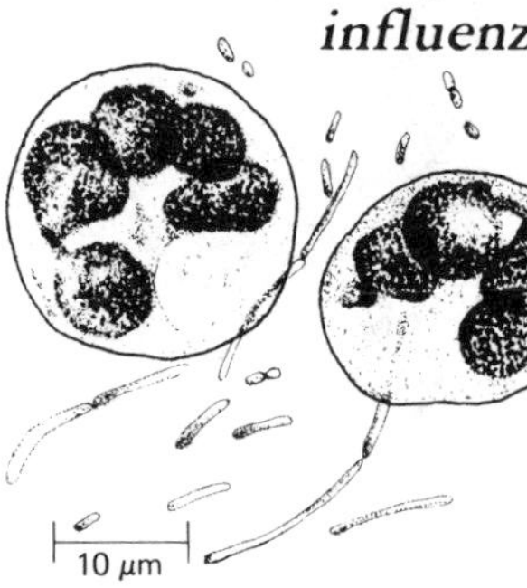

Haemophilus influenzae in CSF

Morphology and Structure

Organisms grown in broth or on agar plates usually show a highly regular shape. The rounded ends of short (1.0–1.5 μm) bacilli make many appear round, hence the term *coccobacilli.* The cells are so small that clear visualization requires optimal light microscopy. In clinical specimens such as sputum, the same morphology is generally seen (Plate O); in cerebrospinal fluid, however, some of the cells may be elongated to several times their usual length.

Serotypes based on polysaccharide capsule

The cell wall has a lipopolysaccharide–protein surface similar to that of other Gram-negative bacteria. *Haemophilus influenzae* may have a polysaccharide capsule, but other species of *Haemophilus* are not encapsulated. Capsulate *H. influenzae* are divided into six serotypes, a–f, based on the capsular polysaccharide antigen. Capsulate strains can be typed with specific antisera by use of the capsule swelling (quellung reaction) test or other serologic procedures for detecting surface antigens. The chemical nature of the capsular polysaccharides is known. For example, type b capsule is made up of a polymer of ribose, ribitol and phosphate, called polyribitol phosphate (PRP). These surface polysaccharides are strongly associated with virulence, particularly in type b *H. influenzae,* which is responsible for most cases of serious systemic infection. Cell wall (somatic) antigens of capsulated and nonencapsulated *Haemophilus* have not been associated with virulence.

Growth

Growth factor requirements: hematin (X) and NAD (V)

In addition to the usual components of enriched culture media, *Haemophilus* species require added blood products for optimal growth (as indicated by the genus name, from the Greek *haema,* blood, and *philos,* loving). This requirement is attributable to the need for hematin and/or nicotinamide adenine dinucleotide (NAD) as growth factors. These growth factors, also termed *X factor* (hematin) and *V factor* (NAD), are both present in eryth-

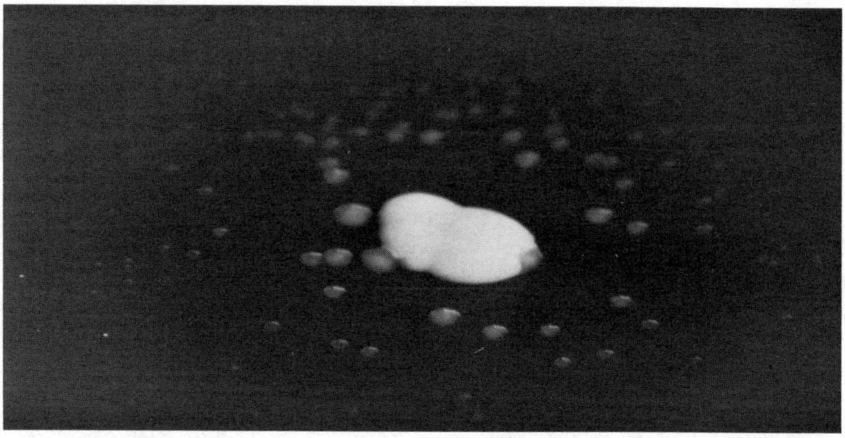

17.1 The satellite phenomenon. This blood agar plate has been evenly spread with *Haemophilus influenzae* and then touched with a wire containing *Staphylococcus aureus.* Note the small colonies appear only around the *S. aureus,* which is producing V factor (NAD). Together with the X factor (hematin) from the blood, the requirement for both X and V factors are met only in this area.

rocytes. In culture medium, optimal concentrations of X and, particularly, V factors are not available to *Haemophilus* from blood unless the red blood cells are lysed by gentle heat (chocolate agar) or some digestion process (Fildes agar). Although erythrocytes are the only convenient source of hematin, the V factor is present in a variety of biologic systems and is produced by some other bacteria and yeast. These conditions are responsible for the "satellite phenomenon," in which *H. influenzae* grows on blood agar only in the vicinity of a colony of *Staphylococcus aureus* that is producing V factor (Figure 17.1).

Satellitism

Cultural characteristics

When their nutritional needs are met, most *Haemophilus* species grow rapidly, producing 1- to 2-mm translucent colonies after overnight incubation under aerobic or anaerobic conditions. Encapsulated strains may produce larger colonies with a glistening mucoid quality. Commonly used broth media lack the X and V factors needed to support growth of *Haemophilus.* When whole blood is added with the inoculum (as in blood cultures) the organisms will grow, but they require 2–3 days and usually do not become sufficiently numerous to produce turbidity. Rapid growth with large numbers of organisms is achieved if the pure growth factors or blood digest supplements are added.

Pathogenesis

carrier rates in health

Various *Haemophilus* species are common inhabitants of the upper respiratory tract. Carrier rates for *H. influenzae* as high as 80% have been found in children and are commonly 20–50% in healthy adults. Most strains are nonencapsulated, but healthy carriers of encapsulated strains are not infrequent. The events that cause these members of the normal flora to initiate disease are poorly understood, and appear to differ for encapsulated and unencapsulated *Haemophilus* strains.

invasive ability of *H. influenzae* type b

Type b *H. influenzae* strains can occasionally multiply and spread into the deeper tissues beyond the nasopharynx. This invasion may involve inflammation and edema of the epiglottis or facial and neck tissues. Invasion of the bloodstream, which is common once the organisms spread beyond the nasopharynx, is probably the mechanism for entry into the central nervous system and for metastatic infections at distant sites such as bones and joints. Host factors probably determine whether meningitis, arthritis, or a more local infection results. Systemic spread is typical only for encapsulated *H.*

influenzae strains, and over 90% of invasive strains are type b. The exact mechanisms of invasion and the unique features of type b versus the other types are unknown.

localized infections with nonencapsulated strains

Nonencapsulated *H. influenzae* and other respiratory *Haemophilus* species produce disease when they gain access to usually protected areas connected to the respiratory tract and are not cleared by the local defenses. Invasion of the middle ear, respiratory sinuses, and bronchi are most common. The infections produced are more superficial than those with type b, and deep invasion and bacteremia are rare.

absence of exotoxins

Haemophilus influenzae produces no known exotoxins or other extracellular products that can be associated with the pathogenesis of infection. Endotoxin is present in the cell wall and may be responsible for some of the manifestations of systemic disease, but endotoxemia is not a feature of *Haemophilus* infections to the extent it is with *Neisseria menigitidis.* The surface capsule contributes to virulence by inhibition of phagocytosis in the same manner as the pneumococcal capsule.

antiphagocytic effect of capsules

Immunity

Anticapsular and bactericidal antibody

type b infections most common at ages when antibody titer is lowest

Immunity to *H. influenzae* infections has been clearly associated with the presence of circulating antibody, which is bactericidal in the presence of complement. The infant is usually protected by passively acquired maternal antibody for the first few months of life. Thereafter the presence of actively acquired antibody increases with age; it is present in the serum of most children by age 10. The peak incidence of *H. influenzae* type b infections is at 6–18 months of age, which corresponds to the nadir of the serum antibody curve (Figure 17.2). This inverse relationship between infection and serum antibody is analogous to that for *N. meningitidis* (Figure 16.2). The major difference is that prevention of infection requires antibody directed against several meningococcal serogroups but against only a single type of *H. influenzae* (type b). Thus, systemic *H. influenzae* infections (meningitis, epiglottitis, cellulitis) are rare in adults. When such infections develop, however, the immunologic deficit is probably the same as that with meningococci: lack of circulating antibody.

poor response to vaccine in early childhood

Recent studies using a vaccine of purified type b PRP have shown age-related differences in ability to respond to this antigen. Infants respond poorly, whereas older children form high levels of antibody. Some infants

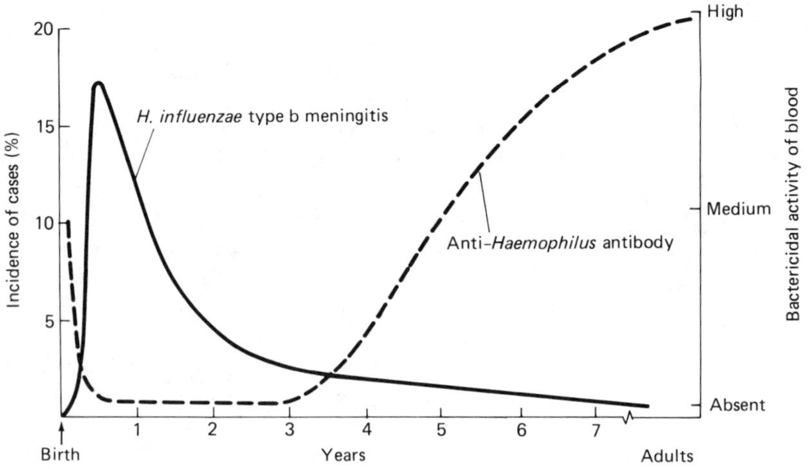

17.2 Relation of age incidence of *H. influenzae* meningitis to the bactericidal activity of blood against *H. influenzae.* (*Adapted from Fothergill and Wright.*)

fail to form anti-PRP antibody after systemic infection and have a second episode of invasive *H. influenzae* disease. A genetic basis for susceptibility to *H. influenzae* type b disease is a possibility that requires further study.

Epidemiology

Age incidence of *H. influenzae* type b meningitis, epiglottitis, and pneumonia

Because it is not a public health requirement to report *H. influenzae* infections, accurate infection rates are not available; the frequency of *H. influenzae* meningitis, however, has been estimated at 8000 cases yearly in the United States. Virtually all of these cases occur in children under 6 and most under 2 years of age. Cases of epiglottitis and pneumonia tend to peak in the 2- to 5-year age range. Evidence indicates that the frequency of systemic type b disease has increased slowly over the past 3–4 decades, and that adult infections are becoming more frequent. The reason for this trend is not known, but changes in the incidence of infection, virulence of the organism, and the impact of antimicrobic usage on development of immunity are possibilities.

increased risk of infection in children who are close contacts

In contrast to meningococcal meningitis, which has long been known to be communicable, *Haemophilus* meningitis was believed to be an isolated endogenous infection. Recent reports of outbreaks in closed populations such as day care centers and careful epidemiologic studies of secondary spread in families, have changed this view. The risk of serious infection for children under 4 years of age living with an index case is more than 500-fold that for nonexposed children. This risk indicates a need for prophylaxis for contacts in the susceptible age group. Although the effectiveness of various antimicrobics as chemoprophylactics has not been clearly established, rifampin is currently recommended for this purpose.

Prophylaxis

Haemophilus influenzae **Infections**

Meningitis

Mortality and morbidity

This is almost invariably caused by type b strains. *Haemophilus* meningitis follows the same pattern as other causes of acute purulent bacterial meningitis (Chapter 61). Meningitis is often preceded by signs and symptoms of an upper respiratory infection, such as nasopharyngitis, sinusitis, or otitis media. Whether these represent a predisposing viral infection or early invasion by the organism is not known. Just as often, meningitis is preceded only by vague malaise, lethargy, irritability, and fever. Mortality is currently 5–10% despite adequate therapy, and roughly one-third of all survivors have significant neurologic damage.

Acute Epiglottitis

respiratory obstruction

Acute epiglottitis is a dramatic infection caused by *H. influenzae* type b in which the epiglottis and surrounding tissues can obstruct the airway. Findings are those of a systemic infection with signs of increasing respiratory difficulty. The onset is sudden, with fever, sore throat, hoarseness, a barking cough, and rapid progression to severe prostration within 24 hr. The prostrated child has air hunger, inspiratory stridor, and retraction of the soft parts of the chest with each inspiration. The hallmark of the disease is an inflamed, swollen, cherry-red epiglottis that protrudes into the airway and can be visualized on lateral x-rays. As with meningitis, this infection is treated as a medical emergency with prime emphasis on maintenance of an airway (tracheostomy). Without an established airway, manipulations, including routine examination or attempting to take a throat swab, can be fatal by triggering acute obstruction.

Cherry-red swollen epiglottis

need for maintaining airway

Cellulitis

A tender, reddish-blue swelling in the cheek or periorbital areas is the usual presentation of *Haemophilus* cellulitis. This disease is also caused by type b strains. Fever and a moderately toxic state are usually present, and the infection may follow an upper respiratory infection or otitis media. A large proportion of cases are bacteremic, and some develop infections at other sites.

Arthritis

most common cause of purulent arthritis in children under 2 years of age

Haemophilus influenzae type b is the leading cause of purulent arthritis in children in the susceptible age range, particularly those under 2 years of age. Infection may follow another *H. influenzae* infection or appear as the primary illness. Local signs of inflammation in single, large, weight-bearing joints with fever and irritability are the usual features. *Haemophilus* arthritis is occasionally the cause of a more subtle set of findings, in which fever occurs without clear clinical evidence of joint involvement. Bacteremia is usually present.

Other Respiratory Infections

Role of noncapsulate strains in otitis media, sinusitis, and bronchitis

Haemophilus influenzae is one of several respiratory organisms that can cause otitis media, acute and chronic sinusitis, and exacerbation of chronic bronchitis. These infections usually result from displacement of the normal flora into normally sterile luminal structures. Thus, most *H. influenzae* infections are caused by nonencapsulated and thus nontypable strains found commonly in the respiratory flora. These infections usually remain localized without bacteremia, but could be a primary risk factor for meningitis and other systemic *H. influenzae* infections when type b strains are involved. This possibility is unproved. Disease may be acute or chronic, depending on the anatomic site and underlying pathology. For example, otitis media is acute and painful because of the small, closed space involved, but usually clears without sequelae after antimicrobic therapy and reopening of the eustachian tube. The association of *H. influenzae* with chronic bronchitis is more complex. There is evidence that *H. influenzae* and other bacteria play a role in inflammatory exacerbations, but a unique cause and effect relationship is difficult to prove. The underlying cause of the bronchitis is usually related to chronic damage resulting from smoking or other factors.

Haemophilus pneumonia may be caused by either encapsulated or nonencapsulated organisms. Encapsulated strains have been observed to produce a disease much like pneumococcal pneumonitis; however, unencapsulated strains may also produce pneumonia, particularly in patients with chronic bronchitis.

Diagnosis

Gram smear

Culture

Demonstration of growth factor requirement

The combination of clinical findings and a typical Gram smear is usually sufficient to make a presumptive diagnosis of *Haemophilus* infection. This diagnosis must then be confirmed by isolation of the organism from the site of infection or from the blood, using appropriate media. In specimens highly suspect for *H. influenzae,* many laboratories inoculate a *Staphylococcus aureus* onto part of the blood agar plate to demonstrate the satellite phenomenon (Figure 17.1) on primary isolation. Gram-negative rods that grow on chocolate agar but not blood agar (except around a staphylococcus colony) strongly suggest *Haemophilus.* Confirmation and speciation depends on demonstration of the requirement for X and V factors. Serotyping, which may be done by slide agglutination or capsular swelling (quellung) techniques, is usually unnecessary for clinical purposes.

Value of blood cultures in systemic infections

Blood cultures are particularly useful in systemic *H. influenzae* infections. It is difficult, except with meningitis, to gain access to the site of infection (epiglottitis, pneumonia) or to obtain a purulent specimen (cellulitis); a large proportion of patients are bacteremic, however, and blood cultures will usually yield the organism.

Detection of type b capsular antigen in body fluids

Haemophilus influenzae type b PRP is released into body fluids and circulates during the course of infection. PRP may be detected in infected body fluid, blood, or urine by methods such as counterimmunoelectrophoresis (Chapter 9). The procedures are not dependent on the presence of live organisms and can be helpful when cultures are negative because of antimicrobial therapy.

Treatment

ampicillin-resistant strains

plasmid-determined β-lactamase

Haemophilus influenzae is usually susceptible in vitro to ampicillin, the newer cephalosporins, chloramphenicol, tetracycline, aminoglycosides, and sulfonamides. It is less susceptible to other penicillins and to erythromycin. *Haemophilus* meningitis has been treated effectively with ampicillin, chloramphenicol, and the newer cephalosporins. Since 1974, the therapy of systemic infections has been complicated by the emergence of ampicillin-resistant strains of *H. influenzae.* These strains produce a potent β-lactamase that is plasmid mediated and identical to that found in other Gram-negative bacteria, such as *Escherichia coli.* These infections do not respond to ampicillin therapy. The frequency of resistant strains varies between 5 and 50% in different geographic areas, but for therapeutic purposes all strains must be considered resistant until proved susceptible. Susceptibility is determined by direct testing for β-lactamase production from colonies and by modifications of standard susceptibility tests that satisfy the growth requirements of *Haemophilus.* Although ampicillin-resistant strains that do not produce β-lactamase have also been described, they are still rare, as are chloramphenicol-resistant *H. influenzae.* Current practice is to start empiric therapy with chloramphenicol or with ampicillin plus chloramphenicol until the results of susceptibility tests are known. Administration of the inappropriate antimicrobic is then discontinued.

Nonencapsulated *Haemophilus* strains have demonstrated ampicillin resistance at about the same rate as the type b organisms. The therapeutic impact of this resistance is less clear, because other organisms may be involved in infections with which they are associated, and a specific etiologic diagnosis is often not established (for example, otitis media). The common use of ampicillin to treat such infections is now questioned, however, and may be responsible in part for the increasing frequency of resistance. The use of sulfonamides and newer cephalosporins resistant to the *Haemophilus* β-lactamase is under increasing consideration.

Prevention

Type b capsular vaccine

Haemophilus influenzae type b PRP has been purified and used as an immunogen for protection against systemic infection. As with meningococcal infections, the vaccine is not consistently effective in children under 18 months of age. Its value is therefore limited, as most cases occur by 2 years of age. Antimicrobial prophylaxis for case contacts is as discussed under Epidemiology.

Other *Haemophilus* Species

Several other *Haemophilus* species exist and are defined by their requirement for X and/or V factor, CO_2 dependence, and other cultural characteristics (Table 17.1). The respiratory species, of which *Haemophilus parainfluenzae* is the most common, have the same biology as the nonencapsulated strains of *H. influenzae.* An organism isolated from outbreaks of conjunctivitis, formerly assigned the name *Haemophilus aegyptius*, is now considered a variant of *H. influenzae.* Most of these species have been reported to cause systemic illness, including pneumonia, meningitis, arthritis, endocarditis, and soft tissue infections. Such cases are rare, as are those with nonencapsulated *H. influenzae.*

Haemophilus ducreyi

rare sexually transmitted disease

Haemophilus ducreyi causes chancroid, a rare venereal disease. The typical lesion of chancroid is a tender papule on the genitalia that develops into a painful ulcer with sharp margins. Satellite lesions may develop by autoinfection, and regional lymphadenitis is common. The incubation period is usually short (2–5 days).

soft chancre

laboratory diagnosis

The diagnosis of chancroid is primarily clinical. It is considered in the differential diagnosis of genital ulcers along with more common causes such as syphilis and genital herpes. In this context, the lack of induration in chancroid has caused the primary lesion to be called *soft chancre* to distinguish it from the primary syphilitic chancre, which is typically indurated and painless. Isolation of *H. ducreyi* is difficult. This difficulty has led to reliance on relatively nonspecific diagnostic techniques, such as Gram staining from specimens inoculated into tubes of clotted rabbit blood. Recent studies show that the organism can be isolated directly from the lesion using chocolate agar, particularly if vancomycin is added to inhibit interfering flora. The bacteria are present in small numbers and may take up to 10 days to grow. Clinical laboratories should be specifically instructed to search for the organism when the disease is suspected.

Table 17.1 Characteristics of *Haemophilus* Species

Species	Growth Factor Requirement		Hemolysis	Enhanced Growth with CO_2	Polysaccharide Capsular Antigen
	X	V			
H. influenzae (encapsulated)	+	+	—	—	Types a–f
H. influenzae (nonencapsulated)	+	+	—	—	—
H. parainfluenzae	—	+	var	var	—
H. haemolyticus	+	+	+	—	—
H. aphrophilus	—	—	—	+	—
H. paraaphrophilus	—	+	—	+	—
H. ducreyi	+	—	—	—	—

Abbreviations: X = hematin; V = nicotinamide adenine dinucleotide; var = variable.

Bordetella pertussis

Bordetella pertussis is a coccobacillus with Gram stain morphology similar to that of *Haemophilus.* The organisms are strict aerobes and nonmotile. Infection of the human tracheobronchial epithelium produces pertussis (whooping cough), a prolonged disease marked by paroxysmal coughing.

Morphology and Structure

small piliated Gram-negative coccobacilli

Bordetella pertussis is a tiny (0.5–1.0 μm), Gram-negative coccobacillus with highly regular staining characteristics. The cell wall has the structure typical of Gram-negative bacteria. Fresh isolates have capsules and pili, but neither have been extensively characterized.

Growth

Bordet–Gengou medium

Bordetella pertussis is a slow-growing organism that requires specialized conditions for growth. Primary media require the addition of fresh blood, albumin, charcoal, starch, or ion exchange resins to an enriched base medium. A widely used medium continues to be Bordet–Gengou agar containing fresh blood in a complex agar base. The function of the additives is not for nutrition but for adsorption of substances toxic to *B. pertussis* that are normally found in culture media. The organism is also very susceptible to environmental changes and survives only briefly outside the human respiratory tract. Isolation requires direct plating onto a specially prepared medium. Aerobic incubation for 3–7 days is required for initial growth, which appears as tiny, glistening, compact colonies with the appearance of bisected pearls or drops of mercury. On media containing blood, a narrow zone of hemolysis is present around the colony. Growth may also be obtained in a suitable enriched broth. Several surface antigens have been identified that tend to change on subculture, a feature of importance in vaccine production, but of unknown significance in disease.

small "drops of mercury" colonies

Toxins

Endotoxin and cell-bound exotoxin

In addition to cell wall endotoxin, *B. pertussis* produces at least one toxin with the biologic characteristics of an exotoxin. However, this protein toxin is closely bound to the organisms and is released only when the cells are disrupted. Experimentally it produces edema and local necrosis with accumulation of lymphocytes and macrophages. Intratracheal administration of this toxin to animals produces lesions histologically similar to those seen in whooping cough. Cultures of *B. pertussis* have also been shown to heighten the sensitivity of animals to histamine and to stimulate marked lymphocytosis. Recently, Bordetella adenylate cyclase production has been shown to depress phagocytic function.

Pathogenesis

Tropism for bronchial epithelium

Immobilization and destruction of ciliated epithelial cells

Bordetella pertussis is a strict pathogen of humans. It has not been isolated from animals or as a member of the normal flora of healthy persons. When introduced into the respiratory tract, the organism has a remarkable tropism for ciliated bronchial epithelium. The bacteria first attach to and immobilize the cilia. This action begins a sequence in which the ciliated epithelial cells are progressively destroyed and extruded from the epithelial border (Figure 17.3). The nonciliated cells are not involved and maintain the integrity of the epithelial lining. All of these events occur without tissue invasion by *B.*

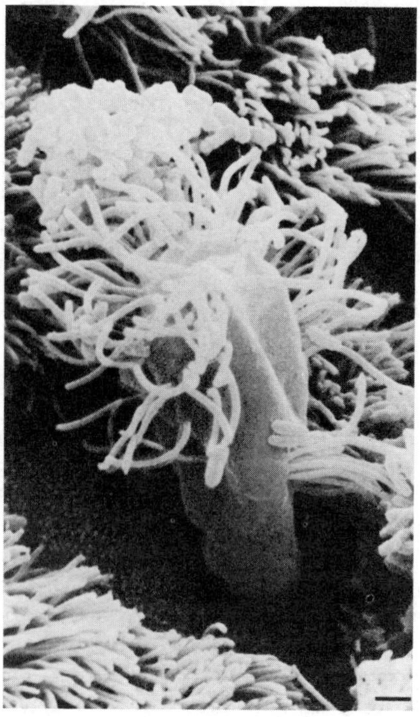

17.3 A tracheal organ culture 72 hr after infection with *B. pertussis.* The organisms have attached to the cilia of some cells and killed them. These balloonlike cells with attached bacteria are extruded from the epithelium. Note the background of uninfected ciliated cells and denuded epithelium where nonciliated cells remain. (*Reproduced with permission from Muse, K.E., Collier, A.M., and Baseman, J.B. 1977. J. Infect. Dis. 136:768–777, Figure 3, copyright 1977 by University of Chicago, publisher.*)

organisms noninvasive

pertussis, although considerable local inflammation and exudate are produced in the bronchi. The initial attachment to the cilia is probably related to the organism's pili, whereas the highly localized destruction is caused by toxin.

Immunity

Although antibodies are produced during the course of pertussis and by immunization, their role in immunity is not well understood. Naturally acquired immunity is not lifelong, although second attacks, when recognized, tend to be mild. The high susceptibility of newborns and infants before immunization may reflect a low level of antibody in adults and thus lack of passive transfer to the infant at birth.

Epidemiology

high infectivity

atypical or subclinical disease in adults

Pertussis is spread by airborne droplet nuclei to those in close contact with a patient in the early stages of illness. It is highly infectious. Secondary spread in families is common; it is not always recognized, however, because of the mildness of symptoms in immunized patients. Such cases, particularly in adults, may serve as a significant reservoir of the organism. Outbreaks in highly susceptible populations such as hospitalized newborns have been traced to hospital employees with pertussis symptoms resembling those of the common cold.

Effectiveness of immunization

The incidence of pertussis has been decreasing since the introduction of immunization in the 1940s. Sporadic epidemics occur, and there is no strong seasonal pattern to the disease. Rates of pertussis have increased when immunization rates have decreased, because of concern of vaccine potency and side effects. Mortality has dropped in accordance with the decreased incidence of disease, but remains highest in infants. Over 70% of fatal cases are in children under 1 year of age, whereas less then 5% are in children over 5 years of age.

Clinical Manifestations

After an incubation period of 7–10 days, pertussis follows a prolonged course consisting of three overlapping stages: 1) catarrhal; 2) paroxysmal coughing; and 3) convalescent.

Catarrhal phase, highly communicable

In the catarrhal stage, the primary feature is a profuse and mucoid rhinorrhea that persists for 1–2 weeks. Nonspecific findings such as malaise, fever, sneezing, and anorexia may also be present. The disease is most communicable at this stage, as large numbers of organisms are present in the nasopharynx and the mucoid secretions.

Paroxysmal phase

inspiratory whoop

high lymphocytosis

The appearance of a persistent cough marks the transition from the catarrhal to the paroxysmal coughing stage. At this time, episodes of paroxysmal coughing occur up to 50 times a day for 2–4 weeks. The characteristic inspiratory whoop follows a series of coughs as air is rapidly drawn through the narrowed glottis. Vomiting frequently follows the whoop. The combination of mucoid secretions, whooping cough, and vomiting causes the child to be miserable, exhausted, and barely able to breathe. Fever is not present unless a complication such as bacterial superinfection or atelectasis develops. Marked leukocytosis, primarily a result of increased levels of circulating lymphocytes, reaches its peak in the paroxysmal stage. Absolute lymphocyte counts of $40{,}000/mm^3$ are typical, and much higher counts have been recorded.

Convalescent phase

During the convalescent stage, which lasts 3–4 weeks, the frequency and severity of paroxysmal coughing episodes gradually diminish. Other features of the disease gradually fade as well.

Partially immune persons and infants under 6 months of age may not show all the typical features of pertussis. Some evolution through the three stages is usually seen, but paroxysmal coughing and lymphocytosis may be absent.

Pulmonary complications

The most common complications of pertussis involve the lung. Pneumonia, usually caused by a superinfecting organism such as *Streptococcus pneumoniae,* is the most serious complication and accounts for the majority of deaths caused by pertussis. Pneumonia typically appears at the height of the paroxysmal coughing stage and, in addition to the usual signs and symptoms, is associated with disappearance of the paroxysms. Atelectasis is also common but may be recognized only by radiologic examination. Other complications, including convulsions, hemorrhage, and hernias, are related to the pressure effects of the paroxysmal coughing and the anoxia produced by inadequate ventilation and apneic spells. Nutritional disturbances and dehydration may also be a problem over the prolonged course of the illness.

Diagnosis

Nasopharyngeal swab

organisms often not present by paroxysmal phase

A clinical diagnosis of pertussis is confirmed by isolation of *B. pertussis* from a nasopharyngeal swab. The organism is not found at distant sites, and bacteremia does not occur. Specimens collected early in the course of disease (during the catarrhal or early paroxysmal stage) provide the greatest chance of successful isolation. Unfortunately, the diagnosis is frequently not considered until paroxysmal coughing has been present for some time, and the number of organisms has decreased significantly. The nasopharyngeal swab is best collected by the pernasal route and plated directly onto either Bordet–Gengou or a special charcoal agar medium. Low concentrations of a penicillin or cephalosporin are usually added to these plates to inhibit members of the normal flora and to allow *B. pertussis* to grow. Characteristic colonies appear after 3–5 days of incubation and the organisms are identified serologically, because *B. pertussis* shows few specific metabolic activities.

Direct immunofluorescence

A direct immunofluorescent technique has been successfully applied to nasopharyngeal smears for rapid diagnosis of pertussis. Smears are stable on transport to the laboratory, whereas the organisms themselves may not survive without special precautions. Positive smears should always be confirmed by culture, if possible.

Treatment

no specific therapy by paroxysmal phase

erythromycin treatment in catarrhal phase

Once the paroxysmal coughing stage has been reached, the treatment of pertussis is primarily supportive. By this stage the bronchial epithelium has already been damaged, and antimicrobial therapy will not reverse it. Antimicrobial therapy is useful at earlier stages and for limiting spread to other susceptible individuals. Some antimicrobics, including penicillin, tetracycline, erythromycin, and chloramphenicol are active in vitro against *B. pertussis.* Of these, erythromycin is preferred because of its clinical effectiveness and relative lack of toxicity. Penicillins, including ampicillin, have not been effective in clearing the organisms from the respiratory tract.

Prevention

Inactivated bacillary vaccine

DPT

Effectiveness and side effects of vaccine

Active immunization is the primary method of preventing pertussis. Vaccines are produced from inactivated whole cell suspensions or from partially purified preparations derived from whole cells. In the United States, the vaccine is combined with diphtheria and tetanus toxoids to produce a triple vaccine, DPT. Three doses given at monthly intervals are begun as early in life as possible (6 weeks) because of the high susceptibility and mortality in infants. Booster doses later in childhood are recommended. Recent immunization reduces the attack rate upon exposure and the severity of disease upon infection. Side effects and vaccine-related complications have been a problem with some pertussis vaccine preparations. Local inflammation and febrile reactions have been common, and occasionally convulsions and brain damage have occurred. Efforts to increase effectiveness and reduce complication rates are continuing with newer vaccine preparations.

Gardnerella (Haemophilus) vaginalis

Small, Gram-variable rods

previously classified with *Haemophilus* and *Corynebacterium*

Gardnerella vaginalis is a small, Gram-variable coccobacillus. Under most conditions, cells are Gram negative and of a size and shape similar to those of *Haemophilus* species. They also have a tendency to arrange in end-to-end or side-by-side pairs, as do corynebacteria, and may show metachromatic granules. Growth is poor on the usual diagnostic media, but small colonies will usually appear on chocolate agar after 24–48 hr. *Gardnerella vaginalis* is facultatively anaerobic, catalase negative, and oxidase negative; it does not possess spores, flagella, or capsules. This species is a taxonomic refugee; it has been classified in various genera, including *Haemophilus* and *Corynebacterium,* only to be removed when more detailed study indicated it was not related to other members of the group. Its current name, *Gardnerella vaginalis,* places it as the sole member of its genus, indicating a lack of relatedness to other genera.

association with "nonspecific vaginitis"

Gardnerella vaginalis has long been associated with nonspecific vaginitis, a syndrome defined by an abnormal vaginal discharge, which occurs in the absence of known genital pathogens (*Neisseria gonorrhoeae* and *Chlamydia* etiologic role uncertain

Clue cells

trachomatis) (Chapter 64). Despite the presence of *G. vaginalis* in many of these cases, its primary role in vaginitis remains to be demonstrated. The organism may be cultured from vaginal discharge if chocolate agar is used, and some selective media have been developed. Vaginal epithelial cells studded with tiny coccobacilli (clue cells) have been observed microscopically; these clue cells are associated with the presence of *G. vaginalis.*

Additional Reading and References

Fothergill, L.D., and Wright, J. 1933. Influenzal meningitis: The relation of age incidence to the bactericidal power of blood against the causal organism. *J. Immunol.* 24:273–284. A classic study, the first to advance the currently accepted concepts of humoral immunity in *Haemophilus influenzae* disease.

Muse, K.E., Collier, A.M., and Baseman, J.B. 1977. Scanning electron microscopic study of hamster tracheal organ cultures infected with *Bordetella pertussis. J. Infect. Dis.* 136:768–777. The unique tropism of *Bordetella pertussis* for ciliated cells and the subsequent destruction of those cells are shown experimentally and visually.

Smith, D.H., Peter, G., Ingram, D.L., Harding, A.L., and Anderson, P. 1973. Responses of children immunized with the capsular polysaccharide of *Haemophilus influenzae* type b. *Pediatrics* 52:637–644. The current dilemma of application of a polyribitol phosphate capsular polysaccharide vaccine is illustrated; that is, many of those who need protection most do not respond.

Ward, J.I., Fraser, D.W., Baraff, L.J., and Plikaytis, B.D. 1979. *Haemophilus influenzae* meningitis: A national study of secondary spread in household contacts. *N. Engl. J. Med.* 301:122–126. This study changed our thinking about the epidemiology of *Haemophilus influenzae* type b infections by elucidating the extent to which they are contagious.

Lawrence Corey

Mycoplasma and *Ureaplasma*

18

Mycoplasma and *Ureaplasma* (formerly called *T-strain Mycoplasma*) are the smallest free-living microorganisms. They comprise the two genera of the family Mycoplasmataceae, members of which resemble other bacteria except in their lack of a cell wall. Species are ubiquitous in nature, and some are pathogens of animals, plants, and humans. DNA base ratio studies indicate that most species are unrelated and have different origins. Numerous *Mycoplasma* species that are associated with humans have been identified (Table 18.1), but only three of these species have been associated with disease. *Mycoplasma pneumoniae* is a lower respiratory tract pathogen. *Mycoplasma hominis* and *Ureaplasma urealyticum* may be involved in genitourinary tract infections.

absence of cell walls

These organisms have diameters of about 0.2–0.3 μm, but they are highly plastic and pleomorphic and may appear as coccoid bodies, filaments, and large multinucleoid forms. They have no cell wall, but are bounded by a single triple-layered membrane (Figure 18.1) that, unlike those of other bacteria, contains sterols. The sterols are not synthesized by the organism, but are acquired as essential components from the media or tissues in which it is growing. *Mycoplasma* stain poorly or not at all with the usual bacterial stains. Because of their lack of cell walls, they are completely insensitive to the penicillins and cephalosporins. Their genome consists of double-stranded DNA with a molecular weight of about 5×10^8 that replicates like that of other bacteria. *Mycoplasma pneumoniae* is an aerobe, but most other species are facultatively anaerobic. All grow slowly in enriched liquid culture media and on special *Mycoplasma* agar to produce minute colonies only after several days of incubation (Plate R). The center of the colony grows into the agar to give an inverted "fried egg" appearance. Growth in culture is inhibited by specific antisera directed at the particular species.

slow growth in specialized artificial media

inhibition of growth by antisera

Differential features

The cell membrane of *M. pneumoniae* has neuraminic acid attachment sites for host cell receptors. The neuraminic acid causes added red blood cells to adhere to colonies on solid media (hemadsorption). Different metabolic properties are characteristic of the various species of *Mycoplasma* and *Ureaplasma* and allow easy differentiation between those of importance in human medicine. The species that infect the respiratory and genital tracts will be considered separately because of their different epidemiologic characteristics.

Table 18.1 Some Mycoplasma and Ureaplasma Species of Humans

Organism	Site	Prevalence	Disease
M. salivarium	Periodontal sulci	Very common	None
M. orale	Upper respiratory tract	Very common	None
M. pneumoniae	Upper and lower respiratory tract	Common	Primary atypical pneumonia
M. fermentans	Genitourinary tract	Rare	None
M. hominis	Genitourinary tract	Common	Postpartum fever; pelvic inflammatory disease
U. urealyticum	Genitourinary tract	Very common	Nongonococcal urethritis
M. genitalium	Genitourinary tract	Undetermined	Unknown

Mycoplasma pneumoniae

Disease Syndromes

Types of infections

Allergic reactions

Mycoplasma pneumoniae is an important respiratory tract pathogen of humans. Several syndromes have been associated with the infection, including pharyngitis, tracheobronchitis, inflammation of the tympanic membrane presenting as bullous myringitis, and pneumonitis. Occasionally, infection caused by *M. pneumoniae* is associated with arthritis, meningoencephalitis, hemolytic anemia, and rash. Allergic reactions (Stevens–Johnson syndrome and erythema multiforme) may develop.

Primary atypical or walking pneumonia

insidious onset

frequent lobar distribution

In most populations, *M. pneumoniae* accounts for approximately 20% of all cases of pneumonia. Classically, it causes a disease less severe than common bacterial pneumonia that has been described as *primary atypical pneumonia* or *walking pneumonia*. Most cases do not require hospitalization. The disease is of insidious onset, with fever, headache, and malaise for 2–4 days before the onset of respiratory symptoms. Pulmonary symptoms generally comprise a nonproductive cough. X-rays reveal a segmental lobar pneumonia, usually in the lower lobes, although multiple lobes are sometimes involved. Small pleural effusions are seen in 25% of cases. Any expectorated

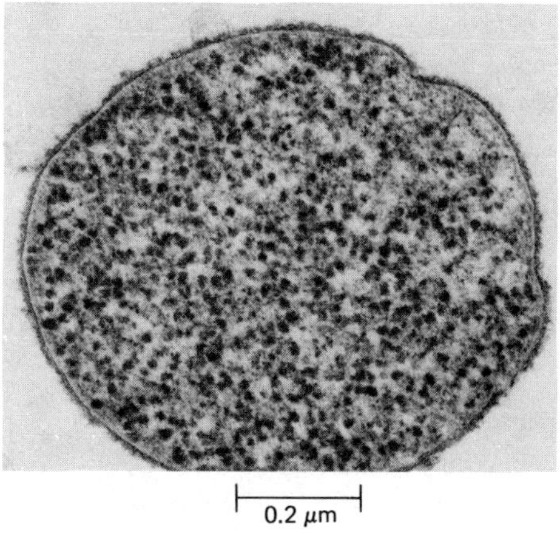

18.1 Electron micrograph of *Mycoplasma*. Note cytoplasmic membrane ribosomes and surface amorphous material with absence of cell wall. (*Kindly provided by Dr. E.S. Boatman.*)

sputum is mucoid, and Gram staining of sputum usually shows some polymorphonuclear cells but a paucity of bacteria, because *M. pneumoniae* are not detectable by this stain.

tracheobronchitis and pharyngitis

A milder tracheobronchitis with fever, cough, headache, and malaise is the most common syndrome associated with acute *M. pneumoniae* infection, although there is usually X-ray evidence of pulmonary involvement. Pharyngitis with fever and sore throat may also occur. The clinical signs and symptoms of *M. pneumoniae* pharyngitis are indistinguishable from those caused by viruses such as Epstein–Barr virus and by the Group A streptococcus.

Bullous myringitis and otitis media

Acute hemorrhagic bullous myringitis is an uncommon but well-described syndrome associated with infection caused by *M. pneumoniae.* Nonpurulent otitis media or myringitis occurs concomitantly in approximately 15% of patients with *M. pneumoniae* pneumonitis. The presence of nonpurulent otitis media and lower respiratory illness in a teenager suggests *M. pneumoniae* infection.

Infection and Pathogenesis

low infecting dose

Infection with *M. pneumoniae* is acquired by droplet spread. In experimental challenge, the human infectious ID_{50} (the dose of organisms required to cause infection in 50% of volunteers) is only one colony-forming unit when inhaled in an aerosol and about 100 colony-forming units by intranasal inoculation.

effect on respiratory epithelium and other pathological manifestations

Initially, the organism attaches to surface protein receptors of the respiratory epithelium. It interferes with ciliary action and leads to desquamation of the involved mucosa and a subsequent inflammatory reaction and exudate. The inflammatory response is at first most pronounced in the bronchial and peribronchial tissue, although the alveoli may also be involved. Lymphocytes, plasma cells, and macrophages then infiltrate and thicken the walls of the alveoli and bronchioles.

prolonged shedding of organisms

Organisms are shed in upper respiratory secretions for 2–8 days before the onset of symptoms, and shedding continues for as long as 14 weeks after infection.

Immune Responses

Both local and systemic specific immune responses occur. Local immunoglobulin A(IgA) antibody is produced, but disappears 2–4 weeks after the onset of the infection. Complement fixing serum antibody titers reach a peak 2–4 weeks after infection and gradually disappear over 6–12 months. Nonspecific immune responses to the glycolypids of the outer membrane of the organism may develop. The most common of these responses involves the production of *cold hemagglutinins*, which are IgM antibodies that react with the I antigen of human red blood cells and cause agglutination at temperatures of 0–4°C. They are seen in about two-thirds of symptomatic patients infected with *M. pneumoniae.* Antibodies to the glycolipids of the outer membrane of the organism, which occasionally result in false-positive reagin tests for syphilis, may include antibody that reacts with a nonhemolytic streptococcus (*Streptococcus MG*).

Complement fixing antibody titers

Cold hemagglutinins

immunity incomplete and reinfection common

Immunity is not complete, and reinfection with *M. pneumoniae* is common. Clinical disease appears to be more severe in older than in younger children, which has led to the suggestion that many of the clinical manifestations of disease are the result of cellular immune responses rather than response to invasion by the organism.

Epidemiology

worldwide endemic infection with intermittent epidemics

most common age incidence 5–15 years

manifestations in family outbreaks

Endemic infections with *M. pneumoniae* occur throughout the year and are worldwide, but they are especially prominent in temperate climates. Epidemics at 4- to 6-year intervals have been noted in both civilian and military populations. The most common age for symptomatic *M. pneumoniae* infection is between 5 and 15 years, and the disease accounts for more than one-third of all cases of pneumonia in teenagers. Infections in children less than 6 months old are uncommon. The disease often appears as a sporadic, endemic illness in families or closed communities because of its relatively long incubation period (2–15 days) and because prolonged shedding in nasal secretions may cause infections to be spread over time. Attack rates in susceptible individuals within families approach 60%. Asymptomatic infections occur, but most studies have suggested that more than two-thirds of infected cases develop some evidence of respiratory tract illness.

Laboratory Diagnosis

diagnosis usually serologic because of slow growth

significance of single high titers

Clinical diagnosis of *M. pneumoniae* infection may be difficult because of the overlap of manifestations with those of other bacterial and viral infections. Direct staining of clinical material is not useful. The organism can be isolated from throat swabs or sputum of infected patients on special enriched culture media; however, because of its relatively slow growth, more than 1 week of incubation is generally required. Thus, serologic tests rather than cultures are usually used for specific diagnosis. A fourfold rise in serum complement fixing antibody during the disease indicates active *M. pneumoniae* infection. A single high titer, such as greater than 1:128, indicates recent or concurrent infection, because complement fixing antibody is of short duration. With the relatively long incubation period and insidious onset of the disease, many patients will have high antibody titers at the time of presentation to the physician.

significance of cold agglutinin titers

In many clinical situations, the demonstration of nonspecific anti-I antibody can be helpful, because more than two-thirds of patients with symptomatic lower respiratory *M. pneumoniae* infection develop high titers of cold hemagglutinins. It must be remembered that cold agglutinins are nonspecific and have been observed in adenovirus infections, infectious mononucleosis, and some other illnesses. The cold agglutinin test is simple, however, and can be performed rapidly in any clinical laboratory or even at the bedside.

Infection by Genitourinary Tract *Ureaplasmas* and *Mycoplasmas*

Ureaplasma urealyticum

urease production

The genus *Ureaplasma* contains a single species, *U. urealyticum*, of which some 14 serotypes have been described. *Ureaplasma* is distinguished from all other members of the order Mycoplasmatales by its production of urease. On special *Ureaplasma* agar media, colonies are small and circular and grow downward into the agar. In liquid media containing urea and phenol red, growth of *Ureaplasma* results in production of ammonia from the urea, with a resultant increase of pH and a change of color in the indicator.

venereal spread

Epidemiology. The main reservoir of human strains of *U. urealyticum* is the genital tract of sexually active men and women; it is rarely found before puberty. Colonization, which probably results primarily from sexual contact, occurs in more than 80% of individuals who have had three or more sexual partners.

association with nongonococcal urethritis

Clinical outline of disease. Because of the high colonization rate, it was difficult to associate specific illness with *Ureaplasma*. However, recent studies suggest that approximately one-half of cases of nongonococcal, nonchlamydial urethritis in men may be caused by *U. urealyticum*. In women, it is less certain that *Ureaplasma* infection causes disease, although chorioamnionitis and postpartum fever have been associated with it.

responsiveness to tetracycline and spectinomycin

Diagnosis and treatment. In the appropriate clinical situation, men with nongonococcal urethritis should be treated on the assumption that *Ureaplasma* infection may be involved. Tetracycline is the treatment of choice because it is also active against chlamydiae. Recently, tetracycline-resistant strains of *Ureaplasma* have been reported that have been associated with recurrences of nongonococcal urethritis in men. In such cases, spectinomycin treatment is also effective.

Mycoplasma hominis

arginine utilization

association with postpartum fever and pelvic inflammatory disease

susceptibility to tetracycline

Mycoplasma hominis is another inhabitant of the genitourinary tract. Although some strains grow on ordinary blood agar as nonhemolytic pinpoint colonies, the organism is best detected on *Mycoplasma* agar, on which it grows rapidly. *Mycoplasma hominis* and *Ureaplasma* can be differentiated by demonstrating arginine utilization by the former and urease activity by the latter. At least seven antigenic variants of *M. hominis* have been described. To date, the major clinical condition associated with *M. hominis* infection is postabortal or postpartum fever. *Mycoplasma hominis* is isolated from the blood of about 10% of women with this condition, and *U. urealyticum* from another 10%. The diseases appears to be self-limiting, although antibiotic therapy may decrease the duration of fever and hospitalization. Recently, serologic studies and animal experiments have indicated that pelvic inflammatory disease syndromes in women may be associated with *M. hominis* infection of the Fallopian tubes. The organism is sensitive to tetracycline, which is the antibiotic of choice. In contrast to *U. urealyticum* and *M. pneumoniae, M. hominis* is resistant to erythromycin.

Additional Reading and References

Clyde, W.A., Jr. 1979. *Mycoplasma pneumoniae* infections of man. In *The Mycoplasmas,* Vol. II. Tully, J.G., and Whitcomb, R.F., Eds. New York: Academic Press, pp. 275–306.

Foy, H.M. 1982. Mycoplasma pneumonia. In *Bacterial Infections of Humans. Epidemiology and Control.* Evans, A.S., and Feldman, H.A., Eds. New York: Plenum, pp. 345–366.

Shepard, M.C., and Masover, G.K. 1979. Special features of ureaplasmas. In *The Mycoplasmas,* Vol. I. Barile, M.F., and Razin, S., Eds. New York: Academic Press, pp. 451–494.

Taylor-Robinson, D., and McCormack, W.M. 1979. Mycoplasmas in human genitourinary tract infections. In *The Mycoplasmas,* Vol. II. Tully, J.G., and Whitcomb, R.F., Eds. New York: Academic Press, pp. 307–366. This and the preceding contributions provide excellent, up-to-date, in-depth reviews of the topics discussed in the present chapter.

Kenneth J. Ryan

Legionella

19

The widely publicized outbreak of pneumonia among attendees of the 1976 American Legion convention in Philadelphia led to the isolation of a new infectious agent, *Legionella pneumophila*. The event was unique in medical history; for months the American public had entertained theories of its cause that ranged from sabotage to viroids, only to find that a previously undescribed Gram-negative rod was responsible. It was an outstanding example of the benefits of pursuing sound epidemiologic evidence until it is explained by equally sound microbiologic findings. We now know the disease has occurred for many years: specific antibodies and organisms have been detected in material preserved from the 1940s, and a mysterious outbreak in 1965 has been solved retrospectively. The primary reasons the organism escaped detection for so long are that it stains poorly or not at all with common methods and will not grow on the usual bacteriologic media.

Morphology

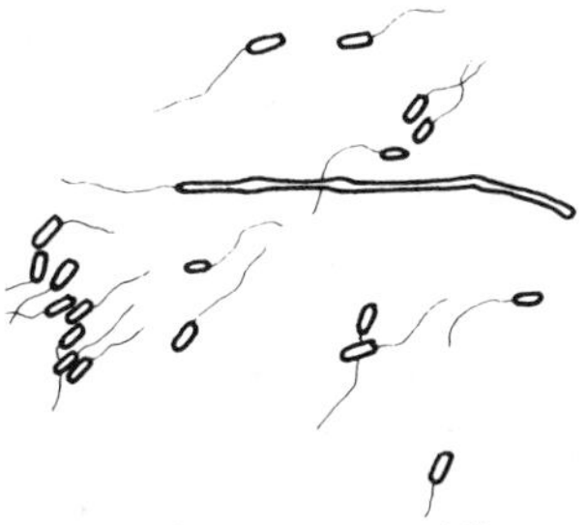
Legionella pneumophila

Staining characteristics

Legionella pneumophila is a thin, pleomorphic, Gram-negative rod 0.5–0.7 μm in width and 2–20 μm or more in length. Elongated, filamentous forms are common. In clinical specimens, the organism stains poorly or not at all by Gram stain or the usual histologic stains; it can be demonstrated, however, by certain silver impregnation methods (Dieterle stain) and by some simple stains that omit decolorization steps. An example of the latter is the *half-Gram*, in which only the first two steps of the standard Gram stain are carried out. It should be emphasized that these staining methods are nonspecific, but suggest *Legionella* when the organism is clearly demonstrable only by such manipulations. Ultrastructurally, *L. pneumophila* has features similar to those of Gram-negative bacteria. Double envelopes are seen, each with a triple-layered unit membrane. Polar, subpolar, and lateral flagella may be present. Lipid-containing inclusion granules are present. Spores are not found.

Growth

Cultural characteristics

Legionella pneumophila grows only on media supplemented by L-cysteine and a source of ferric ions. The latter may be provided by hemoglobin or soluble ferric pyrophosphate. The organism grows optimally at a pH of 6.9, and it is sensitive to major variations from this value. Optimal growth occurs on properly supplemented agar plates under aerobic conditions at 35°C. Colonies, which develop in 3–5 days, have a surface resembling ground glass. Fluid media that permit good growth of *Legionella* are not yet in use. It is interesting to note that good growth has been obtained in broth containing alveolar macrophages and in water containing photosynthetic bacteria, algae, and amoebae.

Classification

Antigenic structure and gas chromatographic patterns

Legionella species are not closely related to any known bacteria. They have been shown to possess catalase, oxidase (weak), gelatinase, and β-lactamase activity, but do not grow or react positively in other taxonomic tests usually used to classify bacteria. Their identification and classification depends largely on antigenic features and chromatographic analysis of cellular fatty acid content. Antisera have been prepared that react specifically with *Legionella*, and the chromatographic profile of cellular branched and unbranched fatty acids is unique. Six serotypes have been defined by immunofluorescent procedures with whole organisms, but the nature of the responsible antigens has not been defined. In addition to *L. pneumophila* types 1–6, a number of similar organisms, originally called *Legionella*-like organisms (LLO), have now been assigned species names within the *Legionella* genus (*L. bozemanii, L. dumoffii, L. micdadei*). These organisms share the poor staining characteristics and growth requirements for primary isolation of *L. pneumophila*, but differ in some cultural and other features. For instance, colonies of the three newly designated species show bright fluorescence under 3.6 Å ultraviolet light. It is likely that more serotypes of *L. pneumophila* and of other species will be discovered as isolation techniques are improved. In the interim, the situation can be confusing because suspected new types or species are given names or alphabetic labels that are later changed or included with another species. A summary of names and disease syndromes is provided in Table 19.1.

Serotypes

Other *Legionella* species

Epidemiology

Pneumonic and nonpneumonic diseases

Two clinically and epidemiologically distinct syndromes are associated with *L. pneumophila*. The first, a severe pneumonia with an incubation period of 2–10 days, is called *Legionnaires' disease* and has mortality as high as 60%. The other, *Pontiac fever* (named for a 1968 Michigan outbreak), is a nonpneumonic febrile illness with an incubation period of 20–48 hr. Pontiac fever is a self-limiting illness that is not life threatening. The attack rate for Legionnaires' disease has been estimated at less than 1% of those exposed, whereas over 90% have had clinical illness in outbreaks of Pontiac fever.

Both syndromes can appear in sporadic or epidemic form. Most outbreaks have occurred in or around large buildings such as hotels, factories, and

Table 19.1 Features of *Legionella* Species

Species	Common Term	Disease Syndrome
L. pneumophila	Legionnaire's agent	Legionnaires' disease Pontiac fever
L. bozemanii	WIGA, Mi-15	Pneumonia[a]
L. dumoffii	NY-23, Tex-KL	Pneumonia[a]
L. micdadei	TATLOCK, HEBA, Pittsburgh pneumonia agent	Pneumonia

[a] Too few cases have been reported to ascertain the clinical spectrum.

Association with humidifying and cooling systems

hospitals. Those outbreaks traced to a source have involved a cooling tower, evaporative condenser, or some other part of the building's air-conditioning system. Organisms contaminating the water are aerosolized and spread either directly or through the air ducts of the system. This method of spread is consistent with the epidemiologic features of all proved outbreaks, although a few have been associated with soil disruption caused by large excavation projects. Person-to-person transmission has not been documented. It is difficult to ascertain the overall incidence of *Legionella* infections, as most information has been from outbreaks. Serologic surveys indicate that outbreaks constitute only a small part of the total cases, many of which currently go undetected. Estimates based on seroconversions suggest approximately 25,000 cases in the United States each year, and that the frequency of pneumonic disease is probably less than that of Pontiac fever. Both serologic and environmental studies indicate that *Legionella* has low virulence for humans.

no person-to-person transmission

most infections subclinical

Water habitats

possible associations with other organisms

Legionella pneumophila has been isolated not only from air-conditioning systems but from freshwater sites such as lakes and ponds, and the organism is known to survive as long as a year in unchlorinated tap water. A potentially important association has recently been discovered between growth of *Legionella* and the presence of prokaryotic blue-green algae or free-living amebas. Given the proper temperature and other conditions, *L. pneumophila* may multiply rapidly in the presence of or even within these free-living forms. This possibility could explain the ready survival in the environment of an organism that is difficult to grow in the laboratory.

Pathogenesis and Pathology

Pulmonary lesions in Legionnaires' disease

association with macrophages

In Legionnaires' disease pathologic changes are limited to the lung and associated structures such as the pleura. The cellular exudate is acute; polymorphonuclear leukocytes and macrophages predominate. Areas of focal necrosis and *Legionella* are generally seen in the alveoli and alveolar septa, but not the bronchi. The organisms are usually found within macrophages, which may explain the good growth observed in vitro in macrophage-containing cultures. The relationship between the possibility of growth in an ameba (for example, living in a humidifier) and multiplication within the alveolar macrophage is intriguing, but has not yet been proved as the link between the environmental reservoir and human pathogenesis. Survival in macrophages is probably enhanced by a toxin, which inhibits the oxidative response during phagocytosis. The sites of multiplication and pathogenic mechanisms involved in the Pontiac fever syndromes are not known; furthermore, there is no evidence to explain the factors determining which illness results from *L. pneumophila* infection, although it has been postulated that inhalation of large numbers of dead organisms may contribute to the disease. Documented infections with the LLO group are still too few to generalize about their pathogenesis.

Other *Legionella* infections

Clinical Features

Legionnaires' disease

Legionnaires' disease is a severe toxic pneumonia that begins with myalgia and headache, followed by a rapidly rising fever. A dry cough may develop and later become productive, but sputum production is not a prominent feature. Chills, pleuritic chest pain, vomiting, diarrhea, confusion, and delirium may all be seen. Radiologically, patchy or interstitial infiltrates with a tendency to progress toward a nodular consolidation are present unilaterally or bilaterally. Liver function tests often indicate some hepatic dysfunction. In the more serious cases the patient becomes progressively ill and toxic over the first 3–6 days, and the disease terminates in shock and/or respiratory failure. The overall mortality is about 15%, but is particularly high in patients with serious underlying disease or immunosuppression. Mortality has been over 50% in some hospital outbreaks.

Mortality

Pontiac fever

Pontiac fever begins similarly with fever and myalgia, and one-half of all patients have a dry cough. The disease does not progress, however, and recovery usually begins after 2–5 days. It would be considered a mild form of Legionnaires' disease were it not for the rather uniform clinical and epidemiologic features in documented outbreaks. In the Pontiac outbreak there were 144 cases with no deaths.

Diagnosis

Specimens

The possibility of Legionnaires' disease should be considered in any patient with severe progressive pneumonia not shown to be caused by another organism. The best means of diagnosis for clinical purposes is direct microscopic examination and culture of infected tissues. For this purpose, a high-quality specimen such as that from a transtracheal aspirate, lung aspirate, or lung biopsy is usually necessary, because the organism is rarely found in sputum. Typically the Gram smear shows no bacteria; the organisms are demonstrated by direct immunofluorescent examination of the same material using *Legionella*-specific conjugates. This method is the most rapid means of diagnosis, but it is positive in only 50% of culture-proved cases.

Direct examination by fluorescence microscopy

Cultures on special media

Cultures should be made on routine media as well as on special agar media that meet the growth requirements of *Legionella*. Currently, the best medium contains charcoal, yeast extract, L-cysteine, ferric pyrophosphate, and a pH buffer. The isolation of morphologically characteristic Gram-negative rods on this medium after 2–5 days, but not on routine culture plates (blood agar, chocolate agar), is presumptive evidence of *Legionella*. These findings are confirmed by direct immunofluorescent staining of smears prepared from the colonies. The medium also allows isolation of most of the LLO group. Occasional cases with positive direct immunofluorescent smears but negative cultures are still seen. These results are probably caused by strains for which cultural conditions for growth remain unmet.

Serodiagnosis

The diagnosis can also be established by demonstrating a significant rise in specific serum antibody titer with an indirect immunofluorescent technique. As with most other serodiagnostic tests, this method requires paired (acute and convalescent) sera to demonstrate a rising titer; it is used primarily for retrospective diagnosis and in epidemiologic studies. In some communities elevated titers in single serum samples have been detected in as much as 25% of the population.

Diagnostic procedures for legionellosis should not be considered routine at present and may not be available in many hospital laboratories. The clinician should always advise the laboratory of the suspicion of Legionnaires' disease before submitting material. Specimens and smears can then, if necessary, be sent to a reference laboratory for processing.

Treatment and Prevention

Erythromycin treatment

The best information on antimicrobial therapy is still provided by the original Philadelphia outbreak. Because the etiology was completely obscure at the time, the cases were treated with many different regimens. Patients treated with erythromycin clearly did better than those given the penicillins, cephalosporins, or aminoglycosides; the poor results with the β-lactam antibiotics may have been caused by the β-lactamase production of *Legionella*. Once the organism was isolated, in vitro susceptibility tests and animal studies confirmed the activity of erythromycin and resistance to most other antibiotics. Tetracycline is also active, but less so than erythromycin. Rifampin has been active in experimental systems, but there is less clinical experience to support its use, and its potential for development of resistance is greater.

Preventive measures

The prevention of legionellosis must involve preventing or minimizing contamination of aerosol sources in cooling towers and in building water supplies. Methods to accomplish these purposes are still under evaluation, although some outbreaks appear to have been aborted by routine cleaning and disinfection or by correcting of malfunctions in air-conditioning systems.

Additional Reading and References

Blackmon, J.A., Chandler, F.W., Cherry, W.B., England, A.C., Feeley, J.C., Hicklin, M.D., McKinney, R.M., and Wilkinson, H.W. 1981. Legionellosis. *Am. J. Pathol.* 103:429–465. A comprehensive review is provided of all aspects of legionellosis, including microbiology, pathology, epidemiology, and clinical features.

Fraser, D.W., Tsai, T.R., Orenstein, W., Parkin, W.E., Beecham, H.J. Sharrar, R.G., Harris, J., Mallison, G.F., Martin, S.M., McDade, J.E., Shepard, C.C., Brachman, P.S., and the Field Investigation Team. 1977. Legionnaires' disease: Descriptions of an epidemic of pneumonia. *N. Engl. J. Med.* 297:1189–1197.

McDade, J.E., Shepard, C.C., Fraser, D.W., Tsai, T.R., Redus, M.A., Dowdle, W.R., and the Laboratory Investigation Team. 1977. Legionnaires' disease: Isolation of a bacterium and demonstration of its role in other respiratory disease. *N. Engl. J. Med.* 297:1197–1203. This study and the report by Fraser et al. describe the 1976 outbreak at the Philadelphia American Legion convention and the methods that led to the discovery of the cause of this "new" disease.

Kenneth J. Ryan

Enterobacteriaceae

20

The Enterobacteriaceae are a large and diverse family of Gram-negative rods, members of which are found free living in nature and as part of the indigenous flora of humans and animals. They grow rapidly under aerobic and anaerobic conditions and are metabolically active, attacking a variety of substrates. Many species are motile, but none forms spores or demonstrates acid fastness. Most species are opportunistic pathogens; some, however, are highly and specifically pathogenic.

Habitat

presence in normal flora of colon

occurrence in respiratory tract of hospitalized patients

Most Enterobacteriaceae are primarily inhabitants of the lower gastrointestinal tract of humans and animals. Many survive readily in nature, and many are found free living where water and minimal energy sources are available. In humans they include the main facultative portion of the bacterial content of the colon. They are also found in the female genital tract and as transient colonizers of the skin. Enterobacteriaceae are often present in small numbers in the respiratory tract of healthy persons; however, they appear in increased numbers in hospitalized patients, particularly those with chronic debilitating diseases. *Escherichia coli* is the most common species of Enterobacteriaceae found among the indigenous flora, followed by *Klebsiella, Proteus,* and *Enterobacter* species. *Salmonella, Shigella,* certain *E. coli* strains, and *Yersinia* species are primarily pathogenic and not part of the normal flora.

Morphology

peritrichous flagella in motile strains

Pili, capsules, and slime layers

The Enterobacteriaceae are among the larger bacteria that colonize humans. In culture or clinical specimens, they are usually 2–4 μm in length and 0.4–0.6 μm in width; the length is variable, however, producing forms that range from large coccobacilli to an elongated, filamentous appearance. The sides of the bacilli are parallel with rounded ends. Motile strains have peritrichous flagella, which have a regular wavelength and extend 1–5 μm beyond the cell wall. Many also have surface fimbriae (pili). Some species (for example, *Klebsiella*) are typically encapsulated. Most have some extracellular surface material, termed the *slime layer,* that is often poorly circumscribed and readily released into the surrounding medium. The cell wall, cell membrane, and internal structure, which are morphologically similar for all Enterobacteriaceae, are as described in Chapter 2 for Gram-negative bacteria.

Growth

rapid growth

Enterobacteriaceae grow readily on simple media, often with only a single carbon energy source. Growth is rapid under both aerobic and anaerobic conditions, producing 2- to 5-mm colonies on agar media and diffuse turbidity in broth after 12–18 hr of incubation. Their simple growth requirements and relative resistance to many substances, such as bile salts and some bacteriostatic dyes, are exploited in selective media and in identification methods. Conversely, their ability to grow under almost any conditions may interfere with the isolation of more fastidious bacteria when clinical specimens also contain Enterobacteriaceae.

Characteristics exploited in selective media

Colonies of Enterobacteriaceae formed on media such as MacConkey agar (Chapter 9) are distinctive for the group and often characteristic for genera. For example, *Klebsiella* typically produces a large, round, pink (acid), mucoid colony on MacConkey agar through its production of a polysaccharide capsule and its fermentation of lactose. These colonial features are useful guides in clinical microbiology laboratories, but are not intrinsically diagnostic because exceptions are common.

Antigenic Structure

Multiple serotypes

The cell wall, capsular slime layer, and flagellar antigens are valuable in identification and in subtyping for epidemiologic purposes. The extent to which these features have been studied and classified varies greatly among the genera. *Escherichia* and *Salmonella* have been divided into hundreds of types based on the presence of various combinations of antigens, whereas other common genera such as *Proteus* have fewer described antigens. The difference in the number of serotypes within different species is probably attributable to the extent to which they have been studied as much as to biologic differences.

flagellar H antigens

Polysaccharide surface K antigens

cell wall O antigen

Core antigen

Flagella are composed of proteins, and their antigenic determinants are designated *H antigens.* Cell surface antigens are generally polysaccharides and are termed *K antigens* (from the Danish *Kapsel,* capsule) regardless of whether they form a well-defined capsule. Specialized designations are given to surface polysaccharides of certain species, such as the Vi antigen of *Salmonella typhi.* Surface protein antigens associated with the fimbriae may also be present but have not been extensively studied. The cell wall lipopolysaccharide (LPS) is described as the *O antigen.* The antigenic specificity of the O antigen is determined by the composition and linkage of the sugars that form the polysaccharide side chains. The remaining antigenic portion of the LPS is a core glycolipid common to Enterobacteriaceae and other Gram-negative bacteria, antibodies to which may give some cross-immunity between species.

Classification

Genera classified by differences in motility and major biochemical characteristics

Because they are among the most metabolically diverse of bacteria, the Enterobacteriaceae are classified into genera according to their motility and biochemical characteristics. All are facultative, all ferment glucose and reduce nitrates to nitrites, and all are oxidase negative. The currently recognized tribes, genera, and species of significant medical importance and their major characteristics are shown in Appendix 20.1. Species designations are based species identified by battery of biochemical tests

on a battery of physiologic characteristics, including most of those discussed in Chapter 9. They include the ability to ferment various carbohydrates, indole production from tryptophan, citrate utilization, amino acid breakdown, and hydrogen sulfide production from sulfur-containing amino acids. These and many other characteristics are used to construct probability tables for assignment of individual isolates to genera and species.

subspecies classified by antigenic structure

bacteriophage and bacteriocin typing

Within species, differences in O, K, and/or H antigens are used for further subdivision into serotypes. For some species, panels of bacteriocins or bacteriophages have been used to establish typing systems in place of, or in addition to, serotyping systems. None of these subtyping systems alone can identify unknown organisms, because cross-reactions are common with organisms from genera other than that for which the system was devised.

For practical reasons, only a portion of the diagnostic tools available for classifying the Enterobacteriaceae are used in clinical laboratories. A battery of 6–12 biochemical reactions is often sufficient to assign a genus identification, and a few more reactions will allow accurate species identification. In some instances, serologic reactions are used to confirm or extend the biochemical identification.

Significance of lactose fermentation

Rapid fermentation of lactose as demonstrated by acid (pink) colonies on MacConkey agar is a useful characteristic for initial differentiation of Enterobacteriaceae. The most common members of the intestinal flora, *Escherichia coli, Klebsiella,* and *Enterobacter,* ferment lactose promptly in more than 90% of cases, whereas many other genera, including the intestinal pathogens *Salmonella* and *Shigella,* are rarely positive.

Toxins

Endotoxin in all species

some produce exotoxins

All Enterobacteriaceae possess the LPS endotoxin, the structure and functional effects of which are discussed in Chapters 2, 7, and 62. Many of the effects of endotoxin such as fever, leukopenia, and activation of blood coagulation factors are seen in human infections, particularly when organisms enter the bloodstream to produce bacteremia. In addition to LPS endotoxin, some Enterobacteriaceae also produce exotoxins, which will be discussed when individual species are considered.

Pathogenicity

some cause specific diseases

many are opportunists

Some species of Enterobacteriaceae have unique pathogenic features that may allow them to produce gastrointestinal or systemic infections in previously healthy individuals. Examples are bacillary dysentery, caused by *Shigella,* and typhoid fever, caused by *S. typhi.* These infections will be discussed as they relate to particular species. Those species that are members of the normal flora, or that exist in the environment, can act as opportunistic pathogens if they are displaced from their normal site or if local or systemic defense mechanisms are damaged. They can produce a variety of infections, the characteristics of which are primarily determined by the organ involved. The most common are urinary tract infections, of which Enterobacteriaceae are the leading causes (Chapter 60), and wound infections (Chapter 53); however, spread beyond the local site may produce more extensive infection, including bacteremia and Gram-negative shock (Chapter 62).

Antimicrobic Susceptibility

marked variation in susceptibility between and within species

Combinations of chromosomal and plasmid-determined resistance (Chapter 10) render Enterobacteriaceae the most variable of all bacteria in their susceptibility to antimicrobial agents. They are usually resistant to high con-

frequent need for in vitro tests

centrations of penicillin G, erythromycin, and clindamycin, but may be susceptible to the broader-spectrum penicillins, cephalosporins, aminoglycosides, tetracycline, chloramphenicol, sulfonamides, nalidixic acid, nitrofurantoin, and the polypeptide antibiotics. As the probability of resistance varies among genera and in different epidemiologic settings, the susceptibility of any individual strain must be determined by in vitro tests. Typical frequencies of resistance for the more common Enterobacteriaceae appear in Chapter 10.

Escherichia coli

Member of normal colonic flora. Motile. Lactose positive

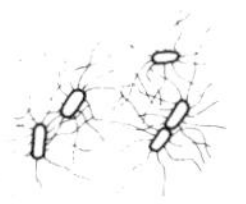

Escherichia coli

multiple serotypes based on O and K antigens

Escherichia coli is the most commonly encountered member of the Enterobacteriaceae in the normal colonic flora and the most common cause of opportunistic infections. Most strains ferment lactose rapidly and produce indole. When grown on blood agar, many strains isolated from infections are hemolytic, a feature uncommon in other Enterobacteriaceae. The hemolysin, an antigenic protein encoded by plasmid genes, has been shown to be toxic in tissue culture and animal experiments. Serotyping systems have been established based on O and K antigens and using agglutination tests. There are over 150 somatic O antigens (for example, 055, 0111, 0144). The *E. coli* K antigens are also designated by number. Thus, the antigenic structure of individual strains is described by designations such as 0111:K58 and 018:K76. In distinguishing O and K antigens, the heat stability of the LPS antigen is exploited: it can withstand boiling for an hour or more, whereas surface K antigens are either destroyed or removed by heating. Approximately 40 flagellar H types have also been defined for *E. coli,* but are used less frequently than O and K antigen types in diagnostic and epidemiologic studies.

Urinary Tract Infections

E. coli most common cause of urinary tract infection; organisms derived from intestine

predominance in women during childbearing years

certain serotypes predominate in urinary infections

Possible role of adherence

Escherichia coli is the most common cause of infections of the urinary bladder, renal pelvis, and kidney (Chapter 60). This finding is explained in part by the large numbers of *E. coli* commonly found in the large intestine and by contamination of the perineum and urethra, particularly in women. Relatively minor trauma or the mechanical effect of sexual intercourse may allow *E. coli* and other organisms from the perineum to enter the bladder. *Escherichia coli* can grow rapidly in urine, typically producing more than 10^5 bacteria per milliliter of urine in clinical infections. The attack rate is highest in sexually active women, and more than 90% of urinary tract infections developing outside hospitals are caused by *E. coli.* In addition to the presence of the organism in the fecal flora, some determinants of virulence appear to be important in the pathogenesis of *E. coli* urinary infections: less than 10 of 150 serotypes are responsible for most cases. Hemolytic strains are common, and strains with certain K surface antigens, particularly K1, predominate in urinary tract infections, probably because they adhere to urinary tract epithelial cells. For example, strains isolated from the urine of patients with pyelonephritis adhere better to uroepithelial cells than do those isolated from asymptomatic bladder infections. Interference with attachment has been shown to decrease the ability of *E. coli* strains to produce bacteriuria in experimental animals. Factors that provide more ready access or delay the exit of *E. coli* from the bladder, such as urinary catheters or urinary obstruction by an enlarged prostate gland, are also associated with infection.

Symptoms

Urinary tract infections vary from asymptomatic to involvement of the entire tract, including the kidney; there are no clinical differences, however, between those caused by *E. coli* and those caused by other organisms (Chapter 60). The most common symptoms are dysuria and urinary frequency. When the renal pelvis and kidney are involved (pyelonephritis), fever and flank pain are common and bacteremia may develop. The duration of symptoms is quite variable, but response to antimicrobial therapy is usually prompt in uncomplicated cases.

Intestinal Infections

epidemiologic association of serotypes with nursery and traveler's diarrhea

It has long been suspected that certain strains of *E. coli* can produce diarrhea. The difficulty of associating the organism with intestinal infections is obvious, however, because multiple strains are present in virtually every stool. Early epidemiologic evidence from outbreaks of diarrhea in nurseries supported the association of *E. coli* with the disease, because identical serotypes were isolated from multiple cases. A list of 10–20 "enteropathogenic" serotypes was developed from epidemiologic studies, but no bacteriologic differences from other strains or pathogenetic mechanisms were noted. Similar evidence incriminated *E. coli* in a form of traveler's diarrhea (*turista*). In a diarrhea outbreak in 1965 among British soldiers after an airlift to the Middle East, sickness was strongly associated with an *E. coli* serotype unknown in England. Later, a technologist in England working with the strain also developed diarrhea.

Enterotoxigenic *E. coli*

LT acts like cholera toxin

More recent experimental animal and volunteer studies have revealed two clear mechanisms by which *E. coli* produces diarrhea. One is through action on the intestinal mucosa of exotoxins (enterotoxins), the elaboration of which is plasmid controlled. Two such toxins, which differ in heat stability and mechanism of action, have been identified. One, a heat-labile toxin (LT), is inactivated by boiling (100°C) and acts in a manner similar to that of cholera toxin (Chapter 21) functionally, structurally, and immunologically. It binds to GM1-ganglioside receptors on mucosal cells and activates adenylate cyclase, causing secretion of water and electrolytes into the intestinal lumen. The other, a heat-stable enterotoxin (ST), resists boiling and causes fluid secretion from mucosal cells; it activates guanylate cyclase, rather than adenylate cyclase, and does not resemble cholera toxin except in its fluid secretion effect. Both toxins are produced in the lumen of the small intestine; they are brought near their site of action with the aid of pili, termed *colonization factors antigens* (CFA) that mediate attachment of the organism to the epithelium. Production of both LT and ST and several immunologically distinct colonization factors are all determined by plasmid genes. A single *E. coli* strain may produce LT, ST, or both, and may or may not possess the colonization factor necessary to colonize the small intestine. Production of disease as a result of toxin requires the ability both to colonize the small intestine and to produce enterotoxin. Strains that produce either or both toxins are collectively called *enterotoxigenic E. coli.*

ST also causes fluid loss

role of colonization factors

enterotoxins and colonization factors plasmid coded

Enteroinvasive *E. coli*

Another mechanism by which certain strains of *E. coli* can cause diarrhea involves direct penetration and destruction of the colonic epithelium. These strains, called *enteroinvasive E. coli,* produce a dysenteric illness with fever, cramps, and pus and blood in the stool. Yet another mechanism for *E. coli* diarrhea has been described recently in which the organisms adhere to the epithelium of the small intestine with disruption of the microvilli. These strains neither invade nor produce known toxins, but may interfere with absorptive and secretory processes via dense colonization.

other mechanisms of virulence

enterotoxigenic strains cause afebrile watery diarrhea

To a large extent, the enterotoxigenic and enteroinvasive mechanisms have been linked with clinical and pathologic findings (Table 20.1). Strains producing either LT or ST usually cause watery diarrhea without fever that lasts only a few days. Some evidence indicates that the diarrhea is more severe if both LT and ST are produced. The enterotoxigenic strains are the

Table 20.1 Features of Intestinal Infections by Various Strains of *Escherichia coli*

Feature	Enterotoxigenic	Enteroinvasive	Enteropathogenic
Pathogenic Mechanism	Heat-labile and/or heat-stable enterotoxin	Epithelial cell invasion	Unknown; ? attachment
Primary site	Small intestine	Large intestine	Unknown
Mucosal pathology	Hyperemia	Necrosis; ulceration; inflammation	Unknown
Epidemiologic	Infant diarrhea; traveler's diarrhea	Sporadic; outbreaks uncommon	? Traveler's diarrhea; ? infant diarrhea
Clinical:			
Diarrhea	Watery	Dysentery	Watery
Fever	—	+	—
White blood cells in stool	—	+	—

major causes of traveler's diarrhea and may produce sporadic endemic diarrhea in any age group. In some nursery outbreaks similar to those associated with specific serotypes in the past, toxigenic strains have been shown responsible; in others, however, they have not. Invasive strains produce a dysenteric colitis rather than watery diarrhea, but are relatively uncommon.

enteroinvasive strains cause dysentery

The importance, and even the existence, of *E. coli* that are enteropathogenic by other mechanisms remains controversial. At the center of the debate is the poor correlation between epidemiologic associations of certain serotypes with diarrhea and direct tests for toxin production or invasiveness. To some, this finding demonstrates the uselessness of serotyping to define pathogenicity; to others, it defines the third category, the *enteropathogenic E. coli* (Table 20.1). It is possible that another toxin exists or that these strains produce disease by simple mucosal adherence; resolution of these questions will require better methods to define pathogenic mechanisms.

Currently, the diagnosis of individual cases of *E. coli* diarrhea requires isolation of the organism and demonstration of its enterotoxigenic or enteroinvasive properties. Although LT can be detected in a tissue culture assay, the test is available in few hospital laboratories, and a negative result does not exclude ST. Isolation of the gene encoding LT by recombinant DNA techniques has provided a probe that readily detects the gene in clinical isolates by hybridization techniques. This approach has great promise for the future. Tests for ST and for enteroinvasive properties still require experimental animals, are cumbersome, and are unavailable in clinical laboratories. At present, serotyping of individual stool isolates is not interpretable; it may still be useful, however, when applied to the study of epidemics.

tissue culture and hybridization techniques to detect LT toxigenicity

Meningitis

Common cause of neonatal meningitis

Escherichia coli is one of the most common causes of neonatal meningitis (Chapter 61). This infection results from *E. coli* colonization of the vagina and contamination of amniotic fluid, failure of protective maternal immunoglobulin M(IgM) antibodies to cross the placenta, and the special sus-

association with K1 antigen

ceptibility of newborns. Fully 75% of cases are caused by strains possessing the surface antigen K1, which appears in less than 10% of normal fecal isolates. Interestingly, it is chemically and antigenically identical to the group B meningococcal polysaccharide. A significant proportion of blood isolates are also K1 strains. The mechanism for enhanced virulence of these *E. coli* strains is not known.

Opportunistic Infections

Predisposing factors

With the exception of urinary tract infections, extraintestinal *E. coli* infections are uncommon. If there is a significant breach in host defenses, however, *E. coli* and other members of the Enterobacteriaceae are potent opportunists. Opportunistic infection may follow mechanical damage, such as a ruptured intestinal diverticulum or intestinal trauma, or involve a generalized impairment of immune function.

The particular diseases that result depend on the sites involved and include many of the syndromes covered in Chapters 53–66. Because of the underlying diseases, opportunistic infections are commonly associated with hospitalized patients and often involve strains resistant to multiple antimicrobics.

Antimicrobial Susceptibility

community-acquired strains often susceptible

hospital isolates often resistant through R plasmids

In the community, *E. coli* strains are commonly susceptible to all agents with potential activity against the Enterobacteriaceae. Sulfonamides are frequently used in uncomplicated urinary tract infections in the community because of the high probability that a susceptible *E. coli* is the cause. Antimicrobial therapy of complicated and opportunistic infections must be guided by susceptibility testing; because of the frequent occurrence of R plasmids, strains acquired in hospitals may be resistant to any combination of potentially effective antimicrobics.

Shigella

Nonmotile; lactose negative

Shigella species are closely related to *E. coli* biochemically and antigenically. Most fail to ferment lactose or to produce gas when fermenting glucose, and all are nonmotile. They are strict pathogens that cause bacillary dysentery, a common disease with worldwide distribution. They do not appear as members of the normal flora, although they may be carried for days or weeks during convalescence.

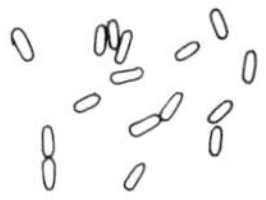

Shigella

Classification

four species; 30 serotypes

The genus *Shigella* is divided into four species, or groups, on the basis of differences in O antigens and some biochemical reactions. They are *Shigella dysenteriae* (group A), *Shigella flexneri* (group B), *Shigella boydii* (group C), and *Shigella sonnei* (group D), as shown in Appendix 20.1. All but *S. sonnei* are further subdivided into a total of more than 30 individual serotypes. *Shigella dysenteriae* type 1, also known as the *Shiga bacillus,* is the cause of classic tropical bacillary dysentery, a disease more serious than those produced by other *Shigella* strains.

Pathogenesis

Strict human pathogens

low infecting dose

All *Shigella* species can be considered strict human pathogens. Significant nonhuman reservoirs do not exist, except in laboratory-maintained primates, and the organism does not survive long after excretion. The organism itself is highly communicable: less than 100 can initiate infection in healthy persons. Transmission is usually by contaminated fingers, food, or water. Mul-

multiplication in small intestine

penetration and ulceration of colonic epithelium

infection localized to colon except occasionally with Shiga bacillus

Uncertain role of toxins

tiplication to high numbers (10^8–10^9 bacteria/ml) in the distal small intestine requires 12 hr or less. Within 1–4 days, the organism invades the large intestine. The primary mechanism of disease production is penetration and destruction of colonic epithelial cells, with subsequent multiplication in the lamina propria, and superficial tissue destruction. This process, which occurs primarily in the lower colon, produces acute inflammation and shallow ulcers scattered along the mucosal surface. Invasion beyond the intestinal mucosa or local lymph nodes is rare, and the organisms are rarely found in deeper tissues or the bloodstream. The Shiga bacillus (*S. dysenteriae* type 1) is more likely than other species to produce bacteremia. All virulent strains of *Shigella* can penetrate epithelial cells; this characteristic has been demonstrated in corneal, conjunctival, and tissue culture cells under experimental conditions. Recent studies with *S. sonnei* have shown that some determinants of virulence, such as invasiveness, are plasmid mediated.

The role of toxins in shigellosis is not certain. In addition to their invasive capacity, Shiga dysentery strains have long been known to produce an exotoxin with neurotoxic properties; more recently, another exotoxin with enterotoxic and cytotoxic properties has been described. The serious nature of Shiga dysentery has been ascribed to the elaboration of these toxins, but experimental studies with toxin-deficient mutants have not clearly supported this concept. Other *Shigella* species have been shown to produce similar toxins, but in smaller amounts. The enterotoxin may account for the initial watery diarrhea, often seen in the early stages of shigellosis, while the organisms are still in the small intestine. The cytotoxic activity may produce the necrosis once cellular penetration has taken place. It is likely that all these reactions represent multiple effects of a single toxin.

Immunity

immunity short-lived, apparently IgA dependent

Shigellosis is usually self-limiting, and infection produces relatively short-lived immunity to reinfection with homologous serogroups. The exact mechanism is not known; however, local IgA production in the intestinal tract is probably more important than humoral immunity. The development of herd immunity through infection and exposure to one serogroup may be responsible for shifts in serogroup prevalence. This hypothesis is suggested by the cyclic patterns of prevalence and serogroup distribution seen over 20- to 30-year periods.

Epidemiology

Fecal–oral spread

high infectivity

Outbreaks of *S. sonnei* in small children

Like other diarrheal infections, shigellosis is strongly associated with poor sanitary practices and poor nutrition. Its fecal–oral mode of spread, from contaminated hands, food, or fomites, usually involves close contact with infected cases; however, flies can be passive vectors.

The low infecting dose and short incubation period facilitate efficient transmission through a population by direct contact. In the past, major outbreaks often occurred during military infantry campaigns through stress and lack of washing or sanitary facilities, and sometimes proved effective peacemakers. Transmission through water and food is responsible for most focal outbreaks. In the United States, 15,000–20,000 cases of shigellosis are reported yearly. Most of these cases are *S. sonnei* infections in children under 10 years of age, with the peak at age 2. Once a case is introduced into a household or day care center, the secondary attack rate by simple hand-to-mouth spread among toddlers may exceed 50%. Organisms are present in stools up to 1 month after an untreated infection. Prolonged carriage is uncommon, but may be the source of a food-borne outbreak.

The most common *Shigella* species in developed countries is *S. sonnei,* followed by *S. flexneri* and *S. boydii. Shigella dysenteriae,* particularly the Shiga bacillus, is rare where hygiene is good, but endemic in tropical, underdeveloped countries. In the mid-1970s, an extensive epidemic of Shiga dysentery occurred in Central America, with occasional cases imported into the United States.

Clinical Features

fever, bloody mucoid stools, and cramping

most infections self-limiting

Shiga dysentery most severe; may be fatal

Shigellosis is an acute diarrheal illness marked by painful passage of bloody, mucoid stools with cramping (dysentery). The stools may initially be watery and voluminous, but quickly become mucoid, bloody, and of smaller volume as the disease localizes in the colon. The typical picture comprises frequent small stools (squirts) with urgency and tenesmus. Although fever is considered a useful feature in differentiating shigellosis from other infectious diarrheas, it is present in less than one-half of cases. The disease is almost always self-limiting; symptoms last a few days to a month, although most cases recover in less than a week without treatment. Except with Shiga dysentery, fatal infections and complications are rare, unless serious underlying disease and/or malnutrition are present. Dysentery caused by the Shiga bacillus is typically more severe; it may occasionally extend beyond the gastrointestinal tract to produce bacteremia. The illness may prove fatal in previously healthy persons, and mortality in epidemics has been as high as 10–20%. With the speed of modern travel, imported cases of Shiga dysentery are possible despite the short incubation period.

Diagnosis

Shigellosis should be suspected in any patient with a diarrheal illness associated with fever, toxemia, or other systemic symptoms. The presence of blood and pus in the stool is suggestive, but not specific; other invasive pathogens (for example, enteroinvasive *E. coli, Campylobacter*), as well as some noninfectious diseases, can also produce this finding. Furthermore, absence of macroscopic or microscopic blood and pus does not exclude shigellosis.

Stool culture on selective media

specimens must be cultured promptly to avoid loss of viability

The only definitive laboratory test is the stool culture. Stool specimens or rectal swabs will yield the organism if promptly plated on appropriate indicator (MacConkey agar) and selective media (Hektoen agar). Enrichment culture techniques are less effective with *Shigella* than with *Salmonella.* Specimens collected early in the course of illness are more likely to be positive, because the organisms are much more numerous. Prompt plating of specimens is important, as the organisms do not survive well outside the body. Non-lactose-fermenting colonies are screened with biochemical tests, and identification is confirmed with serogroup-specific antisera. Typing within the groups is usually available only in reference facilities.

Treatment

treatment may shorten illness and period of excretion

R plasmid-determined resistance

Several antimicrobics have proved effective in the treatment of shigellosis. Because the disease is usually self-limiting, the beneficial effect of treatment is in shortening the illness and the period of excretion of organisms; however, resistance may develop by plasmid transfer. The original discovery of in vivo plasmid transfer involved cases of shigellosis in which the infecting strain acquired multidrug resistance during therapy from an *E. coli* present simultaneously in the bowel. Resistance rates of 5–50% to ampicillin, once considered the treatment of choice, have caused a shift to trimethoprim–sulfamethoxazole in many areas. Tetracycline, nalidixic acid, and oxalinic acid have also been effective against susceptible strains. Mild cases are usually not treated, particularly in adults, who are already improving by the time the organism is isolated. As the diarrhea is not voluminous, fluid replacement can usually be accomplished orally. Antispasmodic agents to control diarrhea may make the patient worse and are not indicated in shigellosis or other invasive diarrheas.

fluid replacement

Prevention

sanitation, insect control, hand washing, cooking

Standard sanitation practices such as sewage disposal and water chlorination are important in preventing the spread of shigellosis. In certain circumstances insect control may also be important, because flies can serve as passive vectors when open sewage is present. Good individual sanitary practices, such as hand washing and proper cooking of food, are highly protective.

Vaccines

Killed parenteral vaccines lead to serum antibody responses, but have not been effective in preventing the disease. Orally administered live attenuated strains are proving more promising. These strains include *Shigella* mutants and *E. coli–Shigella* hybrids that fail to penetrate the mucosa or to multiply after penetration. Although such vaccines have been shown to protect against clinical disease, the relatively short duration of immunity and its serotype specificity complicates their practical application.

Klebsielleae

members of colonic flora or free living

Most ferment lactose

opportunists

Although neither as frequent nor as numerous as *E. coli,* the Klebsielleae, or *Klebsiella–Enterobacter–Serratia* group, are commonly found among the gastrointestinal flora. Many are found free living in nature. Members of the group share similar biochemical features (Appendix 20.1). With the exception of *Serratia* species, they are usually characterized by prompt lactose fermentation. All can be considered opportunistic pathogens, but can neither produce exotoxin nor invade healthy individuals. They are usually associated with nosocomial infections, particularly pneumonia and urinary tract infections. The group as a whole is resistant to ampicillin, and multiresistant strains are common.

Klebsiella

Nonmotile, encapsulated

Multiple capsular types

The most distinctive bacteriologic features of the genus *Klebsiella* are the absence of motility and the presence of a polysaccharide capsule. The latter gives colonies a glistening, mucoid character and forms the basis of a serotyping system. Seventy-two capsular types have been defined; they can be differentiated by precipitin, agglutination, and quellung reactions, although the antisera are usually available only in reference laboratories. Cross-reactions occur between certain *Klebsiella* polysaccharide capsular antigens and those of other encapsulated pathogens, such as *Streptococcus pneumoniae* and *Haemophilus influenzae.* These cross-reactions suggest parallels in the mechanisms of pathogenesis and immunity; the relationship of the *Klebsiella* capsule to virulence, however, has not been demonstrated.

Association with disease

Another similarity to the pneumococcus is the ability of *Klebsiella pneumoniae* to cause classic lobar pneumonia; this association is rare, however, and cases usually involve individuals severely compromised by age or disease. Most *Klebsiella* pneumonias are indistinguishable from those produced by other members of the Enterobacteriaceae. *Klebsiella rhinoscleromatis* has been associated with rhinoscleroma, a chronic granulomatous process of the upper respiratory mucosa, and *Klebsiella ozaenae* with ozena, a form of chronic atrophy of the nasal mucosa. Species associations with disease states are not strict, and any *Klebsiella* can be isolated from a variety of opportunistic infections. *Klebsiella pneumoniae* is by far the most common species and the most frequent cause of infection. *Klebsiellae* are usually resistant to ampicillin and carbenicillin. Plasmid-mediated resistance to other antimicrobics is common.

Enterobacter

Motile

Enterobacter species generally ferment lactose promptly and produce colonies similar to those of *Klebsiella,* although not as mucoid. A differential feature is motility by peritrichous flagella, which are generally present in *Enterobacter* species but uniformly absent in *Klebsiella.* The five species listed in Table 20.1 are all comparable in clinical and epidemiologic significance.

resistance to ampicillin and first-generation cephalosporins

Enterobacter species and infections are less common than those of *Klebsiella.* They are usually found in mixed infections, in which their significance must be decided on clinical and epidemiologic grounds. Several hospital outbreaks traced to contaminated parenteral fluid solutions have implicated *Enterobacter* species. Most isolates are resistant to ampicillin and first-generation cephalosporins, but may be susceptible to second- or third-generation cephalosporins.

Serratia

some yield red colonies; DNAase positive

isolates often highly resistant

Serratia strains ferment lactose slowly (3–4 days), if at all. Some produce distinctive brick-red colonies. All produce a potent extracellular deoxyribonuclease. Although the least commonly isolated of the group, the genus produces the same range of opportunistic infections seen with the rest of the Enterobacteriaceae. *Serratia* strains show consistent resistance to ampicillin and cephalothin, with the frequent addition of plasmid-determined resistance to many other antimicrobics, including the aminoglycosides. Sporadic infections and nosocomial outbreaks with multiresistant strains have often been difficult to control, and some *Serratia* isolates are resistant to essentially all available antimicrobics.

Salmonelleae

Usually lactose negative; motile; produce H_2S

The Salmonelleae tribe includes a range of pathogens that can infect otherwise healthy individuals. Most are associated with disease in a wide range of vertebrates, although *S. typhi,* the cause of typhoid fever, is a strict human pathogen. The organisms are motile by peritrichous flagella. *Salmonella* species do not ferment lactose; some *Arizona* and *Citrobacter* strains, however, may ferment lactose. The ability to produce hydrogen sulfides from sulfur-containing amino acids is a group feature that is used to identify colonies on primary isolation media. As members of the group resemble each other closely, detailed biochemical testing is necessary for differentiation at the species level.

Classification

Three *Salmonella* species

S. enteritidis subdivided into more than 1500 serotypes by O and H antigens

The three species of *Salmonella* (*S. enteritidis, S. choleraesuis,* and *S. typhi*) differ in biochemical, serologic, and pathogenic features. As with the other Enterobacteriaceae, biochemical reactions define the genus and species. *Salmonella typhi* and *Salmonella choleraesuis* each represent a single serotype, but serologic reactions further divide *S. enteritidis* into over 1500 serotypes based on combinations of multiple O and H antigens. More than 80 O antigens

Table 20.2 Antigenic Composition of Some *Salmonella* Species

Species (serotype)	Serogroup	O Antigens	Surface Antigens	Phase of H Antigens 1	2
S. enteritidis (paratyphi B)	B	1,4,5,12	—	b	1,2
S. enteritidis (typhimurium)	B	1,4,5,12	—	i	1,2
S. enteritidis (durban)	D	9,12	—	a	e,n,z_{15}
S. typhi	D	9,12	Vi	d	None
S. choleraesuis	C	6,7	—	c	1,5

have been numerically designated. Several are found in any given strain, and strains with similar combinations of O antigens are organized into nine broad serogroups. There are also multiple flagellar H antigens, more than one of which may be represented on a flagellum. In addition, most *Salmonella* strains show the phenomenon of phase variation of their H antigens; that is, they can synthesize two distinct sets of flagella, termed *phase 1* and *phase 2*. Population shifts between these two phases depend on various cultural and immunologic conditions. Phase 1 and 2 flagellins are coded by genes termed H1 and H2. Expression is controlled by an H2 promoter, which can invert. In one orientation it activates H2 and an H1 repressor. In the other, H2 is not transcribed and H1 is expressed.

Flagellar antigen phase variation

Examples of antigenic formulas for a few serotypes of *S. enteritidis* are shown in Table 20.2. Serotypes are given names such as typhimurium (mouse typhoid), budapest, seminole, tamale, and oysterbeds, which reflect the condition or the place from which they were first isolated. Although this practice causes some confusion between serotype and species, it adds color to the microbiological literature.

Nomenclature of *S. enteritidis* serotypes

Pathogenesis

high infecting dose for *S. enteritidis*

Enterocolitis

Salmonella enteritidis infection usually results from ingestion of numerous organisms in food or occasionally water. Smaller numbers may infect under conditions that decrease gastric acidity or transit time through the stomach (achlorhydria, vagotomy, gastrectomy), presumably because more viable bacteria reach the small intestine. Once in the small intestine, the organisms may multiply and produce an acute enterocolitis with fever, diarrhea, and evidence of inflammation of the bowel; however, infection and colonization may be asymptomatic. *Salmonella enteritidis* has been shown experimentally to penetrate the intestinal mucosa, but this finding alone does not explain the resultant fluid loss. Recently, a *Salmonella* enterotoxin with properties similar to those of *E. coli* LT and cholera toxin was identified. The relative importance of penetration, inflammation, and enterotoxin in the pathogenesis of *S. enteritidis* diarrhea remains to be determined.

Salmonella septicemia associated with *S. choleraesuis*

Salmonella choleraesuis and some serotypes of *S. enteritidis* invade the mucosa and spread to the bloodstream without producing enteritis. Bacteremia is characteristic, and secondary infections can occur at almost any anatomic site. It must be reemphasized, however, that the most common disease caused by *S. enteritidis* is enterocolitis.

Enteric fever usually caused by *S. typhi* (typhoid fever)

Enteric fever represents yet another type of disease. It is usually caused by *S. typhi*, occasionally by certain serotypes of *S. enteritidis*. The infecting dose is less than that required for *Salmonella* enterocolitis, and infection is usually transmitted by fecally contaminated food or water. The disease begins with multiplication of *S. typhi* in the small intestine. The organism penetrates the mucosa without producing enterocolitis, but does not immediately spread to the blood and distant organs. Instead, upon reaching regional lymph nodes, it multiplies within mononuclear cells, then spreads to reticuloendothelial sites in the liver, spleen, and bone marrow through the lymphatic system and blood during the incubation period (approximately 10 days). The intracellular survival of *S. typhi* is associated with inhibition of oxidative metabolism of the host cell during phagocytosis. Continued multiplication results in reseeding of the bloodstream with bacteria, necrosis of reticuloendothelial cells, and onset of clinical enteric fever. In the course of the bacteremia, other sites such as intestinal lymphoid follicles and the biliary tract become infected, leading to reinfection of the intestinal tract. The disease is thus primarily caused by the multiplication of *S. typhi* in the reticuloendothelial system.

Pathogenesis

Involvement of reticuloendothelial system

Bacteremia

infection of intestinal lymphoid follicles and biliary tract

Many of the findings in enteric fever are similar to those caused by Gram-negative endotoxin. The prolonged fever and toxic symptoms in particular tempt one to attribute the disease to continuously circulating endotoxin. Efforts to verify this hypothesis experimentally have been unsuccessful, because endotoxin tolerance develops. Similarly, efforts to correlate symptoms with endotoxin detection in clinical cases have failed. The duration of fever may be attributable to prolonged and diffuse inflammation in the reticuloendothelial system with release of endogenous pyrogen.

Role of endotoxin

Salmonella typhi often possesses a Vi (virulence) surface antigen, which is associated with enhanced capacity to invade the host. The mechanism may involve interference with host phagocytic cells or with serum bactericidal activity. Its presence is not essential for virulence, but appears to lower the infecting dose necessary to produce disease.

S. typhi Vi antigen

Epidemiology

Infections by *S. enteritidis* and *S. choleraesuis* are largely acquired through ingestion of contaminated food or, less often, of water. Direct fecal–oral spread is also possible, particularly in children; this mode of spread is not as efficient as with *Shigella,* however, because the infecting dose of *Salmonella* is much higher. Contamination of foodstuffs is usually from the large reservoir in animals for which *Salmonella* is a primary pathogen. Virtually all species of poultry, mammals, reptiles, and amphibians may be infected. Some serotypes are more adapted to certain animal species, but all are transmissible to humans.

S. enteritidis infection usually from food contamination with animal strains

range of animal hosts

Approximately 20,000–40,000 cases of human *Salmonella* enterocolitis are reported in the United States each year, making it one of the most common bacterial causes of diarrhea. The vehicles of transmission vary according to the animal reservoir; however, they usually involve animal products that are contaminated with *Salmonella* during processing, then handled in ways that allow the bacteria to multiply to levels that increase the probability of infection and disease. This situation usually results when incompletely cooked or uncooked food is allowed to remain warm for a few hours, during which time *Salmonella* can multiply to as many as 10^7–10^9 organisms per gram.

organism multiplies in food to produce infecting dose

The classic example of *S. enteritidis* infection is the church picnic or bazaar, where volunteers prepare poultry, potato salad, and other potential culture media to be eaten later in the day. The source of contamination is often turkey or chicken or the surfaces on which they have been prepared for cooking. Because refrigerators are filled with iced tea, beer, and soda, the food is left out in covered pans. An appropriate incubation temperature is provided by the still-warm contents and the afternoon sun, and the organisms enter logarithmic growth during the softball game. The bacteria usually produce no noticeable change in the food, and those who eat it are stricken the following day in rough proportion to their degree of consumption. This series of events also occurs frequently with other types of bacterial food poisoning (Chapter 59).

common sources of *S. enteritidis*

Approximately one-half of *Salmonella* cases traced to specific vehicles involve poultry or poultry products in fresh, frozen, or dehydrated form. Meat and dairy products are also common vehicles. A recent increase in the popularity of raw milk has been associated with outbreaks of *Salmonella* (and *Campylobacter*) infection. Other sources include some dried egg products and exotic pets such as turtles. Like other enteric infections, *Salmonella* enterocolitis has a seasonal pattern with peaks in the summer months.

S. typhi an exclusively human pathogen

infecting dose may be low

role of chronic carrier

bacteriophage typing of *S. typhi*

As there is no animal reservoir, cases of typhoid fever originate from other human cases or carriers of *S. typhi.* The vehicle of transmission may be water or food contaminated by a preparer carrying the organism. The infecting dose is much lower than that of *S. enteritidis,* and multiplication outside the body before ingestion is usually unnecessary. Most of the 400–500 cases of typhoid fever reported yearly in the United States are now associated with travel to an endemic area or can be traced to a chronic carrier, who may have had the disease many years previously. Water-borne infection is very rare in areas with adequate sewage systems. A typhoid outbreak in 1973 among migrant workers in Florida was traced to leakage of sewage into the water supply, failure of chlorination, and a chronic carrier as the original source. Strains of *S. typhi* can be "fingerprinted" by bacteriophage typing to assist in tracing sources of infection.

Clinical Manifestations of Salmonellosis

incubation period 6–48 hr; constitutional signs of mucosal invasion; diarrhea

disease usually self-limiting

Enterocolitis (food poisoning). Illness begins with nausea, vomiting, and diarrhea of varying severity 8–48 hr after ingestion. Myalgia, headache, fever, and other constitutional symptoms may also develop. The diarrhea is usually intermediate in nature between the voluminous watery diarrhea of cholera (Chapter 21) and the crampy diarrhea of shigellosis. Gross blood and pus are not common, but red and white cells may be seen on microscopic examination of the stool. The diarrhea usually reaches its peak within hours and typically lasts a few hours to a few days. There are considerable variations in severity and duration depending on host factors and inoculum size. Infection tends to be more common, severe, and prolonged in infants, the aged, and the sick than in healthy adults. The usual case is self-limiting without extension beyond the gastrointestinal tract.

incubation period 10–14 days

severe systemic disease lasting 3–4 weeks if untreated; diarrhea often absent

Enteric fever. In contrast to *Salmonella* enterocolitis diarrhea is not a prominent feature of enteric fever and is absent or mild in many cases (Figure 20.1). The illness has an insidious onset 10–14 days after ingestion of the organism, with fever, malaise, headache, and anorexia. Fever and constitutional signs increase over many days. Diarrhea may occur after 1 week, although the patient is often constipated. A maculopapular rash known as *rose spots* may appear on the abdomen in the second or third week, but rarely lasts more than a few days. Abdominal tenderness and distention are common as the disease progresses, and a palpable enlargement of the liver and spleen occurs in up to one-half of cases.

Complications of typhoid

If the illness is not treated, the fever and other findings usually continue

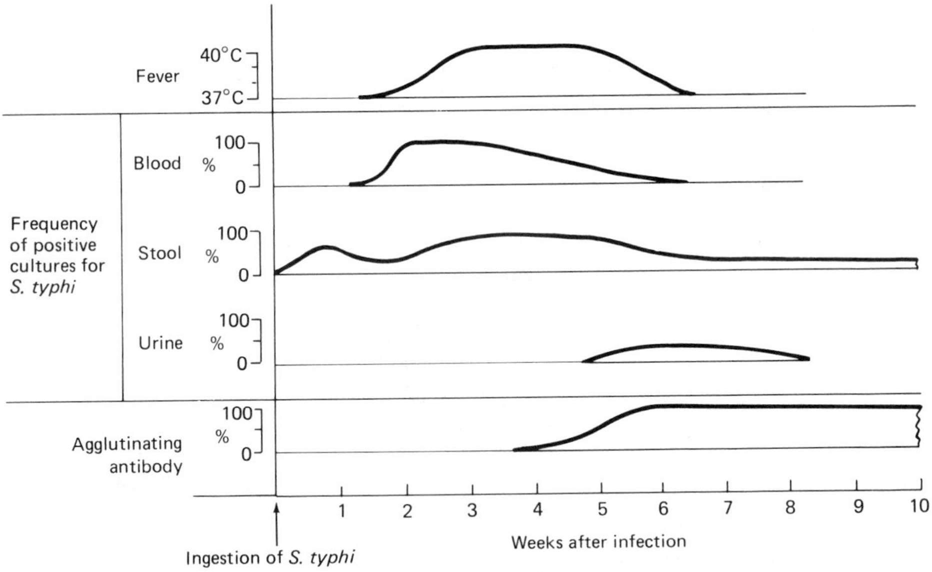

20.1 Natural history of enteric (typhoid) fever. The course of disease without antimicrobial therapy. Fever chart shows time course for typical patient. Culture and agglutinating antibody show timing and probability of positive results in a group of typhoid fever patients.

for 3–4 weeks, then decrease in a gradual stepwise fashion resembling onset in reverse. The primary risk in enteric fever involves its complications. There may be an overwhelming sepsis and toxemia, metastatic infections in other organs (brain, bone, joints, heart valves), or local complications in the gastrointestinal tract. The latter involve infection, hyperplasia, and necrosis of the lymphoid aggregate follicles of the small intestine with ulceration of the intestinal mucosa. Intestinal hemorrhage from the necrotic patch or perforation into the peritoneal cavity is possible. Occasionally the enlarged, friable spleen ruptures. In the preantibiotic era, these complications were responsible for mortality as high as 15% in typhoid fever. With adequate antimicrobial therapy the infection, although still serious, is fatal in less than 1% of cases.

necrosis of lymphoid follicles with hemorrhage or rupture

Other extraintestinal infections. Bacteremia with signs of sepsis may be produced by *S. choleraesuis* or, sometimes, by *S. enteritidis* without associated diarrhea or even positive stool cultures, although the site of invasion is presumably the small intestine. Localization and abscess formation can occur in any anatomic site. Osteomyelitis is noteworthy, because it usually occurs in immunosuppressed patients and those with sickle cell anemia. *Salmonella* bacteremia may be potentiated by the presence of other infectious diseases. In parts of the world where typhus, malaria, and schistosomiasis are endemic, *Salmonella* bacteremia is an important complication of these and other systemic infections.

S. choleraesuis and *S. enteritidis* bacteremia

Osteomyelitis in sickle cell anemia and in the immunocompromised

Carrier State

Excretion of *S. enteritidis* after enterocolitis may continue for a few weeks. Such cases are regarded as convalescent carriers; after 1 month, however, their frequency falls off sharply. Chronic carriage (more than 1 year), which often develops after *S. typhi* infection, is of great epidemiologic significance because carriers are the major reservoir for subsequent cases. The biliary

Typhoid carriage in the biliary tract

tract is the primary site for chronic typhoid carriage, and eradication may be difficult in the presence of biliary tract disease. The presence of gallstones may require cholecystectomy to eliminate the carrier state.

Laboratory Diagnosis

Stool cultures for *S. enteritidis* infection

Salmonella enteritidis enterocolitis is diagnosed by isolation of the causative organism from stool specimens using special indicator and selective media (for example, MacConkey, Hektoen, *Salmonella–Shigella,* and xylose–lysine–deoxycholate). The media used most frequently are appropriate for isolation of both *Salmonella* and *Shigella.* Enrichment broths such as selenite F are generally highly effective in detection of low concentrations of *Salmonella* from stools of cases and carriers. Serologic tests are not useful in the diagnosis or management of *S. enteritidis* infection.

blood cultures positive in early stages of enteric fever; stool cultures positive later

serodiagnostic procedures of limited value

Enteric fever presents a special diagnostic problem because of its complex pathogenesis. As shown in Figure 20.1, the first specimens to yield the organism are blood cultures; stool and sometimes urine cultures become positive later in the clinical course. Most patients with typhoid fever develop agglutinating antibodies to the O and H antigens of *S. typhi* between the second and fourth weeks of illness. Tests for these antibodies (for example, the Widal test) may be used for diagnostic purposes; however, the timing of the antibody response (Figure 20.1), the effects of previous typhoid vaccination, and the occurrence of some false-positive and -negative results limits them to an adjunctive role. The diagnosis is best made by isolation of *S. typhi* from blood and/or stool as early in the illness as possible.

Treatment

antimicrobics in *Salmonella* enterocolitis unhelpful

Uncomplicated enterocolitis rarely requires hospitalization or antimicrobial therapy. Fluid replacement by mouth is usually all that is necessary, unless there is evidence of spread beyond the intestinal tract. Treatment with antimicrobics does not significantly alter the clinical course, and it may cause prolonged excretion of *Salmonella.*

Antimicrobic treatment of enteric fever

Plasmid-mediated resistance

Treatment of chronic typhoid carriers

Enteric fever requires supportive fluid and nutritional therapy as well as an effective antimicrobial agent. *Salmonella typhi* is susceptible in vitro to many antimicrobics, but only chloramphenicol, ampicillin, and trimethoprim–sulfamethoxazole have demonstrated clinical effectiveness. In recent years, therapy has been complicated by plasmid-mediated resistance to these agents, including combined chloramphenicol–ampicillin resistance. Drug selection must be guided by susceptibility tests. Response to treatment is typically gradual, as with natural lysis of the disease. Treatment of the chronic carrier is difficult; for example, high-dose ampicillin therapy for 4–6 weeks is successful in only about 25% of cases without cholecystectomy. Trimethoprim–sulfamethoxazole may be more effective.

Prevention

Typhoid vaccines

Public health sanitary measures, good water and sewage treatment, and education on the proper means of cooking and storing food are the primary ways to prevent *Salmonella* infection. Typhoid vaccines consisting of whole, killed *S. typhi* are available for parenteral administration; the degree of protection is only relative, however, and the vaccines are associated with considerable reactions to their endotoxins. Recent studies with live, attenuated, and genetically engineered oral vaccines promise much more effective prophylaxis in the future.

Arizona

reptiles major reservoir

lactose fermentation common

The genus *Arizona* is very closely related to *Salmonella* both biochemically and serologically, and it has the same serologic complexity. It was originally isolated from lizards and gila monsters in Arizona and was assigned to the *Salmonella* genus. The most important practical difference from *Salmonella* is fermentation of lactose by roughly one-half of strains. Many strains will therefore not be detected in routine stool culture procedures unless the laboratory is told of their possible presence. *Arizona* is an animal pathogen, and its isolation from humans has the same clinical significance as that of *S. enteritidis.*

Citrobacter

enterocolitis

opportunists

The genus *Citrobacter,* although biochemically and serologically related to *Salmonella* and *Arizona,* does not cause typical *Salmonella* enterocolitis or enteric fever. These organisms, which may appear in the normal intestinal flora, are opportunistic pathogens in the same manner as many other Enterobacteriaceae, such as *Enterobacter.* Despite reports of association of *Citrobacter* with diarrheal disease, present evidence does not indicate that the organism should be considered an enteric pathogen.

Proteeae

opportunists

Swarming and nonswarming species

The Proteeae, a group of organisms that includes the genera *Proteus, Morganella,* and *Providencia* (Appendix 20.1), are also opportunistic pathogens found in varying frequencies in the normal intestinal flora. *Proteus mirabilis,* the most commonly isolated member of the group, is one of the most susceptible of the Enterobacteriaceae to the penicillins; this characteristic includes moderate susceptibility to penicillin G. Other Proteeae are regularly resistant to ampicillin and the cephalosporins. *Proteus mirabilis* and *Proteus vulgaris* share the ability to swarm over the surface of enriched media, rather than remaining confined to discrete colonies (Figure 20.2). This characteristic makes them readily recognizable in the laboratory—often with dismay, because the spreading growth covers other organisms in the culture and

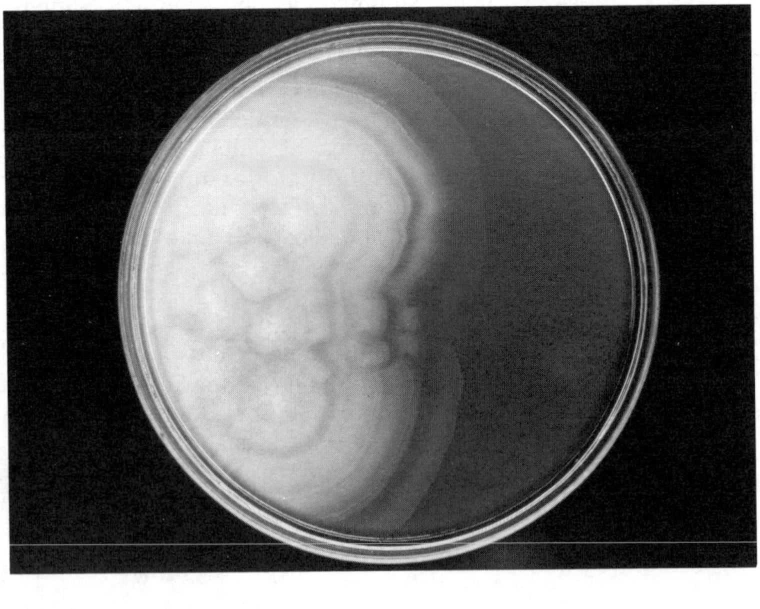

20.2 Swarming *Proteus.* This strain of *Proteus mirabilis* was inoculated at one spot on the blood agar plate. Note the waves of the spreading growth, which have covered the entire plate. On media containing bile salts (MacConkey agar) the swarming is inhibited and discrete colonies are formed.

Proteus and *Morganella* elaborate potent urease

thus delays their isolation. *Proteus* and *Morganella* differ from other Enterobacteriaceae in the production of a very potent urease, which aids their rapid identification. It also leads to production of alkalinity and an ammoniac odor in urinary tract infections. *Providencia* species do not produce urease, are the least frequently isolated, and are generally the most resistant of the group to antimicrobics.

Yersinia

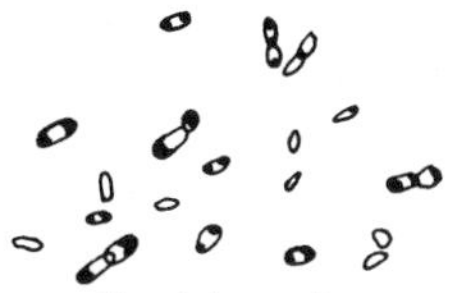
Yersinia pestis

primarily animal pathogens

The genus *Yersinia* has only recently been classified among the Enterobacteriaceae. Of the medically important species of the genus, *Yersinia pestis* and *Yersinia pseudotuberculosis* were previously included in the genus *Pasteurella* and are designated as such in the older literature. *Yersinia enterocolitica* was not described until the 1960s. Morphologically, *Yersinia* tend to be coccobacillary and to retain staining at the ends of the cells (bipolar staining); they otherwise resemble the rest of the Enterobacteriaceae. Their general growth and metabolic characteristics are the same as those of other Enterobacteriaceae, although some strains grow more slowly or have optimal growth temperatures below 37°C. *Yersinia* are primarily animal pathogens, with occasional transmission to humans through direct or indirect contact. *Yersinia pestis* is the cause of plague, one of the great pandemic infectious diseases in human history.

Virulence mechanisms

The virulence of *Yersinia* is related to its invasiveness, endotoxin, and in some instances, production of exotoxin. All three medically important species synthesize protein antigens, termed *V* and *W*, that are necessary for animal pathogenicity and produced only at the temperatures and ionic concentrations found in vertebrate host cells. Thus, they express their greatest virulence after growth within mammalian cells. The function of these proteins is not completely known; however, they interfere with phagocytosis and may provide protection against intracellular leukocyte killing mechanisms and promote growth within host cells. In addition to the V and W proteins, *Y. pestis* also produces a capsular protein antigen termed F1, which has antiphagocytic properties. It is interesting that *Y. pseudotuberculosis* and *Y. enterocolitica* develop motility and certain biochemical reactions only at temperatures below 37°C (Appendix 20.1).

Schemes for serotyping, biotyping, and bacteriophage typing have been developed for *Yersinia*. *Yersinia pestis* is antigenically homogeneous, but *Y. pseudotuberculosis* and *Y. enterocolitica* have multiple O and H antigens (Table 20.1). There are cross-reactions between *Y. pestis* and *Y. pseudotuberculosis.*

Yersinia pestis

Plague

Yersinia pestis causes plague in both man and animals. The pathogenesis, epidemiology, and clinical features of this important disease are covered in Chapter 23.

Yersinia pseudotuberculosis

In animals *Y. pseudotuberculosis* causes pseudotuberculosis, a disease characterized by lesions ranging from local necrosis to granulomatous inflammation in the lymph nodes, spleen, and liver. The organisms have been shown to survive and grow within mammalian cells. In humans the most common manifestation is an acute mesenteric lymphadenitis. The portal of entry is the gastrointestinal tract, and in most cases wild animals are a possible source of infection. The primary clinical manifestations are fever and abdominal pain, often mimicking acute appendicitis. Diagnosis is by isolation of *Y.*

Acute mesenteric lymphadenitis

pseudotuberculosis from lymph nodes or from blood in the small proportion of cases that are bacteremic. The role of antimicrobial therapy in mesenteric lymphadenitis is uncertain, as the disease is usually self-limiting. The organism is usually susceptible to ampicillin, cephalosporins, aminoglycosides, tetracyclines, and chloramphenicol.

Yersinia enterocolitica

Invasive enterocolitis

Other syndromes

Yersinia enterocolitica, a more recently described pathogen, produces a wider variety of infections than other members of the genus. The most common infection is enterocolitis, usually occurring in children and characterized by fever, diarrhea, and abdominal pain. It also causes an acute mesenteric lymphadenitis similar to that produced by *Y. pseudotuberculosis,* terminal ileitis, septicemia, and a polyarthritic syndrome associated with its diarrheal manifestations. In addition to their ability to penetrate cells, *Y. enterocolitica* strains have been shown to produce an enterotoxin with properties similar to *E. coli* ST toxin.

Geographic variation in the frequency of *Y. enterocolitica* infections is marked. The highest rates have been reported from some Scandinavian and other European countries, with much lower rates in the United Kingdom and the United States. Low isolation rates may be partially attributable to the difficulty of growing *Y. enterocolitica* from stool specimens. Few laboratories in the United States routinely screen stools for *Yersinia* because the yield has been low and good selective media are not available.

Yersinia enterocolitica enterocolitis is usually self-limiting, and the influence of antimicrobics on its course is not clear. The organism is susceptible to the same antimicrobics as *Y. psuedotuberculosis,* with the exception of penicillins and cephalosporins, to which it is usually resistant through production of β-lactamases.

Additional Reading and References

Cantey, J.R., Lushbaugh, W.B, and Inman, L.R. 1981. Attachment of bacteria to intestinal epithelial cells in diarrhea caused by *Escherichia coli* strain RDEC-1 in the rabbit: Stages and role of capsule. *J. Infect. Dis.* 143:219–230. This paper provides experimental support for intestinal attachment as virulence mechanism of *Escherichia coli.*

DuPont, H.L., Formal, S.B., Hornick, R.B., Snyder, M.J., Libonati, J.P., Sheahan, D.G., LaBrec, E.H., and Kalas, J.P. 1971. Pathogenesis of *Escherichia coli* diarrhea. *N. Engl. J. Med.* 285:1–9. These in vitro and in vivo studies using human volunteers clearly differentiate the two major mechanisms, invasion and enterotoxin production, by which *Escherichia coli* causes diarrhea.

Gorbach, S.L., Kean, B.H., Evans, D.G., Evans, D.J., and Bessudo, D. 1975. Traveler's diarrhea and toxigenic *Escherichia coli. N. Engl. J. Med.* 292:933–936. This paper is an excellent study of traveler's diarrhea.

Hornick, R.B., Greisman, S.E., Woodward, T.E. et al. 1970. Typhoid fever: pathogenesis and immunologic control. *N. Engl. J. Med.* 283:686–691, 739–746. All aspects of typhoid fever are reviewed in detail, with emphasis on the relationships between pathogenesis and clinical features.

Levine, M.M., DuPont, H.L., Formal, S.B., Hornick, R.B., Takeuchi, A., Gangarosa, E.J., Snyder, M.J., and Libonati, J.P. 1973. Pathogenesis of *Shigella dysenteriae* 1 (Shiga) dysentery. *J. Infect. Dis.* 127:261–270. The relative roles of invasion and toxin are examined in human and animal studies involving wild-type and mutant strains.

Rowe, B., Taylor, J., and Bettelheim, K.A. 1970. An investigation of travellers diarrhea. *Lancet* 1:1–5. The outbreak of traveler's diarrhea among British soldiers, mentioned in the present chapter, is studied. This strain was later shown to produce enterotoxin.

Appendix 20.1 General Characteristics of the Enterobacteriaceae

Organism[a]	Serologic Type (s) (Antigens)	Lactose	Indole	Urease	Hydrogen Sulfide	Motility	Other	Major Disease(s)
		Bacteriologic Features						
ESCHERICHIEAE								
Escherichia coli	150+ (O, K, H)	+	+	—	—	v		Urinary tract infections; diarrhea; opportunistic
Shigella dysenteriae	10 (O)	—	v	—	—	—		Dysentery (type 1, severe)
Shigella flexneri	6 (O)	—	—	—	—	—		Dysentery
Shigella boydii	15 (O)	—	v	—	—	—		Dysentery
Shigella sonnei	1 (O)	—	—	—	—	—		Dysentery
KLEBSIELLEAE								
Klebsiella pneumoniae	72 (K)	+	—	+[b]	—	—	Encapsulated	Pneumonia; opportunistic
K. ozaneae, K. oxytoca, K. rhinoscleromatis								Opportunistic
Enterobacter aerogenes		+	—	—	—	+		Opportunistic
Enterobacter cloacae		v	—	v[b]	—	+		Opportunistic
E. agglomerans, E. sakazakii, E. gergoriae, Hafnia alvei								Opportunistic
Serratia marcescens		—	—	v[b]	—	+	Red pigment	Opportunistic
S. liquefaciens, S. rubidaea								Opportunistic
SALMONELLEAE								
Salmonella enteritidis	1000+ (O, H)	—	—	—	+	+		Diarrhea
Salmonella choleraesuis	1 (O, H)	—	—	—	v	+		Bacteremia
Salmonella typhi	1 (O, H, K)	—	—	—	+	+		Enteric (typhoid) fever
Arizona hinshawii	100+ (O, H)	v	—	—	+	+		Diarrhea; opportunistic
Citrobacter freundei		v	—	v[b]	+	+		Opportunistic
Citrobacter diversus		v	+	v[b]	—	+		Opportunistic
C. amalonaticus								Opportunistic
PROTEEAE								
Proteus mirabilis		—	—	+	+	+	Swarming[c]	Opportunistic
Proteus vulgaris		—	+	+	+	+	Swarming	Opportunistic
Morganella morganii, Providencia rettgeri, P. stuartii, P. alcalifaciens		—	+	v	—	+		Opportunistic
YERSINIEAE								
Yersinia pestis		—	—	—	—	—		Plague
Yersinia pseudotuberculosis	10 (O, H)	—	v	+[b]	—	+[a]		Mesenteric lymphadenitis
Yersinia enterocolitica	50+ (O, H)	—	—	+[b]	—	+[d]		Mesenteric lymphadenitis; enteric fever; diarrhea

Abbreviations: + = more than 90% of strains positive; — = less than 10% of strains positive; V = variable (some strains positive, others negative).

[a] Most common clinical isolates appear in boldface.

[b] Positive reactions weak or delayed compared to those of Proteeae.

[c] Growth swarms over surface of agar plates.

[d] Positive reactions seen at 25°C but not at 37°C.

Kenneth J. Ryan

Vibrio and *Campylobacter*

21

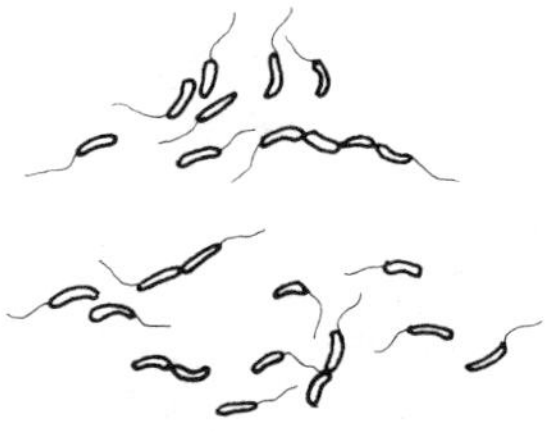

Vibrio cholerae

Vibrio

Vibrios are curved, Gram-negative rods commonly found in water. Cells may be linked end to end, forming S shapes and spirals. They are highly motile with a single polar flagellum, non-spore forming, oxidase positive, and can grow under aerobic or anaerobic conditions. The cell wall and surface structure is similar to that of other Gram-negative bacteria. Some species are pathogenic for humans, causing diarrheal illnesses. *Vibrio cholerae* is the cause of cholera.

Vibrio cholerae

Morphology. Cholera vibrios are slim, short, curved rods, about 0.5 × 3 μm in size. Their motility is extremely rapid.

tolerance for alkaline conditions

facultative anaerobe

Growth. The organism grows readily on the usual broth and solid media used in clinical laboratories. It has a low tolerance for acid, but grows under alkaline (pH 8.0–9.5) conditions that inhibit many other Gram-negative bacteria. It is facultatively anaerobic, but grows best under aerobic conditions.

epidemic cholera limited to serotype 0:1 strains

eltor biotype

Environmental isolates

Differential features. *Vibrio cholerae* is distinguished from other vibrios by its biochemical reactions, O antigenic structure, and production of a potent enterotoxin. From a medical standpoint, the taxonomy is somewhat confused because many strains with essentially the same biochemical reactions may or may not produce enterotoxin and cholera. The strains associated with epidemic cholera are limited to a single serogroup, 0:1, and are further divided into three serologic variants named *Ogawa, Inaba,* and *Hikojima.* A biochemical variant, *V. cholerae* biotype eltor, is sometimes called *Vibrio eltor.* Environmental strains unassociated with epidemic cholera are also termed *V. cholerae,* spawning terms such as *non-0:1 vibrios, nonagglutinable vibrios,* and *noncholera vibrios.* The latter strains have worldwide distribution and are frequently found in water, sewage, and various marine environments. Although they have occasionally been associated with diarrhea and with enterotoxin production, these organisms have not produced epidemic cholera. In the remainder of this chapter, *V. cholerae* will refer only to the serogroup 0:1 strains.

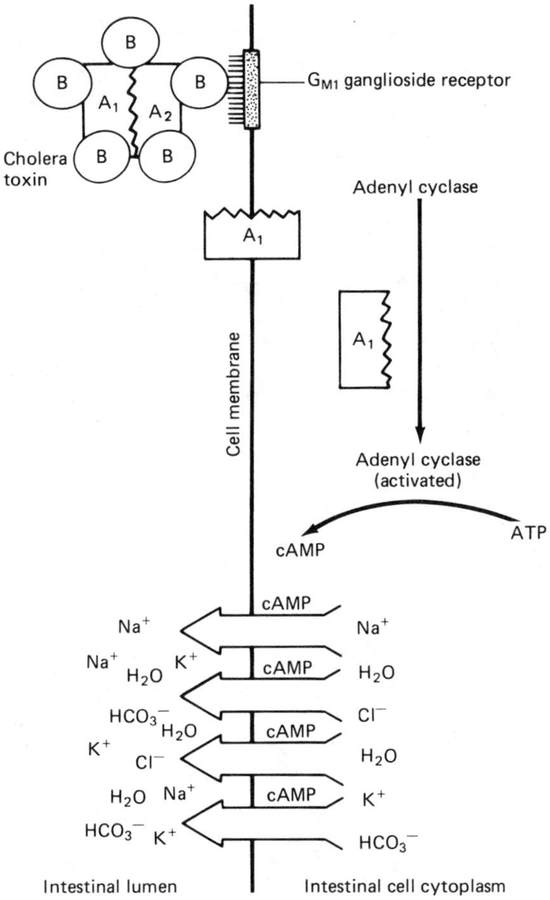

21.1 The action of cholera toxin. The complete toxin is shown binding to the GM1-ganglioside receptor on the cell membrane via the binding (B) subunits. The active portion (A_1) of the A subunit enters the cell and activates adenyl cyclase. The increased adenyl cyclase activity results in accumulation of cyclic adenosine 3′,5′-monophosphate (cAMP) along the cell membrane. The cAMP causes the active secretion of sodium (Na^+), chloride (Cl^-), potassium (K^+), bicarbonate (HCO_3^-), and water out of the cell into the intestinal lumen.

exotoxin with toxic unit and multiple binding units

ganglioside receptor for toxin

toxic unit activates adenyl cyclase

hypersecretion of water and electrolytes from increased cAMP causes diarrhea

Relation of cholera toxin to *E. coli* LT

Toxin. The outstanding feature of *V. cholerae* is the ability of virulent strains to produce a potent enterotoxic exotoxin responsible for the disease cholera. The structure and mechanism of action of this toxin have been studied extensively (Figure 21.1). Its molecule is an aggregate of multiple polypeptide chains organized into a toxic unit (A) and multiple binding units (B). The B units mediate tight binding to a ganglioside receptor on the cell membrane (the GM1-ganglioside). Once bound, the A portion of the active unit enters the cell and activates and stabilizes a membrane-associated enzyme, adenyl cyclase, which in turn stimulates the conversion of adenosine triphosphate to cyclic adenosine 3′,5′-monophosphate (cAMP). The net effect is excessive accumulation of cAMP at the cell membrane, which causes hypersecretion of chloride, potassium, bicarbonate, and associated water molecules out of the cell with consequent diarrhea when the intestinal mucosa is involved. This reaction is not specific for intestinal cells, as adenyl cyclase is found in many other cell types. Understanding the mechanism of action of cholera toxin has acquired additional importance with the discovery that other enterotoxins, such as the heat-labile toxin (LT) of *Escherichia coli* (Chapter 20), utilize the same mechanism. Synthesis of cholera toxin is controlled by a chromosomal gene, whereas the *E. coli* LT gene is located on a plasmid.

large infecting dose

Penetration of mucus and adherence

Pathogenesis. To produce disease, *V. cholerae* must reach the small intestine in sufficient numbers to multiply and colonize. In healthy people, ingestion of large numbers of bacteria is required to offset the acid barrier of the stomach. Colonization is aided by the ability of the organism to penetrate the surface mucus covering of the intestinal mucosa and adhere to the

Colonization of length of intestinal tract

epithelial surface. The mechanisms of adherence for *V. cholerae* have not been well defined. The organism can colonize the entire intestinal tract from the jejunum to the colon and multiply to high numbers.

Extensive fluid, potassium, and bicarbonate loss

The physiologic effects result from the intracellular action of toxin, which is produced at the epithelial surface. Their extent depends on the balance among amount of bacterial growth, toxin production, fluid secretion, and fluid absorption in the entire gastrointestinal tract. In general, an alkaline environment ideal for continued growth of the organism is produced, and fluid loss in the form of voluminous, watery stools results. The outpouring of fluid and electrolytes is greatest in the small intestine, where the secretory capacity is high and absorptive capacity low. The diarrheal fluid can amount to many liters per day, with approximately the same sodium content as plasma but two to five times the potassium and bicarbonate concentrations. The result is dehydration (isotonic fluid loss), hypokalemia (potassium loss), and metabolic acidosis (bicarbonate loss). The diarrheal fluid also contains mucus flecks, giving it a gross appearance called *rice-water stools.* Surprisingly, the intestinal mucosa remains unaltered except for some hyperemia. *Vibrio cholerae* does not invade, and there are no inflammatory or destructive changes.

intestinal mucosa structurally unaffected; no invasion

lower infecting dose in achlorhydria

immunity unassociated with circulating antibody; probably mediated by immunoglobulin A

Immunity. Nonspecific defenses such as gastric acidity, gut motility, and intestinal mucus are important in preventing colonization with *V. cholerae.* For example, in persons who lack gastric acidity (gastrectomy or achlorhydria from malnutrition), the attack rate of clinical cholera is higher. Humoral antibodies against both the O antigens and the toxin appear after immunization and disease, but their association with immunity is not clear. Cholera patients demonstrate resistance to subsequent challenge with *V. cholerae*; however, it is more likely that this resistance is attributable to local than to systemic mechanisms. The immune state has been associated with secretion of immunoglobulin A by lymphocytes in the subepithelial areas of the gastrointestinal tract, but the precise protective mechanism remains to be established. It includes the possibility of local action of antitoxin or of antibody blocking the attachment of the organism.

usual transmission of epidemic cholera through water

Interepidemic maintenance

Epidemiology. Epidemic cholera is spread primarily by contaminated water under conditions of poor sanitation, although other vehicles are clearly important in some instances. During epidemics, numerous vibrios purged from the intestines of infected individuals reach the primary water supply and are then transmitted to others via drinking, food preparation, or bathing. The maintenance of the organism in nature between epidemics is more obscure. It is fragile, surviving only a few days in the environment, but there is growing evidence that *V. cholerae* may be maintained in marine and fresh-water crustaceans. Convalescent human carriage is usually brief, and prolonged carriage very rare.

Spread of eltor biotype

The eltor biotype of *V. cholerae* has a longer survival in nature and is more likely to produce subclinical cases of cholera, both of which would aid its geographic spread and survival. This organism, first discovered in 1905 at El Tor quarantine camp for Mecca pilgrims, has been of increasing importance in the spread of epidemic cholera beyond its previous location in Africa and southern Asia. In the second half of the 20th century, cholera has slowly spread beyond its major endemic focus in the common delta of the Ganges and the Brahmaputra Rivers. This spread has involved Indonesia, south and central Asia, Africa, and western Europe. Recently, endemic cases of cholera caused by the eltor biotype were recognized in the United States. Infection resulted from eating inadequately cooked crabs caught off the Gulf Coast of Louisiana and Texas.

sporadic cases in U.S. associated with eating crabs caught in Southeast extreme watery diarrhea with large fluid loss

disease manifestations from dehydration and electrolyte imbalance

Clinical manifestations. Typical cholera has a rapid onset, beginning with abdominal fullness and discomfort, gurgling, rushes of peristalsis, and loose stools. Vomiting may also occur. The stools quickly become watery, voluminous, almost odorless, and contain mucus flecks. These characteristics account for their description as rice-water stools. There is no pus or blood in the stools, and the patient is afebrile. Other clinical features of cholera result from extensive fluid loss and electrolyte imbalance, which can lead to extreme dehydration, hypotension, and death within hours if untreated.

Stool culture using selective media

Diagnosis. The initial suspicion of cholera depends on recognition of the typical clinical features in an appropriate epidemiologic setting. *Vibrio cholerae* is not the only organism to cause watery diarrhea or rice-water stools, although it produces the most severe disease. A bacteriologic diagnosis is accomplished by isolation of *V. cholerae* from the stool. The organism grows on common clinical laboratory media such as blood agar and MacConkey agar, but its isolation is enhanced by the use of media and growth conditions that favor it selectively. These conditions include the use of an alkaline (pH 9.0) liquid medium and thiosulfate–citrate–bile salt–sucrose agar. Once isolated, the organism is readily identified by biochemical reactions; identification may be confirmed by agglutination with specific antisera, if available. In parts of the world where cholera is not endemic, these procedures are not routinely used in clinical laboratories and must be requested specifically.

Fluid and electrolyte replacement

Treatment. The outcome of cholera is dependent on balancing the diarrheal fluid and ionic losses with adequate fluid and electrolyte replacement. This balance is accomplished by oral and intravenous administration of solutions with near physiologic concentrations of sodium and chloride and higher than physiologic concentrations of potassium and bicarbonate. Exact formulas are available as packets to which a given volume of water is added. Oral replacement, particularly if begun early, is sufficient for all but the most severe cases. Antimicrobial therapy shortens the duration of diarrhea and magnitude of fluid loss. Tetracyclines have been used most frequently, although ampicillin, chloramphenicol, and trimethoprim–sulfamethoxazole have also been effective.

Antimicrobial therapy

hygienic disposal of excreta

water treatment

Vaccines

Prevention. Epidemic cholera, a disease of poor sanitation, does not occur where treatment and disposal of human waste is adequate. As good sanitary conditions do not exist in much of the world, secondary local measures such as boiling or chemical treatment of water during epidemics are required. Vaccines prepared from whole cells, lipopolysaccharide, and cholera toxoid have all been evaluated with variable results. Some preparations are protective, but do not yet confer the long-lasting immunity known to result from natural infection. There is interest in live but avirulent vaccines, but progress has been slow because of the lack of a good animal model and ethical restraints on experimentation in human volunteers.

The occasional cases associated with crustaceans could be prevented by adequate cooking and avoidance of recontamination from containers and surfaces.

Other Vibrios

Halophilic vibrios

Several less common infections have been associated with *Vibrio* species other than *V. cholerae.* Because of their salt requirement and normal habitat in seawater, these species are sometimes called *halophilic vibrios.* Bacteriologically, they resemble *V. cholerae* in many respects, but are readily distinguished on the basis of biochemical and serologic characteristics.

V. parahemolyticus infections from seafood

The most important of these species is *Vibrio parahemolyticus*, which causes an acute illness characterized by severe cramping, abdominal pain, and explosive watery diarrhea. Low-grade fever, chills, and headache are occasionally present. The incubation period is short, typically 24–48 hr after-ingestion. *Vibrio parahemolyticus* is commonly present in coastal waters throughout the world. Infection develops after ingestion of incompletely cooked seafood. In the United States, most cases have been detected in common source outbreaks involving shellfish. In countries such as Japan, where raw fish is commonly eaten, *V. parahemolyticus* accounts for a significant portion of all diarrheal illnesses. The disease is usually self-limiting, and the course is not affected by antimicrobial therapy.

Other halophilic vibrio species may cause infections of cuts and wounds contaminated with seawater. Such infections typically involve seashore bathers or fishermen. A bacteremic illness after ingestion of raw oysters has also been described.

Campylobacter

Similar morphology to vibrios

Campylobacters are small, curved, Gram-negative rods with morphologic features and motility similar to those of vibrios, although often present in pairs to give a "seagull" appearance. Like vibrios, campylobacters are oxidase positive. For many years they were classified as vibrios (*Vibrio fetus*), although their bacteriologic characteristics and DNA sequences are markedly different from those of *V. cholerae.* Campylobacters grow well only on enriched media under microaerophilic conditions (reduced oxygen tension but not strict anaerobiosis). Growth usually requires 2–4 days, sometimes as much as a pylobacters are biochemically inactive. A number of species and subspecies are recognized, two of which are of greatest medical importance: *Campylobacter fetus*, subspecies *fetus*, and *C. jejuni*. The former will be referred to herein as *C. fetus*.

slow growing microaerophiles

Probable zoonotic transmission

Campylobacters are commonly found in the normal gastrointestinal and genitourinary flora of animals, particularly sheep and cattle. Chickens, wild birds, and domestic animals such as dogs may also carry the organisms, and probably play a significant role in transmission to humans.

Campylobacter fetus

Bacteremia in humans

Campylobacter fetus has long been recognized as a common cause of abortion in sheep and cattle and a rare cause of sepsis in humans. The most common human presentation is of intermittent fever without evidence of localized infection. Occasionally the meninges and heart valves may become infected, and thrombophlebitis is considered a typical feature although it occurs in only 10% of cases. The diagnosis is established by isolation of *C. fetus* from the blood.

Campylobacter jejuni

Common cause of infectious diarrhea

Before 1973, *C. jejuni* was not recognized as a cause of human disease. It was not until selective media for its isolation were developed in the late 1970s that its importance was appreciated. This organism is now recognized as one of the most common causes of infectious diarrhea. Studies from various countries have associated *C. jejuni* with 5–10% of all cases of diarrhea, a percentage comparable to those for *Salmonella* and *Shigella.* The illness typically begins with lower abdominal pain, which may be severe enough to mimic acute appendicitis. The abdominal pain is followed by diarrheal

fever and evidence of mucosal invasion

stools containing blood and pus. Fever is commonly present. All of these features suggest an invasive or cytotoxic pathogenic mechanism, but neither has yet been proved.

The illness is typically self-limiting after 3–5 days, but may last 1–2 weeks. The diagnosis is confirmed by isolation of the organism from the stool using a special medium made selective for *Campylobacter* by inclusion of antimicrobics that inhibit the normal facultative flora of the bowel.

Treatment

Susceptibility to erythromycin

Campylobacters are generally susceptible to erythromycin, tetracycline, chloramphenicol, and aminoglycosides, but not to penicillins and cephalosporins. Enteritis caused by *C. jejuni* is usually self-limiting, and the effects of antimicrobics on its course remain unclear. Erythromycin has been suggested for severe cases on the basis of in vitro data and may be effective if given early in the course of the illness. Chloramphenicol, tetracycline, and aminoglycosides have also been cited as useful in treating *C. fetus* infections.

Additional Reading and References

Blake, P.A., Allegra, D.T., Snyder, J.D., Barrett, T.J., McFarland, L., Caraway, C.T., Feeley, J.C., Craig, J.P., Lee, J.V., Puhr, N.D., and Feldman, R.A. 1980. Cholera—A possible endemic focus in the United States. *N. Eng. J. Med.* 302:305–309. This study details the epidemiologic features of cholera cases along the Gulf Coast of Louisiana.

Finkelstein, R.A. 1975. Cholera enterotoxin. In *Microbiology—1975.* Schlessinger, D., Ed. Washington, D.C.: American Society for Microbiology, pp. 236–241. A concise, readable review of cholera toxin and its mechanism of action is provided.

Rettig, P.J. 1979. Campylobacter infections in human beings. *J. Pediatr.* 94:855–864. Both *Campylobacter fetus* and *Campylobacter jejuni* infections are reviewed in detail. The report nicely documents the importance of *C. jejuni* as an intestinal pathogen.

Kenneth J. Ryan

Pseudomonas and Other Opportunistic Gram-Negative Bacilli

22

A number of opportunistic Gram-negative rods of several genera not considered in other chapters are discussed herein. With the exception of *Pseudomonas aeruginosa* they rarely cause disease, and all are frequently encountered as contaminants and superficial colonizers. The significance of their isolation from clinical material thus depends on the circumstance and site of culture and on the clinical situation of the patient.

Pseudomonas aeruginosa

Pseudomonas aeruginosa is an aerobic, motile, Gram-negative rod; its outstanding bacteriologic feature is the production of colorful water-soluble pigments. It is commonly found free living in moist environments but is also a pathogen of plants, animals, and humans. As a cause of infection, it is particularly important in severely burned patients, in those with hematologic and other malignancies, and in the intubated urinary tract. It is also the most consistently resistant of all the medically important bacteria to antimicrobics.

Morphology and Structure

polar flagella

Pseudomonas aeruginosa is generally slimmer and more pale staining than members of the Enterobacteriaceae, but its length is comparable (0.5×2.5 μm). Its flagella are polar, but otherwise morphologic differences from other Gram-negative bacteria are not sufficiently consistent to be diagnostically useful. Ultrastructural features are similar to those of other Gram-negative bacteria. The lipopolysaccharide (LPS) present in the cell wall is structurally similar to that of the Enterobacteriaceae, but differs in some chemical groupings. The composition of the polysaccharide side chains extending from the outer membrane LPS is believed to determine serologic specificity and susceptibility to bacteriocins (pyocins) and bacteriophages. The slime layer has a mixed chemical composition but is primarily polysaccharide. Pili are present on the cell surface.

LPS

slime layer

Growth and Metabolism

aerobes with simple growth requirements

Pseudomonas aeruginosa is an aerobe sufficiently versatile in its growth and energy requirements to utilize simple molecules such as ammonia and carbon dioxide as sole nitrogen and carbon sources. Thus, it does not require enriched media for growth, and it can survive and multiply over a wide temperature range (20–42°C) in almost any environment, including those with a high salt content. The organism uses oxidative energy-producing mechanisms and synthesizes large amounts of cytochrome–oxidase; it is thus oxidase positive. Although an aerobic atmosphere is necessary for optimal growth and metabolism, most strains will multiply slowly in an anaerobic environment if nitrate is present as a hydrogen acceptor.

oxidase positive

Growth on all common isolation media is luxurious, although not as rapid as that of the Enterobacteriaceae. Colonies are well developed after overnight incubation, usually show green pigmentation, and have a delicate, fringed edge. Confluent growth often has a characteristic metallic sheen. Hemolysis may be produced on blood agar. In broth, a surface pellicle is formed, reflecting the organism's preference for aerobic conditions and chemotaxis toward oxygen.

fringed, irregular colonies at 18 hr

surface pellicle in liquid media

Classification

Pseudomonas aeruginosa is one of several oxidase-positive, motile organisms to produce non-lactose-fermenting colonies on MacConkey agar. Its oxidase reaction differentiates it from the Enterobacteriaceae, and its production of blue, yellow, or rust-colored pigments from most other Gram-negative bacteria. The blue pigment, pyocyanin, is produced only by *P. aeruginosa*; its demonstration, however, requires a balance of magnesium, iron, and other ions not found in all media that support its growth. Fluorescin, a yellow pigment that fluoresces under ultraviolet light, is also produced; however, it is not unique to *P. aeruginosa*. The combination of pyocyanin and fluorescin produces a bright green color that diffuses throughout the medium (Plate S). A rust-colored pigment, pyorubrin, is produced by a small proportion of strains. The combination of pyocyanin production and the ability to grow at 42°C is sufficient to distinguish *P. aeruginosa* from other pseudomonads.

no lactose fermentation

Production of blue pyocyanin and yellow fluorescin imparts green color to growth

growth at 42°C

Several systems for subtyping *P. aeruginosa* have been developed; 7–29 serotypes have been defined depending on the particular scheme used. *Pseudomonas* bacteriocins (pyocins) and bacteriophages that lyse *P. aeruginosa* in varying patterns have been isolated and organized into typing systems. The number of types, which depends on the number of indicator strains used, can exceed 30. Various combinations of these typing systems are used for epidemiologic studies. The typing schemes have no particular relation to one another, and individual types have no unique pathogenic or clinical significance.

Serologic, bacteriocin, and phage types

Toxins and Extracellular Products

In addition to the pigments, most strains of *P. aeruginosa* produce extracellular products, including exotoxin A, proteolytic enzymes destructive to tissues, lecithinase, collagenase, and an elastase that digests the elastin found in arterial walls. Hemolysins and a leukocidin have also been described. An enterotoxin produces fluid accumulation in the intestinal tract of animals; it has not been clearly characterized, however, and its role in human disease is uncertain.

Extracellular enzymes

Exotoxin A, the most potent toxic factor, has been studied in greatest detail. It is 10,000 times more toxic to experimental animals than *Pseudomonas* LPS endotoxin and is found in more than 90% of clinical isolates. Mutants that lack exotoxin A have much decreased virulence for experimental animals, and antitoxin protects animals against otherwise fatal challenge with exotoxin A-producing strains. The toxin acts to inhibit protein synthesis by a mechanism identical to that of diphtheria toxin (Chapter 13). It catalyzes

exotoxin A resembles diphtheria toxin

a reaction leading to inactivation of elongation factor 2, an enzyme responsible for sequential elongation of proteins on the ribosome.

Epidemiology

primary habitat environmental

The primary habitat of *P. aeruginosa* and other pseudomonads is environmental. They are found in water, soil, and various types of vegetation throughout the world. *Pseudomonas aeruginosa* has been isolated from the throat and stool of 2–10% of healthy persons. Colonization rates may be higher in hospitalized patients.

can produce invasive infections in immunocompromised hosts

Infection with *P. aeruginosa,* rare in previously healthy persons, is one of the most important causes of invasive infection in compromised patients with serious underlying disease, such as leukemia, cystic fibrosis, and extensive burns. The organism's ability to survive and proliferate in water with minimal nutrients can lead to heavy contamination of any unsterile water, such as that in the humidifiers of respirators. Inhalation of aerosols from such sources can bypass the normal respiratory defense mechanisms and initiate pulmonary infection. Infections have resulted from the growth of *Pseudomonas* in medications, contact lens solutions, and even in some disinfectants. Sinks and faucet aerators may be heavily contaminated and serve as the environmental source for contamination of other items. It is important to recognize, however, that the simple finding of a few *P. aeruginosa* in solutions or sites not normally sterile (for example, drinking water, food) is not in itself abnormal or a cause for alarm. The risk lies in the proximity between items susceptible to contamination and patients uniquely predisposed to infection.

multiplication in humidifiers, solutions, and moist environments

Pathogenesis and Immunity

Need for break in first-line defenses

Although *P. aeruginosa* is an opportunistic pathogen, it is one of particular virulence. The organism usually requires a significant break in first-line defenses (such as a wound) or a route past them (such as a contaminated respirator or intratracheal tube) to initiate infection. Surface pili may facilitate attachment to surfaces, and the slime layer impairs in vitro phagocytosis unless opsonized. The relative roles of the cellular LPS and extracellular enzymes in virulence have been a source of some debate, but current opinion favors the latter as most important, particularly exotoxin A. The toxicity of *Pseudomonas* LPS is weak compared to that of the Enterobacteriaceae; it is a potent immunogen, however, and LPS-directed antibody may decrease the incidence of fatal burn infections. Exotoxin A production is associated with a fatal outcome in bacteremic patients. Antitoxin against it is associated with survival, although the diphtherialike action of exotoxin A does not correlate with the primarily invasive and locally destructive lesions seen in *P. aeruginosa* infections.

Multifactorial nature of virulence

The virulence of *P. aeruginosa* is therefore probably multifactorial. After invasion, the protection from phagocytosis afforded by LPS and slime may provide sufficient time for production of collagenases, elastases, and other enzymes, allowing spread and local tissue destruction. Exotoxin A may be an important contributor to the lethal effects of widespread infection.

Clinical Manifestations

Range of opportunistic infections

Burn infections

Pseudomonas aeruginosa can produce any of the opportunistic extraintestinal infections caused by members of the Enterobacteriaceae, but *Pseudomonas* infections are generally less common. Burn, wound, urinary tract, skin, eye, ear, and respiratory infections all occur. Infection of severe burns is common;

Bacteremia and ecthyma gangrenosum

bacteremia may be a sequel to this or to other severe infection. In some cases of *P. aeruginosa* bacteremia, the cutaneous syndrome of ecthyma gangrenosum develops. It begins with a few painful maculopapular lesions of the skin. As they enlarge over 2–3 days a purple, then black, necrosis develops in the center of the lesion, as a result of direct invasion of blood vessel walls by the organism. *Pseudomonas aeruginosa* is also one of the most common causes of infection associated with injuries in which there is environmental contamination of the wound (for example, osteomyelitis after compound fractures, deep puncture wounds). Such injuries are the major route of deep-seated infection in immunologically normal persons.

Osteomyelitis after wounds

Pneumonia

Pseudomonas aeruginosa pneumonia is a severe infection. It was common after the use of respirators with contaminated humidifiers and occurs in hospitalized patients with granulocytopenia. It is particularly severe and associated with alveolar necrosis, vascular invasion, infarcts, and bacteremia. *Pseudomonas aeruginosa* is also a common cause of otitis externa, particularly the "swimmer's ear" seen in children who spend most of the summer in a pool, and of a rare but life-threatening "malignant" otitis externa in diabetics. Folliculitis of the skin may follow soaking in hot tubs heavily contaminated with the organism.

Otitis externa and folliculitis

Eye infections

The organism can cause conjunctivitis, keratitis, or endophthalmitis when introduced into the eye by trauma or contaminated medication or contact lens solution. Keratitis can progress rapidly and destroy the cornea within 24–48 hr.

Cystic fibrosis infections

Pseudomonas aeruginosa is now the most common bacterial pathogen to complicate the management of patients with cystic fibrosis, an inherited disease of exocrine glands associated with excessive viscid mucus in the smaller respiratory passages. A high proportion of cases become colonized, and the organism may cause or contribute to tracheobronchitis or pneumonia. Pseudomonads isolated from these patients usually produce markedly mucoid colonies because of their extensive matrix of extracellular polysaccharide material. Production of this extracellular polysaccharide probably gives *P. aeruginosa* a survival advantage in the conditions that obtain in the respiratory tract with cystic fibrosis.

Treatment and Prevention

Antimicrobic resistance

Of the pathogenic bacteria, *P. aeruginosa* is the organism most consistently resistant to antimicrobics. It is so regularly resistant to penicillin, ampicillin, cephalothin, tetracycline, chloramphenicol, sulfonamides, and the earlier aminoglycosides (streptomycin, kanamycin) that it is fruitless to perform a susceptibility test with these agents. Much effort has been directed toward the development of antimicrobics with anti-*Pseudomonas* activity. The newer aminoglycosides, gentamicin, tobramycin, and amikacin are all active against most strains despite occasional mutational and plasmid-mediated resistance. Carbenicillin and ticarcillin are active and can be given in high doses, but plasmid-mediated resistance occurs more frequently than with the aminoglycosides. A primary feature of the third-generation cephalosporins (for example, cefotaxime, moxalactam, and cefoperazone) is their activity against *Pseudomonas*. In general, urinary infections may be treated with a single drug; serious systemic *P. aeruginosa* infections, however, are often treated with a combination of an anti-*Pseudomonas* β-lactam antimicrobic and an aminoglycoside, particularly in neutropenic patients. In all cases susceptibility must be confirmed in vitro.

combined therapy

Vaccines

Vaccines incorporating multiple *P. aeruginosa* serotypes have been developed and proved immunogenic in humans. The primary candidates for such preparations are patients with burn injuries, cystic fibrosis, or immunosuppression. Although some protection has been demonstrated, these preparations are still experimental.

Other Pseudomonads

There are a large number of *Pseudomonas* species other than *P. aeruginosa*; however, the total number of infections produced by these species is far less than that produced by *P. aeruginosa* alone. As with other opportunists, they are most frequently seen as colonizers and contaminants. Those of medical importance are shown in Table 22.1. With the exception of the *Pseudomonas pseudomallei* group, the assignment of species names has little clinical importance beyond differentiation from *P. aeruginosa*. Reports vary regarding the frequency of their isolation from cases of bacteremia, arthritis, abscesses, wounds, conjunctivitis, and urinary tract infections. In any individual case the significance of isolating one of these species must be decided on its own merits. In general, unless isolated in pure culture from a high-quality (direct) specimen, it is difficult to attach pathogenic significance to any of the miscellaneous *Pseudomonas* species.

environmental habitat of *P. pseudomallei*

Pseudomonas pseudomallei is not found in the United States. The organism exists as a saprophyte in soil, ponds, rice paddies, and produce in Southeast Asia, the Philippines, Indonesia, and other tropical areas. Infection is acquired by direct inoculation or by inhalation of aerosols or dust containing the bacteria. The disease, melioidosis, is usually an acute pneumonia; however, it is sufficiently variable that subacute, chronic, and even relapsing infections may follow systemic spread. The clinical and radiologic features may resemble tuberculosis. In fulminant cases, rapid respiratory failure may ensue and metastatic abscesses develop in the skin or other sites. Tetracycline, chloramphenicol, sulfonamides, and trimethoprim–sulfamethoxazole have been effective in therapy.

Acute or chronic pulmonary infection

metastatic abscesses

Glanders is a disease of horses and some other mammals caused by *Pseudomonas mallei*. Transmission to humans is extremely rare. The disease manifests as local suppurative or acute pulmonary infections.

Pseudomonas cepacia is an opportunistic organism that has recently been recognized to contaminate reagents, disinfectants, and medical devices in much the same manner as *P. aeruginosa*.

Table 22.1 Pseudomonads Associated with Human Infection

		Bacteriologic Features			
Group	Species	Pyocyanin	Other Pigments	Gentamicin Resistance	Disease
Fluorescent	*P. aeruginosa*	+	+	5–20%	Opportunistic
	P. fluorescens	—	+	Uncommon	Opportunistic
	P. putida	—	+	Uncommon	Opportunistic
Pseudomallei	*P. mallei*	—	—	—	Glanders
	P. pseudomallei	—	—	90%	Melioidosis
	P. cepacia	—	—	90%	Opportunistic
Other	*P. alcaligenes*	—	—	Uncommon	Opportunistic
	P. stutzeri	—	—	Uncommon	Opportunistic
	P. maltophilia	—	+	Uncommon	Opportunistic
	P. putrifaciens	—	—	Uncommon	Opportunistic
	P. acidovarians	—	—	Uncommon	Opportunistic

Acinetobacter

coccoid forms common

The genus *Acinetobacter* comprises Gram-negative coccobacilli that occasionally appear sufficiently round on Gram smears to be confused with *Neisseria.* On primary isolation they closely resemble the Enterobacteriaceae in growth pattern and colonial morphology, but are distinguished by their failure to ferment carbohydrates or reduce nitrates. Although the two major species have well-defined characteristics, the taxonomy has been confused by the use of many names in the past, including *Mima* and *Herellea.* The organism most commonly classified as *Mima* is now termed *Acinetobacter calcoaceticus* var. *lwoffii* (*A. lwoffii*) and *Herellea vaginicola* as *Acinetobacter calcoaceticus* var. *anitratus* (*A. anitratus*).

opportunistic pulmonary, urinary tract, and soft tissue infections

As with most of the organisms discussed in this chapter, the isolation of *Acinetobacter* from clinical material does not define infection, because they appear most frequently as colonizers and contaminants. Pneumonia is the most common infection, followed by urinary tract and soft tissue infections. Nosocomial respiratory infections have been traced to contaminated inhalation therapy equipment, and bacteremia to infected intravenous catheters. Treatment is complicated by frequent resistance to penicillins, cephalosporins, chloramphenicol, and occasionally aminoglycosides.

Moraxella

Moraxella is another genus of coccobacillary, Gram-negative rods that are usually paired end to end. Some species require enriched media, such as blood or chocolate agar. Their morphology, fastidious growth, and positive oxidase reaction can result in confusion with *Neisseria.* The organism now called *Moraxella lacunata,* originally described as a cause of angular conjunctivitis, is an uncommon isolate from any site. All species rarely cause disease. They are susceptible to penicillin.

Aeromonas and *Plesiomonas*

The genera *Aeromonas* and *Plesiomonas* have features similar to those of both the Enterobacteriaceae and *Pseudomonas.* They are aerobic and facultatively anaerobic, attack carbohydrates fermentatively, and demonstrate various other biochemical reactions. Their colonies and growth pattern resemble those of the Enterobacteriaceae. The major taxonomic resemblance to *Pseudomonas* is that both *Aeromonas* and *Plesiomonas* are oxidase positive with polar flagella. Their habitat is basically environmental (water and soil), but they can occasionally be found in the human intestinal tract. In addition to opportunistic infection, some evidence suggests an occasional role in gastroenteritis through production of an enterotoxin. Resistance to penicillins and cephalosporins is common. Most strains show susceptibility to chloramphenicol and tetracycline, with variable susceptibility to aminoglycosides, including gentamicin.

Other Gram-Negative Rods

Nonfermenters

The terms *miscellaneous* or *nonfermenter* are used loosely by bacteriologists to describe Gram-negative rods that do not ferment carbohydrates or that fail to react in many of the tests used to characterize other bacteria. Identification is frequently delayed as additional tests are tried or the organism is sent to a reference laboratory. As the clinical significance of all these organisms is essentially the same, the clinician will usually receive a report of a "nonfermenter" or another descriptive term and a susceptibility test result. The clinical significance of the isolate is then decided on other grounds. The major characteristics of some of these organisms are shown in Table 22.2. All have little inherent virulence and rarely cause infection. The types of

Table 22.2 Characteristics of Miscellaneous Gram-Negative Bacilli

Organism	Usual Habitat	Bacteriologic Features				Infection
		Growth on MacConkey Agar	Oxidase	Motility	Other	
Alkaligenes	Respiratory tract; intestinal tract	+	+	+		Blood; urine; wounds
Cardiobacterium	Respiratory tract; intestinal tract	−	+	−	CO_2 required	Endocarditis
Chromobacterium	Environmental (tropical)	+	+	v	Blue to yellow pigments	Blood; abscesses
Actinobacillus	Oral	−	+	+	CO_2 required	Endocarditis
Flavobacterium	Environmental	−	+	−	Yellow pigment	Meningitis; nosocomial
Eikenella	Respiratory tract	−	+	−	CO_2 required; pits agar	Abscesses; endocarditis

Abbreviations: + = usually positive (more than 90%); − = usually negative (less than 10%); V = variable.

infection listed represent the most common among scattered case reports, and should not be interpreted as typical for each organism.

Some Gram-negative nonfermenters fail to conform to any of the species currently recognized, usually because of insufficient isolates or lack of interest in assigning any unifying bacteriologic or clinical significance. Such strains are usually referred by hospitals to reference centers, such as the Centers for Disease Control (CDC) in Atlanta. They are kept and assigned numbers to aid in comparison with similar past and future strains. Eventually, some are given designations such as "CDC group IIF," which may appear in clinical reports. Much later, a new genus and/or species name may be issued if agreement among taxonomists is sufficient.

Additional Reading and References

Cross, A.S., Sadoff, J.C., Iglewski, B.H., and Sokol, P.A. 1980. Evidence for the role of toxin A in the pathogenesis of infections with *Pseudomonas aeruginosa* in humans. *J. Infect. Dis.* 142:538–546.

Ohman, D.E., Burns, R.P., and Iglewski, B.H. 1980. Corneal infections in mice with toxin A and elastase mutants of *Pseudomonas aeruginosa*. *J. Infect. Dis.* 142:547–555. This paper and the previous reference provide strong evidence for the important role of *Pseudomonas aeruginosa* toxin A in the pathogenesis of both animal and human infections.

Kenneth J. Ryan

Some Bacteria Causing Zoonotic Diseases

23

Many bacterial, rickettsial, and viral diseases are classified as *zoonoses,* because they are acquired by humans either directly or indirectly from animals. This chapter includes organisms causing four zoonotic infections that are not discussed in other chapters. All four, *Brucella, Yersinia pestis, Francisella tularensis,* and *Pasteurella multocida,* are Gram-negative bacilli that are primarily animal pathogens. The diseases that they cause, brucellosis, plague, and tularemia, are rare in humans and develop only after unique animal contact. The full range of zoonoses considered in this chapter and others is shown in Table 23.1.

Brucella and Brucellosis

Three species important in human disease

Brucellosis (sometimes known as *undulant fever* or *Malta fever*) is a genitourinary infection of sheep, cattle, pigs, and other animals caused by several species of *Brucella.* Three are of importance in human medicine: *Brucella abortus, Brucella melitensis,* and *Brucella suis.* Humans become infected directly by occupational contact with these animals (farmers, slaughterhouse workers, veterinarians) or indirectly by consumption of contaminated animal products such as milk. In humans, the reticuloendothelial system is the primary site of infection, producing a prolonged febrile systemic illness.

Microbiology

Gram-negative coccobacilli

Growth requirements

Brucella species are small, coccobacillary, Gram-negative rods that resemble *Haemophilus* and *Bordetella* morphologically (Chapter 17). They are nonmotile, non-acid fast, and non-spore forming. Growth requires an aerobic environment and enriched media such as trypticase soy or blood agar. One species, *B. abortus,* requires enrichment of the atmosphere to 5–10% carbon dioxide. Colonies are not visible on solid media until 2–3 days of incubation, and broth cultures may require more time depending on the size of the inoculum.

slow growth

S to R variation

The antigenic structure of *Brucella* is complex. A smooth (S) even colony form, generally present on primary isolation, is associated with the presence of a small capsule and virulence. Rough (R) colonies have an uneven surface and tend to replace the S form on repeated subculture. They are composed of mutants that have lost their capsules and most of their virulence. Surface protein–lipopolysaccharide surface antigens designated *A* (abortus) and *M*

protein--lipopolysaccharide A and M surface antigens

Table 23.1 Some Important Bacterial and Rickettsial Zoonotic Infections

Disease	Etiologic Agent	Usual Reservoir	Usual Mode of Transmission to Humans	Transmission between Humans	Mode of Transmission between Humans	Special Characteristics
Anthrax	*Bacillus anthracis*	Cattle, sheep, goats	Infected animals or products	No[a]		Resistant spores
Bovine tuberculosis	*Mycobacterium bovis*	Cattle	Milk	No[a]		
Brucellosis	*Brucella* sp.	Cattle, swine, goats	Milk, infected carcasses	No[a]		
Campylobacter infection	*C. fetus, C. jejuni*	Wild mammals, cattle, sheep, pets	Contaminated food and water	Yes	Fecal–oral	
Leptospirosis	*Leptospira* sp.	Cattle, rodents	Water contaminated with urine	No[a]		
Pasteurellosis	*Pasteurella multocida*	Animal oral cavities	Bites, scratches	No[a]		
Plague	*Yersinia pestis*	Rodents	Fleas	Yes	Droplet (pneumonic) spread	Great epidemic potential
Other *Yersinia* infections	*Y. enterocolitica, Y. pseudotuberculosis*	Wild mammals, pigs, cattle, pets	Fecal–oral	Yes	Fecal–oral	
Relapsing fever	*Borrelia recurrentis*	Rodents, ticks	Ticks	Yes	Body louse[b]	Epidemic potential
Salmonellosis	*Salmonella enteritidis*	Poultry, livestock	Contaminated food	Yes	Fecal contamination of food	
Rickettsial spotted fevers	e.g., *R. rickettsii*	Rodents, ticks, mites	Ticks, mites	No[a]		
Murine typhus	*Rickettsia typhi*	Rodents	Fleas	No[a]		
Q fever	*Coxiella burnetii*	Cattle, sheep, goats	Contaminated dust and aerosois	No[a]		

[a] What never? No never. What *never*? Well, hardly ever! (W.S. Gilbert, "H.M.S. Pinafore").
[b] The transmissability of tick-borne relapsing fever between humans by the body louse is uncertain.

(melitensis) are present in different amounts in all three species; A predominates in *B. abortus* and M in *B. melitensis.*

Biochemical characteristics

Species differentiation

Taxonomically, *Brucella* species are not closely related to any other genus, but are homogeneous as judged by analysis of nucleic acid base ratios and DNA homology. All species produce catalase, oxidase, and urease, but do not ferment carbohydrates. They are differentiated by the relative predominance of A and M antigens, CO_2 requirements for growth, hydrogen sulfide production, and the ability of particular concentrations of the dyes thionin and basic fuchsin to inhibit their growth (Table 23.2).

Table 23.2 Characteristic Features of *Brucella* Species

Characteristic	*B. abortis*	*B. melitensis*	*B. suis*
Carbon dioxide requirement	+	−	−
Hydrogen sulfide production	+	−	±
Growth in presence of			
Thionin[a]	−	+	+
Basic fuchsin[a]	+	+	−

[a] Concentration of 1:50,000 in nutrient medium.

Epidemiology

abortion in cattle, goats, and hogs

Brucellosis is an important cause of abortion, sterility, and decreased milk production in cattle, goats, and hogs. It is spread among animals by direct contact with infected tissues and ingestion of contaminated feed and causes chronic infection of the mammary glands, uterus, placenta, seminal vesicles, and epididymis. Although the associations are not absolute, each species is linked to a different animal: *B. abortus* tends to infect cattle, *B. melitensis,* goats, and *B. suis,* hogs.

Unpasteurized milk

Humans acquire the infection by occupational exposure or consumption of unpasteurized dairy products. The organisms may gain access through cuts in the skin, contact with mucous membranes, inhalation, or ingestion. In the United States, the number of cases has dropped steadily from a maximum of more than 6000 per year in the 1940s to the current level of 150–200 per year. Of these cases, 50–60% are in abattoir employees, government meat inspectors, veterinarians, and others who handle livestock or meat products. Consumption of unpasteurized dairy products, which accounts for 8–10% of infections, is the leading source in persons who have no connection with the meat processing or livestock industries. Some recent cases of this type have been associated with "health" foods. In the United States, the distribution of human cases of brucellosis includes virtually every state, but is concentrated in those with large livestock industries (Iowa, Virginia, and Texas).

Pathogenesis and Immunity

Multiplication in macrophages

spread to reticuloendothelial system

activated macrophages inhibit growth

immunity exclusively cell mediated

erythritol in animal placentas

After penetration of the skin or mucous membranes, the organisms are carried within polymorphonuclear leukocytes through the lymph to the systemic circulation by way of the regional lymph nodes and the thoracic duct. Virulent *Brucella* can enter and multiply in macrophages in the liver sinusoids, spleen, bone marrow, and other components of the reticuloendothelial system. Smooth (virulent) *Brucella* strains possess a currently unknown virulence factor that allows some growth despite local macrophage activation and proliferation. The factors that ultimately control infection are complex, although it appears that activated macrophages from infected animals kill virulent organisms more readily than those activated by other stimuli. Thus, intracellular events in the monocyte determine the outcome of a *Brucella* infection, and control is dependent on active T-cell response. Antibodies to *Brucella* antigens can be detected in the sera of patients by a variety of methods, but there is no evidence that they alter the natural history of disease or confer immunity. Exotoxins, capsules, or antiphagocytic components are apparently not involved in virulence. In cows, sheep, pigs, and goats, erythritol, a four-carbon alcohol present in chorionic tissue, markedly stimulates growth of *Brucella.* This stimulation probably accounts for the tendency of the organism to locate in these sites. The human placenta does not contain erythritol.

Granulomas

recurrent bacteremia

If not controlled locally, infection progresses with the formation of small granulomas at the sites of bacterial multiplication and the release of bacteria back into the systemic circulation. These recurrent bacteremic episodes are largely responsible for the recurrent chills and fever of the clinical illness. The entire cycle resembles that of another intracellular pathogen, *Salmonella typhi,* and its disease, typhoid fever (Chapter 20).

Clinical Illness

night sweats

periodic fever

chronic illness and weight loss

splenomegaly

localized infection

Brucellosis starts with malaise, chills, and fever 7–21 days after infection. Drenching sweats in the late afternoon or evening are common, as well as temperatures in the range of 39.4–40°C. The pattern of periodic nocturnal fever (undulant fever) typically continues for weeks, months, or even 1–2 years, and the patient becomes chronically ill with associated body aches, headache, and anorexia. Weight loss of up to 20 kg may occur during prolonged illness. Despite these dramatic effects, physical findings and localizing signs are few. Less than 25% of patients show detectable enlargement of the reticuloendothelial organs, the primary site of infection. Of such findings, splenomegaly is most common, followed by lymphadenopathy and hepatomegaly. Occasionally, localized infection develops in the lung, bone, brain, heart, or genitourinary system. These cases usually lack the pronounced systemic symptoms of the typical illness.

Diagnosis

Cultural diagnosis

Definitive diagnosis requires isolation of *Brucella* from the blood or from biopsy specimens of the liver, bone marrow, or lymph nodes. Supplementation with CO_2 is needed for growth of *B. abortus.* The slow growth of some strains requires prolonged incubation of culture media to achieve isolation. Blood cultures in particular may require 2–4 weeks for growth, although most are positive in 2–5 days.

agglutinins ≥ 1:640

The diagnosis is often made serologically, but is subject to the same interpretive constraints as all serologic tests. Antibodies that agglutinate suspensions of heat-killed organisms typically reach titers of 1:640 or more in acute disease. Lower titers may reflect previous disease or cross-reacting antibodies. Titers return to the normal range within a year after successful therapy.

Treatment and Prevention

tetracycline

control in cattle

pasteurization

Tetracycline is the primary antimicrobic for the treatment of brucellosis. In seriously ill patients, streptomycin or gentamicin may be added. The therapeutic response is not rapid; 2–7 days may pass before patients become afebrile. Up to 10% of cases have relapses in the first 3 months after therapy. Prevention is primarily by control of brucellosis in animals using a combination of immunization and eradication of infected stock. Measures to minimize occupational exposure and the pasteurization of dairy products are important. No human vaccine is used in the United States.

Yersinia pestis and Plague

Plague is an infection of rodents and small mammals caused by *Y. pestis.* It is transmitted to humans by the bite of infected fleas. The disease has two major cycles, urban and sylvatic, and two major clinical forms, bubonic and pneumonic. The combined pathogenic and epidemiologic potential of *Y. pestis* makes it one of the most potent and feared pathogens known.

Microbiology

Yersinia pestis is a nonmotile, non-spore-forming, Gram-negative bacillus with a tendency toward pleomorphism and bipolar staining. It has recently been reclassified as a member of the Enterobacteriaceae. Its biology is discussed in Chapter 20 with that of the other members of the genus *Yersinia.*

Epidemiology

Black Death

The term *plague* is often used generically to describe any explosive pandemic disease with high mortality, although medically it refers only to infections caused by *Y. pestis.* This reputation was justly earned, because *Y. pestis* was the cause of the most virulent epidemic plague of recorded human history, the Black Death of the Middle Ages. In the 14th century, the estimated population of Europe was 105 million; Between 1346 and 1350, 25 million died of plague. Pandemics continued through the end of the 19th and the early 20th century despite elaborate quarantine measures developed in response to the obvious communicability of the disease. Yersin isolated the etiologic agent in China in 1894 and named it after his mentor, Pasteur. Until recently, *Y. pestis* was known as *Pasteurella pestis.*

Urban plague

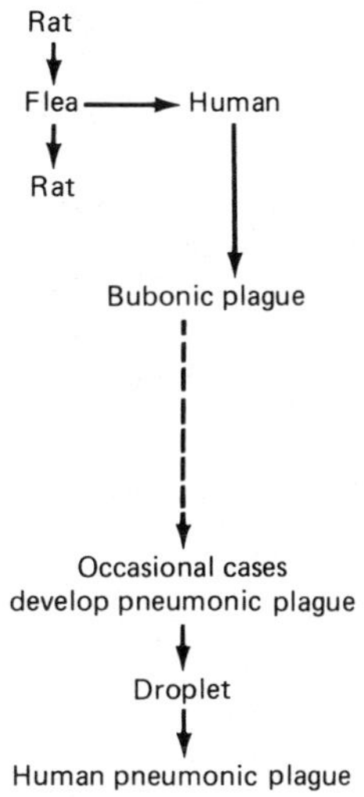

The plagues of the Middle Ages are examples of the urban cycle involving rats and humans. The first step probably involves infection of rats from a sylvatic source. Under poor hygienic conditions and when food sources elsewhere are scarce, rat populations in cities increase, which facilitates rat-to-rat transmission of *Y. pestis* by the rat flea (*Xenopsylla cheopis*). It also brings the primary rat reservoir into contact with humans. When the number of nonimmune rats is sufficient, epizootic plague develops among them with high mortality. As the bacteremic rat dies, its fleas seek a new host, which is usually another rat, but may be a human. The infected flea regurgitates *Y. pestis* from the proventriculus into the bite wound. The probability of transmission to humans is thus greatest when both the rat population and rat mortality are high. The bite of the flea is the first event in the development of a case of bubonic plague, which, even if serious enough to kill the patient, is not normally contagious to other humans. Some patients with bubonic plague, however, develop a secondary pneumonia by bacteremic spread to the lungs. They can then transmit pneumonic plague directly to others by droplet spread. It is not hard to see how rapid spread proceeds in conjunction with crowded unsanitary conditions and continued flea-to-human transmission. An urban plague epidemic is vividly described in Albert Camus' novel *The Plague.*

Sylvatic plague

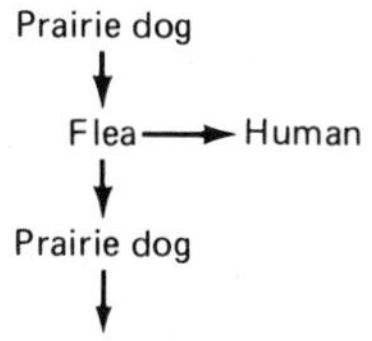

Although urban plague epidemics have been essentially eliminated by rat control and other public health measures, a sylvatic transmission cycle persists in many parts of the world, including North America. This cycle involves nonurban mammals such as prairie dogs, deer mice, rabbits, and wood rats. Transmission between them is accomplished by fleas. Coyotes or wolves may be infected by the same fleas or by ingestion of infected rodents. By their nature, these animals rarely come in contact with humans; when they do, however, the infected fleas they carry can transmit *Y. pestis.* The most common circumstance is a child exploring the outdoors who comes across a dead or dying prairie dog and pokes, carries, or touches it long enough to be bitten by the fleas leaving the animal. The result is a sporadic case of bubonic plague, which occasionally becomes pneumonic.

most human cases in California, Arizona, Utah, New Mexico, and Colorado

Sylvatic plague exists in most continents, but is not found in Western Europe or Australasia. In the United States, the primary enzootic areas are the semiarid plains of the western states. Infected animals and fleas have been detected from the Mexican border to the eastern half of Washington.

increasing incidence in U.S.

Most human cases have occurred in California or the "four corners" area where Arizona, Utah, Colorado, and New Mexico meet. Since the 1950s, the number of cases of plague in the United States has been slowly increasing from a level of 1 per year to 10–15 per year. Data for the first half of 1983 indicate the possibility of an even higher rate.

Pathogenesis and Immunity

Multiplication in flea

Mechanism of virulence

Yersinia pestis multiplies in the infected flea and blocks the foregut. The flea then regurgitates organisms into the next bite wound it produces. The organisms reach the regional lymph nodes of the newly infected individual through the lymphatic vessels. At the temperature of the flea (about 20–25°C), the F1 capsular antigen and the VW antigenic complex responsible for resistance to phagocytosis (Chapter 20), are not synthesized, and plague bacilli engulfed by polymorphonuclear leukocytes are killed. However, those ingested by macrophages survive, produce these virulence determinants within the cell, and emerge fully armed and resistant to subsequent phagocytosis.

bubo

bacteremia

necrotizing pneumonia

cyanosis (Black Death)

In the regional nodes, *Y. pestis* multiplies rapidly and produces a hemorrhagic suppurative necrosis that results in a painful swelling known as a *bubo*. The components of the organism responsible for the necrosis and extreme systemic toxicity remain unclear, although both endotoxin and exotoxins are produced. Further spread leads to bacteremia and seeding of the lungs, liver, spleen, and occasionally the meninges. Pulmonary spread produces a fatal necrotizing hemorrhagic pneumonia known as *pneumonic plague*. Progression of plague pneumonia is rapid and so extensive that a terminal cyanosis is typical (Black Death). Recovery from bubonic plague appears to confer lasting immunity.

Clinical Illness

mortality 50–75% in untreated cases

The incubation period for bubonic plague is 2–7 days after the flea bite. Onset is marked by fever and the painful bubo, usually in the groin (bubo, from the Greek *boubon*, groin) or, less often, in the axilla. Without treatment, 50–75% of patients progress to bacteremia and die in Gram-negative septic shock within hours or days after development of the bubo. About 5% of victims develop pneumonic plague with mucoid, then bloody sputum. Primary pneumonic plague has a shorter incubation period (2–3 days) and begins with only fever, malaise, and a feeling of tightness in the chest. Cough, production of sputum, dyspnea, and cyanosis develop later in the course. Death on the second or third day of illness is common, and survival is rare without specific therapy.

Diagnosis

Direct Gram and immunofluorescent staining

Culture

Gram smears of aspirates from the bubo typically reveal bipolar-staining Gram-negative bacilli. An immunofluorescence technique is available in specialized laboratories for immediate precise identification. *Yersinia pestis* is readily isolated on the media used for other members of the Enterobacteriaceae (blood agar, MacConkey agar), although growth may require more than 24 hr of incubation. The appropriate specimens are bubo aspirate, blood, and sputum. Laboratories must be notified of the suspicion of plague to avoid delay in the bacteriologic diagnosis and to guard against laboratory infection.

Treatment and Prevention

streptomycin and tetracycline

Streptomycin and tetracycline are the preferred antibiotics for treatment of both bubonic and pneumonic plague. Timely treatment reduces the mortality of bubonic plague from more than 50% to 10–15%. Of the 16 human cases of plague reported in the first half of 1983, 4 (25%) died.

rat and flea control

avoidance of sick or dead wild rodents

Urban plague has been prevented by rat control and general public health measures such as use of insecticides. Sylvatic plague is virtually impossible to eliminate because of the size and dispersion of the multiple rodent reservoirs. Disease can be prevented by avoidance of sick or dead rodents and rabbits. Eradication of fleas on domestic pets, which have been known to transport infected fleas from wild rodents to humans, is recommended in endemic areas. The continued presence of fully virulent plague in its sylvatic cycle poses a risk of extension to the urban cycle and epidemic disease in the event of major disaster or social breakdown.

chemoprophylaxis

Chemoprophylaxis with tetracycline is recommended for those who have had close contact with a case of pneumonic plague. It is also used for the household contacts of a case of bubonic plague, because they may have had the same flea contact. A formalin-killed plague vaccine is used only for those in high-risk occupations.

Francisella and Tularemia

Tularemia is a disease of wild mammals caused by *F. tularensis*. Humans become infected by contact with infected animals either directly or through the bite of a vector (tick or deer fly). The illness is characterized by high fever and severe constitutional symptoms. Many features of the epidemiology and clinical infection are similar to those of plague.

Microbiology

Gram-negative coccobacilli

special requirement for -SH compounds

Francisella tularensis is a small, facultative, coccobacillary, Gram-negative organism with much the same morphology as *Brucella*. It is one of the few bacterial species of medical importance that will not grow on the usual enriched media. This characteristic is due to a special requirement for sulfhydryl compounds, and growth occurs best on a cysteine–glucose blood agar medium incubated aerobically. On primary isolation, 2–10 days of incubation are required for appearance of the tiny transparent colonies. The species is antigenically homogeneous and not closely related to any other genus.

Epidemiology

rabbits and ticks

Humans most often acquire *F. tularensis* by contact with an infected rabbit or tick. Many other wild mammals can also be infected, including squirrels, muskrats, beavers, and deer. The most common history is of skinning wild rabbits on a hunting trip. The bite or scratch of a domestic dog or cat, probably after the animal ingested or mouthed an infected rodent or rabbit, has been implicated occasionally. Infected animals may not show signs of infection, because the organism is well adapted to its natural host. Ticks and deer flies are the usual vectors in animals. The tick may also serve as a reservoir of the organism by transovarial transmission to its offspring.

Distribution throughout Northern Hemisphere

Tularemia is distributed throughout the Northern Hemisphere, although there are wide variations in specific regions. It is not found in the British Isles. The number of human cases in the United States has decreased from as many as 10–20 per million in the 1940s to less than 1 per million at the present time.

Pathogenesis and Immunity

low infecting dose

If directly injected or inhaled, the infecting dose of *F. tularensis* is very low (less than 100 organisms). Infection can follow virtually any kind of contact with the skin or mucous membranes, and the organism probably gains access to the tissues through unnoticed breaks in the epithelium.

survival in monocytes

focal necrosis and granulomas

Relatively little is known of the events that occur during the 2–5-day incubation period. The organism infects the reticuloendothelial organs, often forming granulomas, and the disease may sometimes follow a chronic relapsing course. These properties suggest multiplication within macrophages, and *F. tularensis* has been shown to survive in monocytes for long periods. A lesion often develops at the site of infection, which becomes ulcerated. Early bacteremic spread probably occurs although it is rarely detected. Other areas of multiplication are characterized by necrosis or granuloma production, and a mixture of abscesses and caseating granulomas may be seen in the same organ.

cellular immunity

Naturally acquired infection appears to confer long-lasting immunity. Agglutinating antibody titers remain elevated for many years, but cellular immunity probably plays the major role in resistance to reinfection.

Clinical Illness

Ulceroglandular tularemia

oculoglandular

Typhoidal

Pneumonic

After an incubation period of 2–5 days, tularemia may follow a number of courses, depending on the site of inoculation and extent of spread. All begin with the acute onset of fever, chills, and malaise. In the ulceroglandular form, a local papule at the inoculation site becomes necrotic and ulcerative. Regional lymph nodes become swollen and painful. The oculoglandular form which follows conjunctival inoculation, is similar except that the local lesion is a painful purulent conjunctivitis. Ingestion of large numbers of *F. tularensis* (more than 10^8) leads to typhoidal tularemia, with abdominal manifestations and a prolonged febrile course similar to that of typhoid fever. Inhalation of the organisms can result in pneumonic tularemia or a more generalized infection similar to the typhoidal form. Like plague pneumonia, tularemic pneumonia may also develop through seeding of the lungs by bacteremic spread of one of the other forms. Any form of tularemia may progress to a systemic infection with lesions in multiple organs. Without treatment, mortality ranges from 5 to 30%, depending on the type of infection. Ulceroglandular tularemia, the most common form, generally carries the lowest risk of a fatal outcome.

Diagnosis

special media needed for culture

immunofluorescent tests

Because tularemia is rare and *F. tularensis* has unique growth requirements, the diagnosis is easily overlooked. Laboratories must be alerted to the suspicion of tularemia so that specialized media can be prepared and precautions taken against the considerable risk of laboratory infection. An immunofluorescent reagent is available in reference laboratories for use directly on smears from clinical material.

serodiagnosis

Because of the difficulty and risk of cultural techniques, many cases are diagnosed by serologic tests. Agglutinating antibodies are usually present in titers of 1:40 by the second week of illness, rising to 1:320 or greater after 3–4 weeks. Unless previous exposure is known, single high antibody titers are considered diagnostic.

Treatment and Prevention

streptomycin

Streptomycin is the drug of choice in all forms of tularemia. Tetracycline and chloramphenicol have also been effective, but relapses are more common than with streptomycin. Prevention is mainly by the use of rubber gloves and eye protection when handling potentially infected wild mammals. Prompt removal of ticks is also important. A vaccine exists, but is used only in laboratory workers and others who cannot avoid contact with infected animals.

Pasteurella multocida

penicillin sensitive

animal bites or scratches

cellulitis

involvement in bronchiectasis

Pasteurella multocida is one of many species of *Pasteurella* included in the normal respiratory flora of some animals. It is a small, coccobacilliary, Gram-negative organism that grows readily on blood agar but not on MacConkey agar. In addition, it is oxidase positive and ferments a variety of carbohydrates. Unlike most Gram-negative rods, *P. multocida* is highly susceptible to penicillin. Humans are usually infected by the bite or scratch of a domestic dog or cat. Infection develops at the site of the lesion, often within 24 hr. The typical infection is a diffuse cellulitis with a well-defined erythematous border. The diagnosis is made by culture of an aspirate of pus expressed from the lesion. Frequently, too few organisms are present to be seen on a direct Gram smear. *Pasteurella multocida* is by far the most common cause of an infected dog or cat bite. Twenty-one cases were seen in a 30-month period at the Arizona Health Sciences Center. For unknown reasons, *P. multocida* is occasionally isolated from the sputum of patients with bronchiectasis. Infections are treated with penicillin.

Additional Reading and References

Cavanaugh, D.C., and Steele, J.H. 1974. Trends in research in plague immunization. *J. Infect. Dis. (Suppl.)* 129:S1–S120. A report of a symposium on immunity to plague in animals and humans, the ecology of the disease, and aspects of pathogenesis.

Hubbert, W.T., McCulloch, W.F., and Schnurrenberger, P.R., Eds. 1975. *Diseases Transmitted from Animals to Man.* 6th ed. Springfield, Ill.: Charles C Thomas. An excellent multiauthored standard reference text on the subject.

McNeill, W.H. 1976. *Plagues and Peoples.* New York: Anchor Press/Doubleday. An account of the impact of infectious diseases, including zoonoses, on the course of human history.

World Health Organization. 1982. Technical Report Series 682. Bacterial and viral zoonoses. Geneva: World Health Organization. A recent report of an international committee on the health impact and control of zoonotic diseases.

John C. Sherris

Spirochetes

24

The spirochetes are helical organisms; their morphology differs from that of other bacteria in that they have a flexible cell wall around which several fibrils are wound. These fibrils, termed *axial filaments,* are flagellar analogs (Figure 24.1). The cell wall and axial filaments are completely covered by an outer triple-layered membrane similar to the outer membrane of other Gram-negative bacteria. Spirochetes are motile, exhibiting rotation and flexion; this motility is believed to result from movement of the axial filaments, although the mechanism is not clear. Like other bacteria, they divide by transverse fission.

many too slim to be seen by light microscopy

Many spirochetes are very slim (0.15 μm or less) and can only be visualized by dark-field microscopy, electron microscopy, or special staining techniques that effectively increase their diameter to bring them within the resolving power of the light microscope. Others (*Borrelia*) are larger and visible in stained preparations. They are Gram negative, although they are more easily detected by other staining methods.

Treponema, Leptospira, and *Borrelia*

Some spirochetes are free living, some are members of the normal flora of humans and animals, and three genera, *Treponema, Leptospira,* and *Borrelia,* include the causative agents of important human and zoonotic diseases. A recently discovered spirochete that causes Lyme disease has not yet been classified, although, like *Borrelia,* it infects ticks as well as mammals.

some fail to grow in culture

Oxygen requirements

Parasitic spirochetes grow more slowly in vitro than most disease-causing bacteria and some, including the causative agent of syphilis, have not been grown in subculture. Some are strict anaerobes, others require low concentrations of oxygen, and still others are aerobic.

Treponema pallidum and Syphilis

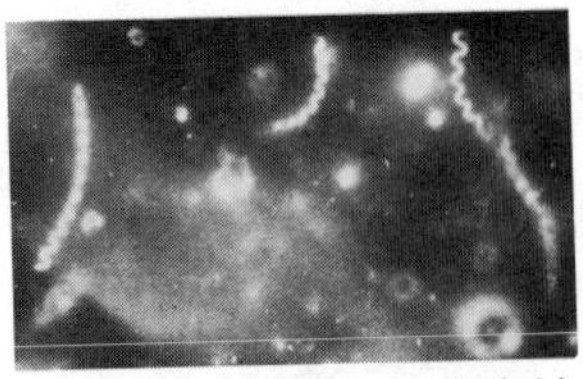

Treponema pallidum. Dark-field microscopy

Treponema pallidum is the causative agent of syphilis, a venereal disease first recognized in the 16th century as an acute and often fatal disease that rapidly spread through Europe as a concomitant of the extensive military campaigns of the century. Over the intervening years, a state of more balanced parasitism developed; the disease is now a more chronic illness, but it can nonetheless have devastating effects.

Morphology

Treponema pallidum is a slim (0.15 μm) spirochete 5–15 μm long with regular spirals of a wavelength of 1 μm and an amplitude of about 0.3 μm. It is not visible by transmitted light under the microscope, because its width is

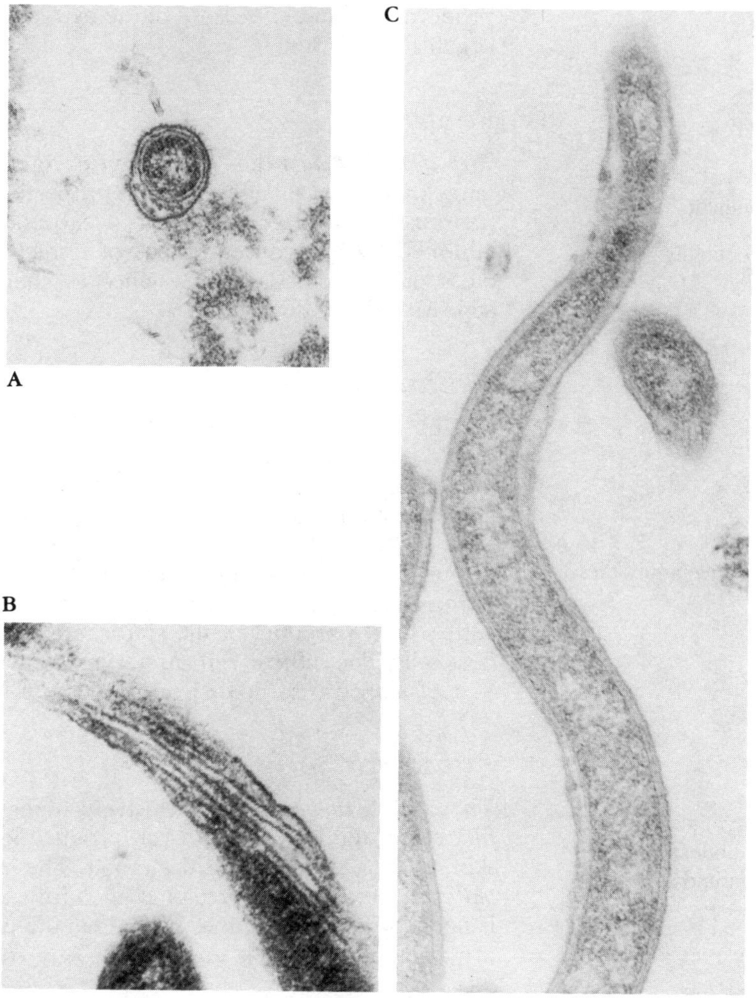

24.1 Spirochete of Lyme disease. Original magnification ×40,000. (**A**) and (**B**) Note flagella. (**C**) Note outer membrane. *(Reprinted with permission from Dr. A.C. Steere and of the N. Engl. J. Med. 1983, 308:736.)*

Fail to stain by routine methods

below the resolving power of the instrument and its refractive index is similar to that of the usual suspending media. It is readily seen by immunofluorescence techniques and by dark-field microscopy, which depends on reflection of light from the surface of particles (Chapter 9). It cannot be visualized with the usual bacteriologic stains; however, its width can be effectively increased by the use of techniques that deposit silver on its surface, and silver impregnation techniques are used to demonstrate it in histologic preparations. Viable *T. pallidum* shows characteristic rotational motility and flexion.

Cultivation

some growth in primary cell culture

probably microaerophilic

Until recently, *T. pallidum* had not been shown to multiply in vitro. Using special tissue culture techniques and careful control of oxygen tension and pH, the organism has now been shown to multiply through several generations in primary tissue cultures, but has not been passed in subculture. It was previously thought that *T. pallidum* was an anaerobe, but it is now known to be capable of carrying out oxidative dissimilation of glucose and to incorporate radiolabeled amino acids in the presence of low concentrations of oxygen. The organism retains viability for considerable periods in liquid medium in the absence of oxygen. Other information about its metabolic properties is limited because of the extreme difficulty in obtaining sufficient organisms for study.

Resistance

rapid death in environment

high susceptibility to penicillin

Treponema pallidum dies rapidly on drying and is readily killed by a wide range of disinfectant agents. These properties account for its almost exclusive transmission by direct contact. It is exquisitely sensitive to penicillin and is inhibited by low concentrations of tetracyclines, erythromycin, and many other antimicrobics. No resistance to chemotherapeutically useful agents appears to have developed.

Antigenic Structure

treponemal antibodies

nontreponemal antibodies

During the course of a syphilitic infection, antibodies develop that react directly with the surface of the spirochete (antitreponemal antibody) and immobilize it in the presence of complement. Different strains appear to be antigenically identical. During infection, antibodies also develop that react with a phospholipid component, cardiolipin (diphosphatidyl glycerol), of normal human and animal tissues that is found in mitochondrial membranes. It remains unclear whether the antigen that stimulates production of this antibody is a product of the spirochete itself or a modified component of host cells. The difficulty in answering this question is compounded, because *T. pallidum* adsorbs lipids from the tissues in which it is multiplying.

Pathogenicity

exclusively human pathogen under natural conditions

experimental rabbit infection

Treponema pallidum is an exclusively human pathogen under natural conditions. In the laboratory, it can produce lesions when inoculated into the skin, cornea, or testicle of the rabbit. The latter yields large numbers of *T. pallidum* which are a source of antigen for serologic tests. Infection in rabbits is nonprogressive and does not mimic the disease in humans. Some degree of passive protection is provided by sera from recovered animals.

Syphilis in Humans

Syphilis is considered in some detail in Chapter 64; thus, only salient clinical features will be considered here.

direct contact with primary or secondary lesion

Transplacental transmission

penetration of epithelia

rapid dissemination

In most cases, *T. pallidum* infection is acquired from direct sexual contact with an individual who has an active primary or secondary syphilitic lesion. Less commonly, the disease may be spread by nongenital contact with a lesion (for example, of the lip) or transplacental transmission to the fetus may occur within approximately the first 3 years of infection (Chapter 63). Occasional cases result from accidental inoculation of infected material. Modern precautions have essentially eliminated blood transfusion as a source of the disease. The spirochete reaches the subepithelial tissues through inapparent breaks in the skin or possibly by passing between the epithelial cells of a mucous membrane. It multiplies locally with a generation time of about 24 hr; although the primary lesion is local, the organism also disseminates rapidly to local lymph nodes, then to other organs by way of the bloodstream.

Primary chancre

highly infectious with numerous spirochetes

The primary lesion develops 2–10 weeks after infection as an indurated swelling at the site of infection. The surface necroses to yield a hard-based ulcerated lesion termed the *chancre,* which is teeming with spirochetes and is highly infectious. The lesion is densely infiltrated with lymphocytes and plasma cells, and the small arterioles show swelling and proliferation of their lesion may be inapparent

endothelial cells, which reduces local blood supply and probably accounts for the necrotic ulceration. Untreated, the lesion heals within 3–8 weeks. The primary lesion is not always apparent, especially when it involves the female genital tract.

Secondary stage

generalized superficial lesions and systemic disease

numerous spirochetes and high infectivity

For reasons that are not understood, the disease is then silent for 2–10 weeks, during which a disseminated secondary stage develops with varying degrees of severity. Lesions are heavily infected with *T. pallidum* and present as a skin rash, as erosions of mucous membranes, and as wartlike condylomata lata in moist areas such as the external female genitalia and perianal areas. The patient often shows systemic manifestations of infection with fever, malaise, enlarged lymph nodes, and patchy loss of hair. This stage may last for several weeks and may relapse. It may be mild, however, and go unnoticed by the patient. Secondary lesions are highly infectious. The factors that control the secondary stage are unclear: humoral antibody has not been shown to play a role, and high titers of both treponemal and nontreponemal antibodies are present throughout.

cure, latency, or tertiary disease

Tertiary gummatous lesions

protean manifestations

absence of readily detectable spirochetes, except in paresis

After the secondary stage, the disease is cured spontaneously in about one-fourth of all cases. In another 25%, the infection becomes latent and produces no further clinical manifestations. The remaining untreated cases develop tertiary manifestations some 2–20 years later. Most late syphilitic manifestations are destructive granulomatous lesions (gummatous lesions), again associated with the characteristic endarteritis of syphilis. They can affect skin, bone, joints, oral and nasal cavities, parenchymatous organs, the cardiovascular system, and the meninges and nervous system. Too few spirochetes are in the lesions to be demonstrated by microscopic techniques, except in general paresis, when large numbers are found in the cerebral cortex. Late disease is not infectious to others. It appears probable that late manifestations involve delayed-type hypersensitivity responses to the spirochete or its products or an autoimmune reaction to host tissues in areas in which spirochetes persist. Once again, however, the processes are unclear.

congenital syphilis

Congenital syphilis may present with the major manifestations of secondary and tertiary syphilis. This illness is considered in Chapters 63 and 64.

Immunity to reinfection

In the early stages of syphilis, the patient rapidly becomes immune to reinfection, but immunity is short-lived if the patient is successfully treated. In the later stages, immunity is more solid.

Laboratory Diagnosis

Dark-field and fluorescent antibody demonstration

Treponema pallidum can be detected in primary and secondary lesions by dark-field microscopy or by treating smears from lesions with fluorescent antitreponemal antibody preparations derived from sera of infected rabbits. Dark-field microscopy requires considerable skill and experience and is prone to misinterpretation in the examination of oral lesions, in which other spirochetes from the normal flora may be numerous.

Nontreponemal cardiolipin serodiagnostic tests

false-positive results

Most cases of syphilis are diagnosed serologically. Nontreponemal tests such as the VDRL and RPR, which depend on immune flocculation of cardiolipin in the presence of lecithin and cholesterol, become positive in the early stages of the primary lesion and are uniformly positive during the secondary stage. They slowly wane in the later stages of the disease (Chapter 64). In neurosyphilis, VDRL tests on cerebrospinal fluid may be positive when the serum VDRL has reverted to negative. This class of test is nonspecific: it may become positive in a variety of autoimmune diseases or in those involving substantial tissue destruction or liver involvement, such as lupus erythematosus, viral hepatitis, infectious mononucleosis, and malaria. False-positive results can also occur occasionally in pregnancy. Nontrepo-

use as screening procedures

nemal tests are thus used as screening procedures for diagnosis and are confirmed by one of the treponemal tests to be described subsequently. They are, however, of substantial value as tests of cure after treatment, because they slowly revert to negative or their titer of reactivity decreases substantially after successful therapy. In contrast, treponemal tests remain positive.

tests of cure

Treponemal serodiagnostic tests

FTA-ABS indirect fluorescence test

Treponemal tests involve direct detection of antibody to *T. pallidum.* The spirochetes used in the tests are derived from rabbit testicular lesions. Two procedures are now used most frequently, the fluorescent treponemal antibody absorption test (FTA-ABS) and the microhemagglutination test for *T. pallidum* antibody (MHA-TP). The FTA-ABS procedure is an indirect immunofluorescent serodiagnostic test (Chapter 9). It involves treatment of the patient's serum with extracts of a cultivated treponema that is not *T. pallidum.* This treatment blocks potential nonspecific cross-reacting antibodies. The treated (absorbed) serum is then applied to a slide to which *T. pallidum* has been fixed. After allowing any specific antibody to react, nonbound constituents of serum are removed by washing, and the presence of antibody on *T. pallidum* is detected by application of a fluorescein-labeled anti-human globulin serum prepared by immunizing rabbits with human immunoglobulin. Positive results are indicated by the bright fluorescence of *T. pallidum* under the ultraviolet microscope.

MHA-TP indirect hemagglutination test

The MHA-TP is simpler than the FTA-ABS procedure, and only slightly less sensitive. It is an indirect hemagglutination test employing *T. pallidum* antigens adsorbed to erythrocytes stabilized by tannic acid and formaldehyde. Appropriate blocking antigens are added to avoid nonspecific reactions.

specificity of treponemal tests

Treponemal tests are considerably more specific than those using cardiolipin, but the titers of positive tests do not decrease significantly with cure. Thus, they are valuable confirmatory tests, but they are not helpful in monitoring therapy.

For consideration of other aspects of syphilis, including its epidemiology, prevention, and treatment, the reader should consult Chapter 64.

Nonvenereal Treponemal Diseases

Three nonvenereal treponematoses, bejel (endemic syphilis), yaws, and pinta, occur in different geographic locations. In each case, the etiologic spirochete is indistinguishable morphologically and antigenically from *T. pallidum,* and the same difficulties have been encountered in attempting to grow them. Patients exhibit serologic responses in nontreponemal and treponemal tests similar to those of patients with syphilis, and it seems probable that each disease, and venereal syphilis itself, is caused by organisms that have diverged in evolution under particular local conditions. It has not been possible to determine which, if any, was the first human disease.

etiologic agents indistinguishable from *T. pallidum*

poor hygienic conditions

Major clinical manifestations

The nonvenereal trematoses all occur in developing countries in which hygiene has been poor, little clothing is worn, and direct skin contact is common, often because of overcrowding. They frequently develop in childhood. The major manifestations of pinta and yaws involve the skin, and infection is transmitted by direct contact. In bejel, primary and secondary lesions usually involve the oral cavity, and spread may occur during suckling, by oral contact, or through fomites. All three diseases have primary and secondary stages, and tertiary manifestations may develop. Their features are summarized in Table 24.1. These infections are rarely transmitted venereally, and congenital infections do not occur. All are susceptible to penicillin. Their manifestations are well recognized by affected populations, and all have been greatly reduced in incidence by public health procedures designed to eradicate them.

Treatment and eradication

Table 24.1 Nonvenereal Treponemata

Disease	Cause	Major Geographic Location	Primary Lesion	Secondary Lesions	Tertiary Lesions
Bejel	*T. pallidum*[a]	Middle East; arid, hot areas	Oral cavity[b]	Oral mucosa	Rare; gummatous lesions of skin, periosteum, bone, and joint[c]
Yaws	*T. pertenue*	Humid, tropical belt	Skin; papillomatous	Systemic; resemble syphilis	Rare; gummatous lesions of skin, periosteum, bone, and joint[c]
Pinta	*T. carateum*	Central and South America	Skin; erythematous papule	Skin; merge into primary lesion; altered pigmentation	Areas of altered skin pigmentation and hyperkeratoses

[a] Probably a variant of that causing venereal syphilis.
[b] Often inapparent.
[c] Neurologic manifestations usually absent.

Leptospira and Leptospirosis

zoonotic disease

animal urine

L. interrogans serogroups and serotypes

Leptospirosis is a worldwide disease of a variety of animal species. It can be transmitted to humans, usually through water contaminated with animal urine. It is caused by *Leptospira interrogans,* the pathogenic member of the genus *Leptospira.* In the past, multiple species of pathogenic leptospires were recognized (for example, *Leptospira icterohaemorrhagiae, Leptospira canicola, Leptospira pomona,* and *Leptospira autumnalis*) based on geographic occurrence, differences in host species, and associated clinical syndromes, as well as antigenic differences. Now, however, 18 serogroups are recognized, many of which bear the names of the previously described species (for example, *L. interrogans,* serogroup pomona), and more than 150 serotypes are recognized within these groups. The clinical syndromes of leptospiroses caused by the different serogroups each have special features, but they show considerable overlap. The distinction between serogroups and serotypes is of epidemiologic and epizoologic importance rather than clinical significance.

Morphology and Cultivation

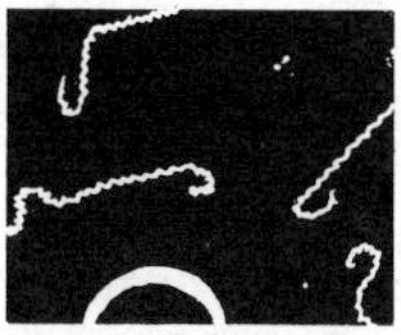

Leptospira. Dark-field microscopy

Leptospira interrogans is a slim (approximately 0.15 μm) spirochete 5–15 μm in length, with fine, closely wound spirals and hooked ends. As it is not visualized with the usual bacteriologic staining procedures, detection is most easily accomplished by dark-field or immunofluorescent microscopy. The organism's fine structure and motility conform to that described for the spirochetes as a group.

Leptospira interrogans is an aerobe and can be grown in certain special enriched semisolid media.

Resistance

survival in water

sensitivity to penicillin

Leptospira interrogans can survive for days or weeks in some waters in the environment at a pH of more than 7.0. Acidic conditions, such as those that may be found in urine, rapidly kill the organism. It is highly sensitive to drying and to a wide range of disinfectants. The organism is also susceptible to a number of antimicrobics, including penicillin and tetracycline.

Antigenic Structure

As indicated previously, *L. interrogans* can be divided into multiple serogroups and serovars (serotypes), although some antigens are common to all members of the species. Seroidentification is accomplished in reference laboratories by agglutination tests using highly specific absorbed antisera against the various antigenic components.

Animal Pathogenicity

chronic renal infections in rodents, cattle, and household pets

The various serogroups of *L. interrogans* are pathogenic to a wide range of wild and domestic animal species, particularly rats, cattle, and dogs. These animals constitute the zoonotic reservoir of the diseases. Infection is often subclinical, with organisms persisting in the renal tubules and being excreted in the urine for many weeks. Guinea pigs and some other small laboratory animals susceptible to intraperitoneal infection have been used to isolate the organism from clinical and environmental sources.

Leptospirosis in Humans

occupational or recreational exposure to contaminated water

Infection usually results from contact with water contaminated with the urine of infected animals or, in the case of the serogroup canicola, by direct contact with canine urine. Sewer workers, miners, farm workers, veterinarians, and slaughterhouse employees are all subject to exposure, although most clinical cases in North America are now associated with recreational exposure to contaminated water (for example, in children playing in irrigation ditches).

infection through upper alimentary tract or skin

bacteremic phase

disease sometimes biphasic

The organism gains entrance to the tissues through small skin lesions, the conjunctiva, or, most commonly, through ingestion and the upper alimentary tract mucosa. Most infections are subclinical and only detectable serologically, but after an incubation period of 7–13 days an influenzalike febrile illness with fever, and muscle pain may develop. This disease is associated with bacteremia. Leptospiras are also found in the cerebrospinal fluid at this stage, but without clinical or cytologic evidence of meningitis. The fever often subsides after about a week, but then recurs with a variety of clinical manifestations depending only partly on the serogroup involved. The disease may present as an aseptic meningitis resembling viral meningitis (Chapter 61) or as a more generalized illness with muscle aches, headache, rash, pretibial erythematous lesions, and/or biochemical evidence of hepatic and renal involvement. In its most severe form (Weil's disease, usually caused by the icterohaemorrhagiae group), there is extensive vasculitis, jaundice, renal damage, and sometimes a hemorrhagic rash. The mortality in such cases is up to 10%.

aseptic meningitis

Weil's disease with hemorrhage, hepatitis, and renal involvement

probable immunologic component to pathogenesis

It appears probable that the second phase of the disease has an immunologic component to its pathogenesis, because antimicrobic therapy does not appear to influence the course of the illness when given at this stage, and the organism is not usually recoverable from the cerebrospinal fluid in cases of leptospiral meningitis. The manifestations of disease may extend for 3 weeks or longer. The disease is blind-ended in humans, and transmission to others is extremely uncommon.

blind-ended infection in humans

Laboratory Diagnosis

blood culture in first week

The leptospire can be isolated from the blood or cerebrospinal fluid during the first week of the disease. Thereafter it can often be isolated from the urine if precautions are taken to initiate cultures immediately after the spec-

urine cultures

serodiagnosis by agglutination tests

imen is collected. Antibodies begin to appear within the first week of clinical disease, and the diagnosis is usually made by agglutination tests using serotypes common in particular regions as antigens. A titer of 1:100 or greater is suggestive of infection in the presence of a compatible clinical picture. A fourfold increase in titer is diagnostic.

Treatment

antimicrobic treatment only effective in first few days

Penicillin and tetracycline treatment appear to modify the course of the disease if given within the first 4 days of the bacteremic phase. Later treatment is ineffective.

Prevention

animal immunization

rodent control and drainage

incidence

Vaccines are used extensively in cattle and household pets to prevent the disease, and this has reduced its occurrence in humans. Other measures include rodent control, drainage of waters known to be contaminated, and care on the part of those subject to occupational exposure to avoid contamination of food or skin lesions. Clinical disease is now unusual in the United States, and fewer than 100 cases are reported annually; however, many cases are probably unreported. It is impossible to eliminate the disease because of its reservoir in rodents. The infection is much more common in developing countries in which exposure to irrigated crops is extensive.

Borrelia recurrentis and Relapsing Fever

Endemic and epidemic diseases

Relapsing fever is a disease transmitted to humans by ticks in the case of endemic relapsing fever, or by body lice in the case of epidemic relapsing fever. The causative agent is *B. recurrentis*, which has remarkable antigenic mutability. In the past, various specific names were given to strains associated with different species of ticks; similarities outweigh differences, however, and all strains are now usually regarded as members of a single species and will be so considered here. The disease is characterized by two or more relapses associated with selection of antigenic variants.

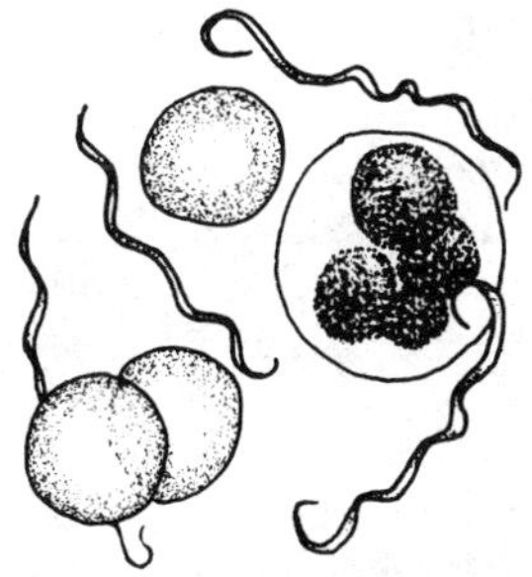

Borrelia recurrentis in blood smear

Morphology, Staining, and Culture

Borrelia recurrentis is a large spirochete 10–30 μm long and approximately 0.3 μm wide. In contrast to those of *Treponema* and *Leptospira*, spirals are irregular, with a wavelength of 2–4 μm. The basic organizational structure of the cell and its motility conform to that of other spirochetes. The organism is Gram negative, but it is seen most readily with Giemsa or Wright staining of smears of blood sampled during the bacteremic phase of the disease.

Borrelia recurrentis is an aerobe and has been successfully grown in artificial cultures.

Antigenic Structure

antigenic variants

The most characteristic antigenic property of *Borrelia* is its mutability. Surface antigens partly responsible for virulence mutate during the course of the disease, and relapses occur because of the failure of these mutants to bind antibody produced in response to the original infection or a previous relapse. Immunity to the disease is largely humoral and appears to involve lysis of the organism in the presence of complement.

Pathogenicity

rodent infection

tick infection

body louse infection

Borrelia recurrentis infects a range of small rodents and other mammals, and it is pathogenic to humans. Ticks of the genus *Ornithodorus* can be infected from the animal reservoir; infected ticks are found in mountainous areas of North America and in other parts of the world in which the endemic disease occurs. The survival of the tick is not influenced by the infection, and the organism can be passed transovarially to subsequent generations. The human body louse can also become infected by ingesting *Borrelia*, but the infection is not transmitted transovarially. The relapsing nature of the disease in humans can be reproduced in susceptible laboratory animals.

Epidemiology

endemic tick-borne infection

transovarial transmission and longevity of ticks

Epidemic louse-borne infection

association with overcrowding, poverty, and war

possible origin of epidemic from endemic disease

Endemic relapsing fever occurs in most areas of the world. It is contracted from the bite of an infected tick and is ultimately derived from the rodent reservoir. Apart from their ability to pass the infection to their progeny, ticks may remain infectious for several years when deprived of hosts. Human cases of endemic relapsing fever are usually sporadic, and in the United States they often develop after exposure to ticks during recreational activities.

Epidemic relapsing fever involves human-to-human spread by the body louse. In this case there is no transovarial spread, and the life span of the infected louse is not longer than 2 months. Infection results from scratching and crushing the infected louse into its bite or other superficial wounds. The disease is associated with overcrowding, war, poverty, and social breakdown, and without treatment the mortality may approach 30%. As the life span of the infected louse is brief and human carriage is not documented, it is quite possible that epidemic relapsing fever can originate from cases of endemic tick-borne relapsing fever. This hypothesis remains to be proved, however, because outbreaks have occurred in areas where the endemic disease is not documented, and there are differences in some pathogenic characteristics of strains isolated from tick or louse borne disease.

Disease in Humans

spirochetemia

endotoxin

relapses

greater severity of epidemic disease

After a mean incubation period of 7 days, massive spirochetemia develops with high fever, rigors, severe headache, muscle pains, and weakness. The organism produces an endotoxin, which probably accounts for some of the manifestations. The febrile period lasts about a week and terminates abruptly with the development of an adequate immune response. The disease relapses 2–4 days later, usually with less severity, but following the same general course. Epidemic relapsing fever is usually limited to two relapses, but with endemic disease three or four may occur.

Epidemic relapsing fever is more severe than endemic disease, possibly because of the social conditions that predispose to it. Fatalities in endemic relapsing fever are rare. Most organs of the body are invaded by *Borrelia* during the disease, and mortality is usually associated with myocarditis.

Laboratory Diagnosis

direct smears

Diagnosis is readily made during the febrile period by Giemsa or Wright staining of blood smears. The appearance of the spirochete among the red cells is characteristic. Cultural and animal inoculation procedures are also used for recovery of the infecting organism. Specific serodiagnostic test are unhelpful; however, patients may develop antibodies to *Proteus* OXK, which can cause problems in differentiating the diagnosis from that of rickettsial disease (Chapter 27).

Treatment

Tetracycline treatment

The disease responds well to tetracycline therapy, and single-dose treatment with this agent can be effective.

Prevention

Prevention of endemic relapsing fever involves attention to deticking and insecticide treatment and rodent control around habitations, such as mountain cabins, shown to be associated with infection.

Epidemic relapsing fever is controlled by delousing, particularly dusting of clothing with appropriate insecticides. Ultimately, improved hygiene will stop an outbreak and prevent further occurrences.

The Spirochete of Lyme Disease

skin lesions

arthritis

Lyme disease has been reported in the United States, Europe, and Australia. It is named for the town in Connecticut in which a cluster of cases was first recognized. It occurs in the summer and is characterized by a migratory chronic erythematous skin rash, fever, muscle and joint pains, and some evidence of meningeal irritation. Later, the patient may develop meningoencephalitis, evidence of myocarditis, and recurrent arthritis, which can be severely disabling and develop over several years.

association with *Ixodes* tick

The disease had been assumed to be an infection because therapy with penicillin or tetracycline in the early stages prevents or modifies later manifestations, which probably have an immunopathologic component. Epidemiologically, the disease is associated with bites of ticks of the genus *Ixodes.*

Characteristics of spirochete

A spirochete was isolated recently from infected cases and from *Ixodes* ticks, and serologic responses to this organism have been shown in other cases. The spirochete resembles *Treponema* (Figure 24.1), but unlike *Treponema* has been grown in special culture media and infects ticks and thus resembles *Borrelia*. The nature of the ultimate reservoir of this organism remains to be determined.

Spirochetes of the Normal Oral Flora and Fusospirochetal Diseases

The oral cavity, particularly the dental crevice, harbors spirochetes of the genera *Treponema* and *Borrelia* as part of its normal flora. As described in Chapter 56, spirochetes from this source, together with fusobacteria (Chapter 15), can cause an anaerobic, synergistic, necrotizing, ulcerative infection of the gums, or similar ulcerations in the oral cavity or pharynx termed *Vincent's infection* or *trench mouth*. This opportunistic infection is usually seen with severe malnutrition, leukemia, or in the immunocompromised host, particularly with deficient phagocytic defenses. It may also follow trauma or complicate herpes simplex infections. The term *trench mouth* was derived from the common occurrence of infections of this type in troops under the appalling conditions that existed in the trenches during World War I, when reasonable oral hygiene could not be maintained.

Predisposing factors

Direct smear examination

Response to penicillin

The disease is readily diagnosed by examining specially stained smears of material taken directly from the ulcerated lesion. Its appearance is illustrated in Figure 24.2 in which the characteristic fusiform and spirochetal

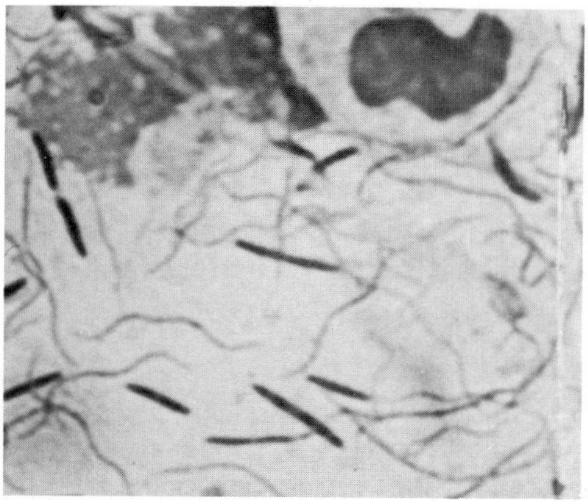

24.2 Fusospirochetal disease. Note the large number of fusiform organisms and spirochetes. *(Reproduced with kind permission from Leon J. Lebeau, Ph.D., Department of Pathology, University of Illinois Medical Center.)*

organisms are seen. Resolution is rapid with penicillin therapy supplemented with careful oral hygiene.

Additional Reading and References

Benach, J.L., Bosler, E.M., Hanrahan, J.P., Coleman, J.L., Habicht, G.S., Bast, T.F., Cameron, D.J., Ziegler, J.L., Barbour, A.G., Burgdorfer, W., Edelman, R., and Kaslow, R.A. 1983. Spirochetes isolated from the blood of two patients with Lyme disease. *N. Engl. J. Med.* 308:740–742. This article and that of Steere et al. are classic studies demonstrating the infectious etiology of a disease caused by a "new" organism.

Johnson, R.C., Ed. 1976. *Symposium: The Biology of Parasitic Spirochetes.* New York: Academic Press.

Schell, R.F., and Musher, D.M. 1983. *Pathogenesis and Immunology of Treponemal Infection. Immunology Series.* Rose, N.B., Ed. New York: Marcel Dekker. This volume is an up-to-date, multiauthored review of present knowledge on the biology of pathogenic treponemata and the pathogenesis of treponemal disease.

Steere, A.C., Grodzicki, R.L., Kornblatt, A.N., Craft, J.E., Barbour, A.G., Burgdorfer, W., Schmid, G.P., Johnson, E., and Malawista, S.E. 1983. The spirochetal etiology of Lyme disease. *N. Engl. J. Med.* 308:733–740.

John C. Sherris

Mycobacteria

25

The mycobacteria are slim, rod-shaped organisms 0.2–0.4 × 2–10 μm in size. They are nonmotile and do not form spores. They have an unusual cell wall structure that contains *N*-glycolylmuramic acid in place of *N*-acetylmuramic acid and has a very high lipid content (60%), which renders the surface hydrophobic and makes mycobacteria difficult to stain with commonly used basic aniline dyes at room temperature. Mycobacteria can be stained with dyes by prolonged application or with heating; once they have taken up the stain, however, they resist decolorization with 1% hydrochloric acid. Some species also resist decolorization with 95% ethanol. These properties, which depend on the integrity of the cell wall, are described as *acid fastness* and *acid–alcohol fastness,* and are exploited in selective stains that allow mycobacteria to be distinguished from other genera and species. For example, the Ziehl–Neelsen stain is commonly applied to cultures or to clinical specimens such as sputum. The method involves flooding the slide with basic fuchsin (a red dye) in 5% phenol as a mordant. The slide is heated gently for several minutes before decolorization with 1% HCl in ethanol. After washing, the preparation is counterstained with methylene blue. Mycobacteria stain red, whereas other genera are decolorized and therefore take the blue color of the counterstain (Plate T). There are various modifications of this procedure, including the use of fluorochromes as the primary stain. In this case, mycobacteria, but not other genera, fluoresce when examined microscopically at the excitor wavelength of the stain.

Acid and alcohol fastness

Ziehl–Neelsen stain

Mycobacteria are strictly aerobic, and the most important pathogen, *Mycobacterium tuberculosis,* shows enhanced growth in 10% carbon dioxide and at a pH of about 6.5–6.8. Nutritional requirements vary among species and range from the ability of some nonpathogens to multiply on the washers of water faucets to the strict intracellular parasitism of *Mycobacterium leprae,* which does not grow in artificial media or tissue culture.

aerobes

Mycobacteria grow more slowly than most human pathogenic bacteria because of their hydrophobic cell surface, which causes them to clump and inhibits permeability of nutrients into the cell. Addition of the surfactant Tween 80 to cultures of *M. tuberculosis* wets the surface and increases the speed of growth.

slow growth of many species

The major distinguishing features among different species of mycobacteria are nutritional and temperature requirements, growth rates, pigmentation of colonies grown in light or darkness, some key biochemical tests, and

distinguishing features

range of pathogenicity in experimental animals. Some of the more important characteristics are summarized in Appendix 25.1. The improved means of in vitro characterization have reduced the need for animal pathogenicity tests.

pathogenicity

Mycobacteria include a wide range of species pathogenic for humans and animals. Some, such as *M. tuberculosis,* occur exclusively in humans under natural conditions. Others, such as *Mycobacterium intracellulare,* can infect various species, including humans, but also appear able to exist in the free-living state. Most nonpathogenic species are widely distributed in the environment.

Diseases caused by mycobacteria tend to develop slowly, follow a chronic course, and elicit a granulomatous response. Infectivity of pathogenic species is quite high, but virulence for healthy humans is low; for example, disease following infection with *M. tuberculosis* is the exception rather than the rule.

hypersensitivity to proteins

Mycobacteria do not produce classic exotoxins or endotoxins, and disease processes are largely a result of delayed-type hypersensitivity reactions to mycobacterial proteins. The hypersensitive state can be detected by intradermal injections of purified proteins from the mycobacteria. Cross-reaction of responses to proteins from different species is considerable.

Mycobacterium tuberculosis

Distinction from *M. bovis*

Mycobacterium tuberculosis is the cause of almost all cases of human tuberculosis in developed countries. In the past a significant number of tuberculous infections were caused by the animal pathogen *Mycobacterium bovis,* usually from drinking milk from infected herds; now, however, the disease has been almost eliminated by eradication programs in cattle and by pasteurization of milk. A variant of *M. tuberculosis* designated *Mycobacterium africanum* causes many tuberculous infections in Africa, but its significance is the same as that of *M. tuberculosis* and it will not be considered separately here.

Morphology, Staining, and Cultural Characteristics

Mycobacterium tuberculosis is a slim, strongly acid–alcohol-fast rod. It frequently shows irregular beading in its staining, appearing as connected series of acid-fast granules. It grows at 37°C, but not at room temperature, and requires enriched or complex media for primary growth from clinical specimens. Growth is enhanced by 5–10% CO_2, but is still very slow, with a mean generation time of more than 6 hr.

complex growth media

Complex media are widely used for primary culture. One, Löwenstein–Jensen medium, is composed of 60% homogenized egg in nutrient base containing a low concentration of malachite green as an inhibitor of non-mycobacterial contaminants. The medium is solidified into slants by heating at 85°C until the egg protein coagulates. Colonies usually appear after 3–6 weeks of incubation. They become raised, warty, and adherent, with a buff pigmentation. They are difficult to emulsify because of their high lipid content. Another commonly used medium is oleic acid–albumin agar, a semisynthetic plating medium that grows *M. tuberculosis* more rapidly. On oleic acid–albumin agar and in liquid medium, virulent strains show "cording" in which multiplying organisms remain attached in parallel bundles and form long intertwining cords or ropes. Cording is caused by a glycolipid termed *cord factor.* Its association with virulence is clear, but its role, if any, as a virulence factor is not. Although complex media are needed for primary isolation, a heavy inoculum of *M. tuberculosis* will grow well on the surface of a liquid medium containing only inorganic salts, asparagine, and glycerol. Under these conditions, the organism appears to produce a substance(s) needed for its own growth that is initially supplied by the heavy inoculum.

slow growth

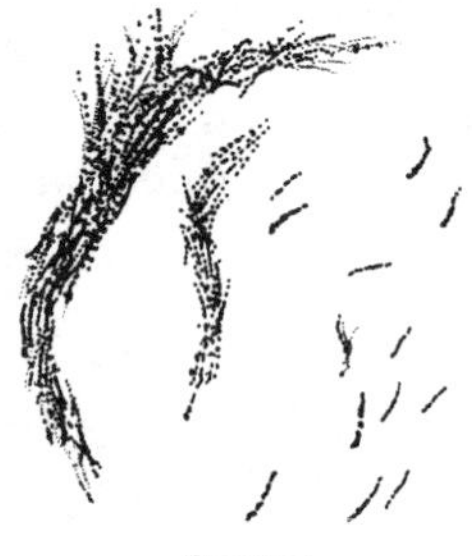

Cording

The major tests for identification of *M. tuberculosis* are summarized in Appendix 25.1. Of particular importance is the ability of *M. tuberculosis* to produce niacin, which is uncommon in other mycobacteria.

Range of Pathogenicity

disease in guinea pigs

Mycobacterium tuberculosis is highly virulent for guinea pigs, but much less so for other commonly used experimental animals; thus, much of our knowledge of the pathogenesis and immunity of tuberculosis has been derived from the guinea pig model. The minimal infecting dose for this animal is usually less than 10 cells, and after subcutaneous or intramuscular injection, a local and systemic infection develops with extensive involvement of lymph nodes, liver, and spleen. Untreated, the animal dies, usually after 6–12 weeks. Monkeys in captivity are also very susceptible to *M. tuberculosis* infection, which they contract from handlers or other infected monkeys. They can pose a serious source of infection to those working with them.

Resistance

Unusual resistance to disinfectants but not to heat

Mycobacterium tuberculosis is unusually resistant to drying, to most disinfectants, and to acids and alkalis. This resistance, attributable to its hydrophobic lipid surface, is exploited in preparing contaminated clinical specimens for culture. Tubercle bacilli are quite heat sensitive; they are killed in milk by pasteurization for 30 min at 62°C.

Antigenic Structure

Mycobacterium tuberculosis has, as do all bacteria, a highly complex antigenic structure, and humoral immune responses are mounted to many of these antigens during the course of a tuberculous infection. Antibody responses do not appear to be involved in immunity to infection, however, and no serologic test has so far proved sufficiently sensitive and specific to be useful as a diagnostic procedure. As there are no consistent antigenic differences between strains of *M. tuberculosis*, there is no practical serologic typing procedure.

Cell-mediated immunity and hypersensitivity

Tuberculin and PPD

Cellular immunity and cell-mediated hypersensitivity to tuberculoproteins develop during the course of tuberculous infection and contribute to both the pathology and the immunity of the disease. The most studied antigens are heat-stable proteins that are liberated into liquid culture media. The original preparation was termed *Old Tuberculin*. Now, a purified protein derivative (PPD) of tuberculin is available for skin testing for hypersensitivity and is standardized according to skin test activity as tuberculin units. Hypersensitivity does not result from repeated PPD injections in those who are skin test negative. It is now recognized, however, that the degree of hypersensitivity may be somewhat increased for a few weeks in those already allergic.

Virulence Mechanisms

lack of toxins

The cells and cellular components of *M. tuberculosis* are remarkably nontoxic to humans and experimental animals not previously sensitized to tuberculin. Two of the cell wall lipids, Wax D and cord factor, will elicit granulomatous lesions, but the amounts required are considerably in excess of those to be expected in a natural lesion. No toxins have been found in the organism, and attempts to isolate single immunizing antigens have been unsuccessful.

ability to multiply in vivo

The organism owes its virulence to its ability to multiply within macrophages and in the physical and chemical conditions (low pH, high lactic acid, high

Table 25.1 Antimicrobics Commonly Used in Treatment of Tuberculosis

First-Line Drugs	Second-Line Drugs[a]
Isoniazid	*para*-aminosalicylic acid
Ethambutol	Ethionamide
Rifampin	Cycloserine
Streptomycin	Kanamycin, etc.

[a] Second-line drugs added to combinations if resistance or toxicity contraindicate first-line agents.

CO_2) that obtain in developing lesions. It is essentially unaffected by the humoral antibody response that it elicits, and it can survive for long periods in macrophages that have been activated by the cellular immune response. Intracellular survival of *M. tuberculosis* appears attributable, at least in part, to inhibition of lysosome fusion to the phagocytic vacuole. This effect is caused by sulfatides in the mycobacterial cell wall. Disease manifestations result primarily from hypersensitivity to tuberculoprotein.

Intracellular survival

Antimicrobic Susceptibility

Isoniazid, ethambutol, rifampin, and streptomycin

Mycobacterium tuberculosis is susceptible to several effective antimicrobics (Table 25.1). Isoniazid, ethambutol, rifampin and streptomycin, and combinations of these agents constitute the primary drugs of choice for treatment of tuberculosis. Isoniazid is bactericidal. It inhibits the synthesis of mycolic acids in the cell wall. Ethambutol is bacteriostatic for some mycobacteria, including *M. tuberculosis,* but its precise subcellular mechanism of action remains uncertain. Rifampin and streptomycin have broader spectra; their modes of action are described in Chapter 10. *Mycobacterium tuberculosis* is also susceptible to other drugs that may be used to replace those of the primary group if they are inappropriate because of resistance or drug toxicity.

mutational resistance and combined therapy

Mutational resistance to all antituberculous drugs occurs at frequencies of 10^{-7}–10^{-10}, and mutants often come to predominate and produce clinical relapse when a single drug is used to treat serious tuberculosis. This resistance develops because organisms in many tuberculous lesions are sufficiently numerous to include resistant mutants, which can grow under the conditions that exist in lesions during treatment and cause clinical relapse. Adequate, continuous treatment with two or three antituberculous drugs with different modes of action greatly reduces this problem, because the chance of a doubly resistant mutant being present among the number of organisms in a lesion is very low. Primary infections with drug-resistant strains continue to occur, and susceptibility tests are indicated for organisms from active cases of tuberculosis.

Tuberculosis

History and prevalence

Tuberculosis is a disease of great antiquity that reached epidemic proportions during the major periods of urbanization in the 18th and 19th centuries: mortality reached 200–400 per 100,000 of the population per year, and morbidity was many times higher. The disease has major sociologic components, flourishing with ignorance, poverty, overcrowding, and poor hygiene and during the social disruptions of war and economic depression. Under these conditions, the poor are the major victims, but all sectors of society are at risk. Chopin, Paganini, Thoreau, Keats, Elizabeth Barrett Browning, and the Brontës, to name but a few, were all lost to the disease in their intellectual prime. With knowledge of its cause and transmission, the disease has rapidly come under control in Western countries, but mortality and morbidity remain at 19th century levels in many countries despite extensive national and international control programs.

Routes of Infection

infection by respiratory route

The great majority of tuberculous infections are first contracted by inhalation of droplet nuclei carrying the causative organism. Epidemiologic data indicate that large doses or prolonged exposure to smaller infecting doses is usually needed to initiate infection in humans. Occasionally, infection occurs through the gastrointestinal tract or the skin.

Primary Tuberculosis

Multiplication in aveolar macrophages

low reactivity and dissemination

Primary tuberculosis is the response to initial infection in an individual not previously infected and sensitized to tuberculoprotein. The infection is usually pulmonary and develops at the periphery of the midzone of the lung. Tubercle bacilli that reach the small bronchi or alveoli with inhaled droplets are engulfed by macrophages. Those that survive continue to multiply within the macrophages and are carried to the hilar lymph nodes that drain the infected site. Multiplication of the organisms is relatively unimpeded, and the inflammatory reaction is minor and nonspecific. Dissemination of some bacilli through the lymphatic vessels and bloodstream is common at this time, and they may be deposited in many organs, including the liver, spleen, kidney, bone, brain, meninges, and other parts of the lung. Symptoms and signs of infection are absent or are manifested as a mild influenzalike disease; however, the primary site of infection and some enlarged hilar lymph nodes can often be detected radiologically.

development of hypersensitivity and cell-mediated immunity

tubercle

arrest of lesion: survival of organisms

Cell-mediated immunity to *M. tuberculosis* and hypersensitivity to tuberculoprotein, both manifestations of the same process, develop 2–6 weeks after infection, with formation of classic histologic tubercles at the sites of bacillary multiplication. These microscopic granulomas consist of a central area of epithelioid cells (modified macrophages), Langhans multinucleate giant cells, and surrounding areas of lymphocytic infiltration (Figure 25.1). Multiplication of *M. tuberculosis* slows or stops, and central necrosis of the lesion often develops as a result of hypersensitivity.

Primary infections are usually handled well by the host, and the lesions in the lung and draining lymph nodes usually fibrose and sometimes calcify

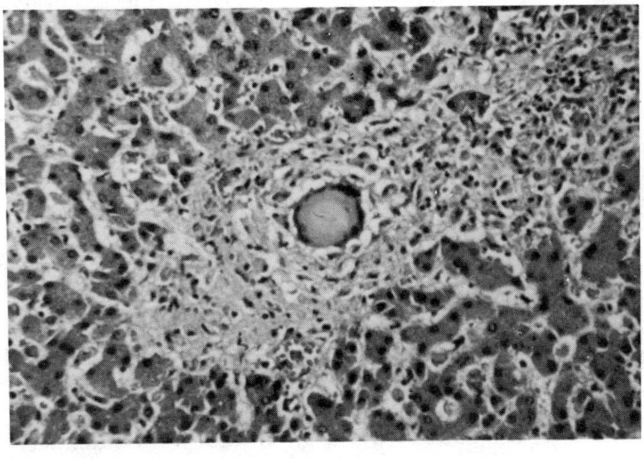

25.1 Microscopic tubercule of liver, showing giant cell and surrounding epithelioid cells and lymphocytes.

Ghon complex

Progressive primary infection

Miliary tuberculosis

to produce the classic Ghon complex on X-ray. Most microscopic lesions in other areas of the body also heal by fibrosis, and the organisms in them slowly die. In others, the tubercle bacilli remain viable for long periods and serve as a potential source of reactivation many months or years later if host defenses weaken. Less commonly, the primary disease is not controlled and merges into the reactivation type of tuberculosis, or it disseminates to many organs to produce active miliary tuberculosis. The latter may result from a necrotic tubercle eroding into a small blood vessel.

Reactivation (Adult) Tuberculosis

reactivation most common in older men

predisposing factors

In Western countries, reactivation of an old, quiescent lesion followed by clinical disease now occurs most often after the age of 50 and is more common in men. Frequently, reactivation is associated with malnutrition, alcoholism, diabetes, old age, and a dramatic change in the individual's life, such as loss of a spouse. When the disease was more common, reactivation tuberculosis was seen more often in young adults of both sexes. Hospital house staff and nurses had a high attack rate, probably because of the long hours and inherent stresses of their jobs superimposed on the virtual inevitability of previous childhood infection at that time.

Apical disease

Caseation

Formation of pulmonary cavities

infectiousness of cavitary tuberculosis

Reactivation usually occurs in body areas of relatively high oxygen tension, most often in the apex of the lung. The lesions show spreading, coalescing tubercles with numerous tubercle bacilli and large areas of caseous necrosis. Necrosis often involves the wall of a small bronchus from which the necrotic material is discharged, resulting in a pulmonary cavity. Frequently, small blood vessels are also eroded. As a result, the sputum in these patients is often bloodstained and contains caseous material and numerous tubercle bacilli. Sputum droplets from such patients are the major source of infection to others. Chronic fever, weight loss, night sweats and productive coughing, often with hemoptysis, are characteristics of the disease. Reactivation tuberculosis can also occur in other organs, such as the kidney, bones, lymph nodes, brain, meninges, bone marrow, and bowel.

Immunity to Tuberculosis

Innate immunity

As discussed previously, humans generally have a rather high innate immunity to development of disease. This immunity was dramatically illustrated in the Lübeck disaster of 1926: as a result of a laboratory error, 249 infants were fed a virulent culture of *M. Tuberculosis* in place of the intended bacillus Calmette–Guérin (BCG) vaccine. Although the dose was very large, 173 of the children developed only minor lesions and survived; 76 children, however, died of acute disease. Among humans, there is excellent epidemiologic and historic evidence for differences in racial immunity. Races with a long history of urbanization and exposure to the epidemics of the 18th and 19th centuries have greater resistance than rural peoples or those whose exposure to infection was recent. Those of urbanized European stock appear to have a high degree of immunity, whereas native Americans and Eskimos, whose exposure was quite recent, are very susceptible and had high morbidity and mortality when the infection was introduced.

Racial immunity

It is impossible to be precise about the extent of the influence of differences in innate immunity on morbidity and mortality, because cultural and environmental differences are also operative. Studies on attack rates in identical and nonidentical twins, however, have clearly shown genetic differences in susceptibility. When one twin is clinically infected, the attack rate in an identical twin is 75%; that in nonidentical twins is 25%.

Acquired immunity and hypersensitivity

Acquired immunity is cell mediated but incomplete. Macrophages are activated and limit both the spread and the multiplication of *M. tuberculosis.* The concomitant delayed-type hypersensitivity to tuberculoprotein plays an important role in immunity to initial infection by mobilizing immune cells and macrophages to the site of deposition of tubercle bacilli. The role of delayed-type hypersensitivity in immunity of established tuberculosis is more complex, because high degrees of sensitivity can precipitate the caseous necrosis that may lead to spread of the disease. Therapy by inoculation with large doses of tuberculin, as attempted at the turn of the century, leads to a systemic tuberculin reaction with hyperemia and even necrosis in tuberculous lesions, marked constitutional signs, and often spread of the disease. This treatment was abandoned rapidly when its effects were recognized.

Systemic tuberculin reaction

The Tuberculin Test

PPD test measures hypersensitivity to tuberculoprotein

The tuberculin skin test measures delayed-type hypersensitivity to tuberculoprotein. Purified protein derivative (PPD), derived from culture filtrates of *M. tuberculosis*, is standardized biologically against an international reference preparation and its activity expressed in tuberculin units (TUs). Most initial skin tests employ 5 TUs (intermediate strength). When an unusually high degree of hypersensitivity or eye or skin tuberculosis is suspected, then 1 TU (first strength) or less is used initially to avoid the risk of an excessive reaction locally or at the site of a mycobacterial lesion.

The test most commonly performed involves intradermal injection of 0.1 ml of PPD containing 5 TU. It is read 48–72 hr later. An area of measured induration of 10 mm or more accompanied by erythema constitutes a positive reaction, although smaller areas of induration and erythema indicate a lesser degree of sensitization to mycobacterial proteins. No induration indicates a negative reaction.

interpretation of PPD test

A positive PPD test indicates that the individual has been infected at some time with *M. tuberculosis* or with a strongly cross-reacting mycobacterium of another species. It carries no implication about the activity of the infection, which may have been simply a primary complex contracted 20 years previously.

A negative PPD test in a healthy individual indicates that he or she has not been infected with *M. tuberculosis,* is in the prehypersensitive stage of a primary infection, or has finally lost tuberculin sensitivity along with disappearance of antigen from an old primary complex. Patients with severe disseminated disease, those on steroid or immunosuppressive drugs, or those with certain other diseases such as measles may also become anergic, lose their tuberculin hypersensitivity, and become more susceptible to the disease.

anergy

Induration below the 10-mm-diameter criterion for positivity indicates low-level sensitization, which may be attributable to *M. tuberculosis* infection or to a cross-reacting mycobacterial infection.

clinical value of PPD test

The clinical value of the PPD test depends on the occurrence of primary infection in different age groups. In earlier years and in many underdeveloped countries, the test had little diagnostic value because primary infection, and thus a high positivity rate, was the rule by late childhood or early adult life. Now, in much of the Western world, primary infection is sufficiently uncommon that a negative test is frequently important in excluding tuberculosis, and a positive test in infancy or childhood has significance in diagnosis and can often be used to trace a household or school source of infection. Epidemiologic surveys of tuberculin reactivity indicate trends in the incidence of infection and constitute the simplest way of monitoring the effectiveness of control measures.

value in case finding

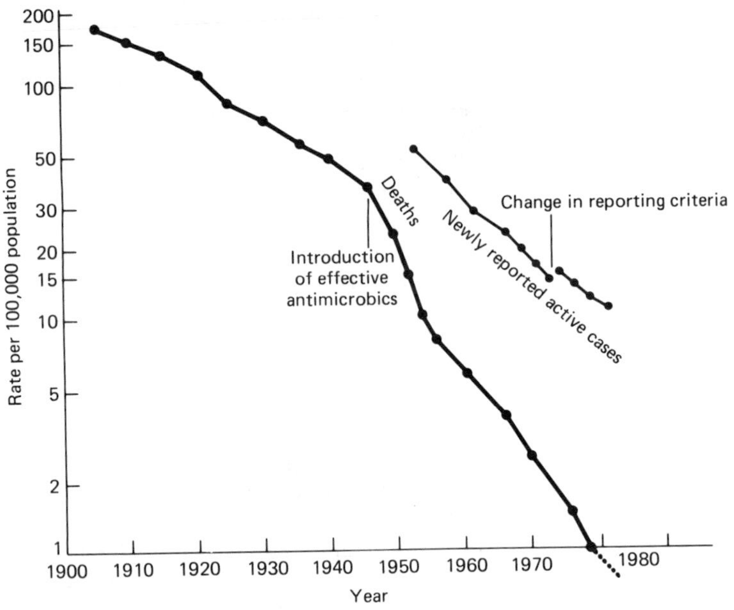

25.2 Morbidity and mortality of tuberculosis in the United States, 1900–1980.

Epidemiology of Tuberculosis

The major factors determining the epidemiology of tuberculosis have already been mentioned. The change in mortality and occurrence of the disease in the United States over the last century is shown in Figure 25.2. As the incidence of infection has decreased, there has been a major shift in the age of tuberculosis patients: now, most are over 50 years old and represent cases in which an old primary lesion, quiescent for decades, has become reactivated. The grandfather who has developed "chronic bronchitis" is a classic source of infection to children.

Single-source epidemics

A few single-source epidemics of tuberculosis occur each year, often involving schoolchildren and a teacher with unrecognized cavitary pulmonary tuberculosis or tuberculous bronchopneumonia. Often the majority of such children exposed over time become PPD positive, and some develop clinical and radiologic evidence of primary infection. Such exposure in childhood is an indication for chemoprophylaxis.

Treatment and Prophylaxis

Combined therapy

Treatment of established tuberculosis always involves double or triple therapy to prevent the selection of resistant mutants. Such treatment with antimicrobics to which the organism is susceptible will usually render the patient noninfectious within a week or two, which has shifted the care of the tuberculous patient from isolation hospitals and sanatoriums to the home or the general hospital. After an initial intense phase of systemic chemotherapy, treatment is usually continued with oral antimicrobics for a year or more. The effectiveness of chemotherapy on most forms of tuberculosis has been dramatic and has greatly reduced the need for surgical procedures such as pulmonary lobectomy. More disabling procedures designed to collapse the affected lung are rarely, if ever, needed. Failure of chemotherapy is often associated with lack of adherence to the regimen by the patient.

prophylactic therapy

Prophylactic chemotherapy, almost always with isoniazid alone, is now used in situations in which known or suspected primary tuberculous infection

Table 25.2 Some Indications for Isoniazid Prophylaxis of Tuberculosis

1. Radiologic evidence of active primary complex.
2. PPD-positive close contact of infectious case.
3. Child who is close contact of infectious case, whether or not PPD positive (retest after 12 weeks).
4. Known recent PPD converter (e.g., laboratory worker who is regularly tested).
5. Patient with skin test, radiologic, or other evidence of primary infection who is immunosuppressed, undergoing corticosteroid treatment, or has a disease causing predisposition to tuberculosis.

Abbreviations: PPD = purified protein derivative.

poses the risk of clinical disease. Some indications for prophylaxis are summarized in Table 25.2. Isoniazid can be used alone in prophylaxis because the load of tubercle bacilli in a subclinical primary lesion is small in relation to that in reactivation tuberculosis, and experience has shown that the development of subsequent clinical disease from isoniazid-resistant strains selected by prophylaxis can be discounted.

Immunoprophylaxis

BCG vaccine

live attenuated derivative of *M. bovis*

The BCG vaccine (named for its originators, Calmette and Guérin) has been used for prophylaxis of tuberculosis in various countries since 1923; administration is usually intradermal. It is a live vaccine derived originally from a strain of *M. bovis* that was attenuated by repeated subculture in a bile-containing medium until it became of markedly reduced virulence, but would still induce tuberculin hypersensitivity. Since then, it has had a checkered history, with results in different controlled trials ranging from ineffectiveness to 80% protection. This disparity arose partly because cultures of BCG maintained in different countries varied in their immunizing ability, partly because of differences in the ages and hypersensitivity status of the trial populations, and partly because some populations already had a baseline immunity from infection with mycobacteria other than *M. tuberculosis.* On the basis of encouraging early trials, massive immunization campaigns sponsored by the World Health Organization were organized in underdeveloped countries.

PPD conversion by BCG

Successful BCG vaccination leads to a minor local lesion, self-limiting multiplication of the organism locally and in draining lymphatic vessels, and development of tuberculin hypersensitivity. The latter results in loss of the PPD test as a diagnostic and epidemiologic tool, and when infection rates are low, as they are now in most Western countries, this loss may offset the possible immunity produced. In general, tuberculosis rates in the West have declined as rapidly in countries that have not used the BCG vaccine as in those that have adopted mass vaccination with its occasional complications. Its potential value is restricted to population groups at particular risk, but its role in developing countries remains a matter of some contention.

Laboratory Diagnosis

Direct smears

Acid–alcohol-fast bacilli can be detected microscopically in clinical specimens if they are present in sufficient numbers (Plate T). About 60% of culture-positive sputum samples show positive direct smears. Direct examination can be done by the Ziehl–Neelsen procedure or one of its modifications, including the fluorescence staining method. These procedures are not specific for *M. tuberculosis* because other mycobacteria may have a similar morphology and may be etiologic agents of disease, members of the normal flora, or external contaminants. Their significance depends on the specimen. Acid-fast bacilli in sputum collected into a container not subject to contamination are highly significant for mycobacterial infection. A clean-voided male urine specimen, on the other hand, is often contaminated with *Mycobacterium smegmatis* from the prepuce, and the finding of acid-fast bacilli does not per se indicate infection. Bronchoscopy equipment and nasotracheal tubes or their lubricants are prone to contamination with free-living mycobacteria, and false conclusions have been drawn from smears of such preparations.

M. smegmatis and contaminating mycobacteria

Specimens for culture

treatment of contaminated material to kill other organisms

Cultural confirmation of a tentative diagnosis of tuberculosis is thus essential, and the organism must be isolated for identification and susceptibility testing. Specimens from protected sites, such as cerebrospinal fluid, bone marrow, pleural fluid, and ureteric urine can be seeded directly to the culture media used for *M. tuberculosis* isolation. Those samples inevitably contaminated with normal flora, such as sputum, gastric aspirations (cultured when sputum is not available, for example, in young children), or voided urine, are treated with alkali, acid, or a detergent germicide under conditions that will kill the normal flora, but allow many mycobacteria to survive because of their resistance to these agents. After neutralization or washing, culture media for *M. tuberculosis* are seeded. The most commonly used treatment now employs *N*-acetylcysteine to dissolve mucus, combined with the antibacterial effect of a weak sodium hydroxide solution.

incubation for 6–8 weeks

Cultures for *M. tuberculosis* are incubated for 6–8 weeks before discarding. Positive cultures rarely show colonies before 3 weeks. Once colonies develop, they are tested for various biochemical activities, including those listed in Appendix 25.1, for speciation.

susceptibility testing

Susceptibility testing is important with newly diagnosed cases. When sufficient numbers of acid-fast bacilli are seen on direct smears, the treated clinical specimen can be seeded directly onto antimicrobic-containing media for susceptibility tests, thereby saving several weeks. If numbers are scanty, the initiation of tests must await primary isolation.

interpretation of test results

Because of the complexity of the laboratory diagnosis of mycobacterial diseases, the clinician and laboratory should cooperate closely in reviewing the progress of specimens and in the interpretation of smear, culture, and susceptibility test results.

Other Mycobacteria Causing Tuberculosislike Diseases

environmental acquisition

pigment production

Mycobacteria causing diseases that often resemble tuberculosis are listed in Appendix 25.1. With the exception of *M. bovis*, they have become relatively more prominent as the incidence of tuberculosis had declined. All have proved or suspected environmental reservoirs, and all of the infections they cause appear to be acquired from these sources. There is no evidence of case-to-case transmission. The organisms grow on the same media as *M. tuberculosis,* but usually more rapidly. Colonies of some species produce yellow or orange pigment in the light (photochromogenic), some in the light and dark (scotochromogenic). Species are distinguished by these characteristics and by biochemical reactions. Environmental mycobacteria that cause tuberculosislike infections are usually more resistant than *M. tuberculosis* to some of the antimicrobics used in the treatment of mycobacterial diseases, and susceptibility testing is often needed as a guide to therapy.

In the past, these organisms were referred to as *atypical* or *anonymous mycobacteria.* Both terms are now inappropriate, because these species are well characterized in their own right.

Mycobacterium kansasii

photochromogen

Distribution

Mycobacterium kansasii is a photochromogenic mycobacterium that usually forms yellow-pigmented colonies after about 2 weeks of incubation in the presence of light. In the United States, infection is most common in Illinois, Oklahoma, and Texas and tends to affect urban residents; it is uncommon in the Southeast. There is no evidence of case-to-case transmission, but the reservoir has yet to be identified.

Diseases

cross-hypersensitivity to PPD from *M. tuberculosis*

Mycobacterium kansasii infections resemble tuberculosis and tend to be slowly progressive without treatment. Cavitary pulmonary disease, cervical lymphadenitis (scrofula), and skin infections are most common, but disseminated infections also occur. Hypersensitivity to proteins of *M. kansasii* develops and cross-reacts almost completely with that caused by tuberculosis. Positive PPD tests may thus result from clinical or subclinical *M. kansasii* infection. Prolonged combined chemotherapy with antimycobacterial drugs, including rifampin, is usually effective.

Mycobacterium scrofulaceum

scotochromogen

Mycobacterium scrofulaceum is an acid-fast scotochromogen that occurs in the environment under moist conditions. It forms yellow colonies in the dark or light within 2 weeks, and it shares several features with the *Mycobacterium avium–intracellulare* complex.

Cervical lymphadenitis

Absence of cross sensitivity to PPD

Mycobacterium scrofulaceum is now one of the more common causes of granulomatous cervical lymphadenitis in young children. It derives its name from *scrofula*, an old descriptive term for tuberculous cervical lymphadenitis. The infection is manifested by an indolent enlargement of one or more lymph nodes with little, if any, pain or constitutional signs. It may ulcerate or form a draining sinus to the surface. It does not cause PPD conversion. Treatment usually involves surgical excision.

Mycobacterium avium–intracellulare Complex

source and pathogenicity

distribution

Mycobacterium avium–intracellulare complex is a group of related acid-fast organisms that grow only slightly faster than *M. tuberculosis* and can be divided into a number of serotypes. Among them are organisms that cause tuberculosis in birds (and sometimes swine), but rarely cause disease in humans. Others may produce disease in mammals, including humans, but not in birds. They are found worldwide in soil and water and in infected animals and birds. In the United States they are most common in the Southeast.

diseases

treatment difficulties

The most common infection in humans is cavitary pulmonary disease, often superimposed on chronic bronchitis and emphysema. Most of those infected are white men aged 50 or more. Cervical lymphadenitis, chronic osteomyelitis, and renal and skin infections also occur. The organisms in this group are substantially more resistant to antituberculous drugs than most other species, and treatment with the three or four agents found to be most active often requires supplementation with surgery. About 20% of cases relapse within 5 years of treatment.

PPD-B

Cross-reactivity with PPD from *M. tuberculosis*

A PPD prepared from a strain of *M. intracellulare* (PPD-B) has been used to detect evidence of previous or present infection as well as in epidemiologic surveys. There is some cross-reaction with PPD from *M. tuberculosis.* Skin test surveys give evidence of a high level of subclinical infection in the population of the southeastern states. Currently, PPD-B is not available for routine use.

Mycobacterium leprae and Leprosy

Leprosy is a rare disease in the United States and other Western countries, and for this reason is considered only briefly. It remains a major problem on a worldwide scale, however, with an estimated 15 million cases. Immigration into the Western countries has increased the number of cases reported there.

failure to grow in culture

Human reservoir

low infectivity

Mycobacterium leprae is an acid-fast bacillus that has not been grown in artificial medium or tissue culture beyond, possibly, a few generations. Its reservoir appears to be infected humans, although armadillos may be infected naturally and, very rarely, cases develop in nonendemic areas without known case contacts. The infectivity of *M. leprae* is low. Most new cases have had prolonged close contact with an infected individual in the past. Transmission probably occurs most commonly by contamination of minor skin lesions with infected nasal secretions from cases of lepromatous leprosy, although biting insects may also be involved. In vivo growth is very slow; as a consequence, the incubation period is measured in years or decades.

slow growth in vivo

Two major forms of the disease are recognized, tuberculoid and lepromatous; intermediate forms are seen, however, and the first form may merge into the second.

Tuberculoid Leprosy

skin and nerve involvement

Few *M. leprae* in lesions

Delayed hypersensitivity and cell-mediated immunity

Tuberculoid leprosy involves the development of macules or large, flattened plaques on the face, trunk, and limbs with raised, erythematous edges and dry, pale, hairless centers. The organism may invade some peripheral sensory nerves, resulting in patchy anesthesia. Few *M. leprae* are seen in tuberculoid lesions, which are granulomatous with extensive epithelioid cells, giant cells, and lymphocytic infiltration. Patients show delayed hypersensitivity to lepromin, a tuberculin analog derived from leprous tissue. They mount an excellent cell-mediated immune response. The disease is indolent, with simultaneous evidence of slow progression and healing.

Lepromatous Leprosy

deficient cell-mediated immunity and anergy to lepromin

many *M. leprae* in lesions

extensive skin lesions

Leonine fascies

In lepromatous leprosy, cell-mediated immunity is deficient and patients are anergic to lepromin. Histologically, lesions show dense infiltration with leprosy bacilli, and large numbers may reach the bloodstream. Skin lesions are extensive, symmetric, and diffuse, particularly on the face, with thickening of the looser skin of the lips, forehead, and ears, resulting in the classic leonine appearance. Damage may be severe, with loss of nasal bones and septum, sometimes of digits, and with testicular atrophy in men. The organism spreads systemically, with involvement of the reticuloendothelial system.

Laboratory Diagnosis

Laboratory diagnosis involves preparation of Ziehl–Neelsen-stained scrapings of infected tissue, particularly nasal mucosa or earlobes. In lepromatous leprosy, large numbers of acid-fast bacilli are seen (Plate U). Tuberculoid leprosy is diagnosed clinically and by histologic appearance or biopsy.

Treatment and Prevention

Sulfones

Treatment has been revolutionized by the development of sulfones such as dapsone, which blocks *para*-aminobenzoic acid metabolism in *M. leprae.* When continued for months or years, this treatment usually controls or cures the disease; however, because of the numerous organisms present, relapse

Combined therapy

may result from mutational resistance. Dual therapy with a sulfone and rifampin reduces the risk of this development. Prevention of leprosy involves recognition and treatment of infectious patients and early diagnosis of the disease in close contacts. Chemoprophylaxis with sulfones has been used for children in close contact with lepromatous cases. Immunization with BCG vaccine has been investigated, with varying results.

A possible diagnosis of leprosy elicits fear and distress in patients and contacts out of all proportion to its risks. Few clinicians in the United States have the experience to make such a diagnosis, and expert help should be sought from public health authorities before reaching this conclusion or indicating its possibility to the patient.

Other Mycobacterial Infections

Mycobacterium fortuitum Complex

rapid growth

abscesses

Mycobacterium fortuitum complex comprises free-living, rapidly growing, acid-fast bacilli that produce colonies within 3 days. Human infections are rare. Abscesses at injection sites in drug abusers are probably the most common lesions. Occasional secondary pulmonary infections develop. Some cases have been associated with implantation of foreign material, for example, breast prostheses and artificial heart valves.

Mycobacterium marinum

fish tuberculosis

infections from swimming pools

skin granuloma

Mycobacterium marinum causes tuberculosis in fish, is widely present in fresh and salt waters, and grows at 30°C but not at 37°C. It occurs in considerable numbers in the slime that forms on rocks or on rough walls of swimming pools, and it can cause skin lesions in humans. Classically, a swimmer who abrades his elbows or forearms climbing out of a pool develops a superficial granulomatous lesion that finally ulcerates. It usually heals spontaneously after a few weeks, but is sometimes chronic. The organism may be sensitive to tetracycline as well as to some antituberculous drugs.

Mycobacterium ulcerans

tropics

severe, progressive ulceration

Mycobacterium ulcerans is a much more serious cause of superficial infection. Cases usually occur in the tropics, most often in parts of Africa, New Guinea, and northern Australia, but have been seen elsewhere sporadically. The source and mode of transmission of the infection are unknown. Those infected develop severe ulceration involving the skin and subcutaneous tissue that is often progressive unless treated effectively. Surgical excision and grafting are usually needed. Antimicrobic treatment is often unsuccessful. Like *M. marinum, M. ulcerans* grows at 30°C, but not at 37°C.

Additional Reading and References

Barksdale, L., and Kim, K-S. 1977. *Mycobacterium. Bacteriol Rev.* 41:217–372. A comprehensive review of mycobacteria and of the immunology and cellular pathogenesis of tuberculosis.

Dubos, R.J., and Dubos, J. 1952. *The White Plague. Tuberculosis, Man, and Society.* Boston: Little Brown and Co. A scholarly and highly readable account of the history and impact of tuberculosis on Western culture.

Lowrie, D.B. 1983. How macrophages kill tubercle bacilli. *J. Med. Microbiol.* 16:1–12. A valuable review of the state of knowledge of intracellular interactions with *M. tuberculosis.*

Wolinsky, E. 1979. Non-tuberculous mycobacteria and associated diseases. *Am. Rev. Resp. Dis.* 119:107–159.

Youmans, G.P. 1979. *Tuberculosis.* Philadelphia: W.B. Saunders Co. A multiauthored text on the subject with a comprehensive reference list.

Appendix 25.1 Mycobacteria of Major Clinical Importance[a]

	Characteristics								
Species	Reservoir	Virulence for Humans	Disease Caused	Case-to-Case Transmission	Growth Rate	Optimum Growth Temperature	Pigment Production[b]	Niacin Production[c]	Virulence for Guinea Pigs[d]
M. tuberculosis	Human	+++	Tuberculosis	Yes	S	37	–	+	+
M. bovis	Animals	+++	Tuberculosis	Rare	S	37	–	–	+
Bacillus Calmette–Guérin	Artificial culture	±	Local lesion	Very rare	S	37	–	–	–
M. kansasii	Environmental	+	Tuberculosislike	No	S	37	Photochromogen	–	–
M. scrofulaceum	Environmental	+	Usually lymphadenitis	No	S	37	Scotochromogen	–	–
M. avium–intracellulare	Environmental; birds	+	Tuberculosislike	No	S	37	±	–	–
M. fortuitum	Environmental	±	Local abscess	No	F	37	±	–	Local abscess
M. marinum	Water; fish	±	Skin granuloma	No	S	30	Photochromogen	–	–
M. ulcerans	Probably environmental; tropical	+	Severe skin ulceration	No	S	30	–	–	–
M. leprae	Human	+++	Leprosy	Yes	NG	NG	NG	NG	–
M. smegmatis	Human, external urethral area	–	None	–	F	37	–	–	–

Abbreviations: S = slow (colonies usually develop in 10 days or more); F = fast (colonies develop in 7 days or less); NG = not grown.

[a] Numerous nonpathogenic environmental mycobacteria exist and may contaminate human specimens.
[b] Yellow-orange pigment. Photochromogen = pigment produced in light; scotochromogen = pigment produced in dark or light.
[c] Many other differential biochemical tests used, e.g., nitrate reduction, catalase production, Tween 80 hydrolysis.
[d] Disease following subcutaneous injection of light inoculum (e.g., 10^2 cells).

Kenneth J. Ryan

Actinomyces and *Nocardia*

26

opportunists

Actinomyces and *Nocardia* are bacteria with filamentous and branching growth, which caused them to be confused with fungi before the fundamental differences between eukaryotic and prokaryotic cells were recognized. They are Gram-positive rods related to the mycobacteria (some species are acid fast), but with a distinctive tendency to grow in a treelike branching network. They are opportunists that can sometimes produce indolent, slowly progressive diseases. A related genus, *Streptomyces,* is of medical importance as a producer of many antibiotics, but rarely causes infections. Important differential features of these groups and of the mycobacteria (Chapter 25) to which they are related are shown in Table 26.1.

Actinomyces and Actinomycosis

Microbiologic Characteristics

Habitat

slow-growing anaerobes

Actinomyces are normal inhabitants of some areas of the gastrointestinal tract of humans and animals from the oropharynx to the lower bowel. They grow only under microaerophilic or strictly anaerobic conditions both in vivo and in vitro, and prolonged incubation (4–10 days) is required before macroscopically visible growth appears in artificial culture. In culture and clinical lesions, the organisms typically appear as elongated Gram-positive rods that branch at acute angles and often show irregular staining. In young broth cultures, shorter forms appear as bent diphtheroids or in X and Y letterlike configurations; in pus, however, the most characteristic form is the *sulfur granule.* This yellow-orange granule, named for its gross resemblance to a grain of sulfur, is a small colony (usually less than 0.3 mm) of intertwined branching *Actinomyces* filaments solidified with elements of tissue exudate. The granule is so dense that the branching bacilli are visible only at the edges in a gram-stained preparation (Plate V).

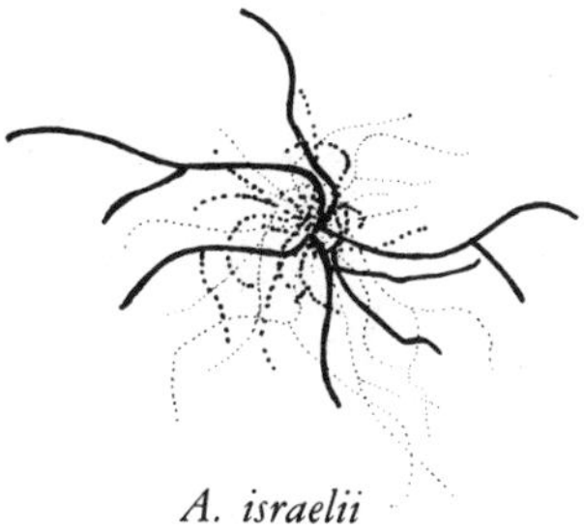

A. israelii

Species of *Actinomyces* are distinguished on the basis of biochemical reactions, cultural features, and cell wall composition. Most human actinomycosis is caused by *Actinomyces israelii,* but other species have been isolated from typical lesions. The related organism *Arachnia propionicus,* originally classified with the *Actinomyces*, can produce clinically similar disease.

Pathogenesis and Pathology

Conditions for growth in tissues

Actinomyces are highly adapted to mucosal surfaces and do not produce disease unless they transgress the epithelial barrier under conditions that produce a sufficiently low oxygen tension for their multiplication. Such conditions

Table 26.1 Some Features of the Family Actinomycetales

Genus	True Branching	Acid Fast	Weakly Acid Fast[b]	Aerobic Growth	Penicillin Susceptible
Mycobacterium[d]	−	+[a]	+	+	−
Actinomyces	+	−	−	−	+
Nocardia	+	−	+[c]	+	−
Streptomyces	+	−	Rare	+	−

[a] Ziehl–Neelsen method for *M. tuberculosis*.
[b] Using weak decolorizer (1% H_2SO_4).
[c] Applies to *N. asteroides* and *N. brasiliensis* only.
[d] See Chapter 25.

usually involve mechanical disruption of the mucosa with necrosis of deeper, normally sterile tissues (for example, following tooth extraction). Once initiated, growth occurs as colonies in the tissues and extends locally through the tissues without regard to anatomic boundaries. The lesion is composed of sinus tracts filled with polymorphonuclear leukocytes surrounded by an indurated fibrous tissue reaction; the sinuses ultimately discharge to the surface. Sulfur granules are present within the pus, but are not numerous. Free *Actinomyces* or small branching units are rarely seen, although contaminating Gram-negative rods are common. As the lesion enlarges, it becomes firm and indurated. If near a cutaneous surface, sinus tracts usually open spontaneously and drain through the skin.

sinus tracts

Pus and sulfur granules

Clinical Manifestations

Cervicofacial actinomycosis

Actinomycosis exists in several forms that differ according to the original site and circumstances of tissue invasion. Infection of the cervicofacial area, the most common site of actinomycosis, is usually related to poor dental hygiene, tooth extraction, or some other trauma to the mouth or jaw. Lesions in the submandibular region and the angle of the jaw give the face a swollen, indurated appearance.

Thoracic actinomycosis

Thoracic actinomycosis is very rare and may involve the lungs, pleura, mediastinal structures, or chest wall. It may follow aspiration of infected material, leading to an actinomycotic lung abscess that can erode through the pleura and even the chest wall. It can also result from sinuses that initiated in actinomycotic lesions above or below the chest.

Abdominal actinomycosis

Abdominal actinomycosis is also rare. It can follow surgery or other trauma to the bowel, as well as perforations of ulcers or diverticula. Diagnosis is usually delayed, because only vague or nonspecific symptoms are produced until a vital organ is eroded or obstructed. The firm, fibrous masses are often initially mistaken for a malignancy.

Pelvic involvement as an extension from other sites also occurs occasionally. It is particularly difficult to distinguish from other inflammatory conditions or malignancies. Recently a more localized chronic endometritis, apparently caused by *Actinomyces,* has been associated with the use of intrauterine contraceptive devices.

Infections with *Actinomyces* are endogenous, and case-to-case transmission does not appear to occur.

Diagnosis

paucity of *Actinomyces* in sinus drainage

A clinical diagnosis of actinomycosis is based on the nature of the lesion, the slowly progressive course, and a history of trauma or of a condition predisposing to mucosal invasion by *Actinomyces.* The etiologic diagnosis can contamination with other species

Collection of pus for sulfur granules

Direct Gram stains

Culture

Biopsy

be difficult to establish with certainty: although the lesions may be extensive, the number of organisms in pus may be few and may remain concentrated in sulfur granule colonies deep in the indurated tissue. The diagnosis is further complicated by heavy colonization of the moist draining sinuses with other bacteria, usually small Gram-negative rods. This contamination not only causes confusion regarding the etiology, but interferes with isolation of the slow-growing anaerobic *Actinomyces.*

Material for direct smear and culture should include as much pus as possible to increase the chance of collecting the diagnostic sulfur granules. Samples may be spread out in a petri dish lid to facilitate location of the granules, or they may be diluted with a large volume of saline; in the latter case, the granules tend to sediment to the bottom of the tube on standing.

Granules crushed between two slides and stained show a dense, Gram-positive center with individual branching rods at the periphery. Granules should also be selected and macerated for culture, because culture of a simple swab from a draining sinus will usually grow only contaminants; thus, detection of any *Actinomyces* is unlikely. Culture media and techniques are the same as those used for other anaerobes (Chapters 9 and 15). Incubation must be prolonged, because some strains require 7 days or more to appear. Identification requires a variety of biochemical tests to differentiate *Actinomyces* from propionibacteria (anaerobic diphtheroids), which may show a tendency to form short branches in fluid culture.

Biopsies for culture and histopathology are useful, but it may be necessary to examine many sections and pieces of tissue before sulfur granule colonies of *Actinomyces* are found. The morphology of the sulfur granule in tissue is quite characteristic with routine hematoxylin and eosin (H&E) or histologic Gram staining. With H&E, the edge of the granule shows amorphous eosinophilic "clubs" formed from the tissue elements and containing the branching actinomycotic filaments.

Treatment

Penicillin therapy

Penicillin G is the treatment of choice for actinomycosis, although a number of other antimicrobics (tetracycline, erythromycin, clindamycin) are active in vitro and have shown some clinical effectiveness. High doses of penicillin must be used and therapy prolonged for 4–6 weeks or more before any response is seen. Although slow, response to therapy is often striking given the degree of fibrosis and deformity caused by the infection. Because detection of the causative organism is difficult, many patients are treated empirically as a therapeutic trial based on clinical findings alone.

Nocardia

Microbiologic Characteristics

aerobes

Habitat

Morphology

Nocardia species are Gram-positive, rod-shaped bacteria that show true branching both in culture and in clinical lesions. In contrast to *Actinomyces,* they are strict aerobes, and the species most common in human infection (*Nocardia asteroides* and *Nocardia brasiliensis*) are weakly acid fast. *Nocardia* species are commonly found in the environment, particularly in soil. They have been isolated in small numbers from the respiratory tract of healthy persons, but are not considered members of the normal human flora.

The microscopic morphology is similar to that of *Actinomyces,* although *Nocardia* tend to fragment more readily and are found as shorter branched units throughout the lesion rather than concentrated in a few colonies or granules. Many strains take the Gram stain poorly, appearing "beaded" with alternating Gram-positive and Gram-negative sections of the same filament. Growth typically appears on ordinary laboratory medium (blood agar) after

Cultural characteristics

2 days. Colonies initially have a dry, chalklike appearance and are usually adherent to the agar, sitting in a craterlike pit. With continued incubation, the colony becomes wrinkled and may develop white to orange pigment. Because of their need for aerobic conditions, colonies form a surface pellicle in broth culture.

Classification

Speciation of *Nocardia* is a tedious process that involves tests for decomposition of substrates such as casein, tyrosine, and xanthine, as well as other tests not usually applied to most bacteria. Although the organism grows in a few days, these tests may require weeks to complete. The species of medical importance are *N. asteroides, N. brasiliensis,* and *Nocardia caviae.*

Pathogenesis and Pathology

Pulmonary nocardiosis

Nocardia produce disease by two distinct routes. The first and most common begins with a pulmonary infection, presumably through inhalation of *Nocardia* present in dust or soil or contaminating mucosal surfaces. This event must be relatively common in comparison to the frequency of disease. Factors leading to disease are poorly understood, although roughly half of all patients with pulmonary nocardiosis have an underlying disease or have undergone treatment known to compromise immune defenses. These conditions include leukemia, lymphoma, chronic pulmonary disorders, and the use of immunosuppressive agents such as corticosteroids. There is evidence that effective cell-mediated immunity is important in host defense against *Nocardia* infection. Increased resistance to experimental *Nocardia* infection in animals has been linked to increased activity of activated macrophages. *Nocardia* are considered opportunists; their infectivity is low, and there is no case-to-case transmission.

Predisposing factors

Immunity

The primary lesions in the lung show acute inflammation with suppuration and destruction of parenchyma to produce multiple, confluent abscesses. Unlike *Actinomyces* infections, there is little tendency toward fibrosis and localization. Dissemination to distant organs, particularly the brain, may occur. In the central nervous system, multifocal abscesses are often produced. The great majority of pulmonary and brain infections are produced by *Nocardia asteroides.*

dissemination to central nervous system

Skin and subcutaneous tissue infections

Another mechanism of infection is direct inoculation of *Nocardia* into the skin or subcutaneous tissues. This mechanism is usually associated with some kind of outdoor activity and with relatively minor trauma, such as a sliver or thorn prick. Infection is usually with *N. brasiliensis,* which produces a superficial pustule at the site of inoculation. If *Nocardia* gain access to the subcutaneous tissues, an infection resembling actinomycosis may be produced, complete with draining sinuses and sulfur granules. This infection may occur with *Nocardia* species or related organisms such as *Actinomadura madurae* (formerly *Nocardia madurae*), a cause of the madura foot syndrome (Chapter 30).

Clinical Manifestations

Bronchopneumonia

Pulmonary infection is usually a confluent bronchopneumonia that may be acute, chronic, or relapsing. Production of cavities and extension to the pleura are common. Symptoms are those of any bronchopneumonia, including cough, dyspnea, and fever. The clinical signs of brain abscess depend on its exact location and size: the neurologic picture can be particularly

Cerebral abscess

confusing when multiple lesions are present. The combination of current or recent pneumonia and focal central nervous system signs is suggestive of *Nocardia* infection. The cutaneous syndrome typically involves a pustule, fever, and tender lymphadenitis in the regional lymph nodes.

Diagnosis

Direct Gram stain

weak acid fastness of *N. asteroides*

The diagnosis of *Nocardia* infection is much easier than that of actinomycosis, because the organisms tend to appear throughout the lesions. Filaments of Gram-positive rods with primary and secondary branches can usually be found in sputum and are readily demonstrated in direct aspirates from skin or other purulent sites. Demonstration of acid fastness, when combined with other observations, is diagnostic of *N. asteroides* or *N. brasiliensis*. The acid fastness of *Nocardia* species differs from that of mycobacteria (Chapter 25), and they are less strongly acid fast. The staining method thus employs a weaker decolorizing agent than that used for mycobacteria. *Nocardia* do not show acid fastness with the regular Ziehl–Neelsen technique; mycobacteria, however, are acid fast by both methods (Table 26.1).

Culture

Culture of *Nocardia* is not difficult if the laboratory is alerted to the possibility of nocardiosis. The organisms grow on routine media used for Gram-positive bacteria (blood agar) or on those used for routine fungal cultures as long as they do not contain antibacterial agents.

Treatment

Sulfonamide therapy and drainage

Nocardia are usually highly sensitive to sulfonamides, but relatively resistant to penicillin. Combination of sulfonamides with drainage and surgery has been successful in treatment of this disease, which rarely enters spontaneous remission. Thus, pulmonary, cutaneous, and central nervous system nocardiosis remains one of the few indications for systemic sulfonamide therapy, although a significant proportion of patients do not respond. Technical difficulties in susceptibility testing have hampered the rational selection and study of other antimicrobics, but various reports support clinical activity of ampicillin, cephalosporins, minocycline, aminoglycosides, cycloserine, and trimethoprim–sulfamethoxazole. Antituberculous agents and antifungal agents such as amphotericin B have no activity against *Nocardia*.

Lawrence Corey

Rickettsiae and Rickettsial Diseases

27

spotted fever
and typhus groups

Members of the genus *Rickettsia* are bacteria that are obligate, intracellular parasites. They multiply by binary fission, contain RNA and DNA, and possess enzymes of the Krebs cycle and ribosomes for protein synthesis. Most rickettsiae have animal reservoirs and are spread by insect vectors, which are prominent components of their life cycles. Pathogenic species are classified into two major groups based on their disease syndromes and vectors. One is the spotted fever group, which includes *Rickettsia rickettsii*, the etiologic agent of Rocky Mountain spotted fever; the other is the typhus group, which includes *Rickettsia prowazekii*, the cause of classic epidemic typhus. An additional rickettsialike organism, *Coxiella burnetii*, causes a distinct systemic disease.

Morphology

small, Gram-negative
coccobacilli

Giemsa stain

Rickettsiae are small bacteria that appear as single coccobacilli or, more commonly, as diplobacilli with tapered ends. The latter usually show a transverse septum between the two bacilli, reflecting division by binary fission. They commonly measure no more than 0.3–0.5 μm. The Gram reaction is negative, but rickettsiae take the usual bacterial stains poorly or not at all. Tissue stains such as Giemsa demonstrate them more clearly, particularly in infected cells. The ultrastructural morphology, which is similar to that of other Gram-negative bacteria, includes a Gram-negative-type cell wall, a plasma membrane, ribosomes, and a nuclear body. Chemically, the cell wall also has the typical Gram-negative peptidoglycan and lipopolysaccharide.

Growth and Metabolism

cytoplasmic growth
in tissue culture

slow growth compared
to most bacteria

induced phagocytosis

Rickettsiae grow only in the cytoplasm of eukaryotic cells, an environment to which they are highly adapted. With one exception, they can be isolated and cultivated in the laboratory using living host cells such as cell cultures or embryonated eggs. Their estimated generation time is much longer than that of bacteria such as *Escherichia coli*, but more rapid than that of *Mycobacterium tuberculosis*. Infection of the host cell begins by induction of a process analogous to phagocytosis, but which requires expenditure of energy by the rickettsiae. The organisms then escape the phagosome to enter the cytoplasm, possibly by elaboration of a phospholipase. Intracytoplasmic growth eventually produces lysis of the cell and infection of another generation of host cells.

exogenous cofactors and ATP required

The obligate intracellular parasitism has several interesting features. Failure to survive outside the cell is apparently related to requirements for nucleotide cofactors (coenzyme A, nicotinamide adenine dinucleotide) and adenosine triphosphate (ATP). In the rickettsia-infected cytoplasm, host cell ATP is exchanged for rickettsial adenosine diphosphate by an exchange transport system similar to that found in mitochondria.

instability outside of cell

Outside the host cell, rickettsiae not only cease metabolic activity, but leak protein, nucleic acids, and essential small molecules. This instability leads to loss of infectivity, because the penetration of another cell requires energy. In summary, rickettsiae have the metabolic capabilities of other bacteria, but must borrow some essential elements from host cells for adequate growth, and thus do not survive well in the environment.

Pathogenesis of Infection

infection of vascular endothelium

Rickettsiae infect the vascular endothelium, usually after the bite of an infected arthropod vector. The organisms multiply within these cells and become disseminated widely throughout the vascular system. Clinically the infection is manifested by fever and headache with widespread focal lesions, the most prominent of which is a rash. In the infected sites there is focal hyperplasia of the infected endothelial cells, inflammation, and thrombosis, leading to obstruction of small blood vessels. An endotoxinlike shock has been demonstrated in animals on injection of whole rickettsial cells, but the nature and role of any toxin in human disease are unknown.

vascular obstruction

possible toxin

pneumonitis without rash in Q fever

Q fever is atypical in its transmission and pathogenesis. The etiologic agent, *C. burnetii*, survives well in the environment and is acquired by inhalation of organisms aerosolized from infected animal tissues. The disease produced is usually a febrile pneumonia without a rash.

Specific Diagnosis of Disease

Weil–Felix serodiagnostic test

In the early 1900s, it was observed that serum from patients with typhus caused agglutination of certain strains of *Proteus vulgaris*. This finding was developed into a serologic testing scheme called the *Weil–Felix test* in which three *Proteus* strains, OX-19, OX-2, and OX-K, have been used as antigens to detect rickettsial antibody (Table 27.1). Recently, more specific serologic tests such as complement fixation have been developed using rickettsial antigens. Isolation of rickettsia in eggs or cell cultures is generally attempted only in reference centers, because the risk of laboratory infection requires special facilities and personnel experienced in handling the organisms.

hazards of attempting isolation

Spotted Fever Group

many tick-borne rickettsioses in different parts of world

A number of spotted fever rickettsioses are found in various parts of the world; the name often reveals the locale (for example, South African tick-bite fever and Queensland tick fever). They are caused by rickettsial species serologically related to, but distinct from, *R. rickettsii*, the cause of the most important rickettsial disease in North America, Rocky Mountain spotted fever. This disease will be used to typify the spotted fevers; another less severe illness that occurs in North America, rickettsialpox, will also be discussed.

Table 27.1 Pathogenic Rickettsiae

Disease	Organism	Geographic Distribution	Zoonotic Cycle: Vector	Zoonotic Cycle: Reservoir	Weil–Felix Serology: OX-19	Weil–Felix Serology: OX-2	Weil–Felix Serology: OX-K
Spotted fever group							
Rocky Mountain	*Rickettsia rickettsii*	North and South America	Tick	Rodents	+	+	−
Rickettsialpox	*Rickettsia akari*	United States; Soviet Union; Korea; Africa	Mite	Mouse	−	−	−
Typhus group							
Epidemic	*Rickettsia prowazekii*	Africa; Asia; South America	Body louse	Man	+	+/−	−
Brill's	*Rickettsia prowazekii*	Worldwide[a]	None[b]	Man	+/−	−	−
Murine	*Rickettsia typhi*	Worldwide (pockets)	Flea	Rodents	+	+/−	−
Scrub	*Rickettsia tsutsugamushi*	South Pacific; Asia	Mite	Rodents	−	−	+
Q fever	*Coxiella burnetii*	Worldwide	None[c]	Cattle; sheep	−	−	−

[a] Related to immigration. [b] Relapsing form of epidemic typhus. [c] Inhalation in humans; animals may have a vector.

Rocky Mountain Spotted Fever

Rocky Mountain spotted fever is a common infection in the United States, with more than 1100 cases reported each year. In the past decade, the number of cases has been increasing, probably because of increased recreational exposure to areas where infected ticks exist. The disease has a significant mortality (7%), although most patients recover spontaneously.

natural infection of ticks

transovarial spread

infected ticks can survive for years without feeding

Habitat. Rickettsia rickettsii is primarily a parasite of ticks. In the western United States, the wood tick (*Dermacentor andersoni*) is the primary vector. In the East the dog tick (*Dermacentor variabilis*) and in the Southwest the Lone Star tick (*Amblyomma americanum*) are the natural carriers and vectors of the disease. As *R. rickettsii* does not kill its arthropod host, the organism is passed through unending generations of ticks by transovarial spread. Rickettsiae acquired transovarially are thus present in the larval, nymph, and adult stages of development. The larval and nymph stages require a blood meal from a small mammal to proceed to the next stage. Adult females require a blood meal to lay eggs. Infected adult ticks have been shown to survive for as long as 4 years without feeding.

Epidemiology. The geographic distribution of Rocky Mountain spotted fever is illustrated in Figure 27.1. The highest attack rates are in the mid-Atlantic states, the Carolinas, and the Virginias. More than two-thirds of cases are in children less than 15 years of age. The illness is generally seen between April and September because of increased exposure to ticks. A history of tick bite can be elicited in approximately 70% of cases.

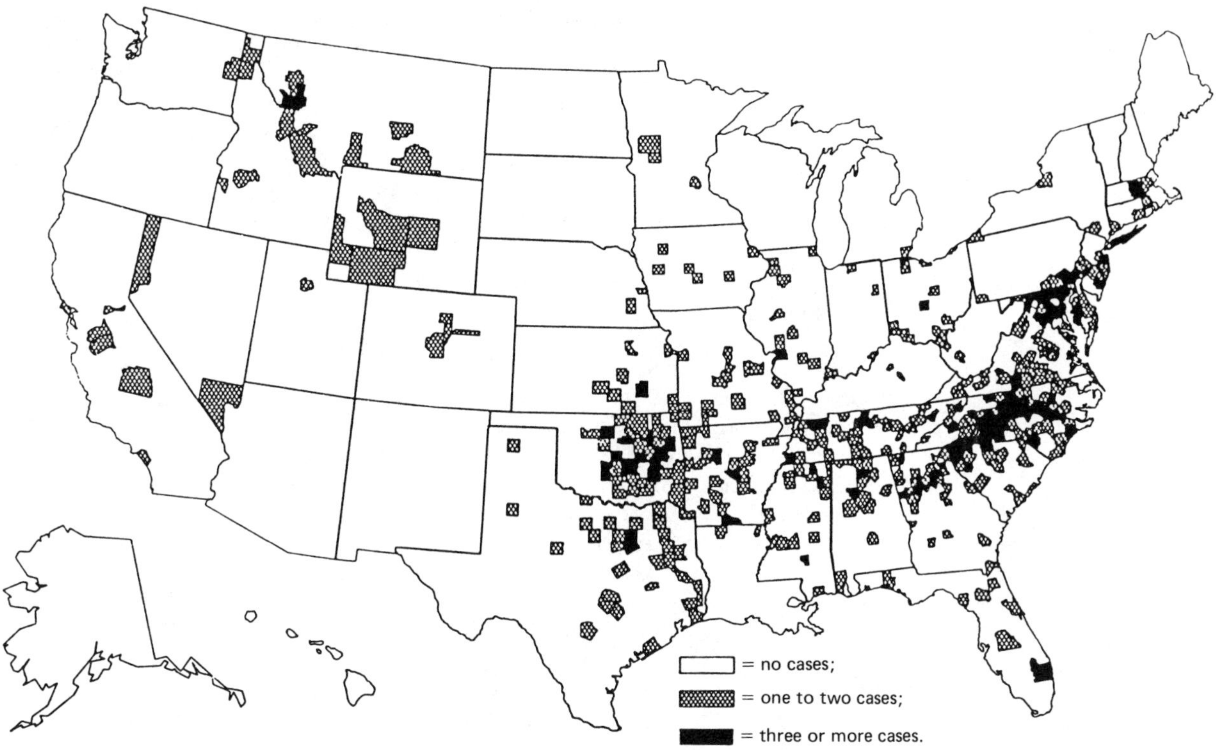

27.1 Rocky Mountain spotted fever. Number of cases reported by county in the United States, 1978. (*Reproduced from Rickettsial Disease Surveillance Summary 1978, Centers for Disease Control, U.S. Department of Health and Human Services.*)

incubation period 2–6 days after tick bite

fever, headache, and rash

spread of rash from extremities to trunk

Disease. The incubation period between the tick bite and the onset of illness is usually 2–6 days, but may be as long as 2 weeks. Fever, headache, rash, toxicity, mental confusion, and myalgia are the major clinical features. The rash is the most characteristic feature of the illness. It usually develops on the second or third day of illness as small erythematous macules that rapidly become petechial. The lesions appear initially on the wrists and ankles, then spread up the extremities to the trunk in a few hours. A diagnostic feature of Rocky Mountain spotted fever is the frequent appearance of the rash on the palms and soles, a finding not usually seen in the maculopapular eruptions associated with viral infections. Muscle tenderness, especially in the gastrocnemius, is characteristic and may be extreme. If untreated, or in occasional cases despite therapy, complications such as disseminated intravascular coagulation, thrombocytopenia, encephalitis, vascular collapse, and renal and/or heart failure may ensue.

Complications

Rickettsial multiplication in endothelial cells causing vasculitis

The primary pathologic lesion is a vasculitis in which rickettsiae multiply in the endothelial cell lining of the small blood vessels. Focal areas of endothelial proliferation and perivascular infiltration lead to thrombosis and leakage of red blood cells into the surrounding tissues, accounting for the rash and petechial lesions; however, vascular lesions occur throughout the body, thus producing the systemic manifestations of the disease. They are obviously most apparent in skin, but most serious in the adrenal glands.

diagnosis and therapy based on clinical manifestations

Diagnosis. No laboratory test is generally available to establish the diagnosis of Rocky Mountain spotted fever early in the course of illness. Specific therapy must be started based solely on clinical signs, symptoms, and epi-

Serodiagnosis: rising OX-19 and OX-2 and complement fixation titers

demiologic considerations. *Rickettsia rickettsii* may be identified by immunofluorescent staining of skin biopsy specimens, but this test is only undertaken in specialized laboratories. Complement fixation and immunofluorescent serologic tests are helpful in confirming the diagnosis, but the patient often does not develop high titers of antibody until late in the course of illness. A fourfold rise in antibody titer between acute and convalescent serum establishes the diagnosis. Rising titers to *Proteus* OX-19 or OX-2 or a single titer of 1:160 or greater in a patient with symptoms similar to Rocky Mountain spotted fever are presumptive evidence of infection. Low titers of antibody to these organisms (1:20 to 1:80) may be found in healthy individuals.

need for treatment during first week

tetracycline or chloramphenicol

Therapy. Appropriate antibiotic therapy is highly effective if given during the first week of illness. If delayed into the second week or when pathologic processes such as diffuse intravascular coagulation are present, therapy becomes progressively less effective. The antibiotics of choice are tetracycline and chloramphenicol. Seriously ill patients and children less than 8 years of age are usually given chloramphenicol. Sulfonamides may enhance the disease process and are thus contraindicated. Before specific therapy became available, the mortality of Rocky Mountain spotted fever was approximately 25%. Treatment has reduced this figure to 5–7%. Death results primarily in patients in whom diagnosis and therapy are delayed into the second week of illness.

frequent deticking

Prevention. The major measure for prevention of Rocky Mountain spotted fever is the avoidance or reduction of tick contact. Frequent deticking in tick-infested areas is important, because ticks generally must feed for 4–6 hr before they can transmit the disease. Tick surveys in the Carolinas have shown infection in about 5% of samples. Killed vaccines prepared from infected ticks, embryonated eggs, and cell cultures have been developed, but none is licensed for clinical use at present.

Rickettsialpox

benign disease transmitted by rodent mites

local eschar

Rickettsialpox was first recognized in New York City in 1946. It is a benign rickettsial illness caused by *Rickettsia akari* and transmitted by a rodent mite. Distinguishing features of the disease include an eschar at the site of the bite, vesicular rash, and the absence of Weil–Felix agglutinins. The house mouse and other semidomestic rodents are the primary reservoir. Humans acquire infection when the mite seeks an alternative host.

fever and rash

tetracycline therapy

Rickettsialpox is a biphasic illness. The first phase is the local lesion at the bite, which starts as a papulovesicle and develops into a black eschar over 3–5 days. Fever and constitutional symptoms appear as the organism disseminates. The second phase of the disease is a diffuse rash distributed randomly in the body, which, like the local lesion, becomes papulovesicular and develops into eschars. Rickettsialpox is self-limiting after 1 week, and no deaths have been reported. Tetracycline therapy shortens the course to 1–2 days.

Typhus Group

Primary Louse-Borne Typhus Fever

severe louse-borne disease

Primary louse-borne typhus fever is an acute, infectious disease caused by *R. prowazekii* that is transmitted to humans by the body louse. Historically, it has appeared during periods of war, famine, and social upheaval, which create conditions favorable to human body lice (crowding, infrequent ba-

Endemic foci

thing, and the like). The last North American epidemic was in Philadelphia in 1893; however, endemic typhus foci persist in Eastern Europe, Asia, Africa, and South America. During both World Wars, louse-borne typhus infected millions and was particularly devastating in concentration camps.

Cycle of infection: not transmitted ovarially in lice

The chain of typhus infection starts with *R. prowazekii* circulating in a patient's blood during an acute febrile infection. The human body louse becomes infected during one of its frequent blood meals and, after 5–10 days of incubation, large numbers of rickettsiae appear in its feces. As the louse defecates while it feeds, the organisms can be rubbed into the louse-bite wounds when the host scratches the site. Dried louse feces are also infectious through the mucous membranes of the eye or respiratory tract. The louse dies of its infection in 1–3 weeks, and the rickettsiae are not transmitted transovarially.

fever, headache, and rash

Complications

Serodiagnosis

Treatment and prevention

Fever, headache, and rash begin 1–2 weeks after the bite. A maculopapular rash appears first on the trunk, then spreads centripetally to the extremities, a pattern opposite to that of Rocky Mountain spotted fever. Headache, malaise, and myalgia are prominent components of the illness. Complications include myocarditis and central nervous system dysfunction. In untreated disease, the fatality rate increases with age from 10% to as high as 60%. The Weil–Felix reaction is positive with *Proteus* OX-19 and less commonly with OX-2 (both are positive in Rocky Mountain spotted fever). As with the spotted fever group, therapy with tetracycline or chloramphenicol is effective. Louse control is the best means of prevention and is particularly important in controlling epidemics. A killed vaccine grown in embryonated eggs is used only in persons at high occupational risk.

relapse of typhus after many years

less severe than epidemic typhus

Brill's disease. Brill's disease is a relapse or recrudescence of louse-borne typhus that occurs years after the primary attack. It is seen primarily in immigrants to other countries from Eastern Europe, whose initial infection often occurred during World War II. Factors triggering the relapse are unknown, but may involve fading immunity to rickettsiae that have remained dormant in reticuloendothelial cells. Because of partial immunity, the recrudescent infection is milder, shorter, and less debilitating than primary typhus. Titers to *Proteus* OX-19 are absent or low. Specific antibodies are of the immunoglobulin G class, in contrast to typhus, which shows a primary immune response predominantly with immunoglobulin M antibodies. Prolonged survival of *R. prowazekii* in the human host is important in the endemic maintenance of the disease.

Murine Typhus

transmitted from rat reservoir

Murine typhus is caused by *Rickettsia typhi* and transmitted to humans by the rat flea (*Xenopsylla cheopis*). Human illness is incidental to the natural transmission of the disease among urban rodents, which serve as the reservoir. Only 40–60 cases of murine typhus are reported in the United States each year. These occur predominantly in the southeastern and Gulf states, especially Texas.

resembles typhus, but less severe

shares antigens with *R. prowazekii*

The pathogenesis and transmission are similar to that of louse-borne typhus. The flea defecates when it takes a blood meal, and the infected feces gain access through the bite wound. After an incubation period of 1–2 weeks, illness begins with headache, myalgia, and fever. The rash is maculopapular, starting on the trunk and then spreading to the extremities in a manner similar to typhus. Serologically, the Weil–Felix reaction is similar in louse-borne and murine typhus. Because of antigens shared by *R. typhi* and *R. prowazekii*, even the complement fixation test may not separate the two diseases. In the untreated patient, fever may last 12–14 days. With tetracycline or chloramphenicol therapy, the course is reduced to 2–3 days. Mortality and complications are rare.

Scrub Typhus

transmitted from natural infection of mites

local eschar

fever, headache, and rash

hepatosplenomegaly

OX-K agglutinins

Scrub typhus is found in the Southwest Pacific, Southeast Asia, and Japan. The causative organism is *Rickettsia tsutsugamushi*, and mites that infest rodents are the reservoir and vectors, transmitting the rickettsiae to their own progeny via infected ova. Humans pick up the mites as they pass by low trees or brush. The mite larvae (chiggers) deposit rickettsiae as they feed.

The typical initial lesion, a necrotic eschar at the site of the bite on the extremities, develops in only 50–80% of cases. Fever increases slowly over the first week, sometimes reaching 40.5°C. Later, headache, rash, and generalized lymphadenopathy follow. The maculopapular rash, which appears after about 5 days, is more evanescent than that seen with louse-borne or murine typhus. Hepatosplenomegaly and conjunctivitis may also appear. The diagnosis is primarily clinical, because the only responses by the Weil–Felix test are to OX-K, and titers are elevated in only one-half of cases. Differentiation from dengue, leptospirosis, malaria, or typhoid fever may be difficult. Both chloramphenicol and tetracycline constitute effective therapy.

Q Fever

zoonosis transmitted by inhalation

Q fever differs from other human rickettsial infections in several ways. It is transmitted from animals to humans by inhalation rather than by arthropod bite. The etiologic agent, *C. burnetii*, is usually stable to drying and survives in the environment quite well; moreover, it does not stimulate any of the Weil–Felix antibodies.

infected livestock

infection of placental tissue

prolonged viability in dust

occupational exposure

Q fever is primarily a zoonosis, affecting cattle, sheep, goats, rodents, and marsupials. Distribution is worldwide. In domestic livestock, the infection is usually inapparent, but as many as 50–75% of animals in a herd may be infected in some areas. *Coxiella burnetii* grows particularly well in placental tissue, where it often attains levels of 10^9 organisms per gram of tissue. At the time of birth, the infected tissues contaminate the ground, where the organisms survive within dry dust particles for months. At 40°C, viability is retained for 1 or more years in dried fomites. This remarkable viability appears related to a sporogenic cycle in the organism. The disease occurs sporadically among those who work with infected animals or their products. Epidemics of Q fever have occurred among workers in abattoirs in which infected animals are slaughtered, producing aerosols with massive contamination of employees. In textile plants, infection may occur among employees who break open bales of wool and do the preliminary washing and sorting. Infection in all of these circumstances is believed to result from inhalation.

systemic infection without rash

lung involvement and hepatosplenomegaly

Diagnosis and treatment

Q fever itself is a systemic infection with or without pneumonia. Little is known of the pathology, as fatal cases are rare. The disease usually begins 9–20 days after inhalation, with abrupt onset of fever, chills, and headache. There may be a mild, dry, hacking cough, and a patchy interstitial pneumonia. There is no typical rash. Hepatosplenomegaly is frequent, and abnormal results of tests of liver function are usual. Complications such as myocarditis, pericarditis, and endocarditis have been reported. The diagnosis is usually made by demonstrating high or rising titers of antibody to Q fever antigen by complement fixation or immunofluorescence methods. The disease responds promptly to tetracyclines and, when treated, death is uncommon. No vaccine is available.

Additional Reading and References

Hattwick, M.A.W., O'Brien, R.J., and Hanson, B.F. 1976. Rocky Mountain spotted fever: Epidemiology of an increasing problem. *Ann. Intern. Med.* 84:732–739. The epidemiology of Rocky Mountain spotted fever is reviewed.

Hattwick, M.A.W., Retailliau, H., O'Brien, R.J., Slutzker, M., Fontaine, R.E., and Hanson, B. 1978. Fatal Rocky Mountain spotted fever. *J. Am. Med. Assoc.* 240:1499–1503. Fatal cases illustrative of delay in diagnosis and rapid clinical course are reviewed.

Lawrence Corey

Chlamydia

28

Members of the genus *Chlamydia* are obligate intracellular parasites that were once believed to be large viruses. They are bacteria, however, because their cells possess both RNA and DNA, have a discrete cell wall similar to that of Gram-negative bacteria, multiply in host cells by binary fission, and are susceptible to several antibacterial antimicrobics. Two species cause diseases in humans, *Chlamydia psittaci* and *Chlamydia trachomatis.*

Morphology and Structure

Gram-negative type of cell wall

Chlamydia species are small, generally rounded organisms that show morphologic variation during their replicative cycle. The cell wall contains peptidoglycan and muramic acid and has a lipid outer layer similar to those of Gram-negative bacteria. They possess ribosomes of the bacterial type and synthesize their own protein. Their DNA genome is about one-fourth the size of that of *Escherichia coli.*

Metabolic Characteristics

inability to synthesize ATP

Chlamydia species are metabolically deficient compared to free-living bacteria, because they are dependent on the host cell for energy generation and cannot synthesize adenosine triphosphate (ATP) or reoxidize reduced nicotinamide adenine dinucleotide phosphate. It is probable that they evolved from free-living bacteria to a state of strict intracellular parasitism.

Replicative Cycle

elementary body infects cell

transforms to initial body, which divides by binary fission

initial bodies produce multiple elementary bodies

The replicative cycle of *Chlamydia* is illustrated in Figure 28.1. A small (0.3 μm) elementary body with an electron-dense center enters a host cell by endocytosis (a process analogous to phagocytosis) within a vacuole derived from the host cell membrane. Metabolic changes that are incompletely understood lead the elementary body to reorganize within about 1 hr into a larger (1 μm) form called the *initial body,* which is less dense than the elementary body. Using the ATP-generating capacity of the host cell, the initial bodies divide by binary fission within the endocytic vacuole. After 24–72 hr, the initial bodies reorganize and condense to yield multiple elementary bodies

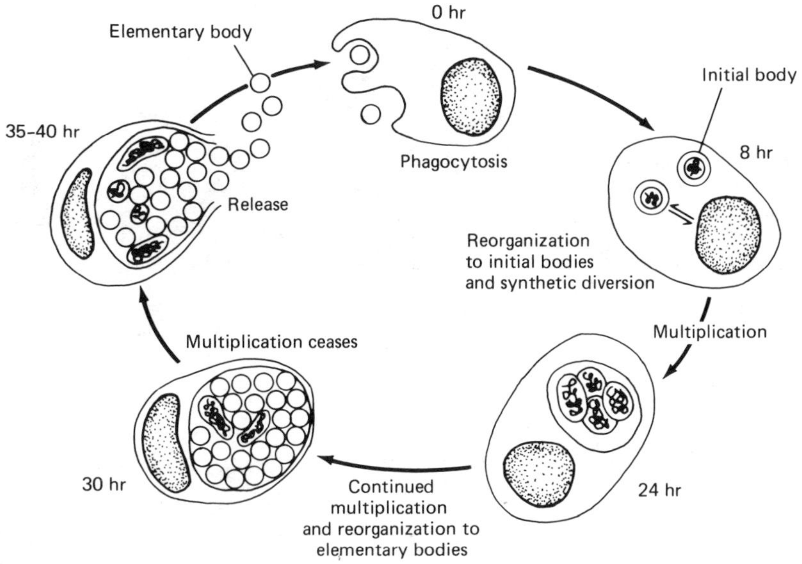

28.1 Reproductive cycle of *Chlamydia. (Reproduced with permission from Alexander, E.R. 1979. Hosp. Pract. July. p.64, drawing by Nancy Lou Gaham.)*

Inclusion bodies

with the capacity to infect other host cells when the infected cell ruptures. One species, *C. trachomatis,* synthesizes large amounts of glycogen, which surrounds the chlamydial cells within the endocytic vacuole. This structure is termed an *inclusion body,* because it is visible on histologic staining as a defined structure that may displace the nucleus of the host cell. Inclusions of the other major species, *C. psittaci,* are more diffuse because glycogen is not synthesized and the vesicle membrane ruptures, resulting in a mass of *Chlamydia* surrounding the nucleus of the host cell.

Growth in the Laboratory

growth in yolk sac of chick embryo and McCoy cells

treatment of McCoy cells for greater chlamydial growth

Chlamydia can be grown in the yolk sac of the developing chick embryo, although it is sometimes difficult with certain strains of *C. trachomatis.* They can also be grown in some tissue culture cells, such as those of the McCoy mouse heteroploid line. Treatment of the cells by irradiation or with idoxuridine (Chapter 10) or cyclohexamide before inoculation inhibits host cell replication and allows *C. trachomatis* to compete better for cell nutrients, and thus to grow better. Chlamydiae may be detected in tissue culture by the development of their characteristic intracytoplasmic inclusions, which are visualized with Giemsa stain or, in the case of *C. trachomatis* (Figure 28.2), with an iodine stain for glycogen. Staining for *Chlamydia* antigen in infected cells using immunofluorescence has also been utilized.

Antigenic Structure

association of specific serotypes with different disease syndromes

Chlamydiae have common lipopolysaccharide antigens and specific cell wall protein antigens by which they are divided into a number of serotypes. Each of the major disease syndromes caused by chlamydiae are associated with different serotypes (Table 28.1). The type-specific antigens elicit protective antibody in experimental animals, but the group antigens do not. Serotyping is performed by a fluorescence antibody procedure, but is not undertaken in routine diagnostic laboratories.

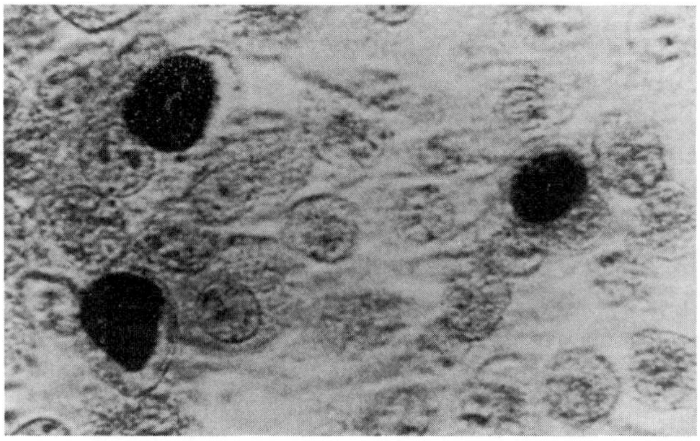

28.2 Iodine-stained inclusions of *C. trachomatis* in McCoy cell culture.

Pathogenesis of Chlamydial Diseases

virulence in mouse

Chlamydia psittaci and some strains of *C. trachomatis* are virulent to varying degrees to mice inoculated by the intravenous or intracerebral route or, in the case of the respiratory pathogen *C. psittaci,* by the intranasal route. *Chlamydia psittaci* is highly infectious to humans by the respiratory route and poses a significant risk to laboratory workers.

prevention of lysosomal fusion

The mechanisms of virulence of *Chlamydia* are incompletely understood. When ingested by phagocytic cells, they prevent lysosomal fusion with the phagocytic vacuole, and thus escape killing by lysosomal enzymes. All species produce heat-labile protein toxins that are lethal to mice on intravenous inoculation and specific to each serotype. Chlamydiae must compete with the host cell for essential nutrients, which may partially account for cell death and consequent tissue damage. *Chlamydia trachomatis* may exist in a latent form and emerge to cause relapses of infection in the immunosuppressed host. The mechanisms of latency are not understood.

competition for nutrients

Susceptibility

failure to survive in environment

Susceptibility to antimicrobics

Chlamydiae are highly susceptible to environmental conditions and survive only briefly outside the body. Thus, transmission involves close contact or, in the case of *C. psittaci,* rapid spread by dust or droplet. They are susceptible to a considerable range of antimicrobics, of which the tetracyclines have been the most effective agents in clinical practice. In contrast to *C. psittaci,*

Table 28.1 Association among Chlamydial Species, Serotypes and Disease

Species	Subtype	Disease
C. psittaci	Many	Psittacosis
C. trachomatis	A, B, C	Trachoma
	D, E, F, H, I, J, K	Nongonococcal urethritis; cervicitis; endometritis; salpingitis; proctitis; epididymitis; inclusion conjunctivitis in newborns; infant syndrome pneumonia
	L_1, L_2, L_3	Lymphogranuloma venerum

Table 28.2 Major Differential Features of *Chlamydia* Species That Cause Human Disease

Feature[a]	*C. psittaci*	*C. trachomatis*
Natural habitat	Birds	Humans
Diseases	Pneumonitis	Conjunctivitis; genital tract infections; lymphogranuloma venereum
Virulence in mouse	High	Variable
Glycogen containing discrete inclusion bodies	No	Yes
Sensitive to sulfonamides	No	Yes

[a] Information regarding serotypes is provided in Table 28.1.

many strains of *C. trachomatis* are sensitive to sulfonamides; this finding indicates that *C. trachomatis* synthesizes its own folic acid, whereas *C. psittaci* uses that provided by the host.

Species Differentiation

Little DNA homology is found between *C. psittaci* and *C. trachomatis,* although they share a common group antigen. Their major differential features are shown in Table 28.2

Infections with *Chlamydia psittaci*

zoonotic respiratory disease from birds

Human psittacosis (ornithosis) is a zoonosis contracted through inhalation of respiratory secretions, or dust from droppings, of infected birds. It was initially described in psittacines such as parrots and parakeets, but was subsequently shown to occur in a wide range of avian species. The disease is usually latent in its natural host but may become active, particularly with the stress of recent captivity or transport; *C. psittaci* is then excreted in large amounts.

association with turkey processing and captive psittacine birds

Psittacosis in humans is now seen mainly as an occupational hazard of poultry workers, especially those associated with processing turkey carcasses. It may also occur in owners of pet psittacine birds. There has been a marked reduction in cases of human psittacosis in the United States during the past 20 years. This decrease has been associated with the use of antimicrobics in poultry feeds and with quarantine regulations for imported psittacine birds.

clinical manifestations of pneumonitis from *C. psittaci*

Clinically, psittacosis in humans is an acute infection of the lower respiratory tract, usually presenting with acute onset of fever, headache, malaise, muscle aches, dry, hacking cough, and X-ray evidence of bilateral interstitial pneumonia. Occasionally, systemic complications such as myocarditis, encephalitis, and hepatitis may develop. The liver and spleen are often enlarged. The diagnosis of psittacosis should be suspected in a patient with acute onset of febrile lower respiratory illness with hepatosplenomegaly who gives a history of close exposure to birds. It must be remembered that spread can occur from both symptomatic and asymptomatic infections of birds. The specific diagnosis is usually made by demonstrating a fourfold rise in the titer of complement fixing antibody to chlamydial group antigen over several days of illness. *Chlamydia psittaci* can be isolated from the blood early in the disease and from sputum. Attempts to do so, however, must be made only in specialized laboratories because of the risk of laboratory infection and

Diagnosis and treatment

spread. Treatment with tetracycline or erythromycin is effective if given early in the course of illness.

Infections with *Chlamydia trachomatis*

Eye Infections

Trachoma and inclusion conjunctivitis

There are two distinct diseases, trachoma and inclusion conjunctivitis, which have some overlap in their clinical manifestations. Trachoma, a chronic infection caused by *C. trachomatis* immunotypes A, B, Ba, and C, is usually seen in less developed countries and often leads to blindness. Inclusion conjunctivitis is a worldwide disease of both adults and newborns. It is characterized as an acute inflammation of the conjunctiva, but is usually not associated with chronicity or permanent eye damage. It is caused by immunotypes D–K.

leading cause of blindness in some developing countries

chronicity

Trachoma. Trachoma, a chronic follicular conjunctivitis, remains one of the leading causes of preventable blindness in the world. It is a major public health problem in North Africa, sub-Saharan Africa, and Central and Southeast Africa. In the United States, pockets of endemic trachoma exist, mainly among Native American populations in the Southwest. It is a complex disease that involves persistent infection and reinfection with *C. trachomatis,* hypersensitivity reactions to the organism, and superinfection with other bacterial species.

usually contracted in early life

eyelid and corneal scarring

The disease is usually contracted in infancy or early childhood from the mother or other close contacts. First exposure results in acute conjunctivitis, which usually resolves. Persistence and reinfections and the associated inflammatory responses provide the stimulus for the major pathologic effects of the disease in untreated cases. Chronic inflammation of the eyelids and increased vascularization of the corneal conjunctiva are followed by severe corneal scarring and conjunctival deformities. Visual loss often occurs 15–20 years after the initial infection.

prevention of reinfection

Treatment

Treatment of trachoma is difficult and generally directed toward prevention of continued reinfection during early childhood. From a public health point of view, improved hygiene appears to be the most effective approach and is aimed at decreasing transmission of infection within families. Treatment with systemic and topical antimicrobial agents such as sulfonamides, tetracycline, and erythromycin is often used to prevent reinfection or to treat persistent infection. Corrective surgery is required for severe corneal and blepharal conjunctival scarring.

common form of neonatal conjunctivitis contracted from maternal genital infection

Inclusion conjunctivitis. Inclusion conjunctivitis is an acute infection of the conjunctiva seen in infants and adults among population groups in which the serotypes causing *C. trachomatis* genital infections are common. It is the most common form of neonatal conjunctivitis in the United States, occurring in 2–6% of newborn infants. The infection results from direct contact with infected cervical secretions of the mother at delivery.

Diagnosis and treatment

Inclusion conjunctivitis usually presents as an acute, copious, mucopurulent eye discharge 2–25 days after birth. The symptoms can resolve spontaneously and may not come to medical attention. Diagnosis can be made most easily by demonstrating characteristic cytoplasmic inclusions in smears of conjunctival scrapings (Figure 28.3). *Chlamydia trachomatis* can be isolated from conjunctival swabs. Topical antimicrobial treatment is effective for controlling eye disease; however, systemic therapy is preferred because the nasopharynx, rectum, and vagina may also be colonized and other forms of disease may develop, such as infant pneumonia syndrome. Inclusion conjunctivitis is less common in adults than in children and is usually associated with concomitant genital tract disease.

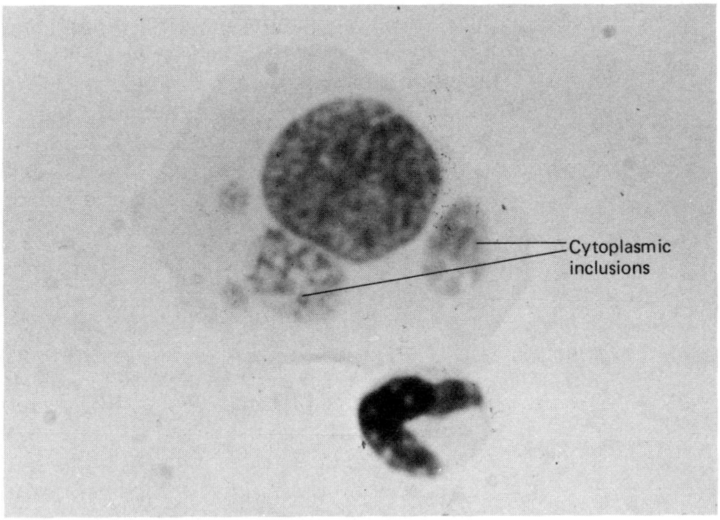

28.3 *Chlamydia trachomatis* cytoplasmic inclusion body in conjunctival epithelial cell.

Genital Tract Infections

The clinical spectrum of sexually transmitted infections with *C. trachomatis* is similar to that of *Neisseria gonorrhoeae. Chlamydia trachomatis* can cause urethritis and epididymitis in men and cervicitis, salpingitis, and urethral syndrome in women. In addition, three serotypes of *C. trachomatis* cause the venereal disease lymphogranuloma venereum.

common cause of nongonococcal urethritis and epididymitis in men

Chlamydia trachomatis has been shown to cause about 40% of cases of nongonococcal urethritis in men in Western industrialized societies, which can be indistinguishable clinically from *N. gonorrhoeae* infection. The patient suffers from dysuria and urethral discharge, and polymorphonuclear leukocytes are seen on Gram stains of the discharge. Chlamydiae are not seen in Gram-stained smears, but can be isolated from urethral swabs. Epididymitis may result, and recent studies in the United States indicate that *C. trachomatis* is more common than *N. gonorrhoeae* as a cause of this disease among sexually active men under 35 years of age.

Diseases in women

In women, *C. trachomatis* has been shown to cause both lower and upper genital tract infections. Infection of the uterine cervix is common and may be asymptomatic. Symptomatic infections present as mucopurulent cervicitis. The prevalence of *C. trachomatis* cervical infections, like those caused by *N. gonorrhoeae,* is highest in young adults, in those from lower socioeconomic groups, and in those with multiple sex partners. In most U.S. populations, *C. trachomatis* has been isolated from 5–10% of women consulting private gynecologists for prenatal examinations. The prevalence among patients at sexually transmitted disease clinics may be as high as 20–25%. Approximately one-third to one-half of all male sexual contacts of women with *C. trachomatis* cervicitis will develop nongonococcal urethritis after an incubation period of 2–6 weeks.

prevalence of cervical infection in different populations and age groups

acute salpingitis

Acute salpingitis (inflammation of the fallopian tubes) can be caused by *C. trachomatis.* Infection appears to ascend the tubes from an infected uterine cervix. In Scandinavia, approximately 20–25% of all proved cases of pelvic inflammatory disease have been shown to be associated with *C. trachomatis* infection.

conjunctivitis in infants of infected mothers

Approximately one-half of all infants born to mothers excreting *C. trachomatis* during labor will develop chlamydial diseases during the first year of life. Most will develop inclusion conjunctivitis. However, 5–10% will

Infant pneumonia syndrome

develop infant pneumonia syndrome. This source accounts for about one-third to one-half of all cases of interstitial pneumonia in infants. The illness usually develops between 6 weeks and 6 months of age and has a gradual onset. The child is usually afebrile, but develops difficulty in feeding, a characteristic staccato (pertussislike) cough, and shortness of breath. Radiography of the chest shows diffuse, bilateral interstitial infiltrates. Laboratory studies usually show a normal white blood cell count, but a slight increase in eosinophils. The disease is rarely fatal, but can be associated with prolonged illness and the need for hospitalization. Treatment with erythromycin or sulfonamides is currently recommended.

Three serotypes cause lymphogranuloma venereum

Lymphogranuloma venereum is a distinct venereal disease caused by three serotypes of *C. trachomatis* that are not associated with other chlamydial infections. It is one of the five "classic" sexually transmitted diseases (Chapter 64) and occurs principally in South America and Africa. The disease is uncommon in North America, but outbreaks have occurred. Lymphogranuloma venereum is one of the few diseases caused by *C. trachomatis* that produces both local and systemic manifestations.

genital ulcer and lymphatic involvement

granulomatous lesions and sinuses

Lymphogranuloma venereum usually begins as a small genital ulcer, often unnoticed by the patient. Marked swelling of the inguinal lymph nodes may develop 2–6 weeks later; they gradually coalesce and become suppurative, often with discharging sinuses. By the time the patient seeks medical help, the original genital ulcer has generally disappeared. Untreated, severe tertiary granulomatous lesions can involve the external genitalia and perineum, especially in women. The diagnosis is usually made by the characteristic clinical appearance. *Chlamydia trachomatis* can be isolated from inguinal node aspirates. In homosexual men, *C. trachomatis* infection of the lower intestinal tract can cause an ulcerative colitislike condition. Genital tract infections caused by *C. trachomatis* are considered further in Chapter 64.

Laboratory Diagnosis

Isolation of *Chlamydia*

Conjunctival inclusions

Isolation of *C. trachomatis,* the best method of diagnosis, is usually achieved by culture using idoxuridine- or cycloheximide-treated McCoy cells. In conjunctivitis, direct staining of scrapings for characteristic cytoplasmic inclusions may be helpful, but will miss about 30% of cases.

Serodiagnosis

Serodiagnostic methods are useful in diagnosis of acute infection. Detection of immunoglobulin (Ig)M antibodies against *C. trachomatis* is particularly helpful in many cases of infant pneumonitis. Because of past infections, single high titers of IgG antibodies in sexually active persons cannot be considered indicative of recent trachomatis infection, and a rising antibody titer must be demonstrated.

Treatment

Effective antimicrobics

Strains of *C. trachomatis* are sensitive to many antimicrobics, of which those most commonly used are the tetracyclines, erythromycin, the sulfonamides, and rifampin. Erythromycin is the preferred systemic agent for pregnant women and infants because of the tooth staining that may result from tetracycline therapy (Chapter 10).

Prevention

At present no effective vaccine is available for the prevention of *C. trachomatis* infection.

use of eyedrops at birth to prevent chlamydial conjunctivitis

Instillation of tetracycline, erythromycin, or chloramphenicol eyedrops at birth decreases the subsequent development of chlamydial conjunctivitis. They are now used increasingly in routine conjunctival prophylaxis for newborns in areas of high prevalence, and they are also effective against most strains of *N. gonorrhoeae* for which prophylaxis is required by law. Silver nitrate eyedrops, which are effective in preventing gonococcal eye infections, are not active against *C. trachomatis.* No conjunctival prophylaxis will prevent colonization of the nasopharynx with *C. trachomatis* or the possible later development of infant pneumonia syndrome.

Additional Reading and References

Mardh, P.-A., Holmes, K.K., Piot, P., Oriel, J.D., and Schachter, J. 1982. *Chlamydia Infections.* New York: Elsevier Biomedical Press. An excellent monograph on recent developments in *Chlamydia trachomatis* infections, with emphasis on sexually transmitted diseases and neonatal diseases.

Schachter, J. 1978. Chlamydial infections. *N. Engl. J. Med.* 298:428–445, 490–495, 540–549. A three-part series reviewing the biology and pathogenesis of chlamydial infections; an excellent in-depth review.

Kenneth J. Ryan

Characteristics of Fungi

29

Fungi are a distinct class of microorganisms, a few of which can produce diseases in humans. These diseases, the *mycoses*, have some unique clinical and microbiologic features. Fungi are eukaryotes with a higher level of biologic complexity than bacteria. They represent a degree of differentiation toward plants. The mycoses vary greatly in their manifestations, but tend to be subacute to chronic diseases with indolent, relapsing features. Acute disease such as that produced by many viruses and bacteria is uncommon in fungal infections.

The Nature of Fungi

Cell structure

The fungal cell has typical eukaryotic features, including a nucleus with chromosomes, a nuclear membrane, and cytoplasmic organelles such as mitochondria and an endoplasmic reticulum. Fungi are usually in the haploid state, although diploid nuclei are formed through nuclear fusion in the process of sexual reproduction. The cell structure includes a cytoplasmic membrane, which contains sterols, and a rigid external cell wall. The cell wall lacks the muramic and teichoic acids of the bacterial cell wall. Instead, it contains hexose and hexosamine polymers, and often a structural macromolecule called *chitin,* which is composed of glucosamine subunits linked in a manner analogous to that found in cellulose, the major structural polymer of plants. Other structural components of some fungi include a glucose polymer (glucan) and a mannose polymer (mannan).

Cell wall

chitin

heterotrophic metabolism

Fungal metabolism is heterotrophic, requiring exogenous organic energy sources. Metabolic diversity is great, but most fungi will grow with only a simple carbon source and ammonium or nitrate ions as a nitrogen source. In nature, nutrients for free-living fungi are derived from decaying organic matter. A major difference between fungi and plants is that fungi lack photosynthetic energy-producing mechanisms. Most are strict aerobes, although some can grow under anaerobic conditions. None are strict anaerobes.

lack of photosynthetic mechanisms

asexual and sexual reproduction

Fungi may reproduce by either asexual or sexual processes. Reproductive elements produced asexually are termed conidia. Those produced sexually are termed spores. Asexual reproduction involves mitotic division of the haploid nucleus and is associated with budding production of spore-like conidia, or separation of hyphal elements. In sexual reproduction, the haploid nuclei of donor and recipient cells fuse to form a diploid nucleus, which then divides by classic meiosis. Some of the four resulting haploid nuclei may be genetic recombinants, and all may undergo further division by mitosis. Highly complex specialized structures may be involved. Detailed study of this process in fungal species such as *Neurospora crassa* has been important in understanding basic cellular genetic mechanisms.

Fungal Growth and Morphology

variations in size

Colonies

The size of fungi varies immensely. A single cell without transverse septa may range from bacterial size (2–4 μm) to a macroscopically visible structure. The morphologic forms of growth vary from a process superficially resembling that of a bacterial colony to the formation of some of the most complex, multicellular, colorful, and beautiful structures seen in nature, such as the mushrooms. The latter can be regarded as complex colonies of fungi showing structural differentiation.

Mycology, the science devoted to the study of fungi, has many terms to describe the morphologic components that make up these structures. Fortunately, the terms and concepts that must be mastered can be limited by considering only the fungi of medical importance and accepting some simplification.

Yeasts

Initial growth from a single cell may follow either of two courses, yeast or mold (Figure 29.1). The first and simplest is the formation of a bud,

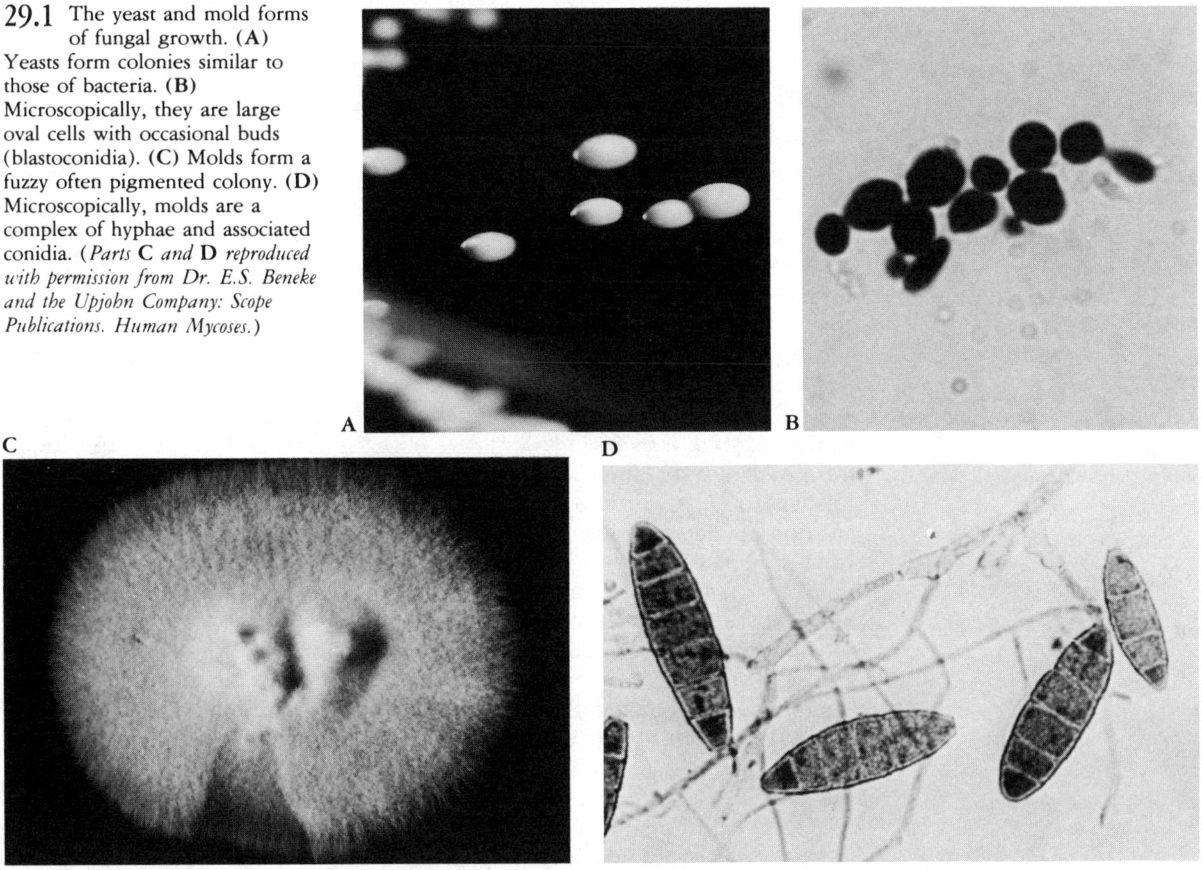

29.1 The yeast and mold forms of fungal growth. (**A**) Yeasts form colonies similar to those of bacteria. (**B**) Microscopically, they are large oval cells with occasional buds (blastoconidia). (**C**) Molds form a fuzzy often pigmented colony. (**D**) Microscopically, molds are a complex of hyphae and associated conidia. (*Parts* **C** *and* **D** *reproduced with permission from Dr. E.S. Beneke and the Upjohn Company: Scope Publications. Human Mycoses.*)

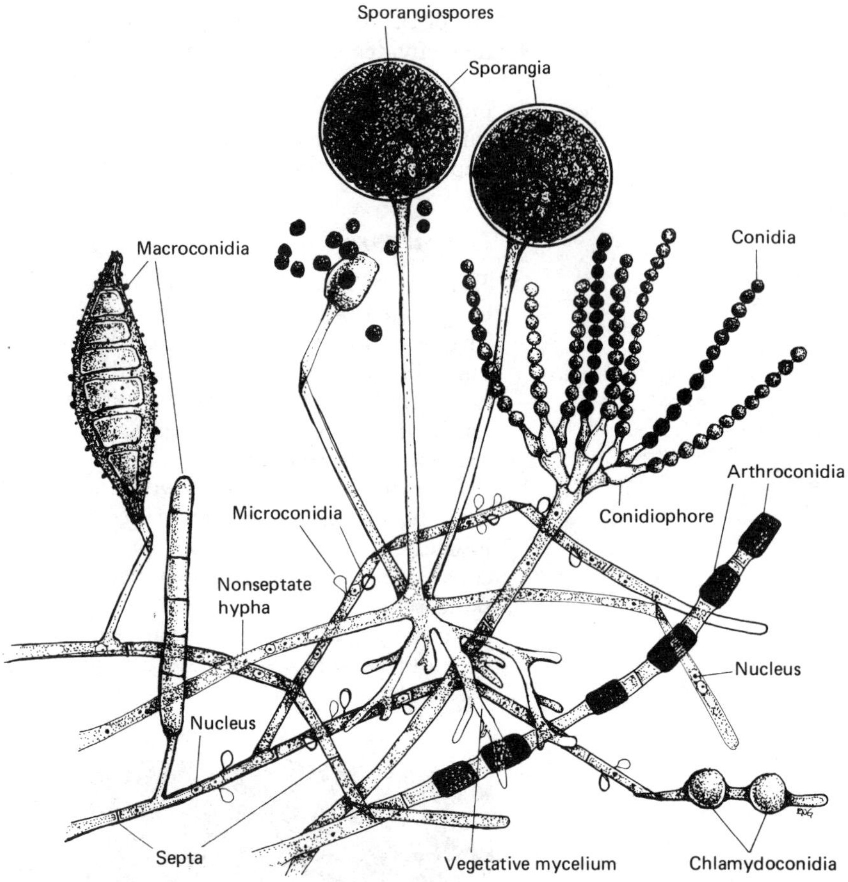

29.2 Forms of molds. The tubelike hyphae form the basic structure of molds. Some of the differentiations and appendages developed from the hyphal wall are shown.

which extends out from a round or oblong parent, constricts, and forms a new cell. These buds are called *blastoconidia* (Figure 29.3) and fungi that reproduce in this manner are called *yeasts.* On plates, yeasts form colonies that often resemble and can be mistaken for those of bacteria. In broth, yeasts produce diffuse turbidity or grow as sediments in unshaken cultures.

blastoconidia

Molds

septate and nonseptate hyphae

vegetative mycelium

aerial mycelium

pseudohyphae

Fungi may also grow through the development of *hyphae* (sing. *hypha*), which are tubelike extensions of the cell with thick, parallel walls. As the hyphae extend, they form an intertwined mass called a *mycelium.* Most fungi form hyphal *septa* (sing. *septum*), which are cross-walls perpendicular to the cell walls that divide the hypha into subunits (Figure 29.2). Some species are nonseptate; they form hyphae and mycelia as a single, continuous cell. In both septate and nonseptate hyphae, multiple nuclei are present with free flow of cytoplasm along the hyphae or through pores in the septa. A portion of the mycelium (vegetative mycelium) usually grows into the medium or organic substrate (for example, soil) and functions, like the roots of plants, as a collector of nutrients and moisture. The more visible surface growth assumes a fluffy character as the mycelium becomes aerial. The hyphal walls are rigid enough to support this highly aerated intertwining network, commonly called a *mold.* The aerial hyphae bear the reproductive structures of this class of fungi. Some fungi form structures called *pseudohyphae* (Figure 29.3), which differ from true hyphae in having recurring budlike constrictions and less rigid cell walls.

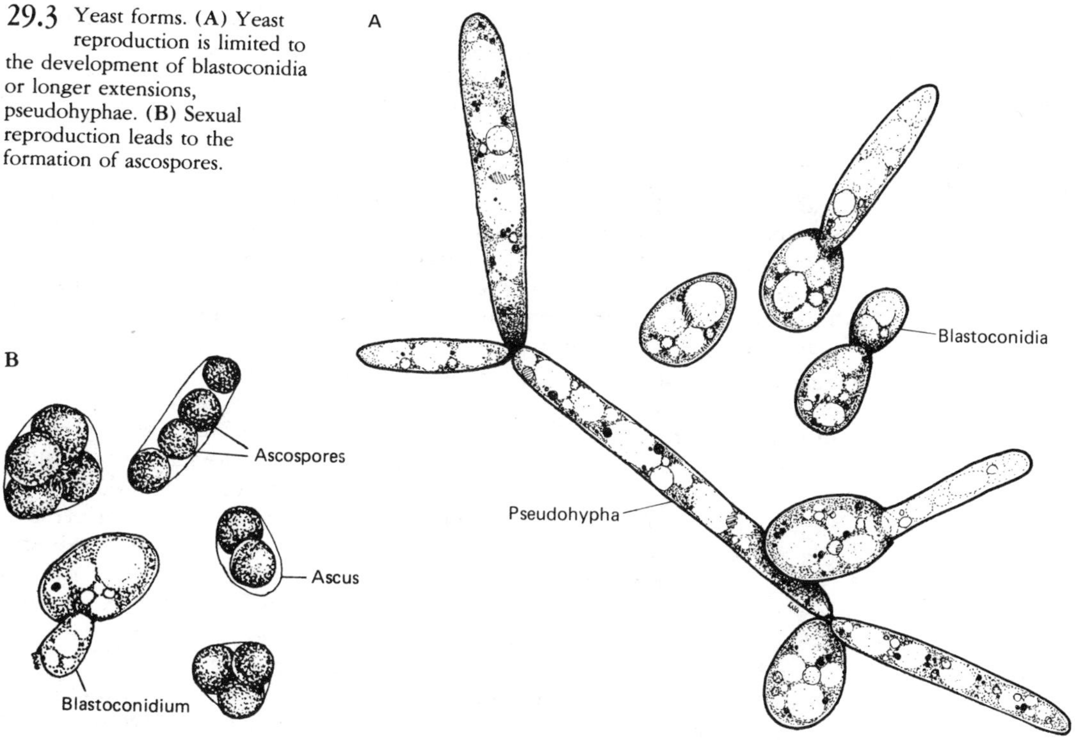

29.3 Yeast forms. (A) Yeast reproduction is limited to the development of blastoconidia or longer extensions, pseudohyphae. (B) Sexual reproduction leads to the formation of ascospores.

reproductive conidia and spores

The reproductive conidia and spores of the molds and the structures that bear them assume a great variety of sizes, shapes, and relations to the parent hyphae, and the morphology of these structures is the primary basis of identification of medically important molds. The mycelial structure plays some role in identification, depending on whether the hyphae are septate or nonseptate, but differences are not sufficiently distinctive to identify or even suggest a fungal species.

conidiophores

Exogenously formed asexual conidia may arise directly from the hyphae, or on a special stalklike structure, the *conidiophore.* Occasionally, terms such as *macroconidia* or *microconidia* are used to indicate the size and/or complexity of these conidia. Conidia that develop within the hyphae are called either *chlamydoconidia* or *arthroconidia.* Chlamydoconidia become larger than the hypha itself; they are round, thick-walled structures that may be borne on the terminal end of the hypha or along its course. Arthroconidia conform more to the shape and size of the hyphal units, forming a series of delicately attached conidia that break off and disseminate when disturbed. The most common sexual spore is termed an *ascospore.* Four or eight ascospores may be found in a saclike structure, the *ascus.* The structures are illustrated in Figures 29.2 and 29.3.

macroconidia, microconidia, chlamydoconidia, and arthroconidia

ascospores

Dimorphism

In general, fungi grow either as yeasts or as molds; mold forms show the greatest diversity. Some species can grow in either a yeast or a mold phase, depending on environmental conditions. These species are known as *dimorphic* fungi. Several human pathogens demonstrate dimorphism: they grow in the yeast phase in infected tissue, but in the mold phase in their environmental reservoir and in culture at ambient temperatures. For most, it is possible to manipulate the cultural conditions to demonstrate both yeast and mold phase in vitro. Yeast phase growth requires conditions similar to those of the parasitic in vivo environment, such as 35–37°C incubation and enriched media. Mold growth requires minimal nutrients and ambient temperatures. The asexual spores produced in the mold phase may be infectious and serve to disseminate the fungus.

Classification

Taxonomy

Although asexual conidia are more readily observed, the taxonomy of fungi depends on the nature of sexual spores and septation of hyphae as its fundamental characteristics. On this basis, four classes—Zygomycetes, Ascomycetes, Basidiomycetes, and Deuteromycetes—are defined as shown in Table 29.1. Some medically important species appear in the Zygomycetes and Ascomycetes, but none in the Basidiomycetes. Most pathogenic species, because they lack a sexual reproductive cycle, have been allocated to the class Deuteromycetes. The mycologist's dislike for this lack of symmetry is indicated by the term *fungi imperfecti,* which is synonymous with Deuteromycetes. It suggests that the sexual spores have been lost during evolution or are so rarely produced that they have not been detected. Indeed, some fungi originally classified in the Deuteromycetes have been transferred to the Ascomycetes on isolation of a sexual (perfect) form. These discoveries do not necessarily simplify classification; for instance, a recently demonstrated sexual stage of *Trichophyton mentagrophytes* was found to be identical to that of an already named ascomycete (*Arthroderma benhamiae*). This type of finding and the morphologic similarity of the asexual forms suggest a close relationship between the classes Ascomycetes and Deuteromycetes.

fungi imperfecti

discovery of sexual phases

Classification by disease states

The grouping of medically important fungi used in the following chapters is based on the type of tissues they parasitize and the diseases they produce, rather than on the principles of basic mycologic toxonomy, because the disease state is how they appear to the clinician. The *superficial* fungi, such as the dermatophytes, cause indolent lesions of the skin and its appendages commonly known as *ringworm* and *athlete's foot.* The *subcutaneous* pathogens characteristically cause infection through the skin, followed by subcutaneous and/or lymphatic spread. The *opportunistic* fungi are those found in the environment or in the normal flora that occasionally produce disease, usually in the compromised host. They may sometimes appear as contaminants on culture media. The *systemic* pathogens are the most virulent fungi and may cause serious progressive systemic disease in previously healthy persons. They are not members of the normal human flora and are rarely, if ever, encountered as contaminants of culture media. Although their major potential is to produce deep-seated visceral infections and systemic spread

superficial fungi

subcutaneous fungi

opportunistic fungi

systemic pathogens

Table 29.1 Taxonomic Classes of Fungi

Class	Hyphae	Reproductive Elements: Sexual	Reproductive Elements: Asexual	Biology
Zygomycetes	Nonseptate	Various types	Sporangioconidia	Saprophytes; rare pathogens[a]
Ascomycetes	Septate	Ascospores	Conidia	Saprophytes; rare pathogens
Basidiomycetes	Septate	Basidiospores	Conidia	Mushrooms, smuts; nonpathogenic
Deuteromycetes (fungi imperfecti)	Septate	None	Conidia	Common pathogens; saprophytes

[a] Pathogenicity for humans. Many fungi are plant pathogens.

(systemic mycoses), they may also produce superficial infections as part of their disease spectrum or as the initiating event. The superficial mycoses do not spread to deeper tissues. As with all clinical classifications, overlaps and exceptions occur. In the end, the organism defines the disease, and it must be isolated or otherwise demonstrated.

Epidemiology

Origin of infection

only dermatophyte infections are communicable

Most fungal infections arise from contact with an environmental reservoir or from the patient's own fungal flora. Some superficial mycoses can be transmitted from person to person by very close contact, such as sharing a comb with a person who has scalp ringworm; others can be acquired from ringworm infections of animals. Other fungal infections are not communicable between humans or animals, and infected patients need not be isolated.

Laboratory Diagnosis of Fungal Infections

Direct examinations

KOH preparation

Gram reaction of yeasts

Histologic preparation

Periodic acid–Schiff and methenamine silver stains

Because of their large size, fungi often demonstrate distinctive morphologic features on direct microscopic examination of infected pus, fluids, or tissues. The simplest method is to mix the specimen with a 10% solution of potassium hydroxide (KOH preparation) and place it under a coverslip. The strong alkali digests or clears the tissue elements (epithelial cells, leukocytes, debris); the rigid cell walls of both yeasts and molds, however, are resistant to the alkali. After digestion of the material, the fungi can be observed under the light microscope with or without staining (Figures 29.1B and 30.1B). Some yeasts will stain with common stains such as the Gram stain, to which they are usually Gram positive. Histopathologic examination of tissue biopsy specimens is widely used and shows the relationship of the organism to tissue elements and responses (blood vessels, phagocytes, granulomatous reactions). Most fungi can be seen in sections stained with the hematoxylin and eosin (H&E) method routinely used in histology laboratories (Figure 29.4B). Specialized staining procedures such as the periodic acid–Schiff and methenamine silver methods are frequently used because they stain almost all fungi. The pathologist should be alerted to the suspicion of fungal infection when tissues are submitted, because special stains and searches for fungi are not made routinely.

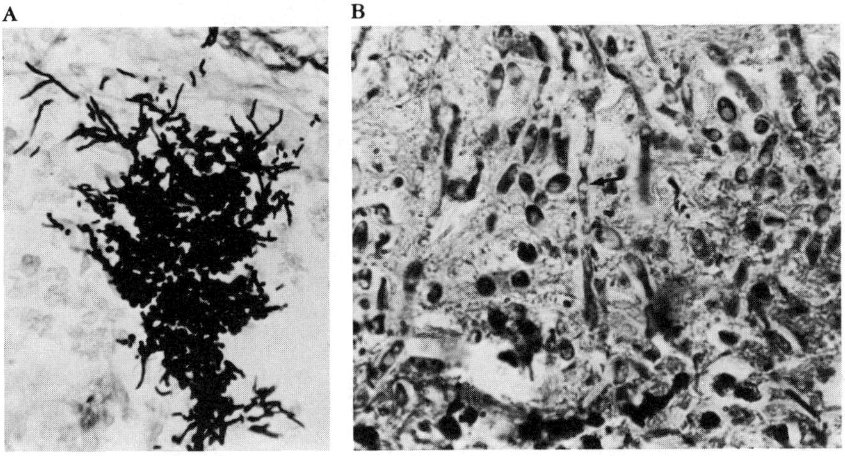

29.4 Direct examinations for fungi. (**A**) Fungi such as *Candida albicans* are large enough to be demonstrated microscopically at low magnification. (**B**) In histologic sections the invasive pseudomycelia (*arrow*) may be seen. (*Part* **A** *reproduced with permission from Dr. E.S. Beneke and from the Upjohn Company: Scope publications. Human Mycoses.*)

Culture

Fungi can be grown by methods similar to those used to isolate bacteria. Growth occurs readily on enriched bacteriologic media commonly used in clinical laboratories (for example, blood agar and chocolate agar). Most fungal cultures, however, require days to weeks of incubation for initial growth; bacteria present in the specimen will grow more rapidly and may interfere with isolation of a slow-growing fungus. Therefore, the culture procedures of diagnostic mycology are designed to favor the growth of fungi over bacteria and to allow incubation to continue for a sufficient time to isolate slow-growing strains.

need for selective media

Sabouraud's agar

The most commonly used medium for cultivating fungi is *Sabouraud's agar*, which contains only glucose and peptones as nutrients. Its pH is 5.6, which is optimal for growth of dermatophytes and satisfactory for that of other fungi. Most bacteria associated with humans fail to grow or grow poorly on Sabouraud's medium.

Other selective media

Blood agar or another enriched bacteriologic agar medium is used when pure cultures would be expected. It is made selective for fungi by the addition of antibacterial antibiotics such as chloramphenicol and gentamicin. Cyclohexamide, which inhibits some saprophytic fungi, is sometimes added to Sabouraud's agar to prevent overgrowth of contaminating molds from the environment, particularly for skin cultures. Media containing these selective agents cannot be relied on exclusively because they can interfere with growth of some pathogenic fungi or because the "contaminant" may be producing an opportunistic infection. For example, cyclohexamide inhibits *Cryptococcus neoformans,* and chloramphenicol may inhibit the yeast forms of some dimorphic fungi. Selective media are not needed for growing fungi from sterile sites such as cerebrospinal fluid or tissue biopsy specimens. In contrast to most parasitic bacteria, many fungi grow best at 25–30°C, and temperatures in this range are used for primary isolation. Paired cultures incubated at 35–37°C may be used to demonstrate dimorphism.

Yeast identification

Once a fungus is isolated, identification procedures depend on whether it is a yeast or mold. Yeasts are identified by biochemical tests analogous to those used for bacteria, including some that are identical (for example, urease production). Some fungi that ordinarily grow as yeast can be induced to form elongated buds called *pseudohyphae.* These differ from true hyphae in their lack of rigid parallel cell walls; they also have a budlike constriction at their origin. Pseudohyphae are particularly common in *Candida* species and are found growing into agar or tissue rather than on the surface.

pseudohyphal formation

Mold identification

Molds are most often identified by the morphology of their asexual conidia and conidiophores. Other features such as the size, texture, and color of the colonies help to characterize molds, but without demonstrating conidiation they are not sufficient for identification. The ease and speed with which various fungi produce conidia vary greatly. Minimal nutrition, moisture, good aeration, and ambient temperature favor conidia development.

slide culture

lactophenol cotton blue preparations

Microscopic fungal morphology is usually demonstrated by methods that allow in situ microscopic observation of the fragile asexual conidia and their shape and arrangement. Morphology may also be examined in fragments of growth teased free of a mold and examined moist in preparations containing a dye called *lactophenol cotton blue.* The dye stains the mycelia and spores. Conidia production may not occur for days or weeks after the initial growth of the mold. It is somewhat like waiting for flowers to bloom, and it can be frustrating when the result has immediate clinical application.

demonstration of dimorphism

It is desirable, but not always possible, to demonstrate both the yeast and mold phases with dimorphic fungi. In some cases, this result can be achieved with parallel cultures at 22°C and 37°C. The tissue form of *Coccidiodes immitis* is not readily produced in vitro.

Serologic tests

Serum antibodies directed against a variety of fungal antigens can be detected in patients infected with those agents. Except for some of the systemic pathogens, the sensitivity and/or specificity of these tests has not been sufficient to recommend them for use in diagnosis or therapeutic monitoring of fungal infections. The tests of value will be discussed in sections on specific agents.

Antimicrobial Susceptibility

Polyene antibiotics

Griseofulvin

Flucytosine

Imidazoles

Fungi are not susceptible to most antimicrobics used to treat bacterial infections, and bacteria are resistant to most antifungal agents. The *polyene antibiotics,* amphotericin B and nystatin, are active against the broadest range of fungi, but their use is limited by their toxicity. They combine with the sterol component of the cytoplasmic membrane, causing permeability changes. Griseofulvin is active against dermatophytes. Flucytosine has activity against *Candida,* cryptococci, and some other yeasts, but not against the systemic pathogens. Recently, a new class of agents, the imidazoles, has been found to have antifungal activity as well as action against some bacteria and parasites. The compounds with greatest antifungal activity are clotrimazole, miconazole, and ketoconazole. Of these agents, ketoconazole shows promise for therapy of systemic infections, but requires further evaluation. Antifungal agents are discussed in more detail in Chapter 10 and in relation to the specific fungi and diseases.

Additional Reading and References

A number of good texts on medical mycology are available. All give more in-depth coverage of the mycologic, epidemiologic, and clinical aspects of mycoses than this book. Several are listed below.

Conant, N.F., Smith, D.T., Baker, R.D., and Calloway, J.L. 1971. *Manual of Clinical Mycology.* 3rd ed. Philadelphia: Saunders. Concise but complete coverage of epidemiologic, diagnostic, and clinical features is provided.

Emmons, C.W., Binford, C.H., Utz, J.P., and Kwon-Chung, K.J. 1977. *Medical Mycology.* 3rd ed. Philadelphia: Lea & Febiger. Coverage of pathologic features is particularly good.

Rippon, J.W. 1982. *Medical Mycology.* 2nd ed. Philadelphia: Saunders. Detailed, comprehensive coverage, including historic aspects, is given.

Wilson, J.W., and Plunkett, O.A. 1965. *The Fungous Diseases of Man.* Berkeley: University of California Press. Excellent photographic material, particularly on the cutaneous manifestations of mycoses, is provided.

Kenneth J. Ryan

Superficial Fungi and Mycoses

30

Dermatophytoses are superficial infections of the skin and its appendages, commonly known as *ringworm, athlete's foot,* and *jock itch.* They are caused by species of the genera *Microsporum, Trichophyton,* and *Epidermophyton,* which are collectively known as *dermatophytes.* These fungi are highly adapted to the nonliving, keratinized tissues of nails, hair, and the stratum corneum of the skin.

Dermatophytes

Microbiology

Dermatophytes are molds that have been classified among the Deuteromycetes (fungi imperfecti). More recently, sexual spores corresponding to two ascomycete genera have been discovered in many of the *Microsporum* and *Trichophyton* species. Dermatophytes are still called by their previous names in the medical literature for reasons of familiarity, and because identification procedures continue to be based on the characteristics of asexual conidia. Many species cause dermatophyte infections, the most common of which are shown in Table 30.1. They require a few days to a week or more to initiate growth. Most grow best at 25°C on Sabouraud's medium, which is usually used for culture. The hyphae are septate, and the conidia may be borne directly on the hyphae or on conidiophores. Small microconidia may or may not be formed; however, the larger and more distinctive macroconidia (Figure 30.1C) are usually the basis for identification.

conidia

best growth at 25°C

septate hyphae

Pathogenesis

Infection

Dermatophytoses begin when minor traumatic lesions come in contact with the fungi. Once the stratum corneum is penetrated the organism can proliferate, but does not invade deeper structures. The course of the infection is then dependent on the anatomic location, the dynamics of skin growth and desquamation, the speed and extent of the inflammatory response, and the infecting species. For example, if the organisms grow very slowly in the stratum corneum, and this layer is turned over by desquamation at a normal rate, the infection will probably be short lived and cause minimal signs and symptoms. Inflammation tends to increase skin growth and desquamation rates and help to limit infection, whereas immunosuppressive agents such as corticosteroids decrease shedding of the keratinized layers and tend to

Balance between growth and desquamation

Table 30.1 Agents of Superficial Mycoses

Fungus	Infection Site(s)	Fungal Growth	
		In Lesion	In Culture (25°C)
Dermatophytes			
Microsporum canis	Hair,[a] skin	Mycelia	Mold
Microsporum audouini	Hair[a]	Mycelia	Mold
Microsporum gypseum	Hair, skin	Mycelia	Mold
Trichophyton tonsurans	Hair, skin, nails	Mycelia	Mold
Trichophyton rubrum	Hair, skin, nails	Mycelia	Mold
Trichophyton mentagrophytes	Hair, skin	Mycelia	Mold
Trichophyton violaceum	Hair, skin, nails	Mycelia	Mold
Epidermophyton floccosum	Skin	Mycelia	Mold
Other mycoses			
Pityrosporium orbiculare	Skin (pink to brown)[b]	Yeast (mycelia)	Yeast
Cladosporium werneckii	Skin (brown-black)[b]	Mycelia	Yeast (mold)
Trichosporon cutaneum	Hair (white)[b]	Mycelia	Mold
Piedraia hortae	Hair (black)[b]	Mycelia	Mold

[a] Specimens fluoresce under ultraviolet light.
[b] Color of clinical lesions.

prolong infection. Most infections are self-limiting, but those in which fungal growth rates and desquamation are balanced and in which the inflammatory response is poor tend to become chronic. The lateral spread of infection and its associated inflammation produce the characteristic sharp advancing margins that were once believed to be the burrows of worms. This characteristic is the origin of the common name *ringworm* and the Latin term *tinea* (worm) that is often applied to the clinical forms of the disease (Figure 30.1A).

Ringworm and tinea

Infection may spread from skin to other keratinized structures, such as hair or nails, or may invade them primarily. The hair shaft is penetrated by hyphae, which extend as arthroconidia either exclusively within the shaft (endothrix) or both within and without the shaft (exothrix). The end result is damage to the hair shaft structure, which often breaks off. Loss of hair at the root and plugging of the hair follicle with fungal elements may result. Invasion of the nail bed causes a hyperkeratotic reaction, which dislodges or distorts the nail.

involvement of hair and nails

endothrix

exothrix

nail bed infection

Epidemiology

There are both ecologic and geographic differences in the occurrence of the various dermatophyte species. Some are primarily adapted to the skin of humans, others to animals. Many wild and domestic animals, including dogs and cats, are infected with certain dermatophyte species and represent a large reservoir for infection of humans. Other pathogenic dermatophytes are found primarily in the soil. There are large differences between temperate and tropical climates in the frequency of cases and isolation from nonhuman sources. Many of these differences are changing with shifts in population.

human, animal, or soil reservoirs

Human-to-human transmission usually requires very close contact with an infected subject or infected materials, because dermatophytes are of low infectivity and virulence. Transmission usually takes place within families or

human-to-human transmission

30.1 Dermatophyte infection of scalp (ringworm). (**A**) Scalp lesions. Note the annular margination. (**B**) Scrapings taken from the edge of the scalp lesion in KOH. Only the hyphal elements are visible. (**C**) Culture. Both hyphae, macroconidia, and microconidia are present. The macroconidia are characteristic for *Trichophyton*. *(Reproduced with permission from Dr. E.S. Beneke and the Upjohn Company: Scope monograph, Human Mycoses.)*

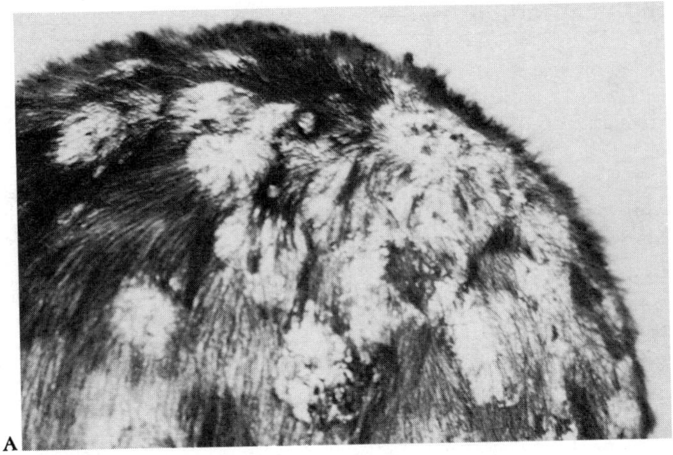
A

B C

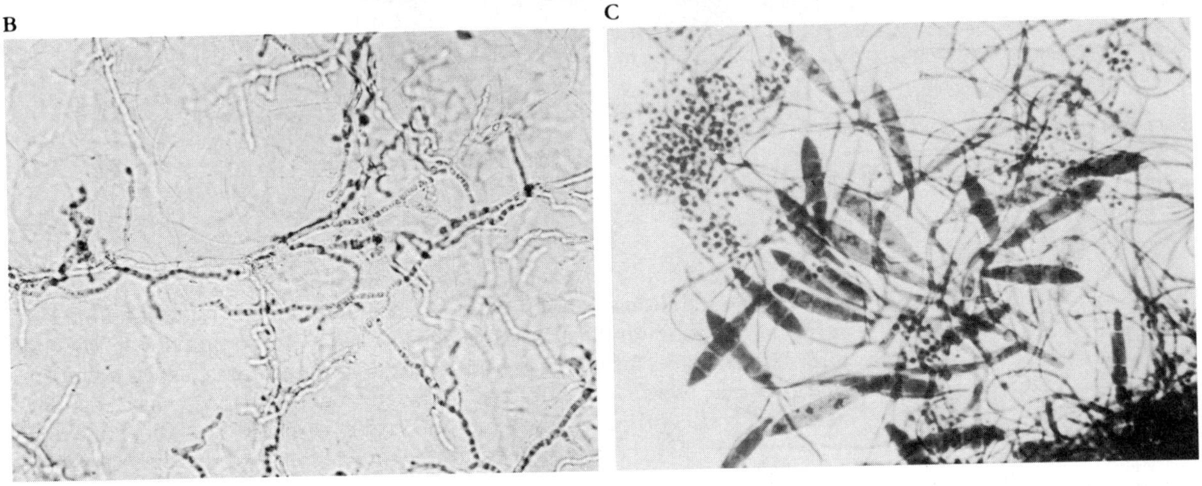

in situations involving contact with detached skin or hair, such as barber shops and locker rooms. No special precautions beyond hand washing need be taken by the medical attendant after contact with an infected patient.

Clinical Manifestations

diversity

Dermatophyte infections range from inapparent colonization to chronic progressive eruptions that last for months or years, causing considerable discomfort and disfiguration.

Clinical syndromes

Dermatologists often give each infection its own "disease" name, for example, *tinea capitis* (scalp), *tinea pedis* (feet, athlete's foot), *tinea manuum* (hands), *tinea cruris* (groin), *tinea barbae* (beard, hair), and *tinea unguium* (nail beds). Skin infections not included in this anatomic list are called *tinea corporis* (body). There are some general clinical, etiologic, and epidemiologic differences between these syndromes, but there is also considerable overlap. The primary differences between etiologic agents that infect different sites are shown in Table 30.1.

Hair infections

Infection of hair begins with an erythematous papule around the hair shaft, which progresses to scaling of the scalp, discoloration, and eventually fracture of the shaft. Spread to adjacent hair follicles progresses in a ringlike fashion, leaving behind broken, discolored hairs and sometimes black dots filled with fungal debris. The degree of inflammatory response markedly effects the clinical appearance and in some cases can cause constitutional symptoms. In most cases symptoms beyond itching are minimal.

Skin infections

Skin lesions begin in a similar pattern and enlarge to form sharply delineated erythematous borders with skin of nearly normal appearance in the center. Multiple lesions can fuse to form unusual geometric patterns on the skin. Lesions may appear in any location, but are particularly common in moist, sweaty skin folds. Obesity and the wearing of tight apparel increase susceptibility to infection in the groin and beneath the breasts. Another form of infection, which involves scaling and splitting of the skin between the toes, is commonly known as *athlete's foot.* Moisture and maceration of the skin provide the mode of entry.

Nail bed infections

Nail bed infections first cause discoloration of the subungual tissue, then hyperkeratosis and apparent discoloration of the nail plate by the underlying infection. Direct infection of the nail plate is uncommon. Progression of hyperkeratosis and associated inflammation cause disfigurement of the nail, but few symptoms until the nail plate is so dislodged or distorted that it exposes or compresses adjacent soft tissue.

Diagnosis

KOH mount of skin scrapings and infected hairs

The goal of diagnostic procedures is to distinguish dermatophytoses from other skin diseases, such as mimicking infections caused by bacteria and other fungi, and from noninfectious inflammatory skin disorders, such as psoriasis and contact dermatitis. The most important step is microscopic examination of material from lesions to detect the fungus. Potassium hydroxide preparations of scales scraped from the advancing edge of a dermatophyte lesion demonstrate septate hyphae (Figure 30.1B). Examination of infected hairs reveals hyphae and arthrospores penetrating the hair shaft. Broken hairs give the best yield. Some species of dermatophyte fluoresce, and selection of hairs for examination can be aided by the use of an ultraviolet lamp (Wood's lamp).

Culture

The same material used for direct examination can be cultured for isolation of the offending dermatophyte. Mild infections with typical clinical findings and positive KOH preparations are often not cultured, because clinical management is not influenced significantly by the identity of the etiologic species. Clinically typical infections with negative KOH preparations require culture. The major reason for false-negative KOH results, however, is failure to collect the scrapings or hairs properly.

Treatment and Prevention

local miconazole or clotrimazole

griseofulvin

Many local skin infections may be treated effectively with topical miconazole or clotrimazole. Scalp, nail bed, and more extensive skin infections require systemic therapy with griseofulvin. Therapy must be continued over weeks to months, and relapses are common.

Dermatophyte infections can usually be prevented simply by observing general hygienic measures. No specific preventive measures such as vaccines exist.

Other Superficial Mycoses

Tinea versicolor

Tinea (pityriasis) versicolor occurs primarily in the tropics; it is characterized by discrete areas of hypopigmentation associated with induration and scaling. Lesions are found on the trunk and arms; some assume pigments ranging from pink to yellow-brown, hence the term *versicolor.* The cause (*Pityrosporum orbiculare*) can be seen in skin scrapings as clusters of budding yeast cells mixed with hyphae. It grows primarily in the yeast form in culture.

Tinea nigra

Tinea nigra, another tropical infection, is characterized by brown to black macular lesions, usually on the hands or feet. There is little inflammation or scaling. The cause (*Cladosporium werneckii*) is a black-pigmented fungus found in soil and other environmental sites. Scrapings of the lesion show brown-black-pigmented septate hyphae. In culture initial growth is in the yeast form, with slow development of hyphal elements.

Piedra

Piedra is an infection of the hair characterized by black or white nodules attached to the hair shaft. White piedra (caused by *Trichosporon cutaneum*) infects the shaft in hyphal forms, which fragment with occasional buds. Black piedra (caused by *Piedraia hortae*) shows branched hyphae and ascopores in sections of the hair.

Kenneth J. Ryan

Candida and Other Opportunistic Fungi

31

The fungi considered in this chapter are usually found as members of the normal flora or as saprophytes in the environment. With breakdown of host defenses they can produce disease ranging from superficial skin or mucous membrane infections to systemic involvement of multiple organs. The most common opportunistic infections are caused by *Candida albicans,* a common member of the skin, gastrointestinal, and genital floras. The diseases caused by *Candida* and other species are summarized in Table 31.1.

Candida

budding yeasts

hyphae

Candida species are usually regarded as yeasts, because they grow as typical 4- to 6-μm, budding, round or oval yeast cells (Figure 29.1) under most conditions and at most temperatures. Under specialized conditions, they can form pseudohyphae or hyphae. Some species form chlamydoconidia. Many *Candida* species have been defined; those most commonly associated with disease in humans are shown in Table 31.2. Species identification is based on a combination of biochemical and morphologic characteristics, such as carbohydrate assimilation and fermentation and the ability to produce germ tubes (hyphae) and chlamydoconidia. Particular attention is given to the differentiation of *C. albicans* from other species, because it is the most frequent cause of disease. Cells of *C. albicans* form germ tubes (Figure 31.1A) within 2–3 hr when incubated at 37°C in serum. The organism also forms terminal thick-walled chlamydoconidia under certain conditions (Figure 31.1B). Other *Candida* species do not have this combination of properties.

C. albicans

germ tube test

chlamydoconidia formation

bacterialike colonies

Most *Candida* species, including *C. albicans,* grow rapidly on Sabouraud's medium and on enriched bacteriologic media. Smooth, white, 2- to 4-mm colonies resembling those of staphylococci are produced on blood agar after overnight incubation. Fluid cultures typically show a deposit at the bottom, but diffuse growth may occur if the broth is well aerated.

Candida albicans Infections

Normal floral organism

local tissue invasion

Pathogenesis. *Candida albicans,* formerly designated *Monilia albicans,* is normally present in small numbers in the oral cavity, lower gastrointestinal tract, and female genital tract. The skin is not usually colonized, but is frequently contaminated from other sites. Under certain conditions *C. albicans* may become locally invasive, sending pseudohyphae down into the tissue and

Table 31.1 Agents of Opportunistic Mycoses

Organism	Infection	Growth: Tissue	Growth: Culture (25°C)	Growth: Culture (37°C)
Candida	Skin, mucous membranes, urinary, disseminated	Yeast (pseudomycelia)[a]	Yeast (mycelia)[a]	Yeast
Aspergillus	Lung, disseminated	Mycelia (septate)	Mold	Mold
Absidia	Rhinocerebral, lung	Mycelia (nonseptate)	Mold	Mold
Mucor	Rhinocerebral, lung	Mycelia (nonseptate)	Mold	Mold
Rhizopus	Rhinocerebral, lung	Mycelia (nonseptate)	Mold	Mold

[a]Less common feature.

producing acute inflammation and tissue destruction (Figure 29.4). The factors that trigger this invasion, beyond some disruption of anatomic barriers or other compromise of host defenses, are not clear. For example, dry, normal skin is resistant to infection, but wet, macerated skin (as in diaper rash) is not. Factors that allow *C. albicans* to increase its relative proportion of the flora (antibacterial therapy) or that compromise the general immune capacity of the host (leukopenia or corticosteroid therapy) are often associated with invasion. Diabetes mellitus creates a general predisposition toward *C. albicans* infection, as well as many other infections. No specific virulence or immunologic factors clearly explain these events, with the exception of those leading to chronic mucocutaneous candidiasis.

host resistance and susceptibility

Dissemination

Disseminated *C. albicans* infections are associated with parenchymal invasion, pseudohyphae production, microabscesses, and, occasionally, chronic granulomatous inflammatory responses. Cases of disseminated disease may begin with superficial infection, but usually involve a major breach of the host's local defenses or general immune responses. Many of the newer technologic devices used in medicine, such as indwelling catheters, monitoring devices, prostheses, and particularly hyperalimentation procedures, can provide a convenient route for *Candida* (and other organisms) to gain

Common sources of infection

Table 31.2 Medically Important *Candida* Species

Species	Germ Tubes[a]	Pseudohyphae	Chlamydoconidia
C. albicans	+	+	+
C. krusei	—	+	—
C. parapsilosis	—	+	—
C. tropicalis	—	+	—[b]
C. guilliermondii	—	+	—
C. (Torulopsis) glabrata	—	—	—

[a] Rapid production (4 hr or less).
[b] Occasional strains produce chlamydoconidia morphologically different from those of *C. albicans*.

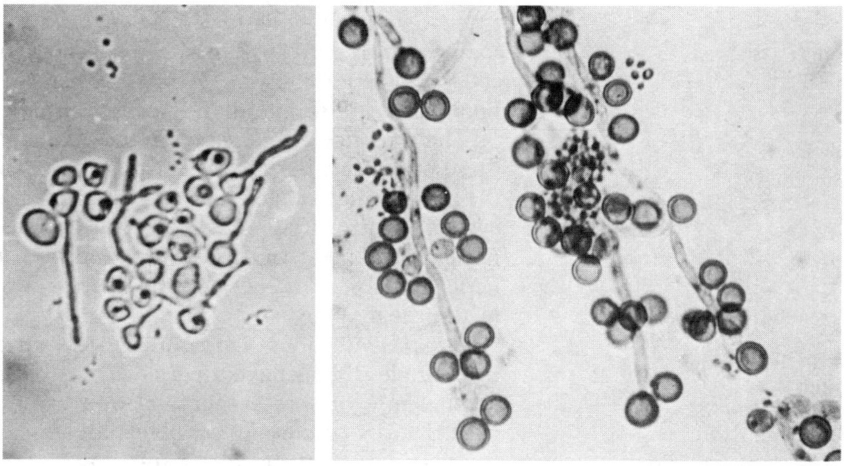

A B

31.1 *Candida ablicans.* (**A**) When incubated at 37°C, *Candida albicans* rapidly forms elongated growths called germ tubes, which are similar to hyphae. (**B**) On specialized media, *Candida albicans* forms thick-walled chlamydoconidia, which differentiate it from other *Candida* species. (*Reproduced with permission from Dr. E.S. Beneke and from the Upjohn Company: Scope Publications, Human Mycoses.*)

access to deeper organs. The organism's resistance to antibacterial drugs and its invasive capacity facilitate production of disease in these circumstances.

Epidemiology. Most *C. albicans* infections are caused by endogenous flora, except in cases of direct mucosal contact with lesions in others (for example, though sexual intercourse). Nosocomial *C. albicans* infections are also derived more frequently from the patient's own flora than from cross-infection; they are often associated with the invasive procedures mentioned previously.

superficial infections

Clinical manifestations. Superficial invasion of the mucous membranes by *C. albicans* produces a white, cheesy plaque that is loosely adherent to the mucosal surface. The lesion is usually painless, unless the plaque is torn away and the raw, weeping, invasive surface is exposed. Oral lesions, called *thrush,* occur on the tongue, palate, and other mucosal surfaces as single or multiple ragged white patches. A similar infection in the vagina, vaginal candidiasis, produces a thick, curdlike discharge and itching of the vulva.

thrush

vaginal candidiasis

Skin infections

Candida albicans skin infections have an appearance similar to that of intertriginous dermatophyte infections and occur in similar circumstances. Crural folds and other areas in which wet, macerated skin surfaces are opposed are the sites most commonly affected. For example, one type of diaper rash is caused by *C. albicans.*

diaper rash

The initial lesions are erythematous papules of confluent areas associated with tenderness, erythema, and fissures of the skin. Infection usually remains confined to the chronically irritated area, but may spread beyond it, particularly in infants. In rare persons with specific T-cell defects in cell-mediated immune defense against *Candida* antigens, a chronic, relapsing form of candidiasis called *chronic mucocutaneous candidiasis* develops. Infections of the skin, hair, or mucous membranes are initially similar to those seen in other patients, but fail to resolve with adequate therapy and management. The mucocutaneous junctions are often involved, with considerable disfigurement and discomfort, particularly when the disease is accompanied by a granulomatous inflammatory response. Although lesions may become extensive, they usually do not disseminate.

Chronic mucocutaneous candidiasis

esophagitis

Inflammatory patches similar to those in thrush may develop in the esophagus with or without associated oral candidiasis. Painful swallowing and substernal chest pain are the most common symptoms. Extensive ulcerations, deformity, and occasionally perforation of the esophagus may ensue. Al-

intestinal candidiasis

though similar lesions may develop in the stomach, they are less frequent than those of the esophagus. Superficial and deep ulcerative lesions of the small and large intestine, which may also occur in immunosuppressed patients, are rare in immunologically normal persons.

urinary candidiasis

The presence of *C. albicans* in the genital flora and anterior urethra allows these organisms to enter the urinary bladder under the same conditions as the more common bacterial causes of urinary infection (Chapter 60). *Candida* cystitis is particularly associated with diabetes mellitus. Infection of the kidneys via the hematogenous or ascending routes may produce acute pyelonephritis, abscesses, perinephric abscess, or expanding fungus ball lesions in the renal pelvis.

Disseminated infection

association with immunocompromise

Candida infections of visceral organs with or without further dissemination to multiple organs have a particularly strong association with immunologic compromise or some other violation of normal defense mechanisms. The organs most commonly involved are the kidneys, brain, heart, and eye. Involvement of many other sites, including the lung, is possible but less frequent. As discussed previously, dissemination may occur from a superficial infection; more commonly, however, the primary mechanism for access to deep tissues involves a medical device, such as an infected intravenous catheter. Multiple organ involvement is typical, particularly if the mechanism of entry causes a continuous fungemia.

central nervous system candidiasis

The clinical findings in disseminated infections are generally not sufficiently characteristic to suggest *C. albicans* rather than bacterial pathogens, which more commonly produce infection of deep organs. Central nervous system infection may appear as meningitis, with a predominantly lymphocytic cell count in the cerebrospinal fluid (CSF), or as multifocal microabscesses. A contaminated ventricular shunt can be a direct route for CSF infection.

enophthalmitis

Candida enophthalmitis has the characteristic funduscopic appearance of a white cotton ball expanding on the retina or floating free in the vitreous humor. Enophthalmitis and infections of other eye structures can lead to blindness.

cardiac infections

A full range of *Candida* cardiac infections may be produced, including pericarditis, myocarditis with microabscesses, and endocarditis. *Candida* endocarditis is particularly associated with cardiac surgery, but is otherwise similar in clinical findings to bacterial endocarditis.

KOH and Gram smears of superficial lesions

Laboratory diagnosis. Superficial *C. albicans* infections are among the easiest to diagnose, but deep organ involvement is very difficult to establish. In addition to their characteristic clinical appearances, superficial infections such as thrush or vaginitis provide ready access to diagnostic material. Exudate or epithelial scrapings are examined by potassium hydroxide or Gram smear. In either case, abundant budding yeast cells are seen (Figure 29.4); if pseudohyphae are present, the infection can be assumed to be caused by *C. albicans,* and culture may not be needed.

methods of obtaining samples in systemic candidiasis

Deep organ involvement is difficult to diagnose because the infected tissues are not accessible for sampling. For example, isolation of *C. albicans* from the sputum of a patient with suspected *Candida* pneumonia is not diagnostic, because the organism is part of the normal flora of the mouth or may come from a superficial oral mucous membrane lesion. Even positive blood cultures may not necessarily be conclusive; they may represent contamination of the intravenous catheters present in patients prone to systemic candidiasis. An invasive sampling procedure, such as a direct aspirate or surgical biopsy, is often required to establish the diagnosis.

Culture and identification

Culture of *Candida* species is not difficult. On isolation, the organisms grow rapidly as yeast on blood or Sabouraud's agar. The primary identification procedure involves presumptive differentiation of *C. albicans* from other *Candida* species with the germ tube test. Germ-tube-negative strains may be further identified or reported as "yeast not *C. albicans*," depending on their apparent clinical significance. Other *Candida* species are much less virulent than *C. albicans*; a possible exception is *Candida tropicalis*, which can be invasive.

blood culture

Candida albicans is readily isolated from the blood in media used for bacteriologic culture, but cultures must be well aerated. The atmospheric conditions present in most commercial blood culture bottles are not satisfactory unless they are vented (aerated) in the laboratory. Growth usually appears in 1–4 days. *Candida* endocarditis represents a special diagnostic problem, because blood cultures have often been negative in established cases. It is likely that the relatively large yeasts are filtered out in the capillary beds and thus prevented from reaching the venous circulation, from which blood samples are collected. Arterial blood cultures, although sometimes successful in this situation, are not a routine procedure.

serodiagnosis

detection of *C. albicans* products

Many serologic tests have been developed for *C. albicans* infection; none has the sensitivity or specificity needed for clinical diagnosis, although *Candida* antibodies can be demonstrated. Chromatographic or immunologic techniques show promise in detection of *Candida* metabolites or cell components such as mannan, but are not yet ready for clinical use.

local treatment

Treatment. *Candida albicans* is usually susceptible to amphotericin B, nystatin, flucytosine, and the imidazoles. Superficial infections are generally treated with topical nystatin, occasionally with amphotericin B. Measures to decrease moisture and chronic trauma are important adjuncts in treating *Candida* skin infections. Deeper *C. albicans* infections may resolve spontaneously with elimination or control of predisposing conditions. Removal of an infected catheter, control of diabetes, or rise in peripheral leukocyte counts are often associated with recovery without antifungal therapy. Persistent relapsing or disseminated candidiasis is treated with amphotericin B, flucytosine, or ketoconozole.

recovery without specific therapy

Amphotericin B, flucytosine, and ketoconozole therapy

Infection with Other Candida Species

Species of *Candida* other than *C. albicans* (Table 31.1) produce infections in circumstances similar to those described previously, but less frequently. When contamination of an indwelling device is the portal of entry, the probability of infection by these other species increases. Both experimental and clinical evidence indicates that *C. tropicalis* has invasive properties equal to or greater than those of *C. albicans*. Infections with this organism, although uncommon, may be particularly serious. Another distinctive organism is *Candida glabrata* (until recently called *Torulopsis glabrata*). This species is a small (2–4 μm) yeast with characteristics similar to those of other *Candida*, with the exception of failure to produce hyphal elements in culture. It is a member of the normal gastrointestinal and genital flora. The most common infections are in the urinary tract, but occasionally other deep tissue involvement and fungemia occur. The organism may appear in the same nosocomial settings as *C. albicans*, including intravenous catheters. In deep tissue infections, the organisms are small enough to be confused with *Histoplasma capsulatum* in histologic preparations. Therapy is similar to that for *C. albicans* infections, although *C. glabrata* is more likely to be resistant to flucytosine on primary isolation.

Aspergillus

Microbiology

Molds

differentiation on basis of conidiophores and conidia

Aspergillus species are rapidly growing molds with septate hyphae and characteristic asexual conidia (Figure 31.2A). Fluffy colonies appear in 1–2 days and by 5 days may cover an entire plate with pigmented growth. Many species in this genus are defined on the basis of differences in the structure of the conidiophore and the arrangement of the conidia. The most important species in human infections are *Aspergillus fumigatus* and *Aspergillus flavus,* but others, such as *Aspergillus niger,* can be involved.

Epidemiology

Environmental organisms

Aspergillus species are widely distributed in nature and found throughout the world. They seem to adapt to a wide range of environmental conditions, and the heat-resistant conidia provide a good mechanism for dispersal. Hospital air and air ducts have received attention as sources of nosocomial *Aspergillus* isolates. Occasionally, building remodeling or other kinds of ma-

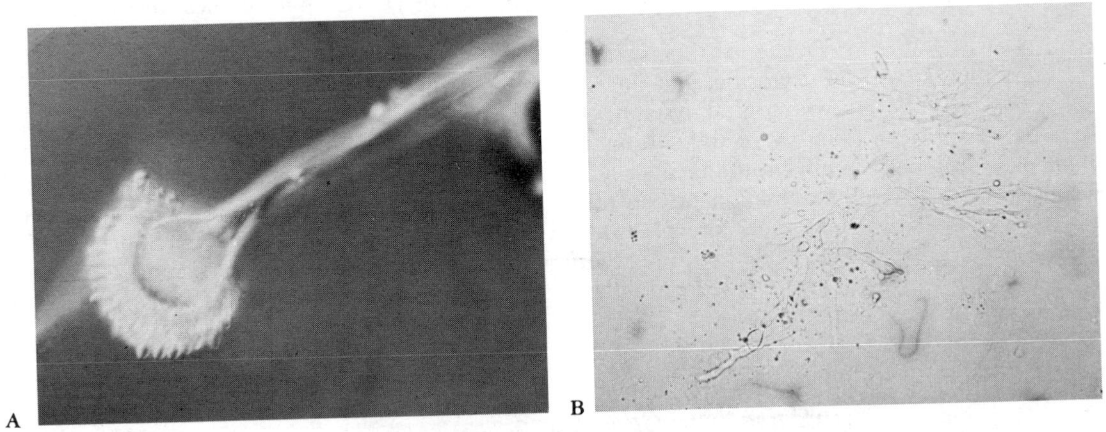

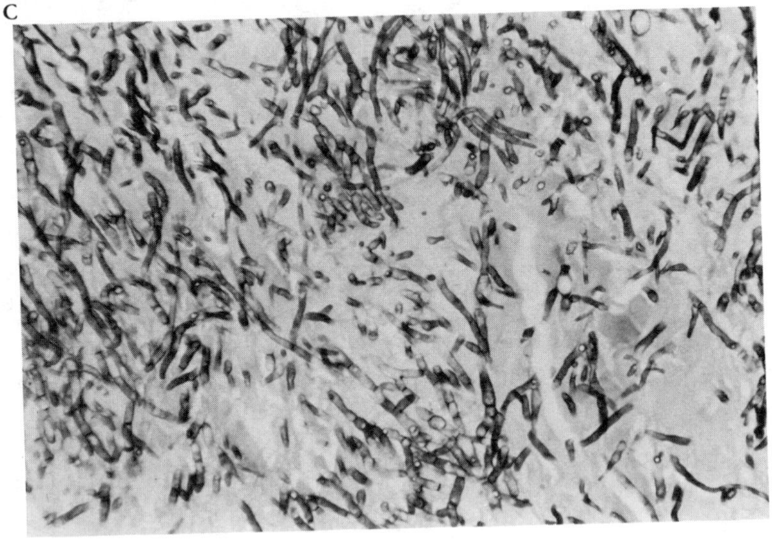

31.2 *Aspergillus.* (**A**) This asexual conidia forming structure is characteristic of *Aspergillus* species. The conidia are borne at the end of the fingerlike extensions at the end of the conidiophore. These structures are rarely produced in vivo. (**B**) This tissue aspirate mixed with KOH shows branching, septate hyphae. (**C**) Histologic sections also show branching, septate hyphae, but because the conidia shown in (**A**) are not seen the findings are not diagnostic of *Aspergillus.* (*Reproduced with permission from Dr. E.S. Beneke and from the Upjohn Company: Scope Publications, Human Mycoses.*)

jor environmental disruption have been associated with increased frequency of *Aspergillus* contamination, colonization, or infection.

Aspergillosis

Allergic aspergillosis

Aspergillus can cause clinical allergies or occasional invasive infection. In both cases, the lung is the organ primarily involved. Allergic aspergillosis, which can be a mechanism of exacerbation in patients with asthma, is characterized by transient pulmonary infiltrates, eosinophilia, and a rise in *Aspergillus*-specific immunoglobulin G. These conditions follow direct inhalation of fungal elements or, more commonly, colonization of the respiratory tract. Areas of the bronchopulmonary tree with poor drainage because of underlying disease or anatomic abnormalities may serve as a site for growth of organisms and continuous seeding with antigen. A particular form of allergic bronchopulmonary disease known as *farmer's lung* is associated with inhalation of large numbers of *Aspergillus* conidia as well as those of other fungi. Acute, recurrent, and chronic pulmonary symptoms are associated with dispersion from haystacks, silos, and similar environments.

Farmer's lung

localized and invasive pulmonary aspergillosis

fungus ball

Invasive aspergillosis occurs in a similar setting of preexisting pulmonary disease (bronchiectasis, chronic bronchitis, asthma, tuberculosis), particularly when dilated bronchi or cavities are present. Colonization with *Aspergillus* can lead to extensive growth, with eventual invasion into the tissue by branching septate hyphae. Mycelial masses can grow to such an extent that they form a radiologically visible *fungus ball* within a cavity. Tissue invasion may involve blood vessels, causing hemoptysis, or erosion into other structures with development of fistulas.

acute pneumonia in immunocompromised host

A more acute form of pneumonia may occur in severely immunosuppressed patients. Multifocal infiltrates expanding to consolidation with high fever are present; this finding, however, is no more characteristic of *Aspergillus* than of many other causes of opportunistic pneumonia in these patients. In contrast to that of the more chronic illness, the prognosis is grave. Dissemination to other organs is common. Invasive aspergillosis outside the lung in nonimmunosuppressed patients is very rare. A few cases of endocarditis have been described, and *Aspergillus* is isolated occasionally from otitis externa and other superficial skin lesions.

Diagnosis

Difficulties in distinguishing infection from contamination

Aspergillus is relatively easy to isolate and identify. Its rapidly spreading mold growth and all too frequent contamination of cultures cause it to be regarded by microbiologists as a kind of weed. The diagnostic problem in aspergillosis is not in isolating the organism, but in distinguishing contamination and colonization with *Aspergillus* from invasive disease. This differentiation cannot be certain without the use of invasive procedures such as lung aspiration or open biopsy. With tissue directly from the lesion, the combination of KOH preparation or histologic findings (large, branching, septate hyphae; Figure 31.2B and C) and culture is diagnostic. The histologic picture alone is suggestive but not diagnostic, because other fungi can have similar appearances. Occasionally the complete fruiting bodies are produced in vivo, creating a striking and diagnostic histologic picture. Serologic methods have been developed to demonstrate *Aspergillus* precipitins. Although they may be helpful in suggesting allergic aspergillosis, their value in invasive disease is unclear.

Histology and culture

Serodiagnostic procedures

Treatment

Amphotericin B is the treatment of choice for invasive or disseminated aspergillosis. The effect in vivo of newer antifungal agents on *Aspergillus* is not yet defined. In cases with pulmonary structural abnormalities and fungus balls, chemotherapy has little effect. Surgical intervention is sometimes needed.

Zygomycosis

zygomycete infections

soil saprophytes

infections in immunocompromised hosts

pulmonary disease

rhinocerebral infections

Zygomycosis (Mucormycosis) is a term applied to infection with any of a group of zygomycetes, the most common of which are *Absidia, Rhizopus,* and *Mucor.* These fungi are ubiquitous saprophytes in soil and are commonly found on bread and many other foodstuffs. They occasionally cause disease in persons with diabetes mellitus and in immunosuppressed patients receiving corticosteroid therapy. Diabetic acidosis has a particularly strong association with mucormycosis.

Pulmonary or rhinocerebral disease is acquired by inhalation of spores. The pulmonary form has clinical findings similar to those of other fungal pneumonias; the rhinocerebral form, however, produces a dramatic clinical syndrome in which agents of mucormycosis show striking invasive capacity. They penetrate the mucosa of the nose, paranasal sinuses, or palate, often resulting in ulcerative lesions. Once beyond the mucosa, they progress through tissue, nerves, blood vessels, fascial planes, and often the vital structures at the base of the brain. The clinical syndrome begins with headache and may progress in less than 2 weeks through orbital cellulitis and hemorrhage, cranial nerve palsy, vascular thrombosis, coma, and death.

nonseptate and non-spore forming in tissues

The pathologic cerebral and pulmonary findings are distinctive: the zygomycetes involved all show large, nonseptate hyphae in tissue, although spores are not seen. As with *Aspergillus,* tissue biopsies are necessary to demonstrate the invasive hyphae, unless they can be seen on scrapings from palatal or nasal ulcers. For reasons that are obscure, biopsy cultures are frequently negative even from tissue containing characteristic hyphae. Therapy involves control of underlying disease, amphotericin B, and occasionally surgery.

Kenneth J. Ryan

Systemic Fungal Pathogens

32

The fungi discussed in this chapter cause a variety of deep-seated infections, all of which can range in severity from mild to progressive and fatal. Growth in environmental sites is an important part of their biology, but they rarely, if ever, contaminate laboratory cultures or colonize healthy humans. Their isolation from clinical material is considered diagnostic of the mycoses described herein.

Cryptococcus neoformans

Microbiology

Yeast with large capsule

Cryptococcus neoformans is a yeast 4–6 μm in diameter that produces a characteristic capsule (Figure 32.1). If included, the capsule extends the overall diameter to 25 μm or more. It is the only pathogenic fungus to form such a capsule. The capsule is composed of polysaccharide, with some differences in antigenic specificity between strains. Cross-reactions with some serotypes of *Streptococcus pneumoniae* have been demonstrated. Other members of the genus *Cryptococcus* are mostly noncapsulate, nonpathogenic, and definitively identified by their biochemical reactions. Cryptococci give a positive test for urease, in contrast to *Candida* and most other yeasts. *Cryptococcus neoformans* grows in 2–5 days at 35–37°C on a variety of media, including blood agar, chocolate agar, and Sabouraud's agar, to produce mucoid, bacterialike colonies. Some strains are inhibited by cyclohexamide, and media containing this selective agent should not be relied on for isolation. A sexual phase has been demonstrated for *C. neoformans.* Under the conditions used in clinical laboratories, however, it grows only in the yeast phase. An older name, *Torula histolytica,* still persists in the literature, and *torulosis* is sometimes used as a synonym for cryptococcosis.

biochemical reactions

growth characteristics

torulosis

Pathogenesis

Infection by inhalation

most infections unrecognized and self-limiting

Cryptococcal infection is usually acquired by inhalation of fungal cells, followed by pulmonary infection or disease. In most instances symptoms and signs must be minimal, because cryptococcal pulmonary infections are rarely seen, or at least rarely diagnosed. In most cases, the inhaled cryptococci are phagocytosed and killed by polymorphonuclear leukocytes or macrophages despite the antiphagocytic effect of the capsule. Occasionally the infection progresses in the lungs or spreads to the central nervous system. Roughly

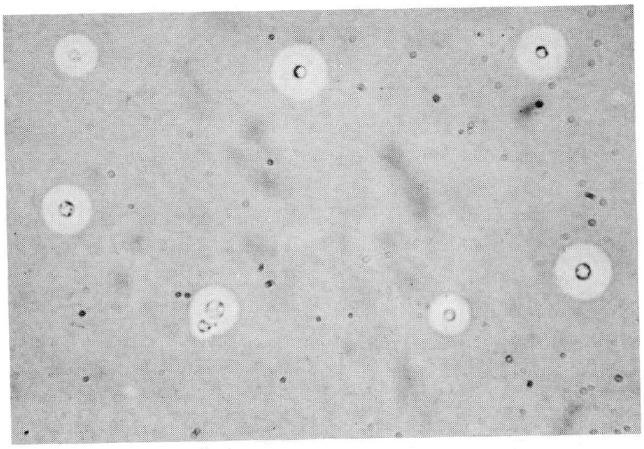

32.1 *Cryptococcus neoformans.* This India ink preparation was made by mixing CSF containing cryptococci with India ink. The yeast cells can be seen within the clear space caused by the large polysaccharide capsule. (*Reproduced with permission from Dr. E.S. Beneke and the Upjohn Company: Scope Monograph, Human Mycoses.*)

Association with other diseases and defects in cellular immunity

half of all such patients have recognized underlying disorders, such as lymphoma or leukemia, that compromise immunity. Various defects of cellular immune function have been demonstrated in other infected patients, but it is not clear whether they are the cause or the result of infection. No toxins, or extracellular enzymes determining virulence, have been recognized in *C. neoformans*.

Tissue reaction to *C. neoformans* may vary from little or none to purulent or granulomatous. Many cases of pulmonary, cutaneous, and even meningeal cryptococcal infection show a remarkable paucity of inflammatory response. Anticryptococcal antibodies are formed in the course of infection, but there is no evidence that they play a role in control of infection.

Epidemiology

reservoir in birds and soil

lack of occupational association

Cryptococcus neoformans is found throughout the world in pigeon or other bird droppings and in soil contaminated with them. The birds themselves do not appear to be infected. Little is known about the mechanism of human infection. Cases appear sporadically, with no particular occupational predisposition. Surprisingly, no increased risk of disease has been found in pigeon fanciers or in those who work with the organism in the laboratory. Case-to-case transmission in humans has not been documented. It is possible that an infectious form, not yet identified, is produced in the environment, but not in vitro.

Clinical Manifestations

Cryptococcal meningitis: chronic course

Central nervous system. Cryptococcal meningitis is the most commonly recognized form of the disease; it usually has a slow, insidious onset with relatively nonspecific findings until late in the course. Intermittent headache, irritability, dizziness, and difficulty with complex cerebral functions appear over weeks or months with no consistent pattern. Behavioral changes have been mistaken for psychoses. Fever is usually, but not invariably, present. Seizures, cranial nerve signs, and papilledema may appear later in the clinical course, as may dementia and decreased levels of consciousness. A more rapid course may be seen in immunosuppressed patients, particularly those receiving steroids.

Cryptococcal pneumonia

Other infections. Cryptococcal pneumonia is often asymptomatic or mild. Sputum production is minimal, and no findings are sufficiently specific to suggest

Other sites of infection

the etiology. Skin and bone are the sites most frequently involved in disseminated disease; skin lesions are sometimes the presenting sign and are often remarkable for their lack of inflammation. The diagnosis is sometimes made when lesions are biopsied as suspected neoplasms.

Laboratory Diagnosis

Cryptococcus neoformans may be demonstrated by direct examination or by cultural isolation. It is important to remember that the number of organisms present may be quite small. Thus, perseverance and attention to detail are important in establishing the diagnosis.

Direct India ink preparation

The typical cerebrospinal fluid (CSF) findings in cryptococcal meningitis are increased pressure, CSF pleocytosis (usually 100 cells or more) with predominance of lymphocytes, and depression of CSF glucose levels. In some cases, one or all of these findings may be absent, yet cryptococci are isolated on culture. *Cryptococcus neoformans* are often demonstrable in CSF by mixing centrifuged sediment with India ink and examining it under the microscope. The yeast and its capsule, which excludes the India ink (Figure 32.1), can often be seen. Some experience is necessary to avoid confusion of lymphocytes with cryptococci. Although this examination is positive in roughly 50% of cases, only a few cryptococci may be present in any single preparation.

Culture

Detection of antigen

Cryptococcus neoformans may be cultured from CSF or other infected sites. The more material cultured, the less the chance of missing cases with small numbers of organisms. In cases with negative cultures, the polysaccharide capsular antigen may be present in the CSF and can be demonstrated immunologically. Test kits containing latex particles coated with antibody to cryptococcal polysaccharide are available for this purpose. The particles agglutinate in the presence of cryptococcal antigens. This method has been the only means of attaining a specific diagnosis in some cases.

Histology

Cryptococcus neoformans stains poorly or not at all with routine histologic stains; thus, it is easily missed unless special fungal stains are used. Once stained, the cells themselves are not distinctive; however, histochemical methods for demonstrating the capsule can differentiate *C. neoformans* from other yeasts.

Treatment

Amphotericin and flucytosine

Amphotericin B, flucytosine, or a combination of both drugs is the usual treatment for systemic cryptococcal disease. Flucytosine alone is effective, but its use is limited by development of resistance during therapy. Although three-fourths of cases of meningitis respond to treatment, a significant portion suffer relapses after antifungal therapy is stopped; many become chronic and require repeated courses of therapy. One-half of those cured have some kind of residual neurologic damage.

Histoplasma capsulatum

Microbiology

Dimorphism

Small yeast cells

Tuberculate macroconidium

Growth

Histoplasma capsulatum is a dimorphic fungus that grows in the yeast phase both in tissue (Figure 32.2A) and in cultures incubated at 37°C. The mold phase grows in cultures incubated at 22–25°C and as a saprophyte in soil. The yeast forms are small for fungi (2–4 μm) and reproduce by budding (blastoconidia). The mycelia are septate and produce microconidia and macroconidia. The diagnostic structure is termed the *tuberculate macroconidium* because of its thick wall and radial, fingerlike projections (Figure 32.2B). Growth is obtained on blood agar, chocolate agar, and Sabouraud's agar,

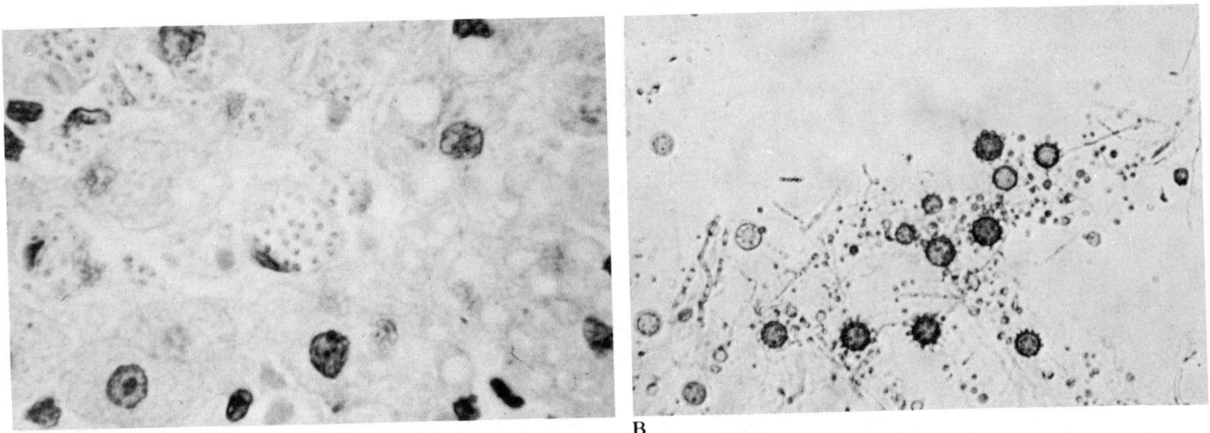

A B

32.2 *Histoplasma capsulatum.* (**A**) Multiple organisms are present within macrophages in the liver. (**B**) The mold is shown with characteristic tuberculate macroconidia. (*Reproduced with permission from Dr. E.S. Beneke and the Upjohn Company: Scope Monograph, Human Mycoses.*)

but may take many weeks to develop. As with *C. neoformans*, a sexual stage has now been discovered, but the older terminology is still used in the medical literature.

absence of capsules

The designation *H. capsulatum* is actually a misnomer, because no capsules are formed: the unstained areas seen around the yeasts in tissue sections (Figure 32.2A) are artifacts of the staining and fixation procedures.

Pathogenesis

Reticuloendothelial system infection

Intracellular habitat

The hallmark of histoplasmosis is infection of the reticuloendothelial system with intracellular growth in phagocytic macrophages. The initial infection is pulmonary, through inhalation of infectious conidia, which convert to the yeast form in the host. This conversion is stimulated by the elevated host temperature (37°C) and associated with a shift in the biochemical pathways used in oxidative metabolism. How this relates to the organism's ability to multiply within monocytes is unknown.

Primary lesion

A primary lesion with lymphatic spread very similar to that seen in tuberculosis (Chapter 25) develops. The vast majority of cases never advance beyond this stage, leaving only a calcified node and a positive histoplasmin skin test as evidence of infection. The extent of spread to the reticuloendothelial system within macrophages during primary infection is unknown, but such spread is presumed to occur and account for the distribution of disseminated disease. Old lesions may reactivate in a small proportion of cases.

Granulomatous response

Pathologically, granulomatous inflammation with necrosis is prominent in pulmonary lesions. *Histoplasma capsulatum* may be difficult to find even with specific fungal stains. Extrapulmonary spread involves the reticuloendothelial system with enlargement of the liver and spleen. Numerous organisms within macrophages may be found in these organs, in lymph nodes, or in bone marrow (Figure 32.2A).

Immunity and hypersensitivity

Histoplasmin

Infection with *H. capsulatum* is associated with the development of cell-mediated immunity to histoplasmin as demonstrated by a positive delayed hypersensitivity skin test. Histoplasmin is a filtrate prepared from mycelial-phase cultures of the fungus. Infection is believed to confer long-lasting immunity, but the relationship of the skin test response to immunity or clinical outcome of infection is not clear. Although relapses have been documented, their overall frequency and their relationship to disseminated disease are not well defined. Infected immunosuppressed persons tend to develop disseminated disease.

Epidemiology

environmental sources

high incidence of infection in central U.S.

Point source outbreaks from bird roosts and bat caves

Histoplasma capsulatum grows in soil containing bird or bat droppings under certain climatic conditions, and disease is acquired from the environment. Although evidence of worldwide distribution is increasing, the greatest concentration by far is in the areas of the United States drained by the Ohio and Mississippi Rivers. Over 50% of residents of states in this area show skin test evidence of previous infection. An African variant with larger yeast-phase cells infects skin and lymph nodes, but rarely produces lung lesions. Disturbances of bird roosts, bat caves, and soil have been associated with point source outbreaks of infection by airborne conidia. The disease is not transmitted from person to person.

Clinical Manifestations

primary infection of respiratory tract

chronic infection

progressive pulmonary disease

Most cases of *H. capsulatum* infection are asymptomatic or show only fever and cough for a few days or weeks. Mediastinal lymphadenopathy and slight pulmonary infiltrates may be seen if X-rays are taken. The histoplasmin skin test becomes positive after about 3 weeks. More severe cases may have chills, malaise, chest pain, and more extensive infiltrates, which usually resolve nonetheless. A residual nodule may continue to enlarge over a period of years, causing a differential diagnostic problem with pulmonary neoplasms. Progressive pulmonary disease occurs in a form similar to that of pulmonary tuberculosis, including the development of cavities, with sputum production, night sweats, and weight loss. The course is chronic and relapsing, lasting many months to years.

Disseminated histoplasmosis

Disseminated histoplasmosis generally appears as a febrile illness with enlargement of reticuloendothelial organs. The central nervous system, skin, gastrointestinal tract, and adrenal glands may also be involved. Painless ulcers on mucous membranes are a common finding. The course is typically chronic with manifestations that depend on the organs involved. For example, chronic bilateral adrenal failure (Addison's disease) may develop when the adrenal glands are involved.

Diagnosis

Direct examination

In most forms of histoplasmosis, the organisms are not readily accessible for demonstration by direct examination or culture. They are rarely present in sputum in primary pulmonary infections, and repeated cultures are necessary to ensure positive findings in chronic cavitary disease. In disseminated disease, smears of a superficial mucous membrane lesion or biopsy samples of a reticuloendothelial organ are the specimens most likely to contain *Histoplasma.* Because of their small size, the yeast cells are difficult to see in potassium hydroxide preparations, and their morphology is not sufficiently distinctive to be diagnostic. Selective fungal stains such as methenamine silver demonstrate the organism, but may not differentiate it from other yeasts. Hematoxylin–eosin (H&E)-stained tissue or Wright-stained bone marrow will often demonstrate the organisms and their intracellular location in macrophages (Figure 32.2A). Specimens must be examined carefully under high magnification (100×, oil immersion).

Culture

Identification

The organism may be grown from tissue, bone marrow, or sputum. The latter poses special problems, as *H. capsulatum* grows slowly in comparison to other bacteria and fungi. Identification requires demonstration of dimorphism and of the asexual conidia. Prolonged incubation may be necessary.

Serologic diagnosis

Complement fixation

Histoplasmin skin test

Serologic tests have been developed using histoplasmin or yeast cell antigens. Antibodies can be detected by immunodiffusion or complement fixation (CF). In histoplasmosis, CF titers typically rise to 1:32 or greater, but false-negative results are common in all clinical forms of the disease. False-positive findings also occur, and definite cross-reactions are found in cases of blastomycosis. The histoplasmin skin test is useful for epidemiologic studies but is often difficult to interpret in clinical situations. Skin testing may stimulate antibodies and thus confuse serologic diagnosis. Neither serologic nor skin test positivity alone is sufficient evidence of disease to initiate therapy. Cultural isolation or clear histologic demonstration is necessary for a firm diagnosis. Specific mycelial antigens can be demonstrated by immunodiffusion once the mold form is isolated (exoantigen test).

Treatment

Amphotericin B is the treatment of choice for histoplasmosis. Its toxicity, however, limits its use to cases of extensive disease, such as progressive pulmonary disease and disseminated histoplasmosis. Primary infections and localized lung lesions require no treatment.

Blastomyces

Microbiology

Dimorphism

large, thick walled yeasts

Blastomyces dermatitidis is a dimorphic fungus with characteristics similar to those of *Histoplasma.* Growth develops in the yeast phase in tissues and in cultures incubated at 37°C. The yeast cells are typically larger (8–15 μm) than those of *H. capsulatum*, with broad-based buds and a thick wall (Figure 32.3). A smaller variant with morphologic characteristics identical to those of *Histoplasma* is occasionally seen. The mold phase appears in culture at 25°C. Hyphae are septate and produce round to oval conidia sufficiently similar to those produced by *H. capsulatum* to cause confusion between the two in young mold cultures. Although older cultures may produce chlamydoconidia, *B. dermatitidis* produces no structure as distinctive as the tuberculate macroconidium of *Histoplasma.*

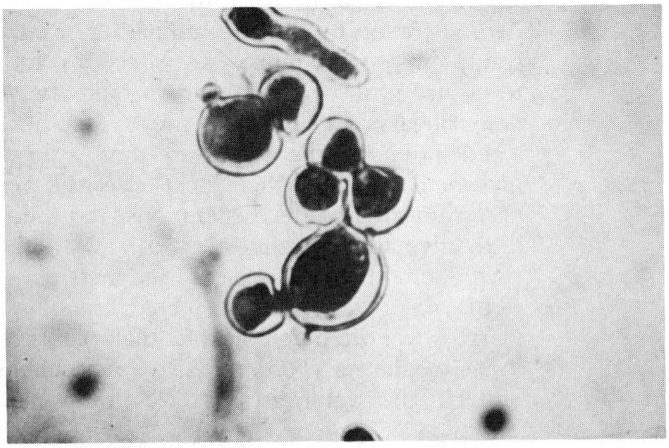

32.3 *Blastomyces dermatitidis.* Large thick-walled yeast are shown. Blastoconidia retain a broad attachment to the mother cell before separating. (*Reproduced with permission from Dr. E.S. Beneke and the Upjohn Company: Scope Monograph, Human Mycoses.*)

Pathogenesis and Epidemiology

Much less is known about blastomycosis than about the other systemic mycoses, such as histoplasmosis and coccidioidomycosis. The lower frequency of disseminated infections and the less satisfactory performance of skin and serologic tests are partly responsible for this lack of information. Much of what is believed to be true of blastomycosis is based on analogy with histoplasmosis.

Pulmonary infection

The primary infection is pulmonary after inhalation of conidia, which are believed to develop in soil. A mixed inflammatory response results, which ranges from neutrophil infiltration to well-organized granulomas with giant cells. The organisms appear as large yeast cells, most of which still have blastospores attached. They appear to have a double wall in H&E sections because of shrinkage of the cytoplasm and dense staining of its periphery. The organism can spread to the skin and less often to bone and viscera. Considerable necrosis and fibrosis can lead to large, expanding lesions at infected sites; slow resolution can occur, however, presumably by immune mechanisms.

Geography

Cases of blastomycosis follow a geographic distribution similar to that of histoplasmosis. Most infections occur in the middle and eastern portions of North America, but cases have been reported in South America and Africa. Again the lack of a specific skin test limits study of the endemic area.

Clinical Manifestations

As mild cases are difficult to diagnose, most infections are recognized at advanced or disseminated stages of the disease. This problem was also posed by the other systemic mycoses before the development of sensitive and specific diagnostic procedures.

Pulmonary blastomycosis

Skin lesions

Bone, urinary and genital tract lesions

Pulmonary infection is evidenced by cough, sputum production, chest pain, and fever. Hilar lymphadenopathy may be present, as well as nodular pulmonary infiltrates with alveolar consolidation. The total picture may mimic a pulmonary tumor, tuberculosis, or some other mycosis. Skin lesions are common and were once considered a primary form of the disease. In contrast to those in histoplasmosis, lesions develop on exposed skin; mucous membrane infection is uncommon. Extensive necrosis and fibrosis may produce considerable disfigurement. Bone infection has features similar to those of other causes of chronic osteomyelitis. The urinary and genital tracts are the most common visceral sites; the prostate is especially prone to infection. Prostatitis is an occasional initial complaint.

Diagnosis

Direct examination

Culture

Direct demonstration of typical large yeasts with broad-based buds (blastoconidia) in KOH preparations is the most rapid means of diagnosis. Biopsy specimens also have a high yield, and the organisms are visible with either H&E or special fungal stains. *Blastomyces dermatitidis* will grow on routine mycologic media, but culture may take as long as 4 weeks. Some strains may be inhibited by cyclohexamide in selective media. Conidia are not particularly distinctive, and demonstration of dimorphism and typical yeast morphology is essential to avoid confusion with other fungi, including *Histoplasma*. The exoantigen test from mycelial-phase cultures is particularly useful in differentiation from strains of *Histoplasma*, which are slow to produce characteristic conidia.

Antigens for CF tests are available, but CF antibodies are absent in up to 50% of cases. Skin tests have no value.

Treatment

Although amphotericin B is the preferred therapy, it is only used for progressive or disseminated disease. As with other systemic mycoses, response to treatment is slow, and relapse is common.

Coccidioides immitis

Microbiology

Dimorphism

Spherule

Endospores

Mold phase

Arthroconidia

Coccidioides immitis is also a dimorphic fungus, but instead of a yeast phase, a large (12–100 μm), distinctive, roundwalled spherule (Figure 32.4A) is produced in the invasive tissue form. Multiple endospores develop within the spherule and are released when the spherule ruptures. They serve as the reproductive unit in vivo. On routine culture, *C. immitis* grows only as a mold at room temperature and 37°C. Growth becomes visible in 2–5 days. Spherules have been cultured in vitro under specialized conditions. The hyphae are septate and produce thick-walled, barrel-shaped arthroconidia (Figure 32.4B), which are the infectious unit in nature and highly infectious when they develop in the laboratory.

Pathogenesis

Respiratory infection

Inflammatory responses

Inhaled arthroconidia bypass the defenses of the upper tracheobronchial tree and lodge in the alveoli. There, the arthroconidia convert to the spherule stage, which begins its slow growth, stimulating a macrophage and neutrophil cellular response. The outer wall of the arthroconidium has antiphagocytic properties, which persist in the early stages of spherule development. As the spherule grows, its size makes effective phagocytosis difficult, although neutrophils are able to digest the wall. Later, as the spherules enlarge and multiply, the overall inflammatory response is granulomatous with some giant cells. Rupture of spherules with release of hundreds of endospores

32.4 *Coccidioides immitis.* (**A**) Tissue with thick-walled spherule containing multiple endospores. (**B**) Mold phase with septate hyphae and arthroconidia. (**C**) KOH preparation of sputum showing thick-walled spherule, which has just burst. (*Reproduced with permission from Dr. E.S. Beneke and the Upjohn Company: Scope Monograph, Human Mycoses.*)

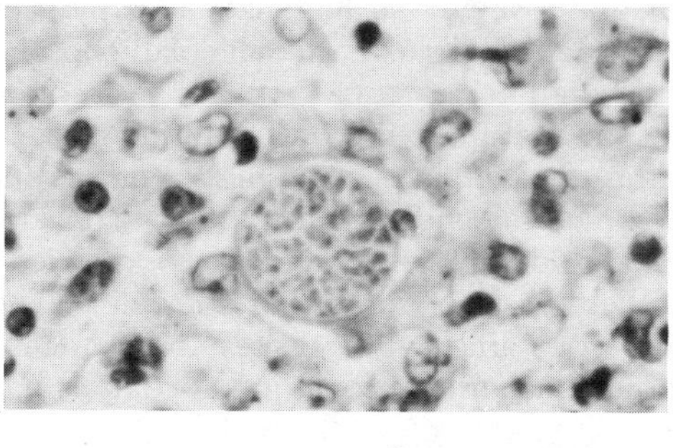

A

B

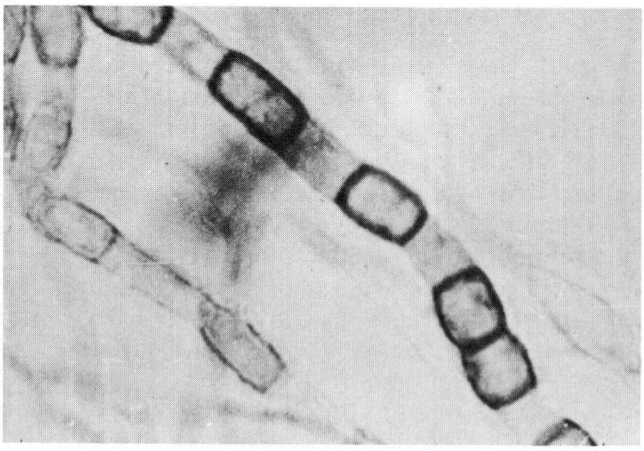

C

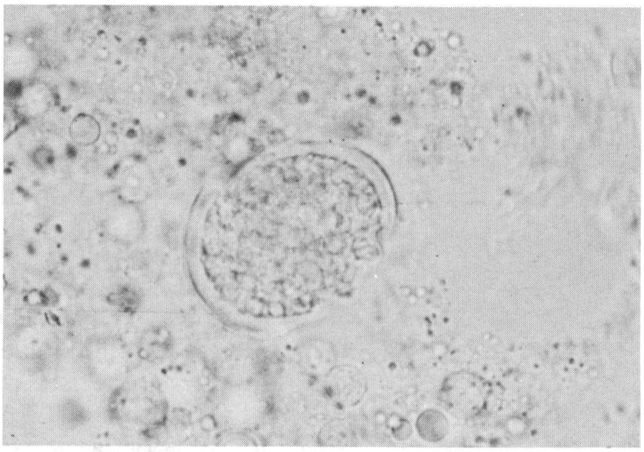

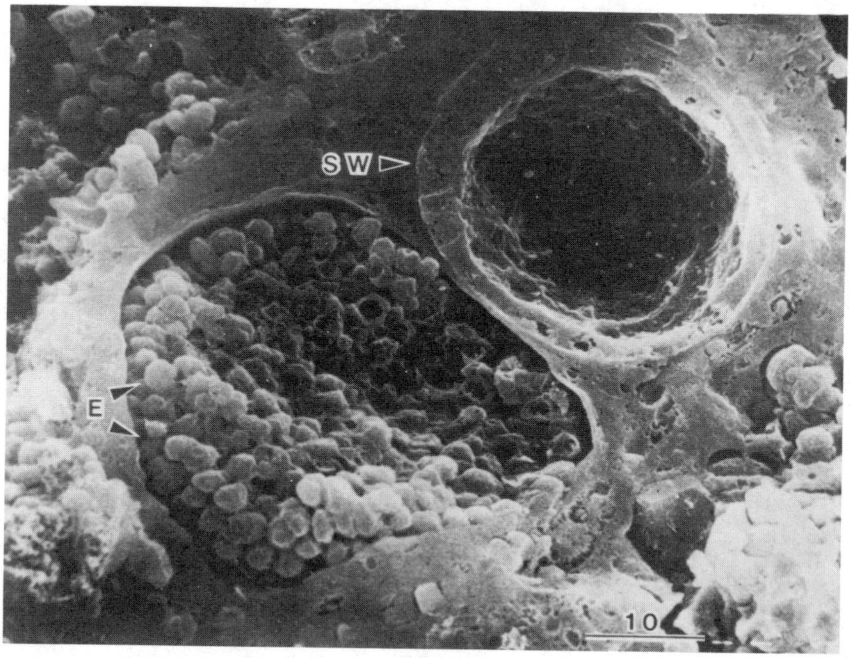

32.5 *Coccidioides immitis.* This electron micrograph of infected mouse lung shows a spherule filled with endospores (E) and one that has discharged its endospores into the surrounding tissue. Note the thickness of the spherule wall (SW). (*Reproduced with permission from Drutz, D.J., and Huppert, M. 1983. J. Infect. Dis. 147: 379, Figure 7. Copyright University of Chicago Publisher.*)

(Figure 32.5) stimulates an acute inflammatory response, which has an uncertain effect. The young endospores are released in packets with a surrounding matrix, which may further protect them from destruction by the host. They then develop into new spherules.

Development of immunity and hypersensitivity

In most cases, this mixed inflammatory response is associated with early resolution of the infection and development of a positive delayed hypersensitivity skin test. In a few cases, the infection is not controlled. These infections may progress to a chronic pulmonary form of the disease or become disseminated to other organs. The mechanism for dissemination is not precisely known, but is believed to involve a subtle defect in cell-mediated immunity to *C. immitis*. In animals, suppression of cellular immunity is associated with more progressive disease, and dissemination in humans is accompanied by skin test anergy.

Progressive and disseminated disease

Cell-mediated immunity

Epidemiology

Geography

Coccidioidomycosis is the most geographically restricted of the systemic mycoses, because *C. immitis* grows only in the semiarid climates known as the Lower Sonoran life zone. These areas are characterized by hot, dry summers, mild winters with few freezes, and annual rainfall of about 10 inches during brief rainy seasons. Areas with these conditions are found scattered throughout the Americas; some are ecologic "islands." The primary endemic zones in the United States are in the southwestern states of Arizona, Nevada, New Mexico, and western Texas and the arid parts of central and southern California. Infection does not normally occur outside the endemic areas, although visits of only a few hours to an endemic zone have resulted in infection. One such anecdote involves a gas station attendant with coccidioidomycosis, whose only contact with an endemic area was changing a flat tire on a truck from California. A recent storm that blew inland dust into the San Francisco Bay area, which is outside the endemic zone, was associated with many cases of coccidioidomycosis. Earth-moving operations and archeologic digs have also been associated with outbreaks.

Dust-borne spread

High infection–low disease rates

Persons living in the endemic areas are at high risk of infection, although disease is much less common. Positive skin test rates of 50–90% occur in longtime residents of highly endemic areas. Coccidioidomycosis is not transmissible from person to person.

Clinical Manifestations

Primary infection

More than one-half of those infected with *C. immitis* suffer no symptoms, or the disease is so mild that it cannot be recalled when skin test conversion is discovered. Others develop malaise, cough, chest pain, fever, and arthralgia 1–3 weeks after infection. This disease, which lasts 2–6 weeks, is known as *valley fever* by the local populations in the United States. Objective findings are few. The chest X-ray is usually clear or shows only hilar adenopathy. Erythema nodosum may develop midway through the course, particularly in women. In most cases, resolution is spontaneous, but only after considerable discomfort and loss of productivity. In over 90% of cases, there are no pulmonary residua. A small number of cases progress to a chronic pulmonary form characterized by cavity formation and a slow relapsing course that extends over years. Less than 1% of all primary infections disseminate to foci outside the lung.

Valley fever

Erythema nodosum

Chronic and disseminated disease

Disseminated disease is more common in men, in dark-skinned races, particularly Filipinos, and in immunosuppressed persons. Evidence of extrapulmonary infection almost always appears in the first year after primary infection. The most common sites are bones, joints, skin, and meninges. Coccidioidal meningitis develops slowly with gradually increasing headache, fever, neck stiffness, and other signs of meningeal irritation. The CSF findings are similar to those in tuberculosis and other fungal causes of meningitis, such as *C. neoformans*. Mononuclear cells predominate in the cell count, but substantial numbers of neutrophils are often present. If untreated, the disease is slowly progressive and fatal.

Racial incidence

Sites of disseminated disease

Meningitis

Diagnosis

Direct examination

With enough persistence, direct examinations are usually rewarding. The thick-walled spherules are so large and characteristic (Figure 32.4A and C) that they are difficult to miss in a KOH preparation. Skin and visceral lesions are most likely to be positive, CSF least. The spherules released into expectorated sputum are often small (10–15 μm) and immature without well-developed endospores. Some experience is necessary to differentiate them from artifacts. Spherules stain well in histologic sections by either H&E or the special fungal stains.

Spherules

Culture

Risk of laboratory infection

Culture of *C. immitis* from sputum, visceral lesions, or skin lesions is not difficult, but must only be undertaken by those with experience and proper biohazard protection. Cultures from CSF are rarely positive. Laboratories must be warned of the possibility of coccidioidomycosis to ensure diagnosis and avoid inadvertent laboratory infection. The latter is particularly significant outside the endemic areas, where routine precautions may not be enforced. Identification requires growth of typical arthroconidia and demonstration of conversion to spherules either in vitro or in animals. The exoantigen immunodiffusion test is also useful for differentation of *C. immitis* from other fungi that produce arthroconidia, and it is more rapid than methods for demonstration of spherules. It is based on the antigenic specificity of the mycelia.

Detection of exoantigen

Skin and serologic tests

Skin and serologic tests are very useful in diagnosis and management of coccidioidomycosis. The skin test usually becomes positive 1–4 weeks after the onset of symptoms of primary infection, and remains so for life. Disseminated disease is frequently associated with anergy, particularly when it is severe. The skin test does not interfere with serologic tests, as it does in histoplasmosis.

IgM response

IgG response

One-half to three-quarters of patients with primary infection will develop serum immunoglobulin M precipitating antibody in the first 3 weeks of illness. These conditions persist for 2–4 months. Immunoglobulin G antibodies detected by the CF test appear somewhat later in symptomatic infections. The amount and duration depend on the extent of disease. Antibodies disappear with resolution and persist with continuing infection. The height of the CF titer is a measure of the magnitude of antigenic stimulation, and thus of the extent of disease. The presence of CF antibody in the CSF is also an important parameter in the diagnosis of coccidioidal meningitis, as cultures are usually negative. The precipitating and CF antibodies may be detected by classic methods or by more recently developed immunodiffusion procedures.

Treatment

Amphotericin B

Ketoconazole

Primary coccidioidomycosis is self-limiting, and no antifungal therapy is indicated. Progressive pulmonary disease and disseminated disease require the use of antifungal agents, usually amphotericin B. The newer imidazoles, particularly ketoconazole, show some promise; and they are less toxic than amphotericin B, but have not yet been proved effective.

Paracoccidioides brasiliensis

Paracoccidioides brasiliensis is the cause of paracoccidioidomycosis (South American blastomycosis), a disease limited to tropical and subtropical areas of Central and South America. The organism is a dimorphic fungus, the most noteworthy feature of which is the production of multiple blastoconidia from the same cell. Characteristic 5- to 40-μm cells covered with budding blastoconidia may be seen in tissue or in yeast-phase growth at 37°C. The disease is primarily manifested by chronic mucocutaneous or cutaneous ulcers. The ulcers spread slowly and develop a granulomatous mulberrylike base. Regional lymph nodes, reticuloendothelial organs, and the lungs may also be involved. Little is known of the pathogenesis, although the route of infection is believed to be inhalation. The disease has a striking predilection for men. Treatment is with sulfonamides, amphotericin B, and, more recently, the imidazole compounds.

Additional Reading and References

Drutz, D.J., and Huppert, M. 1983. Coccidioidomycosis: Factors affecting the host-parasite interaction. *J. Infect. Dis.* 147:372–390. This review of pathogensis is beautifully illustrated with electron micrographs.

Smith, C.E., Saito, M.T., and Simons, S.A. 1956. Pattern of 39,500 serologic tests in coccidioidomycosis. *J. Am. Med. Assoc.* 160:546–552. This study is the basis for the unique application of serologic tests to the diagnosis and prognosis of coccidioidomycosis.

Kenneth J. Ryan

Subcutaneous Fungi and Disease

33

Assignment of fungal organisms to the category of subcutaneous fungi is somewhat arbitrary, because fungal pathogens can produce many subcutaneous manifestations as part of their disease spectrum. Those considered here are introduced traumatically through the skin and mainly involve subcutaneous tissues, lymphatic vessels, and contiguous tissues. They rarely spread to distant organs. The diseases they cause include sporotrichosis, chromoblastomycosis, and mycetoma. Only sporotrichosis has a single specific etiologic agent, *Sporothrix schenckii.* Chromoblastomycosis and mycetoma are clinical syndromes with multiple fungal etiologies (Table 33.1).

Sporotrichosis

Microbiology

cigar-shaped yeast at 37°C

dimorphism

Sporothrix schenckii is a dimorphic fungus that grows as a cigar-shaped, 3- to 5-μm yeast (Figure 33.1A) in tissues and in culture at 37°C. The mold, which grows in culture at 25°C, is presumably the infectious form in nature. The hyphae are thin and septate, producing clusters of conidia at the end of delicate conidiophores (Figure 33.1B).

Epidemiology

saprophye

traumatic infection

occupational incidence

Sporothrix schenckii is a ubiquitous saprophyte found in soil, in decaying organic matter, and on the surfaces of various plants. Infection is acquired by traumatic inoculation through the skin of material containing the organism. Exposure is largely occupational or related to hobbies. The skin of gardeners, farmers, and rural laborers is frequently traumatized by thorns or other material that may be contaminated with spores of *S. schenckii.* An unusual outbreak of sporotrichosis involving nearly 3000 miners was traced to *S. schenckii* in the timbers used to support mine shafts. Infection is occasionally acquired by direct contact with infected pus or through the respiratory tract; these modes of infection, however, are much less common than the cutaneous route.

Pathologic Features

pyogenic and granulomatous lesions

Local multiplication of the organism stimulates both acute pyogenic and granulomatous inflammatory reactions. The infection spreads along lymphatic drainage routes and reproduces the original inflammatory lesions at intervals. The organisms are scanty in human lesions.

Table 33.1 Agents of Subcutaneous Mycoses

Organism	Disease	Growth: Tissue	Growth: Culture (25°C)	Growth: Culture (37°C)
Sporothrix schenckii	Sporotrichosis	Yeast (rare)	Mold	Yeast
Phialophora	Chromoblastomycosis; mycetoma	Mycelia[a]	Mold	Mold
Cladosporium	Chromoblastomycosis	Mycelia[a]	Mold	Mold
Petriellidium	Mycetoma	Mycelia	Mold	Mold

[a] Pigmented, often blunted to form round to oval bodies.

Clinical Features

Skin infection

ulceration

lymphatic spread and involvement

A skin lesion begins as a painless papule that develops a few weeks to a few months after inoculation. Its location can usually be explained by occupational exposure; the hand is most often involved. The papule enlarges slowly and eventually ulcerates, leaving an open sore. Draining lymph channels are usually thickened, and pustular or firm nodular lesions may appear around the primary site of infection or at other sites along the lymphatic drainage route. Once ulcerated, lesions usually become chronic. Multiple ulcers often develop if the disease is untreated. Symptoms are those directly related to the local areas of infection. Constitutional signs and symptoms are unusual.

rare infections in other sites

Occasionally, spread occurs by other routes. The bones, eyes, lungs, and central nervous system are susceptible to progressive infection if the organisms reach them; such spread, however, occurs in less than 1% of all cases. Primary pulmonary sporotrichosis occurs but is also rare.

Diagnosis

frequent failure of direct examination

Direct microscopic examination for fungi is usually unrewarding because there are too few organisms to detect readily with potassium hydroxide preparations. Even specially stained biopsy samples and serial sections are

33.1 *Sporothrix schenckii.* (**A**) The yeast form of *S. schenckii* is typically cigar-shaped but is rarely seen in human lesions. This smear is from infected mouse testis. (**B**) Mold-phase cultures develop delicate hyphae and conidiophores bearing fingerlike clusters of conidia. (*Reproduced with permission from the Scope monograph, Human Mycoses and from Dr. E.S. Beneke and from the Upjohn Company.*)

A

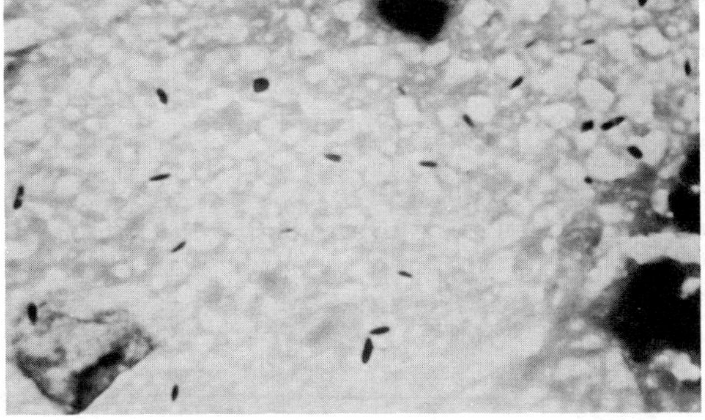

B

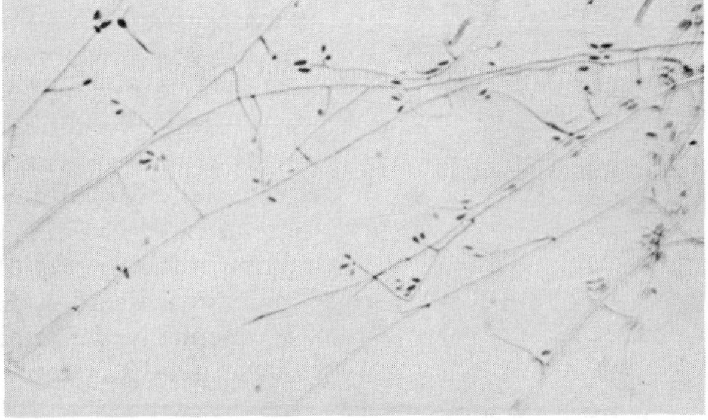

usually negative, although the presence of a histopathologic structure, the asteroid body, is considered diagnostic. This structure is composed of *S. schenckii* yeast cells surrounded by amorphous eosinophilic "rays."

Culture

Definitive diagnosis depends on culture of infected pus or tissue. The organism grows within 2–5 days on all media commonly used in medical mycology. Identification requires demonstration of the typical asexual spores and of dimorphism (Figure 33.1A and B).

Treatment and Prevention

Potassium iodide treatment

Cutaneous sporotrichosis is effectively treated with potassium iodide administered orally. The mechanism of action is unknown, however, as *S. schenckii* is resistant to 10% potassium iodide in vitro. Systemic infections require the use of amphotericin B. There is little therapeutic experience with the newer antifungal agents. Eradication of the environmental reservoir of *S. schenckii* is not usually practical, although the mine outbreak mentioned previously was stopped by applying antifungal agents to the mine shaft timbers.

Chromoblastomycosis

Tropical

Multiple etiologies

Wartlike, pigmented lesions

Chromoblastomycosis is primarily a tropical disease caused by multiple species of two genera of fungi, *Phialophora* and *Cladosporium.* The disease occurs typically on the foot or leg. It appears as papules that develop into scaly, wartlike structures, usually under the feet. Fully developed lesions have been likened to the tips of a cauliflower. Extension is by satellite lesions; it is slow and painless, and does not involve the lymphatic vessels. The organisms are found in the soil of endemic areas, and most infections occur in those who work barefoot.

The outstanding mycologic feature is the presence of brown-pigmented hyphae on direct examination or in culture. Branching septate hyphae, which are often blunted, can be demonstrated in KOH preparations of scrapings or in histologic sections. Cultures grow as molds, but may take weeks to appear and longer for demonstration of characteristic conidia.

difficulties in treatment

Surgery and antifungal therapy have been used in chromoblastomycosis, but results in advanced disease are disappointing. Flucytosine has been the anti-fungal agent most frequently used.

Mycetoma

multiple etiologies

induration and sinuses

Mycetoma is another unusual infection associated with trauma to the foot and inoculation of any of several fungal species. The most common species in nontropical areas is *Petriellidium boydii.* The usual clinical appearance is of massive induration with draining sinuses. Some of the fungi that cause mycetoma are geographically widespread; most cases, however, occur in the tropics, probably because the chronically damp, macerated skin of the feet that causes predisposition toward mycetoma occurs most often in the tropical environment. This finding is illustrated by the case of a college rower in Seattle who developed mycetoma: he was the only member of his shell who insisted on rowing barefoot. Once established, the treatment of mycetoma is difficult. No antimicrobic stands out as particularly helpful.

Microcolonial granules

The precise microbiologic features depend on the agent involved. Hyphae are usually present in tissue, but may be difficult to demonstrate because of a tendency to form microcolonial granules, as in actinomycosis. *Petriellidium* grows relatively rapidly, but some of the other causes may take weeks for initial growth. Identification is by morphology of the asexual conidia.

Actinomycotic mycetoma

Essentially the same disease can be caused by some branching bacteria of the genera *Streptomyces* and *Nocardia* (Chapter 26).

C. George Ray

Respiratory Viruses

34

Respiratory disease accounts for an estimated 75–80% of all acute morbidity in the U.S. population. Most of these illnesses (approximately 80%) are viral. Including episodes not requiring medical attention, the overall average is three to four illnesses per year per person; this average varies among individuals, however, and also inversely with age (the frequency is greater among young children). Seasonality is also a feature; incidence is lowest in the summer months and highest in the winter.

Range of respiratory viruses

The viruses that are major causes of acute respiratory disease (ARD) include influenza, parainfluenza, rhinoviruses, adenoviruses, respiratory syncytial, and respiratory coronaviruses. Reoviruses are of questionable importance, but will also be considered. Others, such as enteroviruses and measles virus, can also cause respiratory symptoms, but are discussed in other chapters.

short incubation period

droplet or manual spread

risk of bacterial superinfection

In addition to the ability to cause a variety of ARD syndromes, this somewhat heterogeneous group of viruses share a relatively short incubation period (1–4 days) and a mode of spread from person to person. Transmission is direct, by infective droplet nuclei, or indirect, by hand contact with contaminated secretions and transfer to nasal or conjunctival epithelium. All of these agents are associated with an increased risk of bacterial superinfection originating in the damaged tissue of the respiratory tract, and all have a worldwide distribution.

Influenza Viruses

Habitat and History

Human, animal and avian strains

Humans are the major hosts of the influenza viruses, and severe respiratory disease is the primary manifestation of infection. Influenza A viruses closely related to those prevalent in humans, however, circulate among many mammalian and avian species. Some of these may undergo antigenic mutation or genetic recombination with human strains and emerge as new human epidemic strains.

Pandemic influenza

Characteristic influenza outbreaks have been described since the early 16th century; since then, outbreaks of varying severity have occurred nearly every year. Severe pandemics with worldwide spread occurred in 1743, 1889–1890, 1918–1919 (the Spanish flu), and 1957 (the Asian flu). These episodes were associated with particularly high mortality; for example, the Spanish flu was thought to have caused at least 20 million deaths. Usually,

Age- and disease-associated mortality

the elderly and those persons of any age group with cardiac or pulmonary disease have the highest death rate.

Group Characteristics

Orthomyxoviruses

types A, B, and C

relative virulence and epidemic spread of different types

Influenza viruses are members of the orthomyxovirus group, which are enveloped, pleomorphic agents possessing single-stranded RNA. They are classified into three major serotypes, A, B, and C, each based on different ribonucleoprotein antigens. Influenza A is the most extensively studied of the three, and much of the following discussion is based upon knowledge of this type. It usually causes more severe disease and more extensive epidemics than the other types and has a greater tendency to undergo significant antigenic changes. Influenza B is somewhat more antigenically stable and usually occurs in more localized outbreaks; influenza C appears to be a minor cause of disease, in contrast to the other types.

enveloped RNA virus

virus-specified glycoproteins

Influenza viruses consist of a nucleocapsid containing RNA, which is enveloped in a glycolipid membrane derived from the host cell plasma membrane. The inner side of the envelope contains a layer of virus-specified protein. Two virus-specified glycoproteins, hemagglutinin and neuraminidase, are imbedded in the outer surface of the envelope and appear as "spikes" over the surface of the virion (Figure 34.1).

Hemagglutinin and viral attachment

The virus-specified glycoproteins are antigenic and have special functional importance to the virus. Hemagglutinin is so named because of its ability to agglutinate red blood cells from certain species (for example, chickens, guinea pigs) in vitro. Its major biologic function is to serve as a point of attachment to mucoprotein receptor sites on human respiratory cell surfaces, which is a critical first step in initiating infection of the cell.

Neuraminidase and viral transport and release from cell

Neuraminidase is an antigenic hydrolytic enzyme that acts on the mucoprotein hemagglutinin receptors by splitting off the terminal neuraminic acid. The result is destruction of receptor activity. Neuraminidase probably serves several functions. It may inactivate a free mucoprotein receptor substance in respiratory secretions that could otherwise bind to viral hemagglutinin and prevent access of the virus to the cell surface. It may be important in fusion of the viral envelope with the host cell membrane as a prerequisite to viral entry. It also aids in the release of newly formed virus particles from infected cells, thus making them available to infect other cells. Type-specific antibodies to neuraminidase appear to inhibit the spread of virus in the infected host and to limit the amount of virus released from host cells.

Viral replication, assembly, and release

After replication of viral components within the cell, virus assembly takes place at the plasma membrane. The complete virus particles are enveloped by the plasma membrane, which by then contains hemagglutinin and neuraminidase. Virus "buds" are formed, and intact virions are released from the cell surface (Figure 34.2).

Viral isolation

culture in embryonated eggs

cell culture

Influenza A viruses were initially isolated in 1933 by intranasal inoculation of ferrets, which developed febrile respiratory illnesses. At present, the viruses are often grown in the amniotic sac of embryonated hen's eggs, where their presence can be detected by the hemagglutination test. Most strains can also be readily isolated in cell culture systems, such as primary monkey kidney cells. Some will cause cytopathic effects in culture; however, the most efficient method of detection is by demonstrating hemadsorption on the infected cell surfaces.

hemadsorption

hemagglutination

Influenza virus can be detected in infected cell cultures by adherence of erythrocytes to infected cells containing hemagglutinin (hemadsorption) or by agglutination of erythrocytes by virus already released into the extracellular fluid (hemagglutination). The virus can then be identified specifically

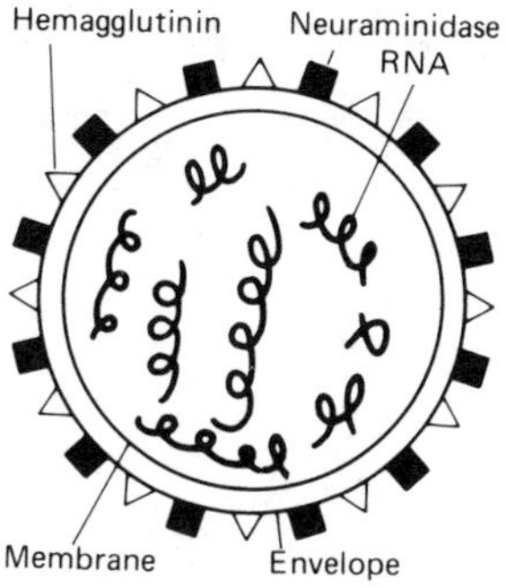

34.1 A diagrammatic view of the influenza A virus, containing eight distinctive segments of single-stranded RNA.

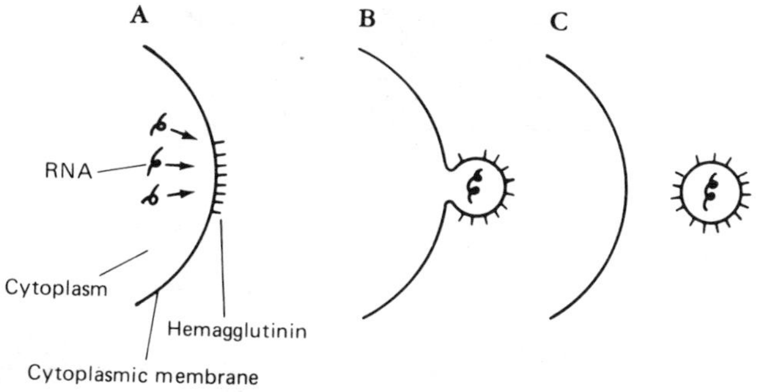

34.2 Late stages in the maturation of an influenza virus. (A) The virus-coded envelope proteins, including hemagglutinin, are assembled and incorporated into the cytoplasmic membrane. (B) Budding begins, with incorporation of the ribonucleoproteins into the contents of the bud. (C) Release of the intact, enveloped virion.

hemadsorption and hemagglutination inhibition

by neutralization or inhibition of these properties by addition of antibody directed specifically at the hemagglutinin. This method is called *hemadsorption inhibition* or *hemagglutination inhibition,* depending upon whether the test is performed on infected cells or extracellular virus, respectively. Also, because the hemagglutinin is antigenic, hemagglutination inhibition tests can be used to detect antibodies in infected subjects. It has been shown that antibody directed against specific hemagglutinin is highly effective in neutralizing the infectivity of the virus.

Detection of antihemagglutinin antibodies in serum

Influenza A

Influenza A will be considered in detail because of its great clinical and epidemiologic importance.

Influenza A genome

The influenza A virion contains at least eight segments of single-stranded RNA with defined genetic responsibilities. These functions include coding for virus-specified proteins and antigens. A unique aspect of influenza A viruses is their ability to develop a wide variety of subtypes through the processes of mutation and recombination. These processes result in antigenic changes called *drifts* and *shifts,* which will be discussed shortly.

Subtypes based on H and N antigens

At least 13 major subtypes of hemagglutinin antigens and 9 subtypes of neuraminidase antigens are known to exist among influenza A viruses. Of these, three hemagglutinins (H_1,H_2, and H_3) and two neuraminidases (N_1 and N_2) appear to be of greatest importance in human infections. These subtypes are designated according to the H and N antigens on their surface, for example, H_1N_1, H_3N_2. Within each subtype there may also be more subtle, but sometimes important, antigenic differences (drifts). These differences are designated according to the major representative virus to which they are most closely related antigenically, using the place of initial isolation, number of isolates, and year of detection. For example, two recent H_3N_2 strains of influenza A viruses that differ antigenically only slightly are called A/Texas/1/77 (H_3N_2) and A/Bangkok/1/79 (H_3N_2).

Antigenic drifts

Antigenic drifts within major subtypes can involve both the H and N antigens and can result from as little as a single mutation in the viral RNA. The mutant may come to predominate under the selective immunologic pressures in the host population. Such drifts have also been observed, but to a lesser extent, with influenza B viruses.

Table 34.1 Major Antigenic Shifts Associated with Influenza A Pandemics, 1947–1977

Year	Subtype	Prototype Strain
1947	H_1N_1	A/FM_1/47
1957	H_2N_2	A/Singapore/57
1968	H_3N_2	A/Hong Kong/68
1977	H_1N_1	A/USSR/77

Major antigenic shifts

Major antigenic changes in the H and N subtypes of epidemic strains can occur rapidly and unpredictably. They may result from recombination, in which different influenza A subtypes simultaneously infect a cell and produce progeny that contain antigens derived from either of the original viruses. For example, a cell infected simultaneously with influenza A (H_3N_2) and A (H_1N_1) may produce a mixture of influenza viruses of the following subtypes: H_3N_2, H_1N_1, H_1N_2, and H_3N_1. This mechanism has been demonstrated in the laboratory and probably occurs in nature, but has not been proved. Alternatively, it is possible that antigenic subtypes become latent in human host tissues, then become reactivated and spread to nonimmune contacts.* Another possibility is that certain subtypes circulate into animal or avian reservoirs, only to reemerge and adapt to human hosts when a sufficient proportion of the population has little or no immunity to the "new" subtypes.

Epidemiology of major antigenic shifts

Major antigenic shifts, which have recently occurred approximately every 8–10 years, have often resulted in serious epidemics or pandemics among populations with little or no preexisting antibody to the new subtypes. Examples include the appearance of an H_1N_1 subtype in 1947, followed by an abrupt shift to an H_2N_2 strain in 1957, which caused the pandemic of Asian flu. A subsequent major shift in 1968 to an H_3N_2 subtype (the Hong Kong flu) led to another, but somewhat less severe epidemic. The Russian flu, which appeared in late 1977, was caused by an H_1N_1 subtype very similar to that which dominated between 1947 and 1957 (Table 34.1).

Role of minor antigenic drifts in maintaining infection

The concepts of antigenic shift and drift in human influenza A virus infections can be roughly summarized as follows: Periodic shifts in the major antigenic components appear, usually resulting in major epidemics in populations with little or no immunologic experience with the subtype. As the population of susceptible individuals is exhausted (that is, subtype-specific immunity is acquired by increasing numbers of people) the subtype continues to circulate for a time, undergoing subtle antigenic drift from season to season, which allows some degree of infection to continue to occur. This infectivity persists because subtype-specific immunity is not entirely protective against drifting strains; for example, an individual may have antibodies reasonably protective against influenza A/Texas/77 (H_3N_2), yet be susceptible in succeeding years to reinfection by influenza A/Bangkok/79 (H_3N_2). Eventually, however, the overall immunity of the population becomes sufficient to minimize the epidemic potential of the major subtype and its drifting strains. Unfortunately, the battle is never entirely won, as the scene

*R.E. Hope-Simpson (*J. Hyg.* 86:35, 1981) suggests that seasonal reactivation in human carrier–hosts may result from seasonal stimuli related to solar radiation.

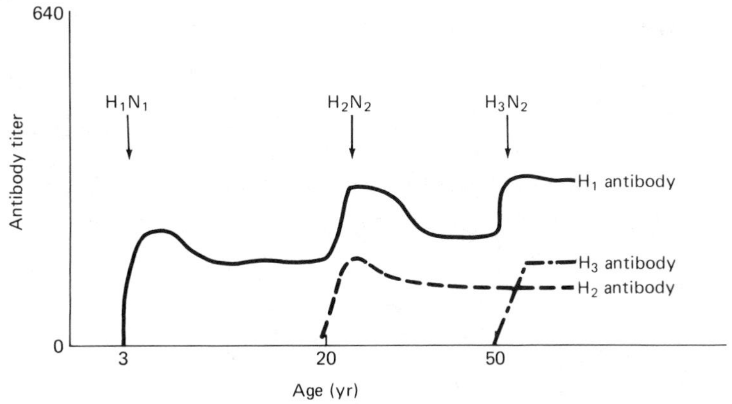

34.3 An illustration of the concept of "original antigenic sin," or "immunologic recapitulation."

is set for the sudden and usually unpredictable appearance of an entirely new subtype that may not have circulated among humans for 20 years or more.

Doctrine of original antigenic sin

continued anamnestic responses to first infecting subtype's antigens

Another important concept essential to understanding the behavior of influenza A virus in humans is the *doctrine of original antigenic sin,* first described by Dr. Thomas Francis and colleagues. This concept is stated as follows: The immune response to all subsequent influenza A infection is dominated by a persistence of antibody to the first virus with which a person has contact through constant anamnestic response. This doctrine primarily describes the antibody response to the hemagglutinin antigen, but there is evidence that it also applies to neuraminidase antigen responses. To clarify the concept, the antibody response to the hemagglutinins is illustrated in the following example (see Figure 34.3): An infant or young child never infected by any influenza A virus is immunologically "virgin" in this respect. The first infection may be with an H_1N_1 subtype, and the patient develops an antibody response to the H_1 antigen. Years later, the patient becomes infected with an H_2N_2 subtype and develops antibodies to the H_2 antigen; in addition, even though the H antigen is different in the second episode, an anamnestic antibody response to the initial (H_1) antigen develops, usually quickly and to high levels. Throughout life, anamnestic "recall" will remain enhanced with regard to the first subtype encountered and, to a lesser extent, to subsequent subtypes, regardless of which influenza A virus later infects the patient.

explanation of age-specific attack rates

This unique immunologic recall response probably accounts for the variability in age-specific attack rates when newer subtypes are introduced into a population. For example, the appearance of the Russian flu (H_1N_1) in 1977–1978 was noteworthy in that a similar subtype had been prevalent during 1947–1956, but then disappeared. Individuals born after 1956 would not have experienced prior infection with the subtype, and the prediction that the highest attack rates would be among those less than 25 years of age turned out to be correct.

Unfortunately, none of these generalizations can be applied with great confidence to the individual patient. People vary in their immune responses to viruses, and other host factors, such as the aging process, can modify susceptibility to infection. Therefore, even though the recent H_1N_1 influenza A subtype was expected primarily to affect younger individuals, it was considered prudent to attempt to protect high-risk groups such as the elderly, who might acquire severe, potentially life-threatening infections.

Infections Caused by Influenza Viruses

Clinical Disease and Outcome

As stated previously, influenza A and B viruses tend to cause the most severe illnesses, whereas influenza C seems to occur infrequently and generally causes milder disease. The typical acute influenzal syndrome will be described here.

short incubation period

Acute disease

The incubation period is brief, lasting an average of 2 days. Onset is usually abrupt, with symptoms developing over a few hours. These include fever, myalgia, headache, and occasionally shaking chills. Within 6–12 hr, the patient is usually at the peak of illness severity, and a dry, nonproductive cough develops. The illness remains severe, sometimes with worsening cough, for 2–5 days, followed by gradual improvement. By a week after onset, the patient feels significantly better. Fatigue, nonspecific weakness, and cough, however, can remain frustrating lingering problems for an additional 2–3 weeks.

Progressive infection

Other complications

Reye's syndrome

Occasional patients develop a progressive infection that involves the tracheobronchial tree and lungs to a greater extent. In these situations pneumonia, which can be lethal, is the result. Other unusual acute manifestations of influenza include central nervous system dysfunction, myositis, and myocarditis. In infants and children, a serious complication known as *Reye's syndrome* may develop 2–12 days after onset of the infection; it is characterized by severe hepatic dysfunction and cerebral edema (encephalopathy with fatty infiltration of the viscera). This syndrome is associated not only with influenza viruses, but with a wide variety of systemic viral illnesses.

Bacterial superinfection

The most common and important complication of influenza virus infection is bacterial superinfection. Such infections usually involve the lung, but bacteremia with secondary seeding of distant sites can also occur. The superinfection, which can develop at any time in the acute or convalescent phase of the disease, is often heralded by an abrupt worsening of the patient's condition after initial stabilization. The bacteria most commonly involved in such superinfections include *Streptococcus pneumonia, Haemophilus influenzae,* and *Staphylococcus aureus.*

Pathogenesis

Effect on infected cells

Inflammatory response

Influenza viruses are lytic: they can switch off host cell protein and nucleic acid synthesis and cause release of lysosomal hydrolytic enzymes. The process of cell death results in the cleavage of complement components, leading to localized inflammation. Early in infection, the primary chemotactic stimulus is directed toward mononuclear leukocytes, which comprise the major cellular inflammatory component.

Viral toxicity

The virus particles are also toxic to tissues. This toxicity can be demonstrated by inoculating high concentrations of inactivated virions into mice, which produces acute inflammatory changes in the absence of viral penetration or replication within cells.

Impairment of host defenses

Several other host cell functions are also severely impaired, particularly during the acute phase of infection. They include polymorphonuclear leukocyte chemotaxis and phagocytic functions, alveolar macrophage activity, ciliated respiratory epithelial cell function (mechanical clearance activity), and immune T-lymphocyte responsiveness.

The net result of these effects is that, on entry into the respiratory tract, the viruses cause cell damage, primarily to the respiratory epithelium, which elicits an acute inflammatory response and impairs mechanical, cellular, and immune host response. This damage renders the host highly susceptible to invasive bacterial superinfection. In vitro studies also suggest that bacterial pathogens such as staphylococci are enhanced in their adherence to the surfaces of influenza virus-infected cells. Viremia is rarely detected, because it usually occurs immediately before onset of symptoms.

Interferon and immune response

Recovery from infection is achieved initially by interferon production, which limits further virus replication, along with the generation of natural killer and cytotoxic T cells, which lyse virus-infected cells. This is followed by the appearance of local and humoral antibody and cellular immunity, and subsequently by repair of tissue damage.

In summary, there are essentially three ways in which influenza may cause patient death:

Causes of mortality

Underlying disease with decompensation. People with limited cardiovascular or pulmonary reserves can be further compromised by any respiratory infection. Thus, the elderly and those of any age with underlying chronic cardiac or pulmonary disease are at particular risk.

Superinfection. Superinfection can lead to bacterial pneumonia and occasionally disseminated bacterial infection.

Direct, rapid progression. Less commonly, direct, rapid progression of the viral infection can lead to severe viral pneumonia with asphyxia.

Immune Responses

Antibody responses

Although cell-mediated immune responses are undoubtedly important in influenza virus infections, humoral immunity has been investigated more extensively. Typically, the patient responds to infection within a few days by the production of antibodies directed toward the group ribonucleoprotein antigen, the hemagglutinin, and the neuraminidase. Antibodies to the first two antigens are detected by complement fixation and hemagglutination inhibition, respectively. Peak antibody titer levels are usually reached within 2 weeks of onset, then gradually wane over the following months to varying low levels. Antibody to the ribonucleoprotein appears to confer little or no protection against reinfection. Hemagglutination inhibition antibody is considered the most protective, as it has the ability to neutralize virus on reexposure; such immunity is relative, however, and quantitative differences in responsiveness exist between individuals. Furthermore, antigenic shifts and drifts often allow the virus to subvert the antibody response on subsequent exposures. Antibody to neuraminidase antigen is not as protective as hemagglutination inhibition antibody, but may play a role in limiting virus spread within the host.

Protective effect of antihemagglutinin

Epidemiology

seasonality

epidemic intervals

increased absenteeism as indicator of epidemic

excess mortality

Direct droplet spread is the most common mode of transmission. Influenza infections in temperate climates tend to occur most frequently during midwinter months. Major outbreaks of influenza A usually occur at 2- to 3-year intervals; influenza B epidemics appear irregularly, usually every 4–5 years. The typical epidemic develops over a period of 3–6 weeks and may involve 10% of the population. Illness rates may exceed 30% among school-aged children, residents of closed institutions, and industrial groups. One major indicator of influenza virus activity is an abrupt rise in school or industrial absenteeism. In severe influenza A epidemics, the number of deaths reported in a given area of the country often exceeds the number expected for that period. This significant increase, referred to as *excess mortality,* is another indicator of severe, widespread illness. Influenza B rarely causes such severe epidemics.

Laboratory Diagnosis

virus isolation and detection

During the acute phase of illness, influenza viruses can be readily isolated from respiratory tract specimens, such as nasopharyngeal and throat swabs. Most strains grow in primary monkey kidney cell cultures or in the amniotic cavity of embryonated hen's eggs, and they can be detected by hemadsorption. The presence of viral hemagglutinin in the amniotic fluid can be demonstrated after 2–3 days of incubation. More recently, diagnosis of infection within 2–3 hr was made possible by direct immunofluorescent detection of viral antigen in epithelial cells from the upper respiratory tract.

direct immunofluorescence

serodiagnosis

Serologic diagnosis is of considerable help epidemiologically and is usually made by demonstrating a fourfold or greater increase in complement-fixing or hemagglutination inhibition antibody titers in acute and convalescent specimens collected 10–14 days apart.

Prevention

Whole virus and "split" vaccines

The best available method of control is by use of killed viral vaccine prepared from those strains related most closely to the antigenic subtypes currently causing infections. These inactivated vaccines may contain whole virions or "split" subunits composed primarily of hemagglutinin antigens. The latter are slightly less capable of inducing a high antibody response, but tend to be less likely to produce local pain and swelling and fever. They are commonly used, in two doses given 1 month apart, for immunizing children who may not have been immunized previously. The whole virus vaccines are usually used for adults, and single annual doses are recommended if the patient has received influenza vaccine in the past. Vaccine efficacy is variable, and annual revaccination is necessary to ensure maximal protection. Used in this way, the whole virus vaccine may be 70–85% effective.

short duration of vaccine immunity

Indications for vaccination

It is recommended that vaccination be directed primarily toward the elderly, individuals of all ages who are at high risk (for example, those with chronic lung or heart disease), and perhaps those in essential jobs, such as medical personnel, police, and the like.

Amantadine prophylaxis for influenza A

Amantadine hydrochloride, a symmetric amine that apparently blocks uncoating of the virus particle on entry into the cell, has been shown to be effective in short-term (several weeks) oral prophylaxis of influenza A infections. It can produce side effects, however, and is recommended only for high-risk patients until vaccine-induced immunity can be achieved. A typical example of its use would be during an epidemic in which an elderly, potentially susceptible patient may become exposed to infection within a short period. Oral amantadine prophylaxis may be initiated concurrently with administration of a vaccine containing the most current antigens and continued for 2 weeks. The immunogenic effect of the vaccine should ensure continued protection. It must be emphasized that amantadine has been proved effective for influenza A virus infections only; it is useless in the management and prevention of infections caused by other influenza types or by any other respiratory virus.

Treatment

nonspecific therapy

The two basic approaches to management of influenzal disease are symptomatic care and anticipation of potential complications, particularly bacterial superinfection. Once the diagnosis has been made, rest, adequate fluid intake, conservative use of analgesics such as aspirin for myalgia and headache, and antitussives for severe cough are commonly prescribed. It must be emphasized that even nonprescription drugs must be used with caution, particularly in children.

Bacterial superinfection

Bacterial superinfection is often suggested by a rapid worsening of clinical symptoms after the patient has initially stabilized. Antibiotic prophylaxis has not been shown to enhance or diminish the likelihood of superinfection, but can increase the risk of acquisition of more resistant bacterial flora in the respiratory tract and make the superinfection more difficult to treat. Ideally, the physician should instruct the patient regarding the natural history of the influenza virus infection and be prepared to respond to bacterial complications, if they occur, with a specific diagnosis and therapy.

Amantadine therapy

When influenza A infection is proved or strongly suspected, 4–5 days of amantadine hydrochloride therapy may also be considered. It has been shown to benefit some patients to a modest degree, as measured by reduction of number of days of confinement to bed, of fever, and of functional respiratory impairment. These beneficial effects, however, have been observed only when the drug is administered early in the illness (within 12–20 hr of onset).

Parainfluenza Viruses

Paramyxoviruses

hemagglutinin and neuraminidase

antigenic stability

There are four serotypes of parainfluenza viruses: parainfluenza 1, 2, 3, and 4. These enveloped viruses belong to the paramyxovirus group, contain single-stranded RNA, and, like the influenza viruses, possess a neuraminidase and hemagglutinin. Their mode of spread and pathogenesis is similar to that of the influenza viruses. They differ from the influenza viruses in that the antigenic makeup of each parainfluenza serotype is relatively stable, and significant antigenic shift or drift does not occur. Each serotype will be considered separately.

Parainfluenza 1

association with croup

Parainfluenza 1 is the major cause of acute croup (laryngotracheitis) in infants and young children, but also causes less severe diseases such as mild upper respiratory illness (URI), pharyngitis, and tracheobronchitis in all age groups. Outbreaks of infection tend to occur most frequently during the fall months.

Parainfluenza 2

Parainfluenza 2 is of slightly less significance than parainfluenza 1 or 3. It has been associated with croup, primarily in children, with mild URI, and occasionally with acute lower respiratory disease. As with parainfluenza 1, outbreaks usually occur during the fall months.

Parainfluenza 3

severe lower respiratory disease in infants

Parainfluenza 3 is a major cause of severe lower respiratory disease in infants and young children. It often causes bronchitis, pneumonia, and croup in children less than 1 year old. In older children and adults, it may cause URI or tracheobronchitis. Infections are common and can occur in any season; it is estimated that nearly one-half of all children have been exposed to this virus by 1 year of age.

Parainfluenza 4

Parainfluenza 4 is the least common of the group and is generally associated with mild upper respiratory illness only.

The parainfluenza viruses are important because of the serious diseases they can cause in infants and young children. Parainfluenza 1 and 3 are particularly common in this regard. Overall, the group is thought to be responsible for 15–20% of all nonbacterial respiratory diseases requiring hospitalization in infancy and childhood. The onset of illness may be abrupt, as in acute spasmodic croup, but usually begins as a mild URI with variable progression over 1–3 days to involvement of the middle or lower respiratory tract. Duration of acute illness can vary from 4 to 21 days but is usually 7–10 days.

Frequency

Duration

Immunity to reinfection is transient; although repeated infections can occur in older children and adults, they are usually milder than the illnesses of infancy and early childhood.

transient immunity

Specific diagnosis is based on virus isolation, usually in monkey kidney cell cultures, or on serology using the hemagglutination inhibition, complement fixation, or neutralization methods on paired sera. Direct immunofluorescence can also be used for rapid detection of antigen in respiratory epithelial cells.

laboratory diagnosis

There is currently no method of control or specific therapy for these infections.

Respiratory Syncytial Virus

Respiratory syncytial virus (RSV) is classified as a pseudomyxovirus, and its name is derived from its ability to produce cell fusion in tissue culture (syncytium formation). It does not agglutinate red cells or cause hemadsorption.

Pseudomyxovirus

syncytium formation

Respiratory syncytial virus is the single most important etiologic agent in respiratory diseases of infancy, and it is the major cause of bronchiolitis and pneumonia among infants under 1 year of age.

Clinical Outline of Disease and Outcome

The usual incubation period is 1–4 days, followed by the onset of rhinitis; severity of illness progresses to a peak within 1–3 days. In infants, this peak usually takes the form of bronchiolitis and pneumonitis, with cough, wheezing, and respiratory distress. Clinical findings include hyperexpansion of the lungs, hypoxemia, and hypercapnea (carbon dioxide retention). Interstitial infiltrates, often with areas of pulmonary collapse, may be seen on chest radiography (Figure 34.4). Fever is variable. The duration of acute illness is often 10–14 days. The fatality among hospitalized infected infants is estimated to be 1–2%. Causes of death include respiratory failure, right-sided heart failure (cor pulmonale), and bacterial superinfection. Death has sometimes resulted from unnecessary procedures in patients in whom RSV infection was not considered. Bronchoscopy, lung biopsy, or overly aggressive therapy with corticosteroids and bronchodilators for presumed asthma can all pose a danger to such patients.

serious bronchiolitis and pneumonitis in infants

Duration and fatality

Older infants, children, and adults are also readily infected. The clinical illnesses in these groups are usually milder and include croup, tracheobronchitis, and URI. Respiratory syncytial virus can also cause acute flareups of chronic bronchitis and trigger acute wheezing episodes in asthmatic children.

Pathogenesis

The virus is spread to the upper respiratory tract by contact with infective secretions. Infection appears to be confined primarily to the respiratory epithelium, with progressive involvement of the middle and lower airways. Viremia occurs rarely.

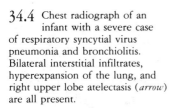

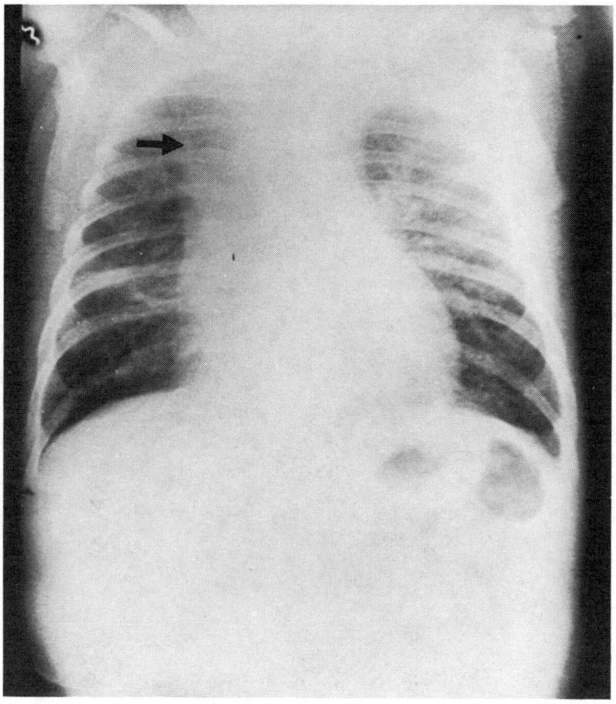

34.4 Chest radiograph of an infant with a severe case of respiratory syncytial virus pneumonia and bronchiolitis. Bilateral interstitial infiltrates, hyperexpansion of the lung, and right upper lobe atelectasis (*arrow*) are all present.

enhancing effect of immune response

It is believed that host-cell-mediated immune responses and perhaps immunoglobulin E also play a role in enhancing severity of disease.

Pathology

The major findings are in the bronchi, bronchioles, and alveoli. These findings include necrosis of epithelial cells, interstitial mononuclear cell inflammatory infiltrates, which sometimes also involve the alveoli and alveolar ducts, and plugging of smaller airways with material containing mucus, necrotic cells, and fibrin (Figure 34.5). Multinucleated syncytial cells with intracytoplasmic inclusions are occasionally seen in the affected tracheobronchial epithelium.

Immune Response

brief immunity to reinfection

Infection results in IgG and IgA antibody responses. Immunity to reinfection is quite tenuous, however, as demonstrated by patients who have recovered from a primary acute episode and have become reinfected with disease of similar severity in the same or succeeding year. Illness severity appears to diminish with increasing age and successive reinfection.

Epidemiology

high attack rate

Community outbreaks of RSV infection occur annually and can commence at any time from late fall to early spring. The usual outbreak lasts 8–12 weeks and can involve nearly one-half of all families with children. In the family setting, it appears that older siblings often introduce the virus into the home, and secondary infection rates can be almost 50%. The usual duration of virus shedding is 3–7 days; young infants, however, may shed virus for 9 days or longer.

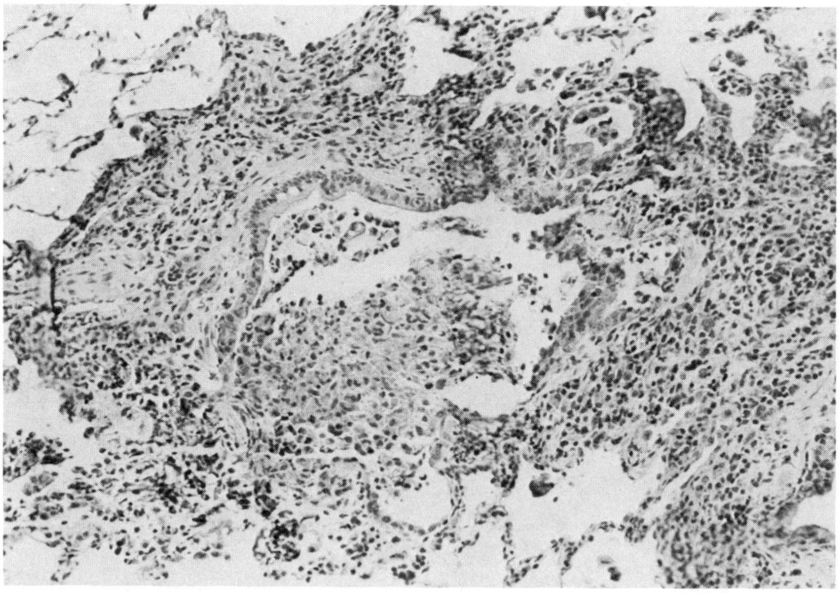

34.5 Photomicrograph illustrating the bronchiolar and surrounding interstitial inflammation in respiratory syncytial virus infection. (Original magnification ×100.)

nosocomial infection

Spread of RSV in the hospital setting is also a major problem. Control is difficult, but includes careful attention to hand washing between contacts with patients, isolation, and exclusion of personnel and visitors to the ward who have any form of respiratory illness. The effectiveness of masks in controlling nosocomial spread is questionable.

Laboratory Diagnosis

direct immunofluorescent antibody detection

cell culture

serodiagnosis

Rapid diagnosis of RSV infection can be made by immunofluorescent antibody detection of viral antigen in the cytoplasm of nasopharyngeal epithelial cells. The virus can also be isolated from the respiratory tract by prompt inoculation of specimens into cell cultures without prior freezing. Syncytial cytopathic effects develop over 2–7 days. The cell cultures of choice are heteroploid cell lines. Serodiagnosis using the complement fixation test may also be employed, but requires acute and convalescent sera and is less sensitive than immunofluorescent antibody or culture.

Prevention and Treatment

No vaccine or specific antiviral therapy is available, although recent experiments suggest that ribaviron aerosol treatment might be effective. Attenuated live virus vaccines are under investigation, but it is uncertain whether they will be of value.

supportive treatment

Treatment is primarily directed at the underlying pathophysiology and includes adequate oxygenation, ventilatory support when necessary, and close observation of complications such as bacterial superinfection or right-sided heart failure.

Adenoviruses

Multiple serotypes naked, double-stranded DNA viruses

Of the almost 100 different serotypes of adenoviruses, 41 are known to affect humans. These viruses are naked, icosahedral, and possess double-stranded DNA. They all share a common group-specific complement-fixing antigen associated with the hexon component of the viral capsid. Adenoviruses are characterized by their ubiquity and their ability to reside in the potential for prolonged infection without disease

host for periods ranging from a few days to several years. Their ability to produce infection without disease is illustrated by the frequent recovery of virus from tonsils or adenoids removed from healthy children (the group name is derived from its discovery in 1953 as a latent agent in many adenoid tissue specimens) and by prolonged intermittent shedding of virus from the pharynx and intestinal tract after initial infection.

Spread and disease

Types 1 and 2 are highly endemic; type 5 is the next most common. Most primary infections with these viruses occur early in life. The spread of the virus can be either respiratory or by fecal–oral contamination.

Overall, only about 45% of adenovirus infections result in disease. Their most significant contribution to acute illness is in children, particularly those under 2 years of age (10.6% of acute febrile illness). They are also major causes of acute respiratory disease in military recruits, usually by types 4 and 7.

Clinical Outline of Disease and Outcome

Upper respiratory infections

Conjunctivitis

More severe disease

The diversity of major syndromes and commonly associated serotypes are summarized in Table 34.2. The acute respiratory syndromes vary in both clinical manifestation and severity. Symptoms include fever, rhinitis, pharyngitis, cough, and conjunctivitis. Adenoviruses are also common causes of nonstreptococcal exudative pharyngitis, particularly among children less than 3 years of age. Acute, and occasionally chronic, conjunctivitis and keratoconjunctivitis have been associated with several serotypes. More severe disease, such as laryngitis, croup, bronchiolitis, or severe pneumonia, may also occur. Occasionally, the illness may be prolonged for several weeks and can clinically resemble pertussis. A syndrome of pharyngitis and conjunctivitis (pharyngoconjunctival fever) is classically associated with adenovirus infection. Adenoviruses can also cause acute hemorrhagic cystitis, in which hematuria and dysuria are prominent findings. More recently, some serotypes that are difficult to cultivate in the laboratory have been recognized as significant causes of gastroenteritis (Chapter 40).

Pathogenesis

Routes of infection

The adenoviruses usually enter the host by inhalation of droplet nuclei or by the oral route. Direct inoculation onto nasal or conjunctival mucosa by hands or by contaminated towels and ophthalmic medications may also occur. The virus replicates in epithelial cells, producing cell necrosis and inflam-

Table 34.2 Clinical Syndromes Associated with Adenovirus Infection

Syndrome	Common Serotypes Found[a]
Childhood febrile illness; pharyngoconjunctival fever	1, 2, *3*, 5, *7*, *7a*
Pneumonia and other acute respiratory illnesses	1, 2, *3*, 5, *7*, *7a*, *7b* (*4* in military recruits)
Pertussislike illness	1, *2*, *3*, 5, *19*, 21
Conjunctivitis	2, 5, *7*, *8*, *19*
Keratoconjunctivitis	*3*, *8*, *9*, *19*
Acute hemorrhagic cystitis	11
Acute gastroenteritis	40, 41

[a] Italicized serotypes are those commonly associated with outbreaks.

Viremic spread and remote disease

mation. Viremia sometimes occurs and can result in spread to distant sites, such as the kidney, bladder, liver, lymphoid tissue (including mesenteric nodes), and occasionally the central nervous system. In the acute phase of infection, the distant sites may also show inflammation; for example, abdominal pain is occasionally seen with severe illnesses and is believed to result from mesenteric lymphadenitis caused by the viruses.

Latency and reactivation

After the acute phase of illness, the viruses may remain in tissues, particularly lymphoid structures such as tonsils, adenoids, and intestinal Peyer's patches, and become reactivated and shed without producing illness for 6–18 months thereafter. This reactivation is enhanced by stressful events (stress reactivation), such as infection by other agents.

Toxic pentons

A potentially important pathogenic feature of the virion is the presence of pentons, which are located at each of the 12 corners of the icosahedron. They are fiberlike projections with knoblike terminal structures and appear to be responsible for a toxic effect on cells, which is manifested by clumping and detachment in vitro.

Pathology

Like that of the viruses described previously, the primary pathology is epithelial cell necrosis with a predominantly mononuclear inflammatory response. In some instances, smudgy intranuclear inclusions may be seen in infected cells (Figure 34.6).

Immune Responses

type-specific immunity

Immunity after infection is serotype specific and usually long lasting. In addition to type-specific immunity, group-specific complement-fixing antibodies appear in response to infection. These antibodies are useful indicators of infection, but do not specify the infecting serotype.

Epidemiology

Infections caused by serotypes 1, 2, and 5 are generally most frequent during the first few years of life. All serotypes can occur during any season of

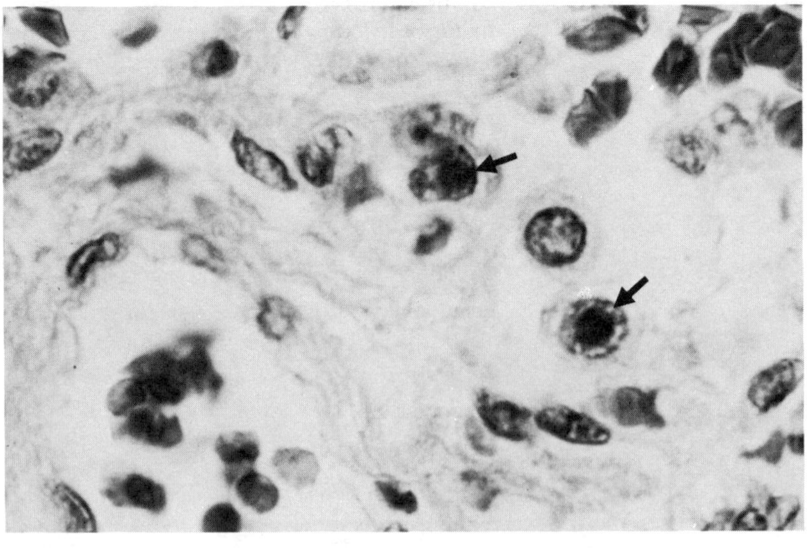

34.6 Lung tissue from a fatal case of adenovirus type 7 pneumonia. (Original magnification ×100.) Large, smudgy intranuclear inclusions in alveolar epithelial cells (*arrows*), which are sometimes seen in adenovirus infections, are present.

swimming pool conjunctivitis

iatrogenic infections

the year, but are encountered most frequently during late winter or early spring. Sharp outbreaks of disease caused by serotypes 3 and 7 have been traced to inadequately chlorinated swimming pools. Conjunctivitis is the illness most commonly associated with these episodes. Other outbreaks of conjunctivitis have been traced to physicians' offices and appear to have been spread by contaminated ophthalmic medications or diagnostic equipment.

Laboratory Diagnosis

Viral isolation

problems of associating isolates with disease

The viruses can be readily isolated in heteroploid cell cultures. There is little difficulty in relating the virus isolate to the illness in question when the isolate has been obtained from a site other than the upper respiratory or gastrointestinal tract (for example, lung biopsy, conjunctival swabs, urine); because of the known tendency for intermittent asymptomatic shedding into the oropharynx and feces, however, isolates from these sites must be interpreted more cautiously. If their significance is questionable, complement fixation tests on acute and convalescent sera may be necessary to confirm the relationship between the virus and the illness in question.

Prevention and Treatment

In the past, killed virus vaccines produced from serotypes 3, 4, and 7 were found effective in reducing illness in military recruits. The vaccine was discontinued, however, when it was found that types 3 and 7 were capable of inducing tumors in newborn hamsters. More recently, a live virus vaccine containing serotypes 4 and 7, enclosed in enteric coated capsules and administered orally, has been used in military recruit groups. The viruses are released into the small intestine, where they produce an asymptomatic, nontransmissible infection. This vaccine has been found effective, but is neither available nor recommended for civilian groups. There is no specific therapy for infection.

Rhinoviruses

more than 100 serotypes

optimum temperature 33°C

The rhinovirus group comprises more than 100 serotypes. They are picornaviruses—small (20–30 nm), naked particles containing single-stranded RNA—and are distinguished from enteroviruses by their acid lability and an optimum temperature of 33°C for in vitro replication. This temperature approximates that of the nasopharynx in the human host. These viruses are most consistently isolated in cultures of human diploid fibroblasts.

Clinical Disease

common cold viruses

Rhinoviruses are known as the *common cold viruses*. They represent the major causes of mild URI syndromes in all age groups, especially older children and adults. Lower respiratory tract disease caused by rhinoviruses is uncommon. The usual incubation period is 2–3 days, and acute symptoms usually last 3–7 days.

Epidemiology

Rhinovirus infections may be seen at any time of the year. Epidemic peaks tend to occur in the early fall or spring months.

Prevention and Treatment

no effective method of prevention

There are no current methods of prevention, either with specific vaccines or with nonspecific measures such as high doses of vitamins. There is also no specific therapy. Prospects for the development of an appropriate vaccine appear dim. The multiplicity of serotypes and their tendency to be type specific in the production of antibodies would demand the development of a potent multivalent vaccine, which would be extremely difficult to accomplish. The present attitude toward these viruses is best summed up by Sir Christopher Andrewes, who pointed out that there is probably no good reason to attempt to control all such virus diseases with vaccines; instead, we should perhaps accept these infections as "one of the stimulating risks of being mortal".*

Coronaviruses

common cold virus

Coronaviruses are enveloped RNA-containing viruses with 13-nm club-shaped projections on the surface. Like the rhinoviruses, they are considered primary causes of the common cold. Based on serologic studies, it is estimated that they may cause as many as 5–10% of common colds in adults and a similar proportion of all lower respiratory illnesses in children.

The number of serotypes is unknown. Two strains (229E and OC43) have been studied to some extent; it is clear that they can cause outbreaks similar to those of the rhinoviruses, and that reinfection with the same serotype can occur.

Reoviruses

The reoviruses (*r*espiratory *e*nteric *o*rphans) are naked virions that contain double-stranded RNA. They are extremely ubiquitous and have been found in humans, simians, rodents, cattle, and a variety of other hosts. Three serotypes are known to infect humans; however, their role and importance in human disease remains uncertain. Sporadic cases of febrile URI, exanthems, pneumonia, hepatitis, encephalitis, and gastroenteritis have all been reported to be associated with these viruses. Asymptomatic shedding of reoviruses also occurs, which makes it difficult to prove association with disease.

Reoviruses can be isolated in cell cultures, particularly primary monkey kidney or human kidney monolayers.

Additional Reading and References

Influenza Viruses

Couch, R.B. 1981. The effects of influenza on host defenses. *J. Infect. Dis.* 144:284–291. An excellent discussion of the possible deleterious effects of influenza viruses, and of how little they are actually understood.

Webster, R.G., Laver, W.G., Air, G.M., et al. 1982. Molecular mechanisms of variation in influenza viruses. *Nature* 296:115–121. An excellent review of "drifts," "shifts," and virulence.

Wright, P.F., Bryant, J.D., Karzon, D.T., et al. 1980. Comparison of influenza B/Hong Kong virus infections among infants, children and young adults. *J. Infect. Dis.* 141:430. The spectrum of illnesses seen in different age groups is illustrated.

*Andrewes, C.H. 1964. The complex epidemiology of respiratory virus infections. *Science* 146:1274.

Respiratory Syncytial Virus

Henderson, F.W., Collier, A.M., Clyde, W.A., et al. 1979. Respiratory-syncytial-virus infections, reinfections, and immunity in young children. *N. Engl. J. Med.* 300:530–534. Examination of the effect of prior exposure on subsequent infection with the same virus suggests that illness upon second infection may be no less severe than that with the first; however, the third reinfection may be modified.

Adenoviruses

Fox, J.P., Hall, C.E., Cooney, M.K., et al. 1977. The Seattle virus watch VII. Observations of adenovirus infections. *Am. J. Epidemiol.* 105:362–386. The epidemiology and problems involved in associating adenoviruses with illnesses are analyzed.

Rhinoviruses

Fox, J.P. 1976. Is a rhinovirus vaccine possible? *Am. J. Epidemiol.* 103:345–354. A good review of the immunologic relationships among the many rhinovirus serotypes.

Gwaltney, J.M., Jr., Moskalski, P.B., Hendly, J.O., et al. 1978. Hand-to-hand transmission of rhinovirus colds. *Ann. Intern. Med.* 88:463–467. An interesting study of the efficiency of spread of rhinoviruses by various routes.

C. George Ray

Viruses of Mumps and Childhood Exanthems

35

The major viruses to be described in this chapter (mumps, measles, and rubella) represent totally different virus families; however, they share several common epidemiologic characteristics: 1) Distribution is worldwide, with a high incidence of infection in nonimmune individuals; 2) humans appear to be the sole reservoir of infection; 3) person-to-person spread is primarily via the respiratory (aerosol) route; and 4) all three diseases are preventable by the use of specific, live, attenuated virus vaccines. Although these viruses are traditionally classified as causes of infection in childhood, the epidemiologic pattern in developed countries has shifted in recent years; currently, the age-specific attack rates for infection are highest among adolescents and young adults. This change is related to the advent and widespread use of potent vaccines during the past 20 years, which has reduced the incidence and transmission among young children; there remains a significant segment of the population, however, that was either unimmunized in infancy or received inadequately protective older vaccines.

respiratory spread

live, attenuated vaccines

changes in age of incidence

As these viruses appear to be restricted to a human reservoir, the possibility exists that, like smallpox, they could be totally eradicated. This prospect appears reasonable in the case of measles, as the disease usually produces symptoms with infection, which aids in readily identifying cases and instituting control measures. Such an expectation is more remote with regard to mumps, as asymptomatic or atypical infections can occur and escape detection. Rubella is the least likely of the three to succumb to extinction: Unlike measles and mumps, rubella can persist in human carriers (for example, congenitally infected infants) who chronically shed infectious virus for months to years; infections can often be subclinical; and the current vaccines may not totally prevent respiratory acquisition and transmission of wild virus by immune subjects.

possibilities for eradication

The other diseases to be discussed in this chapter include roseola infantum and erythema infectiosum, common infections of which little is known concerning cause or pathogenesis.

Mumps

Mumps is a paramyxovirus, and only one antigenic type is known. It shares the morphologic and cultural features of parainfluenza virus type 2; however, there is no apparent cross-immunity between the two viruses.

Paramyxovirus

Clinical Outline of Disease and Outcome

Incubation period

Parotitis

Complications

After an incubation period of 12–29 days (average, 16–18 days), the typical case is characterized by fever and swelling with tenderness of the salivary glands, especially the parotid glands. Swelling may be unilateral or bilateral and persists for 7–10 days. Several complications can occur, usually within 1–3 weeks after onset of illness. All appear to be a direct result of virus spread to other sites and illustrate the extensive tissue tropism of mumps. Complications, which can occur without parotitis, include the following:

1. Meningitis, which approximately 10% of all infected patients develop. It is usually mild, but can be confused with bacterial meningitis. In about one-third of these cases, associated or preceding evidence of parotitis is absent.
2. Encephalitis, which is occasionally severe.
3. Transverse myelitis or polyneuritis (rare).
4. Pancreatitis, which is suggested by abdominal pain and vomiting.
5. Orchitis, which is estimated to occur in 10–20% of infected men. Although there is concern regarding subsequent sterility, it appears that such a sequela is quite rare.
6. Oophoritis, an unusual, usually benign inflammation of the ovarian glands.
7. Other rare and transient complications, including myocarditis, nephritis, arthritis, thyroiditis, thrombocytopenic purpura, mastitis, and pneumonia.

The complications are acute and usually resolve without sequelae within 2–3 weeks; occasional permanent effects have been noted, however, particularly in cases of severe central nervous system infection, where sensorineural hearing loss and other impairment can occur.

Pathogenesis

Viremic phases

Spread to target tissues

Viruria

After initial entry into the respiratory tract, the virus replicates locally. Replication is followed by viremic dissemination to target tissues such as the salivary glands or central nervous system. It is also possible that before development of immune responses, a secondary phase of viremia may result from virus replication in target tissues, for example, initial parotid involvement with later spread to other organs. Viruria is common, probably as a result of direct spread from the blood into the urine as well as active viral replication in the kidney. Virtually all infections are associated with discernible impairment of renal function, usually manifested as a slight decrease in creatinine clearance.

Pathology

The tissue response is that of cell necrosis and inflammation with predominantly mononuclear cell infiltration. In the salivary glands swelling and desquamation of necrotic epithelial lining cells, accompanied by interstitial inflammation and edema, may be seen within dilated ducts.

Immune Responses

lifelong IgG response

As in most viral infections, the early antibody response is predominantly with IgM, which is replaced gradually over several weeks by specific IgG antibody. The latter persists for a lifetime, but can often be detected only by specific neutralization assays. After primary infection, immunity to reinfection is virtually always permanent.

Epidemiology

high infectivity

The highest frequency of infection is observed in the 5- to 15-year age group. Infection is rarely seen in the first year of life. Although about 85% of susceptible household contacts will acquire infection, approximately 30–40% of these contacts will not develop clinical disease. The disease is communicable from approximately 7 days before until 9 days after onset of illness; however, virus has been recovered in urine for up to 14 days following onset. The highest incidence of infection is usually during the late winter and spring months, but can occur during any season.

Laboratory Diagnosis

specimens

cell culture

detection of viral antigen

Mumps virus can be readily isolated early in the illness from the saliva, pharynx, and other affected sites, such as the cerebrospinal fluid. The urine is also an excellent source for virus isolation. Mumps virus grows well in primary monolayer cell culture derived from monkey kidney, producing syncytial giant cells and viral hemagglutinin, and can be isolated in other cell systems as well as in the allantoic cavity of embryonated hen's eggs. Rapid diagnosis can be made by direct detection of viral antigen in pharyngeal cells or urine sediment by direct immunofluorescence.

Complement fixation

V and S antigens

Serologic diagnosis is usually accomplished with the complement fixation test. Two virion antigens can be employed: the S (soluble) nucleocapsid antigen and the V (viral) antigen, which is a component of the viral envelope. Antibody to the S antigen rises as quickly as 3 days after onset of symptoms, then usually disappears in 6–8 months. Antibody to the V antigen rises more slowly; it peaks 2–4 weeks after onset, then remains detectable for years afterward. Other serologic tests may also be used, such as hemagglutination inhibition and neutralization. Of these, the neutralization test is the most sensitive for detection of immunity to infection.

Prevention

live vaccine

Since 1968, a live, attenuated vaccine has been available that is safe and highly effective. It is produced by serial propagation of virus in chick embryo cell tissue cultures. A single dose causes seroconversion in more than 95% of recipients. Duration of immunity, although not yet established, appears to be greater than 10 years and may be lifelong. This vaccine is currently recommended for infants after the first year of life and for adults (particularly men) who may be susceptible and at high risk of exposure.

Treatment

Immune serum globulin or mumps hyperimmune globulin are no longer recommended for the prevention or treatment of mumps. No specific therapy is available.

Measles

Paramyxovirus

Common synonyms for measles include *rubeola, 5-day measles,* or *hard measles.* The virus is classified in the paramyxovirus family, genus *Morbillivirus.* It is enveloped, contains RNA, and possesses hemagglutinin but not neuraminidase. A single antigenic type is known to affect humans. Two antigenically similar viruses, rinderpest of cattle and canine distemper virus, have not been shown to cause human infection.

Clinical Outline of Disease and Outcome

incubation period

prodromal signs

Koplik's spots

Rash

Systemic signs

The incubation period ranges from 7 to 18 days. A typical illness usually begins 9–11 days after exposure, with cough, coryza, conjunctivitis, and fever. One to three days after onset, pinpoint gray-white spots surrounded by erythema (grains-of-salt appearance) appear on mucous membranes. This sign, called *Koplik's spots,* is usually most noticeable over the buccal mucosa opposite the molars and persists for 1–2 days. Within a day of the appearance of Koplik's spots, the typical measles rash begins, first on the head, then on the trunk and extremities. The rash is maculopapular and semiconfluent; it persists for 3–5 days before fading. Fever and severe systemic symptoms gradually diminish as the rash progresses to the extremities. Lymphadenopathy is also common, with particularly noticeable involvement of the cervical nodes.

Severe disease

The disease can be very severe, especially in immunocompromised or malnourished patients. Death may result from overwhelming viral infection of the host, with extensive involvement of the respiratory tract and other viscera, or from other related causes. In underdeveloped countries, mortality of 15–25% has been recorded.

Bacterial superinfection

Bacterial superinfection, the most common complication, occurs in 5–15% of all cases. Such infections include acute otitis media, mastoiditis, sinusitis, pneumonia, and sepsis.

Central nervous system effects

encephalitis

Central nervous system effects are also seen. It is estimated that as many as 50% of uncomplicated cases will develop transient electroencephalographic abnormalities during the acute phase of illness. Whether subtle neurologic injury occurs in these patients remains speculative. Clinical signs of encephalitis will develop in 1 of 500–1000 cases. This complication, which usually occurs 3–14 days after onset of illness, can be extremely severe. The mortality in measles encephalitis is approximately 15%, and permanent neurologic damage among survivors is estimated at 25%.

Thrombocytopenic purpura

Acute thrombocytopenic purpura may also develop during the acute phase of illness, leading to bleeding episodes. Abdominal pain and acute appendicitis can occur secondary to inflammation and swelling of lymphoid tissue.

Depressed cell-mediated immunity

Subacute sclerosing panencephalitis

Both wild and attenuated (vaccine) measles viruses have been shown to depress delayed hypersensitivity and cell-mediated immunity significantly for as long as several weeks. Exacerbation of chronic granulomatous infections such as tuberculosis can result. Measles has also been implicated in a rare, smoldering, usually fatal encephalitis known as *subacute sclerosing panencephalitis.* This disease typically begins in childhood, 2–10 years after measles infection. Further discussion will be provided in Chapter 43.

Pathogenesis

local multiplication

viremic dissemination

After implantation in the upper respiratory tract, viral replication proceeds in the respiratory mucosal epithelium. Replication is followed by viremic and lymphatic dissemination throughout the host to distant sites, including lymphoid tissues, bone marrow, abdominal viscera, and skin. Virus can be demonstrated in the blood, particularly the leukocytes, in the prodromal phase of illness, and viruria persists for up to 4 days after the onset of rash. In addition, virion components can be detected in biopsy specimens of Koplik's spots and vascular endothelial cells in the areas of skin rash.

Role of cell-mediated immunity

Although cell-mediated immune responses to other antigens may be acutely depressed during measles infection, there is evidence that measles virus-specific cell-mediated immunity developing early in infection plays a role in mediating some of the features of disease, such as the rash, and is necessary to promote recovery from the illness. In patients with defects in cell-mediated immunity, including those with severe protein-calorie malnutrition, the infection is prolonged, tissue involvement is more severe, and complications such as progressive viral pneumonia are common.

Pathology

vasculitis

giant cells

inclusions

lesions in encephalitis

In addition to necrosis and inflammatory changes in the respiratory tract epithelium, several other features of measles virus infection are noteworthy. The skin lesions show vasculitis characterized by vascular dilatation, edema, and perivascular mononuclear cell infiltrates. The lymphoid tissues show hyperplastic changes, and large multinucleated giant cells are often observed (Warthin–Finkeldey cells). Some of the giant cells contain intracytoplasmic and intranuclear inclusions. Similar giant cells can be found in the respiratory tract epithelium and urinary sediment.

The major findings in measles encephalitis include areas of edema, scattered petechial hemorrhages, perivascular mononuclear cell infiltrates, and necrosis of neurons. In some cases, perivenous demyelination is also observed, suggesting an autoimmune pathogenesis.

Immune Responses

Lifelong immunity

Specific cell-mediated immunity develops early in the course of infection, helping to control the disease. This immunity is accompanied by a transiently depressed cell-mediated immune response to other antigens. Antibodies to the virus appear in the first few days of illness, peak in 2–3 weeks, then persist at low levels. Immunity to reinfection is lifelong.

Epidemiology

childhood disease

recent increase in infection in young adults

epidemic cycles

high infectivity

The highest attack rates have been in childhood, usually sparing infants less than 6 months of age; however, a shift in age-specific attack rates to greater involvement of adolescents and young adults has been observed recently in the United States. This shift is believed to be attributable to the influence of immunization: younger children may be better immunized to limit spread of the virus, whereas older age groups may have missed effective immunization or earlier infection by the wild virus.

Epidemics tend to occur during the winter and spring in 1- to 3-year cycles. The infection rate among exposed susceptible subjects in a classroom or household setting is estimated at 85%, and over 95% of those infected will become ill. The period of communicability is estimated to be 4 days before appearance of the rash to 5 days afterward.

Laboratory Diagnosis

virus isolation

giant cells in cell culture

rapid diagnosis by fluorescent antibody

serodiagnosis

The typical measles infection can usually be diagnosed on the basis of clinical findings. When the disease is atypical, laboratory confirmation may be necessary. Virus isolation from the oropharynx or urine is usually most productive in the first 5 days of illness. Measles grows on a variety of cell cultures, producing multinucleated giant cells similar to those observed in infected host tissues. If rapid diagnosis is desired, measles antigen may be identified in urinary sediment or pharyngeal cells by direct fluorescent antibody methods. Serologic diagnosis using complement fixation, hemagglutination inhibition, or indirect fluorescent antibody methods is also commonly used and requires acute and convalescent serum samples.

Prevention

live, attenuated vaccine

vaccination after 1 year of age

duration of immunity

contraindications

Live, attenuated measles vaccine is available and highly immunogenic. To ensure effective immunization, the vaccine should be administered to infants after the first year of life (preferred routine immunization is at 13–15 months of age). In children less than 1 year old vaccine efficacy is significantly impaired, probably because of the persistence of maternal antibody and the relatively lower immunologic responsiveness to some antigens early in life. Immunity induced by the vaccine may be lifelong. Reactions to vaccination, usually in the form of fever and occasional rash, are rarely severe. This is no clear evidence of vaccine-caused encephalitis to date. Because the vaccine contains live virus, it should not be administered to immunocompromised patients, and it is not recommended for pregnant women, except in exceptional situations.

Passive protection

Exposed susceptible patients who are immunologically compromised (including small infants) may be given immune serum globulin intramuscularly. This treatment can modify or prevent disease if given within 6 days of exposure, but protection is transient.

dangers of killed vaccines

Killed measles virus vaccines, commonly used before 1965, are no longer available. It has been shown that vaccine virus killed or inadvertently inactivated by improper storage methods is not only a poor immunogen, but may also cause other difficulties: 1) It can sensitize some individuals, who will then develop severe local inflammatory reactions upon subsequent inoculation with live vaccine; and 2) the sensitization may result in severe atypical illness (atypical measles syndrome) when the patient is exposed to the wild virus later in life. This syndrome is characterized by abrupt onset of high fever, often with abdominal pain and pneumonia, and the appearance of a rash, predominantly over the extremities. The rash may be papular, vesicular, or hemorrhagic.

Treatment

No specific therapy is available other than supportive measures and close observation for the development of complications such as bacterial superinfection.

Rubella

enveloped RNA togavirus

hemagglutinins

Teratogenicity

Rubella, commonly known as *German measles* or *3-day measles,* is an enveloped, RNA-containing virus classified as a member of the togavirus family. There is only one serotype, and no extrahuman reservoirs are known to exist. The virus can agglutinate some types of red blood cells, such as those obtained from 1-day-old chicks and trypsin-treated human type O cells.

Rubella was considered a mild, benign exanthem of childhood until 1941, when the Australian ophthalmologist Sir Norman Gregg described the profound defects that could be induced in the fetus as a result of maternal infection. Since 1962, when the virus was first isolated, knowledge regarding its extreme medical importance and biologic characteristics has increased rapidly.

Clinical Outline of Disease and Outcome

mild illness with lymphadenopathy

The incubation period for acquired infection is 14–21 days (average, 16 days). Illness is generally very mild, consisting primarily of low-grade fever, upper respiratory symptoms, and lymphadenopathy, which is most prominent in the posterior cervical and postauricular areas. A macular rash often

Rash

Arthralgia

follows within a day of onset and lasts for 1–3 days. This rash is usually most prominent over the head, neck, and trunk, and may be quite faint. Petechial lesions may also be seen over the soft palate during the acute phase. The most common complication is arthralgia or overt arthritis, which may affect joints of the fingers, wrists, elbows, knees, and ankles. The joint problems, which occur most frequently in women, rarely last longer than a few days to 3 weeks. Other, rarer complications include thrombocytopenic purpura and encephalitis.

mimicking of other viral infections

Because of the rather nonspecific nature of the illness, a diagnosis of rubella cannot be made on clinical grounds alone. More than 30 other viral agents, which will be discussed later in this chapter, can produce a similar illness. Confirmation of the diagnosis requires laboratory studies.

Fetal damage

high risk in first trimester

major lesions

The major significance of rubella is not the acute illness, but the risk of fetal damage in pregnant women, particularly when they contract primary infection during the first trimester. The risk of fetal malformation and chronic fetal infection, which is estimated to be as high as 80% if infection occurs in the first 2 weeks of gestation, decreases to 6–10% by the 14th week. The overall risk during the first trimester is estimated at 20–30%. Clinical manifestations of congenital rubella syndrome vary, but may include any combination of the following major findings: 1) cardiac defects, commonly patent ductus arteriosus and pulmonary valvular stenosis; 2) eye defects such as cataracts, chorioretinitis, glaucoma, coloboma, cloudy cornea, and microphthalmia; 3) sensorineural deafness; 4) hepatosplenomegaly; 5) thrombocytopenia; and 6) intrauterine growth retardation. Other findings include 1) central nervous system defects such as microcephaly, mental retardation, and encephalitis; 2) anemia; 3) transient immunodeficiency; 4) interstitial pneumonia, sometimes chronic; and 5) intravascular coagulation, hepatitis, rash, and other congenital malformations. Late complications of congenital rubella syndrome have also been described, including an apparent increased risk of diabetes mellitis, chronic thyroiditis, and occasionally the development of a progressive, subacute panencephalitis in the second decade of life.

late complications

Some congenitally infected infants may appear entirely normal at birth, and sequelae such as hearing or learning deficits may not become apparent until months later. The spectrum of defects thus varies from subtle to severe.

Pathogenesis

upper respiratory infection

viremic spread

role of cell-mediated immunity and immune complexes

In acquired infection, the virus enters the host via the upper respiratory tract, replicates, then spreads via the bloodstream to distant sites, including lymphoid tissues, skin, and organs. Viremia in these infections has been detected for as long as 8 days before to 2 days after onset of the rash, and virus shedding from the oropharynx can be detected up to 8 days after onset (Figure 35.1). Cellular immune responses and circulating virus–antibody immune complexes are thought to play a role in mediating the inflammatory responses to infection, such as rash and arthritis.

congenital infection

persistent fetal infection

reasons for fetal defects

Congenital infection occurs as a result of maternal viremia, placental infection, and transplacental spread to the fetus. Once fetal infection occurs, it persists chronically. Such persistence is probably related to an inability to eliminate the virus by immune or interferon-mediated mechanisms. There is too little inflammatory change in the fetal tissues to explain the pathogenesis of the congenital defects. Possibilities include placental and fetal vasculitis with compromise of fetal oxygenation, chronic viral infection of cells leading to impaired mitosis, cellular necrosis, and induction of chromosomal breakage. Any or all of these factors may operate at a critical stage

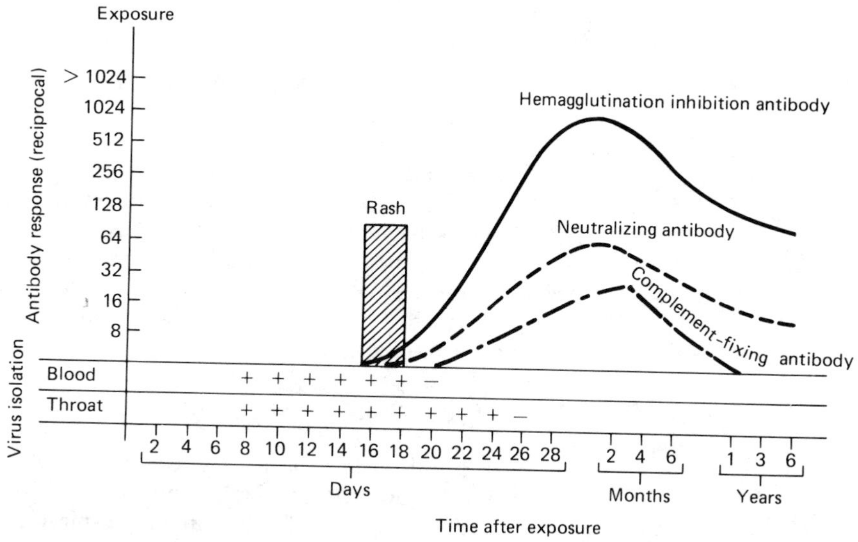

35.1 Antibody response and viral isolation in a typical case of acquired rubella.

of organogenesis to induce permanent defects. Viral persistence with circulating virus–antibody immune complexes may evoke inflammatory changes postnatally and produce continuing tissue damage.

Chronic infection and dissemination after birth

After birth, affected infants continue to excrete the virus in the throat, urine, and intestinal tract (Figure 35.2). Virus may be isolated from virtually all tissues in the first few weeks of life. Shedding of virus in the throat and urine, which persists for at least 6 months in most cases, has been known to continue for as long as 30 months. Virus has also been isolated from lens tissue removed 3–4 years later. These observations underscore the fact that such infants are an important reservoir in perpetuating virus transmission.

The prolonged virus shedding is somewhat puzzling, as it does not represent a typical example of immunologic tolerance. The affected infants are usually able to produce circulating IgM and IgG antibodies to the virus (Figure 35.2), although antibodies may decrease to undetectable levels after 3–4 years. Many infants show evidence of depressed rubella virus-specific cell-mediated immunity during the first year of life.

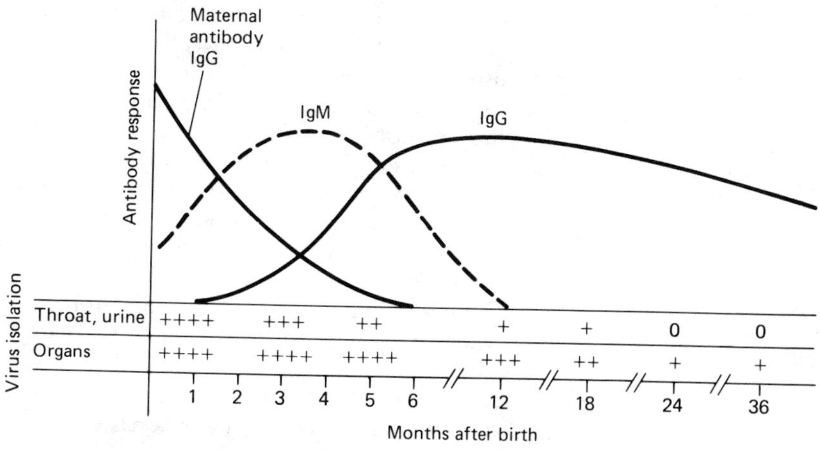

35.2 Persistence of rubella virus and antibody in congenitally infected infants.

Pathology

Postnatal disease

Because postnatally acquired disease is usually mild, little is known about its pathology. Mononuclear cell inflammatory changes can be observed in tissues, and viral antigen can be detected in the same sites (for example, skin, and synovial fluid).

Fetal disease

Congenital infections are characterized primarily by the various malformations. Necrosis of tissues such as myocardium and vascular endothelium may also be seen, and quantitative studies suggest a decrease in cell quantity in affected organs. In severe cases, normal calcium deposition in the metaphyses of long bones is delayed, which creates a "celery-stalk" appearance on a radiograph.

Immune Responses

Antibody response

lifelong immunity

In acquired infection the serum antibody titer rises, with a peak within 2–3 weeks after onset. Natural infection also results in the production of specific secretory IgA antibodies in the respiratory tract. After natural infection, immunity to reinfection is nearly always lifelong; however, reexposure can lead to transient respiratory tract acquisition, with an anamnestic rise in serum IgG and secretory IgA antibodies, but without resultant viremia or illness.

Epidemiology

seasonality

low virulence, high infectivity

duration of infectivity

Infections are usually observed during the winter and spring months. In contrast to measles, which has a high clinical attack rate among exposed susceptible individuals, only 30–60% of rubella-infected susceptible persons will develop clinically apparent disease. Although rubella is highly contagious, an estimated 15% of young adults escape natural infection during childhood. A major focus of concern is the susceptible woman of child-bearing age, who carries a risk of exposure during pregnancy. Disease in patients with primary acquired infections is contagious from 7 days before to 7 days after the onset of rash; as mentioned previously, congenitally infected infants may spread the virus to others for 6 months or more after birth.

Laboratory Diagnosis

cell cultures: rarely used in routine diagnosis

The virus may be isolated from respiratory secretions in the acute phase (and from urine, tissues, and feces in congenitally infected infants) by inoculation into a variety of cell cultures. The cell cultures required are not usually employed routinely in the laboratory, however, and isolation can be expensive, tedious, and time consuming, requiring as long as 2 weeks for the development of interfering or cytopathic effects.

serodiagnosis

hemagglutination inhibition test

Serologic diagnosis is usually employed in acquired infections; paired acute and convalescent samples collected 10–21 days apart are used. The hemagglutination inhibition test is used most often, but complement fixation, indirect fluorescent antibody, enzyme-linked immunosorbent assay, and other tests are available.

value and pitfalls of IgM tests

Determination of IgM-specific antibody is sometimes useful to ascertain whether an infection occurred in the past several months; it has also been used in the diagnosis of congenital infections. Unfortunately, there are certain pitfalls in interpreting this test: Some individuals (less than 5%) with acquired infections may have persistent elevations of IgM-specific antibodies for 200 days or more afterward, and some congenitally infected infants will not produce detectable IgM-specific antibodies. Serial testing for antibodies in suspected congenital infections may be needed to aid in diagnosis.

Serologic tests to detect susceptibility

Serologic testing (usually the hemagglutination inhibition test) is also used to determine potential susceptibility or immunity to infection. The presence of antibodies at or above the threshold level (for example, 1:8 or 1:10 with the hemagglutination inhibition test) indicates a very high probability of immunity (titers of 1:16 or greater are particularly reassuring), whereas titers below the threshold (undetectable) suggest lack of immunity. Such testing is often done to determine which individuals are susceptible, such as female adolescents, who require closer surveillance and consideration for immunization when such a procedure can be safely performed.

Role in preventing or detecting fetal exposure

It is particularly important to determine the immune status of women who are pregnant or contemplating pregnancy, in case exposure should occur subsequently. If the woman has serologic proof of prior immunity, the risk to the fetus if she is accidentally exposed is nil; if not, and exposure occurs during pregnancy, careful serologic monitoring is necessary. Termination of the pregnancy may be considered if there is serologic evidence of primary infection.

Prevention

Live, attenuated rubella vaccine

Since 1969, live attenuated rubella vaccines have been available for routine immunization. The current vaccine virus, grown in human diploid fibroblast cell cultures (RA 27/3), has been shown to be highly effective: it causes seroconversion in approximately 95% of recipients. Interestingly, significant seroconversion is often associated with excretion of the vaccine virus in the pharynx; however, it does not appear to be communicable.

Indications for immunization

Routine immunization is now recommended for infants after the first year of life and for other individuals with no history of immunization and lack of immunity by serologic testing. Target groups include female adolescents and hospital personnel in a high-risk setting.

Complications and contraindications

Complications of the vaccine, although similar to those of the acquired, wild virus disease, are far less frequent and usually milder. They include occasional rash, fever, and joint complaints; the latter are more common in women. The vaccine is contraindicated in immunocompromised patients and in pregnancy. To date, over 80 instances of accidental vaccination of susceptible pregnant women have been reported, with no clinically apparent adverse effects on the fetus; however, it is strongly recommended that immunization be avoided in this setting, and that nonpregnant women avoid conception for at least 3 months after receiving the vaccine.

Duration of artificial immunity

Vaccine-induced immunity may be lifelong. Further follow-up is necessary, however, before any conclusions can be made. Studies to date indicate that the duration of protection is at least 16 years.

Immune serum globulin has not been shown of significant value in postexposure prophylaxis, and it is not routinely recommended.

Treatment

Other than supportive measures, there is no specific therapy for either the acquired or the congenital infection.

Roseola Infantum (Exanthem Subitum)

Roseola infantum is a common, presumably viral disease of infants and children 6 months to 4 years of age. The apparent etiologic agent has been transmitted to human volunteers and monkeys, but has never been isolated in the laboratory.

The illness is characterized by abrupt onset of high fever, sometimes accompanied by brief, generalized convulsions and leukopenia. After 3–5 days, the fever diminishes rapidly, followed in a few hours by a faint, transient, macular rash.

etiologic agent unidentified

Several agents, including adenoviruses, Coxsackie viruses, and echoviruses, have been occasionally noted to cause this syndrome; however, most cases are probably caused by a single, as yet unidentified virus.

Erythema Infectiosum

Like roseola infantum, the causative agent of erythema infectiosum has not been identified. There is some evidence to suggest association with a human parvoviruslike agent, which has also been incriminated in acute aplastic crises among patients with chronic hemolytic anemias. After an incubation period of 5–10 days, a confluent, indurated rash appears on the face, often giving a "slapped-cheek" appearance. The rash spreads in a day or two to other areas, particularly exposed surfaces such as the arms and legs, where it is usually macular and reticular (lacelike). The illness lasts 1–2 weeks, but rash may recur for periods of 2–4 weeks thereafter, exacerbated by heat, sunlight, exercise, or emotional stress. Constitutional symptoms such as fever and malaise are mild or absent. Arthralgia sometimes occurs, especially in female adolescents and women. Complications are extremely rare. The disease tends to occur in small, localized outbreaks, particularly during the spring and early summer.

Although studies of erythema infectiosum have thus far failed to conclusively demonstrate the causative agent, it has been shown that some "classic" cases were caused by echovirus or rubella virus infections. Before a firm diagnosis is made on clinical grounds, especially during outbreaks, it is usually wise to exclude the possibility of atypical rubella infection by appropriate serologic testing.

Other Causes of Rubellalike Rashes

In addition to erythema infectiosum, numerous other agents can mimic rubella clinically. These agents include at least 17 echoviruses, nine Coxsackie viruses, several adenoviral serotypes, arboviruses such as dengue, Epstein–Barr virus, scarlet fever, and toxic drug eruptions, among others. Because of the wide variety of diagnostic possibilities, it is not possible to diagnose or rule out rubella confidently on clinical grounds alone. Therefore, the diagnosis usually requires specific laboratory studies. As rubella is an infection with significant impact on the fetus, laboratory workup is often directed toward serologic study to rule out this possibility.

Additional Reading and References

Mumps

Beard, C.M., et al. 1977. The incidence and outcome of mumps orchitis in Rochester, Minnesota, 1935–1974. *Mayo Clin. Proc.* 52:3–7. Long-term follow-up and incidence and sequelae of mumps orchitis are discussed.

Hayden, G.F., et al. 1978. Current status of mumps and mumps vaccine in the United States. *Pediatrics* 62:965–969. The vaccine and its effectiveness and safety are reviewed.

Lerner, A.M. 1970. Guide to immunization against mumps. *J. Infect. Dis.* 122:116. An excellent review of clinical aspects is presented.

Measles

Fulginiti, V.A., and Helfer, R.E. 1980. Atypical measles in adolescent siblings 16 years after killed measles virus vaccine. *J. Am. Med. Assoc.* 244:804–806. Case reports and bibliography review and illustrate the intriguing effects of killed vaccine.

Hinman, A.R., et al. 1982. Progress in measles elimination. *J. Am. Med. Assoc.* 247:1592–1595. A good historic review is provided, and possibilities for eradication are discussed.

Rubella

Krugman, S. 1980. Rubella immunization: Present status and future perspectives. *Pediatrics* 65:1174–1176. An excellent review of the vaccine and its effect is given, and questions regarding duration of vaccine-induced immunity are raised.

Miller, E., et al. 1982. Consequences of confirmed maternal rubella at successive stages of pregnancy. *Lancet* 2:781–874. A precise analysis of the risks of infection at various times during gestation.

Polk, B.F., et al. 1980. An outbreak of rubella among hospital personnel. *N. Engl. J. Med.* 303:541–545. The contagiousness of the virus and its impact in high-risk settings are illustrated.

Erythema Infectiosum

Brass, C., et al. 1982. Academy rash. A probable epidemic of erythemia infectiosum ("fifth disease"). *J. Am. Med. Assoc.* 248:568–572. Description of an epidemic, clinical features, and discussion of mimicry by viruses such as rubella.

C. George Ray

Poxviruses

36

The poxvirus family includes viruses that infect birds, mammals, and even insects. They are large, brick-shaped or ovoid, DNA-carrying virions (Figure 36.1) measuring approximately $100 \times 200 \times 300$ nm; their structure is complex, and replication occurs in the cytoplasm of infected cells. They possess an envelope, which is not acquired by budding and not essential for infectivity. The agents most important in human disease are variola, vaccinia, molluscum contagiosum, orf, cowpox, and pseudocowpox.

Variola (Smallpox)

Until very recently, smallpox played a significant role in world history with regard to both the serious epidemics recorded since antiquity and the sometimes dangerous measures taken to prevent infection.

Variola major and minor

Two types are known: variola major and variola minor (alastrim). Although the viruses are indistinguishable antigenically, their fatality rates differ considerably (less than 1% for variola minor, 3–35% for variola major). They are also difficult to distinguish in the laboratory; variola major, however, has slightly greater virulence in embryonated hen's eggs.

It is remarkable that, although these viruses are exceedingly infectious, they have been eradicated worldwide. Thus, any discussion of smallpox is now of more historic than practical interest.

Jenner's vaccination experiments

The first major step toward modern prevention and subsequent eradication of smallpox can be credited to Edward Jenner, who noted that milkmaids who develop mild cowpox lesions on their hands appeared immune to smallpox. He published evidence in 1798 indicating that purposeful inoculation of individuals with cowpox material could protect them against subsequent infection by smallpox. The concept of vaccination gradually evolved, with the modern use of live vaccinia virus, a poxvirus of uncertain origin, to produce specific immunity.

human reservoir only

no healthy carriers

In 1967, the World Health Organization launched an ambitious program aimed at eradication of smallpox. This goal was considered realistic for two major reasons: 1) No extrahuman reservoir of the virus was known to exist; and 2) asymptomatic carriage apparently did not occur. The basic approach included intensive surveillance for clinical cases of smallpox, prompt quarantine of such patients and their contacts, and vaccination of contacts to prevent further spread. A tremendous amount of effort was involved, but the results were astonishing—the last recorded case of naturally acquired

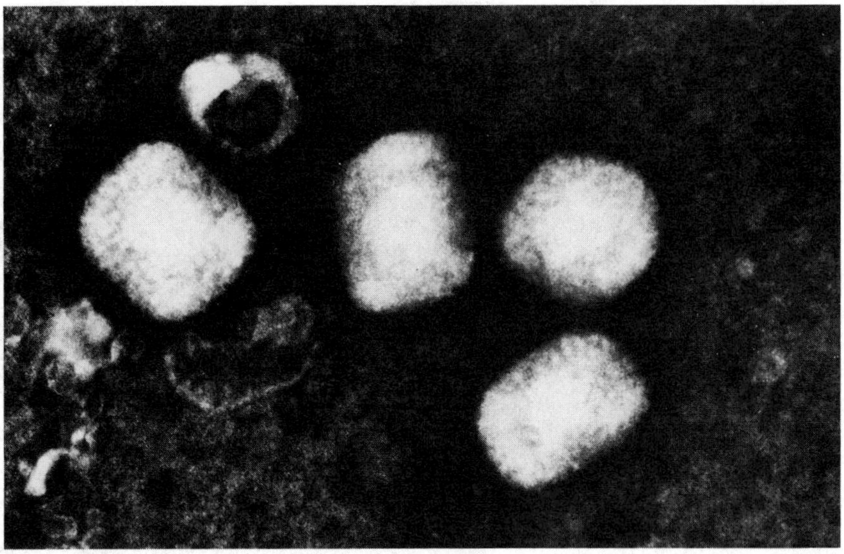

36.1 Electron microscopic appearance of a poxvirus (vaccinia). (Negative stain; original magnification ×60,000). (*Courtesy of Dr. Claire M. Payne.*)

eradication by case finding, quarantine, and immunization

smallpox occurred in Somalia in 1977. After 2 more years of surveillance with discovery of no further infections, global eradiction of smallpox was confirmed in 1979 and accepted by the World Health Organization in May 1980. Global eradication was followed up by destruction of virus kept by laboratories (one tragic episode of laboratory-transmitted smallpox occurred in 1978), with the exception of virus retained by two reference laboratories, one in Atlanta, Georgia and one in Moscow, USSR. Vaccination is therefore no longer deemed necessary, except for the very few laboratory workers who may handle the virus.

Surveillance continues, including studies of poxviruses of animals (for example, whitepox, monkeypox) that are antigenically somewhat similar to smallpox. Some virologists remain legitimately concerned that an animal poxvirus could undergo mutation and become highly virulent to humans, although the probability of such an occurrence seems very low. Also, the possibility of escape of virus from a laboratory source, although highly unlikely, must be considered. Stockpiles of vaccine are maintained by several countries to block spread from any such event.

Clinical Outline of Disease and Outcome

Rash and clinical course

The incubation period of smallpox was usually 12–14 days, although in occasional fulminating cases it could be as short as 4–5 days. The typical onset was abrupt, with fever, chills, and myalgia, followed by a rash 3–4 days later. The rash evolved to firm papulovesicles that became pustular over 10–12 days, then slowly healed. In contrast to varicella, only a single crop of lesions (all in the same stage of evolution) developed; these lesions were most prominent over the head and extremities (Figure 36.2). Some cases of variola major were fulminant, with a hemorrhagic rash ("sledge-hammer" smallpox). Death could result from the overwhelming primary viral infection or from bacterial superinfection. Previous vaccination, usually more than 3 years before the onset of infection, could shorten the evolution of the disease or modify it to a degree that sometimes made diagnosis difficult. The disease was highly contagious, and the virus could survive well

effect of previous vaccination

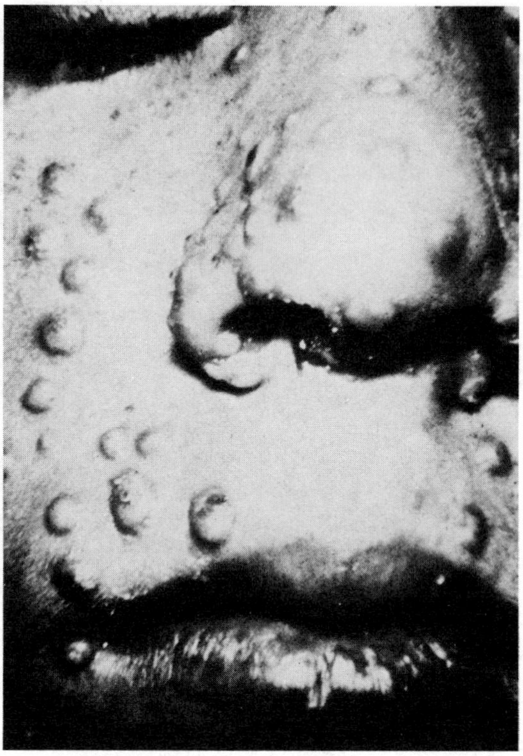

36.2 Close-up of facial lesions of smallpox during the first week of the illness.

respiratory and fomite spread

in the extracellular environment. Acquisition of infection by respiratory spread or by exposure to dried crusts from skin lesions, contaminated articles, and fomites has been well documented.

Laboratory Diagnosis

Variola produces lesions (pocks) on the chorioallantoic membranes of embryonated hen's eggs; it will also infect a variety of cell cultures in vitro. Cytology of lesions shows cytoplasmic inclusions, but neither intranuclear inclusions nor giant cells. Direct electron microscopy and immunoprecipitin tests have also been applied to lesion specimens for rapid diagnosis.

Vaccinia

Origin

Vaccination

Local reactions

Duration of immunity

Severe reactions

Vaccinia virus is serologically related to smallpox, although its exact origin is unknown. Some virologists believe it is a recombinant virus derived from smallpox and cowpox. The virus is usually propagated by dermal inoculation of calves, and the resultant vesicle fluid ("lymph") is lyophilized and used as a live virus vaccine in humans. The vaccine is inoculated into the epidermis and produces a localized lesion, which indicates successful immunization. The lesion becomes vesicular, then pustular, followed by crusting and healing over 10–14 days. The local reaction is sometimes severe and accompanied by systemic symptoms such as fever, rash, and lymphadenopathy.

Vaccinia-produced immunity to smallpox wanes rapidly after 3 years, becoming virtually absent after 20 years.

In addition to the local reactions, several other potentially serious and lethal complications can occur with vaccinia infection. These complications include encephalitis, progressive vaccinia (vaccinia gangrenosum, usually seen in immunocompromised patients), disseminated vaccinia, autoinoculation into the eye or mucous membranes, allergic reactions, and bacterial superinfection. Thankfully, routine use of this agent in the prevention of disease is no longer necessary. In the past, some physicians used vaccinia virus for the treatment of other diseases, such as warts or recurrent herpes simplex infections. Such therapy has no documented efficacy, and its use is considered unwarranted and dangerous.

Molluscum Contagiosum

Infection routes

Molluscum contagiosum is a benign, cutaneous poxvirus disease of humans, spread by direct contact with infected cells. It is usually acquired by inoculation into minute skin abrasions; events that commonly lead to transmission include roughhousing in shower rooms and swimming pools, sharing of towels, and sexual contact.

local lesions

After an incubation period of 2–8 weeks, nodular, pale, firm (pearllike) lesions usually 2–10 mm in diameter develop in the epidermis. These lesions are painless and umbilicated in appearance. A cheesy material may be expressed from the pore at the center of each lesion. Local trauma may cause spread of lesions in the involved skin area. The lesions are not associated with systemic symptoms, and they disappear in 2–12 months without treatment. Specific treatment, if desired, is usually by curettage or careful removal of the central core by expression with forceps.

histology

The pathologic findings, which are limited to the epidermis, include hyperplasia, ballooning degeneration, and acanthosis. The diagnosis, made on clinical grounds, can be confirmed by demonstration of large, eosinophilic cytoplasmic inclusions (molluscum bodies) in the affected superficial epithelial cells.

Orf

Orf is an old Saxon term for a human infection caused by a parapoxvirus of sheep and goats. Synonyms for the infection in animals include contagious pustular dermatitis, ecthyma contagiosum, pustular ecthyma, and "scabby mouth." Humans usually acquire the infection by close contact with young infected animals and accidental inoculation through cuts or abrasions on the hand or wrist. The typical skin lesion is solitary; it begins as a vesicle, then evolves into a nodular mass that later develops central necrosis. Regional lymphadenopathy sometimes develops; dissemination is rare. The average duration of the lesion is 35 days, followed by complete resolution. The diagnosis is usually made on the basis of clinical appearance and occupational history. Serologic confirmation or electron microscopy of the lesion can be done, but are rarely necessary.

Milker's Nodules and Cowpox

Milker's nodules (pseudocowpox) is a cutaneous poxvirus disease of cattle, distinct from cowpox, that can cause local skin infections similar to orf in exposed humans. Healing of the skin lesions may take 4–8 weeks. There is no cross-immunity to cowpox.

Cowpox is now very rare in the United States. It produces a vesicular eruption on the udders of cows and similar, usually localized, vesicular lesions in humans who are accidently exposed.

Additional Reading and References

Breman, J.G., and Arita, I. 1980. The confirmation and maintenance of smallpox eradication. *N. Engl. J. Med.* 303:1263. The circumstances leading to smallpox eradication and concerns for the future are reviewed.

C. George Ray

Enteroviruses

37

Enteroviruses comprise a major subgroup of small RNA viruses (picornaviruses) that readily infect and are shed from the intestinal tract. They include the polioviruses, Coxsackie viruses, echoviruses, and more recently discovered agents that are simply designated enteroviruses. The number of serotypes that can infect humans has grown to a total of nearly 70, and more are likely to be found in the future.

Enteroviruses cause paralytic disease, mild acute aseptic meningitis syndromes, pleurodynia, exanthems, pericarditis, nonspecific febrile illness, and occasional fulminant encephalomyocarditis of the newborn. As more has been learned, it is apparent that the spectrum of disease is even broader. Some infections can lead to permanent damage, and others may trigger chronic, active disease processes.

These viruses, which have many features in common, will first be considered as a group. Some of the special features of important serotypes will be discussed in more detail later in this chapter.

Group Characteristics

Habitat

worldwide occurrence

The enteroviruses of humans and animals are ubiquitous and have been found worldwide. Their name is derived from their ability to infect intestinal tract epithelial and lymphoid tissues and to be shed into the feces.

Morphologic and Biologic Features

small, single-stranded RNA viruses

resistance to inactivation

identification by neutralization tests

As a group, the picornaviruses are extremely small (17–28 nm in diameter), single-stranded RNA viruses with icosahedral symmetry. In contrast to the rhinoviruses, the enterovirus subgroup is resistant to ether, acid pH (4.0), and bile. Another feature is cationic stability; in the presence of magnesium sulfate, the viruses become more resistant to thermal inactivation. They can survive for prolonged periods in sewage and even in chlorinated water if sufficient organic debris is present. Although some of the enterovirus serotypes share complement-fixing antigens, there are no significant serologic relationships between the major classes listed in Table 37.1. Definitive identification of isolates usually requires neutralization tests.

Table 37.1 Human Enteroviruses

Class	Number of Serotypes
Poliovirus	3
Coxsackie virus	
Group A	23
Group B	6
Echovirus	31
Enterovirus	Types 68–72[a]

[a] More recently discovered enteroviruses, which have overlapping biologic characteristics, are identified numerically.

Growth in the Laboratory

growth in primate cell cultures

effects of Coxsackie A and B viruses on newborn mice

Most of these agents can be isolated in primate (human or simian) cell cultures and show characteristic cytopathic effects; some strains, however, particularly several Coxsackie A serotypes, are grown with difficulty in cell cultures, and inoculation of newborn mice may be necessary for detection of virus. The newborn mouse, in fact, is one basis for originally classifying Coxsackie A and B viruses. After inoculation of mice at 24 hr of age or less and observing for 2–12 days, Coxsackie A viruses primarily cause a widespread, inflammatory, necrotic effect on skeletal muscle, leading to flaccid paralysis and death; similar inoculation of Coxsackie B viruses causes encephalitis, resulting in spasticity and occasionally convulsions. Other organs are variably affected, and histopathologic examination is sometimes helpful in distinguishing the two. Echoviruses and polioviruses rarely have an adverse effect on mice, unless special adaptation procedures are first employed. The higher-numbered enteroviruses (types 68–72), which have overlapping, variable growth and host characteristics, have been classified separately. Hepatitis A virus has been classified as enterovirus 72 and is discussed in Chapter 38.

Host Range

Humans are the major natural host for the polioviruses, Coxsackie viruses, and echoviruses. There are enteroviruses of other animals with a limited host range that does not appear to extend to humans. Conversely, viruses thought to be identical or related to human enteroviruses have been isolated from dogs (Coxsackie viruses B_1, 3, and 5; echoviruses 2, 6, and 19) and cats (echoviruses 16 and 19). Whether these agents cause disease in these animals is debatable, and there is no evidence of spread from animals to humans.

Epidemiology

asymptomatic infections common

The enteroviruses have a worldwide distribution, and asymptomatic infection is common. The proportion of infected individuals who will develop illness varies from 2 to 100%, depending upon the serotype or strain involved and the age of the patient. Secondary infections in households are common and range as high as 40–70%, depending upon factors such as family size, crowding, and sanitary conditions.

variation in dominant epidemic strains

In some years, certain serotypes emerge as dominant epidemic strains; they then may wane, only to reappear in epidemic fashion years later. For example, echovirus 16 was a major cause of outbreaks in the eastern United States in 1951 and 1974. Coxsackie B_1 virus was common in 1963, echovirus 9 in 1962, 1965, 1968, and 1969, and echovirus 30 in 1968 and 1969. The emergence of dominant serotypes is quite unpredictable from year to year.

prevalence in summer and fall

All enteroviruses show a seasonal predilection; epidemics are usually observed during the summer and fall months. In subtropical and tropical climates, the duration of greatest transmission sometimes extends into the winter months.

fecal–oral transmission

Direct or indirect fecal–oral transmission is considered the most common mode of spread. After infection, the virus will persist in the oropharynx for 1–4 weeks, and it can be shed in the feces for 1–18 weeks. Thus, sewage-contaminated water, fecally contaminated foods, or insect vectors (flies, cockroaches) may occasionally be the source of infection. More commonly, however, spread is directly from person to person. This mode of transmission is suggested by the high infection rates seen among young children, whose hygienic practices tend to be less than optimal, and in crowded households. Approximately two-thirds of all isolates are from children 9 years of age or younger.

spread usually person to person

most infections in children

Incubation periods

Incubation periods vary, but relatively short intervals (2–10 days) are frequent. Often, illness will be seen concurrently in more than one family member, and the clinical features will vary within the household.

Pathogenesis and Pathology

replication in upper respiratory and gastrointestinal tracts

viremic spread

histopathology

After primary replication in the epithelial cells and lymphoid tissues in the upper respiratory and gastrointestinal tracts, viremic spread to other sites can occur. Potential target organs vary according to the virus strain and its tropism, but may include the central nervous system, heart, vascular endothelium, liver, pancreas, lungs, gonads, skeletal muscles, synovial tissues, skin, and mucous membranes. Histopathologic findings include cell necrosis and mononuclear cell inflammatory infiltrates; in the central nervous system, the inflammatory cells are localized most prominently in perivascular sites. The initial tissue damage is thought to result from the lytic cycle of virus replication; secondary spread to other sites may ensue. Viremia is usually undetectable by the time symptoms appear, and termination of virus replication appears to correlate with the appearance of circulating neutralizing antibody and interferon and mononuclear cell infiltrations of infected tissue. The early antibody response is with immunoglobulin M(IgM), which usually wanes 6–12 weeks after onset to be progressively replaced by IgG-specific antibodies. The important role of antibodies in termination of infection, demonstrated in mouse models of Coxsackie B virus infections, is supported by the observation of persistent echovirus and poliovirus replication in patients with antibody deficiency diseases.

Role of antibody in immunity

Although initial acute tissue damage may be caused by the lytic effects of the virus on the cell, the secondary sequelae may be immunologically mediated. As with any infectious process, the disease and pathology will be determined by both the agent and the host response. Enterovirus-caused poliomyelitis, disseminated disease of the newborn, aseptic meningitis, encephalitis, and acute respiratory illnesses, thought to represent primary lytic infections, can usually be identified through routine methods of virus isolation and determination of specific antibody titer changes. On the other hand, syndromes such as myopericarditis, nephritis, and myositis have been

clinical manifestations from lytic effects of virus

associated with enteroviruses primarily by serologic and epidemiologic evidence. In many of these cases, viral isolation is the exception rather than the rule. The pathogenesis of these latter infections is not clear; however, observations suggest that the acute infectious phase of the virus may be mild or subclinical and often subsides by the time clinical illness becomes evident. Illness probably represents a host immunologic response to tissue injury by the virus or to viral or virus-induced antigens that persist in the affected tissues. Experiments with Coxsackie B viruses in mouse models tend to support this hypothesis. In experimental myocarditis, mononuclear inflammatory cells (monocytes, natural killer lymphocytes) seemed to play a greater role than antibody in termination of infection, and the persistence of inflammation after disappearance of detectable virus or viral antigen appeared to be mediated by cytotoxic T lymphocytes.

Probable immunopathologic manifestations

Immune Responses

Serotype specificity of immunity

Infection by a specific serotype in an immunologically normal host is followed by a humoral antibody response, which can often be detected by neutralization methods for many years thereafter (Figure 37.1). There is relative immunity to reinfection by the same serotype; however, reinfection has been reported, usually resulting in subclinical infection or mild illness. Although there is some antigenic sharing between serotypes in some of the enterovirus classes (for example, Coxsackie B viruses), there is no evidence of significant heterotypic immunity to infection by different serotypes.

Laboratory Diagnosis

viral isolation in acute phase of disease

In acute enterovirus-caused syndromes, diagnosis is most readily established by virus isolation from throat swabs, stool or rectal swabs, body fluids, and occasionally tissues. Viremia is usually undetectable by the time symptoms appear. When there is central nervous system involvement, cerebrospinal fluid cultures taken during the acute phase of the disease may be positive in 10–85% of cases (except in poliovirus infections, in which virus recovery from this site is rare), depending upon the stage of illness and the viral

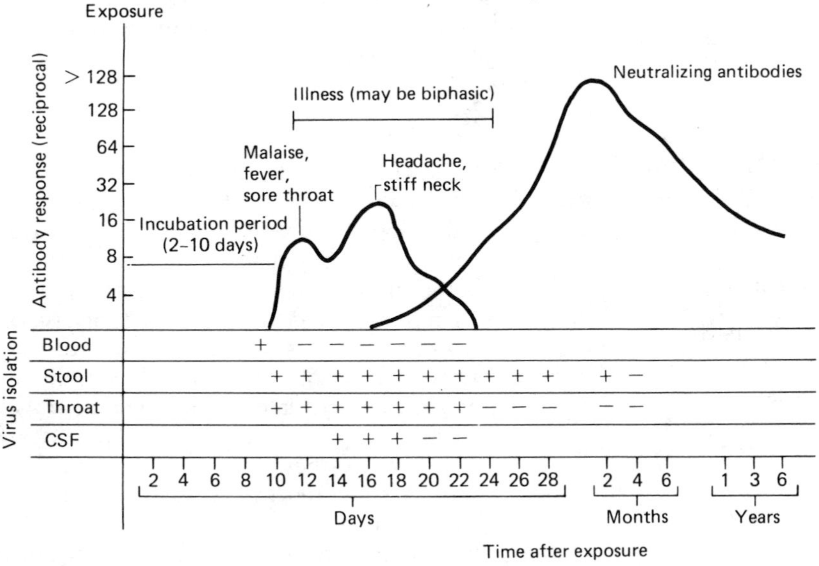

37.1 Antibody response and viral isolation in a typical case of enteroviral infection.

significance of isolates from pharynx and stool

serotype involved. Direct isolation of virus from affected tissues or body fluids in enclosed spaces (for example, pleural, joint, pericardial, or cerebrospinal fluid) usually confirms the diagnosis. Isolation of an enterovirus from the throat is highly suggestive of an etiologic association, as the virus is usually detectable at this site for only 2 days to 2 weeks after infection; isolation of virus from fecal specimens only must be interpreted more cautiously, as asymptomatic shedding from the bowel may persist for as long as 4 months (Figure 37.1).

Limited value of serodiagnosis

The diagnosis may be further supported by fourfold or greater neutralizing antibody titer changes between paired acute and convalescent serum samples. This method is often expensive and cumbersome, however, requiring careful selection of serotypes for use as antigens. Serodiagnosis is generally reserved for critical situations in which the etiology is questioned, such as isolation of a virus only from a peripheral source such as the feces, or in illnesses such as myopericarditis, in which the yield on routine culture is low and number of serotypes that might be expected to be involved is limited. Quantitative interpretations of antibody titers on single serum samples are rarely helpful, because of the wide range of titers to different serotypes that can be found in groups of healthy individuals. In acute poliovirus infections, complement-fixing antibody titer determinations on acute and convalescent sera can aid in diagnosis.

Prevention

Vaccines, which are available only for the prevention of poliovirus infections, will be discussed in detail later in this chapter. Although proper disposal of feces and careful personal hygiene are recommended, the usual quarantine or isolation measures are relatively ineffective in controlling the spread of enteroviruses in the family or community.

Treatment

no specific therapy

None of the currently available antiviral agents or immune serum globulins has been shown effective in treatment or prophylaxis of enterovirus infections. Treatment is entirely symptomatic and supportive. As glucosteroids increase the quantity of virus and extent of ensuing damage in experimental animals, their use is considered contraindicated; they are sometimes employed, however, in the management of established severe myocarditis.

Infections Caused by Major Pathogenic Enteroviruses

Polioviruses

Three serotypes

risk of paralysis from infection increases with age

Worldwide, the most important enteroviruses are the three poliovirus serotypes (types 1, 2, and 3). They first emerged as important causes of disease in developed temperate-zone countries during the latter part of the 19th century, and they have become increasingly important elsewhere as living conditions improve in developing countries. This somewhat paradoxical situation is related to the fact that the risk of paralytic disease resulting from infection increases with age. Improvement of sanitary conditions tends to impede spread of the viruses; thus, individuals may become infected not in early infancy but later in life, when paralysis is more likely to occur.

CNS tropism

The particular tropism of polioviruses for the central nervous system (CNS), which they usually reach by passage across the blood–CNS barrier, is perhaps favored by reflex dilatation of capillaries supplying the affected motor centers of the anterior horn of the brainstem or spinal cord. An alternate pathway is via the axons or perineural sheaths of peripheral nerves. Motor neurons are particularly vulnerable to infection and variable degrees

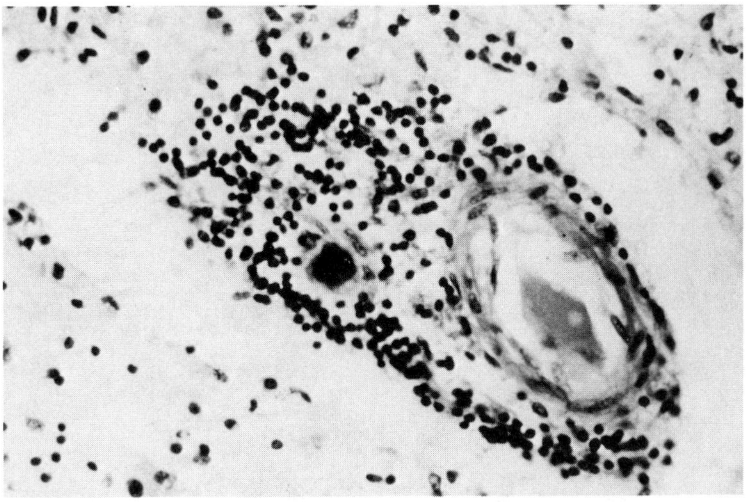

37.2 Section of spinal cord from a fatal case of poliomyelitis, demonstrating perivenous mononuclear cell inflammatory reaction. (*Kindly provided by Dr. Peter C. Johnson.*)

of neuronal destruction. The histopathologic findings in the brainstem and spinal cord include necrosis of neuronal cells and perivascular "cuffing" by infiltration with mononuclear cells, primarily lymphocytes (Figure 37.2).

Subclinical infections

Abortive poliomyelitis

Aseptic meningitis

Paralytic poliomyelitis

Clinical outline of disease and outcome. Most infections (perhaps 90%) are either completely subclinical or so mild that they do not come to attention. When disease does result, the incubation period can be from 4 to 35 days, but is usually between 7 and 14 days. The disease falls into three classes: The first *abortive poliomyelitis,* is a nonspecific febrile illness of 2- to 3-day duration with no signs of CNS localization. In addition to these signs, *aseptic meningitis* (nonparalytic poliomyelitis) is characterized by signs of meningeal irritation (stiff neck, pain, and stiffness in the back). Recovery is rapid and complete, usually within a few days. The third class, *paralytic poliomyelitis,* is the major possible outcome of infection and is often preceded by a period of minor illness, sometimes with 2 or 3 symptom-free days intervening. There are signs of meningeal irritation, but the hallmark of paralytic poliomyelitis is *asymmetric flaccid paralysis,* with no significant sensory loss. The extent of involvement varies greatly from case to case; in its most serious forms, however, all four limbs may be completely paralyzed or the brainstem may be attacked, with paralysis of the cranial nerves and muscles of respiration (bulbar polio). The maximum extent of involvement is evident within a few days after first paralysis. Thereafter, as temporarily damaged neurons regain their function, recovery begins and may continue for as long as 6 months; paralysis persisting after this time is permanent. There is no specific treatment; management involves complete rest during the active phase of the disease, with splinting of affected limbs to avoid muscle contractures, followed by physiotherapy and orthopedic rehabilitation.

flaccid paralysis

recovery phase

Prevention Two types of poliovirus vaccines are currently licensed in the United States: inactivated polio vaccine and live oral attenuated virus vaccine. Each contains the three serotypes of poliomyolitis virus.

Inactivated vaccine

Inactivated polio vaccine (IPV; also known as *killed polio vaccine* or *Salk vaccine*) was introduced in 1955; its use was associated with a dramatic decline in paralytic cases (Figure 37.3). It remains the only vaccine used in some countries, notably Sweden, the Netherlands, and Finland, and its efficacy has been excellent. Vaccination is by subcutaneous injection. Primary vaccination with four doses (three doses 4–8 weeks apart and the fourth 6–12

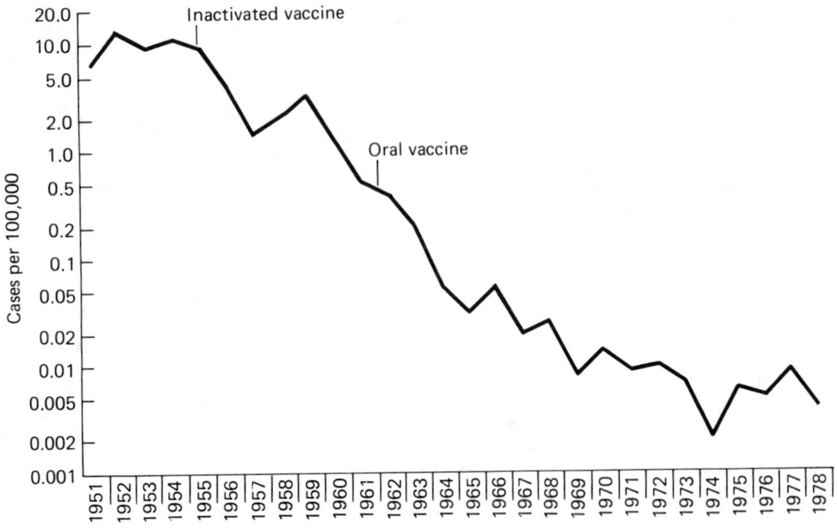

37.3 Reported paralytic poliomyelitis attack rates in the United States, 1951–1978. (*From the Centers for Disease Control, Poliomyelitis Surveillance Summary 1977–1978. Issued December 1980.*)

months later) produces antibody responses in more than 95% of recipients. The current product is considered quite safe, with no significant deleterious side effects.

Live vaccine

Oral polio vaccine [OPV; also known as *poliovirus vaccine, live vaccine, oral trivalent vaccine,* (TOPV), or *Sabin vaccine*] is composed of live, attenuated viruses that have undergone serial passage in cell cultures from humans and subhuman primates. It was first licensed in the United States in 1963. The vaccine is given orally as a primary series of three doses (the first two doses usually 6–8 weeks apart, and the third 8–12 months later) and produces antibodies to all three serotypes in more than 95% of recipients; these antibodies persist for several years. As with IPV, recall boosters are recommended to maintain adequate antibody levels. Like wild poliovirus, OPV viruses infect and replicate in the oropharynx and intestinal tract, and may be shed into the feces for 6 weeks or longer.

Vaccine-associated poliomyelitis

One disadvantage of OPV is the remote risk of vaccine-associated paralytic disease in some recipients, such as immunocompromised persons; susceptible adults also have a slightly higher risk. There is speculation that some instances of vaccine-associated paralytic disease may also be related to reversion of attenuated virus to more virulent characteristics in vivo after serial passage from person to person. The incidence of vaccine-associated paralytic poliomyelitis is estimated at approximately 1 per 3.7 million doses distributed. Of the 76 cases reported in the United States during 1969–1978, 18 were in otherwise healthy vaccine recipients, 47 in healthy close contacts of vaccine recipients, and 11 in persons with immune deficiency conditions.

Effects of oral vaccine on spread of poliovirus

The major advantages of OPV include ease of administration (oral instead of by injection) and secondary immunization of nonimmune contacts through shedding of vaccine virus into the intestinal tract, resulting in more widespread immunity in the population. It is also theorized that during outbreaks, transient vaccine virus colonization and replication results in the induction of mucosal immunity (primarily through secretory IgA), which may interfere with subsequent acquisition and spread of wild poliovirus.

The choice between IPV and OPV for routine primary immunization is still widely debated; however, it is clear that both are highly effective vaccines, and that routine immunization with either agent is important in the prevention and, it is hoped, eradication of this serious disease. Ideally, immunization should commence in infancy.

Although there are no currently recognized areas of wild poliovirus prevalence in the United States, it must be kept in mind that importation of these strains can readily occur from endemic areas in contiguous countries such as Mexico, as well as from developing nations abroad. Once introduced into a community, the virus can spread rapidly among susceptible individuals. Thus, continuing immunization programs are of utmost importance in preventing spread of this disease.

Coxsackie Viruses and Echoviruses

The Coxsackie viruses and echoviruses are widespread throughout the world. The basic features of their epidemiology and pathogenesis appear to be the same as those of the polioviruses. Unlike polioviruses, they have a greater tendency to affect the meninges and occasionally the cerebrum, and only rarely affect anterior horn cells.

most infections subclinical

The consequences of infection with these agents are highly variable and related only in part to virus subgroup and serotype. Up to 60% of infections are subclinical. The main interest in these agents stems from their ability to cause more serious illness, which becomes most evident during epidemics of infection with a particular agent.

Clinical outline of disease and outcome. Inapparent infection is common, but varies with the infecting strain and the host involved. The range of illness manifestations varies from mild to lethal and from acute to chronic. Table 37.2 lists the major syndromes and serotypes commonly associated with each. Considerable overlap occurs, however, and one should not be surprised if an enteroviral serotype found in connection with a specific syndrome differs from that most often encountered. The one generalization that can be made is that the Coxsackie B group appears to have the greatest latitude with regard to tissue tropism.

Table 37.2 Clinical Syndromes and Commonly Associated Enterovirus Serotypes[a]

Syndrome	Coxsackie Virus: Group A	Coxsackie Virus: Group B	Echovirus and Enterovirus (E)
Aseptic meningitis, encephalitis	2, 4, 7, *9*, 10	1, *2, 3, 4, 5*	*4, 6, 9, 11, 16, 30*; E70, E71
Muscle weakness and paralysis (poliomyelitislike disease)	*7, 9*	2, 3, 4, 5	2, 4, 6, 9, 11, 30; *E71*
Cerebellar ataxia	2, 4, *9*	3, 4	4, 6, 9
Exanthems and enanthems	*4, 5, 6, 9, 10, 16*	2, 3, 4, 5	*2, 4, 5, 6, 9, 11, 16, 18, 25*
Pericarditis, myocarditis	4, 16	*2, 3, 4, 5*	1, 6, 8, 9, 19
Epidemic myalgia (pleurodynia), orchitis	9	1, *2, 3, 4, 5*	1, 6, 9
Respiratory	9, 16, *21*, 24	1, 3, 4, 5	*4, 9, 11*, 20, 25
Conjunctivitis	*24*	1, 5	*7; E70*
Generalized disease (infants)	—	1, *2, 3, 4, 5*	3, 6, 9, 11, 14, 17, 19

[a] Serotypes most commonly associated with syndrome are italicized.

aseptic meningitis most common syndrome

In terms of relative frequency and significance, aseptic meningitis is the most important clinical illness associated with enterovirus infections. This syndrome can be mild and self-limiting, lasting 5–14 days; however, it is occasionally accompanied by encephalitis, which can lead to permanent neurologic sequelae, particularly in infants. Overall, enteroviruses cause the majority of all nonbacterial CNS infections now observed in the United States.

myocarditis often associated with Coxsackie B viruses

Acute inflammation of the heart muscle (myocarditis) and/or its covering membranes (pericarditis) can be caused by a variety of viral agents; however, it is estimated that as many as 50% of cases are associated with infection by Coxsackie B viruses. Such infections are usually self-limiting, but can lead to a fatal outcome (arrhythmia or heart failure) or cause chronic heart disease.

exanthems can mimic other diseases

The exanthems may or may not be associated with CNS inflammation. The observed rashes usually resemble rubella, roseola infantum, or adenoviral macular or maculopapular exanthems, but may also appear as vesicular or hemangiomalike lesions. One interesting syndrome is hand-foot-and-mouth disease, which usually affects children and is characterized by a vesicular eruption over the extremities and the oral cavity. Coxsackie A16 virus is the specific enterovirus most frequently implicated, but others, such as enterovirus 71, can cause a similar illness. Herpangina is an enanthematous (mucous membrane) disease characterized by the acute onset of fever and sore throat. Characteristic small vesicles or white papules (lymphonodules) surrounded by a red halo are seen over the posterior half of the palate, pharynx, and tonsillar areas. This mild, self-limiting (1–2 weeks) illness has usually been associated with infection by several different Coxsackie A serotypes.

Hand-foot-and-mouth disease

Herpangina

Epidemic myalgia

Epidemic myalgia (pleurodynia, or Bornholm disease) is characterized by fever and sudden onset of intense upper abdominal or lower thoracic pain, often accompanied by a frontal headache. The pain may be aggravated by movement, such as breathing or coughing, and usually persists for 3–14 days. Coxsackie B viruses are most frequently implicated.

Generalized disease of newborn

Generalized disease of the newborn is a highly lethal expression of enteroviral infection, in which the infant may be overwhelmed by simultaneous virus infection of the heart, brain, liver, and other organs.

Other diseases

It is apparent from Table 37.2 that the spectrum of disease produced by these viruses is enormous, and recent observations suggest that many other illnesses may also result from infections by this subgroup. Recently, epidemics of acute hemorrhagic keratoconjunctivitis associated with enterovirus 70 have been reported in Asia, and localized outbreaks of disease resembling paralytic poliomyelitis caused by enterovirus 71 infection have occurred in Bulgaria and the United States. In addition, there is some recent evidence that certain enteroviruses, particularly Coxsackie B serotypes, may somehow participate in the pathogenesis of at least some cases of insulin-dependent diabetes mellitus, acute arthritis, polymyositis, hemolytic–uremic syndrome, and idiopathic acute nephritis. At the moment, however, such associations between these viruses and the diseases mentioned have not been elucidated; further investigation will be required to establish whether or not they are significant.

Additional Reading and References

Horstmann, D.M. 1982. Control of poliomyelitis: A continuing paradox. *J. Infect. Dis.* 146:540–551. A good discussion of pathogenesis and problems in prevention.

Ray, C.G. 1983. Coxsackievirus and echovirus infections. In *Infectious Diseases.* 3rd ed. P.D. Hoeprich, Ed. New York: Harper & Row, pp. 1289–1299. A review of the clinical and epidemiological features of enteroviral infections.

Lawrence Corey

Hepatitis Virus

38

Viral hepatitis

Hepatitis means inflammation of the liver, and as a disease entity, it has been recognized since the days of Hippocrates. The causes of hepatitis are varied and include viruses, bacteria, and protozoa, as well as drugs and toxins (for example, isoniazid, carbon tetrachloride, and ethanol). The clinical symptoms and course of acute hepatitis can be similar, regardless of etiology, and determination of a specific cause depends primarily on 1) epidemiologic and clinical history; 2) use of laboratory tests for the detection of viruses or other causes; 3) microscopic findings of liver biopsy; and 4) long-term clinical course. The nomenclature *viral hepatitis* has become synonymous with hepatitis A, hepatitis B, and the presumed viral agents of non-A non-B hepatitis; others, however, such as Epstein–Barr virus, cytomegalovirus, varicella-zoster virus, and yellow fever viruses can also cause inflammation of the liver. The major characteristics of the three principal causes of viral hepatitis are summarized in Table 38.1.

Hepatitis A

Biology of the Agent

Virus first detected by immune electron microscopy

Much of our knowledge of the hepatitis A virus (also known as *infectious hepatitis* and *short-incubation hepatitis*) has been derived from the use of immunologic detection methods and by purification of the agent from infected animals or human tissues. In 1973, Feinstone et al., using the technique of immune electron microscopy, examined extracts of stools collected early in the course of infectious hepatitis. Sera from convalescent cases were used as the source of antibody. Antigen–antibody complexes, which involved clumps of viral particles, were demonstrated. Subsequent studies in animals and humans with this technique indicated that this virus was the etiologic agent of the disease now termed hepatitis A.

Unenveloped, small RNA virus of single serotype

Has only been grown in specialized tissue cultures

Hepatitis A virus is an unenveloped RNA-containing virus with cubic symmetry and a diameter of 27 nm (Figure 38.1). It is not inactivated by ether, and it is stable at $-20°C$ and low pH. These properties are similar to those of the picornavirus group, especially the enteroviruses. At present, only one serotype of hepatitis A virus has been demonstrated. Recently the virus has been successfully cultivated in primary marmoset liver tissue cultures and in fetal rhesus monkey kidney cell cultures. However, these cell lines are not available in most clinical virology laboratories.

Table 38.1 Comparison of A, B, and Non-A Non-B Hepatitis

Feature	A	B	Non-A Non-B
Virus type	RNA	DNA	Unknown
Cultured in vitro	Yes	No	No
Incubation period (days)	15–45 (mean, 25)	7–160 (mean, 60–90)	15–160 (mean, 50)
Onset	Usually sudden	Usually slow	Insidious
Age preference	Children, young adults	All ages	All ages
Transmission			
Fecal–oral	+++	+/−	Maybe
Sexual	+	++	Maybe
Transfusion	—	++	+++
Severity	Medium	Often severe	Moderate
Chronicity	None	10%	30% after transfusion
Carrier state	None	Yes	Yes
Immune serum globulin protective[a]	Yes	Yes	Equivocal
Serologic detection methods	Yes	Yes	No

Plus signs indicate relative frequencies.
[a]Hyperimmune globulin more protective.

Human infection

Humans appear to be the major natural hosts of hepatitis A virus. Several other primates (for example, chimpanzees and marmosets), however, are susceptible to experimental infection, and natural infections of these animals may occur.

Clinical Disease

mean incubation period of 25 days

signs and symptoms of acute hepatitis

The most commonly recognized manifestation of hepatitis A virus infection is acute hepatitis. The incubation period of 14–40 days (mean, 25 days) is usually followed by acute onset of fever, anorexia (poor appetite), nausea, pain in the right upper abdominal quadrant, and, within several days, jaundice. Dark urine and clay-colored stools may be noticed by the patient 1–5 days before the onset of clinical jaundice. The liver is enlarged and tender, and serum transaminase and bilirubin levels are elevated as a result of hepatic inflammation and damage.

most cases subclinical

Many persons who have serologic evidence of acute hepatitis A infection are asymptomatic or only mildly ill, without jaundice (anicteric hepatitis A). The infection-to-disease ratio for hepatitis virus is dependent on age; it may

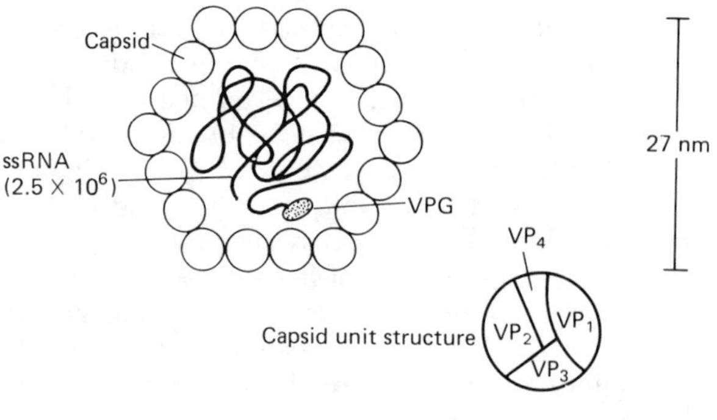

38.1 Diagram of the proposed structure of the hepatitis A virus. The protein capsid is made up of four viral polypeptides (VP_1 to VP_4). Inside the capsid is a single-stranded molecule of RNA (molecular weight 2.5×10^6), which has a genomic viral protein (VPG) on the 5′ end. (*Reproduced by kind permission of Dr. J.A. Hoofnagle and of Abbott Laboratories, Diagnostic Division, North Chicago, Illinois.*)

Does not lead to chronic viral hepatitis

be as high as 20:1 in children and approximately 7:1 in older adults. The vast majority of cases of hepatitis A are self-limiting. Chronic hepatitis such as that seen with hepatitis B or non-A non-B hepatitis has not been described. In rare cases, fulminant fatal hepatitis associated with extensive liver necrosis may occur. Only 7% of all such cases, however, appear to be caused by hepatitis A.

Pathogenesis of Infection

virus replicates in intestinal mucosa during incubation period

viremic spread to liver; hepatic response to infection

The virus is believed to replicate initially in the enteric mucosa. It can be demonstrated in feces by electron microscopy for 10–14 days before onset of disease. In most patients with symptoms of the disease, complete virus is no longer found in fecal specimens; viral antigen, however, has been demonstrated in feces for up to 14 days thereafter. Multiplication in the intestines is followed by a period of viremia with spread to the liver. The response to replication in the liver consists of lymphoid cell infiltration, necrosis of liver parenchymal cells, and proliferation of Kupffer cells. The extent of necrosis often coincides with the severity of disease. A variable degree of biliary stasis may be present.

Immune Response

IgM antibody response develops before symptoms

Antibody to hepatitis A virus can be detected during early illness, when the virus is still found in feces, and most patients with symptoms or signs of acute hepatitis A already have detectable antibody in serum. Early antibody responses are predominantly of the immunoglobulin M(IgM) class, which can be detected by radioimmunoassay for several weeks or months. During convalescence, antibody of the IgG class predominates.

later IgG response; long-term immunity

Detectable levels of IgG antibody to hepatitis A virus persist indefinitely in serum, and patients with anti-hepatitis A virus antibodies are immune to reinfection.

Epidemiology

fecal–oral spread

association with crowding and poor hygiene

no chronic carriers

The major mode of spread of hepatitis A virus is fecal–oral. Inoculation of infectious material intramuscularly can produce disease; transmission through blood transfusion, while possible, is not an important means of spread. Most cases of hepatitis A are not linked to a single contaminated source, but occur sporadically. The disease is common under conditions of crowding, and it occurs at high frequency in mental hospitals and schools for the retarded. As a chronic carrier state has not been observed with hepatitis A, perpetuation of the virus in nature presumably depends on sporadic subclinical infections and person-to-person transmission. Outbreaks of hepatitis A have been linked to the ingestion of uncooked seafood, usually shellfish. In most instances, the water in which the shellfish lived was found to be contaminated with human feces.

variations in attack rates

high incidence in developing countries

The disease is widespread, but seroepidemiologic studies have shown marked variation in infection rates among various population groups. For example, rates are higher among those of lower socioeconomic status and among male homosexuals. Less than one-half of the general population of the United States now has serologic evidence of prior hepatitis A virus infection, however, and age-specific prevalence rates are decreasing, apparently because of better sanitation and less crowding. In contrast, in many underdeveloped countries, more than 90% of the adult population shows evidence of previous hepatitis A infection; in most cases, however, the risk of disease in nonimmune adults

evidence is of asymptomatic infection during childhood. The risk of overt disease is much higher in nonimmune infected adults than in children; travelers from developed countries who enter endemic areas are particularly susceptible.

Laboratory Diagnosis

Serodiagnosis

The most common method of laboratory diagnosis of hepatitis A virus is to demonstrate high titers of specific IgM antibody to the virus in serum drawn during the acute phase of illness. Antigen for the test is derived from infected marmoset liver. Because IgG antibody persists indefinitely, its demonstration in a single serum sample is not indicative of recent infection; a rise in titer between acute and convalescent sera must be documented. Immune electron microscopic identification of the viral antigen in fecal specimens remains a research tool at present.

Prevention

role of passive immunization

The administration of immune serum globulin (ISG) before or during the incubation period of the disease has been shown to be about 80–90% effective in preventing clinically apparent type A hepatitis. In some cases, infection occurs, but disease is ameliorated; that is, the patient develops anicteric, usually asymptomatic, hepatitis A. At present, ISG should be administered to household contacts of hepatitis A patients. Once clinical symptoms have appeared, the host is already producing antibody, and administration of ISG is not indicated. Persons from areas of low endemicity traveling to areas with high infection rates should receive ISG before departure and at 3- to 4-month intervals as long as potential heavy exposure continues.

Treatment

There is no specific treatment for patients with acute episodes of hepatitis A infection. Supportive measures include adequate nutrition and rest.

Hepatitis B

Biology of the Agent

Enveloped DNA virus

Hepatitis B virus is an enveloped DNA virus, unrelated to any other human virus. Recently, an animal virus that causes hepatitis and hepatoma in woodchucks has been shown to have a similar structure. A schematic of the hepatitis B virus is illustrated in Figure 38.2. The complete virion (the Dane particle, named for the worker who first saw it by electron microscopy) is a 42-nm, spherical particle that consists of an envelope around a 27-nm core. The core comprises a nuclear capsid that contains the DNA genome.

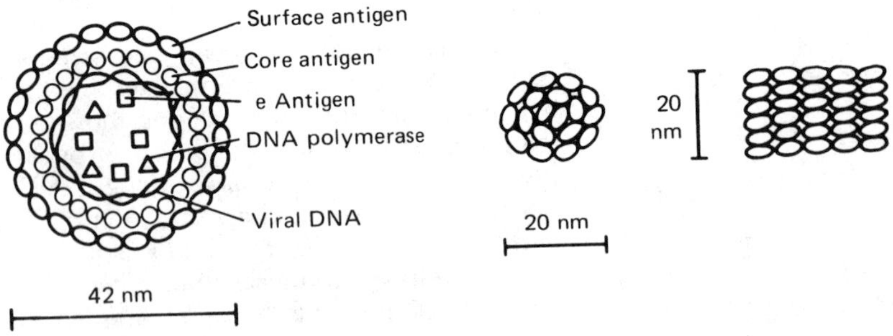

38.2 Schematic diagram of hepatitis B virion. The 42-nm particle is the "Dane particle" or the hepatitis B virus. The 20-nm particles are the filamentous and circular forms of hepatitis B surface antigen or protein coat.

Free nucleocapsids may assume spherical or filamentous shapes with a mean diameter of 22 nm. They are defective particles devoid of DNA.

core comprises DNA genome, DNA polymerase, c and e antigens

The viral genome consists of partially double-stranded DNA with a short, single-stranded piece. It comprises approximately 3000 nucleotides. Closely associated with the viral DNA is a DNA polymerase. Other components of the core are a hepatitis B core antigen (HBcAg) and the hepatitis B e antigen (HBeAg), a glycoprotein believed important in assembling the core and envelope structures of the virus.

envelope antigen, HBsAg

The envelope of the virus contains the hepatitis B surface antigen (HBsAg), formerly called *hepatitis-associated antigen* or *Australia antigen*. This antigen has been shown to possess a group-specific determinant, termed *a*, and two sets of mutually exclusive subtype determinants, *d* and *y* and *w* and *r*. Thus, there are four major subtypes of hepatitis B surface antigen, and adw, ayw, adr, and ayr denote the phenotypes of the virion. These subtypes are important in epidemiologic typing, but not in immunity, because there is antigenic cross-reactivity and cross-protection between subtypes. The HBsAg was the first antigen of the hepatitis B virus to be identified. Aggregates, often found in great abundance in serum, are an indication that intact infectious virions are also present. In infected liver tissue, evidence of HBcAg and HBeAg are found in the nuclei of hepatocytes, whereas HBsAg is found in the cytoplasm.

HBsAg in serum indicates presence of infectious virus

Virus not yet propagated in tissue culture

Despite extensive attempts, hepatitis B virus has not been propagated in the laboratory. Humans appear to be the major host; as with hepatitis A, however, infection of subhuman primates has been accomplished experimentally.

Clinical Disease

variable incubation period (mean, 10 weeks)

Symptoms and signs

The clinical picture of hepatitis B is highly variable. The incubation period may be as brief as 7 days or as long as 160 days (mean, approximately 10 weeks). Acute hepatitis B is usually manifested by the gradual onset of fatigue, loss of appetite, nausea, pain, and fullness in the right upper abdominal quadrant. Early in the course of disease, pain and swelling of the joints and occasionally frank arthritis may occur. Some patients develop a rash. With increasing involvement of the liver, there is increasing cholestasis and, hence, clay-colored stools, darkening of the urine, and jaundice. Symptoms may persist for several months before finally resolving.

course sometimes prolonged

anicteric cases common

can cause chronic hepatitis with HBsAg in serum

In general, the symptoms associated with hepatitis B are more severe and more prolonged than those of hepatitis A; however, anicteric disease and asymptomatic infection occur. The infection-to-disease ratio, which varies according to age and method of acquisition, has been estimated to be approximately 6–7:1. One important difference between hepatitis A and hepatitis B is the development of chronic hepatitis in approximately 10% of patients with hepatitis B infection. This development is associated with ongoing replication of virus in the liver and usually with the presence of HBsAg in serum. Fulminant hepatitis, leading to extensive liver necrosis and death, develops in less than 1% of cases.

Pathogenesis and Pathology of Infection

HBsAg can appear in most body fluids and secretions

In the past, hepatitis B was best known as a form of posttransfusion hepatitis or as hepatitis associated with the use of illicit parenteral drugs (serum hepatitis). Over the past few years, however, it has become clear that the major mode of acquisition is through close contact with infected secretions or blood of acute cases of disease or of chronic carriers of the virus. Hepatitis transmission by blood or close contact with cases or carriers

vertical transmission to infants

B surface antigen has been found in most body fluids, including saliva, semen, and cervical secretions. Transmission by person-to-person contact has been documented, as has vertical mother-to-child transmission, usually at the time of birth. Under experimental conditions, as little as 1/10,000 ml of infectious blood has produced infection. Transmission is therefore possible by vehicles such as inadequately sterilized hypodermic needles or instruments used in tattooing and ear piercing.

rash and arthritis early in disease from immune complexes

anti-HBs Ag protective

role of cell-mediated immunity

The factors determining the different clinical manifestations of acute hepatitis B are largely unknown; however, some appear to involve the immunologic responses of the host. The serum sickness-like rash and arthritis that may precede the development of symptoms and jaundice appear related to circulating immune complexes that activate the complement system. Antibody to the HBsAg is protective and associated with resolution of the disease. Cellular immunity also may be important in the host response, because patients with depressed T-lymphocyte function have a high frequency of chronic infection with the hepatitis B virus. Antibody to the HBcAg, which appears during infection, is present in chronic carriers with persistent hepatitis B virion production. It does not appear to be protective.

hepatic damage and postnecrotic cirrhosis

The morphologic lesions of acute hepatitis B resemble those of hepatitis A and non-A non-B hepatitis. In chronic active hepatitis B, the continued presence of inflammatory foci of infection results in necrosis of hepatocytes, collapse of the reticular framework of the liver, and progressive fibrosis. The increasing fibrosis can result in the syndrome of postnecrotic hepatic cirrhosis.

Antigenemia and Immune Responses

serum HBsAg associated with acute disease and chronic carriage

The nomenclature of hepatitis B antigens and antibodies is shown in Table 38.2. During the acute episode of disease, when there is active viral replication, large amounts of HBsAg can be detected in the serum, as can fully developed virions (Dane particles) and high levels of DNA polymerase and HBeAg. Although HBcAg is also present, antibody against it invariably

Table 38.2 Nomenclature for Hepatitis B Virus

Abbreviation	Description
HBV	Hepatitis B virus; 42-nm double-shelled virus; Dane particle
HBsAg	Hepatitis B surface antigen; found on surface of virus; formed in excess and seen in serum as 22-nm spherical and tubular particles; four subdeterminants (adw, ayw, adr, and ayr) identified
HBcAg	Core antigen (nucleocapsid core); found in nucleus of infected hepatocytes by immunofluorescence
HBeAg	Glycoprotein; associated with core of virus; utilized epidemiologically as marker of serious potential infectivity; seen only when HBsAg is also present
Anti-HBs	Antibody to HBsAg; correlated with protection against and/or resolution of disease
Anti-HBc	Antibody to HBcAg; seen in acute infection and chronic carriers; utilized as marker of past infection; apparently not important in disease resolution
Anti-HBe	Antibody to HBeAg

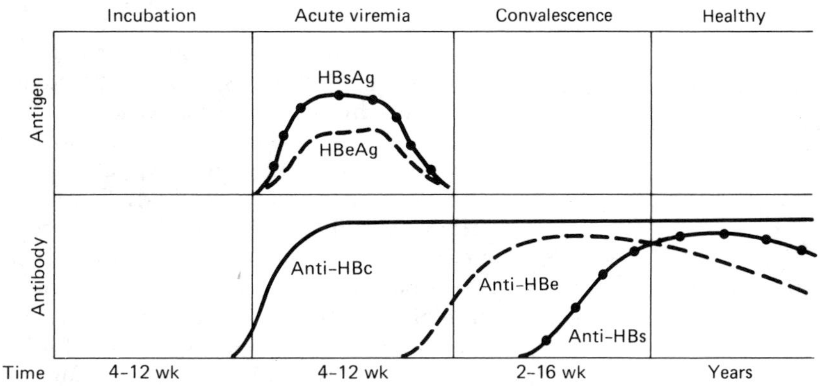

38.3 Sequence of appearance of viral antigens and antibodies in acute cases of hepatitis B. HBsAg = hepatitis B surface antigen; HBeAg = hepatitis B e antigen; anti-HBc = antibody to hepatitis B core antigen; anti-HBe = antibody to HBeAg; anti-HBs = antibody to HBsAg.

anti-HBs associated with elimination of infection and immunity

occurs and prevents its detection. With resolution of acute hepatitis B, HBsAg and HBeAg disappear from serum with the development of antibodies (anti-HBs and anti-HBe) against them. The development of anti-HBs is associated with elimination of infection and protection against reinfection. Anti-HBc is detected early in the couse of disease and persists in serum for years. It is an excellent epidemiologic marker of infection, but is not protective. A schematic diagram of these responses is shown in Figure 38.3.

presence of both HBeAg and HBsAg in chronic carriage suggests continued hepatic damage

In patients with chronic hepatitis B, evidence of viral persistence can be found in serum. As anti-HBs does not develop, HBsAg can be detected throughout the active disease process, which probably accounts for the chronicity of the disease. Anti-HBc is, however, detected. Two types of chronic hepatitis can be distinguished. In one, HBsAg is detected, but not HBeAg; these patients usually show minimal evidence of liver dysfunction. In the other, both antigens are found; the process is more active, with continued hepatic damage that may result in cirrhosis. The occurrence of serum antigen and antibody is shown in Figure 38.4.

Epidemiology

HBsAg-positive carriers main reservoir

Hepatitis B infection is found worldwide, with prevalence rates varying markedly between countries. Chronic carriers of hepatitis B surface antigen (which indicates that intact virus is also present) constitute the main reservoir

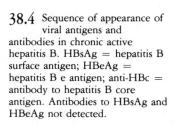

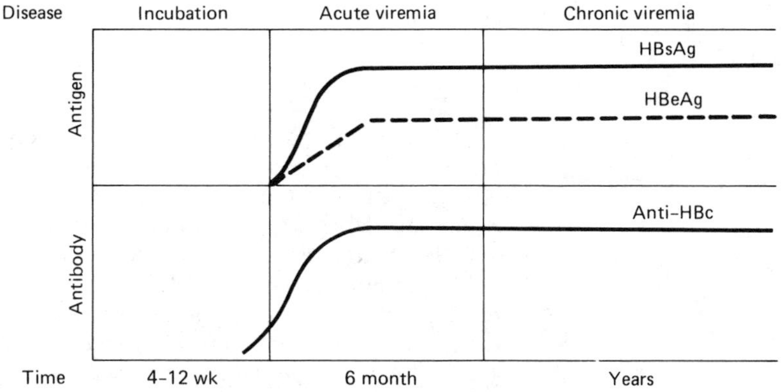

38.4 Sequence of appearance of viral antigens and antibodies in chronic active hepatitis B. HBsAg = hepatitis B surface antigen; HBeAg = hepatitis B e antigen; anti-HBc = antibody to hepatitis B core antigen. Antibodies to HBsAg and HBeAg not detected.

of infection: in some tropical countries as many as 5–15% of all persons are chronic carriers, although most are asymptomatic.

Population groups with higher carrier rates in U.S.

sources of infection

In the United States, it is estimated that 0.1–0.5% of the population comprises chronic carriers of hepatitis B. The occurrence of HBsAg is higher in certain populations, such as male homosexuals, patients on hemodialysis or immunosuppressive therapy, patients with Down's syndrome, and drug addicts using injection methods. Routine screening of blood donors for HBsAg and the elimination of commercial blood banks has markedly decreased the incidence of posttransfusion hepatitis B; 90% of cases developing after transfusion are now caused by non-A non-B hepatitis virus. Some multiple-pool blood products, however, are still significant vehicles of transmission, as are inadequately sterilized, blood-contaminated needles. Exposure to hepatitis viruses from direct contact with blood or other bodily fluids, probably through small lesions, has resulted in sporadic outbreaks of acute viral hepatitis B in medical personnel. Attack rates are also high in spouses and sexual partners of affected patients.

infection at birth associated with development of chronic carriage

Most hepatitis B infection of infants does not appear to be transplacentally transmitted to the fetus in utero, but is acquired by swallowing infected blood or fluids or through abrasions. The rate of virus acquisition is high in infants born to mothers who are suffering from acute hepatitis B infection or carrying HBsAg and HBeAg. Most infants do not develop clinical disease; infection in the neonatal period is associated with failure of antibody production to HBsAg, however, and thus with chronic carriage and epidemiologic perpetuation by transmission in the family setting.

association with hepatic carcinoma

Evidence is strong that persistence of hepatitis B virus can result in the subsequent development of hepatocellular carcinoma. In many parts of Africa and Asia, primary liver cancer accounts for 20–30% of all types of malignancies; this illness has been strongly associated with carriage of hepatitis B virus by serologic tests and by direct detection of viral nucleic acid sequences. In North America, South America, and Europe, primary liver cancer accounts for only 1–2% of all malignancies and tumors.

Laboratory Diagnosis

acute infection and carriage diagnosed by demonstrating serum HBsAg

The laboratory diagnosis of active acute and chronic hepatitis B is best made by demonstrating the HBsAg in serum. Almost all patients who develop jaundice will be HBsAg positive at the time of clinical presentation. In patients with self-limiting anicteric disease, the period of HBsAg detection in serum may be short; other serologic markers, such as antibodies to the core antigen (anti-HBc), may thus help to indicate that the disease was hepatitis B. Past infection with hepatitis B is best determined by detecting anti-HBc, anti-HBs, or both.

Prevention

Passive immunization with HBIG for exposed subjects

Both active and passive prophylaxis of hepatitis B infection can be accomplished. Most preparations of ISG contain only moderate levels of anti-HBs; however, hyperimmune globulin (HBIG) with signficant protective activity is now available. Hyperimmune globulin is prepared from sera of subjects who have high titers of antibody to HBsAg, but are free of the antigen itself. Administration of HBIG soon after exposure to the virus greatly reduces acquisition of symptomatic disease. Currently, it is recommended for prophylaxis in persons who have ingested or been inoculated (for example, by an accidental needle prick) with blood or other materials known or suspected to be HBsAg positive. Administration of HBIG within 48 hr (preferably 2–24 hr) after birth reduces vertical transmission of disease to the infant and may thus eliminate carriage. Second doses of globulin are given after 1 month in adults and 1–3 months in infants.

Prophylaxis for infants of HBsAg-positive mothers

effective vaccine developed from HBsAg

Recently, a hepatitis B vaccine has been developed by purification and inactivation of HBsAg from chronic carriers of the disease. Excellent protection has been shown in studies on homosexual men, medical personnel, and in decreasing vertical transmission. Medical personnel who have frequent contact with blood or blood products should consider receiving hepatitis B vaccine. Recent studies suggest that a combination of passive immunization with HBIG and active immunization with hepatitis B vaccine may be the most effective approach to preventing vertical transmission and for needle stick exposures.

Treatment

Risk of corticosteroid therapy

There is no specific treatment for typical acute viral hepatitis. A high-calorie diet is desirable. Corticosteroid therapy has no value in uncomplicated typical acute viral hepatitis, and recent studies suggest that it may increase the severity of chronic hepatitis caused by hepatitis B virus.

Delta Agent

Recently, a new RNA virus called the Delta agent has been shown to occur in persons with recent or past hepatitis B virus infection. Originally described by Rizetto in Italy, Delta virus infection has been encountered worldwide. The agent is distinct from the hepatitis B virus, but hepatitis B virus infection is a requirement for Delta virus infection. Concomitant infections with both hepatitis B and Delta can occur, but Delta virus infection only occurs alone in those who have chronic or past hepatitis B. Delta virus infection may be asymptomatic or be associated with an exacerbation of hepatitis. The epidemiology of Delta virus infection is similar to that of hepatitis B infection. Parental, nonparental, and vertical transmission have been described.

Non-A Non-B Hepatitis

The curious designation *non-A non-B hepatitis* reflects that little is known about other forms of hepatitis viruses, although 90% of cases of posttransfusion hepatitis are now associated with etiologic agents other than hepatitis A or B. Despite intensive investigation over the past 5 years, the etiologic agent(s) has not been identified.

posttransfusion hepatitis

disease usually mild, but may cause chronic liver damage

Non-A non-B hepatitis is usually insidious in onset, mild, and anicteric, but results in chronic liver disease in many patients. As most transmitters of the disease are asymptomatic, a chronic carrier state is presumed. Transmission to nonhuman primates with development of two distinct pathologic entities has been documented, and two suspected viral candidates have been described. No cross-immunity seems to occur between these two viral candidates.

In addition to its transmission by blood transfusion, non-A non-B hepatitis has occurred in patients undergoing hemodialysis and renal transplantation.

Non-A non-B hepatitis accounts for approximately 20% of cases of sporadic hepatitis presenting for medical evaluation.

probably more than one non-A non-B agent

The occurrence of multiple bouts of non-A non-B hepatitis among drug abusers supports the probability of more than one non-A non-B hepatitis agent. Until further serologic or other experimental markers of infection are developed, knowledge of the pathogenesis, immunology, and epidemiology of the disease(s) will remain incomplete.

Additional Readings and References

Feinstone, S.M., Kapikian, A.Z., and Purcell, R.H. 1973. Hepatitis A: Detection by immune electron microscopy of a viruslike antigen associated with acute illness. *Science* 182:1026–1028. The first description of the hepatitis A virus using immune electron microscopy.

The Hepatitis Knowledge Base: A Prototype Information Transfer System. 1980. *Ann. Intern. Med. (Suppl. 1 Pt. 2)* 93:165–222. A compendium in synoptic form of current knowledge of hepatitis virus.

Krugman, S. 1982. The newly licensed hepatitis B vaccine. Characteristics and indications for use. *J. Am. Med. Assoc.* 247:2012–2015. An up-to-date review of the new hepatitis B vaccine and its use.

Krugman, S., and Gocke, D.J. 1978. Viral hepatitis. In *Major Problems in Internal Medicine.* Vol. XV. Philadelphia: Saunders. A classic monograph by major contributors to knowledge of the disease.

Seeff, L.B., and Hoofnagle, J.H. 1979. Immunoprophylaxis of viral hepatitis. *Gastroenterology* 77:161–182. An excellent consideration of passive immunity in prophylaxis.

Lawrence Corey

Herpesviruses

39

The group *Herpesvirus,* of the family Herpetoviridae, comprises large, enveloped, double-stranded DNA viruses found in both animals and humans. They are ubiquitous and are one of the most commonly acquired infectious agents. The major members of the group to infect humans are two herpes simplex viruses (HSV), cytomegalovirus (CMV), varicella-zoster virus, and Epstein–Barr virus (EBV). Occasionally, the simian herpesvirus, herpes B virus, has caused human disease.

large-enveloped DNA viruses

All herpesviruses are morphologically similar. The nucleic acid core is about 30–45 nm in diameter, surrounded by an icosahedral capsid. The capsid is covered by a glycoprotein envelope. Despite the morphologic similarity between these agents, substantial differences in the molecular composition of the genome are reflected in the structural glycoproteins and polypeptides. Serologic tests can readily differentiate among herpesviruses despite some cross-reactions (for example, between HSV and varicella-zoster viruses).

molecular differences among herpesviruses

Host range differences

The host ranges of these agents under experimental conditions differ considerably. Herpes simplex virus has the widest range; it replicates in numerous animal and human host cells, although it only affects humans in nature. Varicella-zoster is much more restricted; it does not replicate in experimental animals, other than subhuman primates, and is best grown in cells of human origin, although some laboratory-adapted strains can grow in primate cell lines. Human CMV replicates well only in human fibroblast cell lines. Epstein–Barr virus does not replicate in most commonly used cell culture systems, but can be grown in continuous human or primate lymphoblastoid cell cultures.

wide spectrum of diseases

The clinical diseases caused by herpesviruses range from asymptomatic infections to diseases of high morbidity and mortality, such as herpes simplex encephalitis or CMV pneumonia in the immunocompromised patient. Characteristically, all of these agents produce an initial overt infection followed by a period of latent infection in which the genome of the virus is present in the cell, but infectious virus is not recovered (Table 39.1). Reactivation of virus may then result in recurrent infection. Complex host–virus interactions determine the expression of disease. With all of these agents, immunocompromised patients, especially those with altered cellular immunity, have more frequent and severe episodes of disease.

viral latency and disease reactivation

Table 39.1 Major Clinical Syndromes of Herpesviruses in Humans

Virus	Major Clinical Syndrome	Site of Latent Infection
Herpes simplex virus		
Type 1	Gingivostomatitis in children and young adults; recurrent oral–labial infection (cold sores); infection of the cornea (keratitis); herpes encephalitis	Trigeminal nerve root ganglion and autonomic ganglia of superior cervical and vagus nerves
Type 2	Genital herpes; neonatal herpes	Sacral nerve root ganglia
Varicella-zoster	Chickenpox (primary infection); shingles (zoster)	Thoracic nerve root ganglia
Cytomegalovirus	Asymptomatic infection; heterophile-negative mononucleosis; fever hepatitis syndrome in neonates and transplant patients; interstital pneumonia in immunocompromised patients	Leukocytes (neutrophils and lymphocytes)
Epstein–Barr virus	Heterophile-positive mononucleosis	B lymphocytes

Herpes Simplex

Biology of the Agent

HSV-1 and HSV-2

The term *herpes* (from the Greek *herpein,* to creep) and the clinical description of cold sores date back to Hippocrates. Two distinct epidemiologic and antigenic types of HSV exist (HSV-1 and HSV-2). The DNA genomes of both are linear, double-stranded molecules with molecular weights of approximately 10^8. Their nucleic acids demonstrate approximately 50% base-sequence homology, which is considerably greater than that shown between these viruses and other herpesviruses. They share several antigens, including surface glycoproteins and other structural polypeptides. Numerous strains of both HSV-1 and HSV-2 exist. In fact, by restriction endonuclease analysis of the viral genome, most strains of HSV-1 or HSV-2 are found to differ somewhat, except in epidemiologically related cases such as mother–infant or sexual partner transfer.

strain differentiation by restriction endonuclease techniques

Mechanisms of Acute and Latent Infection

HSV viral replication

Herpes simplex virus produces both acute and latent infections, in which the virus–cell interaction and the manifestations of an infection differ. In acute infections, the initial stages entail attachment of the virus to the cell membrane and entry into the cytoplasm. Viral DNA released in the cytoplasm migrates to the nucleus. New viral DNA synthesis and transcription of messenger (m)RNA occurs in the nucleus; mRNA then migrates to the cytoplasm. After translation of virus-specified protein in the cytoplasm, these proteins migrate back to the nucleus, where they encapsulate the viral DNA. The virus "buds" through the nuclear membrane; this process adds the envelope material to the virus particles, which are then released through the cytoplasm.

The molecular events involving synthesis of virus-specific gene products are coordinated and regulated. Three classes of mRNA coding for three groups of virus polypeptides have been identified. The initial products, designated the α-polypeptides, are synthesized 2–4 hr after infection. The exact function of these α-polypeptides, five of which have been identified, is unknown; however, some authorities believe that they may be related to the development of latent infection. The β-polypeptides include virus-specified thymidine kinase and DNA polymerase. These virus-specified enzymes differ from host cell enzymes and are important in chemotherapy, as currently available antiviral drugs inhibit their activity. The synthesis of β-polypeptides shuts off the synthesis of α-polypeptides and induces the synthesis of a third group of polypeptides. The γ-polypeptides, synthesized 12–15 hr after infection, largely represent the structural components of the viral particle.

initially produced α-polypeptides

later β-polypeptides include virus-specified thymidine kinase

γ-polypeptides are structural components of virus

Latent infection of nervous tissue by HSV does not result in the death of the cell; however, the exact mechanism of viral genome interaction with latently infected cells is incompletely understood. As latent infection does not appear to be associated with detectable amounts of β- or γ-polypeptides, antiviral drugs directed at the viral DNA polymerase or thymidine kinase enzymes do not eradicate the virus in its latent state.

latency not associated with detectable β- or γ-polypeptides or whole virions

Diseases Caused by Herpes Simplex Virus, Type 1

Infection with HSV-1 is usually "above the waist." It consists characteristically of grouped or single vesicular lesions that become pustular and coalesce to form single or multiple ulcers. On dry surfaces, these ulcers scab before healing; on mucosal surfaces, they reepithelialize directly. Herpes simplex virus can be isolated from almost all lesions until the crusting stage, but the titer of virus decreases as the lesions progress. Infections generally involve embryonic ectoderm (skin, mouth, vagina, conjunctiva, nervous system). The major clinical manifestations of HSV-1 disease include mucocutaneous superficial infection of the pharynx, skin, and eye and infection of the brain.

vesicular lesions become pustular and ulcerating

Primary infection with HSV-1 is often asymptomatic. When symptomatic, it appears most frequently as gingivostomatitis, usually in 3- to 5-year-old children. There can be fever, irritability, and vesicular or ulcerative lesions involving the buccal mucosa, tongue, gums, and pharnyx. The lesions are quite painful, and the illness usually lasts 5–12 days. After this initial infection, HSV may become latent within sensory nerve root ganglia of the trigeminal nerve.

primary infections often asymptomatic

primary gingivostomatitis in childhood

Lesions usually recur over the anterior buccal mucosa, lips, or perioral area of the face and, because reactivation is usually from a single latent source, are typically unilateral. These lesions are commonly called *cold sores* or *fever blisters*. Symptoms are milder than those with primary infections because of the development of partial immunity. Systemic complaints are unusual, and the episode generally lasts approximately 7 days. It should be noted that HSV may be reactivated and excreted into the saliva with no apparent mucosal lesions present. Herpes simplex virus has been isolated from saliva in 5–8% of children and 1–2% of adults who were asymptomatic at the time.

recurrent cold sores usually unilateral

virus in saliva with asymptomatic reactivation

Herpes simplex virus may also cause pharyngitis, usually in young adults. The disease presents as a sore throat associated with an ulcerative lesion of the posterior pharynx. Pharyngitis is usually a manifestation of primary

Ulcerative pharyngitis

infection; the subsequent history of this infection involves latency in the trigeminal nerve root ganglion, with reactivation of disease manifested by cold sores.

Herpetic whitlow

Herpes simplex virus sometimes infects the finger (Plate Y) and nail area. This infection, termed *herpetic whitlow,* is an occupational hazard of nurses, physicians, and laboratory technicians. It usually results from the inoculation of infected secretions through a small cut in the skin. Painful vesicular lesions of the finger develop and pustulate. These lesions are accompanied by "lymphatic streaking" and epitrochlear and axillary lymphadenopathy. The disease, which often recurs, is frequently misdiagnosed as staphylococcal or streptococcal infection. As with other HSV infections, reactivation and recurrence are possible.

herpetic eye infection and local antiviral treatment

Herpes simplex virus infection of the eye is one of the most common causes of corneal damage and blindness in industrialized nations. Infections usually involve the conjunctiva and cornea, and characteristic dendritic ulcerations are produced. With recurrence of disease, there may be deeper involvement with corneal scarring. Occasionally there may be extension into deeper structures of the eye, especially if topical steroids are used. Debridement of the cornea and topical antiviral therapy with idoxuridine, adenine arabinoside, trifluorothymidine, or acyclovir are effective in ameliorating the course of disease. None of these treatments, however, decreases the rate of recurrence.

Herpes encephalitis

Encephalitis may sometimes result from HSV-1 infection. Herpes encephalitis accounts for approximately 10% of all cases of viral encephalitis in the United States. Only about 1 in 100,000 persons infected with HSV-1, however, will actually develop HSV encephalitis. The pathogenesis of HSV encephalitis is not well understood. Most cases occur in adults with high levels of anti-HSV-1 antibody, suggesting reactivation of latent virus in the trigeminal nerve root ganglion and extension of productive (lytic) infection into the temporal–parietal area of the brain. Alternatively, reinfection with a different strain of HSV with neurotropic spread of the virus from peripheral sites up the olfactory bulb into the brain may also result in parenchymal brain infection. It is unknown why reactivation of disease may result in this devastating complication in a small proportion of latent infections.

encephalitis localized: high mortality if untreated

Classically, the disease affects one temporal lobe, leading to focal neurologic signs and cerebral edema. If untreated, mortality is 70%. Clinically, the disease can resemble brain abscess, tumor, or intracerebral hemorrhage. The virus is easily isolated from brain tissue, and diagnostic brain biopsy remains the most definitive method of diagnosis.

Value of antiviral therapy

Intravenous adenine arabinoside effectively reduces the mortality of the disease. Rapid diagnosis is very important.

Diseases Caused by Herpes Simplex Virus, Type 2

association of HSV-2 with genital herpes

Genital herpes is an important sexually transmitted disease. Both HSV-1 and HSV-2 can cause the disease; however, more than 80% of first episodes of genital HSV infection in the United States are caused by HSV-2. Genital HSV-2 disease is also more likely to recur than genital HSV-1 infection.

Primary genital herpes

Recurrent genital herpes

Primary genital herpes is analogous to primary gingivostomatitis and symptoms such as fever, headache, malaise, and myalgia are commonly present. Characteristically, the patient has multiple (20–30) coalesced, bilaterally distributed, tender lesions of the genital area. Pain, irritation, dysuria, and vaginal or urethral discharge are the predominant local symptoms. In addition, 1–2% of patients develop herpetic aseptic meningitis (Chapter 61). Unlike HSV-1 encephalitis, HSV-2 aseptic meningitis is usually a self-limiting disease with no mortality. Like oral–labial disease, recurrent genital herpes is usually a localized skin infection and lasts for a shorter time than primary infections. Small, vesicular, unilaterally distributed lesions on the genital region are characteristic. The mean duration of viral shedding is 4 days, and lesions usually resolve by 9–12 days after onset. The average number of recurrences seems to be three to five episodes per year. The duration of disease appears to decrease over time.

Neonatal herpes: severe disease with high mortality

Neonatal herpes usually results from transmission of disease during delivery by contact with infected genital secretions from the mother. In utero infection, although possible, is very uncommon. The prevalence rate of neonatal herpes varies greatly depending on the population studied, but is estimated at approximately 1 per 7000 live births in the United States. Because a normal immune response is absent in the neonate, neonatal HSV infection is an extremely severe disease with an overall mortality of more than 60% in untreated subjects. Manifestations may vary; some infants show disseminated vesicular lesions and widespread internal organ involvement. Necrosis of the liver and adrenal glands may occur. The overall mortality of disseminated disease is more than 90%. Some infants, with involvement of the central nervous system only, develop listlessness and seizures; the overall mortality of this syndrome is 50%. Recently, adenine arabinoside has been shown to decrease the mortality of central nervous system neonatal herpes, although the morbidity remains high.

relationship of HSV-2 to carcinoma of the cervix

Epidemiologically, HSV-2 has been associated with cervical carcinoma. A high incidence of HSV-2 antibody in women with cervical carcinoma is found when compared to controls. Viral antigen has been found in the cytoplasm of exfoliated cervical carcinoma cells from preinvasive lesions, virus has been isolated from tissue cultures descended from carcinoma in situ, and HSV-specific mRNA has been detected in tissue specimens of preinvasive cervical carcinoma. All of these data point to an association between HSV-2 and cervical carcinoma; however, whether HSV plays a direct role in its etiology or simply indicates another carcinogenic phenomenon is still unknown.

Pathogenesis of Infection

transmission by contact

initial lesions

Herpes simplex viruses are transmitted through contact with infected lesions or secretions. The incubation period is 2–14 days. Pathologic changes during acute infections consist of development of multinucleated giant cells, ballooning degeneration of epithelial cells, focal necrosis, eosinophilic intranuclear inclusion bodies (Figure 39.1), and an inflammatory response characterized by an initial polymorphonuclear neutrophil infiltrate and a sub-

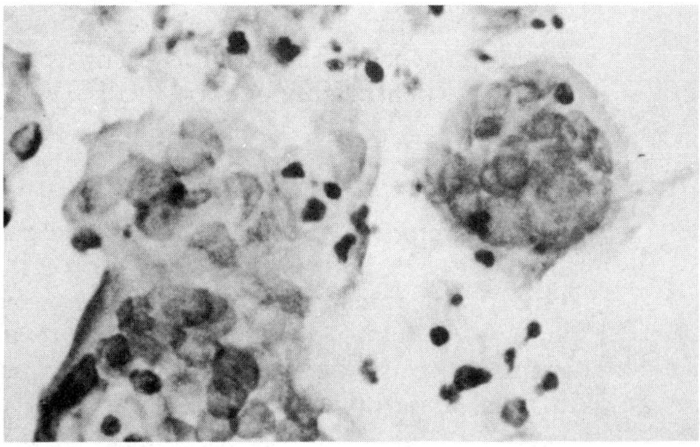

39.1 Multinucleated giant cells from herpes simplex virus lesion.

intraneuronal spread and latent infection

sequent mononuclear cell infiltrate. The virus can spread intra- or interneuronally or through supporting cellular networks of an axon or nerve, resulting in latent infection of sensory and autonomic nervous ganglia. In humans, latent infection by HSV-1 has been demonstrated by cocultivation techniques in trigeminal, superior cervical, and vagal nerve ganglia, and occasionally in the S_2–S_3 dorsal sensory nerve root ganglia. Latent HSV-2 infection has been demonstrated in the sacral (S_2–S_3) region.

Reactivation of latent virus

Reactivation of virus from latently infected ganglionic cells with subsequent release of infectious virions appears to account for most recurrences of both genital and oral–labial infections. The mechanisms by which latent infection is maintained or reactivated are unknown. Two alternative theories have been postulated to explain how latent virus reaches peripheral sites. According to the ganglionic theory, metabolic changes in latently infected cells "switch on" the viral replicative cycle; the virus then travels down the peripheral nerves to the skin, where it replicates in epidermal cells and produces the lesions. An alternative explanation, the skin trigger theory, suggests chronic multiplication of virus in the ganglion with intermittent shedding of the virus through the nerve axon to the skin. Local alterations in host immune status then initiate replication in skin. Precipitating factors that initiate reactivation of herpes simplex are unknown; patients cite sunlight, stress, menstrual periods, and the like as important considerations. Recent data have suggested that occasional episodes of mucocutaneous herpes may be caused by exogenous reinfection with different strains of the same subtype.

ganglionic theory

skin trigger theory

Immunity to Infection

evidence for partial immunity

Host factors have a major effect on clinical manifestations of HSV infection. Many episodes of HSV infection are either asymptomatic or mildly symptomatic. Initial symptomatic clinical episodes of the disease are more severe than recurrent episodes, probably because of the presence of anti-HSV antibodies and immune lymphocytes in persons with recurrent infections. Prior infection with HSV-1 will shorten the duration of symptoms and lessen the severity of first infections with HSV-2.

cell-to-cell transfer in presence of neutralizing antibody

evidence for cell-mediated immunity

Both cellular and humoral immune responses are important in immunity to herpes. Experimentally, neutralizing antibody to HSV can be shown to inactivate extracellular virus; however, the persistence of viral spread through cell-to-cell transfer helps to explain recurrence of HSV in the presence of high titers of neutralizing antibody. Cell-mediated immunity has also been shown to retard viral replication, and recurrences of HSV are clinically of shorter duration and more localized than primary infections. In immunosuppressed patients, especially those with depressed cell-mediated immunity, reactivation of HSV may be associated with prolonged viral excretion and persistence of lesions. Viremia and dissemination through visceral organs has been shown to occur occasionally, even in the presence of detectable neutralizing antibody to HSV.

Epidemiology

contact spread in humans

relationship of spread to socioeconomic status

Herpes simplex viruses have worldwide distribution. There are no known animal vectors, and humans appear to be the only natural reservoir. Direct contact with infected secretions is the principal mode of spread. Seroepidemiologic studies indicate that the prevalence of HSV antibody varies according to the age and socioeconomic status of the population studied. In most underdeveloped countries, 90% of the population have HSV-1 antibody by the age of 30. In the United States, HSV-1 antibody is currently found in approximately 40–60% of middle class populations; among lower socioeconomic groups, however, the percentage approaches 90%.

extent of infection with HSV-2

Detection of HSV-2 antibody before puberty is unusual. The virus is associated with previous sexual activity, and sexual transmission is the major mode of spread. Approximately 20–25% of sexually active adults in Western industrialized countries have HSV-2 antibody. The virus can also be isolated from the cervix and urethra of approximately 5–8% of adults attending sexually transmitted disease clinics; many of these patients are asymptomatic.

Laboratory Diagnosis

Cell culture

Herpes simplex viruses are best demonstrated by isolation from infected secretions or lesions. They grow in a wide variety of cell culture systems and on the chorioallantoic membrane of the chick embryo; most clinical laboratories, however, use diploid fibroblast lines and/or rabbit kidney cells for isolation. The cytopathic effects of HSV, which can usually be demonstrated 24–96 hr after inoculation, are similar for HSV-1 and HSV-2 in most cell systems. Isolates of HSV-1 and HSV-2 can be differentiated presumptively by demonstrating the difference in lesion ("pock") size on the chorioallantoic membranes of the chick embryo: HSV-1 causes small pocks, HSV-2 large pocks. They also differ in their ability to grow in chick embryo monolayers (HSV-2 grows, but not HSV-1) and in their neurotropism in mice (greater for HSV-2 than HSV-1). Definitive separation is serologic, with type-specific antisera, or by restriction enzyme digestion of purified viral DNA, in which each type shows characteristic bands of DNA fragments on agar gel electrophoresis. This technique, which has also revealed numerous subtypes of HSV-1 and HSV-2, can be used to recognize epidemiologically related strains, that is, strains acquired between sexual partners or through mother–infant transmission. Serologic studies can be used to document evidence of past infection. Because of cross-reaction, however, it may be difficult to demonstrate a convincing serologic response to HSV-2 in the presence of high titers of HSV-1 antibody.

Typing procedures

restriction endonuclease analyses

Prevention

Prevention of neonatal infection

No specific form of prevention is available. Avoiding contact with individuals with lesions reduces the risk of spread; however, virus may still be shed asymptomatically from the saliva, urethra, and cervix. Because of the high morbidity and mortality of neonatal infection, special attention must be paid to prevention of spread from infected mothers. In many cases abdominal delivery (cesarean section) may be used to minimize contact of the infant with infected maternal genital secretions. Cesarean section may not be effective if rupture of the membranes precedes delivery.

Treatment

Vidarabine

Several antiviral drugs directed at inhibiting virus-specified enzymes have been developed. Vidarabine (adenine arabinoside) selectively inhibits virus-specified DNA polymerase and hence interferes with viral DNA synthesis. Preferential toxicity for HSV-infected versus noninfected cells has allowed acceptable therapeutic-to-toxic ratios in visceral HSV infections. The drug has been shown to decrease the mortality of HSV encephalitis and, when given systemically, of neonatal infection.

Acyclovir

A recently developed antiviral agent, acyclovir, has been shown to selectively inhibit HSV-1 and -2. Acyclovir is phosphorylated to its monophosphate by HSV specified thymidine kinase, but not cellular kinases. It is then further phosphorylated by cellular kinases to its triphosphate which is a potent inhibitor of the viral DNA polymerase. Recent studies indicate the clinical utility of acyclovir in decreasing the duration of mucocutaneous HSV infections in immunocompromised patients and primary genital HSV infections. To date, no antiviral agents have been developed that decrease the risk of subsequent reactivation of disease.

Varicella-Zoster Virus

Morphologically, varicella-zoster virus is indistinguishable from HSV. In addition, lesions of varicella-zoster may sometimes be confused with those of HSV, and vice versa. As with HSV, pathologic changes in skin consisting of ballooning degeneration of cells, formation of giant cells, and nuclear eosinophilic inclusion bodies are characteristic of the disease. Varicella-zoster virus is more difficult to isolate in cell culture than HSV and grows best in diploid fibroblast cells. Compared with HSV, it has a narrower host range and a slower replicative cycle, and it appears to be less readily released from the cell.

Clinical Disease

Chickenpox virus

Latency and shingles

Varicella-zoster virus produces a primary infection in normal children characterized by a generalized vesicular rash termed *chickenpox.* After clinical infection resolves, the virus may persist for decades in the absence of clinical manifestation. Reactivation of latent virus results in a unilateral vesicular eruption, generally in a dermatomal distribution, that is clinically diagnosed as herpes zoster or "shingles."

Manifestations of chickenpox

The eruptions of varicella generally appear on the back of the head and ears, then spread centrifugally to the face, neck, trunk, and extremities. Involvement of mucous membranes is common, and fever may occur early in the course of disease. Lesions appear in different stages of evolution; this characteristic was one of the major features used to differentiate varicella from smallpox, in which lesions were concentrated on the extremities and appeared at the same stage of disease. Varicella lesions are pruritic (itchy), and the number of vesicles may vary from ten to several hundred.

severe disease in immunocompromised patients

Immunocompromised children may develop progressive varicella, which is associated with prolonged viremia, visceral dissemination, and the development of pneumonia, encephalitis, hepatitis, and/or nephritis. Progressive varicella has an estimated mortality of approximately 20% (Plate Z).

Manifestations of herpes zoster

lesions follow sensory nerve distribution

postherpetic neuralgia

Reactivation of varicella-zoster virus is associated with the disease herpes zoster. Although zoster is seen in patients of all ages, it increases in frequency with advancing age. Clinically, pain in a sensory nerve route distribution may herald the onset of the eruption, which occurs several days to a week or two later. The vesicular eruption is usually unilateral, involving one to three dermatomes (Figure 39.2). New lesions may appear over the first 5–7 days. It is unusual for more than one attack of varicella-zoster to occur in an individual; if recurrent attacks of a vesicular eruption occur in one area of the body, another cause, particularly HSV infections, should be considered. The complications of varicella are varied and depend upon age and host immune factors. Postherpetic neuralgia, which is usually severe pain in the dermatome after resolution of illness, is relatively common in elderly persons. It is not common in younger patients and, although incompletely understood, appears to result from damage to the involved nerve root. Immunosuppressed patients may develop disseminated zoster with visceral

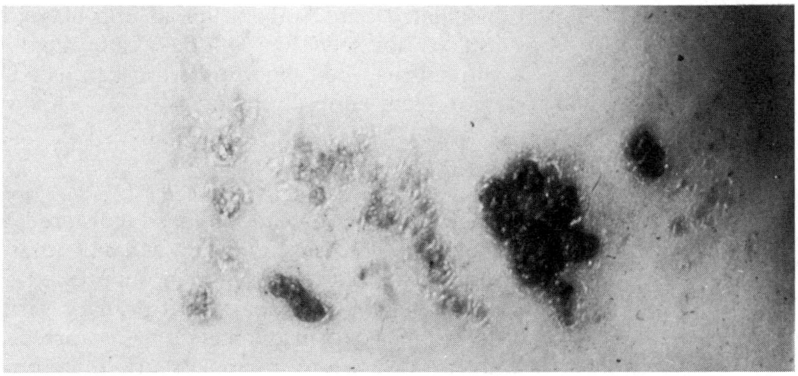

39.2 Herpes zoster lesion of the thorax. Note dermatomal distribution and presence of vesicles, pustules, ulcerated and crusted lesions.

infection, which resembles progressive varicella. Bacterial superinfection is also possible.

Pathogenesis and Immunity

latency of varicella virus in ganglion cells and reactivation to produce zoster

The relationship between zoster and varicella was first described by Von Bokay in 1892, when he observed several instances of varicella in households after the introduction of a case of zoster. On the basis of these epidemiologic observations, he proposed that zoster and varicella were different clinical manifestations of a single agent. The cultivation of varicella-zoster virus in vitro by Weller in 1954 confirmed Bon Bokay's hypothesis: the viruses isolated from chickenpox and from varicella-zoster were identical. Latency of varicella-zoster is believed to occur in the dorsal root ganglia. Unlike herpes simplex, however, varicella-zoster virus has not been "rescued" from ganglion cells by cocultivation techniques. The virus has nonetheless been demonstrated in ganglion and satellite cells by electron microscopy and immunofluorescence at the time of an attack of zoster.

circulating antibody prevents reinfection; cell-mediated immunity controls reactivation

As with HSV, both humoral and cell-mediated immunity are important in varicella-zoster. Circulating antibody prevents reinfection, and cell-mediated immunity appears to control reactivation. In patients with depressed cell-mediated immune responses, especially those with bone marrow transplants, Hodgkin's disease, or lymphoproliferative disorders, zoster infections are more frequent and more severe.

Epidemiology

infection usually by respiratory route and before adulthood

Varicella-zoster infection is ubiquitous. Nearly all persons contract the disease before adulthood, and 90% of cases occur before the age of 10. The virus is highly contagious, with attack rates among susceptible contacts of 75%.

Seasonality, incubation period, and infectivity

Varicella occurs most frequently during the winter and spring months. The incubation period is 11–21 days. The major mode of transmission is respiratory, although direct contact with vesicular or pustular lesions may result in disease. Infectivity is greatest 24–48 hr before the onset of rash and lasts 3–4 days into the rash. Virus is rarely isolated from crusted lesions.

Laboratory Diagnosis

diagnosis usually clinical

Varicella or herpes zoster infection can be readily diagnosed clinically. For confirmation, scrapings of lesions in which to look for multinucleated giant cells may be useful. The virus can be isolated from aspirated vesicular fluid rapid diagnosis with fluorescent antibody

inoculated onto human diploid fibroblasts; however, cytopathic effects are usually not seen for 5–9 days. For rapid viral diagnosis, varicella-zoster antigen may be demonstrated in exfoliated cells from lesions by immunofluorescent antibody staining.

Prevention

passive immunization of exposed immunocompromised children

High-titer immune globulin administered within 72 hr after exposure is useful in decreasing infection and ameliorating disease in patients at risk of serious complications. Immunosuppressed children who are household or play contacts of patients with primary varicella are candidates for immunoprophylaxis. Once infection has occurred, high-titer immune globulin has not proved useful in ameliorating disease or preventing dissemination. In nonimmunosuppressed children varicella is a relatively mild disease, and passive immunization is not indicated. Varicella is a highly contagious disease, and rigid isolation precautions must be instituted in all hospitalized cases. An experimental live vaccine, developed by a group of Japanese workers, is now under investigation. Target populations include children at high risk of complications.

need for isolation of cases in hospital

Treatment

antiviral chemotherapy in immunocompromised patients

Uncomplicated varicella or zoster requires no specific therapy. Analgesics are often required for the severe pain of postherpetic neuralgia. Recently, controlled trials have been undertaken to evaluate the use of vidarabine and interferon in the treatment of herpes zoster in immunocompromised patients. Both studies have indicated that these substances speed healing, decrease the rate of dissemination, and prevent postherpetic neuralgia in these patients. It is not yet clear which of the two products is better. Acyclovir, shown to have potent in vitro activity against varicella-zoster, is also under clinical evaluation. Immunosuppressed patients with zoster and those who develop evidence of visceral dissemination of disease are candidates for antiviral chemotherapy.

Cytomegalovirus

nuclear and perinuclear cytoplasmic inclusions

Human CMV possesses the largest genome of the herpes viruses. It produces cytopathic effects in tissue culture more slowly than varicella-zoster virus and HSV. In addition to the nuclear inclusions characteristic of HSV and varicella-zoster, CMV produces perinuclear cytoplasmic inclusions and can cause latent infection of leukocytes. Clinical manifestations of CMV infection vary with the age, antibody status, and immune response of the patient.

Clinical Syndromes Caused by Cytomegalovirus

teratogenicity of congenital CMV infections

Clinical syndromes associated with CMV are listed in Table 39.2. The most serious is congenital CMV disease. Worldwide, 1% of infants excrete CMV in urine or nasopharynx at delivery as a result of infection in utero. On physical examination, 90% of these infants appear normal; however, long-term follow-up has indicated that 20% will go on to develop sensory nerve hearing loss and/or psychomotor mental retardation. The infants with symptomatic illness (about 0.1% of all births) may have a variety of congenital defects or other disorders (hepatosplenomegaly, jaundice, anemia, thrombocytopenia, low birth weight, microcephaly, and chorioretinitis).

acquired neonatal infection asymptomatic or mild

In contrast to these devastating findings with some congenital infections, acquired neonatal infection appears to be associated with no adverse outcome. Most population-based studies have indicated that 10–15% of all

Table 39.2 Diseases Associated with Cytomegalovirus Infections

Neonatal infection
Congenital infection
Symptomatic
Asymptomatic at birth, subsequent neurologic impairment
Acquired infection (usually asymptomatic)
Infection of children and adults
Heterophile-negative mononucleosis
Interstitial pneumonia
Postperfusion syndrome
Posttransplantation (fever, hepatitis) syndrome
Granulomatous hepatitis
Guillain–Barré syndrome
Rare cases of encephalitis
Genitourinary syndromes
? Cervicitis
? Urethral syndrome

mothers are excreting CMV from the cervix at delivery. Approximately one-third to one-half of all infants born to mothers excreting CMV at delivery will acquire disease. Almost all of these postnatally infected infants have no discernible illness. Infection is only determined if cultures for CMV from urine or nasopharynx are performed. Follow-up of these infants has also shown no incidence of neurologic abnormalities.

CMV pneumonia in immunosuppressed patients

As with intrapartum acquisition of disease, most CMV infections during childhood and adulthood are totally asymptomatic. In young adults, CMV may cause a mononucleosislike syndrome. In immunosuppressed patients, latent CMV may be reactivated, possibly resulting in diffuse involvement of the lung and severe hypoxia (CMV pneumonia). In patients receiving bone marrow transplants, interstitial pneumonia caused by CMV is the leading cause of death (90% mortality).

No effective prevention and/or treatment of CMV exists at present. Studies of interferon for therapy for CMV infections in immunocompromised patients are presently under way.

Epidemiology and Transmission

high infection rates in early childhood and early adulthood

viral latency in leukocyte precursors

transmission by blood transfusion

Cytomegalovirus is ubiquitous, and at least 80% of adults have antibody to it. Age-specific prevalence rates show very high rates of acquisition of infection during the first 5 years of life, after which they level off. The rate subsequently increases during young adulthood, probably through sexual transmission of disease. The virus has been isolated from saliva, cervical secretions, semen and urine, and white blood cells; it may be present and can be isolated from patients with circulating neutralizing antibody. Latent infection, which may reside primarily in leukocytes and their precursors, accounts for transfusion-associated disease. In a recent study, more than one-third of infants born to CMV-negative mothers who received blood from donors with CMV antibody subsequently developed infection. Although most infections from transfusions of CMV-contaminated blood may be asymptomatic, persistent fever, hepatitis, and/or pneumonitis may occur. Granulocyte transfusions may also lead to transmission of CMV. Virus may be excreted in urine or from the cervix for long periods; in infants, high titers have been isolated from urine for more than 5 years after birth. Because of the high prevalence of asymptomatic carriers and the known tendency of CMV to persist for weeks or months in infected individuals, it is frequently difficult to definitely associate a specific disease entity with the isolation of the virus from a peripheral site. Thus, the isolation of CMV from urine of immunosuppressed patients with interstitial pneumonia does not constitute evidence of CMV as the etiology of that illness. The virus must be isolated from the lung.

Laboratory Diagnosis

cell culture, serodiagnosis, and detection of inclusion-bearing cells

Laboratory diagnosis of CMV infection depends on isolating the virus, finding virus particles in body fluid by electron microscopy, or demonstrating a rise in antibody titer. Cytomegalovirus can be grown readily in serially propagated diploid fibroblast cell strains. Demonstration of cytopathic effect generally requires 3–14 days, depending on the concentration of virus in the specimen. The presence of large inclusion-bearing cells in urine sediment may be detected in widespread CMV infection. This technique is insensitive, however, and provides positive results only when large quantities of virus are present in the urine.

Epstein–Barr Virus

etiologic agent of heterophile-positive infectious mononucleosis

cultivation in lymphoblastoid cell lines

EBV-infected cultured cells are transformed

latency and reactivation in epidermal cells

persistent excretion

Epstein–Barr virus is the most recently described of the human herpesviruses. It was discovered in 1964 during the search for a suspected viral etiology of African Burkitt's lymphoma. Infection with EBV is common, worldwide, and usually occurs as a subclinical infection in early childhood. The virus has been established as the etiologic agent of "heterophile-positive" infectious mononucleosis. Although morphologically similar to the other herpesviruses, EBV is unique in that it can be cultured only in lymphoblastoid cell lines derived from B lymphocytes of humans and higher primates. The virus generally does not produce cytopathic effects in infected cells or the characteristic intranuclear inclusions of other herpesvirus infections. After infection with EBV, lymphoblastoid cells containing viral genome can be cultivated continuously in vitro; they are thus transformed, or immortalized. Recent studies suggest that most of the viral DNA in transformed cells remains in circular, nonintegrated form as an episome. Some cell lines produce mature virions, which can be detected by demonstrating capsid antigen with immunofluorescence. Other cell lines, called *nonproducers,* contain no evidence of mature virions, although certain virus-associated antigens may still be detected. Recently, latency has been detected in epidermal cells and reactivation shown to occur in vivo. During episodes of infectious mononucleosis, EBV can be cultured from saliva of some asymptomatic patients. Excretion may persist for weeks or months.

Clinical Disease

widespread asymptomatic infection: disease most common in young adults

infectious mononucleosis syndrome

Infection is widespread. Antibodies to EBV, shown in all population groups studied, are usually found in 90–95% of adults. Most early infections are asymptomatic; clinically apparent EBV infection occurs most frequently in populations in which primary EBV exposure has been delayed until the second decade of life. The disease is thus seen most often in young adults; it consists of a constellation of clinical findings, including fever, lymphadenopathy (especially in the cervical area), sore throat, and fatigue and malaise, which may last from days to several weeks. Laboratory examination reveals a markedly raised lymphocyte and monocyte count with more than 10% atypical lymphocytes, called *Downey cells* (Figure 39.3). Alterations in liver function tests may also occur, and enlargement of the liver and spleen

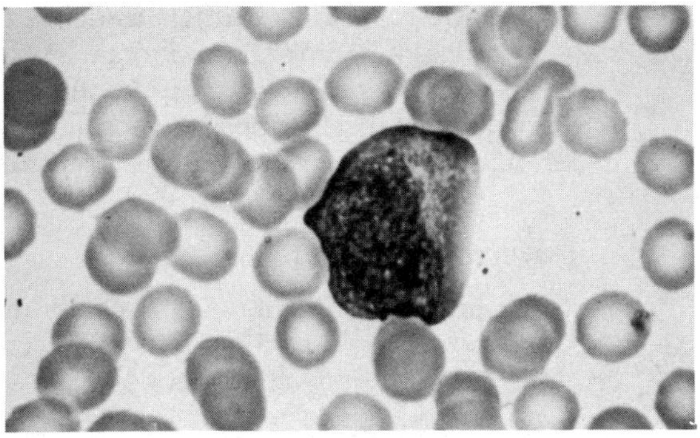

39.3 Atypical lymphocyte (Downey cell) in blood smear from a patient with infectious mononucleosis. Note indented cell membrane.

is a frequent finding. During acute disease, EBV can be isolated from throat washings. Seroconversion and high titers of immunoglobulin M antibody to EBV capsid antigen are usually present.

Immune Response

antiviral and heterophile antibodies

Virus-induced infectious mononucleosis results in the synthesis of circulating antibodies against viral antigens, as well as against unrelated antigens found in sheep, horse, and some beef red blood cells. These heterophile antibodies, a heterogeneous group of predominantly IgM antibodies long known to correlate with episodes of infectious mononucleosis, are commonly used as diagnostic tests for the disease. They do not cross-react with antibodies specific for EBV, and there is no good correlation between the heterophile antibody titer and the severity of illness. Some other immunologic functions are also effected by EBV infection. Cutaneous anergy and decreased cellular immune responses to mitogens and antigens are seen early in the course of mononucleosis.

decreased cellular immune responses

atypical lymphocytes in infectious mononucleosis

The lymphocytosis associated with infectious mononucleosis is caused by an increase in the number of circulating T cells. It has been hypothesized that the atypical lymphocytes are activated cells developed in response to the virus-infected B lymphocytes. With recovery from illness, the atypical lymphocytosis gradually resolves and cell-mediated immune functions return to preinfection levels. The virus may be cultivated intermittently from oropharyngeal washings and blood for 12–18 months after recovery from infectious mononucleosis. Immunosuppressed patients have a higher frequency of EBV in saliva than immunocompetent patients; the virus can be cultured from throat washings from 10–20% of normal healthy adults and from 50% of renal transplant recipients.

viral carriage

Epidemiology

low contagiousness: spread by repeated contact

The most likely route of initial EBV infection is via the oropharynx; large numbers of EBV are present in throat washings from patients with infectious mononucleosis. The virus is a widespread agent of low contagiousness; most cases of infectious mononucleosis are contracted after repeated contact between susceptible persons and those asymptomatically shedding the virus. Secondary attack rates of infectious mononucleosis are low (less than 10%), because most family or household members already have antibody to the agent. Infectious mononucleosis has also been transmitted by blood transfusion, and infections have developed after open heart surgery. Most transfusion-associated mononucleosis syndromes, however, are attributable to CMV virus.

secondary attack rates low

Involvement of EBV in Burkitt's lymphoma and nasopharyngeal carcinoma

Epidemiologic studies strongly associate EBV with African Burkitt's lymphoma and nasopharyngeal carcinoma. The exact relationship between EBV and these neoplasms is currently undefined, because host genetic and environmental factors also appear to account for some of the varied incidences, manifestations, and associations between these illnesses.

Laboratory Diagnosis

Heterophile antibody test

Tests for heterophile antibodies, recently modified as the *Monospot test,* are used most commonly for diagnosis of infectious mononucleosis. In the heterophile antibody test, the patient's serum is first absorbed with guinea pig kidney homogenate to remove cross-reacting antibodies that may develop in other situations, such as serum sickness. With infectious mononucleosis, heterophile antibody is still present and is usually detected by agglutination of sheep red blood cells. The heterophile antibody titer is the highest dilution of the absorbed serum to agglutinate these erythrocytes.

Tests for antiviral antibodies

Virus-specific antibodies to the EBV viral capsid antigen or nuclear antigen can also be determined. These antibodies are specific for the virus and can be utilized to document infection. The most commonly used test is antibody to the viral capsid antigen. Titers to the EBV capsid antigen rise quickly in disease and persist for life. Antibodies to the nuclear antigen rise later in disease (after about 1 month) and also persist in low titers for life. Thus, a high titer to viral capsid antigen and no titer to nuclear antigen are indicative of recent EBV infection, whereas antibody titers to both antigens are indicative of past infection. In the last few years, virus specific serologic diagnosis of EBV infections has been used increasingly. This test is especially important in young children (less than 6 years of age), who do not produce heterophile antibodies with acute EBV infections.

Treatment and Prevention

Treatment of infectious mononucleosis is largely supportive. More than 95% of patients recover uneventfully. In a small percentage of patients, splenic rupture may occur; thus, restriction of contact sports or heavy lifting during the acute illness is recommended. Specific antiviral chemotherapy against EBV is currently unavailable. The DNA polymerase enzyme of EBV has been shown to be sensitive to acyclovir, and acyclovir can decrease the amount of replication of EBV in tissue culture. Viral replication increases once administration of the drug is discontinued. No vaccine is available.

Additional Reading and References

Herpes Simplex Virus

Corey, L. 1982. The diagnosis and treatment of genital herpes. *J. Am. Med. Assoc.* 248:1041–1050. A recent review of genital herpes and antiherpes therapy.

Overall, J.C., Jr. 1979. Viral dermatologic diseases. In *Antiviral Agents and Viral Diseases of Man.* G.J. Galasso, T.C. Merigan, and R.A. Buchanan, Eds. New York: Raven, pp. 305–384. An overview of herpes simplex viral epidemiology and pathogenesis.

Cytomegalovirus

Ho, M. 1982. *Cytomegalovirus, Biology and Infection.* New York: Plenum. An up-to-date monograph on cytomegalovirus.

Epstein–Barr Virus

Kieff, E., Dambaugh, T., Hellers, M., et al. 1982. The biology and chemistry of Epstein–Barr virus. *J. Infect. Dis.* 146:506–517.

C. George Ray

Viruses of Diarrhea

40

Acute diarrheal disease is an illness, usually of rapid evolution (within several hours), that lasts less than 3 weeks. A variety of infectious agents can be responsible; overall, bacteria and protozoa have been implicated as etiologic agents in approximately 20–25% of cases. In many of the remaining cases, viruses have been considered as the cause. Unfortunately, investigations have been hampered because most of these viruses cannot be readily cultivated in the laboratory. Viruses that can be cultivated, such as enteroviruses and many adenoviruses, replicate in the intestinal tract; however, epidemiologic studies have failed to implicate them as primary, important causes of acute gastrointestinal disease.

most cultivated with difficulty or not at all

Until the past decade, proof of viral causation of acute diarrhea was usually based on exclusion of known bacterial or protozoan causes and supported by feeding cell-free filtrates of diarrheal stools to human volunteers in an attempt to reproduce the disease. As might be expected, the results of such experiments were variable, and the methods were not applicable to routine laboratory diagnosis.

One aspect of such infections that proved of great help was that many were associated with abundant excretion of virus particles during the acute phase of illness. Particle numbers in excess of 10^8 per gram of diarrheal stool are relatively common; these particles can often be readily visualized with an electron microscope. In recent years, direct electron microscopy and immune electron microscopy have been employed to detect and identify the presumed causative viruses; the latter method can also be used to detect humoral antibody responses to infection.

many viral particles in stool

visualization by electron microscopy

Visualization of a specific virus in the stools of symptomatic patients is not sufficient to establish the role of the virus in causing disease. Other criteria to be fulfilled include the following: 1) establish that the virus is detected in ill patients significantly more frequently than in asymptomatic, appropriately matched controls, and that virus shedding temporally correlates with symptoms; 2) demonstrate significant antibody responses (seroconversion from negative to positive, or a fourfold or greater antibody increase) in acute and convalescent sera from patients shedding the virus; 3) reproduce the disease by experimental inoculation of nonimmune human or animal hosts (usually the most difficult criterion to fulfill); and 4) exclude other known causes of diarrhea, such as bacteria, bacterial toxins, and protozoa. Using these criteria, two groups of viruses have been clearly estab-

Criteria for establishing etiologic relationship

Table 40.1 Biologic and Epidemiologic Characteristics of Viruses Causing Diarrhea

Special Features	Rotavirus	Parvo/picornavirus
Biologic		
Nucleic acid	Double-stranded RNA	Unknown
Diameter, shape	70 nm, naked, double-shelled capsid	24–28 nm, naked, round
Replication in cell culture	Incomplete, poor	None
No. of serotypes	4, perhaps 5	3, perhaps many more
Pathogenetic		
Site of infection	Duodenum; jejunum	Jejunum
Mechanism of immunity	Local intestinal IgA	Unknown (?genetic factors)
Epidemiologic		
Epidemicity	Epidemic or sporadic	Family and community outbreaks
Seasonality	Usually winter	Usually winter
Ages primarily affected	Infants, children < 2 yr old	Older children and adults
Method of transmission	Fecal–oral	Fecal–oral; contaminated water and shellfish
Incubation period (days)	1–3	1–2
Major diagnostic tests	EM, RIA, ELISA	EM, IEM, RIA

Rotaviruses, parvo/picornaviruses, and adenoviruses

Other "candidate" viruses

lished as important causes of gastrointestinal disease: the rotaviruses, the parvo/picornaviruses (Norwalklike agents), and some adenovirus serotypes. Other viruses have also been implicated; as all of the above criteria have not been fulfilled, however, they are currently regarded only as "candidate" causes of gastrointestinal disease.

The currently established and candidate viruses are listed in Table 40.1, in which it can be seen that much remains unknown about most of these viruses. All have several features in common, including a tendency toward brief incubation periods, fecal–oral spread by direct or indirect routes, and production of vomiting, which generally precedes or accompanies the diarrhea. The latter feature has influenced physicians to use the term *acute viral gastroenteritis* to describe the syndrome associated with these agents.

Rotaviruses

Habitat

most common cause of winter gastroenteritis in children < 2 years old

The human intestinal rotaviruses were first found in 1973 by electron microscopic examination of duodenal biopsy specimens from infants with diarrhea. Since then, they have been found worldwide, and they are believed to account for 40–60% of cases of acute gastroenteritis occurring during the cooler months in infants and children less than 2 years of age. Thus far, these viruses have been detected only in intestinal contents and in tissues from the upper gastrointestinal tract.

Group Characteristics

Double-stranded RNA viruses

The rotaviruses belong to the family Reoviridae. They are naked, spherical particles 65–75 nm in diameter (smaller forms have also been described) that contain double-stranded RNA and a double-shelled outer capsid. Their

Table 40.1 *(continued)*

Astrovirus	Calicivirus	Coronaviruslike	Adenovirus
Unknown	Single-stranded RNA	Unknown	Double-stranded DNA
28–38 nm, naked, star shaped	29–33 nm, naked, cuplike surfaces	80–300 nm, enveloped, pleomorphic	70–90 nm, naked, icosahedral
None	None	None	None or incomplete
Unknown	Unknown	Unknown	Unknown
?Small intestine	?Small intestine	?Small intestine	?Small intestine
Unknown	Unknown	Unknown	Unknown
Sporadic	Sporadic	Sporadic	Sporadic
None known	None known	None known	None known
Infants, children	infants, children	Neonates, immunocompromised children and adults	Infants, children
?Fecal–oral	?Fecal–oral	?Fecal–oral; ?Perinatal	Fecal–oral
?1–2	?1–2	?1–2	8–10
EM	EM	EM	EM

Abbreviations: IgA = immunoglobulin A; EM = electron microscopy; IEM = immune electron microscopy; RIA = radioimmunoassay; ELISA = enzyme-linked immunosorbent assay.

name is derived from the Latin *rota* (wheel) because of the outer capsid, which resembles a wheel attached by short spokes to the inner capsid and core (Figure 40.1). At least four serotypes, based on type-specific antigens on the outer capsid, are known to affect humans. Rotaviruses can replicate in the cytoplasm of infected cell cultures in the laboratory, but are difficult to propagate because the replicative cycle is usually incomplete; that is, mature, infectious virions are not produced. However successful propagation of human strains in vitro has been achieved in some instances.

antigenic types based on capsid structure

Animal rotaviruses

interspecies spread not demonstrated in nature

Rotaviruses of animal origin are also highly prevalent and produce acute gastrointestinal disease in a variety of species. The very young, such as calves, suckling mice, piglets, and foals, are particularly susceptible. The animal rotaviruses can often replicate in cell cultures, and infection across species lines has been accomplished experimentally; there is no evidence, however, that such interspecies spread occurs in nature (for example, animal rotaviruses are not known to affect humans, and vice versa). Animal and human rotaviruses share a common group-specific antigen believed to reside on the inner layer of the double-shelled capsid.

Human Rotavirus Infections

short incubation period

vomiting, diarrhea

Clinical outline of disease and outcome. After an incubation period of 1–3 days, there is usually an abrupt onset of vomiting, followed within hours by watery, brown, copious, frequent stools. In severe cases, the stools may become clear; the Japanese refer to the disease as *hakuri,* the white stool diarrhea. Fever, usually low grade, is often present. Vomiting may persist for 1–3 days, and diarrhea for 5–8 days.

The major complications result from severe dehydration, occasionally associated with hypernatremia. This complication can lead to death, particularly in very small or malnourished infants.

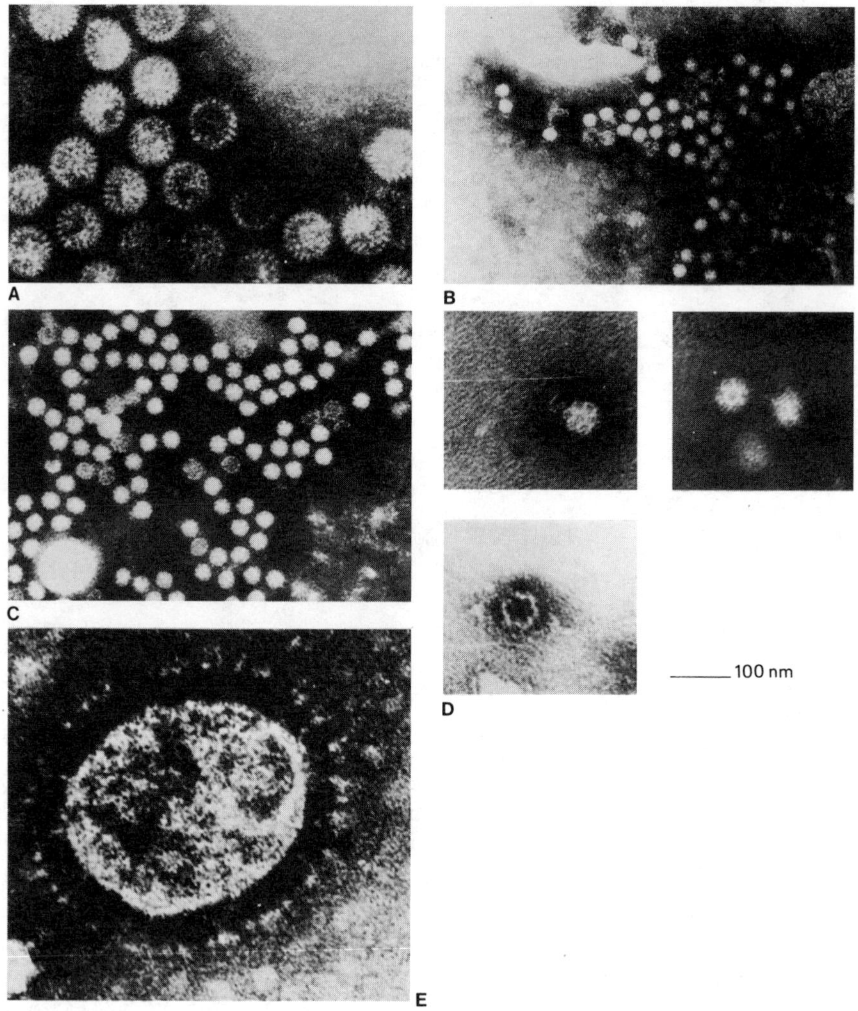

40.1 Viruses of diarrhea. (A) Rotavirus. (B) Parvo/picornavirus. (C) Astrovirus. (D) Calicivirus. (E) Coronaviruslike particle. (*Kindly provided by Claire M. Payne.*)

upper intestinal involvement

Pathogenesis and pathology. Rotaviruses appear to localize primarily in the duodenum and proximal jejunum, causing destruction of villous epithelial cells with blunting (shortening) of villi and variable, usually mild infiltrates of mononuclear and a few polymorphonuclear inflammatory cells within the villi. The gastric and colonic mucosa are unaffected; however, for unknown reasons, gastric emptying time is markedly delayed. The primary pathophysiologic effects are 1) a decrease in absorptive surface in the small intestine, and 2) decreased production of brush border enzymes, such as the disaccharidases. The net result is a transient malabsorptive state, with defective handling of fats and sugars. It may take as long as 3–8 weeks to restore the normal histologic and functional integrity of the damaged mucosa.

transient malabsorptive state

Duration of viral excretion

Viral excretion usually lasts 2–12 days but can be greatly prolonged, with persistent symptoms, in malnourished or immunodeficient patients.

Type-specific humoral and IgA antibodies

Immune responses. Patients with rotavirus infection respond with production of type-specific humoral antibodies that appear to last for years, perhaps a lifetime. In addition, type-specific secretory immunoglobulin A antibodies protective role of breast-feeding

are produced in the intestinal tract. The latter antibodies seem to correlate best with immunity to reinfection. Breast-feeding also seems to play a protective role against rotavirus disease in young infants. This protection is thought to be due to the presence of IgA antibodies to rotaviruses in colostrum and their continued secretion in breast milk for several months post partum.

seasonality and age incidence

Epidemiology. Outbreaks of rotavirus infection are common, particularly during the cooler months, among infants and children 1–24 months of age. Older children and adults can also be affected, but attack rates are usually much lower. Recently, outbreaks among elderly, institutionalized patients have also been recognized.

infection of infants without disease

Although newborn infants can be readily colonized with the virus, such infections often result in little or no clinical illness. This finding is illustrated by reported colonization rates of 32–49% in some neonatal nurseries, but mild illness in only 8–28% of the infants. It is unclear whether this transiently decreased susceptibility to disease is a result of host maturation factors or transplacentally conferred immunity.

most older children and adults immune

Seroepidemiologic studies have been useful in demonstrating the ubiquity of these viruses, and perhaps help to explain the age-specific attack rates. By the age of 4 years, over 90% of individuals have humoral antibodies, suggesting a high rate of virus infection early in life.

Electron microscopic or serologic detection of virus

Laboratory diagnosis. Diagnosis of acute rotavirus infection is usually by detection of virus particles in the stools during the acute phase of illness. Detection can be accomplished by direct examination of the specimen by electron microscopy or by immunologic detection of antigen with enzyme-linked immunosorbent assay or radioimmunoassay methods. In the latter techniques, unlabeled specific antirotavirus antibody is used to "capture" the viral antigen on a solid surface. The antigen is then demonstrated by addition of enzyme- or radioisotope-labeled specific antibody, which attaches to the antigen and can be detected by the presence of a color change when an appropriate substrate for the enzyme is added, or by radioactivity.

Fluid and electrolyte replacement

Treatment and prevention. There is no specific treatment. Vigorous replacement of fluids and electrolytes, often required in severe cases, can be lifesaving.

The rotaviruses are highly infectious and can spread quickly in family and institutional settings. Control consists of rigorous hygienic measures, including careful hand washing, and adequate disposal of enteric excretions.

Theoretically, vaccines could be developed to aid in prevention of these infections. First, however, more must be learned about the immunologic determinants of resistance to infection, and methods must be developed to improve propagation of the viruses in the laboratory.

Parvo/picornaviruses

Although the parvo/picornaviruses were the first to be clearly associated with outbreaks of gastroenteritis, considerably less is known about their biology than about that of the rotaviruses. They were first associated with an outbreak in Norwalk, Ohio, in 1968, and their role was confirmed by production of disease in human volunteers fed fecal filtrates. The original virus was thus called the *Norwalk agent,* and subsequent, similar viruses have been given names such as Hawaii agent, Montgomery County agent, Ditchling agent, and so on. The group is sometimes termed the *Norwalklike viruses.*

Group Characteristics

small, circular viruses

nucleic acid category unknown

several serotypes

not yet grown

The viruses are small, naked, round particles 24–28 nm in diameter; their appearance is similar to that of the DNA-containing parvoviruses and hepatitis A virus (Figure 40.1). At present, their nucleic acid content is unknown; thus, they are temporarily known as parvo/picornaviruses. The viruses appear to be extremely hardy; their infectivity persists after exposure to acid, ether, and heat.

Several different serotypes have been demonstrated by immune electron microscopy with convalescent sera from affected patients. Knowledge of the antigenic characteristics and biology of these viruses has been seriously hampered by the current inability to grow them in the laboratory and by their lack of known pathogenicity for animals.

Infections Caused by Parvo/picornaviruses

clinical picture similar to that of rotavirus infection

Clinical outline of disease and outcome. The incubation period is 1–2 days, followed by abrupt onset of vomiting and diarrhea—a syndrome clinically indistinguishable from that caused by rotaviruses. Respiratory symptoms rarely coexist, and the duration of illness is relatively brief (usually 1–2 days).

Pathogenesis and pathology. Both the pathogenesis and the pathology are similar to those described for rotaviruses. The mucosal changes usually revert to normal within 2 weeks after onset of illness. Virus shedding in the feces generally lasts no more than 3–4 days.

reinfection can occur

Immune responses. Patients and experimentally infected volunteers respond to infection with the production of humoral antibodies, which persist indefinitely; their role in protection from reinfection, however, appears minimal. Reinfection and illness with the same serotype occurs, and the role of local antibody has not been well defined. It is possible that other nonimmune or genetic factors are essential for protection.

seasonal incidence

Winter vomiting disease

older children and adults usually affected

Epidemiology. Family and community outbreaks are common, particularly during the cooler months. The high infectivity, sharp outbreaks, clinical symptoms, and seasonal predilection have given rise to the term *winter vomiting disease.* Unlike rotaviruses, the parvo/picornaviruses are a much more common cause of gastrointestinal illness in older children and adults. This difference in age-specific predilection is perhaps reflected in serosurveys, which have shown that the prevalence of antibodies to Norwalk agent rises slowly, reaching approximately 50% by the fifth decade of life—a striking contrast to the frequent acquisition of antibodies to rotaviruses early in life. Transmission is primarily fecal–oral; outbreaks have also been associated with consumption of contaminated water and shellfish.

diagnostic tests similar to those for rotavirus infection

Laboratory diagnosis. These viruses can be detected by electron microscopy or immune electron microscopy in stools during the acute phase of illness. In addition, radioimmunoassay methods have been developed for detection of antigen as well as for measurement of humoral antibody responses to infection.

Prevention and treatment. As with rotavirus infection, there is no specific treatment other than fluid and electrolyte replacement. Prevention requires good hygienic measures.

Adenoviruses and Candidate Viruses

Some adenoviruses, most of which are exceedingly difficult to cultivate in vitro (in contrast to those associated with respiratory diseases), are now recognized as significant intestinal pathogens. They may account for an estimated 5–15% of all viral gastroenteritis in young children. These include serotypes 38, 40 and 41.

Other viruses associated with gastrointestinal diseases include astroviruses, caliciviruses, coronaviruslike agents, and some coxsackie A viruses (the latter primarily cause gastrointestinal symptoms in severely immunocompromised patients). Characteristics of the major ones are listed in Table 40.1. This list may grow in the future, and some of the candidates are rapidly becoming accepted as definite causes of such diseases; however, much remains to be learned about their biology and epidemiologic behavior.

Additional Reading and References

Blacklow, N.R., and Cukor, G. 1981. Viral gastroenteritis. *N. Engl. J. Med.* 304:397–406. An excellent review of the viruses involved, with extensive references, is provided.

C. George Ray

Arthropod-Borne and Other Zoonotic Viruses

41

include members of several virus families

The arboviruses (arthropod-borne viruses) comprise more than 400 agents with worldwide distribution. Their name is taken from their mode of transmission, which is primarily by infected bloodsucking insects such as mosquitoes, ticks, and phlebotomus flies (sandflies). Many of these viruses appear to be involved primarily in infections of lower vertebrates; others have not yet been associated with disease in any host. Members of this group are from diverse taxonomic families, including primarily the Togaviridae, Bunyaviridae, Rhabdoviridae, and Reoviridae.

This chapter will describe the arboviruses of greatest importance in human disease; in addition, non-arthropod-borne viruses considered to be of zoonotic origin will be discussed.

Arboviruses

Range of diseases

On a worldwide basis, the most important arboviruses (in terms of amount and seriousness of disease caused) include yellow fever, dengue, Japanese B encephalitis, St. Louis encephalitis, western equine encephalitis, eastern equine encephalitis, Russian spring–summer encephalitis, West Nile fever, and sandfly fever. In addition to dengue and yellow fever, other agents cause outbreaks of severe hemorrhagic disease; however, these latter agents are important only in very restricted areas. They include the viruses of Kyasanur forest disease in India and Omsk hemorrhagic fever in Russia.

Arboviral infections in U.S.

The western equine, eastern equine, St. Louis, and California encephalitis viruses are the most important arboviral agents in the United States. Dengue and yellow fever are present in many tropical areas, including the Caribbean, and Venezuelan equine encephalitis is endemic in Central America. As appropriate vectors still exist, these viruses can and occasionally have spread into nearby areas of the southern United States.

The arboviruses can produce disease ranging from simple, febrile, influenzalike illness to hemorrhagic disease or encephalitis. Representative viruses, their classification, their vectors, and the primary diseases they cause are summarized in Table 41.1.

General Virology

Taxonomy

Most arboviruses are members of the families Togaviridae and Bunyaviridae. In general, the viruses are named according to location of initial isolation (for example, St. Louis encephalitis) or on the basis of disease produced

Table 41.1 Selected Arboviruses of Major Importance to Humans

Family and Genus Member	Major Geographic Distribution	Primary Arthropod Vector	Usual Disease Expression
TOGAVIRIDAE			
Alphavirus			
Western equine encephalitis	North America	Mosquito	Encephalitis
Eastern equine encephalitis	North America	Mosquito	Encephalitis
Venezuelan equine encephalitis	Central and South America	Mosquito	Encephalitis
Chikungunya	Africa and Asia	Mosquito	Febrile illness
Flavirus			
St. Louis encephalitis	North America	Mosquito	Encephalitis
Dengue	All tropical zones	Mosquito	Febrile illness or hemorrhagic fever
Yellow fever	Africa, South America, and Caribbean	Mosquito	Hemorrhagic fever
West Nile fever	Africa	Mosquito	Febrile illness
Murray Valley encephalitis	Australia	Mosquito	Encephalitis
Russian Spring–Summer encephalitis	Eastern Soviet Union and Central Europe	Tick	Encephalitis
Powassan	Canada	Tick	Encephalitis
Japanese B encephalitis	Japan, Korea, and Philippines	Mosquito	Encephalitis
BUNYAVIRIDAE			
Bunyavirus			
California	North America	Mosquito	Encephalitis
Bunyamwera	Africa	Mosquito	Febrile illness
Rift Valley fever	Africa	Mosquito	Febrile illness
Sandfly fever	Mediterranean	Phlebotomus	Febrile illness
REOVIRIDAE			
Orbivirus			
Colorado tick fever	North America	Tick	Febrile illness

(for example, yellow fever). It has been possible, however, to assign most to one or another virus family on the basis of morphologic and biochemical features, and some to genera within the families on the basis of antigenic relationships. For example, the St. Louis encephalitis and dengue viruses are both members of the family Togaviridae, and they share antigens common to the genus *Flavivirus.* These antigenic similarities can be detected by serologic tests such as complement fixation or hemagglutination inhibition. The following sections provide a general description of the families represented by major arboviruses of importance in human disease.

Single-stranded RNA enveloped virion

Togaviridae. Togaviruses are enveloped virions containing single-stranded RNA and measuring 40–70 nm in external diameter. The envelope contains a hemagglutinin and lipoproteins. The lipid of the envelope is an essential component, and lipid solvents such as ether and deoxycholate can readily inactivate these viruses. They replicate in the cytoplasm of infected cells and mature by budding from cytoplasmic membranes. Replication can occur in cells of infected arthropods and vertebrate hosts.

The two genera of togaviruses in which most arthropod-borne viruses are classified are *Alphavirus* and *Flavivirus*; rubella virus (*Rubivirus*) is also a togavirus, but it is not arthropod-borne. Viruses within each of these genera are serologically related to one another, but not to other togaviruses. Representatives are listed in Table 41.1.

Single-stranded RNA enveloped virion

Bunyaviridae. Bunyaviruses are enveloped and contain single-stranded RNA. They are spherical, measuring approximately 90–100 nm in external diameter. Like the togaviruses, they replicate in the cytoplasm of infected cells; however, they mature by budding into smooth-surfaced vesicles in or near the Golgi region. The LaCrosse and snowshoe hare antigenic subtypes of California virus are the most important bunyaviruses in North America.

Double-stranded nonenveloped virion

Reoviridae. The most important North American arbovirus of the family Reoviridae is Colorado tick fever. A member of the genus *Orbivirus*, it possesses double-stranded RNA in a nonenveloped virion of cubic symmetry that measures about 80 nm in diameter.

Growth in the Laboratory and Diagnosis

intracerebral inoculation of newborn mice

The arboviruses may be isolated in various culture systems; for most agents, however, intracerebral inoculation of newborn mice is used, which often results in encephalitis and death.

virus from blood and infected tissue

The viruses may be found in the blood (viremia) from a few days before onset of symptoms through the first 1–2 days of illness; attempts at isolation from blood, however, are generally useful only when viremia is more prolonged, as in dengue, Colorado tick fever, and some of the hemorrhagic fever viruses. Virus is not present in the stool and is rarely found in the throat; viral recovery from cerebrospinal fluid is also unusual. Virus can be isolated readily from affected tissue during the acute phase of illness, but this approach is seldom practical in diagnosis. Specific diagnosis is usually accomplished by serologic techniques, using acute and convalescent sera. Various tests have been utilized, including hemagglutination inhibition, complement fixation, and virus neutralization methods. Other serologic tests, such as precipitin and enzyme-linked immunosorbent assay techniques, have also been employed in selected instances.

serodiagnosis

Pathogenesis and Pathology

Arthropod infection and transmission

As noted previously, the arboviruses can infect cells of arthropods, humans, and a variety of lower vertebrate hosts. Infection in the arthropod usually does not appear to harm the insect; a period of virus multiplication (extrinsic incubation period) is required, however, to enhance the capacity to transmit infection by bite. The consequences of infection transmitted from the arthropod to suceptible vertebrate hosts are variable; some will develop illness of varying severity, with transient viremia, whereas others will become viremic without clinical disease. Vertebrate hosts can be a source of further spread of the virus by *amplification*, in which noninfected arthropods feeding

Virus amplification in vertebrate hosts

on viremic hosts acquire the virus, thereby increasing the risk of transmission. Transient viremia is often insufficient, however, to sustain transmission of the viruses for an appreciable length of time; those affected, including humans and higher vertebrates (for example, horses and cattle), are often referred to as *blind-end hosts.*

blind-ended infections

significance of vertebrate reservoir

In contrast, if viremia is sustained for longer periods (for example, a week or longer in dengue, yellow fever, and Colorado tick fever in humans; weeks to months in a variety of togavirus and bunyavirus infections in lower vertebrates), the vertebrate host becomes highly important as a reservoir for continuing transmission.

Mechanisms of overwintering in arthropods

Obviously, the usual arthropod vectors are rarely present during all seasons. The question then arises of how the arboviruses survive between the time the vector disappears, then reappears in subsequent years. Several mechanisms can operate to sustain the virus between transmission periods (often referred to as *overwintering*): 1) Sustained viremia in lower vertebrates such as small mammals, birds, and snakes, from which newly mature arthropods can be infected when taking a blood meal; 2) hibernation of infected adult arthropods that survive from one season to the next; and 3) transovarial transmission, whereby the infected female arthropod can transmit virus to its progeny.

viremia

localization in target organs

Infection of the human by a biting arthropod is followed by viremia, which is apparently amplified by extensive virus replication in the reticuloendothelial system and vascular endothelium. After replication the virus becomes localized in various target organs, depending upon its tropism, and illness results. The viruses produce cell necrosis with resultant inflammation, which leads to fever in nearly all infections.

CNS infection with aseptic meningitis or encephalitis

If the major viral tropism is for the central nervous system, virus reaching this site by crossing the blood–brain barrier or along neutral pathways can cause meningeal inflammation (aseptic meningitis) or neuronal dysfunction (encephalitis). The central nervous system pathology consists of meningeal and perivascular mononuclear cell infiltrates, degeneration of neurons with neuronophagia, and occasionally destruction of the supporting structure of neurons.

Liver tropism and hemorrhage in yellow fever

In some infections, especially yellow fever, the liver is the primary target organ. Pathologic findings include hyaline necrosis of hepatocytes, which produces cytoplasmic eosinophilic masses called *Councilman bodies.* Degenerative changes in the renal tubules and myocardium may also be seen, as well as microscopic hemorrhages throughout the brain. Hemorrhage is a major feature of yellow fever, largely because of the lack of liver-produced clotting factors as a result of liver necrosis.

Other hemorrhagic fevers

Effect of dengue virus on vascular system

increased vascular permeability and DIC

Hemorrhagic fevers other than those related to primary hepatic destruction have a somewhat different pathogenesis, which has been studied most extensively in dengue infections. In uncomplicated dengue fever, which is associated with a rash and influenzalike symptoms, there are changes in the small dermal blood vessels. These alterations include endothelial cell swelling and perivascular edema with mononuclear cell infiltration. More severe infection (dengue hemorrhagic fever [DHF], often complicated by shock) is characterized by widespread effusions into serous cavities such as the pleura, hemorrhage, and perivascular edema. The spleen and lymph nodes show hyperplasia of lymphoid and plasma cell elements, and there is focal necrosis in the liver. The pathophysiology seems related to increased vascular permeability and disseminated intravascular coagulation, which is further complicated by liver and bone marrow dysfunction (for example, decreased platelet production, decreased production of liver-dependent clotting factors). The major vascular abnormalities may be provoked by circulating

Immune-complex contribution to disease

virus–antibody complexes (immune complexes), which mediate activation of complement and subsequent release of vasoactive amines. The precise reason for this phenomenon is not clear; it may be related to the intrinsic virulence of the virus strain involved and to host susceptibility factors. Two hypotheses are based on the existence of four distinct but antigenically related serotypes of dengue virus, any of which can generate group-specific cross-reacting antibodies, which are not necessarily protective against other serotypes. One possibility is that preexisting group specific antibody at a critical concentration serves as "enhancing" rather than neutralizing antibody. In the presence of enhancing antibody, virus antibody complexes are more efficiently adsorbed to and engulfed by leukocytes and macrophages. Subsequent replication leads to spread throughout the host. Alternatively, or in concert with this, activation of previously sensitized T cells by viral antigen present on the surfaces of macrophages may result in release of lymphokines, which mediate the development of shock and hemorrhage.

possible enhancing effect of antibody on the infection

possible effects of lymphokines

Immune Responses

The usual humoral antibody responses (hemagglutination inhibition, complement fixation, neutralization, precipitation) in relation to onset of illness are illustrated in Figure 41.1. One exception to this general pattern is Colorado tick fever, in which increases in complement fixation antibody titer may be delayed by 3–6 weeks. The rise in antibody titer generally correlates with recovery from infection. Neutralizing antibodies, which are the most serotype specific, generally persist for many years after infection. Hemagglutination inhibition and complement fixation antibodies to togaviruses and bunyaviruses are group specific; that is, they do not always clearly distinguish between members of a specific genus, such as the flaviviruses. Hemagglutination inhibition antibodies may persist for several years after infection, whereas complement fixation antibodies are relatively short-lived; the presence of the latter suggests relatively recent infection (within 1–2 years). Immunity to reinfection is serotype specific and appears to be permanent.

Epidemiology

Most are zoonoses involving lower vertebrates and arthropods

With the possible exception of urban dengue and sandfly fever, all arbovirus diseases are zoonoses; that is, their basic reservoir mechanism involves both arthropods and lower vertebrates, which typically experience only subclinical

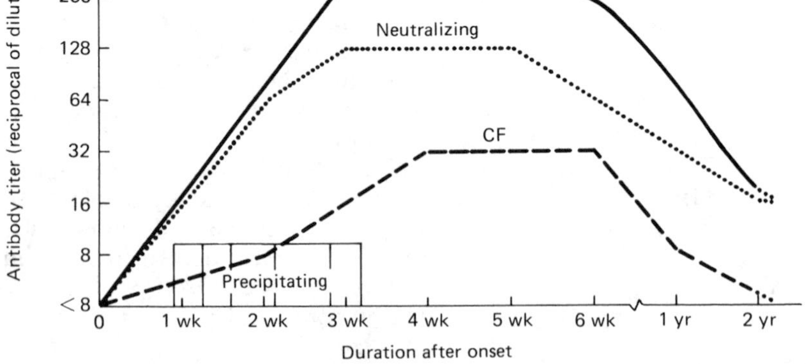

41.1 Typical patterns of antibody response after arbovirus infection. HI = hemagglutination inhibition antibodies; CF = complement fixation antibodies; precipitating = precipitating antibodies detected by immunodiffusion (sometimes used in diagnosis of California virus encephalitis).

infections. For most, human infection is a blind end in the chain of transmission.

Seasonal incidence

In temperate climates such as the United States, arboviruses are major causes of disease during the summer and early fall months, the season of greatest activity of the arthropod vectors (usually mosquitoes or ticks). When climatic conditions and ecologic circumstances (for example, swamps and ponds) are optimal for arthropod breeding and egg hatching, arbovirus amplification may begin.

Amplification

An example of amplification is provided by western equine encephalitis. When the mosquito vectors become abundant, the level of transmission among the basic reservoir hosts (birds and small mammals) increases, and the mosquitoes also turn to other susceptible species such as domestic fowl. These hosts experience a rapidly developing asymptomatic viremia, which permits still more arthropods to become infected upon biting. At this point, spread to blind-end hosts such as humans or horses becomes likely, with the development of clinical disease. This occurrence depends upon the accessibility of the host to the infected mosquito and on mosquito feeding preferences, which for unknown reasons vary from one season to another.

The several basic cycles of arbovirus transmission are as follows.

Examples of cycles

Urban. As the term suggests, the urban cycle is favored by the presence of relatively large numbers of humans living in close proximity to arthropod (usually mosquito) species capable of virus transmission. The cycle is

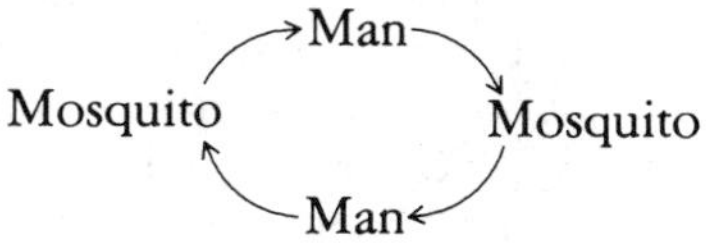

Examples of this cycle include urban dengue, urban yellow fever, and the occasional urban outbreaks of St. Louis encephalitis.

Sylvatic or jungle. In the sylvatic cycle, a single nonhuman vertebrate reservoir may be involved as follows:

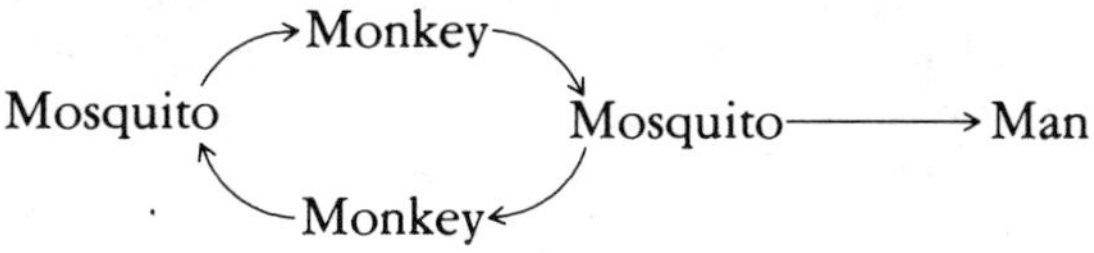

In this situation the human, who becomes a tangential host through accidental intrusion into a zoonotic transmission cycle, is not important in maintaining the infection cycle. An example of this cycle is jungle yellow fever.

In contrast, multiple vertebrate reservoirs may be involved in this cycle:

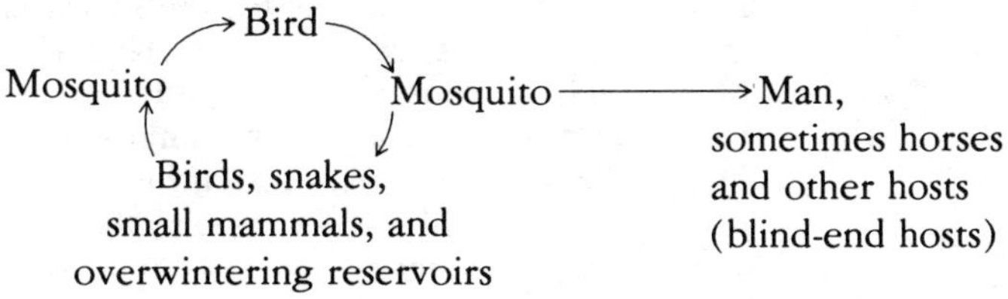

Examples of this cycle include the western equine encephalitis, eastern equine encephalitis, and California viruses. In some situations, such as St. Louis encephalitis and yellow fever, the urban and sylvatic cycles may operate concurrently.

Arthropod sustained. Arthropods, expecially ticks, may sustain the reservoir by transovarial transmission of virus to their progeny, with abetment of the cycle by spread to and from small mammals:

$$\text{Small mammals} \Longleftrightarrow \begin{matrix} \text{Tick} \\ \downarrow \\ \text{Tick} \\ \downarrow \\ \text{Tick} \end{matrix} \mapsto \left\{ \begin{matrix} \text{Man} \\ \text{Cattle} \\ \text{Goats} \\ \text{(Blind-end} \\ \text{hosts)} \end{matrix} \right\} \longrightarrow \begin{matrix} \text{Man (via milk,} \\ \text{an aberrant} \\ \text{pathway)} \end{matrix}$$

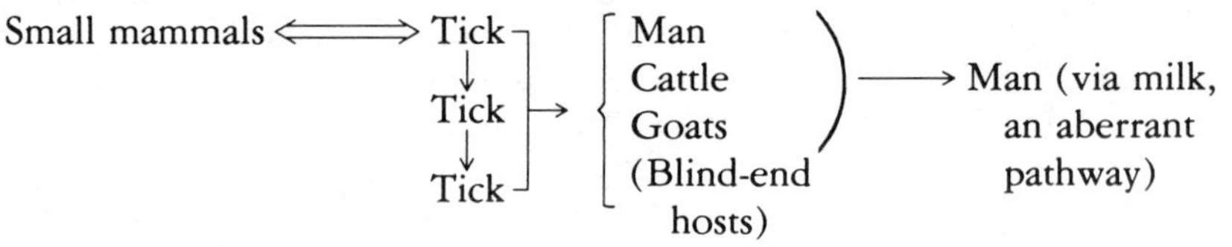

Tick-borne encephalitis in the Soviet Union is transmitted by this cycle.

Treatment and Prevention

Arthropod
vector control

Other than supportive care, there is no specific treatment for arboviral infections. Prevention is primarily by avoidance of contact with potentially infected arthropods, a task that can be extremely difficult, even with the use of adequate screening and insect repellents. In some settings, vector control can be accomplished by elimination of arthropod breeding sites (pools and the like) and sometimes by attempts to eradicate the arthropods with careful use of insecticides. Such measures have been highly effective in the control of urban yellow fever, in which elimination of urban breeding sites and attempts to eradicate the principal mosquito vector species (*Aëdes aegypti*) have been used. Those viruses maintained in complex sylvatic cycles, however, are considerably more difficult to control without risking major environmental disruption and inestimable expense.

Equine
encephalitis
vaccines

Live attenuated
yellow fever vaccine

Vaccines are available for immunization of horses against western and Venezuelan equine encephalitis virus infections; the latter vaccine has also been used for some laboratory personnel who work with the virus. The only other arbovirus vaccine in general use for humans is a live, attenuated yellow fever virus vaccine (17-D strain), which is used to protect rural populations exposed to the sylvatic cycle and for international travelers to endemic areas. In fact, many countries in tropical Africa, Asia, and South America require proof of yellow fever vaccination before allowing travelers to enter. A single subcutaneous dose results in the appearance of antibodies that persist for at least 16–19 years, which correlates well with protective immunity. If booster doses are desired, they need not be given more than once every 10 years to maintain protection.

Specific Arboviruses of Major Importance

Western United
States and
midwest

Western equine encephalitis. The agent that causes western equine encephalitis is prevalent in the western United States, particularly in the central valley of California, eastern Washington (Yakima Valley), Colorado, and Texas. It has also been responsible for outbreaks in midwestern states (Minnesota, Wisconsin, Illinois, Missouri, and Kansas) and as far east as New Jersey. Horses and humans represent blind-end hosts; both are susceptible to infection and illness, commonly manifested as encephalitis. Although human infection in endemic areas is commonplace, overall only 1 of 1000 infections results in clinical illness. In young infants (under 1 year of age), however, 1 of every 25 infections may produce severe illness. The attack rates are therefore far higher in young infants than in other groups.

infection in
humans common:
disease rare

Aseptic meningitis:
encephalitis

The disease spectrum may range from mild, nonspecific febrile illness to aseptic meningitis or severe, overwhelming encephalitis. Mortality is estimated at 5% for cases of encephalitis. It is a very serious disease in infants severity in infants

less than 1 year of age: as many as 60% of survivors have permanent neurologic impairment.

Atlantic seaboard of United States

mosquito, bird, horse cycle

major morbidity in children

Eastern equine encephalitis. The eastern equine encephalitis virus is largely confined to the Atlantic seaboard states from New England down the coast of Florida, although it may extend down the Atlantic coast of Central and South America. The mosquito vector generally restricts its feeding to horses and birds, although occasional outbreaks among humans have occurred. The virus can cause severe encephalitis in horses and also in wild pheasants. The attack rate in humans is highest in infants and children; the mortality in this group is estimated at 20% or greater, and the incidence of severe sequelae among survivors is high.

major morbidity and mortality in adults

St. Louis encephalitis. The St. Louis encephalitis virus is a major cause of arbovirus encephalitis in the United States. Although its geographic distribution is similar to that of western equine encephalitis, it has been much more active in eastern states, Texas, Mississippi, and Florida. It infects but causes no disease in horses. The disease spectrum is similar to that of western equine encephalitis, but the major morbidity and mortality as well as the highest attack rates are among adults over 40 years of age. Infants and young children are relatively spared.

major occurrence in midwest

highest attack rates age 5–18

California virus. Although California virus was first isolated in that state, its major distribution in the United States has been in the Midwest; outbreaks are particularly prevalent in Wisconsin, Ohio, Minnesota, and Indiana. Studies elsewhere in North America and throughout the world, however, indicate that California virus or closely related agents are present nearly everywhere. In the upper midwestern states of Wisconsin and Minnesota, California virus is considered the most important cause of encephalitis. Both the primary mosquito vector (*Aëdes triseriatus*) and human hosts are commonly encountered in suburban or rural environments. Unlike those of the western equine, eastern equine, and St. Louis encephalitis viruses, the highest attack rates are seen in those aged 5–18 years. Infection is often characterized by abrupt onset of encephalitis, often with seizures.

Central and South America and Africa

Nonencephalitic systemic disease involving liver

Yellow fever. Geographically, yellow fever is distributed throughout the Caribbean, Central America, the Amazon Valley in South America, and a broad central zone in Africa from the Atlantic coast to the Sudan and Ethiopia. It continues to be a potential threat to the southeastern United States because of the presence of an urban vector (*Aëdes aegypti*) in that area.

The clinical disease is characterized by abrupt onset of fever, chills, headache, and hemorrhage; it may progress to severe vomiting (sometimes with gastric hemorrhage), bradycardia, jaundice, and shock. If the patient recovers from the acute episode, there are no long-term sequelae.

Middle East, Africa, Far East, and Caribbean

Nonencephalitic systemic disease, sometimes hemorrhagic

Dengue. There are four related serotypes of dengue, any of which may exist concurrently in a given endemic area. These agents are widespread throughout the world, particularly in the Middle East, Africa, the Far East, and the Caribbean Islands, and they have invaded the United States in the past. The vector (*Aëdes aegypti*) is the same as the domestic vector of yellow fever. The known transmission cycle is man–mosquito–man, although a sylvatic cycle involving monkeys may also exist.

The characteristic clinical illness usually results in fever, severe pain in the back, head, muscles, and joints, and erythematous rash. Especially in the Far East (the Philippines, Thailand, and India), the disease has periodically assumed a severe form characterized by shock, pleural effusion, and hemorrhage (DHF), often followed by death.

Japanese B encephalitis. The *Flavivirus* species that causes Japanese B encephalitis is prevalent on the eastern coast of Asia, on its offshore islands (Japan, Taiwan, and Indonesia), and in India. Its transmission cycle resembles that of the St. Louis encephalitis and western equine encephalitis viruses. A high proportion of human infections are subclinical, especially in children; when encephalitis does develop, however, it is severe and often fatal.

Powassan virus. Powassan virus is the only known tick-borne *Flavivirus* species of North America. First isolated in Ontario from a fatal case of encephalitis, it has been found in infected ticks in Ontario, British Columbia, and Colorado. Its significance to humans is not yet established, as only a few cases of encephalitis proved to be caused by this agent have been described. Serologic evidence, however, suggests that the virus is prevalent in many areas of North America.

Tick-borne encephalitis

Colorado tick fever. The tick-borne *Orbivirus* species that causes Colorado tick fever has been found throughout the western United States, including Washington, Oregon, Colorado, and Idaho, and also on Long Island. It is frequently found in *Dermacentor andersoni,* which are also vectors for *Rickettsia rickettsii.* The typical illness, which occurs 3–6 days after the tick bite, is characterized by a sudden onset with headache, muscle pains, fever, and occasionally encephalitis. It is estimated that no more than one clinical illness occurs for every 100 infections with this agent.

Arenaviruses

Enveloped single-stranded RNA virions containing host ribosomes

The family Arenaviridae comprises enveloped spherical or pleomorphic viruses containing single-stranded RNA in several segments and measuring 50–300 nm in diameter. They mature by budding from host cell cytoplasmic membranes and contain host cell ribosomes in their interior. These ribosomes confer a granular appearance to the viruses, hence their name (from the Latin *arenosus,* sandy). They can be isolated by inoculation of clinical specimens (blood, cerebrospinal fluid, and the like) into mice, hamsters, guinea pigs, and a variety of tissue cultures.

reservoir in small rodents

vertical transmission

A common feature of the arenaviruses is their zoonotic reservoir, particularly small rodents, in which they may be sustained for long periods. Primary infection of mature rodents often results in disease and death, whereas intrauterine or perinatal infection (vertical transmission) usually leads to chronic lifelong viremia with persistent shedding of virus into the feces, urine, and respiratory secretions. Although chronically infected rodents are somewhat tolerant to the virus (that is, infection is persistent without causing illness), they do produce antibodies, and evidence of deleterious effects can be found in older hosts, usually in the form of immune-complex glomerulonephritis. The viruses are perpetuated by vertical transmission from infected mothers to their offspring. When environmental contact becomes close, spread from the rodent reservoir to humans (and, in some instances, subhuman primates) can occur via aerosols, through exposure to infective urine, feces, or tissues, or directly by rodent bites.

spread to humans

Lymphocytic Choriomeningitis Virus

human chronic meningititis or meningoencephalitis from contact with rodents

Infection with lymphocytic choriomeningitis virus is particularly common in hamsters and mice. In the United States, most human illnesses have been traced to contact with rodent breeding colonies in research or pet supply centers and to pet hamsters in the home. The illness usually consists of fever, headache, and myalgia, although meningitis or meningoencephalitis also occurs occasionally. Such central nervous system infections, which may persist for as long as 3 months, have been associated with transient hydrocephalus; cerebrospinal fluid lymphocytosis (sometimes with eosinophils), elevated protein levels, and transiently decreased glucose values are also common.

The diagnosis is suggested by a history of rodent contact. The virus may be isolated in the early stages of disease by intracerebral inoculation of blood or cerebrospinal fluid into weanling mice or young guinea pigs. More commonly, the diagnosis is confirmed by serologic testing of acute and convalescent sera using complement fixation, indirect immunofluorescence, or neutralization tests. No person-to-person transmission of infection has been documented.

Arenaviruses Associated with Hemorrhagic Fevers

transmission from rodent reservoir or by body fluids

The agents of hemorrhagic fevers are transmitted from infected rodents to humans, although person-to-person spread via contact with secretions and body fluids can also occur readily. The viruses in this group include the South American hemorrhagic fever agents (Junin virus, the cause of Argentinian hemorrhagic fever, and Machupo virus, the cause of Bolivian hemorrhagic fever) and Lassa virus, the cause of Lassa fever in West Africa.

systemic diseases with high mortality

These viruses have pathogenic and pathologic features similar to those described for the arboviruses that cause hemorrhagic fevers; however, the mechanisms involved in the coagulation abnormalities are not understood. All are characterized by fever, usually accompanied by hemorrhagic manifestations, shock, neurologic disturbances, and bradycardia. Lassa fever also frequently causes hepatitis, myocarditis, and exudative pharyngitis. Mortality is estimated to be 10–50% for Lassa fever and 5–30% for the others. All are considered highly dangerous in terms of infectivity. Importation of cases to nonepidemic areas has occurred, with significant risk of spread to medical and laboratory personnel.

risk of nosocomial infection of medical and laboratory staff

The diagnosis is suggested primarily by the recent travel history of the patient and the clinical syndromes. Although virus isolation and serologic diagnosis can be done, *these procedures should not be attempted in a hospital diagnostic laboratory.* Any patient suspected of having such an infection should be immediately isolated and public health authorities notified. Because of the high risk of spread of infection from body fluids and excreta, even routine laboratory studies are best deferred until the diagnosis and proper disposition of specimens can be resolved. Viremia can persist for 1 month, and virus shedding in the urine may continue for more than 2 months after the onset of illness.

Treatment is primarily supportive. Anecdotal reports of the apparent beneficial effects of transfusing immune plasma from donors who have survived the illness have not been confirmed in controlled trials.

Other Viruses of Apparent Zoonotic Origin

Marburg and Ebola Viruses

Marburg virus transmitted from infected monkey

The association of the Marburg virus with serious disease did not become apparent until 1967, when 26 cases of hemorrhagic fever occurred among persons in Germany and Yugoslavia who were handling a group of African green monkeys imported from central Uganda. The agent was later identified as Marburg virus, apparently transmitted by the infected monkeys. In 1975 it was associated with a similar disease in three travelers in South Africa, and in 1980 in Kenya.

Ebola virus outbreaks in Zaire and Sudan

In 1976, severe outbreaks of hemorrhagic fever occurred in northern Zaire and the southern Sudan. The illnesses were similar to those described for Marburg virus. They were later shown, however, to be caused by an antigenically different agent now known as *Ebola virus,* named after a small river in Zaire. Two distinct antigenic types are now recognized.

Ebola virus produces disease in humans and subhuman primates; onset is within 4–6 days of inoculation. The reservoir, although uncertain, is thought to be in small mammals, perhaps rodents.

high mortality during epidemics

Serosurveys of humans residing in the areas where outbreaks have occurred suggest that human infection may be relatively common; as much as 7% of the survey group had antibodies, indicating past infection. In symptomatic infections, the mortality for both Marburg and Ebola viruses is extremely high (30–80%).

Filamentous viral particles

The viruses have a similar appearance in cell cultures; they produce filamentous particles averaging 100 nm in diameter and 300–1500 nm in length as they bud from cell membranes. Both have been tentatively classified as members of the new family Filoviridae.

person-to-person spread of Ebola virus

As with the arenavirus-associated hemorrhagic fevers, the diagnosis of infection by these agents is suggested by a similar syndrome and recent travel history. Person-to-person transmission similar to that described for Lassa fever occurs in Ebola virus infections and may be possible with Marburg virus. Diagnosis can be confirmed by isolation of virus in Vero cells (a continuous line of African green monkey kidney), mice, and guinea pigs, as well as by serologic methods employing indirect immunofluorescence. As with the arenavirus-associated hemorrhagic fevers, however, utmost care in isolation precautions and *prompt* notification of public health authorities is mandatory for suspected cases *before* any diagnostic attempts are made. There is no specific therapy for the infections.

Vesicular Stomatitis Virus

A rhabdovirus that causes outbreaks of disease in cattle, pigs, and horses and can be transmitted by arthropods is vesicular stomatitis virus. Human infection acquired by contact with infected animals is unusual; it consists of a self-limited febrile illness and occasional herpeslike eruptions over the lips and oral mucosa.

Korean Hemorrhagic Fever and Related Agents

As its name implies, Korean hemorrhagic fever (KHF) is endemic to Korea and surrounding areas in the Far East. It is an important cause of hemorrhagic fever, often complicated by varying degrees of acute renal failure. The first reported isolation of KHF was in 1978, when the antigen was detected in the lung tissues of wild rodents (*Apodemus* species) by indirect immunofluorescence using convalescent sera from affected patients. No illness was apparent in the rodents, suggesting a reservoir mechanism and mode of transmission similar to those described for the arenaviruses. Additional work using the Hantaan virus (a prototype strain serially propagated in a continuous cell line from a human pulmonary carcinoma) suggests that the agent is probably a member of the genus *Bunyavirus.* Several different serotypes probably exist.

Recently, evidence has accumulated indicating that an agent (or agents) with a close antigenic similarity to KHF virus is responsible for hemorrhagic–renal syndromes occurring throughout northern Eurasia, including the Soviet Union, eastern Europe, Finland, and Scandinavia. These syndromes have been given a variety of names, including nephropathia epidemica (NE). Methods similar to those used to detect KHF antigen have detected the NE antigen in the lungs of small rodents (bank voles) in Finland. Recently, antigens and antibodies of a Hantaan-like virus have been detected in urban rat species, both in Korea and Baltimore, Maryland. Thus there is a possibility that human infection with disease may occur in the United States. There is no evidence of human-to-human transmission, but some investigators believe that arthropod vectors are possible.

Additional Reading and References

Bowen, E.T.W., Lloyd, G., Harris, W.J., et al. 1977. Viral haemorrhagic fever in southern Sudan and northern Zaire. *Lancet* 1:571–573. A good description of Ebola disease is provided; accompanying articles in the same issue are also useful in describing the virus.

Brummer-Korvenkontio, M., Vaheri, A., Hovi, T., et al. 1980. Nephropathia epidemica: Detection of antigen in bank voles and serologic diagnosis of human infection. *J. Infect. Dis.* 141:131–134. Knowledge of KHF-like diseases and their possible common cause is extended.

Hinman, A.R., Fraser, D.W., Douglas, R.G., et al. 1975. Outbreak of lymphocytic choriomeningitis virus infections in medical center personnel. *Am. J. Epidemiol.* 101:103–110. A good description of disease and epidemiology is provided.

Johnson, K.M. 1979. Arthropod-borne viral fevers. In *Cecil Textbook of Medicine.* 15th ed. P.B. Beeson, et al., eds. Philadelphia: Saunders, p. 276. A review of the clinical and epidemiologic aspects of arboviruses.

Lee, H.W., Lee, P.W., Johnson, K.M., et al. 1978. Isolation of the etiologic agent of Korean hemorrhagic fever. *J. Infect. Dis.* 137:298–308. Disease importance and methods used to detect the causative agent are described.

Pang, T. 1983. Delayed-type hypersensitivity: Probable role in the pathogenesis of dengue hemorrhagic fever/dengue shock syndrome. *Rev. Infect. Dis.* 5:346–352. An excellent discussion of dengue pathogenesis (including work of Dr. Scott Halstead), which may eventually apply to our knowledge of some other infectious disease processes.

Zweighaft, R.M., Fraser, D.W., Hattwick, M.A., et al. 1977. Lassa fever: Response to an imported case. *N. Engl. J. Med.* 297:803–807. The extreme concern regarding infectivity and diagnosis of hemorrhagic fever viruses is illustrated.

Lawrence Corey

Rabies

42

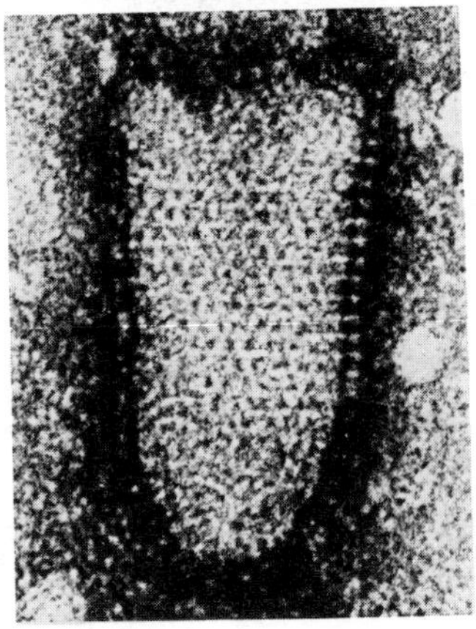

Rabies virus *

Rabies is an acute viral illness of the central nervous system. It can affect all mammals and is transmitted between them by infected secretions, usually saliva.

Agent

The rabies virus is a bullet-shaped, enveloped, single-stranded RNA virus of the rhabdovirus group. Other human pathogens in this group include Marburg virus, Ebola virus, Mokola virus, and vesicular stomatitis virus (Chapter 41). Rabies virus is large, with a diameter of about 180 × 70 nm. Knoblike glycoprotein excrescences, which elicit neutralizing and hemagglutination inhibition antibodies, cover the surface of the virion.

The virus, which can be grown in tissue culture, produces rapid encephalitis when injected intracerebrally into laboratory rodents. In the past, a single antigenically homogeneous virus was believed responsible for all rabies. However, some differences in tissue culture growth characteristics of isolates from different animal sources, some differences in virulence for experimental animals, and recent work using monoclonal antibodies have indicated some antigenic differences in strains from various animal species. These studies may help to explain some of the biologic differences noted, as well as the occasional case of "vaccine failure."

Clinical Manifestations

encephalitic manifestations; survival rare

Rabies in humans presents as an acute, fluminant, fatal encephalitis; human survivors have been reported only occasionally. The disease begins as a nonspecific illness marked by fever, headache, malaise, nausea, and vomiting. Abnormal sensations at or around the site of viral inoculation occur frequently and probably reflect local nerve involvement. The onset of encephalitis is marked by periods of excess motor activity and agitation. Hallucinations, combativeness, muscle spasms, signs of meningeal irritation, seizures, and focal paralysis appear. Periods of mental dysfunction are interspersed with completely lucid periods; as the disease progresses, however,

*Rabies virus particle figure reproduced with permission of Dr. K. Hummuler. Hummuler, K., Koprowski, M., and Wiktor, T.J. 1967. *J. Virol.* 1:152–170.

the patient lapses into coma. Autonomic nervous system involvement often results in increased salivation. Brainstem and cranial nerve dysfunction is characteristic, with double vision, facial palsies, and difficulty in swallowing. The combination of excess salivation and difficulty in swallowing produces the traditional picture of "foaming at the mouth." Hydrophobia, the painful, violent, involuntary contractions of the diaphragm and accessory respiratory, pharyngeal, and laryngeal muscles initiated by swallowing liquids, is seen in about 50% of cases. Involvement of the respiratory center produces respiratory paralysis, the major cause of death. The median survival after onset of symptoms is 4 days, with a maximum of 20 days unless artificial supporting measures are instituted.

hydrophobia

brief course with development of respiratory paralysis

Occasionally rabies may appear as an ascending paralysis resembling Guillain–Barré syndrome.

Pathogenesis

routes of infection

initial replication in muscle followed by spread from nerves to brain

centrifugal spread in autonomic nerves; salivary gland involvement

factors influencing incubation period

The essential first event in human or animal rabies infection is the introduction of virus through the epidermis, usually as a result of an animal bite. Inhalation of heavily contaminated material, such as bat droppings, can also cause infection. Rabies virus first replicates in striated muscle tissue at the site of inoculation. It then enters the peripheral nervous system at the neuromuscular junctions and spreads up the nerves to the central nervous system, where it replicates exclusively within the gray matter. It then passes centrifugally along autonomic nerves to reach other tissues, including the salivary glands, adrenal medulla, kidneys, and lungs. Passage into the salivary glands in animals facilitates further transmission of the disease by infected saliva. The incubation period ranges from 10 days to a year, depending on the amount of virus introduced, the amount of tissue involved, the host immune mechanisms, and the distance the virus must travel from the site of inoculation to the central nervous system. Thus, the incubation period is generally shorter with face wounds than with leg wounds. Immunization early in the incubation period frequently aborts the infection.

Pathology

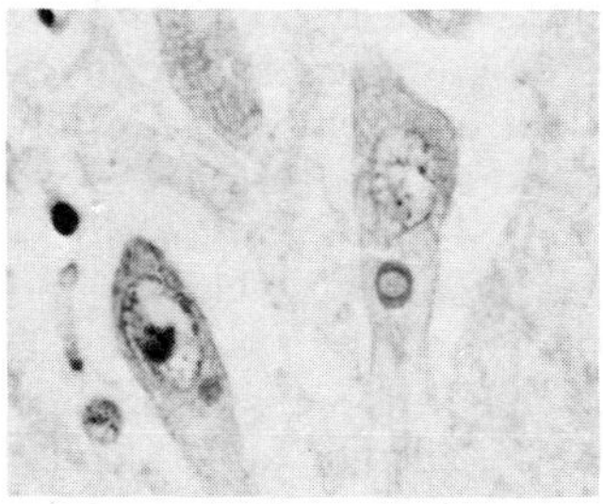

Negri body in cytoplasm of neuron*

The neuropathology of rabies resembles that of other viral diseases of the central nervous system, with infiltration of lymphocytes and plasma cells into central nervous system tissue and nerve cell destruction. The pathognomic lesion is the Negri body, an eosinophilic cytoplasmic inclusion distributed throughout the brain, particularly in the hippocampus, cerebral cortex, cerebellum, and dorsal spinal ganglia. As Negri bodies are not seen in at least 20% of rabies victims, and their absence does not rule out the diagnosis.

Laboratory Diagnosis

Intracerebral inoculation of suckling mice

Demonstration of Negri bodies

Laboratory diagnosis of rabies is accomplished by indirect or direct demonstration of virus. Intracerebral inoculation of infected brain tissue or secretions into suckling mice results in death in 3–10 days. Histologic examination of their brain tissue shows Negri bodies; both Negri bodies and rhabdovirus particles may be demonstrated by electron microscopy. Viral antigen can be demonstrated by immunofluorescent procedures. Specific

*Negri bodies figure provided by Dr. Daniel P. Perl.

antibodies to rabies virus can be detected, but generally only late in the disease.

Epidemiology and Epizoology

Urban and sylvatic animal rabies

infection of cattle and humans are blind-ended

most human cases from infected dogs or cats

Rabies exists in two epizoologic forms: urban, which is associated with unimmunized dogs or cats; and sylvatic, which occurs in wild skunks, foxes, wolves, racoons, mongooses, and bats. Human infection, or the much more common infection of cattle, is incidental, blind-ended, and does not contribute to maintenance or transmission of the disease. In the United States, more than 75% of reported cases of rabies in animals occur among wildlife. Most human exposure, however, is from bites by unimmunized dogs or cats. Infection in domestic animals usually represents a spillover from infection in wildlife reservoirs. Human infection tends to occur where animal rabies is common and where there is a large population of unimmunized domestic animals. Worldwide, the occurrence of human rabies is estimated to be about 15,000 cases per year, with the highest attack rates in southeast Asia, the Philippines, and the Indian subcontinent. In the United States, one to three cases of human rabies are reported yearly. A recent addition to the epidemiology of rabies in the United States has been the transmission of disease through transplantation of infected corneal tissue from a recently deceased but undiagnosed case.

Bat rabies in United States

In most areas of the world, the dog is the most important vector of the rabies virus to humans. Other important sources of disease are the wolf in eastern Europe, the mongoose in Africa, the fox in western Europe, and the bat in Latin America and the United States.

Prevention and Treatment

Prevention is the mainstay of controlling human rabies. Intensive supportive care has resulted in two or three long-term survivals; despite the best modern medical care, however, the mortality still exceeds 90%. In addition, because of the infrequency of the disease, many cases die without definitive diagnosis.

Pasteur's vaccine

In the late 1800s Pasteur, noting the long incubation period of rabies, suggested that a vaccine to induce an immune response before the development of disease might be useful in prevention. He apparently successfully vaccinated Joseph Meister, a boy severely bitten and exposed to rabies with multiple injections of a crude vaccine made from dried spinal cord of rabies-infected rabbits. This treatment emerged as one of the best known and noteworthy accomplishments in the annals of medicine.

preexposure prophylaxis

human diploid cell culture vaccine

Currently, the prevention of rabies virus is divided into preexposure and postexposure prophylaxis. Preexposure prophylaxis is recommended for individuals at high risk of contact with rabies virus, such as veterinarians, spelunkers, laboratory workers, and animal handlers. Two types of vaccine are currently licensed in the United States for preexposure prophylaxis. The newest and best vaccine employs an attenuated rabies virus grown in human diploid cell culture. It is more immunogenic than the older duck embryo vaccine (DEV). Both the human diploid tissue culture and DEV are inactivated virus preparations. In general, DEV is less immunogenic and has a higher rate of side effects than the human diploid vaccine. Preexposure therapy consists of two subcutaneous injections of vaccine given 1 month apart, followed by a booster dose several months later.

Postexposure proplylaxis

Postexposure prophylaxis requires careful evaluation and judgment. Every year more than one million Americans are bitten by animals, and in factors influencing decision to immunize after possible exposure

each instance a decision must be made whether to initiate postexposure rabies prophylaxis. In this decision the physician must consider 1) whether the individual came into physical contact with saliva or another substance likely to contain rabies virus; 2) whether there was significant wounding or abrasion; 3) whether rabies is known or suspected in the animal species and area associated with the exposure; 4) the circumstances surrounding the exposure (that is, whether the bite was provoked or unprovoked); and 5) whether the animal is available for laboratory examination. Any wild animal or ill, unvaccinated, or stray domestic animal involved in a possible rabies exposure, such as an unprovoked bite, should be captured and killed. The head should be sent immediately to an appropriate laboratory, usually at the State Health Department, for search for rabies antigen by immunofluorescence. If examination of the brain by this technique is negative for rabies virus, it can be assumed that the saliva contains no virus and that the exposed person requires no treatment. If the test is positive, the patient should be given postexposure prophylaxis. It should be noted that rodents and rabbits are not important vectors of rabies virus.

Postexposure prophylaxis is based on 1) local wound debridement; 2) local passive immunization by instillation around the wound site of human rabies immune globulin, a hyperimmune globulin containing antirabies antibody; and 3) active immunization with antirabies vaccine. With human diploid vaccine, six doses of vaccine given on days 1, 3, 7, 14, 30, and 90 are recommended. With DEV, daily doses for 21 days are recommended, with a booster dose at 30 and 90 days. An algorithm illustrating the approach to postexposure prophylaxis is shown in Figure 42.1.

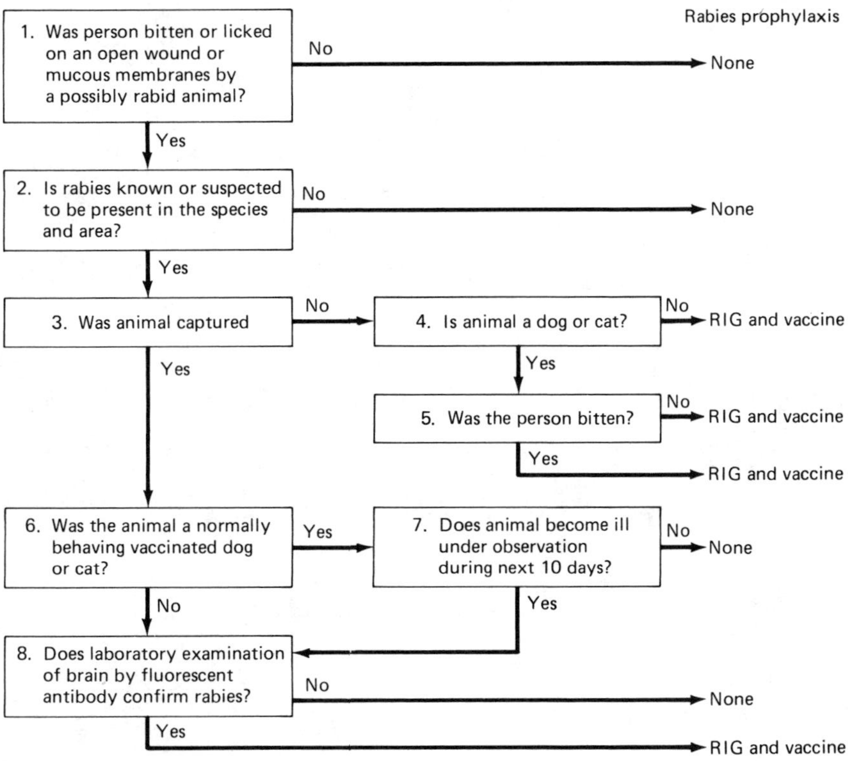

42.1 Postexposure rabies prophylaxis algorithm. RIG = rabies immune globulin; vaccine of choice is human diploid cell culture vaccine. *(Adapted from Corey, L., Hattwick, M.A.W. 1975. J. Am. Med. Assoc. 232:272.)*

need for consultation

The physician in private practice in the United States, should always seek the advice of the local health department when the question of rabies prophylaxis arises.

Additional Reading and References

Anderson, L.J., Winkler, W.G., Hafkin, B., et al. 1980. Clinical experience with a human diploid cell rabies vaccine. *J. Am. Med. Assoc.* 244:781–784. A review of the use of the new diploid cell rabies vaccine.

Hattwick, M.A.W. 1974. Human rabies. *Public Health Rev.* 3:229–274. A comprehensive review with valuable consideration of clinical manifestations.

Lawrence Corey

Slow Viruses and Tumor Viruses

43

Slow Viruses and Slow Virus Diseases

The past 25 years have brought the recognition that a variety of progressive neurologic diseases in both animals and humans appear to be caused by viral agents (Table 43.1). These illnesses have been termed *slow virus diseases*; the slowness being not necessarily a feature of the pathogen, but of the delayed and insidious onset of clinical signs in the host. Slow virus infections of the central nervous system can be classified as 1) diseases associated with "conventional" viral agents, which contain nucleic acid, induce immune responses, and may be grown in cell culture systems; and 2) diseases associated with "unconventional" viruses, which are small, filterable infectious agents that are transmissible in animal model systems but do not appear to be associated with discernible immune responses and have not yet been cultivated in cell culture.

Diseases Associated with Conventional Agents

Disease of children

Subacute sclerosing panencephalitis. Subacute sclerosing panencephalitis is a progressive neurologic disease of children. It is characterized by insidious onset of personality change, poor school performance, progressive intellectual deterioration, development of myoclonic jerks (periodic muscle spasms), and motor dysfunctions such as spasticity, tremors, loss of coordination, and ocular abnormalities, including cortical blindness. Neurologic and intellectual deterioration generally progresses over 6–12 months, with the child eventually becoming bedridden and stuporous. Dysfunctions of the autonomic nervous system, such as difficulty with temperature regulation, may develop. Progressive inanition, superinfection, and metabolic imbalances eventually lead to death.

Pathologic features

Most of the pathologic features of the disease are localized to the central nervous system and retina. Both the gray and the white matter of the brain are involved, the most noteworthy feature being the presence of intranuclear and intracytoplasmic inclusions in oligodendroglial and neuronal cells.

chronic measles virus infection

Subacute sclerosing panencephalitis results from chronic measles virus infection of the central nervous system. Evidence for this conclusion includes 1) elevated measles antibody titers in the cerebrospinal fluid (CSF); 2) intranuclear and intracytoplasmic inclusions characteristic of a paramyxovirus in brain cells; 3) demonstration of measles-specific antigen by immunoflu-

Table 43.1 Slow Virus Infections

Disease	Agent
Conventional Viruses	
Subacute sclerosing panencephalitis	Measles virus
Progressive panencephalitis after congenital rubella	Rubella virus
Progressive multifocal leukoencephalopathy	Papovaviruses, J.C. virus, SV40-like agent
Unconventional Viruses[a]	
Kuru	
Creutzfeld–Jakob disease	
Scrapie (sheep and goats)	
Transmissible mink encephalopathy	

[a] Subacute spongiform encephalopathies.

orescent testing in brain cells; and 4) isolation of measles virus from brain tissue and lymph nodes by cocultivation rescue techniques. Recently, patients with subacute sclerosing panencephalitis have been shown to fail to respond immunologically to the M (matrix) protein of the measles virus. The M protein gene product is an internal membrane protein (one of six major proteins of measles) with a key role in virus assembly, probably in nucleocapsid alignment beneath the cytoplasmic membrane before budding. It tends to disappear as measles infection progresses in the central nervous system. As a result, restriction of M protein synthesis in the brain leads to a lack of virus assembly, and subsequently to a defective immunologic response. The latter may account for the inability to eradicate the virus from the central nervous system.

Rarely, a similar progressive, degenerative neurologic disorder may be related to persistent rubella virus infection of the central nervous system. This condition is seen most often in adolescents who have had congenital rubella syndrome. Rubella virus has been isolated from brain tissue in these patients, again using cocultivation techniques.

Diagnosis: findings in CSF

A characteristic clinical course in a child with an elevated measles antibody titer in the CSF is the mainstay of diagnosis. The CSF is usually abnormal, showing a small increase in lymphocytes, an elevated protein level, and a normal glucose level. Levels of immunoglobulin G in the CSF are increased. The electroencephalogram may also show a characteristic pattern. Definitive diagnosis is made from typical pathologic changes in brain tissue, demonstration of measles virus antigen in brain, or isolation of measles virus from brain tissue.

Epidemiology

reduced incidence after introduction of measles vaccine

The mean annual incidence of subacute sclerosing panencephalitis in the United States is 3.5 cases per 10 million persons less than 20 years of age. The disease appears to be twice as frequent in male as in female subjects and four times more frequent in white than in black subjects. Marked geographic variations in the prevalence of the disease in the United States have been noted; the attack rate is highest in children in rural, particularly farming, areas. Its occurrence in the United States has decreased markedly over the past 10 years with the widespread use of live measles vaccine.

At present, there is no accepted effective therapy of subacute sclerosing panencephalitis. The antiviral and immune modulating drug isoprinosine is believed by some to reduce disease activity, but controlled evaluations have not been made.

progressive neurologic disease of adults

Progressive multifocal leukoencephalopathy. Progressive multifocal leukoencephalopathy is a rare, subacute, degenerative disease of the brain found

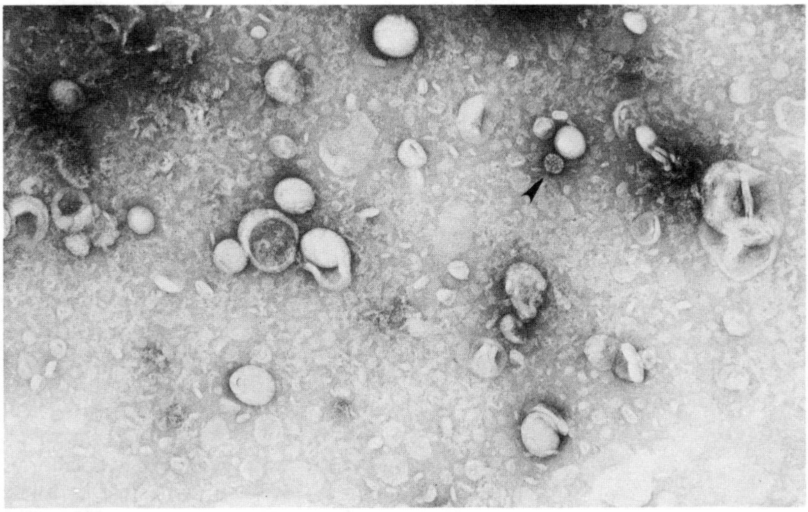

43.1 J.C. virus (*arrow*) among debris of cells from a brain biopsy of a case of progressive multifocal leukoencephalopathy. (*Reprinted with permission from Palmer, E. and Martin, M.L. 1982. An atlas of mammalian viruses. CRC Press, Inc. Boca Raton, Fl. Copyright 1982 by CRC Press, Inc.*)

primarily in adults with other chronic diseases, especially malignancy. The disease is characterized by the development of impaired memory, confusion, and disorientation, followed by a multiplicity of neurologic symptoms and signs that includes hemiparesis, visual disturbances, incoordination, seizures, and visual abnormalities. The disease is progressive, with death usually occurring 3–6 months after onset of symptoms. The CSF is often normal, although some patients show a slight increase in lymphocytes, and elevated protein levels may be present. Pathologically, foci of demyelination are found, surrounded by giant, bizarre astrocytes containing intranuclear inclusions. Although the clinical diagnosis is confusing, these pathologic features are relatively pathognomonic of the disease. Electron microscopic studies have demonstrated papovaviruslike particles within the nuclei of oligodendrocytes. In addition, papovavirus antigen has been demonstrated by immunofluorescence, and two types of papovaviruses have been isolated from brain tissue of patients with the disease. One of these agents is related to the SV40 virus of primates. The other virus has been called the *J.C. virus* (the initials are those of the patient from whom it was first isolated) (Figure 43.1). The J.C. virus has been grown in primary human fetal glial culture cells and isolated from the urine of some immunosuppressed patients. Seroepidemiologic studies have indicated that antibody to J.C. virus can be found in about 70% of adults in the United States, although no defined clinical symptoms have been associated with the infection that occurred. It appears that progressive multifocal leukoencephalopathy is a rare manifestation of infection with these agents.

Pathologic features

association with papovaviruses, including J.C. virus

Diseases Caused by Unconventional Viral Agents

Subacute spongiform encephalopathies in humans and animals

Within the last two decades, a group of progressive degenerative diseases of the central nervous system called the *subacute spongiform encephalopathies* have been shown to be caused by infectious agents with unusual physical and chemical properties. Two of these illnesses, kuru and Creutzfeldt–Jakob disease, occur in humans; two others, scrapie in sheep and goats and progressive encephalopathy in mink (Table 43.1), occur in animals. Although the pathogenesis of these four illnesses is not well understood, they have similar features. There are varying degrees of neuronal loss, spongiform neurologic changes, and astrocyte proliferation. The incubation periods are

Table 43.2 Biologic and Physical Properties of Unconventional Viruses

Chronic progressive pathology without remission or recovery.
No pathologic evidence of an inflammatory response.
Filterable to estimated diameter of $\leq$5nm.
No virionlike structures visible by electron microscopy.
Replication to high titers in susceptible tissue.
Transmissible to experimental animals.
No alteration in pathogenesis by immunosuppression or immunopotentiation.
No interferon production or interference by other viruses.
Infectious nucleic acid or viral antigens not detected.
Unusual resistance to ultraviolet radiation.
Resistance to inactivation by alcohol, 10% formalin, β-propiolactone, boiling water, proteases, and nucleases.
Can be inactivated by 5% sodium hypochlorite, 1N sodium hydroxide, and autoclaving and partially inactivated by acetone and ether.

transmissible to animal models

months to years. The diseases have a protracted and inevitably fatal course. All four have been transmitted to animals by inoculation of infected tissues.

unusual characteristics of infectious agents

The nature of these unconventional agents is still obscure. They are small and filterable to diameters of 5nm or less, have wide host ranges, multiply to high titers in the reticuloendothelial system and brain, produce characteristic infections, and can remain viable even in formalinized brain tissue for many years. They are resistant to ionizing radiation, boiling, and many common disinfectants. Recognizable virions have not been found in tissues, and the agents have not been grown in cell culture. Treatment of infectious material with proteases and nucleases does not decrease infectivity. Neither humoral nor cellular immunity develops in natural or experimental infections, and interferon is not produced. Some authorities have suggested the agents may be prions, that is, proteinaceous agents that exist without nucleic acids. Their relationship to these encephalopathies remains speculative, and their motor replication is unknown. The major characteristics of the agents are listed in Table 43.2.

Absence of immune response

possible relationship to prions

occurrence in women and children of the Fore people of New Guinea

Kuru. Kuru is a subacute, progressive neurologic disease of the Fore people of the Eastern Highlands of New Guinea. Although the illness is localized and decreasing in incidence, its study has thrown light on the transmissibility and infectious nature of similar transmissible encephalopathies. In the local Fore dialect, *kuru* means "to tremble with fear or to be afraid." The disease was brought to the attention of the Western world by Drs. Carleton Gadjusek and Vincent Zigas in the mid-1950s. Epidemiologic studies indicated that kuru usually afflicted adult women or children of either sex. The disease was rarely observed outside of the Fore region, and outsiders in the region did not contract the disease. The symptoms and signs were ataxia, hyperreflexia, and spasticity, which led to progressive starvation and death. Mental alertness was unaffected until the late stages of illness. Pathologic examination revealed changes only in the central nervous system, with diffuse neuronal degeneration and spongiform changes of the cerebral cortex and basal ganglia. No inflammatory response was noted. Inoculation of infectious brain tissue into primates produced a disease that caused similar neurologic symptoms and pathologic manifestations after an incubation period of approximately 40 months. Epidemiologic studies indicated that transmission of the disease in humans was associated with ritual cannibalism, practiced mainly by women and young children and occasionally by men. This ritual

Clinical and pathologic features

Transmissibility to primates

association with cannibalism

involved the handling and ingestion of organs of deceased relatives. Inoculation through lesions in the skin and mucous membranes was shown to be the most likely mode of transmission, with clinical disease developing 4–20 years after exposure. Since the elimination of cannibalism from the Fore culture, kuru has disappeared.

progressive disease of the elderly

Creutzfeldt–Jakob disease. Creutzfeldt–Jakob disease is a progressive, fatal illness of the central nervous system that is seen most frequently in the sixth and seventh decades of life. The initial clinical manifestations are a change in cerebral function, usually diagnosed initially as a psychiatric disorder. Forgetfulness and disorientation progress to overt dementia, with the development of changes in gait, increased tone in the limbs, involuntary movement, and seizures. The disorder runs a course of 12 months to 4–5 years, eventually leading to death.

Pathologic features and transmission to animals

The pathology of Creutzfeldt–Jakob disease is essentially identical to that of kuru. It has been transmitted to chimpanzees, mice, and guinea pigs by inoculation of infected brain tissue, leukocytes, and certain organs. High levels of infectious agent have been found, especially in the brain, where they may reach 10^{-7} infectious doses per gram of brain tissue. Nonpercutaneous transmission of disease has not been observed, and there is no evidence of transmission by direct contact or airborne spread.

Epidemiology: natural mode of acquisition unknown

Creutzfeldt–Jakob disease is found worldwide, with an incidence of disease of one case per million per year. Most cases are sporadic, although 20% develop in family members. The mode of acquisition is unknown.

Nosocomial infections

Nosocomial infection has been observed to develop in one individual from an infected corneal transplant and in another from contact with infected electrodes used in a neurosurgical procedure. In these cases, the incubation period of the disease was approximately 15–20 months. Other evidence suggests that a longer latency may follow natural infection.

prevention of nosocomial infections from transplants or instruments

There is no effective therapy of Creutzfeldt–Jakob disease, and all cases have been fatal. The risk of nosocomial infection can be greatly reduced. Stereotactic neurosurgical equipment, especially that used in patients with undiagnosed dementia, should not be reused. In addition, organs from patients with undiagnosed neurologic disease should not be used for transplants. The agent of Creutzfeldt–Jakob disease has not been transmitted to animals by inoculation of body secretions, and no increased risk of disease has been noted in family members or medical personnel caring for patients. Disinfection of potentially infectious material can be accomplished by treatment for 1 hr with 0.5% sodium hypochlorite solution or by autoclaving at 121°C for 1 hr.

Tumor Viruses

The topic of tumor viruses is one of intense interest at present, because molecular biologic studies of interactions between tumor viruses and cells have provided major clues to the general pathogenesis of tumors. It is also of great importance that, after many years of searching, a human leukemia virus has been closely associated with a rare type of T-cell leukemia. The subject will not be discussed in depth because it is beyond the scope and purpose of the book, but the following provides an overview of the present state of knowledge.

Historic Perspectives

The concept that infectious agents may be involved etiologically in cancer was advanced as early as 1908 by Ellerman and Bang, who observed that the mode of transmission of leukemia in fowl was similar to that of an infectious disease. Shortly thereafter, Rous demonstrated that an infectious agent in avian sarcomas could pass through a filter that would not permit passage of bacteria. In 1932, Shope reported that a filterable agent transmitted a wartlike growth in wild cottontail rabbits, and in 1938, Bittner discovered the "milk factor," a virus associated with mammary gland tumors in mice that passed from mother to offspring during suckling. Since then, numerous viral agents have been isolated that cause many kinds of cancer in a variety of animals.

association with latent infections

The mechanism by which a virus can induce tumors has been one of intensive study and interest. In our discussions of most viral infectious diseases we have focused on the "lytic" interaction between viruses and cells, a process involving the multiplication of a virus and the destruction of the host cell. Certain viruses, however, can interact with cells in a manner in which virus multiplication is repressed and the host cell is not destroyed (that is, the virus establishes a latent infection). With some viruses, viral DNA or DNA transcripts of viral RNA become associated with the cell's genetic apparatus, thereby giving rise to a new entity, the transformed cell. Transformed cells contain either the whole or part of the genome of the virus that causes the transformation, and it may be integrated into the cell's nuclear DNA or exist in a free plasmidlike state. The extent to which viral genetic information is expressed varies from full expression to complete silence.

viral genome in transformed cells

Properties of transformed cells

tumorigenicity

Some cells transformed with viruses in vitro will lead to tumors of the same cell type when injected into animals, particularly those with immunodeficiency or immunosuppression. Some of these tumors are highly invasive. Morphologically, transformed cells may differ from normal cells in cell culture in that they are rounder and tend to orient themselves randomly, unlike the regular patterns of normal cells. They may show more rapid and extensive growth than untransformed cells. For example, most types of normal cells grow in vitro to a certain cell density; cell division is inhibited by contact with other cells and slows greatly when a monolayer or uniformly spread cell sheet is formed. The ability to respond to contact helps to ensure that any given cell grows only in its appropriate location within living tissues. In contrast, transformed cells continue to divide, yielding very high cell densities. Cell transformation increases membrane transport; simple sugar and nutrients are thus transported more rapidly, resulting in more rapid growth. Transformed cells sometimes demonstrate the acquisition of new or altered surface antigens, the presence of which may cause their recognition as foreign antigens by the host. The altered karyotype of transformed cells can include deletion or duplication of portions of chromosomes. The finding that nonvirally induced transformed cells often exhibit the same deletions and duplications prompted the formulation of a theory that some genes promote malignancy, whereas others tend to suppress it.

morphologic changes and lack of contact inhibition

increased membrane transport of nutrients

acquisition of new antigens

altered karyotype

DNA Tumor Viruses

Several different DNA viruses have been shown to be associated with the development of tumors. They include the papovavirus family, the herpesviruses, and the adenoviruses of animals.

Papilloma viruses

The papilloma viruses have been shown to cause a variety of both benign and malignant tumors in a wide range of animals, and different genotypes of human papilloma viruses have been associated with a variety of warts. The DNA from human papilloma virus types 3 and 5 has also been found in a rare skin tumor called epidermodysplasia verruciformis. Recently, human papilloma viruses have been found to occur more frequently in women with cellular abnormalities of the uterine cervix (cervical dysplasia) than in those with normal cervical biopsy results. These data suggest that human papilloma viruses may also play a role in the development of tumors in humans. Further work in this area is needed to clarify the relationship between these infections and the subsequent development of tumors.

Polyoma viruses: SV40 and J.C. viruses

A primate polyoma virus, the SV40 virus, has been associated with production of lymphocytic leukemia and a variety of reticuloendothelial cell sarcomas in baby hamsters. In humans, however, no association between cancer and SV40 virus infection has been noted on follow-up of recipients of an early poliomyelitis vaccine that contained live SV40 from contaminated monkey kidney cell cultures. Several different human polyoma viruses related to SV40 also produce tumors in animals, but not in humans. The J.C. virus produces brain tumors in more than 80% of infected hamsters, and another polyoma virus termed BK is also weakly oncogenic in animals.

From a biologic point of view, the polyoma viruses are particularly interesting because they can interact with different cells in a variety of ways. In some cells, the virus can multiply and cause lytic infection and cell death. In others that do not permit viral multiplication, they can cause transformation. In still others, defective virus particles with deletions in the viral genome and replication processes can develop upon repeated passage of the agent and subsequently produce cell transformation. In transformation with polyoma virus, viral DNA becomes stably integrated into the DNA of the host cell.

defective particles

Adenoviruses and herpesviruses

Adenoviruses can also transform animal cells in vitro, and some serotypes can cause tumors when injected into newborn animals. No human neoplasms have been found that contain adenovirus DNA. In contrast, some members of the herpesvirus family have been shown to be oncogenic in animals, and some have been epidemiologically associated with tumors in humans. Epstein–Barr virus causes a lymphoma in marmosets and transforms human peripheral blood leukocytes, which normally cannot multiply in vitro, into lymphoblastlike cells with an indefinite life span. Such cells do not produce fully replicating Epstein–Barr virus, but can be stimulated to do so. The DNA of Epstein–Barr virus is present in Burkitt's lymphoma, a malignant tumor encountered in parts of Africa, at a rate of approximately 1–10 viral genome equivalents of DNA per cell. This viral DNA may be integrated into the host genome or exist in a circular plasmidlike form. Epstein–Barr viral DNA has also been detected in cells of patients with nasopharyngeal carcinoma, which occurs with rather high frequency among the southern Chinese. Herpes simplex virus can transform a variety of cells, particularly if the virus is first inactivated with ultraviolet light to prevent the development of a lytic virus–cell interaction. Naked herpesvirus DNA can also transform cells. By restriction endonuclease analysis, the transforming sequence has been traced to a small segment of viral DNA. Epidemiologically there is evidence of a higher incidence of carcinoma of the cervix in women infected with herpes simplex virus type 2, and portions of this viral genome have been demonstrated in cells of precancerous lesions of the cervix by in situ hybridization techniques. It is not known whether this relationship is etiologic or simply an association.

Epstein–Barr virus, Burkitt's lymphoma, and nasopharyngeal carcinoma

RNA Tumor Viruses or Retroviruses

The RNA tumor viruses can cause transformation of many cells. They are found in almost all vertebrate species, and in animals they may cause tumors primarily of connective tissues (sarcomas) or the hematopoietic system. They have also been implicated in certain carcinomas, such as those caused by mouse mammary tumor virus.

For many years after the discovery that certain tumor viruses contain

RNA rather than DNA, it was not understood how cells transformed by an RNA tumor virus could produce silent virus for generation after generation. In 1964, Temin proposed that upon infection, the viral RNA genome was transcribed into DNA by reversal of the usual flow of information transfer. This DNA was integrated into the host genome, and the progeny viral genome was transcribed from it. The hypothesis implied that the RNA present in the virus was not the viral genome, but the messenger RNA of a genome that could exist only intracellularly in the host cell. The discovery of reverse transcriptase independently by Temin and Baltimore in 1970 proved this hypothesis correct. The replication of an RNA tumor virus thus requires successful absorption and penetration into the cell, where the RNA is transcribed by reverse transcriptase into linear double-stranded DNA often termed *proviral DNA*. The mechanism of tumorigenesis by retroviruses appears to be as follows: they either carry an oncogene that is under the control of a promoter and transcribed at excessive levels, or they simply provide the promoter, which leads to excess production of the product of an oncogene already present in the cell. In either case, the protein for which the oncogene codes mediates cell transformation. Recent studies suggest that a simple amino acid substitution (point mutation) into an encoded protein may be sufficient to confer transforming properties to a cell.

reverse transcriptase

retroviruses and oncogene activation

Morphology: A–D particles

Morphologically, there are four groups of RNA tumor viruses, which are labeled A–D. The most common appearance is that of the C-type particle, which is characteristic of most leukemia and sarcoma viruses. This virus particle possesses an electron-dense nucleus surrounded by two shells. The B-type particles are RNA tumor viruses with an eccentric nucleocapsid and prominent glycoprotein spikes not seen in the C-type viruses. The B-type particle is characteristic of mammary tumor viruses. The A type appears to be an intracytoplasmic, unenveloped precursor of the B- and C-type particles. The appearance of the D-type particles is intermediate between those of the B- and C-type particles. The D-type virus particles have been isolated from subhuman primates such as rhesus monkeys and from human tumor cell lines such as HeLa cells.

horizontal and vertical transmission

There are two major classes of RNA tumor viruses based on their modes of transmission. Some are transmitted horizontally from animal to animal, like other infectious agents; examples include the Rous sarcoma virus of chickens and the simian sarcoma virus. Those of the second class are transmitted vertically as dominant genetic traits, like cellular genes, and exist only in provirus form covalently linked into the host DNA. These agents are often termed *endogenous* RNA tumor viruses. Their expression appears to be controlled by the host's regulatory mechanisms.

repression and derepression of proviral RNA viruses

Proviral RNA viruses appear to be present in all animal species. In most animal populations, the expression of such endogenous RNA tumor viruses is usually repressed. Strains of animals have been produced by inbreeding in which the mechanism for control of endogenous virus expression has been derepressed. As a result, RNA tumor viruses are present in high titer and tumors occur at high frequency. For example, some strains of mice have large numbers of C-type particles in their bloodstreams and frequently develop leukemia between 6 and 12 months of age. Others have low rates of RNA tumor virus viremia and lower rates for the subsequent development of leukemia. Some strains of mice, which have had endogenous viruses and proviruses bred out of them, rarely develop the disease. As with other families of viruses, there may be great variability in the oncogenicity of different strains of the same RNA tumor viruses. For example, one strain of mouse mammary tumor virus occurs in large numbers in lactating tissue and milk; it is passed readily to the progeny, in which it produces mammary adenocarcinoma with high frequency early in life. Other strains of this tumor virus express themselves far less readily in these strains of mice, are not present in milk, and are only transmitted vertically. They are much less oncogenic and cause tumors with lower frequency later in life.

role in human tumors

Although primates have been shown to have C- and D-type RNA tumor viruses, the relationship between endogenous RNA tumor viruses and tumors in humans is still unclear. Recently, however, human retroviruses (RNA tumor viruses) called HTLV-I and HTLV-II have been isolated from forms of leukemia or lymphoma that affect T lymphocytes. Human T-cell leukemia/lymphoma is most prevalent in southern Japan, although sporadic cases are seen throughout the world, including the United States. Recent studies have strongly implicated a third member of this family (HTLV-III) as a probable cause of acquired immune deficiency syndrome (AIDS). Intensive investigation of the relationship between the agent and the development of other human tumors and AIDS is under way. It seems probable that other retroviruses will be found to play some role in certain tumors of humans.

Additional Reading and References

Bishop, J.M. 1980. The molecular biology of RNA tumor viruses: A physician's guide. *N. Engl. J. Med.* 303:675–682. An excellent description is provided of the replication of retroviruses and the means by which they cause cell transformation.

Gajdusek, D.C. 1977. Unconventional viruses and the origin and disappearance of kuru. *Science* 197:943–960. This article, the lecture that Dr. Gajdusek delivered when he received the Nobel Prize in Physiology and Medicine in 1976, is a fascinating, authoritative review of the biology, epidemiology, and state of the art of the subacute spongiform encephalopathies. It is recommended reading for all.

Howley, P.M. 1983. The molecular biology of papillomaviruses transformation. *Am. J. Pathol.* 113: 414–421. A description of the use of molecular biologic techniques to explore the mechanisms of transformation by a virus-type that does not integrate into the host chromosome but exists as circular multicopy plasmids.

Logan, J., and Cairns, J. 1982. The secrets of cancer. *Nature* 300:104. Recent discoveries in oncogenesis, including its relationship to retrovirus tumor induction; are discussed.

Papovick, M., Sarngadharan, M.G., Read, E., and Gallo, R.C. 1984. Detection, isolation, and continuous production of cytopathic retroviruses (HTLV-III) from patients with AIDS and pre-AIDS. *Science* 224: 497–500. This and three companion papers summarized the findings that suggest an association between HTLV-III and future prospects for prevention.

James J. Plorde

Introduction to Pathogenic Parasites

44

This chapter provides an overview of parasitic diseases. The student may find it valuable to reread it after studying the subsequent chapters in this section.

Eukaryotic single-celled protozoa and multicellular macroscopic helminths

most are free living

Disease-producing species usually obligate parasites

Definition. Within the context of this section, the term *parasite* will refer to organisms belonging to one of two major taxonomic groups: *protozoa* and *helminths.* The former are microscopic, single-celled eukaryotes superficially resembling yeasts in both size and simplicity. The helminths, in contrast, are macroscopic, multicellular worms possessing differentiated tissues and complex organ systems; they vary in length from a meter to less than a millimeter. The majority of both protozoa and helminths are free living, play a significant role in the ecology of the planet, and seldom inconvenience the human race. The less common disease-producing species are typically obligate parasites, dependent on vertebrate and/or arthropod hosts for their survival. When their level of adaptation to a host is high, their presence typically produces little or no injury. Less complete adaptation leads to a more serious disturbance of the host and, occasionally, to death of both host and parasite.

Significance of Human Parasitic Infections

The relative infrequency of parasitic infections in the temperate, highly sanitated societies of the industrialized world has sometimes led to the parochial view that knowledge of parasitology has little relevance for physicians practicing in these areas. This attitude has been reflected in a dramatic decline in both the time allocated to the teaching of clinical parasitology and the amount of research funds devoted to the study of tropical illness.

major causes of disease and death

In fact, parasitic diseases remain among the major causes of human misery and death in the world today and, as such, are important obstacles to the development of the economically less-favored nations (Table 44.1). Moreover, a number of recent medical, socioeconomic, and political pheonomena have combined to produce a dramatic recrudescence of several parasitic diseases with important consequences to both the United States and the developing world.

Malaria

Currently, over a billion people live in malarious areas, and of these, approximately 200 million are infected at any given time. At least a million children die of malaria each year. *Plasmodium falciparum,* the most deadly

Table 44.1 Prevalence of Parasitic Infections in 1982

Disease	Estimated Population Involved
Amebiasis	10% of world population
Malaria	
Population at risk	> 1 billion
Population infected	177 million
Annual deaths	1 million
African trypanosomiasis	
Population at risk	35 million
New cases/year	≥ 10,000
American trypanosomiasis	
Population at risk	35 million
New cases/year	≥ 10,000
Schistosomiasis	> 200 million
Opisthorciasis	19 million
Paragonimiasis	3.2 million
Fasciolopsiasis	10 million
Filiariasis	250 million
Onchocerciasis	> 20 million
Dracunculiasis	50–80 million
Ascariasis	650 million
Hookworm	450 million
Trichuriasis	350 million
Strongyloidiasis	35 million
Cestodiasis	65 million

resistance of parasite to chemotherapeutic agents

resistance of insect vectors to insecticides

recent increases in incidence

of the malarial organisms, has developed resistance to a major category of antimalarial agents, and resistant strains are now found throughout Southeast Asia, parts of the Indian subcontinent, large areas of tropical America, and, most recently, limited areas of Africa. Growing resistance of the mosquito vector of malaria to the less toxic and less expensive insecticides has resulted in a cutback of many malaria control programs. In countries such as India, Pakistan, and Sri Lanka, where eradication efforts had previously interrupted parasite transmission, the disease incidence has increased 100-fold in recent years. In tropical Africa, the intensity of transmission defies current control measures. Of direct interest to American physicians is the spillover of this phenomenon to the United States. During 1980, the number of cases of imported malaria increased 213% to nearly 2000 cases, almost half the number seen at the height of the Vietnam War.

Amebic dysentery

Entamoeba histolytica, an intestinal protozoan, infects 10% of the world's population, including 2–3% in the United States. Invasive strains produce amebiasis, a disease characterized by intestinal ulcers and liver abscesses. It is more commonly seen in the poorly sanitated areas of the world, but occurs in the United States as well, particularly in institutions for the mentally retarded and among migrant workers and male homosexuals.

Trypanosomiasis

In Latin America, *Trypanosoma cruzi* infects an estimated 10 million individuals annually, leaving many with the characteristic heart and gastrointestinal lesions of Chagas' disease. In Africa, from the Sahara Desert in the north to the Kalahari in the south, a related organism, *Trypanosoma brucei,* causes one of the most lethal of human infections, sleeping sickness. Animal

Leishmaniasis

Parasitic worm infections

Schistosomiasis

Filariasis

Parasitic diseases common in the United States

strains of this same organism limit food supplies by making the raising of cattle economically infeasible.

Leishmaniasis, a disease produced by another intracellular protozoan, is found in parts of Europe, Asia, Africa, and Latin America. Clinical manifestations range from a self-limiting skin ulcer, known as *oriental sore,* through the mutilating mucocutaneous infection of espundia, to a highly lethal infection of the reticuloendothelial system (kala azar).

In 1947 Stall, in an article entitled "This Wormy World," estimated that between the tropics of Cancer and Capricorn there were many more intestinal worm infections than people. The prevalence was judged to be far lower in temperate climates. Warren, however, recently estimated that 27% of the American population harbored worms. The most serious of the helminthic diseases, schistosomiasis, affects an estimated 200 million individuals in Africa, Asia, and the Americas. Individuals with heavy worm levels develop bladder, intestinal, and liver disease, which may ultimately result in death. Unfortunately, the disease is frequently spread as a consequence of rural development schemes. Irrigation projects in Egypt, the Sudan, Ghana, and Nigeria have significantly increased the incidence of the disease in these areas, often mitigating the economic gains of the development program itself.

Two closely related filarial worms, *Wucheria bancrofti* and *Burgia malayi,* which are endemic in Asia and Africa, interfere with the flow of lymph and can produce grotesque swellings of the legs, arms, and genitals. Another filaria produces onchocerciasis (river blindness) in millions of Africans and Americans, leaving thousands blind.

Toxoplasmosis, giardiasis, trichomoniasis, and pinworm infections are four cosmopolitan parasitic infections well known to American physicans. The first, a protozoan infection of cats, infects possibly one-third of the world's human population. Although it is usually asymptomatic, infection acquired in utero may result in abortion, stillbirth, prematurity, or severe neurologic defects in the newborn. Asymptomatic infection acquired either before or after birth may subsequently produce visual impairment. Immunosuppressive therapy may reactivate latent infections, producing severe encephalitis.

Biology, Morphology, and Classification

Protozoa

Morphology. Protozoan protoplasm consists of a true membrane-bound nucleus and cytoplasm. The former contains clumped or dispersed chromatin and a central nucleolus or karyosome. The shape, size, and distribution of these structures may be used to distinguish protozoan species from one another.

The cytoplasm is frequently divided into an inner endoplasm and a thin outer ectoplasm. The granular endoplasm is concerned with nutrition and often contains food reserves, contractile vacuoles, and undigested particulate matter. The ectoplasm is organized into specialized organelles of locomotion. In some species, these organelles appear as blunt, dynamic extrusions known as *pseudopods.* In others, highly structured threadlike cilia or flagella arise from intracytoplasmic basal granules. Flagella are longer and less numerous than cilia and possess a structure and a mode of action distinct from those seen in prokaryotic organisms.

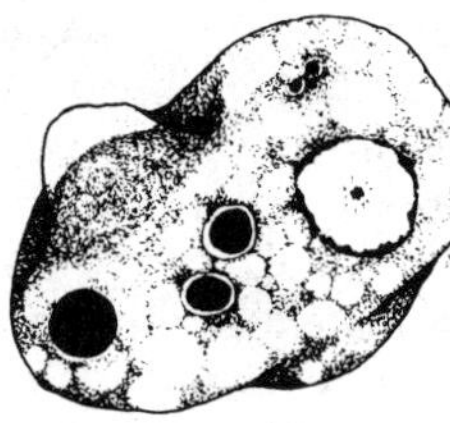

Prototypic rhizopod

Classification. Mode of reproduction and type of locomotive organelle are used to divide the protozoa into four major classes (Table 44.2). Although most rhizopods (amebas) are free living, several are found as commensal

Table 44.2 Classes of Protozoa

Class	Organelles of Locomotion	Method of Reproduction
Rhizopods (amebas)	Pseudopods	Binary fission
Ciliates	Cilia	Binary fission
Flagellates	Flagella	Binary fission
Sporozoa	None	Schizogony/sporogony

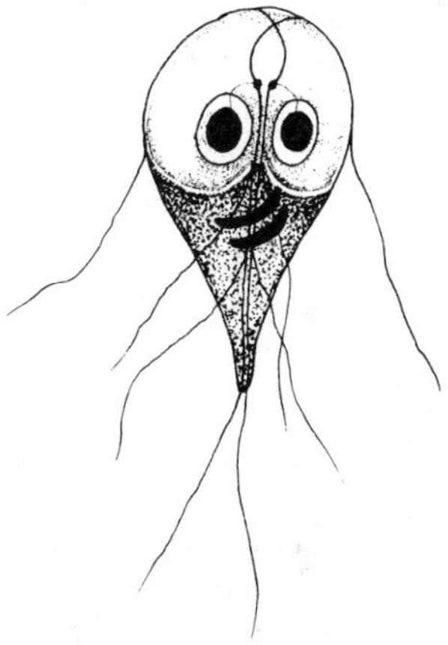

Prototypic flagellate

inhabitants of the intestinal tract in humans. One of these organisms, *E. histolytica,* may invade tissue and produce disease. Occasionally, free-living amebas may gain access to the body and initiate illness. The majority of ciliates are free living and seldom parasitize humans. Flagellates of the genera *Trypanosoma* and *Leishmania* are capable of invading the blood and tissues of humans, where they produce severe chronic illness. Others, such as *Trichomonas vaginalis* and *Giardia lamblia,* inhabit the urogenital and gastrointestinal tracts and initiate disease characterized by mild to moderate morbidity but no mortality. Sporozoan organisms, in contrast, produce two of the most potentially lethal diseases of humankind, malaria and toxoplasmosis.

facultative anaerobes

nutrients engulfed by phagocytosis or pinocytosis

extrusion of wastes

Physiology. Most parasitic protozoa are facultative anaerobes. As they lack photosynthetic capacity, they must assimilate organic nutrients. This assimilation is accomplished by engulfing soluble or particulate matter in digestive vacuoles, processes termed *pinocytosis* and *phagocytosis,* respectively. In some species, food is ingested at a definite site, the peristome or cytostome. Food may be retained in special intracellular reserves, or *vacuoles.* Undigested particles and wastes are extruded at the cell surface by mechanisms that are the reverse of those used in ingestion.

Protozoal cysts

reproduction

Survival is ensured by highly developed protective and reproductive techniques. Many protozoa, when exposed to an unfavorable milieu, become less active metabolically and secrete a cyst wall capable of protecting the organism from physical and chemical conditions that would otherwise be lethal. In this form, the parasite is better equipped to survive passage from host to host in the external environment. Reproduction is accomplished primarily by simple *binary fission.* In one class of protozoa, the *Sporozoa,* a cycle of *multiple fission* (schizogony) alternates with a period of sexual reproduction (sporogony).

Helminths

great variation in size

differentiated organs: no circulatory system

Morphology and classification. Worms are elongated, bilaterally symmetric animals that vary in length from less than a millimeter to a meter or more. The body wall is covered with a tough acellular cuticle, which may be smooth or possess ridges, spines, and tubercles. At the anterior end there are often suckers, hooks, teeth, or plates used for the purpose of attachment. All helminths have differentiated organs. Primitive nervous and excretory systems and a highly developed reproductive system are characteristic of the entire group. Some have alimentary tracts; none possesses a circulatory system.

The common helminthic parasites of humans can be placed in one of three classes on the basis of body and alimentary tract, configuration, nature

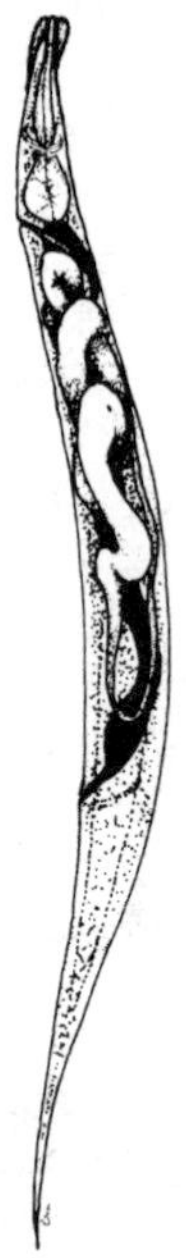

Prototypic nematode
(roundworm)

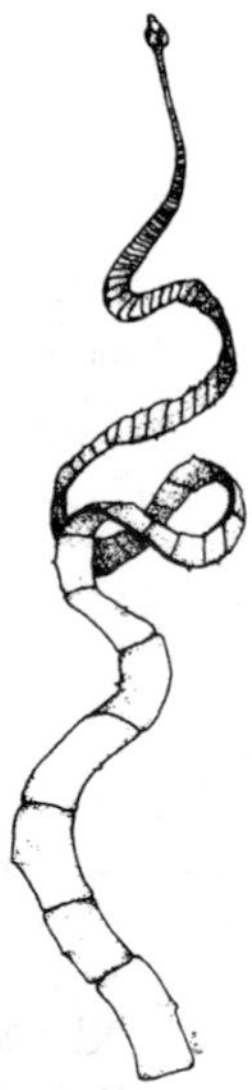

Cestode
(tapeworm)

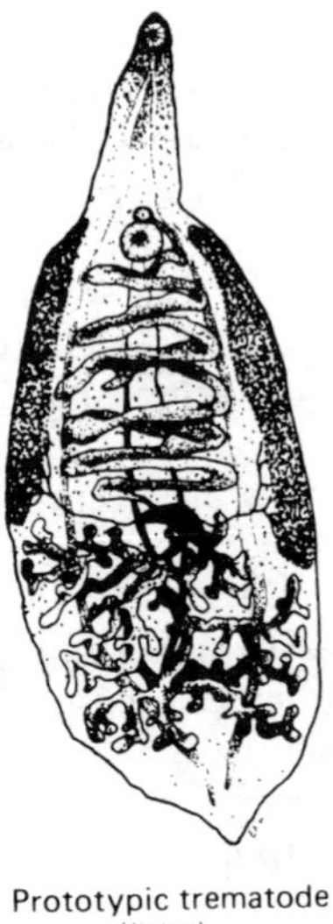

Prototypic trematode
(flukes)

Table 44.3 Classification of Helminthic Parasites of Humans

Characteristic	Roundworm (Nematode)	Tapeworm (Cestode)	Fluke (Trematode)
Morphology	Spindle shaped	Head with segmented body (proglottids)	Leaf shaped with oral and ventral suckers
Sex	Separate sexes	Hermaphroditic	Hermaphroditic[a]
Alimentary tract	Tubular	None	Blind
Intermediate host	Variable[b]	One[c]	Two[d]

[a] *Schistosoma* group has separate sexes.
[b] Tissue nematodes have intermediate hosts; intestinal nematodes do not.
[c] *Diphyllobothrium* group has two.
[d] *Schistosoma* group has one.

of the reproductive system, and need for more than a single host species for the completion of the life cycle (Table 44.3).

Roundworms, or nematodes, have a cylindric fusiform body and a tubular alimentary tract that extends from the mouth at the anterior end to the anus at the posterior end. The sexes are separate, and the male worm is typically smaller than the female. These worms can be divided into those that dwell within the gastrointestinal tract and those that parasitize the blood and tissues of humans. Unlike the latter, those in the gastrointestinal tract generally do not require intermediate hosts.

Tapeworms, or cestodes, have flattened, ribbon-shaped bodies. The anterior end, or scolex, is armed with suckers and frequently with hooklets, which are used for attachment. Immediately behind the head is a neck that generates a chain of reproductive segments, or proglottids. Each segment contains both male and female gonads. The worm lacks a digestive tract and presumably absorbs nutrients across its cuticle. One or sometimes two intermediate hosts are required for the completion of the life cycle.

Flukes, or trematodes, are leaf-shaped organisms with blind, branched alimentary tracts. Particulate waste is regurgitated through the mouth. Two suckers, one surrounding the mouth and the second located more distally on the ventral aspect of the body, serve as organs of attachment and locomotion. Most are hermaphroditic and require two intermediate hosts. The blood-dwelling schistosomes, however, are unisexual and require but a single intermediate.

anaerobic respiration of adult worm

Physiology. Helminthic parasites are nourished by ingestion or absorption of the body fluids, lysed tissue, or intestinal contents of their hosts. Carbohydrates are rapidly metabolized, and the glycogen concentration of the worms is high. Respiration is primarily anaerobic, although larval offspring frequently require oxygen. A large part of the energy requirement is devoted to reproductive needs. The daily output of offspring can be as high as 200,000 for some worms. Typically, helminths are oviparous (excrete eggs), but a few species are viviparous (give birth to living young).

high fertility

protection from environment

longevity

Protection from the host's digestive and body fluids is afforded by the tough cuticle and the secretion of enzymes. Some worms, such as the schistosomes, can protect themselves from immunologic attack by the incorporation of host antigens into their cuticles. The life span of the adult helminth is often measured in weeks or months, but some, such as the hookworms, filaria, and flukes, can survive within their hosts for decades.

Life Cycles, Transmission, and Distribution

Single-Host Parasites

As is evident from the previous discussion, many parasites require but a single host species for the completion of their life cycles. The method by which the parasite is transmitted from individual to individual within that species is determined in large part by its viability in the external environment and, in the case of helminths, by the conditions required for the maturation of offspring. The mode of transmission, in turn, determines the social, economic, and geographic distribution of the parasite. A few illustrative examples are summarized in Table 44.4.

direct contact transmission

The protozoan *T. vaginalis* does not produce protective cyst forms. Although its vegetative, or trophozoite, form is relatively hardy, it can survive only a few hours outside of its normal habitat, the human genital tract. Thus, for all practical purposes, transmission requires the direct genital contact of sexual intercourse. As a result, trichomoniasis is cosmopolitan, occurring wherever human hosts engage in sexual activity with multiple partners.

Fecal–oral transmission

survival of cysts

Another protozoan, *E. histolytica,* inhabits the human gut and produces hardy cysts that are passed in the stool. Transmission occurs when another individual ingests these cysts. Like *T. vaginalis,* the organism can be passed by direct physical contact, in this case by oral–anal sexual activity. This mode of transmission, in fact, accounts for the high incidence of amebic infections in male homosexuals. Unlike *T. vaginalis,* however, the cysts can survive for prolonged periods of time in the external environment, where they may eventually contaminate food or drinking water. Thus, in environments such as mental institutions, where the level of personal hygiene is low, or in populations in which methods for the sanitary disposal of human wastes are not available, amebiasis is common.

fecal–oral transmission with infectivity developing in soil

The intestinal helminth *Ascaris lumbricoides* illustrates still another transmission pattern. In this infection, highly resistant eggs are passed in the human stool. Unlike the situation with *E. histolytica* described previously, the eggs are not immediately infective, but must incubate in soil under certain conditions of temperature and humidity before they are fully embryonated and infectious. As a result, this parasite cannot be transmitted directly from host to host. The organism spreads only when indiscriminate human defecation results in deposition of eggs on soil and subsequent exposure of that soil to the climatic conditions required for embryonation of the eggs. For this reason, *Ascaris* infections are most prevalent in poorly sanitated areas of the tropics and subtropics.

Table 44.4 Transmission and Distribution

Organism	Infective Form	Mechanism of Spread	Distribution
Trichomonas vaginalis	Trophozoite	Direct (venereal)	Worldwide
Entamoeba histolytica	Cyst/trophozoite Cyst	Direct (venereal) Indirect (fecal–oral)	Worldwide Areas of poor sanitation
Ascaris lumbricoides	Egg	Indirect (fecal–oral)	Areas of poor sanitation
Plasmodium falciparum	Sporozoite	*Anopheles* mosquito	Tropical and subtropical areas

Multiple-Host Parasites

Definitive and intermediate hosts

A few protozoa and many helminths require two or more host species in their life cycle. To avoid confusion, it is customary to refer to the species in which the parasite reproduces sexually as the *definitive host*; that in which asexual reproduction or larval development takes place is the *intermediate host.* When there is more than one intermediate, they are known simply as the first or second intermediate hosts. In some cases, such as that of *Taenia saginata,* the beef tapeworm, both host species are vertebrates; humans serve as the definitive host and cattle as the intermediate. Among parasites that inhabit the blood and tissues of humans, it is more common for a blood-feeding arthropod to serve as a second host and as the transmitting vector. An example is malaria, in which the causative plasmodium is transmitted from person to person by the bite of an infected female mosquito of the genus *Anopheles.* In this particular instance, sexual reproduction occurs in the mosquito, making it the definitive host and relegating the human host to the role of a mere intermediate.

Influence of distribution of nonhuman hosts on disease occurrence

The distribution of parasites requiring a nonhuman host is limited to the ecologic niche occupied by this second host. Thus, the areas in which malaria is endemic are restricted by the distribution of *Anopheles.* The area of disease distribution is, in fact, generally smaller than that of the nonhuman host, because conditions favoring parasite transmission may also differ. For example, both the abundance of *Anopheles* and the speed with which the malarial parasite completes its development within them are directly related to the ambient temperature and humidity. Among temperate-zone *Anopheles,* the number of infected mosquitoes may be insufficient to sustain parasite transmission. In tropical areas, transmission is more likely to be constant and intense. In another more obvious example, infections with *T. saginata* are found only in areas where cattle are raised for human consumption and, within those areas, only where indiscriminate human defecation and the ingestion of raw or undercooked beef are common.

Pathogenesis

Humans as definitive and intermediate hosts

most adult helminths do not multiply within host

significance of reinfection and worm loads

In helminthic infections, humans may serve as the definitive host to the sexually mature adult worms (for example, *T. saginata*) or as the intermediate host to the larval stages (for example, *Echinococcus granulosus*). Occasionally, humans serve as both the definitive and the intermediate host to the same worm (for example, *Trichinella spiralis, Taenia solium*). Unlike protozoan parasites, most adult helminths are incapable of increasing their numbers within their definitive host. As a result, the severity of clinical illness is related to the total number of worms acquired by the host over time. Most small worm loads are, in fact, asymptomatic and may not require therapy. Many worms are long-lived, however, and repeated infections can result in very high worm loads with subsequent disability.

Some pathogenetic mechanisms

The pathogenesis of both protozoan and helminthic disease is variable. The fish tapeworm *Diphyllobothrium latum* competes with the host for nutrients. The protozoan *G. lamblia* and the helminth *Strongyloides stercoralis* interfere with the absorption of food across the intestinal mucosa. Hookworm infections cause loss of iron, an essential mineral. Other helminths, such as *Clonorchis sinensis* and *Schistosoma haematobium,* compromise the function of important organs by obstruction, secondary bacterial infection, and induction of carcinomatous changes. Occasionally, as in the case of echinococcosis, disease results from pressure and displacement of normal tissue by the slow growth of the parasitic cyst. In malaria, the primary pathogenic mechanism appears to be the invasion and subsequent alteration and/or destruction of human erythrocytes. Similarly, many helminthic larvae are capable of tissue invasion and destruction. *Entamoeba histolytica* can destroy host cells without actual cellular invasion. Finally, immunologic mechanisms are responsible for tissue damage and clinical manifestations in many parasitic diseases, including the nephrotic syndrome in malaria and schistosomiasis.

Diagnosis

need to consider indigenous and imported infections

Although parasitic diseases are not as common in the United States as elsewhere, they do occur and may, at times, be life threatening. In addition, the continuous arrival of travelers and immigrants from endemic areas necessitates consideration of these diseases in differential diagnoses. Unfortunately, the clinical manifestations of parasitic infections are seldom sufficiently characteristic to raise this possibility in the clinician's mind. Moreover, routine laboratory tests are seldom of aid. Although eosinophilia has been recognized as an important clue to the diagnosis of parasitic disease, this phenomenon is characteristic only of helminthic infection, and even in these cases it is frequently absent. Eosinophilia, which presumably reflects an immunologic response to the complex foreign proteins possessed by worms, is most marked during tissue migration. Once migration ceases, the eosinophilia may decrease or disappear entirely. Thus, the clinician must usually rely on a detailed travel, food intake, transfusion, and socioeconomic history to raise the possibility of parasitic disease.

variable eosinophilia in helminthic infections

demonstration and identification of intestinal parasites

Once considered, diagnosis is usually straightforward. Typically, it rests upon the demonstration and morphologic identification of the parasite or its progeny in the stool, urine, sputum, blood, or tissues of the human host.

Stool concentration techniques for intestinal parasites

In intestinal infections, a simple wet mount and/or stained smear of the stool is often adequate. Some parasites, however, are passed in the feces intermittently or in fluctuating numbers, and repeated specimens are needed. Ova of worms and cysts of protozoa may be concentrated by sedimentation or flotation techniques to increase their numbers for diagnosis. Occasionally, specimens other than stool must be examined. In the case of small-bowel infections such as giardiasis and strongyloidiasis, aspirates of the duodenum or a small-bowel biopsy may be required to establish the diagnosis. Similarly, the recovery of large-bowel parasites such as *E. histolytica* and *Schistosoma mansoni* may require proctoscopy or sigmoidoscopy with aspiration or biopsy of suspect lesions. Eggs of pinworms (*Enterobius*) and tapeworms (*Taenia*) may be found on the perineal skin when they are absent from the stool.

Demonstration and identification of blood and tissue parasites

Parasites dwelling within the tissue and blood of the host are more difficult to identify. Direct examination of the blood is useful for the detection of malarial parasites, leishmania, trypanosomes, and filarial progeny (microfilariae). The concentration of organisms in the bloodstream often fluctuates, however, requiring the collection of multiple specimens over several days. Both wet mount and stained preparations of thin and thick blood smears (Chapter 45) are used. Lung flukes and occasionally other helminths discharge their offspring in the sputum and may be found there with appropriate concentration techniques. In others, larvae can be recovered with skin (onchocerciasis) or muscle (trichinosis) biopsy.

Serologic tests

In some infections, parasite recovery is uncommon. Reliable serologic tests have been developed for several, including toxoplasmosis, amebiasis, South American trypanosomiasis, trichinosis, echinococcosis, and *Toxocara* infections. The recent introduction of purified homologous antigens and the adaptation of enzyme-linked immunosorbent assays to detection of parasitic infections will undoubtedly increase the number of useful tests in the near future.

Control and Treatment

The control of diseases spread by the fecal–oral route depends upon the improvements in personal hygiene and sanitation that accompany general economic development. In contrast, efforts at preventing the spread of multihost parasites is usually focused on the control or elimination of the nonhuman host.

Toxicity of many antiparasitic drugs

Many drugs used to treat parasitic disease are potentially toxic. For this reason, the decision to treat must be based on the morbidity and mortality of the parasitic disease in question. In helminthic infections, in which disability is usually related to the intensity of infection, worm load should be estimated before treatment is undertaken. In many intestinal infections, estimates of the worm load can be made by determining the concentration of eggs in the stool. Minor infections are treated only when small numbers of worms may be dangerous, as in the case of *A. lumbricoides,* or when the anthelmintic agent required is free of serious side effects.

Additional Reading and References

Desowitz, R.S. 1981. *New Guinea Tapeworms and Jewish Grandmothers: Tales of Parasites and People.* New York: Norton. A delightful look at the host–parasite relationship.

Dorozynski, A. 1976. The attack on tropical disease. *Nature* 262:85. A brief look at the World Health Organization's efforts to relieve mankind of one of its major burdens.

James J. Plorde

Sporozoan Infections

45

intracellular protozoa with alternating sexual and asexual cycles

malaria and toxoplasmosis major diseases

Sporozoa are a unique class of intracellular protozoa distinguished by their alternating cycles of sexual and asexual reproduction. Asexual multiplication occurs by a process of multiple fission termed *schizogony.* In it, the nucleus of a trophozoite divides into several parts, forming a multinucleated *schizont.* Cytoplasm then condenses around each nuclear portion to form new daughter cells, or *merozoites,* which burst from their intracellular location to invade new host cells. After the completion of one or more of these asexual cycles, some merozoites differentiate into male and female gametocytes, initiating the cycle of sexual reproduction known as *sporogony.* The gametocytes mature and effect fertilization, forming a *zygote.* Upon encysting, the zygote is known as an *oocyst. Sporozoites* formed within the oocyst are released, penetrate host tissue cells, and begin another asexual cycle as trophozoites.

Two sporozoan infections, malaria and toxoplasmosis, are common diseases of humans; together, they affect more than one-third of the world's population and kill or deform perhaps a million neonates and children each year.

MALARIA

Plasmodia: The Malarial Parasites

> Of all infectious diseases there is no doubt that malaria has caused the greatest harm to the greatest number. . . .
>
> Laderman, 1975

Sexual phase in mosquito

Asexual phase in humans

Species of malarial parasite

Definition. The plasmodia are sporozoa in which the sexual and asexual cycles of reproduction are completed in different host species. The sexual phase occurs within the gut of mosquitoes. These arthropods subsequently transmit the parasite while feeding upon a vertebrate host. Within the red cells of the vertebrate, the plasmodia reproduce asexually; they eventually burst from the erythrocyte and invade other uninvolved red cells. This event produces periodic fever and anemia in the host, a disease process known as *malaria.* Of the many species of plasmodia, four are known to infect humans and will be considered here: *Plasmodium vivax, Plasmodium ovale, Plasmodium malariae,* and *Plasmodium falciparum.*

Life Cycle of Malarial Parasites

Sexual cycle in mosquito

Sporogony, or the sexual cycle, begins when a female mosquito of the genus *Anopheles* ingests circulating male and female gametocytes while feeding upon a malarious human. In the gut of the mosquito, the gametocytes mature and effect fertilization. The resulting zygote penetrates the gut wall, lodges beneath the basement membrane, and vacuolates to form an oocyst. Within this structure thousands of sporozoites are formed. The enlarging cyst eventually ruptures, releasing the sporozoites into the body cavity. Some penetrate the salivary glands, rendering the mosquito infectious for humans. The time required for the completion of the cycle in mosquitoes varies from 1 to 3 weeks, depending upon the species of insect and parasite as well as on the ambient temperature and humidity.

sporozoites reach mosquito salivary glands

humans infected by mosquito bite

Hepatic asexual cycle in humans

Schizogony, the asexual cycle, begins when the infected *Anopheles* again takes a blood meal. Sporozoites from the mosquito's salivary glands are injected into the human's subcutaneous capillaries and circulate in the peripheral blood. Within one hour they invade liver cells (hepatocytes). In *P. vivax* and *P. ovale* infections, some of the sporozoites enter a dormant state immediately after cell invasion. The remaining sporozoites initiate *exoerythrocytic* schizogony, each producing about 2,000 to 40,000 daughter cells, or merozoites. One to two weeks later, the infected hepatocytes rupture, releasing merozoites into the general circulation.

Erythrocytic asexual cycle in humans

The erythrocytic phase of malaria starts with the attachment of a released hepatic merozoite to a specific receptor on the red cell surface. After attachment, the merozoite invaginates the cell membrane and is slowly endocytosed. The intracellular parasite initially appears as a ring-shaped trophozoite, which enlarges and becomes more active and irregular in outline. Within a few hours, nuclear division occurs, producing the multinucleated schizont. Cytoplasm eventually condenses around each nucleus of the schizont to form an intraerythrocytic cluster of 6–24 merozoite daughter cells. About 48 (*P. vivax, P. ovale,* and *P. falciparum*) to 72 (*P. malariae*) hr after initial invasion, infected erythrocytes rupture, releasing the merozoites and producing the first clinical manifestations of disease. The newly released daughter cells invade other red cells, where most repeat the asexual cycle. Other daughter cells are transformed into sexual forms or gametocytes. These latter forms do not produce red cell lysis and continue to circulate in the peripheral vasculature until ingested by an appropriate mosquito. The recurring asexual cycles continue, involving an ever increasing number of erythrocytes until finally the development of host immunity brings the erythrocytic cycle to a close. The dormant hepatic sporozoites of *P. vivax* and *P. ovale* survive the host's immunologic attack and may, after a latent period of months to years, resume intrahepatic multiplication. This leads to a second release of hepatic merozoites and the initiation of another erythrocytic cycle, a phenomenon known as *relapse.* The life cycle of malarial parasites is summarized in Figure 45.1.

cyclical rupture and reinfection of erythrocytes

Some gametocytes formed; mosquito ingests gametocytes with blood meal

intrahepatic dormancy and relapses with *P. vivax* and *P. ovale*

Morphology

The morphology of the stained intraerythrocytic parasites is shown following color Plate DD. Three characteristic features are noted: red nuclear chromatin; blue cytoplasm; and brownish-black malarial pigment, or hemozoin, thought to be denatured hemoglobin. The change in the shape of the cytoplasm and the division of the chromatin at different stages of parasite development are obvious. Gametocytes can be differentiated from the asexual forms by their large size and lack of nuclear division. Some of the

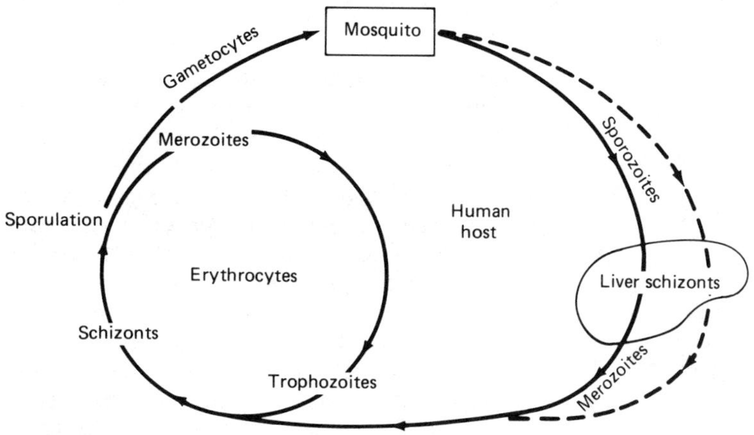

45.1 Malarial parasite cycle. — — — = dormancy in liver (*Plasmodium vivax, Plasmodium ovale*).

infected erythrocytes develop membrane invaginations, which appear in the stained cell as pink cytoplasmic granules.

Morphologic differences between intraerythrocytic parasites

The appearance of each of the four species of plasmodia that infect humans is sufficiently different to allow their differentiation in stained smears. The parasitized erythrocyte in *P. vivax* and *P. ovale* infections is pale, enlarged, and contains numerous small granules known as *Schüffner's dots.* All asexual stages (trophozoite, schizont, merozoite) may be seen simultaneously. Cells infected by *P. ovale* are elongated and frequently irregular or fimbriated in appearance. In *P. malariae* infections, the red cells are not enlarged and contain no granules. The trophozoites often present as "band" forms, and the merozoites are arranged in rosettes around a clump of central pigment. In *P. falciparum* infections, the rings are very small and may contain two rather than a single chromatin dot. There is often more than a single parasite per cell, and parasites are frequently seen lying against the margin of the cell. Intracytoplasmic granules known as *Maurer's dots* may be present, but are often cleft shaped and fewer in number than Schüffner's dots. Schizonts and merozoites are not present in the peripheral blood. Gametocytes are large and banana shaped. These characteristics are summarized in Table 45.1 and illustrated in the color plate.

Table 45.1 Differential Characteristics of *Plasmodium* Species

Characteristics	*P. vivax*	*P. ovale*	*P. malariae*	*P. falciparum*
Erythrocyte				
Enlarged, pale	+	+	—	—
Oval, fimbriated	—	+	—	—
Schüffner's dots	+	+	—	—
Maurer's dots	—	—	—	+
Parasite				
All asexual stages seen	+	+	+	—
Band forms	—	—	+	—
Double infections	—	—	—	+
Double chromatin dots	—	—	—	+
Banana-shaped gametocytes	—	—	—	+

Physiology

parasites vary in ability to attack subpopulations of erythrocytes

Species of plasmodia differ significantly in their ability to invade subpopulations of erythrocytes; *P. vivax* and *P. ovale* attack only immature cells (reticulocytes), whereas *P. malariae* attacks only senescent cells. During infection with these species, therefore, no more than 1–2% of the cell population is involved. *Plasmodium falciparum,* in contrast, invades red cells *regardless of age* and may produce very high levels of parasitemia. In part, these differences may be related to the known differences in the red cell receptor sites available to the individual *Plasmodium* species. In the case of *P. vivax,* the site is closely related to the Duffy blood group antigens (Fy^a and Fy^b). Duffy-negative individuals, who constitute the majority of people of West African ancestry, are therefore resistant to vivax malaria. The receptors in the other species have not yet been defined.

Relation of Duffy antigen to *P. vivax* receptor

Effect of sickle cell trait on intensity of *P. falciparum* infection

Certain red cell abnormalities may also effect parasitism. The altered hemoglobin (hemoglobin S) associated with the sickle cell trait limits the intensity of the parasitemia caused by *P. falciparum* and thereby provides a selective advantage to individuals who are heterozygous for the sickle cell gene. As a result, the sickle cell gene, which would otherwise be disadvantageous, is found at high frequency in populations living in malarious areas. A similar protective effect may be exerted by hemoglobins C, D, and E, thalassemia, and glucose 6-phosphate dehydrogenase (G6PD) or pyridoxal kinase deficiencies, as these abnormalities have also been found more frequently in malarious areas. The mechanisms of protection have not been clearly defined; however, infected red cells heterozygous for hemoglobin S develop a sickle form more readily in vitro than do noninfected cells, and if this occurs in vivo the cells may be more readily phagocytosed and destroyed. In thalassemia, the protection may be related in part to the production of fetal hemoglobin, which retards maturation of *P. falciparum.*

Changes in erythrocytes

Once invasion has occurred, malarial parasites may induce changes in erythrocytic membranes. In addition to invaginations or clefts, elevated knobs or excrescences may form on the surface, particularly in *P. falciparum* infections. These outgrowths have been shown to fuse with endothelial cell membranes, suggesting that they may play a role in the known tendency of *P. falciparum*-infected cells to sequester in the capillaries of the deep organs, where they can produce obstruction and microinfarcts. Malarial parasites may also alter the lipid composition of the erythrocytic membrane, and proteins from the parasite may modify both its osmotic properties and its susceptibility to immunologic attack.

association with microinfarcts

Metabolism of malarial parasites

Malarial parasites generate energy by metabolism of glucose. They appear to satisfy their protein requirements by the degradation of hemoglobin, resulting in the formation of the malarial pigment (hemozoin) mentioned previously. It has been estimated that the average plasmodium destroys between 25 and 75% of the hemoglobin of its host erythrocyte. Unlike their vertebrate hosts, malarial parasites synthesize folates de novo. As a result, antifolate antimicrobics such as pyrimethamine are effective antimalarious agents.

Growth in the Laboratory

Continuous in vitro cultivation of plasmodia in human erythrocytes has been achieved recently. The technique, which employs dilute cultures with low initial parasite densities in a reduced oxygen atmosphere, provides new opportunities for studying the biology, immunology, and chemotherapy of human malaria. Its most immediate impact has been on the development of methods for testing the sensitivity of *P. falciparum* to chemotherapeutic agents.

Malaria Infections

Epidemiology

Distribution

Malaria has a worldwide distribution between 45°N and 40°S latitude, generally at altitudes below 1800 m. *Plasmodium vivax* is the most widely distributed of the four species and, together with the uncommon *P. malariae,* is found primarily in temperate and subtropical areas. *Plasmodium falciparum* is the dominant organism of the tropics. *Plasmodium ovale* is rare and found principally in Africa.

Factors influencing intensity

Clinical manifestations muted with hyperendemicity

The intensity of malarial transmission in an endemic area depends upon the density and feeding habits of suitable mosquito vectors and the prevalence of infected humans, who serve as parasite reservoirs. In hyperendemic areas, transmission is usually constant, and disease manifestations are moderated by the development of immunity. Mortality is largely restricted to infants and to nonimmune adults who migrate into the region. When the prevalence of disease is lower, transmission is typically intermittent. In this situation, solid immunity does not develop and the population suffers repeated, often seasonal, epidemics, the impact of which is shared by people of all ages.

Extent and mortality of malaria

At the present time, malaria infects over 125 million inhabitants of 104 countries throughout Africa, Asia, Latin America, and Oceania (Figure 45.2). One million children, primarily Africans, die of the disease each year.

45.2 Status of malaria, 1979. (*Reproduced from Health Information for International Travel, Supplement, Morbidity and Mortality Weekly Report, Vol. 30, 1981, U.S. Government Printing Office.*)

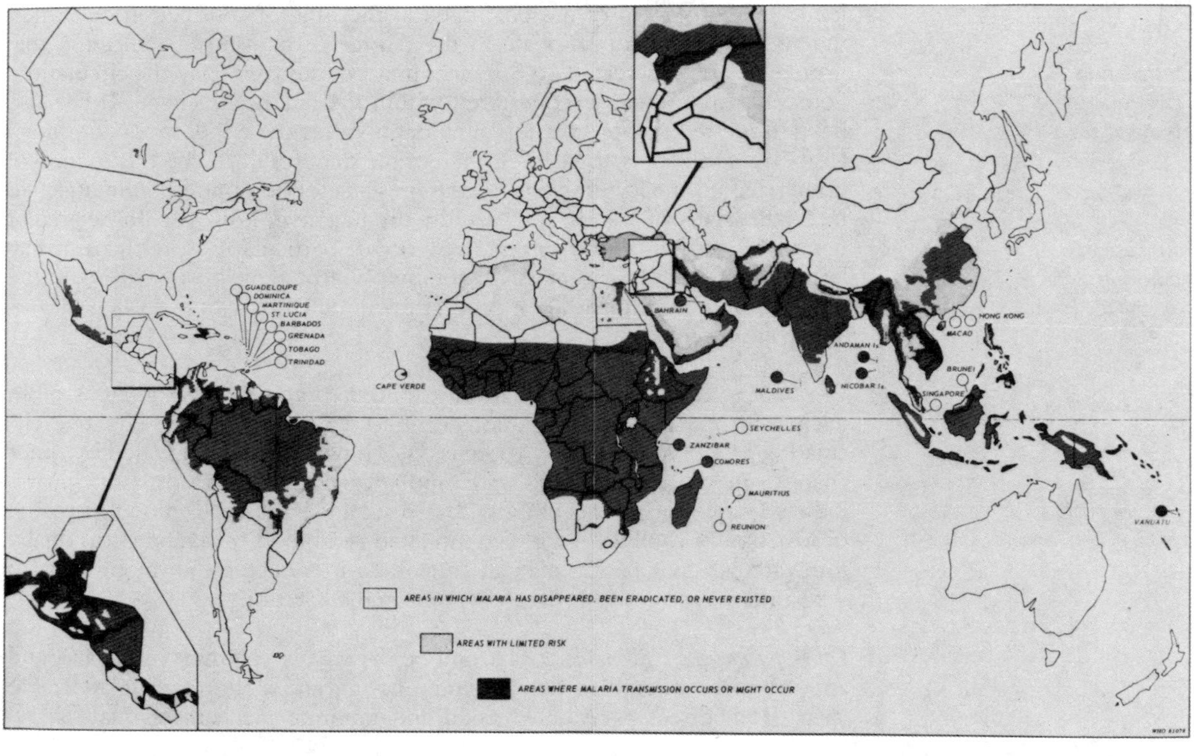

Imported malaria

Although endemic malaria disappeared from the United States three decades ago, imported cases continue to be reported, and the recent worldwide resurgence of malaria combined with an increase in international travel has resulted in an increase in their numbers. Approximately 50% of imported cases acquire the disease in Asia, 30% in Africa, and 10% in the Caribbean or Latin America. Clinical manifestations typically develop within 6 months of arrival of cases in the United States; however, one-third of cases caused by *P. vivax* are delayed beyond that time. Approximately 20% of imported cases and almost all associated fatalities have been caused by the virulent *P. falciparum.* Tragically, most of these cases could have been prevented or successfully treated.

Pathogenesis and Pathology

The fever, anemia, circulatory changes, and immunopathologic phenomena characteristic of malaria are all the result of erythrocytic invasion by the plasmodia.

Fever associated with red cell rupture

Fever. Fever, the hallmark of malaria, appears to be initiated by the process of red cell rupture that leads to the liberation of a new generation of merozoites (sporulation). It seems likely that a pyrogenic substance released during this process is responsible for the fever; to date, however, all attempts to detect the presence of a circulating pyrogen have been unsuccessful. Early in malaria, red cells appear to be infected with malarial parasites at several different stages of development, each inducing sporulation at a different time. The resulting fever is irregular and hectic. Eventually one population dominates, sporulation is synchronized, and fever occurs in distinct paroxysms at 48-hr or, in the case of *P. malariae,* 72-hr intervals.

Synchronization of sporulation

Phagocytosis of parasitized erythrocytes

Anemia. Parasitized erythrocytes are phagocytosed by a stimulated reticuloendothelial system or are destroyed at the time of sporulation. At times, the anemia is disproportionate to the degree of parasitism, indicating that normal as well as infected erythrocytes may be removed from the circulation. Some are undoubtedly sequestered within the enlarging spleen. It has also been suggested that production of autoantibodies and adherence of antigen–antibody complexes to the cell membrane may result in the destruction of uninfected erythrocytes. Tests for the presence of immunoglobulin attached to erythrocytes (Coombs' test) are usually negative, however. Intravascular hemolysis, although uncommon, may occur, particularly in falciparum malaria. When hemolysis is massive, hemoglobinuria develops, resulting in the production of dark urine. This process in conjunction with malaria is known as *blackwater fever.*

Destruction of normal erythrocytes

Intravascular hemolysis and blackwater fever

Decreased blood flow to vital organs

Circulatory changes. The high fever results in significant vasodilatation. In falciparum malaria, vasodilatation leads to a decrease in the effective circulating blood volume and hypotension, which may be aggravated by other changes in the small vessels and capillaries. Localized vasospasm, kinase-induced capillary permeability with a resultant increase in blood viscosity, obstruction of capillaries with agglutinated red blood cells, and occasionally intravascular coagulation may all contribute to a decrease in blood flow to vital organs, resulting in tissue hypoxia and infarction.

Other pathogenetic phenomena. Thrombocytopenia is common in malaria and appears to be related to both splenic pooling and a shortened platelet life span. Both direct parasitic invasion and immune mechanisms may be responsible. There may be an acute transient glomerulonephritis in falciparum malaria and progressive renal disease in chronic *P. malariae* malaria. These phenomena probably result from the host immune response, with deposition on immune complexes in the glomeruli.

Immunity. Once infected, the host quickly mounts an immunologic response that typically limits parasite multiplication and moderates the clinical manifestations of disease. There follows a prolonged recovery period marked by recurrent exacerbations in both symptoms and number of erythrocytic parasites. With time, the recrudescences become less severe and less frequent, eventually stopping altogether.

evidence for antibody-mediated immunity

The exact mechanisms involved in this recovery are uncertain. In simian and probably in human malaria, recovery is known to require the presence of both T and B lymphocytes. It is probable that the T cells have a helper effect on antibody production. Some authorities have suggested that they may also play a more direct role by stimulating effector cells to release nonspecific factors capable of inhibiting intraerythrocytic multiplication. The B lymphocytes begin production of strain-specific antiplasmodial antibodies within the first 2 weeks of parasitemia. With the achievement of high levels of antibodies, the number of circulating parasites decreases. The infrequency with which malaria occurs in young infants has been attributed to the transplacental passage of such antibodies. It is uncertain whether they are directly lethal, act as opsonizing agents, or block merozoite invasion of red cells.

evidence for antigenic variation of malarial parasites

In simian malaria, the parasite can undergo antigenic variation and thereby escape the suppressive effect of the antibodies. This antigenic variation leads to cycles of recrudescent parasitemia but, ultimately, to production of specific antibodies to the variants, and cure. It seems probable that similar changes occur in humans, leading to the eventual disappearance of erythrocytic parasites. With *P. falciparum* and *P. malariae,* which have no persistent hepatic forms, this results in cure. In the former, the disease typically does not exceed 1 year, but with *P. malariae* the erythrocytic infection can be extremely persistent, lasting in one case up to 53 years. How erythrocytic parasites circulating in numbers too small to be detected on routine blood films escape immunologic destruction remains a puzzle. In a closely related simian malaria, splenectomy results in rapid cure, suggesting that suppressor T cells in the spleen may play a protective role. In infection with *P. vivax* and *P. ovale,* latent hepatic infection may result in the discharge of fresh merozoites into the bloodstream after the disappearance of erythrocytic forms. This phenomenon, known as relapse, is capable of maintaining infection for 3–5 years.

possible role of suppressor cells in maintenance of erythrocytic parasites

Clinical Manifestations

Incubation period

The incubation period between the bite of the mosquito and the onset of disease is approximately 2 weeks; that with *P. malariae* and with strains of *P. vivax* in temperate climates, however, is often more prolonged. Individuals who contract malaria while taking antimalarial suppressants may not experience illness for many months. In United States, the interval between entry into the country and onset of disease exceeds 1 month in 25% of *P. falciparum* infections and 6 months in a similar proportion of vivax cases.

malarial paroxysm: cold, hot, and wet stages

The clinical manifestations vary with the species of plasmodia, but typically include chills, fever, splenomegaly, and anemia. The hallmark of disease is the malarial paroxysm. This manifestation begins with a *cold stage,* which persists for 20–60 min. During this time, the patient experiences continuous rigors and feels cold. With the consequent increase in body temperature, the rigors cease and vasodilatation commences, ushering in a *hot stage.* The temperature continues to rise for 3–8 hr, reaching a maximum of 40–41.7°C (104–107°F) before it begins to fall. The *wet stage* consists of a decrease in fever and profuse sweating. It leaves the patient exhausted but otherwise well until the onset of the next paroxysm. Typical paroxysms first appear in the second or third week of fever, when parasite sporulation becomes synchronized. In falciparum malaria, synchronization may never take place, and the fever may remain hectic and unpredictable. The first attack is often severe and may persist for weeks in the untreated patient. Eventually the paroxysms become less regular, less frequent, and less severe. Symptoms finally cease with the disappearance of the parasites from the blood.

typical paroxysms when sporulation is synchronized

In falciparum malaria, capillary blockage can lead to several serious complications. When the central nervous system is involved (cerebral malaria), the patient may develop delirium, convulsions, paralysis, coma, and rapid death. Blockade of the pulmonary circulation may result in cough, blood-streaked sputum, and difficult breathing. Pulmonary manifestations frequently accompany cerebral malaria. When splanchnic capillaries are involved, the patient may experience vomiting, abdominal pain, and diarrhea with or without bloody stools. Jaundice and acute renal failure are also common in severe illness. These pernicious syndromes generally appear when the intensity of parasitemia exceeds 100,000 organisms per cubic millimeter of blood.

Cerebral malaria and other severe systemic manifestations with *P. falciparum*

Laboratory Diagnosis

Thick and thin blood smears

Malarial parasites can be demonstrated in stained smears of the peripheral blood in virtually all symptomatic patients. Typically, capillary or venous blood is used to prepare both thin and thick smears, which are stained with Wright or Giemsa stain and examined for the presence of erythrocytic parasites. Thick smears, in which erythrocytes are lysed with water before staining, concentrate the parasites and allow detection of very mild parasitemia. Nonetheless, it may be necessary to obtain several specimens before parasites are seen. Artifacts are numerous in thick smears, and correct interpretation requires experience. The morphologic differences among the four species of plasmodia allow their speciation on the stained smear by the skilled observer.

Serologic tests for malaria are available, but are used primarily for epidemiologic purposes. They are occasionally helpful in speciation and detection of otherwise occult infections.

Treatment

need to destroy all forms of the parasite

The adequate treatment of malaria requires the destruction of three parasitic forms: the erythrocytic schizont, the hepatic schizont, and the erythrocytic gametocyte. The first terminates the clinical attack, the second prevents relapse, and the third renders the patient noninfectious to *Anopheles* and thus breaks the cycle of transmission. Unfortunately, no single drug accomplishes all three goals. The present strategy of chemotherapy is shown in Table 45.2.

chloroquine-resistant strains

Termination of acute attack. Several agents can destroy asexual erythrocytic parasites. Chloroquine, a 4-aminoquinalone, is that most commonly used. It is rapidly effective against all four species of plasmodia and, in the dosage used, is free of serious side effects. Strains of *P. falciparum* resistant to this agent are present in Latin America, Sóutheast Asia, and East Africa. They are treated with combinations of quinine, antifolates, and sulfonamides.

Table 45.2 Chemotherapy of Malaria

Stage of Parasite	Clinical Goal	Drug
Erythrocytic schizont	Treat clinical attack	
	All species	Chloroquine
	CRFM	Quinine, antifolates, sulfonamides
	Suppress clinical attack	
	All species	Chloroquine
	CRFM	Antifolates, sulfonamides
Erythrocytic gametocyte	Prevent transmission	
	Relapsing malaria	Chloroquine
	Falciparum malaria	Primaquine
Hepatic schizont	Radical cure	
	Relapsing malaria	Primaquine
	Falciparum malaria	None required

Abbreviation: CRFM = chloroquine-resistant falciparum malaria.

Radical cure. In *P. vivax* and *P. ovale* infections, hepatic schizonts persist and must be destroyed to prevent reseeding of circulating erythrocytes with consequent relapse. Primaquine, an 8-aminoquinalone, is used for this purpose. Unfortunately, it may induce hemolysis in patients with glucose 6-phosphate dehydrogenase deficiency. Persons of Asian, African, and Mediterranean ancestry should thus be screened for this abnormality before treatment.

Destruction of circulating gametocytes. Chloroquine destroys the gametocytes of *P. vivax, P. ovale,* and *P. malariae,* but not those of *P. falciparum.* Primaquine is, however, effective for this species.

Prevention

Mosquito control

Chemoprophylaxis

Personal protection. In endemic areas, mosquito contact can be minimized through the use of house screenings, mosquito netting around beds, and insect repellents. In addition, it is possible to suppress clinical manifestations of infection, should it occur, with a weekly dose of chloroquine. In areas where chloroquine-resistant strains are common, pyrimethamine plus sulfadoxine can be taken orally at the same interval. On leaving an endemic area, it is necessary to eradicate residual hepatic parasites with primaquine before discontinuing suppressive therapy.

Attempts at eradication

General. Malaria control measures are directed toward reducing the infected human and mosquito populations to below the critical level necessary for sustained transmission of disease. The techniques employed include those mentioned previously, treatment of febrile patients with effective antimalarial agents, chemical or physical disruption of mosquito breeding areas, and use of residual insecticide sprays. An active international cooperative program aimed at the eradication of malaria resulted in a dramatic decline in the incidence of the disease between 1956 and 1968. Eradication was not achieved, however, as mosquitoes became resistant to some of the chemical agents used, and today malaria still infects 125 million inhabitants of Africa, Latin America, and Asia. Tropical Africa alone accounts for 100 million of the afflicted and for most of the 1 million deaths that occur annually as a result of this disease. The long-term hope for progress in these areas now depends upon the development of new technologies. Work on a malaria vaccine is continuing, and it is hoped that effective preparations may become available in this century.

TOXOPLASMOSIS

Toxoplasma

Asexual and sexual cycles in felines

Spectrum of disease

Definition. Like the plasmodia, *Toxoplasma gondii,* the cause of toxoplasmosis, is an obligate intracellular sporozoan. It differs from *Plasmodium* in that both sexual and asexual reproductive cycles occur within the gastrointestinal tract of felines, the definitive host. The disease is transmitted to other host species by the ingestion of oocysts passed in the feces of infected felines.

Toxoplasma can infect most warm-blooded animals, both domestic and wild; they are thus the most cosmopolitan of parasites. Approximately one-half of the human population of the United States has been infected. In the overwhelming majority the infection is chronic, asymptomatic, and self-limiting. Clinical disease presents in three major forms: 1) self-limiting febrile lymphadenopathy; 2) highly lethal infection of immunocompromised patients; and 3) congenital infection of infants.

Life Cycle

infection in cat ileal cells

fusion of gametes leads to oocyst formation; shed in feces

Sporulation in external environment

Definitive host. Sexual reproduction of *T. gondii* occurs only in the intestinal tract of felines. Production of oocysts has been demonstrated in ocelots, bobcats, cougars, and leopards, in addition to the domestic cat. Ingested parasites enter the epithelial cells of the ileum by mechanisms that remain poorly defined. Intracellularly, the trophozoites reside within a membrane-bound vacuole and undergo schizogony. With cell rupture, merozoites are released. The merozoites infect adjacent epithelial cells; they then repeat another asexual cycle or eventually differentiate into gametocytes, initiating sexual reproduction. Fusion of the mature male and female gametes leads to the formation of an oval, thick-walled oocyst that is then shed in the feces. In the typical infection, millions of these structures are released daily for 1–3 weeks. The oocysts are immature at the time of shedding and must complete sporulation in the external environment. In this process, two sporocysts, each containing four sporozoites, develop within each oocyst. The time required for sporulation varies from 1 day to 3 weeks, depending upon the ambient temperature and moisture. Once mature, the resistant oocyts may remain viable and infectious for as long as a year.

Mature oocysts infect hosts orally

released sporozoites invade macrophages

development of cysts

Infection from cysts in meat

Intermediate hosts. After ingestion by a susceptible warm-blooded animal, sporozoites are released from the disrupted oocyst and enter macrophages. Within these cells they are transported through the lymphohematogenous system to all organ systems. Continued intracellular schizogony results in macrophage rupture and release of new parasites, which may invade any adjacent nucleated host cell and continue the asexual cycle. With the development of host immunity, many of the parasites are destroyed. Within the cells of certain organs, particularly the brain, heart, and skeletal muscle, the trophozoites produce a membrane that surrounds and protects them: within this tissue cyst, multiplication continues at a more leisurely pace. Eventually, cysts that measure up to 200 μm in diameter and contain more than a thousand organisms are produced. These cysts may persist intact for the life of the host or rupture, producing parasitologic relapse. If they are ingested by a carnivore, they survive the digestive enzymes and initiate infection in the new host.

Description of Organism

General. *Toxoplasma gondii* was first demonstrated in 1908 in the gondi, an African rodent, by Nicolle and Marceaux. Its name, derived from the Greek *toxo* (arc), is based on the characteristic shape of the organism. All strains of this parasite appear to be closely related antigenically. The major morphologic forms of the parasite are the oocyst, trophozoite, and tissue cyst.

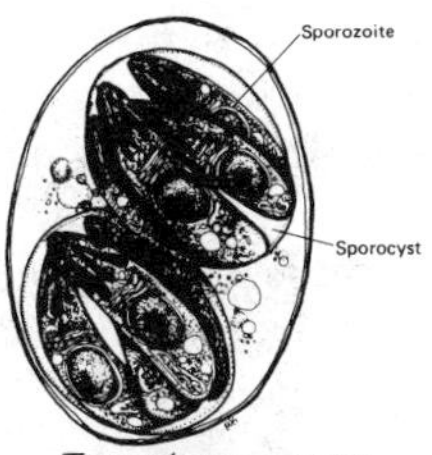

Toxoplasma oocyst

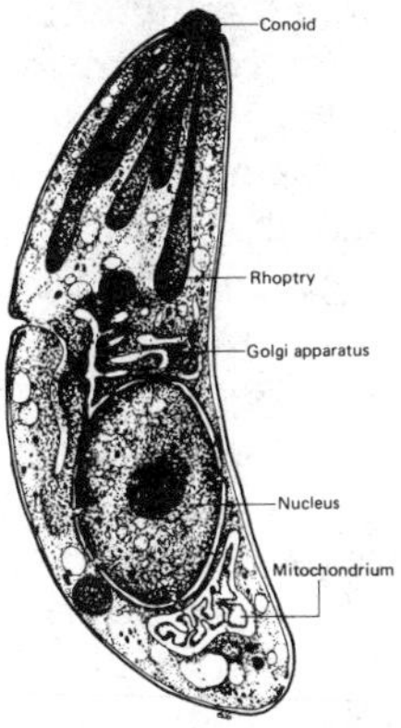

Toxoplasma tachyzoite (trophozoite)

Oocyst. The oocyst is ovoid, measures 10–12 μm in diameter, and possesses a thick wall that makes it resistant to most environmental challenges. It may be destroyed by heat in excess of 66°C, and chemicals such as iodine and formalin. In its immature form, the center of the cyst lacks internal structure. With maturation two sporocysts appear, and later four sporozoites may be discerned within each sporocyst. Sporulation does not occur at temperatures below 4°C or above 37°C. This form is responsible for the spread of the parasites from felines to other warm-blooded animals via the fecal–oral route.

Trophozoite. The term *trophozoite* is used in its broadest sense to refer to the asexual proliferative forms responsible for cell invasion. In different stages of the asexual cycle it is referred to by several other terms, including merozoites, endozoite, schizont, and tachyzoite. It is crescent or arc shaped, and measures 3 × 7 μm, and can invade all nucleated cell types. Although trophozoites are obligate intracellular organisms, they may survive extracellularly in a variety of body fluids for periods of hours to days. They cannot, however, survive the digestive activity of the stomach, and therefore are not infective on ingestion.

Tissue cysts. Cysts measure 10–200 μm in diameter. The contained organisms are similar to but smaller than trophozoites. Tissue cysts are resistant to digestive enzymes; thus, they are infectious to the animal that ingests them. They survive normal refrigerator temperatures, but are killed by freezing and thawing and by normal cooking temperatures.

Toxoplasma Infections

Prevalence and Distribution

Toxoplasmosis is a cosmopolitan disease that invades almost all mammals and many birds. Human infections are found in every region of the globe; in general the incidence is higher in the tropics and lower in cold, arid regions. In the United States, the prevalence of positive serologic test results for the disease increases with age. By adulthood, approximately 50% of Americans can be shown to have circulating antibodies against *T. gondii.*

Transmission

Although it is known that humans may acquire toxoplasmosis in a variety of ways, data on their relative frequency are both meager and conflicting. It is likely that the route of transmission varies from population to population and, perhaps, from age to age within any given area. The most important transmission mechanisms are discussed below.

significance of feline infections

Ingestion of oocysts. Felinophobes are inclined to the view that the deposition of oocysts in the feces of cats and their subsequent ingestion by the unsuspecting owner is the most frequent way in which humans acquire this important infection. Disease epidemics associated with exposure to infected cats have been reported. Unfortunately, data from studies relating the frequency of feline exposure to the prevalence of positive serologic tests are conflicting. Acutely infected cats shed oocysts for only a few weeks. It has been shown, however, that chronically infected felines can reshed oocysts, and prevalence studies have demonstrated that 1% of domestic cats excrete oocysts at any given time. The large number of these structures passed during active shedding and their prolonged survival in the external environment greatly enhance their chance of transmission. Particularly at risk are individuals such as children at play, who may come in close contact with areas likely to be contaminated with cat feces, and adults responsible for changing kitty litter. It is also possible that insects can mechanically transfer oocysts to human food.

special hazard to children

Ingestion of tissue cysts. Tissue cysts have been frequently demonstrated in meat produced for human consumption. They are most common in pork (25%) and mutton (10%), less so in beef and chicken (less than 1%). Although such cysts are killed at normal (well done) cooking temperatures, an impressive array of epidemiologic information links the handling and/or ingestion of raw or undercooked meat with serologic and, occasionally, clinical evidence of disease. Confounding these data is an Indian study that demonstrated no difference between meat eaters and vegetarians in the incidence of positive serologic tests.

cysts killed by normal cooking

Congenital. Approximately 1 of every 500 pregnant women acquires acute toxoplasmosis, and in one-half of all such cases the infection spreads to the fetus. The risk of transplacental transmission is independent of the clinical severity of the disease in the mother, but does correlate with the stage of gestation at which she is exposed. Fetal involvement occurs in 17% of first trimester and 65% of third trimester infections. Conversely, the earlier a fetal infection is acquired, the more severe it is likely to be. Overall, 20% of fetuses experience severe consequences; a similar proportion develop mild disease. The remainder are asymptomatic.

Transplacental transmission

Miscellaneous. In addition to causing congenital infection, trophozoites have been responsible for disease transmission in a number of other situations, including laboratory accidents, transfusions of whole blood and leukocytes, and organ transplantation. As trophozoites may survive for several hours in body fluids or exudates of acutely infected humans, it is possible for infection to occur after contact with such materials.

Laboratory accidents

Blood and organ transplantation

Immunity and Pathogenesis

In the primary infection, the proliferation of trophozoites results in the death of involved host cells and the stimulation of a mononuclear inflammatory reaction. In immunodeficient hosts, rapid organism proliferation continues, producing numerous widespread foci of tissue necrosis. The consequences are most serious in organs such as the brain, where the potential for cell regeneration is limited.

dissemination in immunosuppressed subjects

In normal hosts, however, acute infection is rapidly controlled with the development of humoral and cellular immunity. Extracellular parasites are destroyed, intracellular multiplication is hindered and tissue cysts are formed. With the exception of the destruction of extracellular parasites, cell-mediated immunity appears to play the principal role in this process. Immunity appears to be lifelong, possibly because of survival of the parasite in the tissue cysts.

The cysts, which are found most frequently in the brain, heart, and skeletal muscle, normally produce little or no tissue reaction. The suppression of cell-mediated immunity that accompanies serious illness, or the administration of immunosuppressive agents may lead to the rupture of a cyst and the release of trophozoites. Their subsequent proliferation and the intense immunologic reaction to their presence results in an acute exacerbation of the disease.

Clinical Manifestations

In the vast majority of patients, infection with *T. gondii* is completely asymptomatic. Clinical manifestations, when they do appear, vary with the type of host involved. In general, they may be grouped into one of the three syndromes listed below.

severe manifestations of infection in utero

Congenital toxoplasmosis. Immune mechanisms are poorly developed in utero. As a result, a large proportion of fetal infections result in clinical illness. If the infection spreads to the central nervous system, the outcome is often catastrophic. Abortion and stillbirth are the most serious consequences. Liveborn children may demonstrate microcephaly, hydrocephaly, cerebral calcifications, convulsions, and psychomotor retardation. Disease of this severity is usually accompanied by evidence of visceral involvement, including fever, hepatitis, pneumonia, and skin rash. Infants infected later in prenatal development demonstrate milder disease. Many appear healthy at birth, but develop epilepsy, retardation, or strabismus months or years later. Probably the most common delayed manifestation of congenital toxoplasmosis is chorioretinitis. This condition, which is thought to result from the reactivation of latent tissue cysts, typically presents during the second or third decade of life as recurrent bouts of eye pain and loss of visual acuity. The lesions are usually bilateral but focal. If the retinal macula is not involved, vision improves as the inflammation subsides. This manifestation accounts for one-quarter of all cases of granulomatous uveitis seen in the United States.

Chorioretinitis

can mimic infectious mononucleosis

Normal host. The most common clinical manifestation of toxoplasmosis acquired after birth is asymptomatic localized lymphadenopathy. The cervical nodes are most frequently involved, but nontender enlargement of other regional groups, including the retroperitoneal nodes, also occurs. At times, the adenopathy is accompanied by fever, sore throat, rash, hepatosplenomegaly, and atypical lymphocytosis, thus mimicking the clinical and laboratory manifestations of infectious mononucleosis. Occasionally the normal host will develop severe visceral involvement, which may be manifested as meningoencephalitis, pneumonitis, myocarditis, or hepatitis. Chorioretinitis following postnatally acquired infection, although documented, is highly unusual. Unlike congenitally acquired ocular disease, it occurs during midlife and is generally unilateral.

Immunocompromised host. In the immunocompromised host, toxoplasmosis is a serious, often fatal disease. If primary infection is acquired while a patient is undergoing immunosuppressive therapy for malignancy or organ transplantation, widespread dissemination of the infection with necrotizing pneumonitis, myocarditis, and encephalitis may occur. More commonly, acute disease in this population results from the activation of chronic, latent infection by the immunosuppressive therapy. Encephalitis occurs in 50% of such cases and in more than 90% of fatal cases.

reactivation of latent infections with severe manifestations

Laboratory Diagnosis

Demonstration of parasite

The diagnosis may be established by a variety of methods. In acute toxoplasmic lymphadenitis, the histologic appearance of the involved nodes is often pathognomonic. The trophozoite may be demonstrated in tissue with Wright or Giemsa stain. Electron microscopy and indirect fluorescent antibody techniques have also been used successfully on brain tissue obtained by biopsy. Although tissue cysts are selectively stained by periodic acid–Schiff, their presence is not indicative of acute disease. Isolation of the organism can be accomplished by inoculating blood or other body fluids into mice or tissue cultures. Inoculation of other tissues is not usually helpful, as a positive result may only reflect the presence of latent tissue cysts.

Serodiagnosis

Serologic procedures are the primary method of diagnosis. To establish the presence of acute infection, it is usual to demonstrate a fourfold rise in the IgG antibody titer between acute and convalescent serum specimens. As peak titers are often reached within 4–8 weeks, the acute serum must be collected early in the course of illness. Of the many tests developed for the detection of IgG antibodies, the Sabin–Feldman dye test and the indirect fluorescent antibody test are those most frequently used; they both are sensitive and highly specific. With these tests, titers of 1:1000 or more are usually detected after an acute infection. These levels gradually fall, but may remain high for many years.

Significance of IgM antibody

The detection of IgM antibodies provides a more rapid confirmation of acute infection. As detected by an indirect fluorescent antibody technique, these antibodies arise within the first week of infection, peak in 2–4 weeks, and quickly revert to negative. It also appears that IgM antibodies are produced after reactivation of latent disease. A single high titer (1:80 or more) therefore establishes the presence of acute infection or reactivation. Unfortunately, this test has been difficult to standardize, lacks sensitivity in neonates and immunocompromised hosts and is not widely available. A recently developed enzyme-linked immunosorbent assay for IgM antibody may circumvent many of these difficulties.

Treatment and Prevention

Combined sulfonamide and pyrimethamine therapy

Normal patients do not require therapy unless symptoms are particularly severe and persistent or unless vital organs, such as the eye, are involved. Immunocompromised and pregnant women, however, should be treated if acute infection (or reactivation) is documented (Table 45.3). Routine serial serologic testing of immunocompromised patients and pregnant women would allow early detection of patients and enhance the prospects of a successful outcome. At present, the only proved therapeutic regimen avail-

Table 45.3 Treatment of Toxoplasmosis[a]

Serologic Criteria	Clinical Criteria
Elevated IgM titers	Pregnant woman
Fourfold rise in IgG titers	Neonate
Very high IgG titers (greater than 1:1000)	Immunocompromised patient: severe constitutional symptoms
	Vital organ involvement (including active chorioretinitis)

[a]Must satisfy one serologic plus one clinical criterion.

able in this country is the combination of sulfonamides and pyrimethamine. Unfortunately, the latter drug is teratogenic and should not be used in the first trimester of pregnancy.

Prevention should be directed primarily at pregnant women and the immunologically compromised host. Hands should be carefully washed after handling uncooked meat. Cysts in meat can be destroyed by proper cooking (56°C for 15 min) or by freezing to −20°C. Cat feces should be avoided, particularly the changing of kitty litter.

Additional Reading and References

Bruce-Chwatt, L.J. 1979. Man against malaria: Conquest or defeat. *R. Soc. Trop. Med. Hyg.* 73:605–617. The world's leading malariologist reviews the successes and failures of the WHO-sponsored Malaria Eradication Program.

Desowitz, R.S., and Miller, L.H. 1980. A perspective on malaria vaccines. *Bull. WHO* 58:897–908.

Dubey, J.P., Miller, N.L., and Frenkel, J.K. 1970. The *Toxoplasma gondii* oocyst from cat feces. *J. Exp. Med.* 132:636–662. The first demonstration of a sexual form of *T. gondii,* thus establishing its definitive host, method of transmission, and taxonomic status as a coccidian.

Frenkel, J.K., and Ruiz, A. 1981. Endemicity of toxoplasmosis in Costa Rica. Transmission between cats, soil, intermediate hosts and humans. *Am. J. Epidemiol.* 113:254–269. This article is the most comprehensive study on the role of cats in the transmission of toxoplasmosis. It suggests that humans are infected primarily from soil contaminated with cat feces, rather than direct contact.

Langer, H. 1963. Repeated congenital infection with *Toxoplasma gondii. Obstet. Gynecol.* 21:318–329.

Molineaux, L., and Gramiccia, G. 1980. *The Garki Project. Research on the Epidemiology and Control of Malaria in the Sudan Savanna of West Africa.* Geneva: World Health Organization. The most comprehensive study ever undertaken of malaria transmission in holoendemic areas.

James J. Plorde

Rhizopod Infections

46

Rhizopods, or amebas, are the most primitive of the protozoa. They multiply by simple binary fission and move by means of cytoplasmic organelles called *pseudopodia.* These projections of the relatively solid ectoplasm are formed by streaming of the inner, more liquid endoplasm. They move the ameba forward and, incidentally, engulf and internalize food sources found in its path. Most amebas, when faced with a hostile environment, can produce a resistant, external wall that surrounds and protects them. These inactive cysts may survive for prolonged periods under conditions that would rapidly destroy the motile trophozoite.

Free-living amebas

The majority of amebas belong to free-living genera. They are widely distributed in nature, being found in literally all bodies of standing fresh water. Few free-living amebas produce human disease, although two genera, *Naegleria* and *Acanthamoebae*, have been implicated occasionally as causes of meningoencephalitis.

Parasitic amebas

Several genera of amebas including *Entamoeba, Endolimax,* and *Iodamoeba,* are obligate parasites of the human alimentary tract and are passed as cysts from host to host by the fecal–oral route. Several are devoid of mitochondria, presumably because of the anaerobic conditions under which they exist in the colon. Only one, *Entamoeba histolytica,* regularly produces disease.

Entamoeba histolytica

Description of Organism

Morphology and physiology. Entamoeba histolytica possesses both trophozoite and cyst forms. The trophozoites are microaerophilic, dwell in the lumen or wall of the colon, feed on bacteria and tissue cells, and multiply rapidly in the anaerobic environment of the gut. When diarrhea occurs, the trophozoites are passed unchanged in the liquid stool. Here they can be recognized by their size (12–20 μm in diameter), directional motility, and sharply demarcated, clear ectoplasm with fingerlike pseudopods. Appropriate stains reveal a nucleus with a small central karyosome or nucleolus and fine regular granules evenly distributed around the nuclear membrane (peripheral chromatin). Invasive strains tend to be larger and may contain ingested erythrocytes within their cytoplasm (Figure 46.1).

trophozoites passed in diarrheal stools; may contain ingested erythrocytes

With normal stool transit time, trophozoites usually encyst before leaving the gut. Initially, a cyst contains a single nucleus, a glycogen vacuole, and one or more large, cigar-shaped inclusions known as *chromatoid bodies.* With

resistant mature quadrinucleate cysts

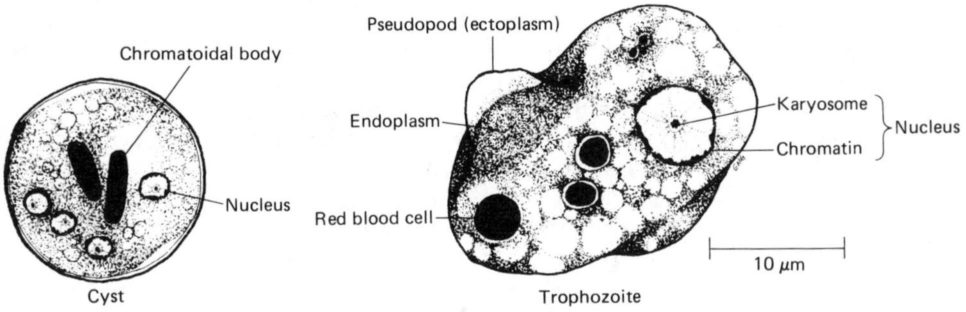

46.1 *Entamoeba histolytica.*

maturation, these cytoplasmic inclusions are absorbed and the cyst becomes quadrinucleate. In contrast to the fragile trophozoite, mature cysts can survive environmental temperatures up to 55°C, chlorine concentrations normally found in municipal water supplies and normal levels of gastric acid. *Entamoeba histolytica* can be differentiated from the other amebas of the gut by its size, nuclear detail, and cytoplasmic inclusions (Table 46.1).

human-to-human infection by ingested cysts

cyst releases trophozoites in jejunum

trophozoites colonize cecum and rectosigmoid

Life cycle. Humans are the principal hosts and reservoirs of *E. histolytica.* Transmission from person to person occurs when a parasite passed in the stool of one host is ingested by another. Because the trophozoites die rapidly in the external environment, successful passage is achieved only by the cyst. After passage through the stomach, the cyst eventually reaches the distal small bowel. Here the cyst wall disintegrates, releasing the quadrinucleate parasite, which divides to form eight small trophozoites that are carried to the colon. Trophozoites can effect colonization in the cecum and rectosigmoid, where fecal stasis is common.

Factors influencing invasiveness and virulence

Pathogenicity. Normally, *E. histolytica* exists as a commensal organism. Occasionally it becomes invasive, producing clinical disease. The factors that initiate invasiveness are poorly understood, but include changes in host resistance and organism virulence. High-carbohydrate diets, corticosteroid

Table 46.1 Some Differential Characteristics of *Entamoeba* Species

Characteristic	*E. histolytica*	*E. hartmanni*	*E. coli*
TROPHOZOITES			
Cytoplasm	Differentiated[a]	Differentiated	Undifferentiated
Nucleus			
Peripheral chromatin	Fine	Fine	Coarse, irregular
Karyosome	Small, central	Small, central	Large, eccentric
Ingested particles			
Bacteria	No	—	Yes
Red blood cells	Yes	No	No
Size	> 12 μm	< 12 μm	> 12 μm
CYSTS			
Nuclei[b]	1–4	1–4	1–8
Chromatoid bodies	Rods	Rods	Splinters
Size	> 10 μm	< 10 μm	> 10 μm

[a]Sharp differentiation between ectoplasm and endoplasm.
[b]Fine structure similar to that of trophozoites.

administration, and pregnancy all render the host more susceptible to invasion. Virulence appears to be an unstable characteristic. It may be lost by continued in vitro culture and enhanced by animal passage. Generally, strains in the tropical zone are more virulent than those isolated in more temperate areas. Possibly the poor sanitation characteristic of these regions results in more frequent passage through humans, thus enhancing virulence. Recently, it has been shown that invasive strains belong exclusively to 2 of 18 distinctive zymodemes. The factors directly responsible for the virulence of these strains remain undefined.

Although *E. histolytica* produces a cytotoxic enterotoxin and a variety of enzymes that could conceivably play a role in tissue invasion, there is no certain correlation between the presence of these substances and the virulence of individual strains. Virulent strains are, however, uniquely capable of producing lysis of tissue cells after direct cell-to-cell contact.

Laboratory growth. Trophozoites are facultative anaerobes that require complex media for growth. Most require the addition of live bacteria for successful isolation. Sterile culture techniques have been developed, however, and are essential for the preparation of the purified antigens required for serologic testing. The value of culture procedures in the diagnosis of amebiasis remains unproved.

Amebiasis

mucosal ulceration; little inflammatory response

Pathology. Amebas contact and lyse colonic epithelial cells, producing small mucosal ulcerations. There is little inflammatory response other than edema and hyperemia, and the mucosa between ulcers appears normal. Trophozoites are present in large numbers at the junction between necrotic and viable tissue. Once the lesion penetrates below the superficial epithelium, it meets the resistance of the colonic musculature and spreads laterally in the submucosa, producing a flasklike lesion with a narrow mucosal neck and a large submucosal body. It eventually compromises the blood supply of the overlying mucosa, resulting in sloughing and a large necrotic ulcer. Extensive ulceration leads to secondary bacterial infection, formation of granulation tissue, and fibrotic thickening of the colon. Occasionally, the granulation tissue is organized into large tumorlike masses known as *amebomas.* The major sites of involvement, in order of frequency, are the cecum, ascending colon, rectum, sigmoid, appendix, and terminal ileum. Amebas may also enter the portal circulation and be carried to the liver or, more rarely, to the lung, brain, or spleen. In these organs, liquefaction necrosis leads to the formation of abscess cavities.

flasklike lesion of submucosa

Amebomas and metastatic amebic abscesses

immunity incomplete, does not correlate with antibody response

Immunity. Although animal studies have demonstrated the existence of protective immunity, reinfections are noted frequently in the human population. This finding suggests that immunity develops slowly, is incomplete, and serves to limit, rather than prevent, reinfection. Invasive disease produces high levels of circulating antibodies of various types, but there appears to be no correlation between the titer of such antibodies and immunity. It is therefore likely that immunity, if and when it occurs, is cell mediated.

relationship usually commensal

Clinical manifestations. Individuals who harbor *E. histolytica* are usually clinically well. In most cases, particularly in the temperate zones, the organism is avirulent, living in the bowel as a normal commensal inhabitant. Spontaneous disappearance of amebas is common among such patients, occurring at the rate of 15% per annum. Serologic data, however, suggest that some asymptomatic carriers possess virulent strains and incur minimal tissue invasion. In this population, the infection may eventually progress to produce overt disease.

Symptoms and signs of intestinal amebiasis

chronic ulceration with mucus and blood in stool

Diarrhea, flatulence, and cramping abdominal pain are the most frequent complaints of symptomatic patients. The diarrhea is intermittent, alternating with episodes of normality or constipation over a period of months to years. Typically, the stools consist of one to four loose to watery, foul-smelling passages that contain mucus and blood. Physical findings are limited to abdominal tenderness localized to the hepatic, ascending colonic, and cecal areas. Sigmoidoscopy reveals the typical ulcerations with normal intertwining mucosa.

fulminating amebic dysentery

Fulminating amebic dysentery is less common. It may occur spontaneously in debilitated or pregnant individuals or be precipitated by corticosteroid therapy. Its onset is often abrupt, with high fever, severe abdominal cramps, and profuse, bloody diarrhea and tenesmus. Severe abdominal tenderness and tender hepatomegaly are common. Sigmoidoscopy reveals extensive rectosigmoid ulceration. Trophozoites are numerous in stools and ulcer aspirates. A number of complications may accompany fulminant disease, including massive hemorrhage and bowel perforation with resulting peritonitis. Amebomas may project into the lumen of the bowel, where they may be mistaken for adenocarcinoma, or extend circumferentially around the colon, producing partial obstruction. If tissue destruction is extensive the colon may be left scarred and irritable despite eradication of the organism, resulting in so-called *postdysenteric colitis.*

Postdysenteric colitis

Hepatic abscess

Hepatic abscess presents either acutely or insidiously with fever and tender hepatic enlargement. Most commonly, abscesses occur singly and are localized to the upper outer quadrant of the right lobe of the liver. This localization results in the development of point tenderness overlying the cavity and elevation of the right diaphragm. Liver function is usually well preserved. Isotopic or ultrasound scanning confirms the presence of the lesion. Needle aspiration results in the withdrawal or reddish-brown, odorless fluid free of bacteria and polymorphonuclear leukocytes; trophozoites may be demonstrated in the terminal portion of the aspirate.

complications of hepatic abscess

Approximately 5% of all patients with symptomatic amebiasis present with a liver abscess. Ironically, fewer than one-half can recall significant diarrheal illness, and *E. histolytica* is demonstrated in the stools of less than one-third. Complications relate to the extension of the abscess into surrounding tissue, producing pneumonia, empyema, or peritonitis. Extension of an abscess from the left lobe of the liver to the pericardium is the single most dangerous complication. It may produce rapid cardiac tamponade and death or, more commonly, a pericardial disease that may be confused with congestive cardiomyopathy or tuberculous pericarditis.

Worldwide infection; highest rates in warmer climates

Epidemiology. Amebiasis has a worldwide distribution. Infection rates are higher in warmer climates and may exceed 50% in areas where the level of sanitation is low. Stool surveys in the United States indicate that 1–5% of the population harbors *E. histolytica,* although the virulence of these strains is often uncertain. Invasive disease is both less common and less widely distributed. Reports of amebic liver abscess, for instance, emanate primarily from Mexico, western South America, South Asia, and West and South Africa. For reasons apparently unrelated to exposure, symptomatic illness is much less common in women and children than in men.

In the United States, the incidence of invasive amebiasis has decreased invasive disease rare in United States

sharply over the past few decades. Today, most cases are acquired outside the country. Invasive amebiasis, however, is still seen in institutions for the mentally retarded, Indian reservations, and migrant labor camps.

fecal–oral spread

other modes of transmission

Epidemics

Symptomatic amebiasis is usually sporadic, the result of direct person-to-person fecal–oral spread under conditions of poor personal hygiene. Venereal transmission appears to be particularly common among male homosexuals, presumably the result of oral–anal sexual contact. Food- and water-borne spread occur, occasionally in epidemic form. Such outbreaks, however, are seldom as explosive as those produced by pathogenic intestinal bacteria.

Stool examination for trophozoites and cysts

Laboratory diagnosis. The diagnosis of intestinal amebiasis depends upon the identification of the organism in stool or sigmoidoscopic aspirates. As trophozoites appear predominantly in liquid stools or aspirates, a portion of such specimens should be fixed immediately to ensure preservation of these fragile organisms for stained preparations. The specimen may then be examined in wet mount for typical motility, concentrated to detect cysts, and stained for definitive identification of *E. histolytica.* Three or more specimens may be required for diagnosis. If protozoa or cysts are seen, they must be carefully differentiated from those of the commensal parasites, particularly *Entamoeba hartmanni* and *Entamoeba coli* (Table 46.1).

Serodiagnosis of extraintestinal amebiasis

The diagnosis of extraintestinal amebiasis is more difficult, as the parasite usually cannot be recovered from stool or tissue. Serologic tests are therefore of paramount importance. Typically, results are negative in asymptomatic patients, suggesting that tissue invasion is required for antibody production. Most patients with symptomatic intestinal disease and more than 90% with hepatic abscess have diagnostic titers. Unfortunately, these titers may persist for months to years after an acute infection, making the interpretation of a postive test difficult in endemic areas. At present, the indirect hemagglutination test and the enzyme-linked immunosorbent assay appear to be the most sensitive. Several rapid tests, including latex agglutination and counterimmunoelectrophoresis, are available to smaller laboratories.

Primary role of metronidazole

Treatment. Treatment is directed toward relief of symptoms, blood and fluid replacement, and eradication of the organism. The drug of choice for eradication is metronidazole. It is effective against all forms of amebiasis, but should be combined with a second agent, such as diiodohydroxyquin or tetracycline, to improve cure rates in intestinal disease and diminish the chance of recrudescent disease in hepatic amebiasis. Specific contraindications to the use of metronidazole are given in Chapter 47 in the section on treatment of *Trichomonas vaginalis.*

Prevention. As the disease is transmitted by the fecal–oral route, efforts should be directed toward sanitary disposal of human feces and improvement in personal hygienic practices among institutionalized patients. Male homosexuals should be made aware that certain sexual practices substantially increase their risk of this and other infections.

Primary Amebic Meningoencephalitis

Naegleria and *Acanthamoeba*

Primary amebic meningoencephalitis is caused by free-living amebas belonging to the genus *Naegleria* or *Acanthamoeba.* The disease produced by the former has been better defined; it affects children and young adults, appears to be acquired by swimming in fresh water, and is almost always fatal. *Acanthamoeba* meningoencephalitis is a milder and more chronic illness. *Naegleria* species are found in large numbers in shallow fresh water, particularly during warm weather. *Acanthamoeba* species are found in soil and in fresh and brackish water, and they have been recovered from the oropharynx of asymptomatic humans.

Naegleria Infections

associated with freshwater swimming

Approximately 100 cases of *Naegleria* meningoencephalitis have been reported, primarily in Great Britain, Czechoslovakia, Australia, and the United States. Serologic studies suggest that inapparent infections are much more common. Most cases in the United States have occurred in the southeastern states. Characteristically, the patients have fallen ill during the summer after swimming or water skiing in small, shallow, freshwater lakes. The Czechoslovakian cases followed swimming in a chlorinated indoor pool, and several have occurred after bathing in hot mineral water. A recent report suggests the disease may have been acquired by inhaling airborne cysts during the dry, windy season in sub-Saharan Africa.

passage to central nervous system across cribriform plate

Histologic evidence suggests that *Naegleria* traverses the nasal mucosa and the cribriform plate to the central nervous system. Here the organism produces a severe hemorrhagic inflammatory reaction that extends perivascularly from the olfactory bulbs to other regions of the brain. The infection is characterized by rapid onset and a brief fatal course.

purulent bloody cerebrospinal fluid containing *Naegleria* trophozoites

A careful examination of the cerebrospinal fluid often provides a presumptive diagnosis of *Naegleria* infection. The fluid is usually bloody and demonstrates an intense neutrophilic response. The protein level is elevated and the glucose level decreased. No bacteria can be demonstrated on stain or culture. Early examination of a wet mount preparation of unspun spinal fluid will reveal typical trophozoites. Staining with specific fluorescent antibody confirms the identification. To date, only two patients have survived a *Naegleria* infection. Both were diagnosed early, and one was treated with amphotericin B, the other with amphotericin B, miconazole, and rifampin.

Acanthamoeba Infections

affects older immunocompromised subjects

The epidemiology of *Acanthamoeba* infections has not been clearly defined. Infections usually involve older, immunocompromised persons, and a history of freshwater swimming is generally absent. The ameba probably reaches the brain by hematogenous dissemination from an unknown primary site, possibly the respiratory tract or skin. Metastatic lesions have been reported.

granulomatous lesions

Histologically, *Acanthamoeba* infections produce a diffuse, necrotizing, granulomatous encephalitis with cysts as well as trophozoites in the lesions.

more chronic disease with spontaneous recovery

The clinical course of *Acanthamoeba* disease is more prolonged than that of *Naegleria* infection and often ends in spontaneous recovery, although fatal disease has occurred in immunocompromised hosts. Skin lesions, uveitis, and corneal ulcerations have all been reported. The spinal fluid usually demonstrates a mononuclear response. *Acanthamoeba* species are sensitive to a variety of agents, including sulfonamides, clotrimazole, 5-fluorocytosine, and polymyxin. Studies of clinical efficacy have not been done.

Additional Reading and References

Adams, E.B., and MacLeod, I.N. 1977. Invasive amebiasis. *Medicine (Baltimore)* 56:315–334. A review of amebiasis by the Amebiasis Research Unit in Durban, South Africa, the leading center in the world for the study of this disease.

Chesley, A.J., Craig, C.F., Fishbein, M., et al. 1934. Amebiasis outbreak in Chicago. Report of a special committee. *J. Am. Med. Assoc.* 102:369–372. A description of the best known outbreak of amebiasis in the United States. Fourteen hundred clinical infections and 100 deaths resulted from an inadvertent connection between the water supply and sewage in two Chicago hotels.

Duma, R.J., Helwig, W.B., and Martinez, A.J. 1978. Meningoencephalitis and brain abscess due to a free-living amoeba. *Ann. Intern. Med.* 88:468–473. A recent case report and discussion regarding the taxonomic criteria used to identify free-living amebas producing human disease.

Elsdon-Dew, R. 1968. The epidemiology of amoebiasis. *Adv. Parasitol.* 6:162. An exhaustive review.

Ochsner, A., and DeBakey, M. 1943. Amebic hepatitis and hepatic abscess. An analysis of 181 cases with review of the literature. *Surgery* 13(3):460–493, 13(4):612–649. One of the early classics on amebiasis.

James J. Plorde

Flagellate Infections

47

Like their amebic cousins, flagellate protozoa are widespread in nature, multiply by binary fission, and move about by means of cytoplasmic organelles of locomotion. Motility, however, is distinctly more vigorous among this group of organisms because of the efficiency of their locomotive apparatus, the flagellum. This organelle arises from an intracellular focus known as a *blepharoplast,* extends to the cell wall as a filamentous *axoneme,* and continues extracellularly as the *free flagellum.* In some species, the blepharoplast is paired with a second cytoplasmic structure known as a *parabasal body.* This structure is believed to be composed of modified mitochondria responsible for the control of flagellar movement. Both structures stain with nucleic acid stains, and they are known collectively as the *kinetoplast.*

Undulating membranes

In many flagellates the axoneme, before exiting from the cell, lifts a segment of external wall into a longitudinal fold. This *undulating membrane* is thrown into movement as the organism progresses, often imparting to it a characteristic rotary motion.

The long, whiplike free flagella may be single or multiple. The number is distinctive for individual species. When more than one is present, each has its own associated blepharoplast and axoneme.

Invasive and noninvasive pathogenic flagellates

Although a number of flagellate genera parasitize humans, only four, *Giardia, Trichomonas, Leishmania,* and *Trypanosoma,* commonly induce disease. The first two comprise noninvasive organisms that inhabit the lumina of the genitourinary or gastrointestinal tract and are spread without benefit of an intermediate host. Disease is of low morbidity and cosmopolitan distribution. *Leishmania* and *Trypanosoma,* on the other hand, are invasive blood and tissue parasites that produce highly morbid, frequently lethal diseases. These *hemoflagellates* require an intermediate insect host for their transmission. As a result, their associated disease states are limited to the semitropical and tropical niches of these intermediate hosts.

Luminal Flagellates

Luminal flagellates can be found in the mouth, vagina, or intestine of almost all vertebrates, and it is common for an animal host to harbor more than one species. Humans may serve as host and reservoir to eight (Table 47.1), but only two cause disease. Of these, *Giardia lamblia* inhabits the intestinal tract and *Trichomonas vaginalis* inhabits the vagina and genital tract.

Table 47.1 Luminal Flagellates Infecting Humans

Flagellate	Pathogenicity to Humans	Site
Giardia lamblia	+	Intestine
Dientamoeba fragilis	?	Intestine
Chilomastix mesnili	—	Intestine
Enteromonas hominis	—	Intestine
Retortamonas intestinalis	—	Intestine
Trichomonas hominis	—	Intestine
Trichomonas tenax	—	Mouth
Trichomonas vaginalis	+	Vagina

These organisms are elongated or oval in shape and typically measure 10–20 μm in length. They often possess a rudimentary cytostome and organelles such as sucking discs or axostyles, which assist them to maintain their intraluminal position. They are readily recognized in body fluid or excreta by their rapid motility, and some can be specifically identified in unstained preparations. All can be cultivated on artificial media.

Some luminal flagellates, most notably *T. vaginalis,* possess only a trophozoite stage and are passed from host to host by direct physical contact. Most, including *G. lamblia,* possess both trophozoite and cyst forms. The latter, which is the infective form, is transmitted via the fecal–oral route. Human-to-human infection is thus found in populations where inadequate sanitation or poor personal hygiene favors spread.

Trichomonas vaginalis

Organism. Three members of the genus *Trichomonas* parasitize humans (Table 47.1), but only *T. vaginalis* is an established pathogen. The three species closely resemble one another morphologically, but confusion in identification is rare because of the specificity of their habitats.

The *T. vaginalis* trophozoite (Figure 47.1) is oval and typically measures 7 × 15 μm. Organisms up to twice this size are occasionally seen. In stained preparations, a single, elongated nucleus and a small cytostome are observed anteriorly. Five flagella arise nearby. Four immediately exit the cell. The fifth bends back and runs posteriorly along the outer edge of an abbreviated undulating membrane. A conspicuous supporting rod or axostyle bisects the trophozoite longitudinally and protrudes through its posterior end. It is thought that the pointed tip of this structure is useful for attachment, and it may be responsible for the tissue damage produced by the parasite. In unstained wet mounts, *T. vaginalis* is identified by its axostyle and jerky, nondirectional movements.

In vitro cultivation

The organism can be grown on artificial media under anaerobic conditions at pH 5.5–6.0. It is capable of utilizing a variety of carbohydrates with the production of acid and gas. Bacteria, leukocytes, and occasionally erythrocytes may be ingested through any area of its cell surface. Although it lacks

Resistance

a cyst form, the trophozoite can survive outside of the human host for 1–2 hr on moist surfaces. In urine, semen, and water, it is viable for up to 24 hr, making it one of the most resistant of protozoan trophozoites. Attempts to infect laboratory animals have met with limited success.

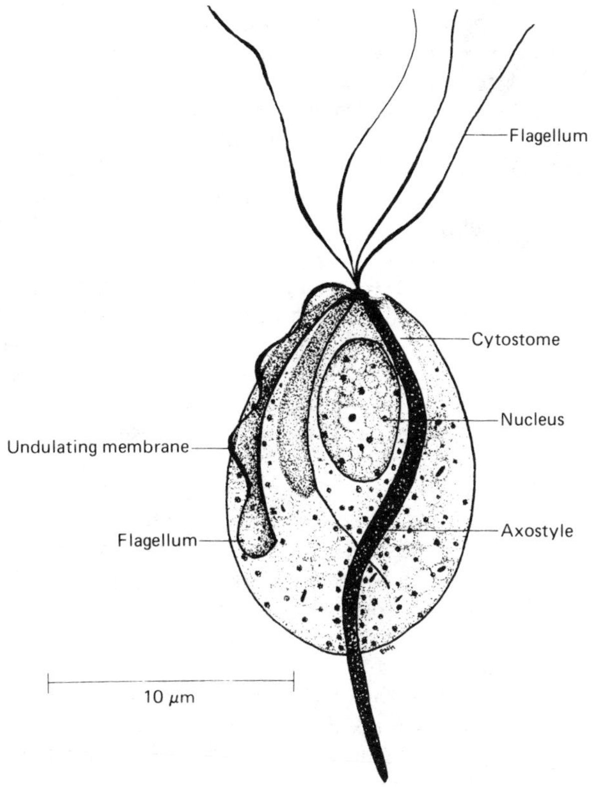

47.1 *Trichomonas vaginalis.*

Trichomoniasis

transmission usually sexual

Epidemiology. Trichomoniasis is a cosmopolitan disease usually transmitted by sexual intercourse. It is estimated that 3 million women acquire this disease annually in the United States, and 25% of sexually active women are infected at any given time. Presumably, men are similarly involved, but data on this point are lacking. As would be expected, the likelihood of acquiring the disease correlates directly with the number of sexual contacts. Infection is rare in adult virgins, whereas rates as high as 70% are seen among prostitutes, sexual partners of infected patients, and individuals with other venereal diseases.

nonvenereal transmission

neonatal infection

Nonvenereal transmission is uncommon. Transfer of organisms on shared washcloths may explain, in part, the high frequency of infection seen among institutionalized women. Female neonates are occasionally noted to harbor *T. vaginalis,* presumably acquiring it during passage through the birth canal. High levels of maternal estrogen produce a transient decrease in the vaginal pH of the child, rendering it more susceptible to colonization. Within a few weeks, estrogen levels drop, the vagina assumes its premenarchal state, and the parasite is eliminated.

Chronic vaginitis

vaginitis worsens during pregnancy

Clinical manifestations. In women, *T. vaginalis* produces a persistent vaginitis. Approximately 75% of recently infected women develop a discharge, which is typically accompanied by vulvar itching or burning, dyspareunia, dysuria, and a disagreeable odor. Although fluctuating in intensity, symptoms usually persist for weeks or months. Commonly, manifestations worsen during menses and pregnancy, presumably because of the alkaline shift in the pH of

Clinical manifestations

the vagina that accompanies these events. Eventually, the discharge subsides, even though the patient may continue to harbor the parasite. In symptomatic patients, physical examination reveals reddened vaginal and endocervical mucosa. In severe cases, petechial hemorrhages and extensive erosions are present. A red, granular, friable endocervix (strawberry cervix) is a characteristic, but uncommon, finding. An abundant discharge is generally seen pooled in the posterior vaginal fornix. Although classically described as thin, yellow, and frothy in character, the discharge more frequently lacks these characteristics.

urethritis and prostatitis in men usually asymptomatic

The urethra and prostate are the usual sites of infection in men; the epididymis may be involved on occasion. Infections are usually asymptomatic, possibly because of the efficiency with which the organisms are removed from the urogenital tract by voided urine. Symptomatic men complain of recurrent dysuria and scant, nonpurulent discharge. Acute purulent urethritis has been reported rarely.

Wet mount examination for motile trophozoites

Diagnosis. The diagnosis of trichomoniasis rests on the detection and morphologic identification of the organism in the genital tract. Identification is accomplished most easily by examining a wet mount preparation for the presence of motile organisms. In women, a drop of vaginal discharge is the most appropriate specimen; in men, urethral exudate or urine sediment after prostate discharge may be used. Although highly specific when positive, wet mounts are often negative in asymptomatic or mildly symptomatic patients and in women who have douched in the previous 24 hr. Giemsa and Papanicolaou stained smears provide little additional help. Cultures of urogenital specimens may increase the number of detected cases. Unfortunately, this procedure is not generally available in clinical laboratories and requires several days to complete.

positive cases should be tested for other venereal diseases

Patients in whom wet mount or culture yields positive results for trichomoniasis should be examined carefully for other venereal disease.

Metronidazole: Precautions against teratogenic effects

Treatment. Oral metronidazole (Flagyl) is extremely effective in recommended dosage, curing more than 95% of all infections. Simultaneous treatment of sexual partners may minimize recurrent infections, particularly when single-dose therapy is employed for the index case. Because of metronidazole's disulfiramlike activity, alcohol consumption should be suspended during treatment. Because of its potential teratogenic activity, the drug should never be used during the first trimester of pregnancy. Use in the last two trimesters is unlikely to be hazardous, but should be reserved for patients whose symptoms cannot be adequately controlled with vinegar douching. High-dose long-term metronidazole treatment has been shown to be carcinogenic in rodents. No association with human malignancy has been described to date, and in the absence of a suitable alternative drug, metronidazole continues to be used.

Giardia lamblia

Organism. Giardia lamblia was first described by Anton von Leeuwenhoek 300 years ago when he examined his own diarrheal stool with one of the first primitive microscopes. It was not until this past decade, however, that the cosmopolitan flagellate became widely regarded in the United States as a pathogen. Of the six other flagellated protozoans known to parasitize the alimentary tract of humans, only one, *Dientamoeba fragilis,* has been credibly associated with disease. Definitive confirmation or refutation of its pathogenicity will, it is hoped, not require the passage of another three centuries.

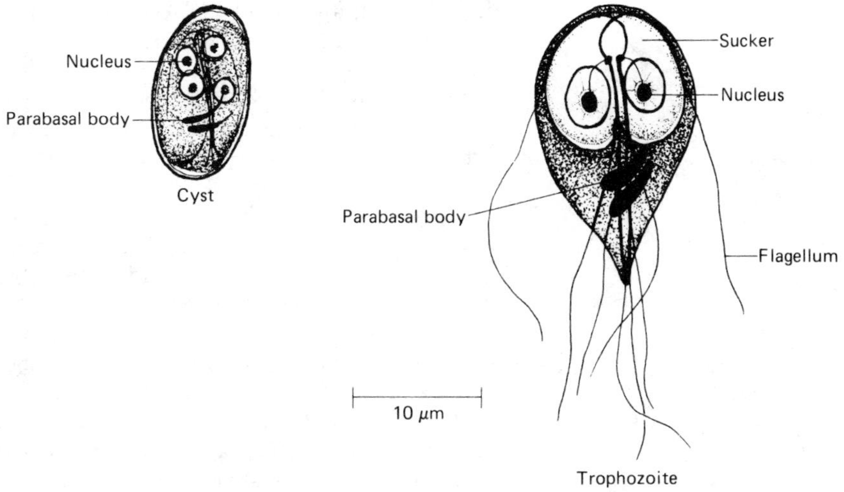

47.2 *Giardia lamblia.*

Unlike *T. vaginalis, Giardia* possesses both a trophozoite and a cyst form (Figure 47.2). It is a sting-ray-shaped trophozoite 9–21 μm in length, 5–15 μm in width, and 2–4 μm in thickness. When viewed from the top, the organism's two nuclei and central parabasal bodies give it the appearance of a face with two bespectacled eyes and a crooked mouth. Four pairs of flagella—anterior, lateral, ventral, and posterior—reinforce this image by suggesting the presence of hair and chin whiskers. These distinctive parasites reside in the duodenum and jejunum, where they thrive in the alkaline environment and absorb nutrients from the intestinal tract. They move about with a peculiar tumbling or "falling leaf" motility and, with the aid of a large ventral sucker, attach themselves to the brush border of the intestinal epithelium. Unattached organisms may be carried by the fecal stream to the large intestine. In the descending colon, if transit time allows, the flagella are retracted into cytoplasmic sheaths and a smooth, clear cyst wall is secreted. These forms are oval and somewhat smaller than the trophozoites. With maturation, the internal structures divide, producing a quadrinucleate organism harboring two sucking discs, four parabasal bodies, and eight axonemes (Figure 47.2). When fixed and stained, the cytoplasm pulls away from the cyst wall in a characteristic fashion. The mature cysts, which are the infective form of the parasite, are transmitted from host to host by the fecal–oral route. In the duodenum of a new host, the cytoplasm divides to produce two binucleate trophozoites.

tumbling motility

attach to mucosa of small intestine

resistant cysts transmitted from host to host

Organisms of the genus *Giardia* are among the most widely distributed of intestinal protozoa; they are found in fish, amphibians, reptiles, birds, and mammals. At first, it was assumed that *Giardia* species found in different animals were host specific, and at least 40 different species were described. It is now known that at least some strains can infect more than a single host species. Unfortunately, there is no general agreement on organism characteristics to be used to define species.

wide distribution in animal kingdom

Giardiasis

Epidemiology. Giardiasis has a cosmopolitan distribution; its incidence is highest in areas with poor sanitation and among populations unable to maintain adequate personal hygiene. In the United States, *G. lamblia* is found in 4% of stools submitted for parasitologic examination, making it the most fre-

transmission facilitated by poor hygiene

quently identified intestinal parasite. All ages and economic groups are represented, but young children and young adults are preferentially involved. Children with immunoglobulin deficiencies are more likely to acquire the flagellate, possibly because of a deficiency in intestinal immunoglobulin A. Giardiasis is also common among attendees of day-care nurseries. Attack rates of over 90% have been seen in the ambulatory non-toilet-trained population (age, 1–2 years) of these institutions, suggesting direct person-to-person transmission of the parasite. The frequency with which secondary cases are seen among family contacts reinforces this probability. Undoubtedly, direct fecal spread is also responsible for the high infection rate among male homosexuals. In several recent studies, the prevalence of giardiasis and/or amebiasis in that population has ranged from 11 to 40% and is correlated closely with the number of oral–anal sexual contacts. Waterborne and, less frequently, food-borne transmission of this organism has also been documented and probably accounts for the frequency with which American travelers to Third World nations acquire infection. Unlike the typical bacterial diarrhea syndrome seen in travelers, the diarrhea begins late in the course of travel and may persist for several weeks. More than 20 waterborne outbreaks of giardiasis have also been reported in the United States. The sources have included untreated pond or stream water, sewage-contaminated municipal water supplies, and chlorinated but inadequately filtered water. In a few of these outbreaks, epidemiologic data have suggested that wild mammals, particularly beavers, served as the reservoir hosts.

high attack rates in day-care centers

giardiasis among male homosexuals

water- and food-borne outbreaks

Beavers and other mammals possible sources

Malabsorption syndrome

Pathology and pathogenesis. Disease manifestations appear related to intestinal malabsorption of fat and carbohydrates. Disaccharide deficiency with lactose intolerance, altered levels of peptide hydrolase, enteropeptidase, and decreased vitamin B_{12} absorption have been demonstrated. The precise pathogenetic mechanisms responsible for these changes remain poorly understood. Mechanical blockade of the intestinal mucosa by large numbers of *Giardia,* damage to the fuzzy coat of the microvilli by the parasite's sucking disc, organism-induced deconjugation of bile salts, altered intestinal motility, accelerated turnover of mucosal epithelium with functional immaturity of transport systems, and mucosal invasion have all been suggested; none correlates well with clinical manifestations. Patients with severe malabsorption have jejunal colonization with enteric bacteria or yeasts, suggesting that these organisms may act synergistically with *Giardia.* Eradication of the associated microorganism, however, has not resulted in clinical improvement. Jejunal biopsies sometimes reveal a flattening of the microvilli and an inflammatory infiltrate. Generally, both malabsorption and the jejunal lesions have been reversed with specific treatment.

Predisposing factors

Susceptibility to giardiasis has been related to several factors, including strain virulence, inoculum size, achlorhydria or hypochlorhydria, and immunologic abnormalities. In one experimental study, humans were challenged with varying doses from as few as 10 cysts. They were uniformly parasitized when 100 or more were ingested. Several workers have noted the frequency with which giardiasis occurs in achlorhydric and hypochlorhydric individuals. Although reinfection is common, the frequent occurrence of giardiasis in patients with immunologic diseases, plus the rarity with which it is seen in older adults, suggests that protective immunity, albeit incomplete, does develop in humans. Animal studies suggest that both humoral and cellular mechanisms are operative.

Occurrence in immunocompromised subjects

Subclinical and acute infections

Clinical manifestations. Infection is frequently subclinical. Symptoms, when they do occur, begin 1–3 weeks after exposure; they typically include diarrhea, which is sudden in onset and explosive in character. The stool is foul smelling, greasy in appearance, and floats on water. It is devoid of blood or mucus. Upper abdominal cramping is common. Large quantities of intestinal gas produce abdominal distention, sulfuric eructations, and abundant flatus. Nausea, vomiting, and low-grade fever may be present. The acute illness generally resolves in 1–4 weeks; in children, however, it may persist for months, leading to significant malabsorption and weight loss.

Subacute and chronic infections

In many adults, the acute phase is often followed by a subacute or chronic phase characterized by intermittent bouts of mushy stools, flatulence, and "heartburn" and weight loss that persist for weeks or months. At times, patients presenting in this fashion deny having experienced the acute syndrome described previously. In the majority, symptoms and organisms eventually disappear spontaneously. It is not uncommon for lactose intolerance to persist after eradication of the organisms. This condition may be confused with an ongoing infection, and the patient may be subjected to unnecessary treatment.

lactose intolerance

search for trophozoites and cysts in stool

Laboratory diagnosis. The diagnosis is made by finding the cyst in formed stool or the trophozoite in diarrheal stools, duodenal secretions, or jejunal biopsy specimens. In acutely symptomatic patients, the parasite can usually be demonstrated by examining one to three stool specimens, providing appropriate concentration and staining procedures are used. In chronic cases, excretion of the organism is often intermittent, making parasitologic confirmation more difficult. Many of these patients can be diagnosed by examining specimens taken at weekly intervals over 4–5 weeks. Alternatively, duodenal secretions can be collected and examined for trophozoites in trichrome or Giemsa stained preparations. The organism can be grown in culture, but the methods are not currently adaptable to routine diagnostic work. The value of serologic tests is under investigation.

duodenal aspirates

several drugs available

Treatment and prevention. Three drugs are currently available for the treatment of giardiasis in the United States: quinacrine hydrochloride, metronidazole, and furazolildone. The latter drug is used by pediatricians because of its availability as a liquid suspension, but it has the lowest cure rate. Quinacrine and metronidazole are somewhat more effective (70–95%) and are preferred for patients capable of ingesting tablets. Because of the potential of giardiasis for person-to-person spread, it is important to examine and, if necessary, treat close physical contacts of the infected patient, including playmates at nursery school, household members, and sexual contacts. If possible, treatment should be withheld from pregnant women because of the potential teratogenicity of available drugs.

examination of close contacts

Hikers should avoid ingestion of untreated surface water, even in remote areas, because of the possibility of contamination by feces of infected animals. Adequate disinfection can be accomplished with halogen compounds.

avoidance of drinking untreated surface water

Blood and Tissue Flagellates

Leishmania and *Trypanosoma*

Life cycle includes insect host stage

Of the many genera of hemoflagellates, two are pathogenic to humans: *Leishmania* and *Trypanosoma*. They reside and reproduce within the gut of specific insect hosts. When these vectors feed on a susceptible mammal, the parasite penetrates the feeding site, invades the blood and/or tissue of the new host, and multiplies to produce disease. The life cycle is completed when a second insect ingests the infected mammalian blood or tissue fluid. During the course of their passage through insect and vertebrate hosts, flagellates undergo developmental change. Within the gut of the insect (and in culture media) the organism assumes the promastigote (*Leishmania*) or epimastigote (*Trypanosoma*) form (Figure 47.3). These protozoa are motile,

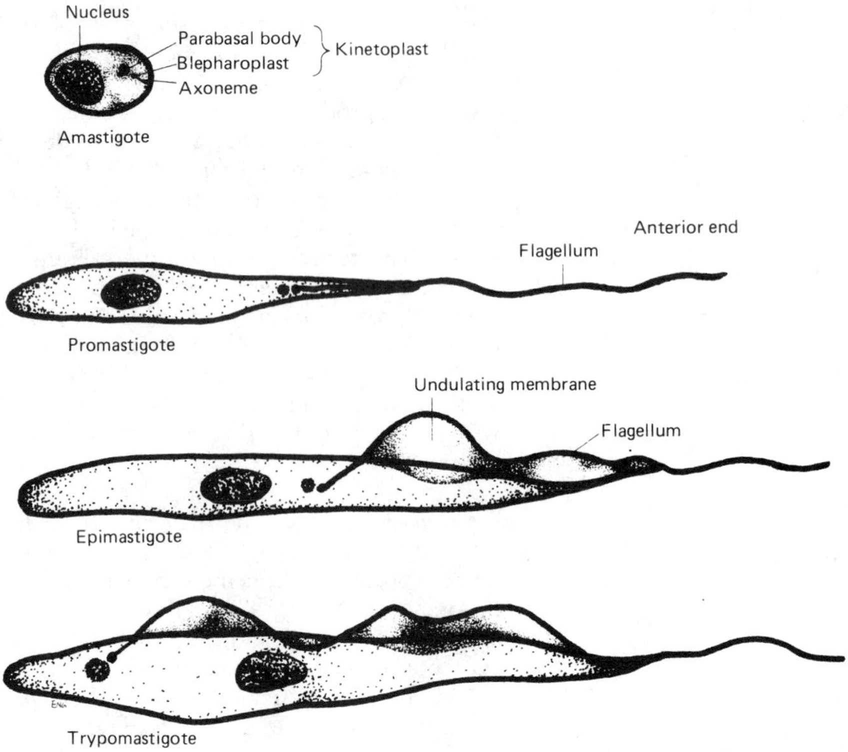

47.3 Stages in the life cycle of the hemoflagellates (Trypanosomidae).

promastigote and epimastigote forms in insects

fusiform, and have a blunt posterior end and a pointed anterior from which a single flagellum projects. They measure 15–30 μm in length and 1.5–4.0 μm in width. In the promastigote, the kinetoplast is located in the anterior extremity and the flagellum exits from the cell immediately. The kinetoplast of the epimastigote, in contrast, is located centrally, just in front of the vesicular nucleus. The flagellum runs anteriorly in the free edge of an undulating membrane before passing out of the cell. In the mammalian host, hemoflagellates appear as trypomastigotes (*Trypanosoma*) or amastigotes (*Leishmania*, *Trypanosoma cruzi*). The former circulate in the bloodstream and closely resemble the epimastigote form, except that the kinetoplast is in the posterior end of the parasite. The amastigote stage is found intracellularly. It is round or oval, measures 1.5–5.0 μm in diameter, and contains a clear nucleus with a central karyosome. Although it has a kinetoplast and an axoneme, there is no free flagellum.

trypomastigote and amastigote forms in humans

The flagellated forms move in a spiral fashion, and all reproduce by longitudinal binary fission. The flagellum itself does not divide; rather, a second one is generated by one of the two daughter cells. The organisms utilize carbohydrate obtained from the body fluids of the host in aerobic respiration.

Leishmania

Taxonomy

Organism. Leishmania species are obligate intracellular parasites of mammals. Several strains can infect humans; they are all morphologically identical, resulting in some confusion over their proper speciation. At present, they are differentiated into four major groups based on their serologic, biochemical, cultural, nosologic, and behavioral characteristics. In this chapter, they will be discussed as individual species. Each, however, contains a variety of strains that have been accorded separate species or subspecies status by some authorities.

Disease associations

Disease and transmission. *Leishmania tropica* in the Old World and *Leishmania mexicana* in the New World produce a localized cutaneous lesion or ulcer, known popularly as *oriental sore* and *chiclero ulcer.* *Leishmania braziliensis* is the cause of American mucocutaneous leishmaniasis (espundia), and *L. donovani* is the etiologic agent of kala azar, a disseminated visceral disease.

all four species transmitted by nocturnally feeding sandflies

All four species are transmitted by phlebotomine sandflies. These small, delicate, short-lived insects are found in animal burrows and crevices throughout the tropics and subtropics. At night, they feed on a wide range of mammalian hosts. Amastigotes ingested in the course of a meal assume the flagellated promastigote form, multiply within the gut, and eventually migrate to the buccal cavity. When the fly next feeds on a human or animal host, the buccal promastigotes are injected into the skin of the new host and invade the cytoplasm of mononuclear phagocytes. Here, they lose their flagella and multiply as the rounded amastigote form. In stained smears, they take on a distinctive appearance and are termed *Leishman–Donovan* bodies. Continued multiplication leads to the rupture of the phagocyte and release of the daughter cells. Some may be taken up by a feeding sandfly; most invade neighboring mononuclear cells. (Figure 47.4).

promastigotes injected by fly invade macrophages

amastigotes released from macrophages can infect feeding sandfly

Continuation of this cycle results in extensive histiocytic proliferation. The course of the disease at this point is determined by the species of parasite and the host's immune response. In the localized cutaneous forms of leishmaniasis, a vigorous cellular immune response results in the development of a positive delayed skin (leishmanin) reaction, lymphocytic infiltration, reduction in the number of parasites, and, eventually, spontaneous disappearance of the primary skin lesion. In infections with *L. braziliensis,* this sequence may be followed weeks to months later by mucocutaneous metastasis. These secondary lesions are highly destructive, presumably as a result of the host's hypersensitivity to parasitic antigens.

cellular immune responses in localized disease with spontaneous cure

metastic lesions in *L. braziliensis* infections

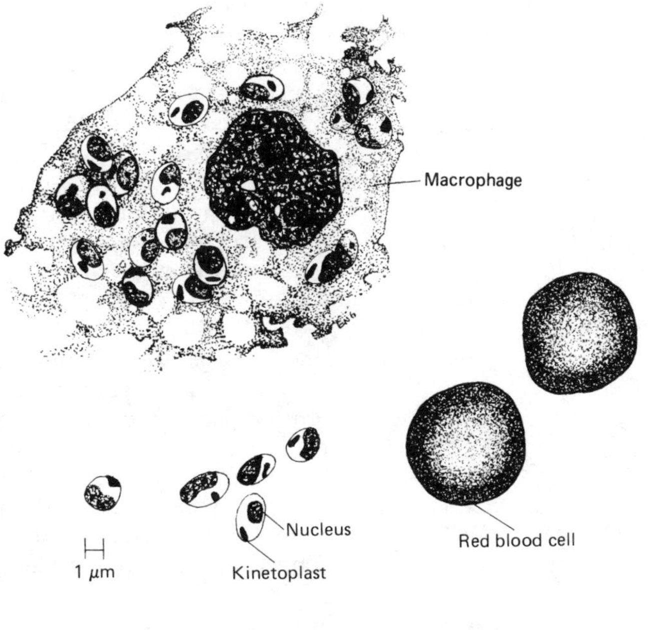

47.4 *Leishmania* within a mononuclear cell.

Table 47.2 Immune Response to Leishmaniasis

Human Disease	Parasite	Leishmanin Skin Test	Number of Lymphocytes	Number of Parasites	Prognosis	Humoral Antibody Titer
Localized skin ulcer (oriental sore, chiclero ulcer, uta)	*L. tropica*	Positive	Many	Few	Good	Low
Mucocutaneous lesions (espundia)	*L. braziliensis*	Positive	Many	Few	Poor	Low
Disseminated cutaneous						
Ethiopian American	*L. aethiopica* *L. mexicana*	Negative	Few	Many	Poor	High
Disseminated visceral (kala azar)	*L. donovani*	Negative	Few	Many	Poor	High

lack of cellular immune response in disseminated and chronic infections

Some strains of *L. tropica* and *L. mexicana* fail to elicit an effective immune response in certain hosts. Consequently, there is no infiltration of lymphocytes or decrease in the number of parasites. The skin test remains negative, and the skin lesions disseminate and become chronic (diffuse cutaneous leishmaniasis). In infections with *L. donovani,* there is a similar failure of cellular immunity; in this case the organisms disseminate to the visceral organs, rather than the skin. Although dissemination is associated with the development of circulating antibodies, they do not appear to serve a protective function and may, via the production of immune complexes, be responsible for the development of glomerulonephritis. The immune responses in different forms of leishmaniasis are summarized in Table 47.2

Localized Cutaneous Leishmaniasis

Geographic distribution of rodent reservoir and transmission to humans

Epidemiology. The disease is a zoonotic infection of tropical and subtropical rodents. It is particularly common in areas of China, India, Asia Minor, Africa, the Mediterranean littoral, and Central America. In the latter area, *L. mexicana* infects several species of arboreal rodents. Humans become involved when they enter forested areas to harvest chicle for chewing gum and are bitten by infected sandflies. In the eastern hemisphere, the desert gerbil serves as the reservoir host of *L. tropica.* Human infection occurs when rural inhabitants come in close contact with the burrows of these animals. In the Mediterranean area and in India, human disease involves urban dwellers, primarily children. In this setting, the domestic dog serves as the reservoir, although sandflies may also transmit *L. tropica* directly from human to human.

canine reservoir in urban areas in the Mediterranean

chronic, self-limiting skin ulceration

Clinical manifestations. Lesions usually appear on the extremities or face (the ear in cases of chiclero ulcer) 1–2 months after the bite of the sandfly. They first appear as pruritic papules, often accompanied by regional lymphadenopathy. In a few months the papules ulcerate, producing painless craters with raised erythematous edges, sharp walls, and a granulating base. Satellite lesions may form around the edge of the primary sore and fuse with it. Multiple primary lesions are seen in some patients. Spontaneous healing occurs in 3–6 months, leaving a pitted, depigmented scar. Occasionally the strain-specific immunity

lesions fail to heal, particularly on the ears, leading to progressive destruction of the pinna. A permanent strain-specific immunity follows healing.

Search for Leishman–Donovan bodies and culture

Management. In endemic areas, the diagnosis is made on clinical grounds and confirmed by the demonstration of the organism in the advancing edge of the ulcer. Material collected by biopsy, curettage, or aspiration is smeared and/or sectioned, stained, and examined microscopically for the pathognomonic Leishman–Donovan bodies. Material should also be cultured on special media. The skin test becomes positive early in the course of the disease and remains so for life.

Pentavalent antimonial agents, amphotericin B, and cycloguanil pamoate have all proved effective chemotherapeutic agents, but are generally reserved for extensive or multiple ulcerations. Secondary bacterial infections are treated with appropriate antibiotics.

Prophylactic measures include the control of the sandfly vector by use of insect repellents and fine mesh screening on dwellings.

Mucocutaneous Leishmaniasis

rodent reservoir of *L. braziliensis*

Epidemiology. Leishmania braziliensis causes a natural infection in the large forest rodents of tropical Latin America. Sandflies transmit the infection to humans engaged in opening jungle areas for new settlements.

Primary progressive lesion

Destructive oral and nasal lesions

Clinical manifestations. A primary skin lesion similar to oriental sore develops 1–4 weeks after sandfly exposure. Occasionally it undergoes spontaneous healing. More commonly, it progessively enlarges, often producing large vegetative lesions. After a period of weeks to years, painful, destructive, metastatic lesions of the mouth and nose appear in 2–50%. Sometimes, decades pass and the primary lesion totally resolves before the metastases manifest themselves. Destruction of the nasal septum produces the characteristic *tapir nose.* Erosion of the hard palate and larynx may render the patient aphonic. In blacks, the lesions are often large, hypertrophic, polypoid masses that deform the lips and cheeks. Fever, anemia, weight loss, and secondary bacterial infections are common.

Management. The diagnosis is made by finding the organisms in the lesions as described for localized cutaneous leishmaniasis. Growth characteristics in culture help to differentiate *L. braziliensis* from *L. mexicana.* The leishmanin skin test yields positive results, and most patients have detectable antibodies.

Treatment is accomplished with pentavalent antimonial agents or amphotericin B, as described for kala azar. Advanced lesions are often refractory, and relapse is common. Cured patients are immune to reinfection. Control measures, other than insect repellents and screening of dwellings, are impractical because of the sylvatic nature of the disease.

Diffuse Cutaneous Leishmaniasis

Skin lesions resemble lepromatous leprosy; no cellular immune response

Diffuse cutaneous leishmaniasis is an unusual disease seen primarily in Ethiopia and Venezuela, where it is caused by variants of *L. tropica* and *L. mexicana* that do not stimulate a cellular immune response in the host. Massive dissemination of skin lesions results. The clinical picture bears a striking resemblance to that of lepromatous leprosy. The lesions contain large numbers of organisms, making the diagnosis quite simple. In contrast to all other forms of cutaneous leishmaniasis, the results of the leishmanin skin test are negative. The disease is progressive and very refractory to treatment. Pentamidine and amphotericin B may produce remissions, but cure is rare.

Disseminated Visceral Leishmaniasis (Kala Azar)

Geographic differences in reservoirs and severity

Epidemiology. Kala azar, which is caused by *L. donovani,* occurs in the tropical and subtropical areas of every continent except Australia. Its epidemiologic and clinical patterns vary from area to area. In Africa, rodents serve as the primary reservoir. Human cases occur sporadically, and the disease is often acute and highly lethal. In Eurasia and Latin America, the domestic dog is the most common reservoir. Human disease is endemic, primarily involves children, and runs a subacute to chronic course. In India, the human is the only known reservoir, and transmission is carried out by anthropophilic species of sandflies. The disease recurs in epidemic form at 20-year intervals, when a new cadre of nonimmune children and young adults appears in the community.

parasites invade macrophages of reticuloendothelial system

Pathogenesis and pathology. After the host is bitten by an infected sandfly, the parasites disseminate in the bloodstream and are taken up by the macrophages of the spleen, liver, bone marrow, lymph nodes, skin, and small intestine. Histiocytic proliferation in these organs produces enlargement with atrophy or replacement of the normal tissue.

delayed onset; recurrent fever; chronic disease; diarrhea

severe systemic manifestations

Immune complex glomerulonephritis

Clinical manifestations. Symptoms appear 3–12 months after acquisition of the parasite. Fever, which is usually present, may be abrupt or gradual in onset. It persists for 2–8 weeks and then disappears, only to reappear at irregular intervals during the course of the disease. A double-quotidian pattern (two fever spikes in a single day) is a characteristic, but uncommon, finding. Diarrhea and malabsorption are frequent in Indian cases, resulting in progressive weight loss and weakness. Physical findings include enormous splenomegaly, lymphadenopathy, hepatomegaly, and edema. In light-skinned individuals, a grayish pigmentation of the face and hands is commonly seen, which gives the disease its name (kala azar = black disease). Anemia with resulting pallor and tachycardia are typical in advanced cases. Thrombocytopenia induces petechial formation and mucosal bleeding. The peripheral leukocyte count is usually less than $4000/mm^3$; agranulocytosis with secondary bacterial infections contributes to lethality. Serum immunoglobulin G levels are enormously elevated, but play no protective role. Circulating antigen–antibody complexes are present and are probably responsible for the glomerulonephritis seen so often in this disease.

search for Leishman–Donovan bodies

Management. The diagnosis is made by demonstrating the presence of the organism in aspirates taken from the bone marrow, liver, spleen, or lymph nodes. In the Indian form of kala azar, *L. donovani* is also found in circulating monocytes. The specimens may be smeared, stained, and examined for the typical Leishman–Donovan bodies (amastigotes in mononuclear phagocytes) or cultured in artificial media and/or experimental animals. Serologic tests are available, but lack sensitivity and specificity. Results of the leishmanin skin test are negative during active disease, but become positive after successful therapy.

high mortality without treatment

The mortality in untreated cases of kala azar is 75–90%. Treatment with pentavalent antimonial drugs lower this rate dramatically. Initial therapy, however, fails in up to 30% of African cases, and 15% of those that do respond eventually relapse. Resistant cases are treated with the more toxic pentamidine or amphotericin B.

Control measures are directed at the *Phlebotomus* vector, with the use of residual insecticides, and at the elimination of mammalian reservoirs by treating human cases and destroying infective dogs.

African Trypanosomiasis (Sleeping Sickness)

West and East African sleeping sickness

Definition. African trypanosomiasis is a highly lethal meningoencephalitis transmitted to humans by bloodsucking flies of the genus *Glossina.* It occurs in two distinct clinical and epidemiologic forms: West African or Gambian sleeping sickness and East African or Rhodesian sleeping sickness. Nagana, a disease of cattle caused by a closely related trypanosome, renders over 10 million square kilometers of Central Africa unsuitable for animal husbandry.

three recognized subspecies of *T. brucei*

Development cycle in tsetse fly

trypomastigote forms in bloodstream of mammalian host

Antigenic variation of glycoprotein coat of trypomastigotes

Organism. The trypanosomes that produce these diseases are morphologically and serologically identical. Accordingly, they are considered varieties of a single species, *Trypanosoma brucei.* The three subspecies, known as *T. brucei gambiense, T. brucei rhodesiense,* and *T. brucei brucei,* can be distinguished by their biologic and enzymatic characteristics and mitochondrial morphology. All undergo similar development changes in the course of their passage from insect to mammalian host. Upon ingestion by the tsetse fly (*Glossina* sp.) and after a period of multiplication in the midgut, they migrate to the insect's salivary glands and assume the epimastigote form. After a period of weeks they are transformed into trypomastigotes, which renders them infectious to mammals. When the fly again takes a blood meal, the parasite is inoculated with the fly's saliva. In the mammal, they continue to multiply and eventually invade the bloodstream. During the initial stages of parasitemia, the trypomastigotes elongate to become graceful, slender organisms 30 μm or more in length. Eventually multiplication slows, and some forms lose their flagella and assume a short, stumpy appearance. Near the end of the episode of parasitemia, both morphologic types may be seen in a single blood specimen. Regardless of their morphology, all trypomastigotes possess a highly immunogenic glycoprotein surface coat. In the presence of specific antibody, individual strains of *T. brucei* can change the antigenic character of this coat in a sequential and, at times, predictable fashion. The antigenic repertoire of an individual trypanosomal genotype appears both large and distinctive, suggesting that expression of alternate genes, rather than genetic mutation, accounts for this variability.

humans major reservoir of West African sleeping sickness; chronicity ensures maintenance

Epidemiology. The tsetse fly, and consequently sleeping sickness, is confined to the central area of Africa by that continent's two great deserts, the Sahara in the north and the Kalahari in the south. Riverine tsetse flies found in the forest galleries that border the streams of West and Central Africa serve as the vectors of the Gambian disease. Although these flies are not exclusively anthropophilic, humans are thought to be the major reservoir of the parasite. The infection rate in humans is affected by proximity to water, but seldom exceeds 2–3% in nonepidemic situations. Nevertheless, the extreme chronicity of the human disease ensures its continued transmission.

savanna antelopes are reservoirs of East African trypanosomiasis; humans infected incidentally

Rhodesian sleeping sickness, in contrast, is transmitted by flies indigenous to the great savannas of East Africa that feed on the blood of the small antelope inhabiting these areas. The antelope serves as the major parasite reservoir, although human-to-human and cattle-to-human spread has been documented. Humans typically become infected only when they enter the savanna to hunt or to graze their domestic animals.

local chancre at site of inoculation and enlarged lymph nodes

intermittent parasitemia with antigenic shifts

parasites localize in blood vessels of heart and central nervous system with local vasculitis

Pathology and pathogenesis. Multiplication of the trypomastigotes at the inoculation site produces a localized inflammatory lesion. After the development of this chancre, organisms spread through lymphatic channels to the bloodstream, inducing a proliferative enlargement of the lymph nodes. The subsequent parasitemia is typically low grade and recurrent. As host antibody is produced to the surface antigen characteristic of a particular parasitemic wave, the trypomastigotes disappear from the blood, reappearing 3–8 days later as new antigenic variants arise. The recurrences gradually become less regular and frequent, but may persist for weeks to years before finally disappearing. During the course of the parasitemia, trypanosomes localize in the small blood vessels of the heart and central nervous system. This localization results in endothelial proliferation and a perivascular infiltration of plasma cells and lymphocytes. In the brain, hemorrhage and a demyelinating panencephalitis may follow.

high levels of immunoglobulin M

circulating immune complexes may cause vasculitis

The mechanism by which the trypanosomes elicit vasculitis is uncertain. The infection stimulates the production of large quantities of immunoglobulin M (typically 8–16 times the normal limit). In part, this reaction represents specific protective antibodies that are ultimately responsible for the control of the parasitemia. The bulk, however, consists of nonspecific heterophile antibodies and rheumatoid factor. Antibody-induced destruction of trypanosomes releases nuclear and cytoplasmic antigens with the production of circulating immune complexes. Many authorities believe that these complexes are largely responsible for the vasculitis seen in this disease.

local lesion at site of inoculation

parasitemic manifestations 2–3 weeks later

CNS involvement

manifestations of meningoencephalitis, fatal if untreated

Clinical manifestations. The trypanosomal chancre appears 2–3 days after the bite of the tsetse fly as a raised, reddened nodule on one of the exposed surfaces of the body. With the onset of parasitemia 2–3 weeks later, the patient develops recurrent bouts of fever, tender lymphadenopathy, skin rash, headache, and impaired mentation. In the Rhodesian form of disease, myocarditis and central nervous system involvement begin within 3–6 weeks. Heart failure, convulsions, coma, and death follow in 6–9 months. Gambian sleeping sickness progresses more slowly. Bouts of fever often persist for years before central nervous system manifestations gradually appear. Spontaneous activity progressively diminishes, attention wavers, and the patient must be prodded to eat or talk. Speech grows indistinct, tremors develop, sphincter control is lost, and seizures with transient bouts of paralysis occur. In the terminal stage, the patient develops a lethal intercurrent infection or lapses into a final coma.

trypomastigotes sought in lymph node aspirates, blood, and cerebrospinal fluid

animal inoculation

Laboratory diagnosis. The diagnosis is made by microscopically examining lymph node aspirates, blood, or cerebrospinal fluid for the presence of trypomastigotes. Often the actively motile organisms can be seen in a simple wet mount preparation; definitive identification requires examination of an appropriately stained smear. If these tests prove negative, they are repeated after concentrating the organisms by centrifugation or filtration. Inoculation of rats or mice can also prove helpful in diagnosing the Rhodesian disease. The patient may also be screened for elevated levels of immunoglobulin M in the blood and spinal fluid or specific trypanosomal antibodies.

Selection of drugs dependent on whether central nervous system is involved

Treatment. Lumbar puncture must always be performed before initiation of therapy. If the specimen reveals evidence of central nervous system involvement, agents that penetrate the blood–brain barrier must be included. Unfortunately, the most effective agent of this type is a highly toxic arsenical, melarsoprol (Mel B). Although this agent occasionally produces a lethal hemorrhagic encephalopathy, the invariably fatal outcome of untreated central nervous system disease warrants its use. If the central nervous system is not yet involved, less toxic agents such as suramin or pentamidine can be used. In such cases, the cure rate is high and recovery complete.

Prevention. Although a variety of tsetse fly control measures, including the use of insecticides, deforestation, and the introduction of sterile males into the fly population have been attempted, none has proved totally practicable. Similarly, eradication of disease reservoirs by the early detection and treatment of human cases and the destruction of wild game has had limited success. Attempts to develop effective vaccines are currently under way, but are complicated by the antigenic variability of most trypomastigotes. A degree of personal protection can be achieved with insect repellents and protective clothing. Although prophylactic use of pentamidine was once advocated, enthusiasm for this treatment has waned.

American Trypanosomiasis (Chagas' Disease)

Transmission of *T. cruzi* by reduviid bugs

Definition. American trypanosomiasis is a disease produced by *T. cruzi* and transmitted by true bugs of the family Reduviidae. Clinically, the infection presents as an acute febrile illness in children and a chronic heart or gastrointestinal malady in adults.

mammalian cycle with nondividing extracellular trypomastigotes and dividing intracellular amastigotes

Organism. The trypomastigotes of *T. cruzi* closely resemble those of *T. brucei*, and, like them, disseminate from the site of inoculation to circulate in the peripheral blood of their mammalian hosts. Their developmental cycle, however, differs in several respects. Most significant, *T. cruzi* does not multiply extracellularly. The circulating trypomastigotes must invade tissue cells, lose their flagella, and assume the amastigote form before binary fission can occur. Continued multiplication leads to distention and eventual rupture of the tissue cell. Released parasites revert to trypomastigotes and regain the bloodstream. This new generation of trypomastigotes may invade other host cells, thus continuing the mammalian cycle. Alternatively, they may be ingested by a feeding reduviid and develop into epimastigotes within its midgut. Upon completion of the invertebrate cycle, the parasites migrate to the hindgut and are discharged as infectious trypomastigotes when the reduviid defecates in the process of taking another blood meal. This process can recur at each feeding for as long as 2 years. Infection in the new host is initiated when the trypomastigotes contaminate either the feeding site or the mucous membranes.

invertebrate cycle in bug

bug may remain infectious for up to 2 years

Trypanosoma cruzi comprises a number of strains, each with its own distinct geographic distribution, tissue preference, and virulence. They may be distinguished from one another with specific antisera and by differences in their isoenzyme and DNA restriction patterns. All are morphologically identical. In blood specimens, the trypomastigotes can be distinguished from those of *T. brucei* by their characteristic C or U shape, narrow undulating membrane, and large kinetoplast.

Geographic distribution of Chagas' disease

Epidemiology. Chagas' disease affects over 7 million people living in South and Central America. *Trypanosoma cruzi* has been found in both vertebrate and invertebrate hosts in the southwestern United States, and serologic evidence suggests that human infections are not uncommon in this area. To date, however, few have been clinically apparent.

nocturnal transmission in rural areas

Transmission occurs almost exclusively in rural areas where the reduviid can find harborage in animal burrows and in the cracked walls and thatch of poorly constructed buildings. This large (3 cm) winged insect leaves its hiding place at night to feed on its sleeping hosts. Its predilection to bite near the eyes or lips have earned this pest the nicknames of "kissing bug" and "assassin bug."

"kissing bug"

other reservoirs and modes of transmission

In addition to humans, a number of wild and domestic animals, including rats, cats, dogs, opossums, and armadillos, serve as reservoirs. The close association of many of these hosts with human dwellings tends to amplify the incidence of disease in humans and the difficulty involved in its control. Congenital and transfusion-related infections are rapidly increasing problems in endemic areas.

local lesion at site of inoculation

Pathogenesis and pathology. Multiplication of the parasite at the portal of entry stimulates the accumulation of neutrophils, lymphocytes, and tissue fluid, resulting in the formation of a local chancre or chagoma. The subsequent dissemination of the organism with invasion of tissue cells produces a febrile illness that may persist for 1–3 months and result in widespread organ damage. Any nucleated host cell may be involved, but those of mesenchymal origin, especially the heart, skeletal muscle, smooth muscle, and glial nerve cells, are particularly susceptible. Intracellular multiplication results in formation of a *pseudocyst,* a greatly enlarged and distorted host cell containing masses of amastigotes. With the rupture of the pseudocyst, many of the released organisms disintegrate, eliciting an intense imflammatory reaction with destruction of surrounding tissue. The development of an antibody-dependent, cell-mediated immune response leads to the eventual destruction of the *T. cruzei* parasites and the termination of the acute phase of illness. Unfortunately, many of the antibodies produced cross-react with muscle tissue, initiating a sustained autoimmune inflammatory reaction in the absence of systemic manifestation of illness. In the heart, this reaction leads to loss of muscle tissue, interstitial fibrosis, and degenerative changes in the mycocardial conduction system. In the digestive tract, loss of both ganglionic nerve cells and smooth muscle results in dilatation and loss of peristaltic movement, particularly of the esophagus and colon.

dissemination and invasion of tissue cells

Pseudocysts

Immunity and immunologic damage to heart

loss of ganglionic and smooth muscle cells in digestive tract

most infections asymptomatic; acute disease usually in children

Clinical manifestations. Serologic studies suggest that most infections remain asymptomatic. Acute manifestations, when they occur, are seen primarily in children. They begin with the appearance of the nodular, erythematous chagoma 1–3 weeks after the bite of the reduviid. If the eye served as a portal of entry, the patient will present with Romaña's sign: reddened eye, swollen lid, and enlarged preauricular lymph node. The onset of parasitemia is signaled by the development of a sustained fever, enlargement of the liver, spleen, and lymph nodes, and the appearance of peripheral edema or a transient skin rash. Heart involvement results in tachycardia, electrocardiographic changes, and occasionally arrhythmia and enlargement. Newborns may experience acute meningoencephalitis. Clinical manifestations persist for weeks to months. In 5–10% of untreated patients, severe myocardial involvement or meningoencephalitis leads to death.

Myocardial and central nervous system signs

chronic disease in adults

Chronic disease, the result of end-stage organ damage, is usually seen only in adulthood. Ironically, the majority of patients with late manifestations deny a history of acute illness. The most serious of the late manifestations is heart disease, which may present as arrhythmia, heart block, enlargement with congestive heart failure, and cardiac arrest. In some areas of rural Latin America, as much as 10% of the adult population may show cardiac man-

Cardiac manifestations

Dilatation of esophagus and colon

ifestations. Megaesophagus and megacolon, which are less devastating than the heart disease, are typically seen in more southern latitudes. This geographic variation in clinical manifestations is thought to be attributable to a difference in tissue tropism between individual strains of *T. cruzi.* Megaesophagus leads to difficulty in swallowing and regurgitation, particularly at night. Megacolon produces severe constipation with irregular passage of voluminous stools.

Search for trypomastigotes

Xenodiagnosis

Culture

Laboratory diagnosis. The diagnosis of acute Chagas' disease rests on finding the trypomastigotes from the peripheral blood and their morphologic identification at *T. cruzi.* The methods are similar to those described for diagnosis of African trypanosomiasis. If results are negative, a laboratory-raised reduviid can be fed on the patient, then dissected and examined for the presence of parasites, a procedure known as *xenodiagnosis.* Alternatively, the blood may be cultured in a variety of artificial media or experimental animals. In the diagnosis of chronic disease, recovery of the organisms is the exception rather than the rule, and diagnosis depends upon the clinical, epidemiologic, and serologic findings.

Treatment. The role of treatment in Chagas' disease remains unsettled. Until recently, no effective chemotherapeutic agent was available. At present, nitrofuramox is used to treat acute disease; however, whether this agent is curative or simply suppresses *T. cruzi* is debatable. It appears to have a negligible effect on chronic disease.

Prevention. The reduviid vector can be controlled by applying residual insecticides to rural buildings at 2- or 3-month intervals. Transfusion-induced disease in endemic areas can be prevented by adding gentian violet to all blood packs before use or by screening potential donors serologically for Chagas' disease. Immunoprophylaxis is not available at present.

Additional Reading and References

Adler, S. 1959. Darwin's illness. *Nature* 184:1102. The author describes Charles Darwin's 40-year illness and offers convincing arguments that it represented Chagas' disease acquired during Darwin's round-the-world expedition on H.M.S. *Beagle.*

Black, R.E., Dykes, A.C., Sinclair, S.P., and Wells, J.G. 1977. Giardiasis in day-care centers: Evidence of person-to-person transmission. *Pediatrics* 60:486. This article constitutes the first report of giardiasis in day-care centers.

Fouts, A.C., and Kraus, S.J. 1980. *Trichomonas vaginalis*: Reevaluation of its clinical presentation and laboratory diagnosis. *J. Infect. Dis.* 141:137–143. This report asserts that many of the characteristics thought to be typical of trichomoniasis are, in fact, shared by other causes of vaginitis.

Jordan, A.M. 1979. Trypanosomiasis control and land use in Africa. *Outlook Agric.* 10:2123. This article discusses the impact of animal trypanosomiasis on the utilization of land in tropical Africa.

Lainson, R., and Shaw, J.J. 1978. Epidemiology and ecology of leishmaniasis in Latin America. *Nature* 273:595.

Moore, G.T., Cross, W.M., McGuire, D., et al. 1969. Epidemic giardiasis at a ski resort. *N. Engl. J. Med.* 281:402–407. This and the report by Walzer et al. are two of the early studies to document the pathogenicity of *Giardia lamblia* and its transmission via water supplies.

Phillips, S.C., Mildvan, D., William, D.C., et al. 1981. Sexual transmission of enteric protozoa and helminths in a venereal-disease clinic population. *N. Engl. J. Med.*

305:603–606. These authors establish that homosexual men have a high prevalence of infections with *Entamoeba histolytica* and *Giardia lamblia* and that the association between these infections and oral–anal sex is significant.

Teixeira, A.R.L. 1979. Chagas' disease: Trends in immunological research and prospects for immunoprophylaxis. *Bull. WHO* 57:697. The current state of knowledge regarding the immunopathogenesis of chronic Chagas' disease is lucidly recapitulated.

Vickerman, K. 1978. Antigenic variation in trypanosomes. *Nature* 273:613. This report provides the best discussion currently available on the complex and important phenomenon of antigenic variation seen in African trypanosomiasis.

Walzer, P.D., Wolfe, M.S., and Schultz, M.G. 1971. Giardiasis in travelers. *J. Infect. Dis.* 124:235–237.

James J. Plorde

Pneumocystis carinii Infections

48

Pneumocystosis is a highly lethal pneumonitis of immunocompromised patients and premature infants caused by *Pneumocystis carinii*, an organism of uncertain classification. It is now seen most frequently in patients undergoing cancer chemotherapy, organ transplant recipients receiving suppressive therapy, and in homosexual males with acquired immunodeficiency syndrome.

Organism

taxonomic status uncertain

cyst and trophozoite forms

Methods of demonstrating parasite

Animal strains

Growth in cell culture

Although widely believed to be a protozoan, the taxonomic position of *P. carinii* remains unsettled. Both cyst and trophozoite forms have been described. The former are round or oval, measure 5–8 μm in diameter, and contain two to eight small "sporozoites." The cysts often occur in clumps and, at points of contact, their walls are typically flattened, producing a characteristic honeycomb appearance. Rupture of the cysts results in release of mature trophozoites. These pleomorphic forms possess a single eccentric nucleus, a reticular cytoplasm, and a poorly differentiated cell membrane (Figure 48.1). Electron microscopic studies suggest the capacity for oxidative metabolism and protein synthesis. Both cysts and trophozoites can be demonstrated in tissue with phase or fluorescent microscopy, as well as with a number of special stains. Methenamine silver and toluidine blue O stain the cyst wall, whereas Giemsa, Wright, and Gram–Weigert stains preferentially color sporozoites and trophozoites. Hematoxylin–eosin visualizes neither. Organisms morphologically identical to the human parasite have been found in the lungs of several lower animals. Immunologic studies have revealed significant antigenic differences, suggesting the existence of separate strains or species.

In vitro cultivation, a necessary prerequisite to detailed study of any microbe, has only recently been accomplished for *P. carinii.* It can now be grown in a variety of cell culture lines.

Pneumocystosis

Epidemiology

Latent infection

Latent pulmonary infection occurs worldwide in a broad spectrum of animal life. Serologic and histologic evidence suggests a similar pattern in humans. Specific antibodies, detected by indirect immunofluorescence, are present in more than two-thirds of normal children, and autopsy studies have demonstrated organisms in the lung tissue of patients without clinical evidence

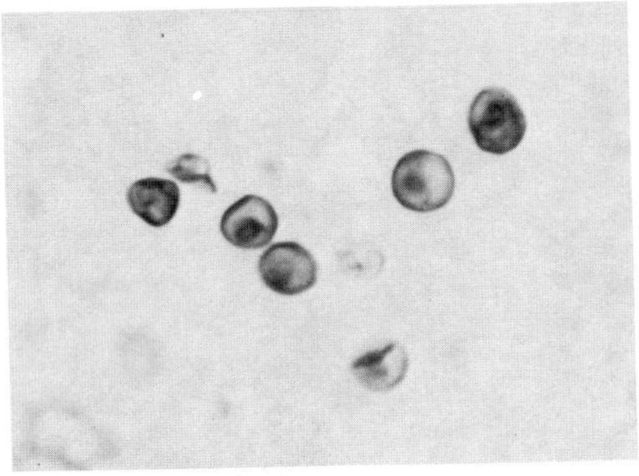

48.1 Trophozoites of *Pneumocytis carinii* in bronchial lavage fluid stained with methenamine silver.

of disease. Manifest illness, when it occurs, may appear in either an epidemic or a sporadic pattern.

Occasional epidemic infection in infants

Epidemics of pneumocystosis were first documented in Europe after World War II, when nursery outbreaks of interstitial pneumonia involving debilitated and premature infants were ultimately proved to be caused by *P. carinii.* Clinical and serologic data collected at that time suggested that the disease was contagious, possibly spreading from person to person via aerosols. With economic recovery and improvement in infant nutrition, the epidemic form of disease disappeared from Europe; however, it continues to be reported occasionally from other parts of the world, most recently in orphanages in Southeast Asia. In contrast, cases in the United States have occurred sporadically among immunocompromised patients. In infants the disease is associated with congenital immunodeficiencies; in older children and adults, it occurs as a complication of lymphoreticular malignancy, autoimmune or collagen vascular disease, renal failure, and organ transplantation. Recently, a cluster of cases of pneumocystosis among male homosexuals has been reported. These otherwise healthy individuals have demonstrated impaired cellular immunity and evidence of past or current cytomegalovirus infection. A few have developed Kaposi's sarcoma, a malignant skin condition. As both cytomegalovirus infection and Kaposi's sarcoma occur more frequently in immunosuppressed hosts, the association of these three relatively uncommon problems in male homosexuals is intriguing, but not presently explainable. Pneumocystosis has also been reported occasionally in the absence of underlying disease.

Sporadic cases in immunocompromised hosts

Occurrence in homosexual men

Origin of sporadic cases

It is generally believed that the sporadic cases in immunocompromised patients represent activation of latent infection. However, secondary cases in the families of some patients and the occasional clustering of cases in cancer wards suggest that this form of the disease may also be contagious.

Pathogenesis and Pathology

Opportunistic pathogen

Pneumocystis carinii is evidently an organism of low virulence that seldom produces disease in a normal host. In experimental animals, progressive infection can be initiated with starvation or corticosteroid administration, presumably by activating a latent infection. Concurrent viral, bacterial, fungal, and protozoan infections are found frequently in human cases, suggesting that *P. carinii* may require the presence of another microbial agent for its multiplication.

Predisposing conditions

Histology and development of pulmonary lesions

Histologically, latent infections are characterized by the presence of scattered, isolated cysts forms within normal-appearing alveolar septa of the lung. In clinically manifest disease, the alveoli are filled with desquamated

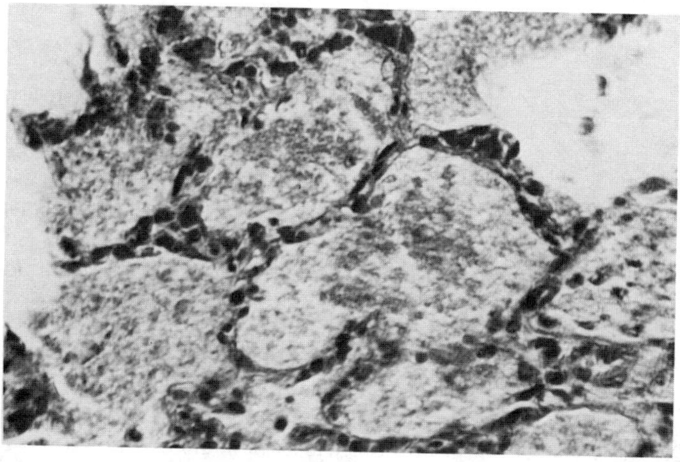

48.2 Lung biopsy specimen from *Pneumocystis carinii* infection, showing "foamy" contents of alveoli.

alveolar cells, monocytes, organisms, and fluid, producing a distinctive foamy appearance (Figure 48.2). Hyaline membranes may be present, and round cell infiltrates are visible in the septa. Fibrosis, when present, is usually minimal. These changes are generally reversible with therapy, although calcification and persistent fibrosis have been documented occasionally. Lesions outside the lung have been noted, but are extremely rare.

Clinical Manifestations

progressive, diffuse pneumonitis

In the immunocompromised host, the disease presents as a progressive, diffuse pneumonitis. Illness may begin after discontinuation or a sudden decrease in the dose of corticosteroids or, in the case of acute lymphatic leukemia, during a period of remission. In infants the onset is typically insidious, and the clinical course is 3–4 weeks in duration. Fever is mild or absent. In older individuals and patients on high doses of corticosteroids, the onset is more abrupt, and the course is both febrile (38–40°C) and abbreviated. In both populations, the cardinal manifestation is progressive dyspnea and tachypnea; cyanosis and hypoxia eventually supervene. A nonproductive cough is present in one-half of all patients. Clinical signs of pneumonia are usually absent, despite the presence of infiltrates on x-ray. These infiltrates are alveolar in character and spread out symmetrically from the hili, eventually affecting most of the lung. Pleural effusions are uncommon. Death occurs by progressive asphyxia.

progressive difficulty in breathing and hypoxia

Diagnosis

Bronchial lavage and biopsy

Lung biopsy

Definite diagnosis depends upon finding organisms of typical morphology in appropriate specimens. Although the organism has been found in sputum, tracheal aspirates, and gastric contents, the yield from such specimens is low. Bronchial lavage and endobronchial brush biopsies have been found more helpful. Percutaneous needle aspiration of the lung, needle biopsy, and open lung biopsy, although somewhat more sensitive techniques, are accompanied by more complications, including pneumothorax and hemothorax.

Several tests have been developed to detect circulating antibodies, but none to date has been sufficiently sensitive and specific to warrant routine application. More promising are methods currently being developed for the detection of circulating antigens.

Treatment and Prevention

Trimethoprim–sulfamethoxazole treatment

Patients with acquired immunodeficiency syndrome excepted, appropriate management of this disease can reduce mortality from 100 to 30%. Oxygen therapy must be administered to maintain adequate oxygenation. In some patients, mechanical ventilatory assistance may be required. The organism is inhibited by trimethoprim–sulfamethoxazole, which should be given orally or intravenously for 14 days. It has been shown recently that long-term, low-dose administration of trimethoprim–sulfamethoxazole will significantly decrease the incidence of *P. carinii* pneumonia in high-risk patients.

Additional Reading and References

Burke, B.A., and Good, R.A. 1973. *Pneumocystis carinii* infection. *Medicine* (*Baltimore*) 52:23–51. A classic review.

Gottlieb, M.S., et al. 1981. *Pneumocystis carinii* pneumonia and mucosal candidiasis in previously healthy homosexual men. *N. Engl. J. Med.* 305:1425–1431. This report is one of a series of recent papers describing the simultaneous presence of *Pneumocystis carinii* pneumonia, cytomegalovirus infection, and Kaposi's sarcoma in a group of homosexual men.

Hughes, W.T., et al. 1977. Successful chemoprophylaxis for *Pneumocystis carinii* pneumonitis. *N. Engl. J. Med.* 297:1419–1426. The first controlled study demonstrating the effectiveness of trimethoprim–sulfamethoxazole treatment in preventing *P. carinii* infections in cancer patients is reported.

James J. Plorde

Intestinal Nematodes

49

The intestinal nematodes have cylindric, fusiform bodies covered with a tough acellular cuticle. Sandwiched between this integument and the body cavity are layers of muscle, longitudinal nerve trunks, and an excretory system. A tubular alimentary tract consisting of a mouth, esophagus, midgut, and anus runs from the anterior to the posterior extremity. Highly developed reproductive organs fill the remainder of the body cavity. The sexes are separate; the male worm is generally smaller than his mate. The female, which is extremely prolific, can produce thousands of offspring, generally in the form of eggs. Typically, the eggs must incubate or embryonate outside of the human host before they become infectious to another person; during this time, the embryo repeatedly segments, eventually developing into an adolescent form known as a *larva.* In some species of nematodes, offspring develop to the larval stage in the uterus of the worm. The duration and site of embryonation differ with each worm species and determine how it will be transmitted to the new host. In many cases, eggs of nematodes that dwell within the human gastrointestinal tract are carried to the environment in the feces and embryonate on the soil for a period of weeks before becoming infectious. The egg may then be ingested with contaminated food. In some species, the egg hatches outside of the host, releasing a larva capable of penetrating the skin of a person who comes in direct physical contact with it. Obviously, intestinal nematodes are principally found in areas where human feces are deposited indiscriminately or used for fertilizer.

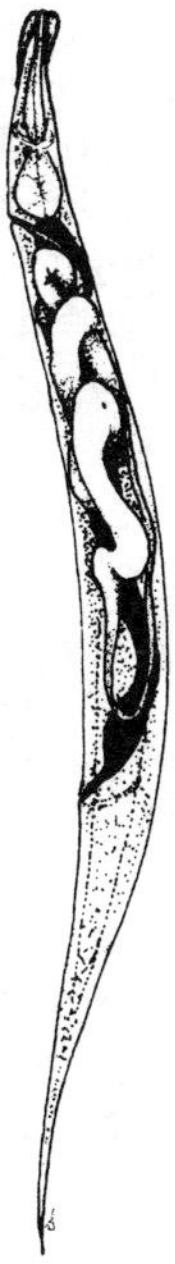

Nematode

significance of duration and site of embryonation

There are six intestinal nematodes that commonly infect humans: *Enterobius vermicularis* (the pinworm), *Trichuris trichuria* (the whipworm), *Ascaris lumbricoides* (the large roundworm), *Necator americanus* and *Ancylostoma duodenale* (the hookworms), and *Strongyloides stercoralis* (Table 49.1). Together they infect more than one-quarter of the human race, producing embarrassment, discomfort, malnutrition, anemia, and occasionally death. Other closely related nematodes of animals that may occasionally infect humans are also listed in Table 49.1 but will not be discussed here.

Members of group

The adults of each of the six nematodes listed previously can survive for months or years within the lumen of the gut. The severity of illness produced by each depends upon the level of adaptation to the host it has achieved. Some species have a simple life cycle that can be completed without serious consequences to the host. Less well-adapted parasites, on the other hand, have more complex cycles, often requiring tissue invasion and/or production of enormous numbers of offspring to ensure their continued survival and

long survival in gut lumen

relationship of parasitic adaptation to disease

Table 49.1 Intestinal Nematodes

Human Parasite	Animal Parasite	Human Disease
Enterobius vermicularis (pinworm)		Enterobiasis
Trichuris trichuria (whipworm)		Trichuriasis
	Capillaria philippinensis	Intestinal capillariasis
Ascaris lumbricoides (large roundworm)		Ascariasis
	Ascaris suum	Ascariasis
	Anisakis sp.	Anisakiasis
	Toxocara canis, *Toxocara cati*	Toxocariasis (visceral larva migrans)
Necator americanus (hookworm) *Ancylostoma duodenale* (hookworm)		Hookworm disease
	Ancylostoma braziliense	Cutaneous larva migrans
Strongyloides stercoralis		Strongyloidiasis

Importance of worm load and repeated infection

immune response slow and incomplete

dissemination. Within a given species, disease severity is related directly to the number of adult worms harbored by the host. The greater the worm load or worm burden, the more serious the consequences. As nematodes do not multiply within the human, small worm loads may remain asymptomatic and undetected throughout the life span of the parasite. Repeated infections, however, will progressively increase the worm burden and, at some point, induce symptomatic disease. Although humans can mount an immune response that will eventually lead to the expulsion of worms, it is slow to develop and incomplete. It is therefore the frequency and intensity of reinfection, more than the host's immune response, that determine the worm burden.

Life Cycles

The life cycles of the intestinal nematodes are summarized in Table 49.2 and considered in greater detail below.

Table 49.2 Life Cycle of Intestinal Nematodes

Parasite	Route of Infection	Migration in Body	Diagnostic Form	Site of Embryonation	Infective Form	Free-Living Cycle
Enterobius vermicularis	Mouth	Intestinal	Egg	Perineum	Egg	No
Trichuris trichuria	Mouth	Intestinal	Egg	Soil	Egg	No
Ascaris lumbricoides	Mouth	Pulmonary	Egg	Soil	Egg	No
Necator americanus[a]	Skin	Pulmonary	Egg	Soil	Filariform larvae	No
Stronglyoides stercoralis[b]	Skin	Pulmonary	Rhabditiform larvae	Soil; intestine[b]	Filariform larvae	Yes

Reproduced with permission from Plorde, J.J. in Isselbacher et al. *Harrison's Principles of Internal Medicine*, 9th ed. 1980. McGraw-Hill, Inc. Table 206–3, p. 891.

[a]Also *Ancylostoma duodenale*. [b]Intestine only in cases of autoinfection.

Enterobius vermicularis

female traverses anus at night; eggs deposited, causing pruritis

eggs ingested by patient or others

maturation to adult within gut

Enterobius vermicularis, the best adapted of the intestinal nematodes, has the simplest life cycle. The adult male and female lie attached to the mucosa of the cecum. After copulation, the gravid female migrates down the colon, slips unobserved through the anal canal in the dark of night, and deposits approximately 20,000 sticky eggs on the host's perianal skin, bedclothes, and linens. The eggs are near maturity at the time of deposition and become infectious shortly thereafter. Handling of bedclothes or scratching of the perianal area to relieve the associated itching results in adhesion of the eggs to the fingers and subsequent transfer to the oral cavity during eating or other finger–mouth maneuvers. Alternatively, the eggs may be shaken into the air (for example, during making of the bed), inhaled, and swallowed. The eggs subsequently hatch in the upper intestine and the larvae migrate to the cecum, maturing to adults in the process. The entire adult-to-adult cycle is completed in only 2 weeks.

Trichuris trichuria

female releases eggs in gut lumen

eggs mature in soil

Trichuris trichuria, the next best adapted of the gut worms, has a life cycle that differs from that of the pinworm only in its external phase. The gravid female does not leave her home in the cecum, but releases her eggs into the gut lumen. They pass out of the body with the feces and, in poorly sanitated areas of the world, are deposited on soil. The eggs are immature at the time of passage and must incubate for at least 10 days (longer if conditions of temperature and moisture are suboptimal) before they become fully embryonated and infectious. Once mature, they are picked up on the hands of children at play or agricultural workers and passed to the mouth. In areas where human feces are used as a fertilizer, raw fruits and vegetables can be contaminated and later ingested.

no direct person-to-person transmission

Although the differences between the life cycle of *Enterobius* and that of *Trichuris* are minor, they have profound epidemiologic ramifications. Unlike the pinworm, the whipworm cannot be passed directly from person to person. Transmission occurs only in populations that practice indiscriminate defecation and live in climates suitable for the maturation of the eggs in the soil.

Ascaris lumbricoides

eggs mature in soil

larvae from ingested eggs enter bloodstream, pass through alveoli and to gastrointestinal tract via respiratory tract and esophagus

Ascaris lumbricoides is a large roundworm that may measure more than a foot in length. It is less well adapted to its human host than the smaller pinworm and whipworm. It lives high in the small intestine and deposits hundreds of thousands of eggs daily into the fecal stream. The development of these progeny outside of the host is identical to that of *T. trichuria.* The similarity ends, however, upon ingestion of the eggs by the host. After hatching from the eggs, the larvae penetrate the intestinal mucosa and invade the portal venules. They are carried to the liver, where they are still small enough to squeeze through that organ's capillaries and exit in the hepatic vein. They are then carried to the right side of the heart and subsequently pumped out to the lung. In the course of this migration, the larvae increase in size. By the time they reach the pulmonary capillaries, they are too large to pass through to the left side of the heart. Finding this route blocked, they rupture into the alveolar spaces, are coughed up, and are subsequently swallowed. After they regain access to the upper intestine, they become sedentary, mature to adults, and spend the remainder of their lives in the safety of the intestinal lumen.

Hookworms

eggs mature and release rhabditiform larvae in soil

infected larvae penetrate human skin, then follow same path as *Ascaris* larvae to gut

For all practical purposes, the life cycles of the two hookworms, *N. americanus* and *A. duodenale,* are identical; they differ from that of *Ascaris* in only one significant way. Their mature eggs hatch while still in the soil, releasing active, free-feeding *rhabditiform larvae.* These larvae molt, become infective *filariform larvae,* and penetrate the skin of any human that comes in contact with them. The larvae are carried by the lymphohematogenous system to the right side of the heart and onward to the lungs. Here they rupture into the alveolar spaces and, like *Ascaris,* are coughed up, swallowed, and passed into the small intestine, where they mature to adulthood.

Strongyloides stercoralis

Three possible developmental cycles

1. resembles hookworm cycle, except that hatched larvae are passed in stool

2. internal and external autoinfection with increasing worm load

3. free-living propagation of worms with production of infective larvae

The adaption of *S. stercoralis* is the least satisfactory of the intestinal nematodes and, in an evolutionary sense, appears to have occurred quite recently. It may utilize any one of three developmental cycles. The first is similar to that of the hookworm, except that the eggs are deposited and hatch in the submucosa of the gut. The rhabditiform larvae penetrate back into the gut, and they, rather than the eggs, are passed in the feces. In the second (autoinfection) cycle, the rhabditiform larva's passage through the colon to the outside world is delayed by constipation or other factors, allowing it to transform into a filariform larva while still within the body of its host. This larva may then invade the intestinal mucosa (internal autoinfection) or perianal skin (external autoinfection) directly without an intervening soil phase. Thus, *S. stercoralis,* unlike any of the other intestinal nematodes, has the capacity to multiply within the body of the host. The worm burden may increase dramatically and the infection persist indefinitely in the absence of external reinfection, often with dire consequences to the host. In the third cycle, the rhabditiform larvae, after passage in the stool and deposition on the soil, develop into free-living adult males and females. These adults may propagate several generations of free-living worms before infective filariform larvae are again produced. This cycle creates a soil reservoir that may persist even without continued deposition of feces.

Parasites and Diseases

Enterobiasis

Organism. The adult female is a 10-mm-long, cream-colored worm with a sharply pointed tail, characteristics that have given rise to the common name *pinworm.* Running longitudinally down both sides of the body are small ridges that widen anteriorly to finlike alae. The seldom seen male is smaller (3 mm) and possesses a ventrally curved tail and copulatory spicule. The clear, thin-shelled, ovoid eggs are flattened on one side and measure 25 × 50 μm (Figure 49.1).

infects 30–40 million in U.S.

Epidemiology. The pinworm is the oldest and most widespread of the helminths. Eggs have been found in a 10,000-year-old coprolith, making this nematode the oldest demonstrated infectious agent of humans. It has been estimated to infect at least 200 million people worldwide, 30–40 million in the United States alone. Infection is more common among the young and poor, but may be found in any age or economic class. The incidence in white individuals is significantly higher than that in blacks.

resistant infective eggs

The eggs are relatively resistant to desiccation and may remain viable in linens, bedclothes, or house dust for several days. Once infection is introduced into a household, other family members are rapidly infected.

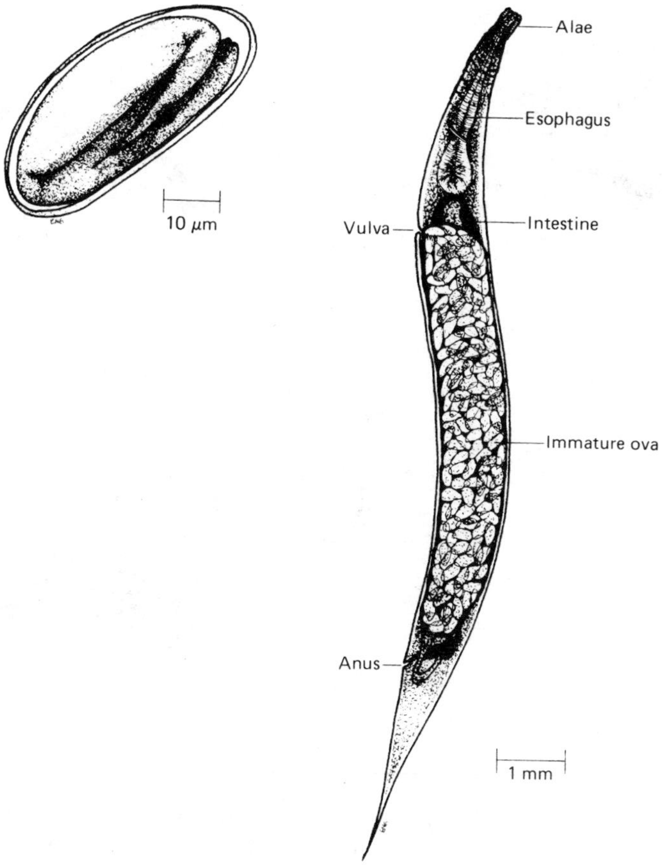

49.1 Female pinworm (*Enterobius vermicularis*) and embryonated egg.

nocturnal pruritis ani

Clinical manifestations. Enterobius vermicularis seldom produces serious disease. The most frequent symptom is pruritis ani (anal itching). This symptom is most severe at night and has been attributed to the migration of the gravid female. It may lead to irritability and other minor complaints. In severe infections, the intense itching may lead to scratching, excoriation, and secondary bacterial infection. In female patients, the worm may enter the genital tract, producing vaginitis, granulomatous endometritis, or even salpingitis. It has also been suggested that migrating worms might carry enteric bacteria into the urinary bladder in young women, inducing an acute bacterial infection of the urinary tract. Although this worm is frequently found in the lumen of the resected appendix, it is doubtful that it plays a causal role in appendicitis. Perhaps the most serious effect of this common infection is the psychic trauma suffered by the economically advantaged when they discover that they, too, are subject to intestinal worm infection.

occasional infection of female genitourinary tract

Anal cellophane tape test for ova

Laboratory diagnosis. The diagnosis is suggested by the clinical manifestations and confirmed by the recovery of the characteristic eggs from the anal mucosa. Identification is accomplished by applying the sticky side of cellophane tape to the mucocutaneous junction, then transferring the tape to a glass slide and examining the slide under the low-power lens of a microscope. Occasionally, the adult female will be seen by a parent of an infected child or recovered with the cellophane tape procedure.

Treatment and prevention. Several highly satisfactory agents, including pyrantel pamoate and mebendazole, are available for treatment. Many author-

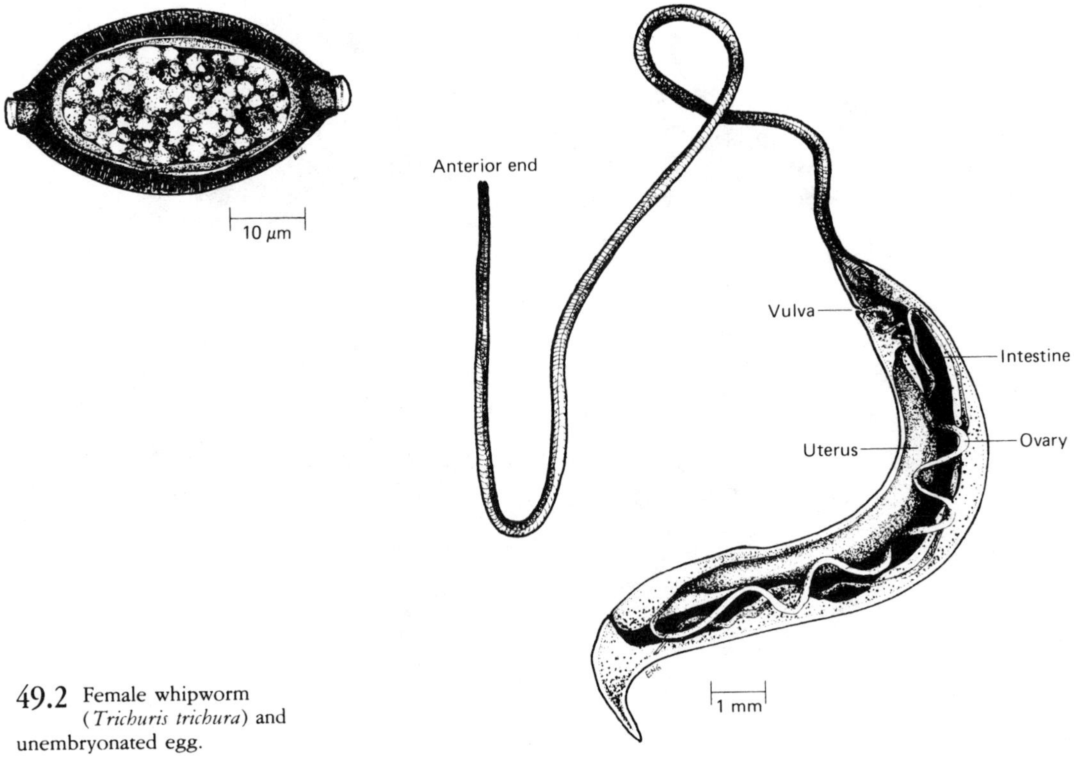

49.2 Female whipworm (*Trichuris trichura*) and unembryonated egg.

all family members may need treatment

reinfection common

ities believe that all members of a family or other cohabiting group should be treated simultaneously. In severe infections, retreatment after 2 weeks is recommended. Although cure rates are high, reinfection is extremely common. It need not be treated in the absence of symptoms.

Trichuriasis

Organism. The adult whipworm is 30–50 mm in length. The anterior two-thirds is thin and threadlike, whereas the posterior end is bulbous, giving the worm the appearance of a tiny whip. The tail of the male is coiled, that of the female straight. The female produces 3000–10,000 oval eggs each day. They are of the same size as pinworm eggs, but have a distinctive thick brown shell with translucent knobs on both ends (Figure 49.2).

occurs with defecation on soil and warm, humid climate

Epidemiology. Although it is less widespread than the pinworm, the whipworm is a cosmopolitan parasite, infecting approximately 1 billion people throughout the world. It is concentrated in areas where indiscriminate defecation and a warm, humid environment produce extensive seeding of soil with infectious eggs. In tropical climates, infection rates may be as high as 80%. Although the incidence is much lower in temperate nations, trichuriasis is found throughout the rural areas of the southeastern United States. Here it occurs primarily in family and institutional clusters, presumably maintained by the poor sanitary habits of toddlers and the mentally retarded. Although the intensity of infection is generally low, adult worms may live 4–8 years.

Longevity of worms

colonic damage with severe infection

Clinical manifestations. Light infections are asymptomatic. With moderate worm loads, damage to the intestinal mucosa may induce nausea, abdominal pain, and diarrhea. Occasionally, a child may harbor 800 worms or more.

In these situations, the entire colonic mucosa is parasitized, with significant mucosal damage, blood loss, and anemia. The shear-force of the fecal stream on the bodies of the worms may produce prolapse of the colonic or rectal mucosa through the anus, particularly when the host is straining at defecation or childbirth. The sudden appearance of a prolapsed rectum teeming with hundreds of wriggling whipworms has been known to produce nausea and lightheadedness in uninitiated obstetricians.

Colonic or rectal prolapse

Laboratory diagnosis. In light infections, stool concentration methods may be required to recover the eggs. Such procedures are almost never necessary in symptomatic infections, as they inevitably produce more than 10,000 eggs per gram of feces, a density readily detected by examining 1–2 mg of emulsified stool with the low-power lens of a microscope.

Stool examination for eggs

Treatment. Infections should not be treated unless they are symptomatic. Mebendazole is the drug of choice. Although the cure rate is only 60–70%, more than 90% of the adult worms are usually expelled, rendering the patient asymptomatic. Prevention requires the improvement of sanitary facilities.

Ascariasis

Organism. Ascaris lumbricoides, a short-lived worm (6–18 months), is the largest and most common of the intestinal helminths. Measuring 150–350 mm in length, it dwarfs its fellow gut roundworms and brings an unexpected richness to our mental image of a parasite. Its firm, creamy cuticle and more pointed extremities differentiate it from the common earthworm, which it otherwise resembles in both size and external morphology. The male is slightly smaller than the female and possesses a curved tail with copulatory spicules. His mate passes 200,000 eggs daily, whether she is fertilized or not. Eggs are elliptic in shape, measure 35×55 μm, and have a rough, mammilated, albuminous coat over their chitinous shells. They are highly resistant to environmental conditions and may remain viable for up to 6 years in mild climates (Figure 49.3).

prolonged viability of eggs

Epidemiology. More than 1 billion of the world's population, including 4 million Americans, are infected. Like trichuriasis, with which it is coextensive, ascariasis is a disease of warm climates and poor sanitation. It is maintained by small children who defecate indiscriminately in the immediate vicinity of the home and pick up infectious eggs on their hands during play. Geophagia is common and may result in massive worm loads. The parasite may also be acquired through ingestion of egg-contaminated food by the host; in dry, windy climates, eggs may become airborne, and be inhaled and swallowed. In tropical areas, the entire population may be involved. Isolated infected family clusters are more common in temperate climes.

epidemiology similar to that of *Trichuris*

Clinical manifestations. Clinical manifestations may result from either the migration of the larvae through the lung or the presence of the adults in the intestinal lumen. Pulmonary involvement is usually seen in communities where transmission is seasonal; the severity of symptoms is related to the degree of hypersensitivity induced by previous infections and the intensity of the current exposure. Fever, cough, wheezing, and shortness of breath are common. Laboratory studies reveal eosinophilia, oxygen desaturation, and migratory pulmonary infiltrates. Death from respiratory failure has been noted occasionally.

Pulmonary reactions to larval migration

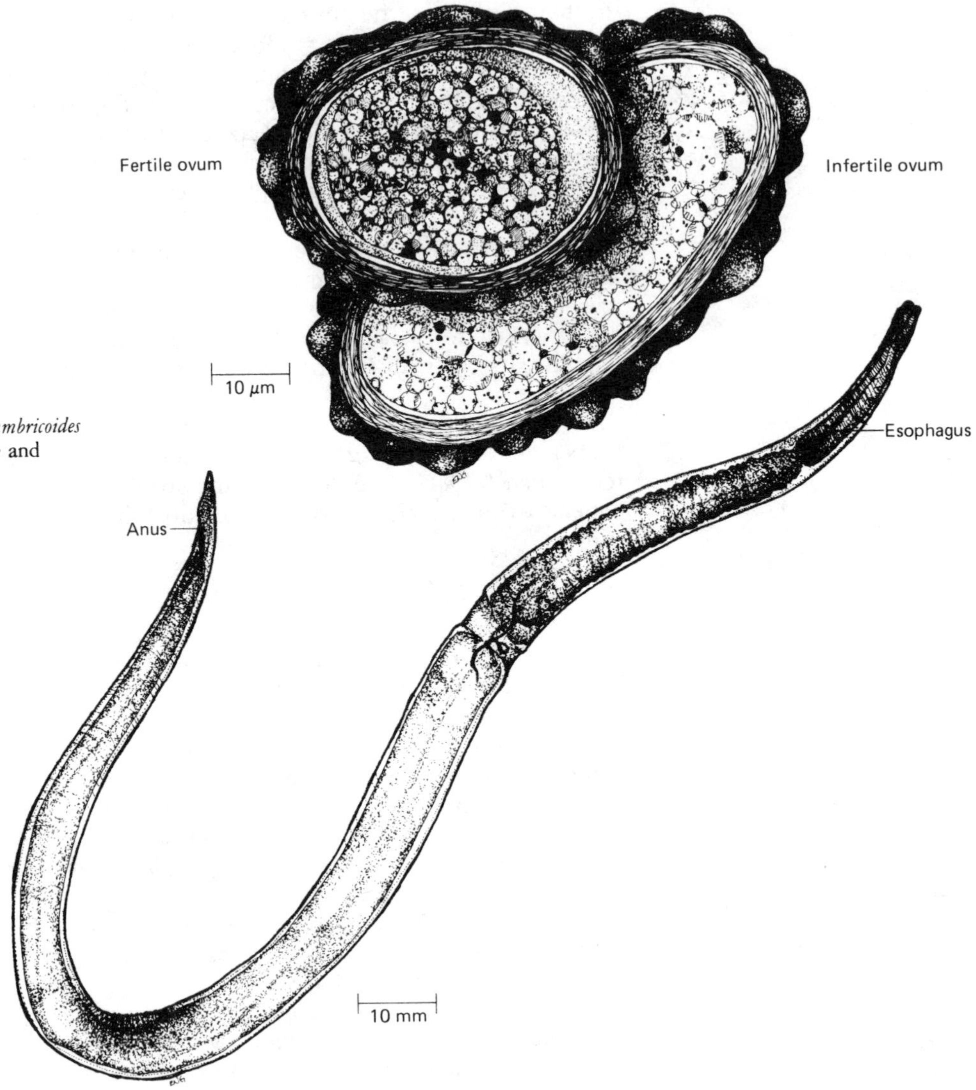

49.3 Female *Ascaris lumbricoides* worm and fertile and infertile eggs.

Asymptomatic infections with small worm loads

If the worm load is small, infections with adult worms may be completely asymptomatic. They come to clinical attention when the parasite is vomited up or passed in the stool. This situation is most likely during episodes of fever, which appear to stimulate the worms to increase motility. Most physicians who have worked in underdeveloped countries have had the disconcerting experience of observing an ascarid crawl out of a patient's mouth, nose, or ear during an otherwise uneventful evaluation of fever. Occasionally an adult worm will migrate to the appendix, bile duct, or pancreatic duct, causing obstruction and inflammation of the organ. Heavier worm loads may produce abdominal pain and malabsorption of fat, protein, carbohydrate, and vitamins. In marginally nourished children, growth may be retarded. Occasionally a bolus of worms may form and produce intestinal obstruction, particularly in children. Worm loads of 50 are not uncommon, and as many as 2000 worms have been recovered from a single child. In the United States, where worm loads tend to be modest, obstruction occurs in 2 per 1000 infected children per year. The mortality in these cases is 3%.

Malabsorption and occasional obstruction with heavy worm loads

Stool examination for eggs

Laboratory diagnosis The diagnosis is generally made by finding the characteristic eggs in the feces. The extreme productivity of the female ascarid generally makes this task an easy one, except when the atypical-appearing unfertilized eggs predominate. The pulmonary phase of ascariasis is diagnosed by the finding of larvae and eosinophils in the sputum.

Treatment and prevention. Pyrantel pamoate and mebendazole are both highly effective; the latter is preferred if *T. trichuria* is also present. Communitywide control of ascariasis can be achieved with mass therapy administered at 6-month intervals. Ultimately, control requires adequate sanitation facilities.

Hookworm Infections

N. americanus and *A. duodenale* infect humans

feed on blood

Organism. Two species, *N. americanus* and *A. duodenale,* infect humans. Adults of both species are pinkish-white and measure about 1 cm in length (Figure 49.4). The head is often curved in a direction opposite that of the body, giving these worms the hooked appearance from which their common name is derived. The males have a unique fan-shaped copulatory bursa, rather than the curved, pointed tail common to the other intestinal nematodes. The two species can be readily differentiated by the morphology of their oral cavity. *Ancylostoma duodenale,* the Old World hookworm, possesses four sharp toothlike structures, whereas *N. americanus,* the New World hookworm, has dorsal and ventral cutting plates. With the aid of these structures, the hookworms attach to the mucosa of the small bowel and suck blood. Each adult *A. duodenale* extracts 0.2 ml of blood daily, *N. americanus* 0.03 ml. Part of the blood loss is related to the tendency of the worms to migrate

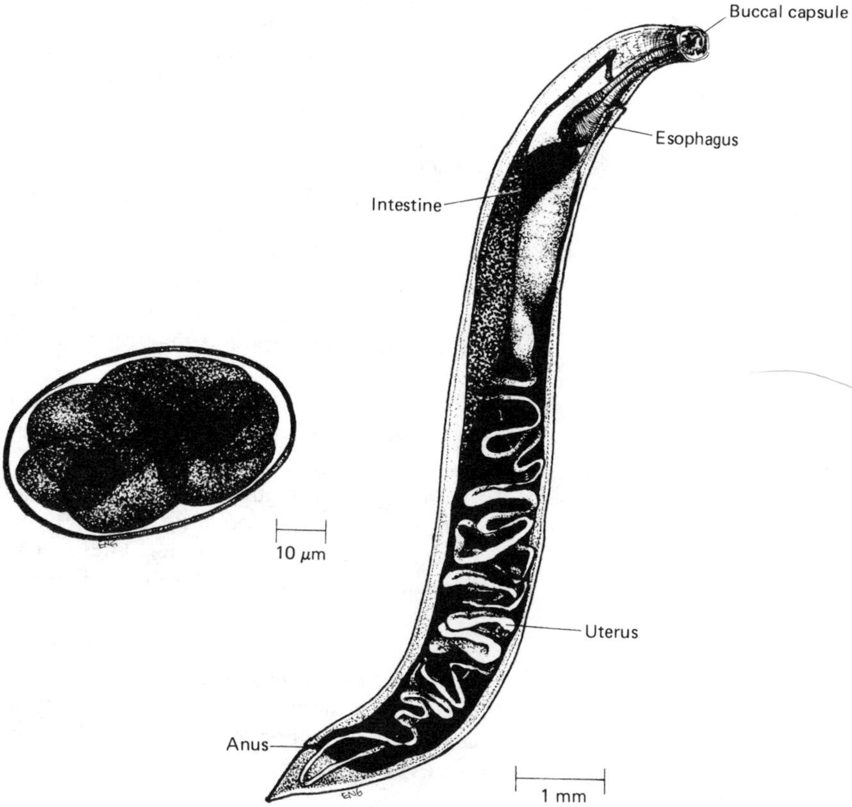

49.4 Female hookworm (*Necator americanus*) and egg.

within the intestine, leaving bleeding points at old sites of attachment. As the adults may survive 2–14 years, the accumulated blood loss may be enormous. The fertilized female releases 10,000–20,000 eggs daily. They measure 40 × 60 μm, possess a thin shell, and are usually in the two- to four-cell stage when passed in the feces (Figure 49.4).

deposition of eggs on soil

larvae hatch under moist conditions and traverse skin

Geographic distribution

Epidemiology. Hookworm infection is found worldwide between the latitudes of 45° N and 30° S. Transmission requires deposition of egg-containing feces on shady, well-drained soil, development of larvae under conditions of abundant rainfall and high temperatures (23–33°C), and direct contact of unprotected human skin with resulting filariform larvae. Infections become particularly intense in closed, densely populated communities, such as tea and coffee plantations. *Necator americanus* is found in the tropical areas of Asia, Africa, and America, as well as the southern United States, where it was introduced with the African slave trade. *Ancylostoma duodenale* is seen in the Mediterranean basin, the Middle East, northern India, China, and Japan. It has been estimated that together these two worms extract over 7 million liters of blood each day from 700 million individuals scattered around the globe.

most infections asymptomatic

pruritis at site of skin penetration

Clinical manifestations. In the overwhelming majority of infected patients, the worm burden is small and the infection asymptomatic. Clinical manifestations, when they do occur, may be related to the original penetration of the skin by the filariform larva, the migration of the larva through the lung, and/or the presence of the adult worm in the gut. Skin penetration may produce a pruritic erythematous rash and swelling, popularly known as *ground itch.* This manifestation is more common in infection with *N. americanus,* generally occurs between the toes, and may persist for several days. It is probably the result of prior sensitization to larval antigens.

Pulmonary manifestations

iron deficiency anemia caused by blood loss from intestinal worms

Pulmonary manifestations may mimic those seen in ascariasis, but are generally less frequent and less severe. In the gut, the adult worm may produce epigastric pain and abnormal peristalsis. The major manifestations, however—anemia and hypoalbuminemia—are the result of chronic blood loss. The severity of the anemia depends upon the worm burden and intake of dietary iron. If iron intake exceeds iron loss resulting from hookworm infection, a normal hematocrit will be maintained. Commonly, however, dietary iron is ingested in a form that is poorly absorbed. As a result, severe anemia may develop over a period of months or years. In children, this condition may often precipitate heart failure or kwashiorkor. Mental, sexual, and physical development may be retarded.

Detection of eggs in stool

Laboratory diagnosis. The diagnosis is made by examining direct or concentrated stool for the distinctive eggs. As they are identical in the two species, precise identification of the causative worm is generally not attempted. Quantitative egg counts can permit accurate estimation of worm load. If the stool is allowed to stand too long before it is examined, the eggs may hatch, releasing rhabditiform larvae. These larvae closely resemble those of *S. stercoralis* and must be differentiated from them.

Treatment and prevention. The anemia must be corrected. When it is mild or moderate, iron replacement is adequate. More severe anemia may require blood transfusions. The two most widely used anthelmintic agents, pyrantel pamoate and mebendazole, are both highly effective. Prevention requires improved sanitation.

Strongyloidiasis

Organism. Strongyloides stercoralis may measure only 2 mm in length, making it the smallest of the intestinal nematodes. The male, which is seldom seen, is probably eliminated from the gut soon after copulation; some authorities believe that the female can conceive parthenogenetically. Be that as it may, the gravid female penetrates the mucosa of the duodenum, where she deposits her eggs. In severe infections, the biliary and pancreatic ducts, the entire small bowel, and the colon may be involved. The eggs hatch quickly, releasing rhabditiform larvae that reenter the bowel lumen and are subsequently passed into the stool. These larvae, which measure about 16 × 200 μm, can be distinguished from the similar larval stage of the hookworms by their short buccal cavity and large genital primordium (Figures 49.5 and 49.6).

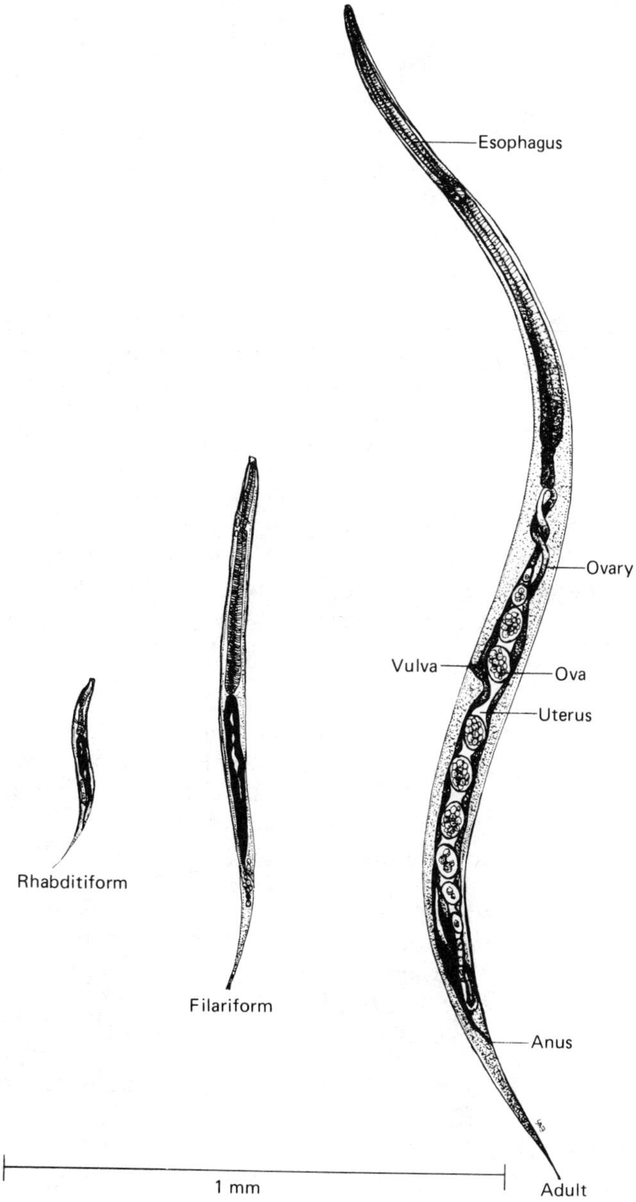

49.5 *Strongyloides stercoralis* worm and rhabditiform and filariform larvae.

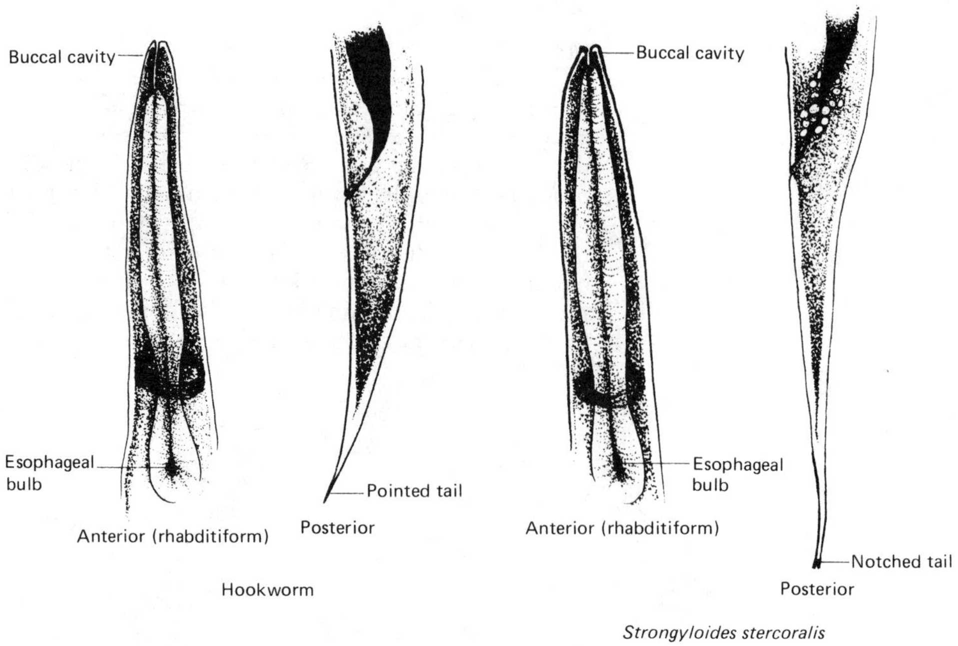

49.6 Anterior and posterior ends of hookworm and *Strongyloides stercoralis.*

distribution and penetration of skin like that of hookworm

Epidemiology. The distribution of *S. stercoralis* parallels that of the hookworms, although it is less prevalent in all but tropical areas. It is found throughout the rural areas of Puerto Rico and the southeastern sections of the continental United States. Although, like hookworm infection, it is generally acquired by direct contact of skin with soil-dwelling larvae, infection may also follow ingestion of filariform-contaminated food. Transformation of the rhabditiform larvae to the filariform stage within the gut can result in seeding of the perianal area with infectious organisms. These larvae may be passed to another person through direct physical contact or autoinfect the original host. In debilitated and immunosuppressed patients, transformation to the filariform stage occurs within the gut itself, producing extreme autoinfection or hyperinfection.

autoinfection and infection by ingestion of filariform larvae also occurs

Pulmonary and intestinal manifestations

Clinical manifestations. Patients with strongyloidiasis do not generally give a history of ground itch. They do, however, manifest the pulmonary disease seen in both ascariasis and hookworm infection. The intestinal infection itself is usually asymptomatic. With heavy worm loads, however, the patient may complain of epigastric pain and tenderness, often aggravated by intake of food. In fact, peptic-ulcer-like pain associated with peripheral eosinophilia strongly suggests the diagnosis of strongyloidiasis. With widespread involvement of the intestinal mucosa, vomiting, diarrhea, paralytic ileus, and malabsorption may be seen.

External autoinfection

External autoinfection produces transient, raised, red, serpiginous lesions over the buttocks and lower back that reflect larval invasion of the perianal area. If the patient is not treated, these lesions may recur at irregular intervals over a period of decades; they are particularly common after recovery from a febrile illness.

Hyperinfection in immunosuppressed host

Massive hyperinfection may occur in immunosuppressed patients, producing severe enterocolitis and widespread dissemination of the larvae to extraintestinal organs, including the heart, lungs, and central nervous system. The larvae may carry enteric bacteria with them, producing Gram-negative bacteremia and occasionally Gram-negative meningitis. Unrecognized and untreated, it usually results in death.

Rhabditiform larvae in stool or duodenal aspirates

Laboratory diagnosis. The diagnosis is usually made by finding the rhabditiform larvae in the stool. Preferably, only fresh specimens should be examined to avoid the confusion induced by the hatching of hookworm eggs with the release of their look-alike larvae. The number of larvae passed in the stool varies from day to day, often requiring the examination of several specimens before the diagnosis of strongyloidiasis can be made. When absent from the stool, larvae may sometimes be found in duodenal aspirates or jejunal biopsy specimens. If the pulmonary system is involved, the sputum should be examined for the presence of larvae.

treatment essential

Special precautions with immunosuppressed host

Treatment and prevention. All infected patients should be treated to prevent the buildup of the worm burden by autoinfection and the serious consequences of hyperinfection. The drug of choice is thiabendazole. In hyperinfection syndromes, therapy must be extended for a week. The cure rate is significantly less than 100%, and stools should be checked after therapy to see if retreatment is indicated. Patients who have resided in an endemic area at some time in their lives should be examined for the presence of this parasite both before and during steroid treatment or immunosuppressive therapy. Medical personnel caring for patients with hyperinfection syndromes should wear gowns and gloves, as stool, saliva, vomitus, and body fluids may contain infectious filariform larvae.

Additional Reading and References

Blumenthal, D.S. 1977. Intestinal nematodes in the United States. *N. Engl. J. Med.* 297:1437–1439.

Marsden, P.D. 1978. Other nematodes. *Clin. Gastroenterol.* 7:219–229. Several nematode infections of animals that may involve humans are reviewed.

Stevens, D.P. 1978. Quantitative techniques. *Clin. Gastroenterol.* 7:231–238. The relationship of worm burden to severity of disease and need for therapy is discussed.

James J. Plorde

Tissue Nematodes

50

The nematodes discussed in this chapter induce disease through their presence in the tissues and lymphohematogenous system of the human body. They are a heterogenous group. Two of them, *Toxocara canis* and *Trichinella spiralis*, are natural parasites of domestic and wild carnivores. Although capable of infecting humans, they cannot complete their life cycle in this host. Humans therefore serve only as injured bystanders, rather than major participants, in the life cycle of these parasites (Table 50.1).

The remaining four major nematodes, *Wuchereria bancrofti, Brugia malayi, Loa loa*, and *Onchocerca volvulus*, are members of a single superfamily (Filarioidea), and all utilize humans as their natural definitive host (Table 50.1). The thin, threadlike adults live for years in the subcutaneous tissues and lymphatic vessels, where they discharge their liveborn offspring or *microfilariae*. These progeny circulate in the blood or migrate in the subcutaneous tissues until they are ingested by a specific bloodsucking insect. Within this vector, they transform into filariform larvae capable of infecting another human when the invertebrate host again takes a blood meal.

The nematodes considered, the diseases caused, and the usual routes of infection in humans are listed in Table 50.1.

Toxocariasis

Organism

cycle in canines resembles ascariasis in humans

transplacental infection of puppies

Toxocara canis is a large, intestinal ascarid of canines, including dogs, foxes, and wolves. Each female worm discharges approximately 200,000 thick-shelled eggs daily into the fecal stream. After reaching the soil, these eggs embryonate for a minimum of 2–3 weeks. Thereafter, the eggs are infectious to both canines and humans and, in moist soil, may remain so for months to years. When ingested by a dog, the larvae exit from the eggshell, penetrate the intestinal mucosa, and migrate through the liver and the right side of the heart to the lung. Here, like the offspring of *Ascaris lumbricoides*, they burst into the alveolar air spaces and are coughed up and swallowed; thereafter, they mature in the small bowel. In fully grown dogs, some of the migrating larvae can pass through the pulmonary capillaries and reach the systemic circulation. These larvae eventually filter out and encyst in the tissues. Hormonal changes in the pregnant bitch stimulate the larvae to migrate; some penetrate the placenta to infect the unborn pups. Approximately 4 weeks after parturition, both the puppies and the lactating mother begin to pass large numbers of eggs in their stools.

Table 50.1 General Characteristics of Tissue Nematodes

Parasite	Disease	Usual Source of Human Infection
Toxocara canis	Toxocariasis (visceral larva migrans)	Ingestion of ova from canine stools
Trichinella spiralis	Trichinosis	Ingestion of improperly cooked pork
Major filarial worms		
Wuchereria bancrofti, Brugia malayi	Lymphatic filariasis (elephantiasis)	Mosquito
Onchocerca volvulus	Onchocerciasis (river blindness)	*Simulium* flies
Loa loa (eye worm)	Loiasis (Calabar swellings)	Deer flies

Transmission to humans by ingestion of ova; larvae do not reach maturity

When humans ingest infectious eggs, the liberated larvae are small enough to pass through the pulmonary capillaries and reach the systemic circulation. Rarely does the organism break into the alveoli and reach the intestine to complete its maturation to adulthood. Larvae in the systemic circulation continue to grow. When their size exceeds the diameter of the vessel through which they are passing, they penetrate its wall and enter the tissue.

Epidemiology

extent of contamination of soil with ova

Age incidence of disease

disease underreported

Toxocara canis is a cosmopolitan parasite. The infection rate in the 50 million dogs inhabiting the United States is very high; over 80% of puppies and 20% of older animals are involved. As "man's best friend" deposits more than 3500 tons of feces daily in the streets, yards, and parks of America, there is a real health risk to our sons and daughters. In areas where studies have been done, between 10 and 30% of soil samples taken from public parks have contained viable *Toxocara* eggs. Moreover, serologic surveys of humans indicate that approximately 4–20% of the population has ingested these eggs at some time. The incidence of infection appears to be higher in the southeastern sections of the country; presumably the warm, humid climate prolongs survival of the eggs, thereby increasing exposure. The presence of puppies in the home increases the risk of infection. Clinical manifestations occur predominantly among children 1–6 years of age; many have a history of geophagia, suggesting that disease transmission results from direct ingestion of eggs in the soil. Most infections are subclinical, and the incidence of overt disease, although difficult to assess, is certainly underreported. Serious ocular infection by larvae is frequently seen by ophthalmologists.

Clinical Manifestations

Tissue invasion by larvae

disease caused by mechanical effects and hypersensitivity

Larvae that reach the systemic circulation may invade any tissue of the body, where they can induce necrosis, bleeding, and the formation of eosinophilic granulomas. The liver, lungs, heart, skeletal muscle, brain, and eye are involved most frequently. The severity of clinical manifestations is related to the number and location of these lesions and the degree to which the host has become sensitized to larval antigens. In 1953, investigators fed 200 embryonated eggs to each of two severely retarded young children. During the subsequent 14 months of observation, the children remained well, but demonstrated a persistent eosinophilic leukocytosis. Children with more intense infection may have fever and an enlarged, tender liver. Those who are seriously ill may develop a skin rash, an enlarged spleen, asthma, recurrent pulmonary infiltrates, behavioral changes, focal neurologic defects, and convulsions. Illness often persists for weeks to months. Death may result from respiratory failure, cardiac arrhythmia, or brain damage. In older children and adults, systemic manifestations are uncommon. Ocular invasion by larvae is more common. Typically, unilateral strabismus (squint) or decreased visual acuity causes the patient to consult an ophthalmologist. Examination reveals granulomatous endophthalmitis, which is usually a reaction to a larva that is already dead; it is sometimes mistaken for malignant retinoblastoma, and an unnecessary enucleation is performed.

Ocular manifestations

Laboratory Diagnosis

Biopsy

Eosinophilia

Serodiagnosis

Stool examination is not helpful, as the parasite seldom reaches adulthood in humans. Definitive diagnosis requires demonstration of the larva in a liver biopsy specimen or at autopsy. A presumptive diagnosis may be made based on the clinical picture, on eosinophilic leukocytosis, and on elevated antibody titers to blood group antigens, particularly the group A antigen. Recently, an enzyme-linked immunosorbent assay utilizing larval antigens was developed, providing clinicians for the first time with a reasonably sensitive and specific serologic test. Unfortunately, many patients with related ocular infections remain seronegative.

Treatment and Prevention

role of corticosteroids

need for worming of dogs

Corticosteroid treatment may be lifesaving if the patient has serious pulmonary, myocardial, or central nervous system involvement. The efficacy of specific anthelmintic therapy is still uncertain. Prevention requires control of indiscriminate defecation by dogs and repeated worming of household pets. Worming must begin when the animal is 3 weeks of age and be repeated every 3 months during the first year of life and twice a year thereafter.

Trichinosis

Organism

parasite of many flesh-eating animals

The adult *T. spiralis* lives in the duodenal and jejunal mucosa of flesh-eating animals, particularly swine, rodents, bears, canines, felines, and marine mammals. The tiny (1.5 mm) male copulates with his outsized (3.5 mm) mate and, apparently spent by the effort, dies. Within a week, the inseminated female begins to discharge offspring. Unlike those of most nematodes, these progeny undergo intrauterine embryonation and are released as second-stage larvae. The birthing continues for the next 6 weeks, resulting in the generation of some 1500 larvae, each measuring 6×100 μm. From their submucosal position, they find their way into the vascular system and pass from the right side of the heart through the pulmonary capillary bed to the systemic circulation, where they are distributed throughout the body. Larvae penetrating tissue other than skeletal muscle disintegrate and die. Those finding their way to striated muscle, however, continue to grow, molt, and gradually encapsulate over a period of several weeks. Calcification of the cyst wall begins 6–18 months later, but the contained larvae may remain viable for 5–10 years. The muscles invaded most frequently include the extraocular muscles of the eye, the tongue, the deltoid, pectoral, and intercostal muscles, the diaphragm, and the gastrocnemius. If a second animal

larvae reach striated muscle and encapsulate

eating of infected flesh spreads disease

feeds on the infected flesh of the original host, the encysted larvae are freed by gastric digestion and mature in the intestinal lumen.

Epidemiology

infection of swine

human infection from undercooked pork

Infection from bear and walrus meat

Trichinosis is widespread in carnivores. Among domestic animals, swine are most frequently involved. They acquire the infection by eating rats or garbage containing cyst-laden scraps of uncooked meat. Human infection, in turn, results largely from the consumption of improperly prepared pork products. In the United States, most outbreaks have been traced to ready-to-eat pork sausage prepared in the home or in small, unlicensed butcheries. Disease incidence is highest in Americans of Polish, German, and Italian descent, presumably because of their custom of producing and eating such sausage during holidays. Outbreaks have also followed feasts of wild pig in California and Hawaii. At present, approximately 10% of human cases, particularly those in Alaska and other western states, have been attributed to consumption of bear meat. One recent outbreak among Alaskan Eskimos followed the ingestion of *Trichinella*-infected walrus. Each year, a few cases are acquired from ground beef intentionally but illegally adulterated with pork.

human infections still widespread, most subclinical

Human infections are found worldwide, with the exception of Asia and Australia. In the United States, the prevalence of cysts found in the diaphragms of patients at autopsy has declined from 16.1 to 4.2% over a period of 30 years. This decline has been attributed to decreased consumption of pork and pork products, federal guidelines for the commercial preparation of such foodstuffs, and legislation requiring the thorough cooking of any meat scraps to be used as hog feed. Nevertheless, it is estimated that more than 1.5 million Americans carry live *Trichinella* in their musculature and that 150,000–300,000 acquire new infection annually. Fortunately, the overwhelming majority are asymptomatic, and only about 100 clinically recognized cases are reported annually to federal officials.

Pathogenesis and Pathology

larvae in muscle, heart, and central nervous system

acute inflammatory reaction

Eosinophilia

The pathologic lesions of trichinosis are related almost exclusively to the presence of larvae in the striated muscle, heart, and central nervous system. The muscle cells enlarge, lose their cross-striations, and undergo a basophilic degeneration. Surrounding the involved cell is an intense inflammatory reaction consisting of neutrophils, lymphocytes, and eosinophils. With the development of specific immunoglobulin G antibodies, eosinophil-mediated destruction of the larvae begins. A vasculitis demonstrated in some patients has been attributed to deposition of circulating immune complexes in the walls of the vessels.

Clinical Manifestations

initial diarrhea

extent of larval invasion of muscle

fever, muscle pain, and swollen eyelids

One or two days after the host has ingested tainted meat, the newly matured adults penetrate the intestinal mucosa, producing nausea, abdominal pain, and diarrhea. In mild infections, these symptoms may be overlooked, except in a careful retrospective analysis; in more serious infections, they may persist for several days and render the patient prostrate. Larval invasion of striated muscle begins approximately 1 week later and initiates the longer (6 weeks) and more characteristic phase of the disease. Patients in whom 10 or fewer larvae are deposited per gram of tissue are usually asymptomatic; those with 100 or more generally develop significant disease; and those with 1000–

More severe complications

5000 have a very stormy course that occasionally ends in death. Fever, muscle pain, muscle tenderness, and weakness are the most prominent manifestations. Patients may also display eyelid swelling, a maculopapular skin rash, and small hemorrhages beneath the conjunctiva of the eye and the nails of the digits. Hemoptysis and pulmonary consolidation are common in severe infections. If there is myocardial involvement, electrocardiographic abnormalities, tachycardia, or congestive heart failure may be seen. Central nervous system invasion is marked by encephalitis, meningitis, and polyneuritis. Delirium, psychosis, paresis, and coma can follow.

Laboratory Diagnosis

Eosinophilia

The most consistent abnormality is an eosinophilic leukocytosis that appears during the second week of illness and persists for the remainder of the clinical course. The eosinophilia typically ranges from 15 to 50% and in some patients may induce extensive damage to the cardiac endothelium. In severe or terminal cases, the eosinophilia may disappear altogether.

Serodiagnosis

There are a number of valuable serologic tests, including complement fixation, indirect fluorescent antibody, and bentonite flocculation. Significant antibody titers are generally absent before the third week of illness, but may then persist for years. Recently, an ELISA capable of detecting specific antibody formation during the first week of illness was developed.

Muscle biopsy

Biopsy of the deltoid or gastrocnemius muscle during the third week will usually reveal encysted larvae.

Treatment

Corticosteroids

Patients with severe edema, pulmonary manifestations, myocardial involvement, or central nervous system disease are treated with corticosteroids. The value of specific anthelmintic therapy remains controversial; it is possible that mebendazole may shorten the clinical course. The mortality of symptomatic patients is 1%, rising to 10% if the central nervous system is involved.

Prevention

Pork should be cooked to an internal temperature of at least 60°C, frozen at −15°C for 3 weeks, or thoroughly smoked before it is ingested.

Lymphatic Filariasis

Definition

Lymphatic filariasis encompasses a group of diseases produced by certain members of the superfamily Filarioidea that inhabit the lymphatic system of humans. Their presence induces an acute inflammatory reaction, lymphatic blockade, and, in some cases, grotesque swellings of the extremities and genitalia known as *elephantiasis.*

Organisms

adult worms in lymphatic vessels

The two agents most commonly responsible for lymphatic filariasis are *W. bancrofti* and *B. malayi.* Both are threadlike worms that lie coiled in the lymphatic vessels, male and female together, for the duration of their decade-long life span. The female *W. bancrofti* measures 100 mm in length, the male, 40 mm. *Brugia malayi* adults are approximately half these sizes. The gravid females produce large numbers of embryonated eggs. At oviposition,

Microfilariae

the embryos uncoil to their full length (200–300 μm) to become microfi-

Table 50.2 Differentiation of Microfilariae

Parasite	Location	Sheath	Size (μm)	Nuclei of Tail	Periodicity
Wuchereria bancrofti	Blood	Yes	360	None	Usually nocturnal
Brugia malayi	Blood	Yes	220	Two	Nocturnal
Loa loa	Blood	Yes	275	Continuous	Diurnal
Onchocerca volvulus	Skin	No	300	None	None

lariae. The shell of the egg elongates to accommodate the embryo and is retained as a thin, flexible sheath. Although the offspring of the two species resemble each other, they may be differentiated on the basis of length, staining characteristics, and internal structure (Table 50.2). The microfilariae eventually reach the blood. In most *W. bancrofti* and *B. malayi* infections, they accumulate in the pulmonary vessels during the day. At night, in response to changes in oxygen tension, they spill out into the peripheral circulation, where they are found in greatest numbers between 9 PM and 2 AM. A Polynesian strain of *W. bancrofti* displays a different periodicity, the peak concentration of organisms occurring in the early evening. Periodicity has an important epidemiologic consequence, as it determines the species of mosquito to serve as vector and intermediate host. Within the thoracic muscles of the mosquito, microfilariae are transformed first into rhabditiform and then into filariform larvae. These larvae actively penetrate the feeding site when the mosquito takes its next meal. Within the new host, the parasite migrates to the lymphatic vessels, undergoes a series of molts, and reaches adulthood in 6–12 months.

periodicity of microfilariae in peripheral blood

mosquito essential vector

Epidemiology

Geographic distribution

Transmission

Lymphatic filariasis currently infects about 250 million individuals in Africa, Latin America, the Pacific Islands, and Asia; more than three-quarters of these cases are concentrated in the latter continent. *Wuchereria bancrofti,* transmitted primarily by mosquitoes of the genus *Culex,* is the more cosmopolitan of the two species; it is found in patchy distribution throughout the poorly sanitated, densely crowded urban areas of all three continents. A small endemic focus once existed near Charleston, South Carolina, but died out in the 1920s. Moreover, some 15,000 *W. bancrofti* infections were acquired by American servicemen during World War II.

Brugia malayi, transmitted by mosquitoes of the genus *Mansonia,* is confined to the rural coastal areas of Asia and the South Pacific. Strains with an unusual periodicity have been found in animals. For *W. bancrofti,* however, humans are the only known vertebrate host.

Pathology and Pathogenesis

acute lymphangitis, fibrosis, and lymphatic obstruction

lymphatic blockade with repeated infection

Pathologic changes, which are confined primarily to the lymphatic system, can be divided into acute and chronic lesions. In acute disease, the presence of molting adolescent worms and dead or dying adults stimulates infiltration of lymphocytes, plasma cells, and eosinophils, hyperplastic changes in the lymphatic endothelium, and thrombus formation (that is, acute lymphangitis). These developments are followed by granuloma formation, fibrosis, and permanent lymphatic obstruction. Repeated infections eventually result in massive lymphatic blockade. The skin and subcutaneous tissues become edematous, thickened, and fibrotic. Dilated vessels may rupture, spilling lymph into the tissues or body cavities. Bacterial cellulitis often supervenes and contributes to tissue damage.

Clinical Manifestations

Lymphadenitis and lymphangitis

Mild infections often go unnoticed. With a larger worm load, the patient experiences onset of fever, lymphadenitis, and lymphangitis 8–12 months after exposure. The fever is typically low grade; in more serious cases, however, temperatures as high as 40°C, chills, muscle pains, and other systemic manifestations may be seen. Classically, the lymphadenitis is first noted in the femoral area as an enlarged, red, tender lump. The inflammation spreads centrifugally down the lymphatic channels of the leg. The vessels become enlarged and tender, the overlying skin red and edematous. Frequently the lymphatic vessels of the spermatic cord are also involved, producing a painful orchitis, epididymitis, and funiculitis; inflamed retroperitoneal vessels may simulate acute abdomen. Epitrochlear, axillary, and other lymphatic vessels are involved less frequently. The acute manifestations last a few days and resolve spontaneously, only to recur periodically over a period of weeks to months. With repeated infection, permanent lymphatic obstruction develops in the involved areas. Edema, ascites, pleural effusion, hydrocele, and joint effusion result. The lymphadenopathy persists and the palpably swollen lymphatic channels may rupture, producing an abscess or draining sinus. Rupture of intraabdominal vessels may give rise to chylous ascites or urine. In patients heavily and repeatedly infected over a period of decades, elephantiasis may develop. Such patients may continue to experience acute inflammatory episodes.

Relapse

effects of repeated infection

Elephantiasis

Tropical eosinophilia syndrome

In India, Pakistan, Sri Lanka, Indonesia, and Southeast Asia an aberrant form of filariasis is seen. This form, termed *tropical eosinophilia,* is characterized by an intense eosinophilia, high titers of filarial antibodies, the absence of microfilaria from the circulating blood, and a chronic clinical course marked by massive enlargement of the lymph nodes and spleen (children) or chronic cough, nocturnal bronchospasm, and pulmonary infiltrates (adults). Microfilariae have been found in the tissues of such patients, and the clinical manifestations may be terminated with specific antifilarial treatment. It has been suggested that this syndrome represents a hypersensitivity reaction to circulating microfilariae. This results in the trapping of microfilariae in various tissue sites where they incite an eosinophilic inflammatory response, granuloma formation, and fibrosis.

hypersensitivity manifestations

Laboratory Diagnosis

Eosinophilia is usually present during the acute inflammatory episodes, but definitive diagnosis requires the demonstration of microfilariae in the blood or lymphatic, acitic, or pleural fluid. They are sought in Giemsa- or Wright-stained thick and thin smears. The major distinguishing features of these and other microfilariae are listed in Table 50.2. As the appearance of the microfilariae is usually periodic, specimen collection must be properly timed. If this procedure proves difficult, the patient may be challenged with the antifilarial agent diethylcarbamazine. This drug stimulates the migration of the microfilariae from the pulmonary to the systemic circulation and enhances the possibility of their recovery. If the parasitemia is scant, the specimen may be concentrated before it is examined. Once found, the microfilariae must be differentiated from those produced by other species of filariae. Tropical eosinophilia is diagnosed as described previously.

Timing of search for microfilariae

Treatment

killing of microfilariae may stimulate allergic response

Diethylcarbamazine eliminates the microfilariae from the blood and kills or injures the adult worms, resulting in long-term suppression of the infection or parasitologic cure. Frequently, the dying microfilariae stimulate an allergic reaction in the host. This response is occasionally severe, requiring the use of antihistamines and corticosteroids. The tissue changes of elephantiasis are irreversible, but the enlargement of the extremities may be ameliorated with pressure bandages or plastic surgery. Control programs combine mosquito control with mass treatment of the entire population.

Onchocerciasis

Definition

Onchocerciasis or *river blindness,* produced by the skin filaria *O. volvulus,* is characterized by subcutaneous nodules, thickened, pruritic skin, and blindness.

Organism

Infection of subcutaneous tissue, skin, and eye

Transmitted by *Simulium* fly

The 20- to 50-mm adults lie in coiled masses within fibrous subcutaneous nodules. The female gives birth to more than 2000 microfilariae each day of her 15-year life span. These progeny lose their sheaths soon after leaving the uterus, exit from the fibrous capsule, and migrate for up to 2 years in the subcutaneous tissues, skin, and eye. Ultimately they die or are ingested by black flies of the genus *Simulium,* which breed along the banks of fast-moving streams. After transformation into filariform larvae, they are transmitted to another human host. There they molt repeatedly over 6–12 months before reaching adulthood and becoming encapsulated.

Epidemiology

important cause of blindness in affected areas

Onchocerciasis infects approximately 50 million persons, rendering 5% of them blind. Most of the afflicted live in tropical Africa, but foci of infection are also located in Yemen and Latin America. It has been suggested that the disease was introduced into South America by West Africans enslaved and transported to the New World for the purpose of mining gold in the mountain streams of Venezuela and Columbia. The Central American foci date from Napoleon III's use of Sudanese troops to support his invasion of Mexico in 1862. The disease still persists on the high slopes of the Sierra, where coffee plantations lie along the rapidly flowing streams that serve as breeding places for *Simulium* species.

Clinical Manifestations

Subcutaneous nodules

The subcutaneous nodules that harbor the adult worms can be located anywhere on the body. In Mexico and Guatemala, where the fly vector typically bites the upper part of the body, they are concentrated on the head; in South America and Africa, they are found primarily on the trunk and legs. Although nodules may number in the hundreds, most infected individuals have less than 10. They are firm, freely movable, and measure 1–3 cm in diameter. Unless the nodule is located over a joint, pain and tenderness are unusual. Of greater consequence to the patient are the side effects of the presence of microfilariae in the tissues. Sensitization to antigens released by the parasites results in a chronic inflammatory reaction. In the skin, this reaction is manifested as a papular or erysipelaslike rash with severe itching.

Hypersensitivity reactions to microfilariae

Ocular lesions

In time, the skin thickens and lichenifies. As subepidermal elastic tissue is lost, wrinkles and large skin folds or *hanging grains* are formed. In parts of Africa, infection may result in elephantiasis. Invasion of the eye, however, causes the most devastating lesions. Punctate keratitis, iritis, and chorioretinitis can lead to a decrease in visual acuity and, in time, total blindness. In Central America, eye lesions may be seen in up to 30% of infected patients. In certain communities in West Africa, 85% of the population has ocular lesions and one-half of the adult male population is blind.

Laboratory Diagnosis

The diagnosis is made by demonstrating the microfilariae in a thin skin sample taken from an involved area. When the eye is involved, the organism may sometimes be seen in the anterior chamber with the help of a slit lamp.

Treatment and Prevention

Treatment-induced hypersensitivity reactions

Diethylcarbamazine is used to kill the microfilariae. Treatment is begun with very small doses to prevent rapid parasite destruction and the attendant allergic consequences. This consideration is particularly important when the eye is involved, as a treatment-induced inflammatory reaction can damage it further. Unfortunately, diethylcarbamazine does not destroy the adult worms, which must be removed by surgical excision or killed with a second, more toxic agent, suramin. No satisfactory methods of control have yet been developed. Application of insecticides to the vector's breeding waters must be sustained for decades to disrupt transmission permanently, as the parasite is so long-lived within humans. Mass therapy is precluded by the serious allergic reactions that accompany unsupervised treatment.

Loiasis

adults migrate through subcutaneous tissues

Calabar swellings and subconjunctival migration

Loiasis is a filarial disease of West Africa produced by the eye worm, *L. loa.* The long-lived adults migrate continuously through the subcutaneous tissues of humans at a maximum rate of about 1 cm per hour. During migration, they produce localized areas of allergic inflammation termed *Calabar swellings.* These egg-sized lesions persist for 2–3 days and may be accompanied by fever, itching, urticaria, and pain. At times, the adult worms may cross the eye subconjunctivally, producing intense tearing, pain, and alarm.

The female produces sheathed microfilariae, which are found in the bloodstream during daytime hours. Deer flies of the genus *Chrysops* serve as vectors.

Demonstration of adult in eye or microfilaria in blood

The diagnosis is made by recovering the adult worm from the eye or by isolating the characteristic microfilariae from the blood or Calabar swellings. Eosinophilia is constant. Diethylcarbamazine destroys both adults and microfilariae, but must be administered cautiously to avoid marked allergic reactions.

Additional Reading and References

Barrett-Connor, E., Davis, C.F., Hamburger, R.N., and Kagan, I. 1976. An epidemic of trichinosis after ingestion of wild pig in Hawaii. *J. Infect. Dis.* 133:473–477.

Edeson, J.F.B. 1972. Filariasis. *Br. Med. Bull.* 28:60–65. A brief, succinct review of a complicated subject.

Margolis, H.S., Middaugh, J.P., and Burgess, R.D. 1979. Arctic trichinosis: Two Alaskan outbreaks from walrus meat. *J. Infect. Dis.* 139:102–105. A report of two unusual outbreaks of trichinosis.

James J. Plorde

Cestode Infections

51

Cestodes are long, ribbonlike helminths that have gained the common appellation of *tapeworm* from their superficial resemblance to sewing tape. Their appearance, number, and exaggerated reputation for inducing weight loss have made them the best known of the intestinal worms. Although improvements in sanitation have dramatically reduced their prevalence in the United States, they continue to inhabit the bowels of many of its citizens. In some parts of the world, indigenous populations take purgatives monthly to rid themselves of this, the largest and most repulsive of the intestinal parasites.

Morphology

absence of gut

Scolex, neck, and segmented body

Attachment mechanisms

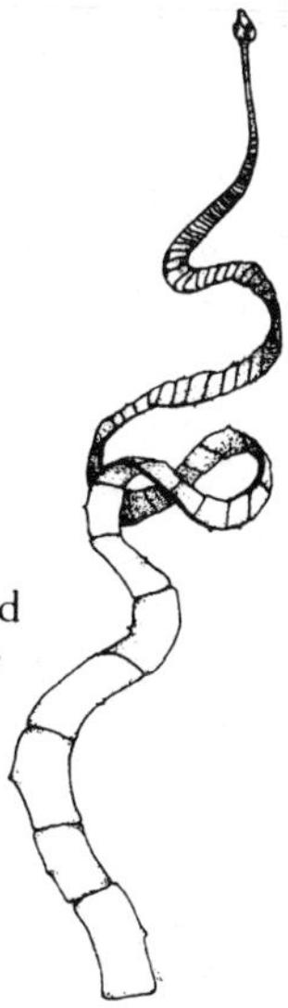

Cestode

each proglottid a hermaphroditic unit

Like all helminths, tapeworms lack vascular and respiratory systems. In addition, they are devoid of both gut and body cavity. Food is absorbed across a complex cuticle, and the internal organs are embedded in a solid parenchyma. The adult is divided into three distinct parts: the "head" or *scolex*; a generative *neck*; and a long, segmented body, the *strobila*. The scolex typically measures less than 2 mm in diameter and is equipped with four muscular sucking discs used to attach the worm to the intestinal mucosa of its host. (In one genus, *Diphyllobothrium*, the discs are replaced by two grooves, or *bothria*.) As a further aid in attachment, the scolex of some species possesses a retractable protuberance, or *rostellum*, armed with a crown of chitinous hooks. Immediately posterior to the scolex is the neck from which individual segments, or *proglottids*, are generated one at a time to form the chainlike body. Each proglottid is a self-contained hermaphroditic reproductive unit joined to the remainder of the colony by a common cuticle, nerve trunks, and excretory canals. Its male and female gonads mature and effect fertilization as the segment is pushed further and further from the neck by the formation of new proglottids. When the segment reaches gravidity, it releases its eggs by rupturing, disintegrating, or passing them through its uterine pore. The eggs of the genus *Taenia* possess a solid shell and contain a fully developed, six-hooked (hexacanth) embryo. Those of *Diphyllobothrium latum*, in contrast, are immature and have an operculate shell.

Life Cycle

eggs of *Taenia* ingested by intermediate host

infectious cysts of *Taenia* form in tissues of intermediate

With the exception of that of *Hymenolepis nana,* further development of all cestodes requires the passage of the larvae through one or more intermediate hosts. Eggs of the genus *Taenia* pass in the stool of their definitive host, reach the soil, and are ingested by the specific intermediate. They hatch within its gut, and the released embryos penetrate the intestinal mucosa, find their way through the lymphohematogenous system to the tissues, and encyst therein. From the germinal lining of this cyst, immature scolices or *protoscolices* are formed. A cyst with a single such structure is known as a *cysticercus* (or, in the case of *H. nana,* a cysticercoid); a cyst with multiple protoscolices is known as a *coenurus.* In some species of tapeworm, daughter cysts, each containing many protoscolices, are formed within the mother or *hydatid* cyst. The cycle for all is completed when the definitive host ingests the cyst-ridden flesh of the intermediate host. After digestion of the surrounding meat in the stomach, the cyst is freed, and the protoscolex everts to become a scolex. Following attachment to the mucosa, a new strobila is generated.

definitive host ingests cysts in flesh of intermediate hosts to yield adult intestinal worms

D. latum requires two intermediates, a copepod and a freshwater fish, to complete cycle

Diphyllobothrium latum, whose eggs are immature upon release, requires two intermediates to complete its larval development. The egg must reach fresh water before the operculum opens and a ciliated, free-swimming larva or *coracidium* is released. The coracidium is then ingested by the first intermediate host, a copepod, in which it is transformed into a larva (*procercoid*). When the copepod is, in turn, ingested by a freshwater fish, the larva penetrates the musculature of the fish to form an elongated and infectious larva, the *plerocercoid.* Life cycles and characteristics of important intestinal and tissue tapeworms infecting humans are summarized in Table 51.1.

Clinical Disease

The clinical consequences of tapeworm infection in humans depend on whether the patient serves as the primary or the intermediate host. In the

Table 51.1 Intestinal and Tissue Tapeworms

Stage	*Diphyllobothrium latum*	*Taenia saginata*
Adult		
Definitive host	Humans, cats, dogs	Humans
Location	**Gut lumen**[a]	**Gut lumen**
Length (m)	3–10	4–6
Attachment device	Grooves	Discs
Mature segment	Broad	Elongated
Egg		
Maturation status	Nonembryonated	Embryonated
Distinguishing characteristic	Operculate	Radial striations
Larval development in humans	No	No
Larva		
Intermediate host	Copepods, fishes	Cattle
Location	Tissue	Tissue
Form	Procercoid (copepod) Plerocercoid (fish)	Cysticercus

[a]Sites of human infection appear in boldface.

clinical effects depend on whether humans are definitive hosts or intermediate hosts,

former case, the adult worm is confined to the lumen of the gut, and the consequences of the infection are typically minor. Taeniasis saginata and diphyllobothriasis are prime examples. In contrast, when the patient serves as the intermediate host (for example, for *Echinococcus granulosus*), larval development produces tissue invasion and frequently serious disease. The capacity of *H. nana* and *Taenia solium* to utilize humans as both primary and intermediate hosts is unique.

Beef Tapeworm Infection

Organism

T. saginata inhabits human jejunum

gravid proglottids passed in stool

eggs ingested by herbivore intermediates

cysticerci in bovine striated muscle

humans infected by eating inadequately cooked infested meat

Taenia saginata, the beef tapeworm, inhabits the human jejunum, where it may live for up to 25 years and grow to a maximum length of 10 m. Its 1-mm scolex lacks hooklets, but possesses the four sucking discs typical of most cestodes (Figure 51.1A). The creamy white strobila consists of 1000–2000 individual proglottids. The terminal segments are longer (20 mm) than they are wide (5 mm) and contain a large uterus with 15–20 lateral branches; these characteristics are useful in differentiating them from those of the closely related pork tapeworm, *T. solium* (Figure 51.1B). When fully gravid, strings of terminal proglottids break free from the remainder of the strobila and are passed intact with the stool. Proglottids reaching the soil eventually disintegrate, releasing their distinctive eggs. These eggs are 30–40 μm in diameter, spherical, and possess a thick, radially striated shell (Figure 51.1C). In appropriate environments, the hexacanth embryo may survive for months. If ingested by cattle or certain other herbivores, the embryo is released, penetrates the intestinal wall, and is carried by the vascular system to the striated muscles of the tongue, diaphragm, and hindquarters. Here it is transformed into white, ovoid (5×10 mm) cysticerci *(Cysticercus bovis).* When present in large numbers, they impart a spotted or "measley" appearance to the flesh. Humans are infected when they ingest inadequately cooked meat containing these larval forms.

Table 51.1 (*continued*)

Taenia solium	*Hymenolepis nana*	*Echinococcus granulosus*	*Echinococcus multilocularis*
Humans	Humans, rodents	Dogs, wolves	Foxes
Gut lumen	**Gut lumen**	Gut lumen	Gut lumen
2–4	0.02–0.04	0.005	0.005
Discs, hooklets	Discs, hooklets	Discs, hooklets	Discs, hooklets
Elongated	Broad	Elongated	Elongated
Embryonated	Embryonated	Embryonated	Embryonated
Radial striations	Polar filaments	Radial striations	Radial striations
Yes	Yes	Yes	Yes
Swine, humans	Humans, rodents	Herbivores, humans	Field mice, humans
Tissue	**Gut mucosa**	**Tissue**	**Tissue**
Cysticercus	Cysticercoid	Hydatid cyst	Hydatid cyst

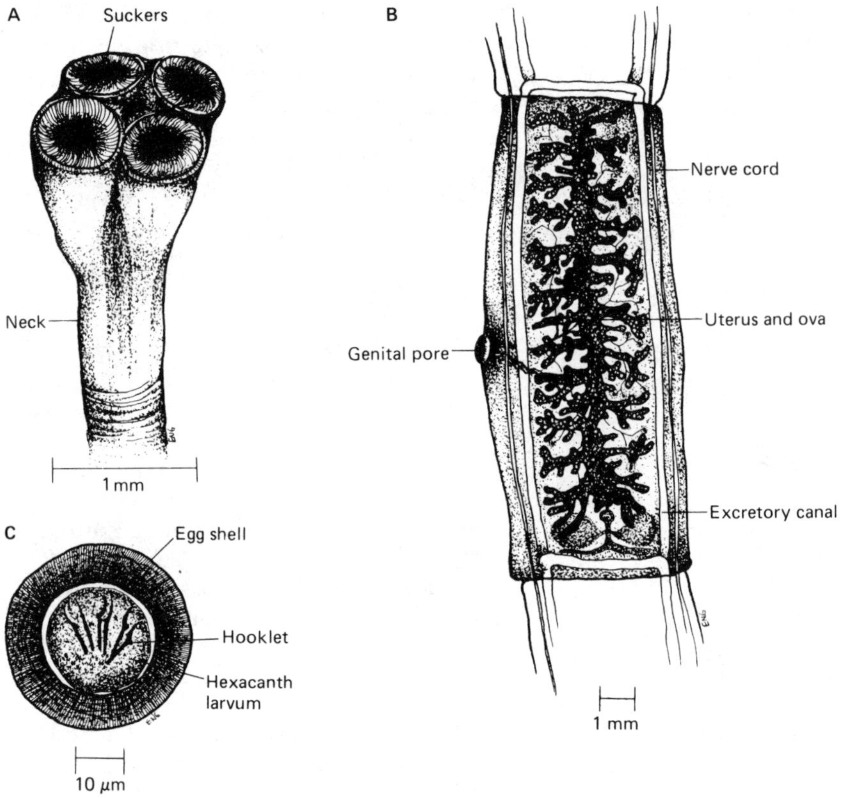

51.1 *Taenia saginata.* (**A**) Scolex. (**B**) Gravid proglottid. (**C**) Ovum.

Epidemiology

indigenously acquired disease rare in U.S.

In the United States, sanitary disposal of human feces and federal inspection of meat have precluded transmission of *T. saginata* almost entirely. At present, less than 1% of examined carcasses are infected. Nevertheless, the parasite can still be acquired in some parts of the country, particularly the West and Northeast. In countries where sanitary facilities are less comprehensive and undercooked or raw beef is eaten, *T. saginata* is highly prevalent. Examples include Kenya, Ethiopia, the Middle East, Yugoslavia, and parts of the Soviet Union and South America.

Clinical Manifestations

clinical symptoms usually mild

Most infected patients are asymptomatic and become aware of the infection only through the spontaneous passage of proglottids. The proglottids may be observed on the surface of the stool or appear in the underclothing or bed sheets of the alarmed host. Passage may occur very irregularly and can be precipitated by excessive alcohol consumption. Some patients report epigastric discomfort, nausea, irritability (particularly after passage of segments), diarrhea, and weight loss. Occasionally the proglottids may obstruct the appendix, biliary duct, or pancreatic duct.

Laboratory Diagnosis

The diagnosis is made by finding eggs or proglottids in the stool. Eggs may also be distributed on the perianal area secondary to rupture of proglottids during anal passage. The adhesive cellophane tape technique described for adhesive cellophane tape technique and stool examination for eggs and proglottids

pinworm can be used to recover them from this area. With this procedure, 85–95% of infections are detected, in contrast to only 50–75% by stool examination. As the eggs of *T. solium* and *T. saginata* are morphologically identical, it is necessary to examine a proglottid to identify the species correctly.

Treatment

The drug of choice is niclosamide, which acts directly on the worm. It is a highly effective single-dose oral preparation. A second effective agent, mebendazole, has not yet been approved for treatment of taeniasis.

Prevention

sewage disposal, meat inspection, and adequate cooking

Ultimately, control is best effected through the sanitary disposal of human feces. Meat inspection is helpful, as the cysticerci are readily visible. In areas where the infection is common, thorough cooking is the most practical method of control. Internal temperatures of 56°C or more for 5 min or longer will destroy the cystecerci. Salting or freezing for 1 week at −15°C or less is also effective.

Pork Tapeworm Infection

Organism

T. solium strobila shorter than in *T. saginata*

Like the beef tapeworm, which it closely resembles, *T. solium* inhabits the human jejunum, where it may survive for decades. It can be distinguished from its close relative only by careful scrutiny of the scolex and proglottids; the former possesses a rostellum armed with a double row of hooklets (Figure 51.2A). The strobila is generally smaller than that of *T. saginata*, seldom exceeding 5 m in length or containing more than 1000 proglottids. Gravid segments measure 6 × 12 mm and thus appear less elongated than those of the bovine parasite (Figure 51.2B). Typically, the uterus has only 8–12 lateral branches. Although the eggs appear morphologically identical to those

51.2 *Taenia solium.* (A) Scolex. (B) Gravid proglottid. (C) Ovum.

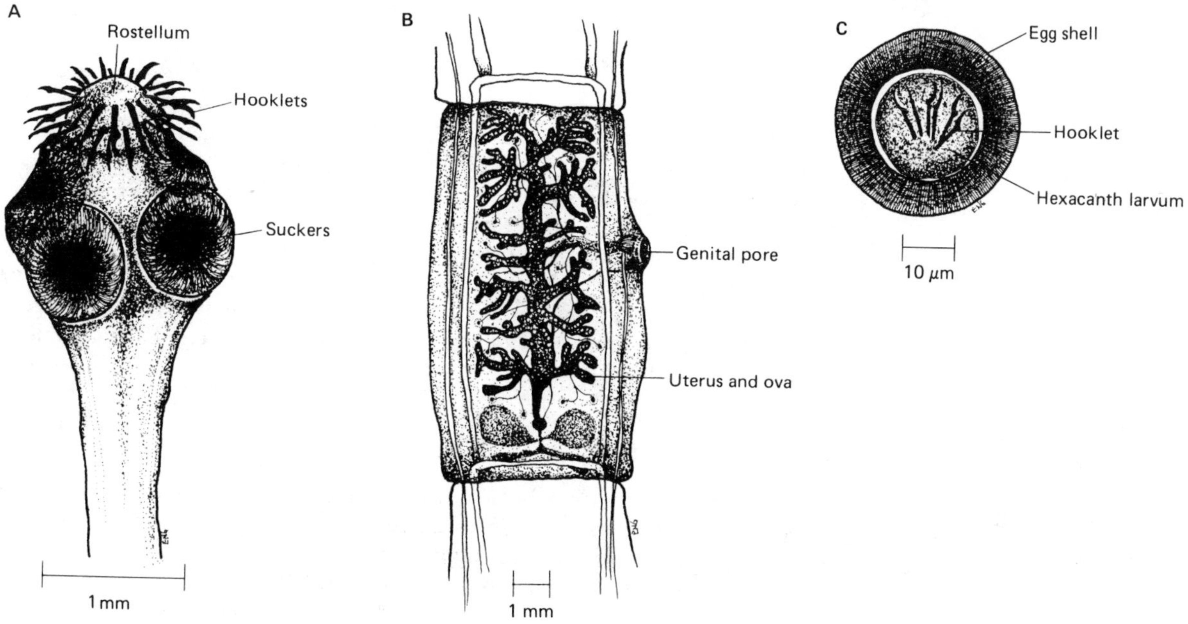

eggs infective to swine and to humans by autoinfection

of *T. saginata,* they are infective only to swine and, perhaps reflecting a genetic proximity we would prefer to overlook, humans. Both pigs and people become intermediate hosts when they ingest food contaminated with viable eggs. Some authorities have suggested that humans may be autoinfected when gravid proglottids are carried backward into the stomach during the act of vomiting, initiating the release of the contained eggs. It seems more likely to this author that autoinfection results from the transport of the eggs from the perianal area to the mouth on contaminated fingers.

tissue cysticerci in humans and swine

Regardless of the route, an egg reaching the stomach of an appropriate intermediate host hatches, releasing the hexacanth embryo. The embryo penetrates the intestinal wall and is carried by the lymphohematogenous system to all tissues of the body. Here it develops into a 1-cm, white, opalescent cysticercus over 3–4 months. The cysticercus may remain viable for up to 5 years, eventually infecting humans when they ingest undercooked and "measley" flesh. The scolex everts, attaches itself to the mucosa, and develops into a new adult worm, thereby completing the cycle.

Epidemiology

T. solium no longer found in U.S.

Transmission of the parasite no longer occurs in the United States. It is, however, widely distributed throughout much of the world, and is particularly common in eastern Europe, Asia, Africa, and Latin America.

Clinical Manifestations

major clinical manifestations caused by reaction to cysticerci

The signs and symptoms of infection with the adult worm are similar to those of taeniasis saginata. Clinical manifestations are totally different when humans serve as intermediate hosts. Cysticerci develop in the subcutaneous tissues, muscles, heart, lungs, liver, brain, and eye. As long as the number is small and the cysticerci are viable, tissue reaction is moderate and the patient asymptomatic. The death of the larva, however, stimulates a marked inflammatory reaction, fever, muscle pains, and eosinophilia. Patients with lesions of the central nervous system may present with meningoencephalitis, epilepsy, and other neurologic or psychiatric manifestations.

Eosinophilia

Laboratory Diagnosis

presence of adult worm diagnosed from proglottids

Biopsy for cysticerci

Infection with the adult worm is diagnosed as described for *T. saginata.* Cysticercosis is suspected when an individual who has been in an endemic area presents with neurologic manifestations or subcutaneous nodules. Roentgenograms of the soft tissues often reveal calcified cysticerci. Similarly, multiple small brain masses may be detected by computed tomography, radioisotope scanning, or ultrasonography. The diagnosis is confirmed by demonstrating the larva in a biopsy sample of a subcutaneous nodule or specific antibodies in the circulating blood. Unfortunately, the available serologic tests lack sensitivity and may yield false-positive results in a number of other helminthic infections.

Treatment and Prevention

surgery occasionally needed for cysticercosis

Infection with the adult worm is approached in the manner described for *T. saginata.* At present, no approved medical therapy is available for cysticercosis, although clinical trials suggest that praziquantel is effective. Surgery may be required in some cases of cerebral and ocular cysticercosis.

Fish Tapeworm Infection

D. *latum* has broad proglottids

Organism

The adult *D. latum* attaches to the ileal mucosa with the aid of two sucking grooves (bothria) located in an elongated fusiform scolex (Figure 51.3A). In life span and overall length, it resembles the *Taenia* species discussed previously. The 3000–4000 proglottids, however, are uniformly wider than they are long, accounting for one of this cestode's common names, the broad tapeworm. The gravid segments contain a centrally positioned, rosette-shaped uterus unique among the tapeworms of humans. Unlike those of the *Taenia* species, ova are released through the uterine pore. Over 1 million oval (55 × 75 μm) operculate eggs are released daily into the stool (Figure 51.3B).

eggs release coracidia in water

crustacean and fish intermediates

humans infected by ingesting inadequately cooked fish

On reaching fresh water they hatch, releasing ciliated, free-swimming larvae or coracidia. If ingested within a few days by small freshwater crustaceans of the genus *Cyclops* or *Diaptomus,* they develop into procercoid larvae. When the crustacean is ingested by a freshwater fish, the larvae migrate into the musculature of the fish and develop into infectious plerocercoid larvae. Humans are infected when they eat improperly prepared freshwater fish containing such forms.

Epidemiology

Worldwide distribution

worm found in Alaska, Midwest, and Florida

Fish tapeworms are found wherever raw, pickled, or undercooked freshwater fish is eaten by humans who defecate in the same lakes and streams from which the fish was obtained. Human infections have been described in the Baltic and Scandinavian countries, Russia, Switzerland, Italy, Japan, and Chile. The worm, brought to North America by Scandinavian immigrants, is now found in Alaska, Canada, the midwestern states, and Florida. It was shown recently that infectious plerocercoid larvae may develop in anadromous salmon, and human cases have been traced to the ingestion of such fish taken from Alaskan waters. The increasing popularity of raw fish dishes such as Japanese sushi and sashimi may lead to increased prevalence of this disease in the United States. Among Ontario Indians, infection is acquired by eating fresh salted fish. Even when fish is appropriately cooked, individuals may become infected by sampling the flesh during the process of preparation.

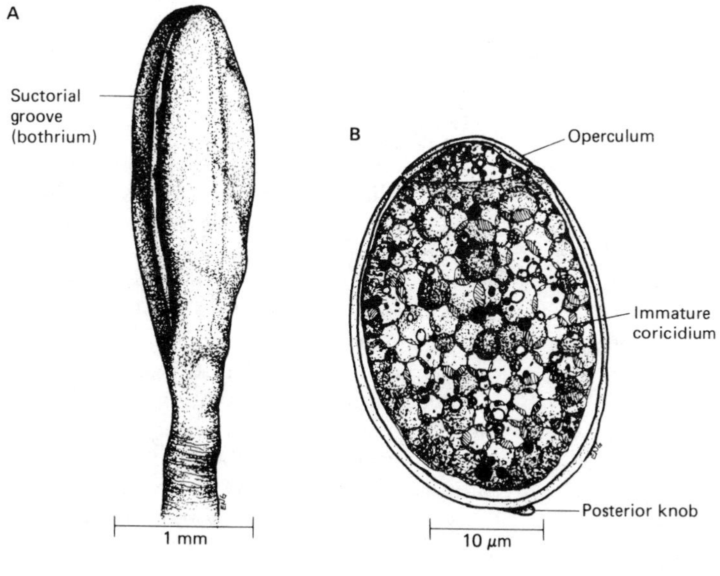

51.3 *Diphyllobothrium latum.* (**A**) Scolex. (**B**) Ovum.

Clinical Manifestations

occasional intestinal obstruction

vitamin B_{12} deficiency

Most infected patients are asymptomatic. On occasion, however, they have complained of epigastric pain, abdominal cramping, vomiting, and weight loss. Moreover, the presence of several adult worms within the gut has been known to precipitate intestinal obstruction. Forty percent of fish tapeworm carriers demonstrate low serum levels of vitamin B_{12}, apparently as a result of the competition between the host and the worm for ingested vitamin. Recent studies have shown that a worm located high in the jejunum may take up 80–100% of vitamin B_{12} given by mouth. Approximately 0.1–2% of patients develop macrocytic anemia. They tend to be elderly, to have impaired production of intrinsic factor, and to have worms located high in the jejunum. In many, folate absorption is also diminished, which may contribute to the anemia. Neurologic manifestations of vitamin B_{12} deficiency occur, sometimes in the absence of anemia. They include numbness, paresthesia, loss of vibration sense, and, rarely, optic atrophy with central scotoma.

Laboratory Diagnosis

Demonstration of eggs in stool

The diagnosis is established by finding the typical eggs in the stool. As *D. latum* produces large numbers of ova, identification is usually accomplished without the need for concentration techniques.

Treatment and Prevention

fish rendered noninfectious at −10°C for 48 hr

Treatment is carried out as described for *T. saginata* infections. When anemia or neurologic manifestations are present, parenteral administration of vitamin B_{12} is also indicated. Personal protection can be accomplished by thorough cooking of all salmon and freshwater fish. Devotees of raw fish may choose to freeze their favorite dish at −10°C for 48 hr before serving. Ultimately, control of diphyllobothriasis is accomplished only by prohibiting the discharge of untreated sewage into lakes and streams.

Hydatid Disease

Definition

Hydatid disease or echinococciasis is a tissue infection of humans caused by larvae of *E. granulosus* and *Echinococcus multilocularis.* The former, the more common infection, is that discussed herein.

Organism

adult in canines

wide range of herbivores, and humans, serve as intermediates

larvae from ingested eggs penetrate to portal circulation

The adult *E. granulosus* inhabits the small bowel of dogs, wolves, and other canines, where it survives for a scant 12 months. The scolex, like that of the genus *Taenia,* possesses four sucking discs and a double row of hooklets. The entire strobila, however, measures only 5 mm in length and contains but three proglottids; one immature, one mature, and one gravid. The latter segment splits either before or after passage in the stool, releasing eggs that appear identical to those of *T. saginata* and *T. solium.* A number of mammals may serve as intermediates, including sheep, goats, camels, deer, caribou, moose, and, most important, humans. When one of these hosts ingests eggs, they hatch, and the embryos penetrate the intestinal mucosa and are carried by the portal blood to the liver. Here, many are filtered out in the hepatic sinusoids. The rest traverse the liver and are carried to the lung, where most lodge. A few pass through the pulmonary capillaries, enter the systemic circulation, and are carried to the brain, heart, bones, and other tissues.

cysts and daughter cysts develop in tissues

cycle completed with ingestion of cysts by canine

Many of the larvae are phagocytosed and destroyed. The survivors form a cyst wall composed of an external laminated cuticle and an internal germinal membrane. The cyst fills with fluid and slowly expands, reaching a diameter of 1 cm over 5–6 months. Secondary or daughter cysts form within the original hydatid. Within each of these daughter cysts, new protoscolices are produced from the germinal lining. Some break free, dropping to the bottom of the cyst to form *hydatid sand.* When hydatid-containing tissues of the intermediate host are ingested by a canine, thousands of scolices are released in the intestine to develop into adult worms.

Epidemiology

pastoral infections maintained by dogs feeding on viscera of herbivores

hand-to-mouth infection of humans

Sylvatic cycle in Alaska and western Canada

There are two major epidemiologic forms of echinococciasis, pastoral and sylvatic. The more common pastoral form has its highest incidence in Australia, New Zealand, South and East Africa, the Middle East, Central Europe, and South America, where domestic herbivores such as sheep, cattle, and camels are raised in close contact with dogs. Although approximately 200 human cases are reported each year in the United States, most were acquired elsewhere. Indigenous cases do occur, however, particularly among Basque sheep farmers in California, southwestern Indians and some Utah shepherds. Animal husbandry practices that permit dogs to feed on the raw viscera of slaughtered sheep allow the cycle of transmission to continue. Shepherds become infected while handling or fondling their dogs. Eggs retained in the fur of these animals are picked up on the hands and later ingested.

Sylvatic echinococciasis is found principally in Alaska and western Canada, where wolves act as the definitive host and moose or caribou as the intermediate. In two counties in California, a second cycle involving deer and coyotes has been described. When hunters kill these wild deer and feed their offal to accompanying dogs, a pastoral cycle may be established.

Clinical Manifestations

disease caused by mechanical effects of cysts after many years

pulmonary cysts predominate in sylvatic disease, hepatic in pastoral

cysts may attain large size

rupture leads to hypersensitivity manifestations and dissemination

The enlarging hydatid cysts produce tissue damage by mechanical means. The clinical presentation depends on their number, site, and rate of growth. Typically, there is a latent period of 5–20 years between acquisition of infection and subsequent diagnosis. Intervals as long as 75 years have been reported occasionally.

In sylvatic infections, two-thirds of the cysts are found in the lung, the remainder in the liver. Most patients are asymptomatic when the lesion is discovered on routine chest X-ray or physical examination. Occasionally, the patient may present with hemoptysis, pain in the right upper quadrant of the abdomen, or a tender hepatic mass. Significant morbidity is uncommon, and death extremely rare. In the pastoral form of disease, 60% of the cysts are found in the liver, 25% in the lung. One-fifth of all patients show involvement of multiple sites. The hydatid cysts, which grow more rapidly (0.25–1 cm per year) than the sylvatic lesions, may reach enormous size. Twenty percent eventually rupture, inducing fever, pruritis, urticaria, and, at times, anaphylactic shock and death. Release of thousands of scolices may lead to dissemination of the infection. Rupture of pulmonary lesions also induces cough, chest pain, and hemoptysis. Liver cysts may break through the diaphragm or rupture into the bile duct or peritoneal cavity. The majority, however, present as a tender, palpable hepatic mass. Intrabiliary extrusion of calcified cysts may mimic the signs of acute cholecystitis; complete obstruction results in jaundice. Bone cysts produce pathologic fractures, severe effects of cerebral cysts

whereas lesions in the central nervous system are often manifest as blindness or epilepsy. Cardiac lesions are associated with embolic metastases. A recent study has suggested that circulating antigen–antibody complexes may be deposited in the kidney, initiating membranous glomerulonephritis.

Laboratory Diagnosis

Radiologic and tomographic appearance

aspiration of cysts contraindicated

Serologic diagnosis

On chest X-ray, pulmonary lesions present as slightly irregular, round masses of uniform density devoid of calcification. In contrast, more than one-half of hepatic lesions display a smooth, calcific rim. Computer tomography scanning may reveal either a simple fluid-filled cyst or daughter cysts with hydatid sand. Because of the potential for an anaphylactoid reaction and dissemination of infection, diagnostic aspiration is contraindicated. In patients with ruptured pulmonary cysts, however, scolices may be demonstrated in the sputum. In most cases, confirmation of the diagnosis requires serologic testing. Unfortunately, current procedures are not totally satisfactory. The indirect hemagglutination and latex agglutination tests are positive in 90% of patients with hepatic lesions and 60% of those with pulmonary hydatid cysts. The presence of an "arc 5" in the immunoelectrophoresis test appears to be more specific. An adaption of this test to an enzyme-linked immunoelectrodiffusion technique is presently being studied and, if successful, could provide a rapid, sensitive diagnostic test.

Treatment

Surgical extirpation

The only definitive therapy available at this time is surgical extirpation. Patients with pulmonary hydatid cysts of the sylvatic type and small calcified hepatic lesions require surgery only if they become symptomatic or the cysts increase dramatically in size over time. All other lesions should be excised or drained and sterilized. Medical therapy using high-dose mebendazole is experimental, but may be considered when surgery is contraindicated.

Prevention

Infected dogs should be wormed, and infected carcasses and offal burned or buried. Hands should be carefully washed after contact with infected dogs.

Additional Reading and References

Jones, T.C., 1978. Cestodes. *Clin. Gastroenterol.* 7:105. An extensive review.

Wilson, J.F., Diddams, A.C., and Rausch, R.L., 1968. Cystic hydatid disease in Alaska. *Am. Rev. Respir. Dis.* 98:1–15. The unique characteristics of sylvatic *Echinococcus granulosus* infections in Alaska are discussed.

James J. Plorde

Trematode Infections

52

Morphology

inch worm locomotion

reproductive systems

eggs hatch in freshwater to release miracidia which infects snails

snail releases cercariae in water

Schistosoma cercariae infect humans through skin. *Paragonimus* and *Clonorchis* cercariae have second intermediate host

Of the myriad relationships that have developed between helminth and human over the millennia of our mutual existence, none has proved more destructive to our health and productivity than that forged with the indomitable flukes. Typically, the adults live for decades within human tissues and vascular systems, where they resist immunologic attack and produce progressive damage to vital organs. Morphologically, trematodes are bilaterally symmetric, vary in length from a few millimeters to several centimeters, and possess two suckers from which they derive their name. One surrounds the oral cavity; the other is located on the ventral surface of the worm. These organs are used for both attachment and locomotion; movement is effected in a characteristic "inchworm" fashion. The digestive tract begins at the oral sucker and continues as a muscular pharynx and esophagus before bifurcating to form lateral ceca that end blindly near the posterior extremity of the worm. Undigested food is vomited out through the oral cavity. The excretory system consists of a number of "flame cells" connected by ducts to a posterior excretory pore.

The reproductive systems vary and serve as a means for dividing the trematodes into two major categories: the hermaphrodites and the schistosomes. The adult hermaphrodite contains both male and female gonads and produces operculate eggs. The schistosomes have separate sexes, and the fertilized female deposits only nonoperculated offspring. The two groups have similar life cycles. The major differential features are summarized in Table 52.1. Eggs are excreted from the human host and, if they reach fresh water, hatch to release ciliated larvae called *miracidia.* These larvae find and penetrate a snail host specific for the trematode species. In this intermediate host, they are transformed by a process of asexual reproduction into thousands of tail-bearing larvae or *cercariae,* which are released from the snail over a period of weeks and swim about vigorously in search of their next host. In the case of schistosomal cercariae, this host is the human. When they come in contact with the skin surface, they attach, discard their tails, and invade, thereby completing their life cycle. The cercariae of the hermaphroditic flukes encyst in or upon an aquatic plant or animal, where they undergo a second transformation to become infective *metacercariae.* Their cycle is completed when the second intermediate host is ingested by a human. Of the many trematodes that infect humans, only five will be discussed: the

Table 52.1 General Characteristics of Trematodes

Characteristic	Trematode Type: Blood	Trematode Type: Tissue/Intestinal
Genus	*Schistosoma*	*Paragonimus, Clonorchis*
Morphology		
Adult	Oral and ventral suckers Blind gastrointestinal tract Slender, wormlike	Oral and ventral suckers Blind gastrointestinal tract Flat, leaflike
Egg	Nonoperculate	Operculate
Biology		
Sexes	Separate	Hermaphroditic
Intermediates	One	Two
Life span	Long	Long

lung (*Paragonimus* species) and liver (*Clonorchis sinensis*) flukes, which are hermaphroditic; and the blood flukes, all of which are members of the genus *Schistosoma* (*S. mansoni, S. haematobium*, and *S. japonicum*) (Figure 52.1).

Paragonimiasis (Lung Fluke Infection)

Organism

adults encapsulate in lung

Several *Paragonimus* species may infect humans. *Paragonimus westermani*, which is widely distributed in East Asia, is the species most frequently involved. The short, plump (10 × 5 mm), reddish-brown adults are characteristically found encapsulated in the pulmonary parenchyma of their definitive host. Here they deposit operculate, golden-brown eggs, which are distinguished from similar structures by their size (50 × 90 μm) and prominent periopercular shoulder. When the capsule erodes into a bronchiole, the eggs are coughed up and spat out or swallowed and passed in the stool. If they reach fresh water, they begin to embryonate several weeks before the ciliated miracidia emerge through the open opercula. After invasion of an appropriate snail host, 3–5 months pass before cercariae are released. These larval forms invade the gills, musculature, and viscera of certain crayfish or freshwater crabs, in which, over 6–8 weeks, they transform into metacercariae. When the flesh of these second intermediate hosts is ingested by humans, the metacercariae encyst in the duodenum and burrow through the gut wall into the peritoneal cavity. The majority continue their migration through the diaphragm and reach maturity in the lungs 5–6 weeks later. Some organisms, however, are retained in the intestinal wall and mesentery or wander to other foci such as the liver, pancreas, kidney, skeletal muscle, subcutaneous tissue, or central nervous system.

capsule erodes into bronchiole, eggs coughed up; cycle continues if eggs reach water with susceptible snail

crayfish and freshwater crabs second intermediate hosts

Nonhuman definitive hosts

In addition to humans, other carnivores, including the rat, cat, dog, and pig, may serve as definitive hosts. Immature ectopic adults in the striated muscles of the pig may infect humans after ingestion of undercooked pork.

Epidemiology

infected snails often found in mountain streams

Although concentrated in Far Eastern nations such as Korea, Japan, China, Taiwan, the Philippines, and Indonesia, paragonimiasis has recently been described in India, Africa, and Latin America. Infection of the snail host, which is typically found in small mountain streams located away from human habitation, is probably maintained by animal hosts other than humans. Hu-

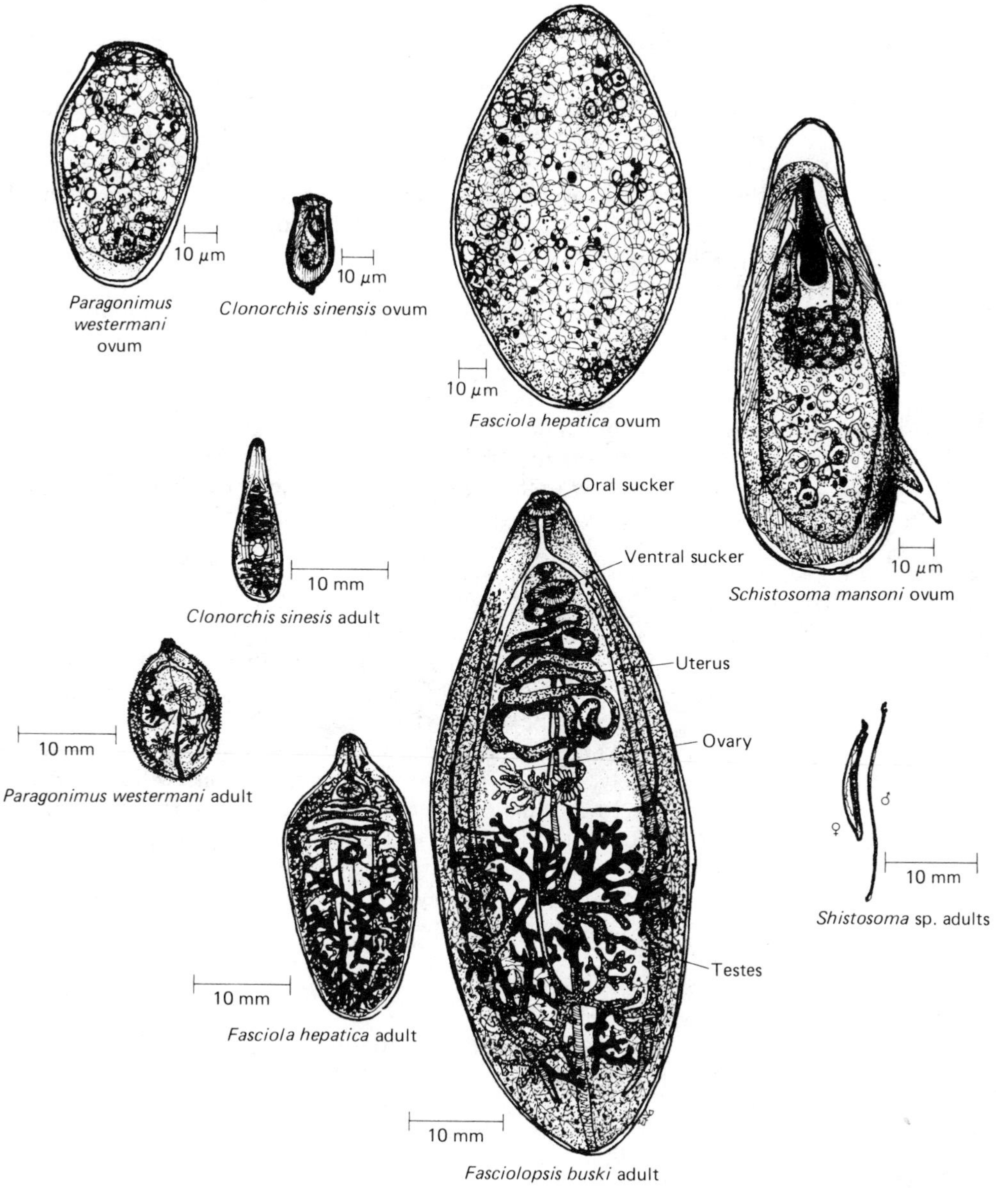

52.1 Adult flukes and eggs.

humans infected by ingesting infected crustaceans

man disease occurs when food shortages or local customs expose individuals to infected crabs. When these crustaceans are prepared for cooking, juice containing metacercariae may be left behind on the working surface and contaminate other foods subsequently prepared in the same area. Fresh crab juice, which is used for the treatment of infertility in the Cameroons and of measles in Korea, may also transmit the disease. In the Orient, crabs are frequently eaten after they have been lightly salted, pickled, or immersed briefly in wine (drunken crab), practices that are seldom lethal to the metacercariae. Children living in endemic areas may be infected while handling or ingesting crabs during the course of play.

Clinical Manifestations

formation of lung cysts

secondary infection of ruptured cysts

chronic pulmonary abscess

Other infected sites

The presence of the adult worm in the lung elicits an eosinophilic inflammatory reaction and, eventually, the formation of a 1- to 2-cm fibrous capsule that surrounds and encloses the parasite. With the onset of oviposition, the capsule swells and erodes into a bronchiole, resulting in expectoration of the brownish eggs, blood, and an inflammatory exudate. Secondary bacterial infection of the evacuated cysts is common, producing a clinical picture of chronic bronchitis or bronchiectasis. When cysts rupture into the pleural cavity, chest pain and effusion can result. In severe infection, the patient may develop chronic pneumonia or a nonresolving lung abscess, a clinical picture closely resembling that of pulmonary tuberculosis. The confusion is compounded by the frequent coexistence of the two diseases. Adult flukes in the intestine and mesentery produce pain, bloody diarrhea, and, on occasion, palpable abdominal masses. In approximately 1% of Oriental cases, parasites lodge in the brain and produce a variety of neurologic manifestations, including epilepsy, paralysis, homonymous hemianopsia, optic atrophy, and papilledema.

Laboratory Diagnosis

search for eggs in sputum, pleural fluid, and feces

Serodiagnosis

Eggs are usually absent from the sputum during the first 3 months of overt infection; however, repeated examinations will eventually demonstrate them in more than three-quarters of infected patients. When a pleural effusion is present, it should be checked for eggs. Stool examination is frequently helpful, particularly in children who swallow their expectorated sputum. Approximately 50% of patients with brain lesions will demonstrate calcification on X-ray films of the skull. The cerebrospinal fluid in such cases shows elevated protein levels and eosinophilic leukocytosis. A diagnosis in these cases, however, often depends on the detection of circulating antibodies. Their presence usually correlates well with acute disease and disappears with successful therapy.

Treatment and Prevention

The disease responds well to bithionol or praziquantel therapy. Control requires the adequate preparation of shellfish before ingestion.

Clonorchiasis (Liver Fluke Infection)

Organism

adults in biliary tract

eggs in feces

snails first intermediate host, fish second

Flukes of the genera *Fasciola, Opisthorchis*, and *Clonorchis* may all infect the human biliary tract and, at times, produce manifestations of ductal obstruction. *Clonorchis sinensis*, the Chinese liver fluke, is the most important and is discussed herein. The small, slender (5 × 15 mm) adult survives up to 50 years in the biliary tract of its host by feasting on the rich mucosal secretions. A cone-shaped anterior pole, a large oral sucker, and a pair of deeply lobular testes arranged one behind the other in the posterior third of the worm serve to distinguish it from other hepatic parasites. Approximately 2000 tiny (15 × 30 μm) ovoid eggs are discharged daily and find their way down the bile duct and into the fecal stream. The exquisite urn-shaped shells have a discernible shoulder at their opercular rim and a tiny knob on the broader posterior pole. On reaching fresh water, they are ingested by their intermediate snail host, transformed into cercariae, and released to penetrate the tissues of freshwater fish, in which they encyst to form metacercariae. If the latter host is ingested by a fish-eating mammal, metacercariae from ingested fish migrate to biliary system

the larvae are released in the duodenum, ascend the common bile duct, migrate to the bile capillaries, and mature to adulthood over 30 days.

In addition to humans, rats, cats, dogs, and pigs may serve as definitive hosts.

Epidemiology

Geography

Mechanism of transmission to humans

high attack rate

ingestion of uncooked fish

Clonorchiasis is endemic in the Far East, particularly in Korea, Japan, Taiwan, the Red River Valley of Vietnam, the Southern Chinese province of Kwantung, and Hong Kong. In previous years, parasite transmission was perpetuated by the practice of fertilizing commercial fish ponds with human feces. Recent improvements in the disposal of human waste have diminished acquisition of the disease in most countries. However, the extremely long life span of these worms is reflected in a much slower decrease in the overall infection rate. In some villages in southern China, the entire adult population is infected. A recent survey of stool specimens from immigrants from Hong Kong to Canada showed an infection rate of more than 15% overall and 23% in adults between 30 and 50 years of age. The disease is acquired by eating raw, frozen, dried, salted, or pickled fish. Commercial shipment of such products outside of the endemic area may result in the acquisition of worms far from their original source.

Clinical Manifestations

light infection usually asymptomatic

Severe hepatic and biliary manifestations from heavy worm loads

Migration of the larvae from the duodenum to the bile duct may produce fever, chills, mild jaundice, eosinophilia, and liver enlargement. The adult worm induces epithelial hyperplasia, adenoma formation, and inflammation and fibrosis around the smaller bile ducts. In light infection, clinical disease seldom results. However, numerous reinfections may produce worm loads of 500–1000, resulting in the formation of bile stones and sometimes cholangiocarcinoma in patients with severe, long-standing infections. Calculus formation is often accompanied by asymptomatic biliary carriage of *Salmonella typhi*. Dead worms may obstruct the common bile duct and induce secondary bacterial cholangitis, which may be accompanied by bacteremia, endotoxin shock, and hypoglycemia. Occasionally, adult worms are found in the pancreatic ducts, where they can produce ductal obstruction and acute pancreatitis.

Laboratory Diagnosis

search for eggs in feces and duodenal aspirates

eosinophilia common in acute disease

Definitive diagnosis requires the recovery and identification of the distinctive egg from the stool or duodenal aspirates. In mild infections, repeated examinations may be required. As most patients are asymptomatic, any individual with clinical manifestations of disease in whom *Clonorchis* eggs are found must be evaluated for the presence of other causes of illness. In acute symptomatic clonorchiasis, there is usually leukocytosis, eosinophilia, elevation of alkaline phosphatase levels, and abnormal radioisotopic and ultrasonographic liver scans. Cholangiograms may reveal dilatation of the intrahepatic ducts and small filling defects compatible with the presence of adult worms.

Treatment and Prevention

Praziquantel, an experimental agent currently undergoing clinical trials, shows promise as an effective therapeutic agent. Prevention requires thorough cooking of freshwater fish and sanitary disposal of human feces.

Schistosomiasis (Blood Fluke Infection)

Organism

inhabit portal vascular system

The schistosomes are a group of closely related flukes that inhabit the portal vascular system of a number of animals. Of the five species known to infect humans, three—*Schistosoma mansoni, Schistosoma haematobium*, and *Schistosoma japonicum*—are of primary importance, infecting over 200 million individuals worldwide. The remaining two are found only in limited areas of Africa (*Schistosoma intercalatum*) and Southeast Asia (*Schistosoma mekongi*) and will not be discussed in detail.

sexually differentiated

The adults of these species can be distinguished from the hermaphroditic trematodes by the anterior location of their ventral sucker, by their cylindric bodies, and by their reproductive systems (that is, separate sexes). They are differentiated from one another only with difficulty. The 1- to 2-cm male possesses a deep ventral groove, or *gynecophoral canal*, in which he carries the longer, more slender female in life-long copulatory embrace. After mating in the portal vein, the conjoined couple utilize their suckers to ascend the mesenteric vessels against the flow of blood. Guided by unknown stimuli, *S. japonicum* enters the superior mesentery vein, eventually reaching the venous radicals of the small intestine and ascending colon; *S. mansoni* and *S. haematobium* are directed to the inferior mesenteric system. The destination of the former is the descending colon and rectum; the latter, however, passes through the hemorrhoidal plexus to the systemic venous system, ultimately coming to rest in the veins of the bladder and other pelvic organs. On reaching the submucosal venules, the worms initiate oviposition. Each pair deposits 300 (*S. mansoni*) to 3000 (*S. japonicum*) eggs daily for the remainder of its 4- to 35-year life span. Enzymes secreted by the enclosed miracidium diffuse through the shell and digest the surrounding tissue. Ova lying immediately adjacent to the mucosal surface rupture into the lumen of the bowel (*S. mansoni, S. japonicum*) or bladder (*S. haematobium*) and are passed to the outside in the excreta. Here, with appropriate techniques, they may be readily observed and differentiated. The eggs of *S. mansoni* are oval, possess a sharp lateral spine, and measure 60 × 140 μm. Those of *S. haematobium* differ primarily in the terminal location of their spine. The eggs of *S. japonicum*, in contrast, are more nearly circular, measuring 70 × 90 μm. A minute lateral spine can be visualized only with care.

S. mansoni reaches colon and rectum and *S. haematobium* reaches veins of bladder and pelvis

eggs deposited submucosally, rupture to lumina, and pass outside

miracidia invade snail

cercariae from snail become schistosomula, traverse human skin and vascular system to portal vein

When the eggs are deposited in fresh water, the miracidia hatch quickly. Upon finding a snail host appropriate for their species, they invade and are transformed over 1–2 months into thousands of forked-tailed cercariae. When released from the snail, these infectious larvae swim about vigorously for a few days. Cercariae coming in contact with human skin during this time attach, discard their tails, and penetrate. The resulting *schistosomula* enter small venules and find their way through the right side of the heart to the lung. After a delay of several days, the parasites enter the systemic circulation and are distributed to the gut. Those surviving passage through the intestinal capillary bed return to the portal vein, where they mature to sexually active adults over 1–3 months.

Epidemiology

most important of helminthic infections

The widespread distribution and extensive morbidity of schistosomiasis makes it the single most important helminthic infection in the world today. Currently, more than 200 million individuals in 71 countries are infected. The continued presence of the parasite depends upon the disposal of infected human excrement into fresh water, the availability of appropriate snail hosts, and the exposure of humans to water infected with cercariae. The construction of modern sanitation and water purification facilities would break this cycle of transmission, but exceeds the economic resources of most endemic nations. Paradoxically, several massive land irrigation projects launched over the past two decades for the express purpose of speeding economic development have resulted in the dispersion of infected humans and snails to previously uninvolved areas.

spread to areas served by new irrigation projects

Geographic distribution

Schistosoma mansoni, the most widespread of the blood flukes, is the only one present in the Western Hemisphere. Originally introduced by African slaves, it is now found in Venezuela, Brazil, Puerto Rico, the Dominican Republic, St. Lucia, and several other Caribbean islands. As a suitable snail host is lacking, transmission does not occur within the continental United States; however, nearly half a million individuals residing there have acquired schistosomiasis elsewhere. Puerto Rican, Yemenite, and Southeast Asian populations are those predominantly involved. In the Eastern Hemisphere, the prevalence of *S. mansoni* infection is highest in the Nile Delta and the tropical section of Africa. Isolated foci are also found in East and South Africa, Yemen, Saudi Arabia, and Israel.

dependence on snail host

Schistosoma haematobium is largely confined to Africa and the Middle East, where its distribution overlaps that of *S. mansoni. Schistosoma japonicum* affects the agricultural populations of several Far Eastern countries, including Japan, China, the Philippines, and the Celebes. The closely related *S. mekongi* is found in the Mekong and Mun River valleys of Vietnam, Thailand, Cambodia, and Laos.

Age-related susceptibility

Within endemic areas, there are wide variations in both infection rates and worm loads. In general, both peak in the second decade of life and then decrease with advancing age. This finding has been explained in part by changes in the intensity of water exposure and in part by the slow development of immunity. Most infected patients carry fewer than 10 pairs of worms in the vascular system and, accordingly, lack clinical manifestation of disease. Individuals who develop much heavier loads as a result of repeated infections may experience serious morbidity or mortality.

Pathogenesis and Clinical Manifestations

There are three major clinicopathologic stages in schistosomiasis: The first stage is initiated by the penetration and migration of the schistosomula. The second or intermediate stage begins with oviposition and is associated with a complex of clinical manifestations. The third or chronic stage is characterized by granuloma formation and scarring around retained eggs.

local and systemic hypersensitivity reactions

Early stage. Within a few hours of penetrating the skin, a large proportion of the schistosomula die. Immediate and delayed hypersensitivity to parasitic antigens results in an intensely pruritic papular skin rash. As the viable schistosomula begin their migration to the liver, the rash disappears and the patient experiences fever, headache, and abdominal pain for 1–2 weeks.

serum sickness-like illness

Intermediate stage. One to two months after primary exposure, patients with severe *S. mansoni* or *S. japonicum* infections experience the onset of an acute febrile illness that bears a striking resemblance to serum sickness. It has been suggested that the onset of oviposition leads to a state of relative antigen excess and the formation of soluble immune complexes. Indeed, high levels of such complexes have been demonstrated in the peripheral blood and correlate well with the severity of illness. In addition to the fever, patients experience cough, urticaria, arthralgia, lymphadenopathy, splenomegaly, abdominal pain, and diarrhea. Sigmoidoscopic examination reveals eosinophilia

an inflamed colonic mucosa and petechial hemorrhages; typically, marked peripheral eosinophilia is present. This symptom complex is commonly termed the *Katayama syndrome;* it may persist for 3 months or more and occasionally results in death.

inflammatory and fibrotic reactions to retained eggs cause chronic disease

Chronic schistosomiasis. Approximately one-half of all deposited eggs reach the lumen of the bowel or bladder and are shed from the body. Those retained induce inflammation and scarring, initiating the final and most morbid phase of schistosomiasis. Soluble antigens excreted by the eggs stimulate the formation of a T-cell-mediated eosinophilic granuloma and the proliferation of fibroblasts. Early in the infection, the inflammatory response is vigorous, producing lesions more than 100-fold larger than the inciting egg itself. Obstruction of blood flow is common. As the fibroblasts lay down scar tissue, the obstruction may become permanent. As would be expected, the severity of tissue damage is directly related to the total number of eggs retained.

bladder lesions with *S. haematobium*

In *S. haematobium* infection, the bladder mucosa becomes thickened, papillated, and ulcerated. Hematuria and dysuria result; repeated hemorrhages produce anemia. In severe infections the muscular layers of the bladder are involved, with loss of bladder capacity and contractibility. Vesicoureteral reflux, ureteral obstruction, and hydronephrosis may follow. Progressive obstruction leads to renal failure and uremia. Calcification of the bladder wall is occasionally seen, and approximately 10% of patients harbor urinary tract calculi. Secondary bacterial infections are common. Chronic *Salmonella* bacteruria with recurrent bouts of bacteremia have been reported from Egypt. In the same country, bladder carcinoma is frequently seen as a late complication of disease.

chronic urinary carriage of *Salmonella*

bowel, liver, and pulmonary damage in *S. mansoni* and *S. japonicum* infections

In *S. mansoni* and *S. japonicum* infections, the bowel mucosa is congested, thickened, and ulcerated. Polyposis has been reported from Egypt, but not elsewhere. Patients experience abdominal pain, diarrhea, and blood in the stool. Eggs deposited in the larger intestinal veins may be carried by the portal blood flow back to the liver, where they lodge in the presinusoidal capillaries. The resulting inflammatory reaction leads to the development of periportal fibrosis and hepatic enlargement. The frequency and severity with which the liver is involved are genetically determined and associated with the HLA type of the patient. In most cases, liver function is well preserved. Infected individuals who subsequently acquire hepatitis B virus develop chronic active hepatitis more frequently than those free of schistosomes. The presinusoidal obstruction to blood flow can result in the serious manifestations of portal obstruction. Eggs carried around the liver in the portosystemic collateral vessels may lodge in the small pulmonary arterioles, where they may produce interstitial scarring, pulmonary hypertension, and right ventricular failure. Occasionally, eggs may be deposited in the central nervous system, where they may cause epilepsy or paraplegia.

Some differences between the clinical presentation of schistosomiasis mansoni and that of schistosomiasis japonicum have been noted. Manifestations of the latter disease typically occur earlier in the course of the infection and tend to be more severe. When involvement of the central nervous system develops, it is more likely to occur in the brain than the spinal cord. On the other hand, immune complex nephropathy and recurrent *Salmonella* bacteremia are more likely to be seen in hepatosplenic *S. mansoni* infections. The latter phenomenon is apparently related to the ability of *Salmonella* to parasitize the gut and integument of the adult fluke, providing a persistent bacterial focus within the portal system of the infected patient. This focus cannot be eradicated without treatment of the schistosomal infection.

recurrent *Salmonella* bacteremia in *S. mansoni* infection

Immunity

major manifestations from effects of cell-mediated immunity

The major clinicopathologic manifestations of schistosomiasis result from the host's cell-mediated immune response to the presence of retained eggs. With time, the intensity of this reaction is muted; granulomas formed in the later stages of infection are smaller and less damaging than those formed early. The mechanisms responsible for this modulation are not fully understood. Present evidence suggests that both suppressor T-cell activity and antibody blockade are involved. The correlation in humans between HLA types A1 and B5 and the development of hepatosplenomegaly suggests that the extent of the immunoregulation is influenced, at least in part, by the genetic background of the host.

antigenic disguise by adult parasite

As evidenced by their prolonged survival, the adult worms are remarkably well tolerated by their hosts. In part, this tolerance may be attributable to the ability of the developing parasites to disguise themselves with host molecules, including immunoglobulins, blood group glycolipids, and histocompatibility complex antigens. Antibodies formed against the immature worms before they have acquired host antigens, however, are effective in protecting the host from reinfection. Schistosomula that penetrate the skin after the primary infection are coated with specific antibody, bound to eosinophils, and destroyed. Although protection is not complete, the 60–80% kill rate is highly effective in controlling the intensity of parasitism. This condition, in which adult worms from a primary infection can survive in a host resistant to reinfection, has been termed *concomitant immunity.* It may be experimentally reproduced by exposing subjects to irradiated cercariae incapable of reaching full maturity.

Concomitant immunity

Laboratory Diagnosis

search for *S. haemotobium* eggs in urine

Definitive diagnosis requires the recovery of the characteristic eggs in urine, stool, or biopsy specimens. In *S. haematobium* infections, eggs are most numerous in urine samples obtained at midday. When examination of the sediment yields negative results, eggs may sometimes be recovered by filtering the urine through a membrane filter. Cystoscopy with biopsy of the bladder mucosa may be required for the diagnosis of mild infection. Eggs of *S. mansoni* and *S. japonicum* are passed in the stool. Concentration techniques such as formalin–ether or gravity sedimentation are necessary when the ova are scanty. Results of rectal biopsy may be positive when those of repeated stool examinations are negative.

S. mansoni and *S. japonicum* eggs in stool; rectal biopsy

Determination of egg viability

Because dead eggs may persist in tissue for a long time after the death of the adult worms, active infection is confirmed only if the eggs are shown to be viable. This confirmation may be obtained by observing the eggs microscopically for movement or by hatching them in water. Quantitation of egg output is useful in estimating the severity of infection and in the following response to treatment.

Currently available skin and serologic tests lack sensitivity and specificity and cannot be used to confirm or exclude the presence of active infection.

Treatment

Treatment of hypersensitivity reactions

No specific therapy is available for the treatment of schistosomal dermatitis or the Katayama syndrome. Antihistamines and corticosteroids may be helpful in ameliorating their more severe manifestations. In the late stage of schistosomiasis, therapy is directed at interrupting egg deposition by killing or sterilizing the adult worms. As the severity of clinical and pathologic manifestations is related to the intensity of infection, therapy is usually reserved for patients with moderate or severe active infections.

Anthelmintic drugs

Several anthelmintic agents may be used. Praziquantel, which is active against all three species of schistosomes, is the agent of choice for *S. japonicum.* In addition to praziquantel, metrifonate may be used for *S. haematobium* and oxamniquine for *S. mansoni.*

Control and Prevention

sanitary disposal of feces

It has proved both difficult and expensive to control this deadly disease. Programs aimed at interrupting transmission of the parasite by the provision of pure water supplies and the sanitary disposal of human feces are often beyond the economic reach of the nations most seriously affected. Similarly, measures to deny snails access to newly irrigated lands are expensive. Chemical molluscicides have been shown effective in limited trials, but have been less successful when used over large areas for prolonged periods. Mass therapy of the infected human population has, until recently, been severely limited by the toxicity of effective agents. It is possible that the agents developed most recently will prove more suitable for this purpose. At present, programs that have incorporated all of these control measures have been the most successful.

Molluscicides

Vaccines

Currently, there is intense interest in developing a vaccine suitable for human use. A vaccine made from irradiated *Schistosoma bovis* cercariae, developed for cattle, appears to confer a significant degree of protection against infection. It seems likely that some time will pass before a similar human vaccine suitable for mass therapy is available.

Additional Reading and References

Seah, S.K. 1978. Digenetic trematodes. *Clin. Gastroenterol.* 7:87–104. A number of trematode infections are discussed.

Warren, K.S. 1978. The pathology, pathobiology and pathogenesis of schistosomiasis. *Nature (Parasitol. Suppl.)* 273:609.

Warren, K.S. 1980. The relevance of schistosomiasis. *N. Engl. J. Med.* 303:203–206. Schistosomiasis as both a major global problem and an intriguing challenge to medical research is described briefly.

John C. Sherris

Skin and Wound Infections

53

Skin Infections

Microbial infections of the skin can result from invasion from an external source by certain bacteria, viruses, fungi, or parasites or from such organisms reaching the skin through the bloodstream as part of a systemic disease. Blood-borne involvement may be evidenced by rashes in many viral and bacterial infections, such as measles, varicella, meningococcal septicemia, and secondary syphilis, or may yield more chronic skin lesions in granulomatous diseases, such as blastomycosis, tuberculosis, and syphilis. Skin lesions remote from sites of infection can be produced by some bacterial toxins, such as the erythrogenic toxin of *Streptococcus pyogenes* and the exfoliatin of some strains of *Staphylococcus aureus,* or result from immunologic responses to microbial antigens that have reached the skin. Thus, there are manifold skin manifestations of infections; however, this chapter will be restricted to the discussion of *direct* infections that are common in the western hemisphere.

The skin is an organ system with multiple functions, including protection of the tissues from external microbial invasion. Its keratinized stratified epithelium prevents direct microbial invasion under normal conditions of surface temperature and humidity, and its normal flora, pH, and chemical defenses tend to inhibit colonization by many pathogens (Chapters 6 and 7). However, the skin is subject to repeated minor traumas that are often unnoticed, but that destroy its integrity and allow organisms to gain access to its deeper layers from the exernal environment. The surface is also penetrated by ducts to pilosebaceous units and sweat glands, and microbial invasion can occur along these routes, particularly if the ducts are obstructed.

Infections in Hair Follicles, Sebaceous Glands, and Sweat Glands

Staphylococcal folliculitis

Folliculitis, a minor infection of the hair follicles, is usually caused by *S. aureus.* As it is often associated with areas of friction and of sweat gland activity, it is seen most frequently on the neck, face, axillae, and buttocks. Blockage of ducts with inspissated sebum, as in acne vulgaris, predisposes to this condition. Folliculitis can also be caused by *Pseudomonas aeruginosa,* and this form of the disease has become more common in recent years with the popularity of hot tubs and whirlpool baths. Unless these facilities are thoroughly cleansed and adequately chlorinated, they can grow large num-

Pseudomonas folliculitis

bers of pseudomonads at their normal operating temperatures, causing extensive folliculitis on areas of the body that have been immersed. The lesions subside rapidly when the insult is discontinued.

Acne vulgaris also involves inflammation of hair follicles and associated sebaceous glands. The comedo of acne results from multiplication of *Propionibacterium acnes,* the predominant anaerobe of the normal skin, behind and within inspissated sedum. Organic acids produced by this organism are believed to stimulate an inflammatory response and thus contribute to the disease process. The primary cause of the disease, however, is hormonal influences on sebum secretion that occur at puberty, and the disease usually resolves in early adult life.

Staphylococcal furuncles

Furuncles. The furuncle is a small staphylococcal abscess that develops in the region of a hair follicle. Furuncles may be solitary or multiple and may constitute a troublesome recurrent disease. Spread of infection to the dermis and subcutaneous tissues can result in a more extensive multiloculated abscess, the carbuncle. These lesions and their treatment are considered in Chapter 11. Occasionally folliculitis and associated furuncles may be caused by infection with *Candida albicans.* Such cases are particularly common in immunocompromised hosts.

Candida furuncles

Treatment. Folliculitis and individual furuncles are normally treated locally by measures designed to establish drainage without the use of antibiotics. Chronic furunculosis may require attempts to eliminate nasal carriage of *S. aureus,* which is sometimes the source of the infection. Antimicrobics are not usually required unless surrounding cellulitis develops. Severe acne can often be treated effectively with topical drying agents and prolonged administration of low oral doses of tetracycline. The reason for the therapeutic response is uncertain.

Infections Often through Minor or Inapparent Skin Lesions

Minor or inapparent skin lesions serve as the route of infection in many localized skin infections and in some systemic diseases, such as syphilis and leptospirosis.

keratin utilized by dermatophytes

Infection of keratinized layers. The only organisms that can utilize the keratin on cells, hairs, and nails are the dermatophyte fungi and *C. albicans* (Chapters 30 and 31). The dermatophytes are particularly well adapted to these sites, cannot grow at 37°C, and fail to invade deeper layers. The clinical manifestations of these infections result from the inflammatory and delayed hypersensitivity responses of the host, and the desquamation induced by these processes is a major factor in the ultimate control of the infection by removing infected skin. In candidiasis, control involves cell-mediated immune mechanisms, and chronic *Candida* skin and nail infections are often associated with defects in cellular immunity. The clinical manifestations of these diseases are described in Chapters 30 and 31.

effect of desquamation

cell-mediated immunity in candidiasis

Streptococcal pyoderma

Infection of other skin layers. Pyoderma, also termed *impetigo,* is a common, sometimes epidemic skin lesion. This disease is caused by *S. pyogenes,* although the lesion frequently becomes secondarily infected with *S. aureus.* The initial lesion is often a small vesicle that develops at the site of invasion and ruptures with superficial spread characterized by skin erosion and a serous exudate, which dries to produce a honey-colored crust. The exudate and crust contain numerous infecting streptococci.

Epidemic impetigo is most common in childhood and under conditions of heat, humidity, poor hygiene, and overcrowding. The infection may be spread by fomites such as shared clothing and towels. It is often caused by nephritogenic strains of *S. pyogenes,* particularly in the tropics, and acute glomerulonephritis may result. Rheumatic fever is not associated with streptococcal lesions of the skin. Treatment is usually local with topical antimicrobics such as bacitracin or skin antiseptics such as chlorhexidine or povidone–iodine.

Staphylococcal bullous impetigo and exfoliatin

Bullous impetigo is a distinct disease caused by strains of *S. aureus* (usually phage type 71) that produce exfoliatin. It is most common in small children, but may occur at any age. The infection is characterized by large serum-filled bullae (blisters) within the skin layers at the site of infection. Minor infections are treated topically; bullous impetigo in infants, however, is a serious disease that usually requires systemic antimicrobic treatment. Epidemic spread may occur under conditions similar to those described for streptococcal impetigo.

S. pyogenes erysipelas

Erysipelas is a rapidly spreading infection of the deeper layers of the dermis that is almost always caused by *S. pyogenes.* It is associated with edema of the skin, marked erythema, pain, and systemic manifestations of infection, including fever and lymphadenopathy. As the infection is intradermal, *S. pyogenes* cannot usually be isolated from the skin surfaces. The disease can progress to septicemia or local necrosis of skin. It is serious and requires immediate treatment with penicillin or another β-lactam antibiotic with high activity against streptococci. Erythromycin is an alternative agent; however, erythromycin-resistant strains of *S. pyogenes* have become common in areas in which the antimicrobic has been widely used.

risk of septicemia

cellulitis caused by pyogenic cocci

Cellulitis is not a skin infection per se, but can develop by extension from skin or wound infections. It usually presents as an acute inflammation of subcutaneous connective tissue with swelling and pain and often with marked constitutional signs and symptoms. It can be caused by many pathogenic bacteria, but *S. aureus* and *S. pyogenes* are most common. Enteric Gram-negative rods, clostridia, and other anaerobes may also cause cellulitis as a complication of wound infections, particularly in the immunocompromised host and the uncontrolled diabetic.

H. influenzae cellulitis

A relatively uncommon but important form of cellulitis that also involves the dermis is caused by *Haemophilus influenzae* type b. The infection develops most often in children. It is manifested by a warm, painful, bluish swelling that advances rapidly and is associated with fever and considerable toxicity. Sepsis or meningitis may develop subsequently. Infections caused by ampicillin-sensitive strains respond rapidly to that antimicrobic, but resistant strains are becoming more common. Chloramphenicol is effective in almost all cases.

Skin Ulcers and Granulomatous Lesions

Many acute and subacute skin infections are characterized by ulceration or a granulomatous response. Some are sexually transmitted and are discussed in Chapter 64. Others derive from systemic infection and are not direct infections of skin. A few examples of direct infections, which pose special diagnostic problems are considered herein.

Herpetic paronychia

Herpes simplex virus can invade through the skin to produce a local vesicular lesion followed by ulceration. The lesion may then recur in the infected area. Primary herpetic lesions of the finger (Plate Y) can mimic staphylococcal paronychia very closely, as well as produce lymphangitis and local and lymph node enlargement with pain and fever. The lesions are sterile on bacterial culture.

Skin diphtheria

Skin diphtheria, which remains common in some tropical areas, also occurs endemically among the transient population of the West Coast of the United States. The organism gains access through a wound or insect bite and causes chronic erosion and ulceration of the skin, sometimes with evidence of the systemic effects of diphtheria toxin.

Swimmer's granuloma

Mycobacterium marinum produces a self-limiting granuloma, usually of the forearms and knees. The organism enters through abrasions as they occur or upon contamination. Infections with *Mycobacterium ulcerans* are more serious and produce progressive ulceration, but are limited to tropical areas and do not occur in the United States or Europe.

Necrotic ulcerations in immunocompromised host

Bacterial synergistic gangrene

Several rare forms of necrotic spreading skin ulceration tend to develop in immunosuppressed hosts, in diabetics, and as complications of abdominal surgery. These lesions include bacterial synergistic gangrene, apparently caused by a peptostreptococcus and *S. aureus,* streptococcal gangrene associated with *S. pyogenes* infection, and infection with a variety of opportunistic fungi. Variants of these conditions produce extensive and spreading necrotic cellulitis. Although unsuccessful at times, the major form of treatment is to excise the infected tissues widely and supplement such surgery with massive chemotherapy.

Fungal and parasitic ulcerations

Several primary fungal diseases are associated with cutaneous ulceration or cellulitis, including mycetoma and chromoblastomycosis, which involve the feet, and sporotrichosis, in which ulceration often develops from infected subcutaneous lymph nodes and vessels. Likewise, some parasites directly infect and ulcerate the skin, as in cutaneous leishmaniasis and cutaneous amebiasis. These latter two diseases are not contracted in the United States.

Wound Infections

Wounds subject to infection can be classified as surgical, traumatic, or physiologic. The latter include the endometrial surface, after separation of the placenta, and the umbilical stump. Traumatic wounds comprise such diverse damage as deep cuts, compound fractures, frostbite necrosis, and thermal burns.

Sources of infection

Sources of infection include 1) the patient's own normal flora; 2) infectious material from carriers or other infected individuals that may reach the wound (for example, on fomites, on the hands of attendants, or through the air); and 3) pathogenic organisms from the inanimate environment that can contaminate the wound through soil, clothing, and other foreign material. Examples of such infections include contamination of a penetrating stab wound to the abdomen by colonic flora, contamination of a clean surgical wound in the operating room with *S. aureus* spread by dust from the clothing of a perineal carrier, and introduction of spores of *Clostridium tetani* into the tissues on a splinter.

Classification of Wounds

Surgical and traumatic wounds can be classified according to the extent of potential contamination. This criterion corresponds to the risk of infection and carries important implications regarding surgical treatment and chemoprophylaxis.

Clean, clean contaminated, and dirty wounds

Clean wounds are surgical wounds made under aseptic conditions that do not traverse infected tissues or extend into sites with a normal flora. Clean contaminated wounds are operative wounds that extend into sites with a normal flora (except the colon) without known contamination. Contaminated wounds include fresh surgical and traumatic wounds with a major risk of contamination, such as incisions entering nonpurulent infected tissues.

Dirty and infected wounds include old, infected traumatic wounds, wounds substantially contaminated with foreign material, and wounds contaminated with spillage from perforated viscera.

Infection rates in clean surgical wounds without chemotherapy should be less than 1%, whereas untreated dirty wounds have a high probability of infection. Similar considerations apply to the chance of infection developing in a placental site or on the umbilicus. A normal delivery without retained products will rarely be followed by endometrial infection. A prolonged delivery after rupture of the membranes with retained placental fragments poses an increased risk of infection. In some rural cultures in Africa, soil is applied to the umbilical stump, and neonatal tetanus is common, whereas it is almost unknown in the Western world.

Factors Contributing to Infection Probability

Various factors, in addition to those indicated previously, contribute to the probability of a wound becoming infected.

contaminating dose

The contaminating dose of microorganisms and their virulence can be critical and, all other things being equal, the chance of infection developing increases progressively with the contaminating dose.

vascular integrity in wound

The physical and physiologic condition of the wound also influences the probability of infection. Areas of necrosis, vascular strangulation from excessively tight sutures, hematomas, excessive edema, poor blood supply, and poor oxygenation all compromise normal defense mechanisms and substantially reduce the dose of organisms needed to initiate infection. Thus, removal of necrotic tissue and the surgeon's skill, gentleness, and attention to detail are major factors in preventing the development of infection.

nutritional and immunologic status and inflammatory response

The general health, nutritional status, and ability of the patient to mount an inflammatory response are also major determinants of whether a wound infection develops. Infection rates are higher in the elderly, the obese, uncontrolled diabetics, and those on immunosuppressive or corticosteroid therapy. Nutritional deficiencies enhance the risk of infection, and new approaches to avoid protein-calorie malnutrition in patients with severe burns, for example, have led to substantial reductions in severe clinical infections.

critical period of contamination

There is strong evidence that the critical period determining whether contamination of surgical wounds proceeds to infection lies within the first 3 hr after contamination. It is for this reason that prophylactic chemotherapy of some surgical wounds and procedures can be restricted to the immediate perioperative period.

Etiologic Agents

Staphylococcal infections

increasing proportion of opportunistic Gram-negative infections

S. pyogenes infection

Staphylococcus aureus remains the single most common source of infection of clean surgical wounds; however, the number of infections caused by opportunistic Gram-negative organisms is now increasing. This finding reflects the extension of surgical intervention to more patients whose defenses are compromised or who would have been unacceptable surgical risks before the introduction of new technical and therapeutic procedures. Infections with *S. pyogenes* are now uncommon; however, because of their tendency to spread and cause septicemia, wound or puerperal infections by this organism can be devastating if not treated rapidly.

Anaerobic Gram-negative wound infections have been reported increasingly in the last decade or so as a result of the higher incidence of such infections in immunocompromised patients and better laboratory recognition. Most infecting organisms derive from normal floral sites. The majority of these infections are caused by *Bacteroides fragilis* or *Bacteroides melaninogenicus*, often in combination with anaerobic Gram-positive cocci and facultative aerobic bacteria. They tend to be associated with necrosis, which may spread subcutaneously, and with thrombophlebitis, which may lead to bacteremia with the possible development of metastatic hepatic, pulmonary, or cerebral abscesses. Most postpartum uterine infections are now caused by Gram-negative anaerobes or anaerobic Gram-positive cocci; they can range from self-limiting infections associated with little or no constitutional symptoms to severe infections of the uterus with pelvic thrombophlebitis. Human bite wounds are particularly subject to anaerobic infections.

Bacteroides and anaerobic Gram-positive cocci

Burn infections and *P. aeruginosa*

Burns and areas of necrosis resulting from vascular stasis or insufficiency are subject to infection with the same organisms that predominate in postsurgical wound infections; *P. aeruginosa* causes particularly serious infections in burns, however, with loss of skin grafts and a high risk of septicemia and death. If the fluid electrolyte and nutritional deficiencies of a burned patient can be controlled, the greatest hazard to life is infection.

Clostridial infections: tetanus and gas gangrene

Tetanus remains a threat to the unimmunized or inadequately immunized individual, particularly from heavy contamination of puncture wounds or introduction of foreign bodies such as splinters, soil, or clothing into the subcutaneous tissues. The pathogenesis, treatment, and prevention of the disease are discussed in Chapter 15. It is worth repeating that a low oxidation–reduction potential in the tissue as a result of necrosis or the presence of foreign material is essential for the multiplication of *C. tetani*, that the organism never spreads beyond the site of the local lesion, and that adequate circulating antibody from tetanus toxoid immunization will prevent the development of the disease.

Gas gangrene (clostridial myositis) is also discussed in some detail in Chapter 15. It can develop within a few hours and lead to rapid death. *Clostridium perfringens* is the most common contributor to the infection, and its α-toxin is the major cause of the spreading tissue damage and muscle death. Other aerobic and anaerobic bacteria are invariably present and sometimes play an important etiologic role. The disease is always associated with muscle trauma and necrosis, which provide the conditions for anaerobic multiplication. Compound fractures, gunshot wounds, and similar extensive injuries that allow entry of clostridial spores set the stage for the disease. Prevention involves surgically debriding all necrotic or potentially necrotic tissue as soon as possible, leaving the wound unsutured, and administering high-dose chemoprophylaxis, in which penicillin is the agent of choice.

Prevention and Treatment

Immunization and prevention of wound and burn infections

Epidemiologic approaches to the prevention of wound infection and the appropriate uses of chemoprophylaxis are considered in Chapters 10 and 66. Recently, however, there has been increasing interest in the possibilities of immunization against the types of organisms that may infect a particular patient, for example, one who has suffered a burn recently or is to undergo certain types of major surgery. Some degree of protection from *P. aeruginosa* infection has been achieved with both active and passive immunization, and the degree of toxicity and risk of septicemia are reduced. It was shown recently that immunization with the common antigen of *Escherichia coli*, an antigen it shares with many other Gram-negative organisms, provides a broad range of increased immunity to Gram-negative (including *P. aeruginosa*) infections in experimental animals. Initial clinical trials appear promising.

Severe wound infections are almost always treated with a combination of surgical and chemotherapeutic approaches. Necrotic tissue and contaminated foreign bodies, such as sutures, must be removed, pockets of pus opened, and drainage established. This approach permits access of the appropriate antibiotics to viable tissues in which they can act.

Additional Reading and References

Hunt, T.K., and Dunphy, J.E. 1979. *Fundamentals of wound management.* Norwalk, Conn.: Appleton-Century-Crofts. An authoritative consideration of the factors contributing to wound infections and their management.

Lennard, E.S., and Dellinger, E.P. 1981. Prophylactic antibiotics in surgery. *J. Fam. Pract.* 12:464–467. A valuable review of indications for prophylaxis and factors determining its duration.

Ziegler, E.J., et al. 1982. Treatment of Gram-negative bacteremia with human serum to a mutant *Escherichia coli. N. Engl. J. Med.* 307:1225–1230. Provides evidence of cross-protection with antibodies against the core antigen of endotoxin and their ameliorating effects on serious Gram-negative infections in humans.

C. George Ray

Bone and Joint Infections

54

Infections of bones and joints may exist separately or together. Both are most common in infancy and childhood. They are usually caused by bloodborne (hematogenous) spread to the infected site, but can also result from local trauma with secondary infection. Sometimes there may be local spread from a contiguous soft tissue infection, often associated with the presence of a foreign body at the site of the primary wound.

The local effect of such infections can be devastating if they are inadequately treated, because inflammation and resultant tissue necrosis may produce irreparable damage. The presence of pus under pressure can compromise normal blood flow and even cause destruction of blood vessels with avascular necrosis of tissue. When this condition develops a *sequestrum* can result, in which a part of the cartilage or bone becomes totally separated from its blood supply and cannot be incorporated into the healing process. In some patients, sequestrum formation can lead to a smoldering chronic infection with draining sinuses and loss of functional integrity. Normal growth of the affected site can be severely impaired in the infant or child, particularly when the epiphysis is involved.

sequestrum formation

chronic infection with draining sinuses

growth impairment in children

bacteremia and metastatic spread

In the acute phase of infection, bacteremia may also cause sepsis and metastatic infections in sites such as the lungs and heart. The result may be fatal.

Osteomyelitis

Clinical signs of acute hematogenous osteomyelitis

Spread from local infections

The onset of acute hematogenous osteomyelitis is usually abrupt, but can sometimes be quite insidious. It is classically characterized by localized pain, fever, and tenderness to palpation over the affected site. More than one bone or joint may be involved as a result of blood spread to multiple sites. With progression, the classic signs of heat, redness, and swelling may develop. Laboratory findings often include leukocytosis and elevated acute-phase reactants, such as the sedimentation rate. Osteomyelitis caused by a contiguous focus of infection is usually associated with the presence of local findings of soft tissue infection, such as skin abscesses and infected wounds.

Extension to joint

When osteomyelitis occurs in close proximity to a joint, septic arthritis may develop by direct spread through the epiphysis (usually in infants) or by lateral extension through the periosteum into the joint capsule. Such extension is particularly common in hip and elbow infections.

Table 54.1 Common Causes of Acute Osteomyelitis

Situation	Usual Causative Organism
Age group	
Neonates (< 1 mo)	*Staphylococcus aureus*; group B streptococci; Gram-negative rods (e.g., *Escherichia coli, Klebsiella, Proteus, Pseudomonas*)
Older infants, children, adults	*Staphylococcus aureus*
Special problems	
Chronic hemolytic disorders (e.g., sickle cell disease)	*Staphylococcus aureus; Streptococcus pneumoniae; Salmonella* species
Infection after trauma or surgery	*Staphylococcus aureus; Streptococcus pyogenes;* Gram-negative aerobic or anaerobic bacteria
Infection after puncture wound of foot	*Pseudomonas aeruginosa; Staphylococcus aureus*

Etiologic Agents

Age-related etiologies

The most common causes of acute osteomyelitis and those associated with special circumstances are shown in Table 54.1. It is clear that age plays a significant role in influencing the relative frequency of the various infective agents, particularly in early infancy; however, most infections at any age are caused by *Staphylococcus aureus.*

Chronic granulomatous osteomyelitis

In low-grade smoldering infections, chronic granulomatous processes may require consideration, including tuberculosis, coccidioidomycosis, histoplasmosis, and blastomycosis. These manifestations usually result from systemic dissemination of infection, and the lesions develop slowly over a period of months. Occasionally bone tumors or cysts and leukemia must also be considered in the differential diagnosis.

General Diagnostic Approaches

Blood cultures, direct aspirates, and bone scans

The primary goals of diagnosis are to establish the existence of infection and to determine its cause. The following procedures are generally employed:

1. Blood cultures, because many infections are associated with bacteremia.
2. Radionuclide bone scanning to demonstrate evidence of localized infection.
3. Direct staining, culture and histology of needle aspirates, or biopsy of periosteum or bone.
4. X-rays of affected sites, which often appear normal in the early stages of infection. The first changes seen are swelling of surrounding soft tissues, followed by periosteal elevation. Demineralization of bone and calcification of the periosteum and surrounding soft tissues may not become apparent for 2 weeks or more after the onset of symptoms.

X-rays may be normal in early stages of infection

General Principles of Management

Bactericidal antibiotics

In acute infections, early intervention is important. Management includes vigorous use of bactericidal antibiotics, which must often be continued for several weeks to ensure a bacteriologic cure. Surgical drainage is also essential if there is significant pressure from the localized, purulent process.

prolonged therapy for chronic osteomyelitis

In chronic osteomyelitis, sequestrum formation is frequent and sinuses may develop that drain the bone abscess to the surface. The infection is persistent, and treatment becomes extremely difficult. Such patients often require long-term antibiotic treatment (months to years) combined with surgical procedures to drain the abscesses and remove necrotic, infected tissues in an attempt to control infection while preserving the integrity of the affected bone.

Septic Arthritis

Clinical signs of arthritis

The usual clinical features of septic arthritis include onset of pain, which is often abrupt and accompanied by fever. Single or multiple joints may be involved. Tenderness and swelling of the affected joints and frequently other signs of local inflammation are present. Attempts to move the joints, either actively or passively, result in severe pain. In infants, the symptoms may be somewhat nonspecific; local swelling or excessive irritability with unwillingness to move the affected extremity (pseudoparalysis) may be the only clues to the diagnosis.

Common Etiologic Agents

Age-related etiologies

The major causes of septic arthritis are listed in Table 54.2. Although *S. aureus* infection can occur at any age, there are some significant age-specific relationships to other bacterial causes. There is a high frequency of group B streptococcal infections in neonates, whereas in children between 1 month and 4 years of age, *Haemophilus influenzae* type b accounts for up to 75% of all cases. *Neisseria gonorrhoeae* is implicated in most cases of septic arthritis in young adults.

Tuberculous and fungal arthritis

Subacute or chronic septic arthritis should prompt consideration of tuberculosis, syphilis, and deep mycosis such as coccidioidomycosis or *Candida* infection. Arthritis attributable to *Candida* infection is particularly likely in immunocompromised patients.

Self-limiting viral or *Mycoplasma*-associated arthritis

Viruses and *Mycoplasma* can also cause acute arthritis in single or multiple joints. Such illnesses have been associated with rubella, hepatitis B, mumps, varicella, Epstein–Barr virus, Coxsackie virus, and adenovirus infections, as well as with *Mycoplasma pneumoniae,* and *Mycoplasma hominis.* These arthri-

Table 54.2 Common Causes of Septic Arthritis

Age Group	Usual Causative Organism
Neonate (<1 mo)	*Staphylococcus aureus;* group B streptococci; Gram-negative rods (e.g., *Escherichia coli, Klebsiella, Proteus, Pseudomonas*)
1 mo–4 yr	*Haemophilus influenzae* type b; *Staphylococcus aureus; Streptococcus pyogenes; Streptococcus pneumoniae; Neisseria meningitidis*
4–16 yr	*Staphylococcus aureus*
16–40 yr	*Neisseria gonorrhoeae; Staphylococcus aureus*
>40 yr	*Staphylococcus aureus*

tides are usually self-limiting and rarely require specific therapy. Some bacterial infections of sites other than joints may be associated with noninfectious (reactive) arthritis, possibly resulting from deposition of circulating immune complexes and complement in synovial tissues, leading to inflammation. Examples include intestinal infections caused by *Yersinia enterocolitica, Campylobacter jejuni,* and some *Salmonella* species.

Arthritis associated with intestinal infections

Noninfectious causes of arthritis must also be considered in the differential diagnosis. They can closely mimic septic arthritis. Examples include inflammatory collagen vascular disease such as rheumatoid arthritis, gout, traumatic arthritis, and degenerative arthritis.

General Diagnostic Approaches

Blood culture

Needle aspiration

Characteristics of synovial fluid

In acute cases, blood cultures are often useful because bacteremia may be present. The definitive diagnosis is established by examination of synovial fluid removed from the joint by needle aspiration (arthrocentesis). As other noninfectious causes must be considered, it is important to analyze the chemical and cellular characteristics of the fluid in addition to performing a Gram stain and culture. Table 54.3 summarizes the major findings in synovial fluid in normal and various disease states. Septic bacterial arthritis is usually associated with grossly purulent fluid containing more than 25,000 white blood cells per cubic millimeter, predominantly polymorphonuclear cells. The glucose level in the synovial fluid is usually less than 25% of that in the blood.

In viral, tuberculous, and fungal arthritis, as well as in partially treated bacterial arthritis, cell counts are usually lower, and mononuclear cells may constitute a greater proportion of the inflammatory cells. Occasionally, biopsy of the synovial membrane may be required to resolve the diagnosis. Histologic examination and culture of the tissue are particularly helpful in distinguishing granulomatous from rheumatoid disease.

Gonococci may be difficult to isolate from joint fluid

In most cases of acute septic arthritis, the blood culture and/or synovial fluid culture will yield the specific etiologic agent. One major exception is *N. gonorrhoeae,* which can be difficult to isolate from these sources. When this organism is suspected, it is often wise to include cultures of other sites of potential infection or colonization, such as the urethra, cervix, rectum, and pharynx, as well as skin lesions.

Table 54.3 Findings in Synovial Fluid in Various Forms of Arthritis

Laboratory Test	Normal	Septic Bacterial Arthritis	Trauma, Degenerative Joint Disease	Rheumatoid Arthritis, Gout
Clarity and color	Clear	Opaque, yellow to green	Clear, yellow	Translucent, yellow; or opalescent
Viscosity	High	Variable	High	Low
White blood cells/mm^3	<200	25,000–100,000	200–2000	2000–20,000
Polymorphonuclear cells (%)	<25	>75	25–50	≥50
Glucose level (relative to simultaneous blood glucose level)	Nearly equal	>25%	Nearly equal	50–80%

General Principles of Management

Prompt, vigorous, systemic antimicrobial therapy is required as soon as diagnostic tests suggest a bacterial cause. This treatment usually must be continued for 3–6 weeks, depending upon the etiologic agent and the clinical response to therapy.

Drainage of pus under pressure is also an important aspect of management. In cases of hip joint involvement, open surgical drainage is often necessary because collateral blood supply to the hip joint is relatively small, and pus under pressure can lead to irreversible avascular necrosis of the tissues and permanent crippling. It is also difficult to evaluate the amount of pus that may be present because of the extensive overlying muscle. Other joints can usually be managed by simple aspiration of pus whenever it reaccumulates significantly during the acute phase of infection.

C. George Ray

Eye, Ear, and Sinus Infections

55

Eye Infections

Ocular infections can be divided into those that primarily involve the external structures—eyelids, conjunctiva, sclera, and cornea—and those that involve internal sites.

Defenses of the eye

The major defense mechanisms of the eye are the tears and the conjunctiva, as well as the mechanical cleansing that occurs with blinking of the eyelids. The tears contain secretory immunoglobulin A antibodies and lysozyme, and the conjunctiva possesses numerous lymphocytes, plasma cells, neutrophils, and mast cells, which can respond quickly to infection by inflammation and production of antibody and interferon. The internal eye is protected from external invasion primarily by the physical barrier imposed by the sclera and cornea. If these are breached (for example, by a penetrating injury or ulceration), infection becomes a possibility. In addition, infection may reach the internal eye via blood-borne mechanisms to the retinal arteries and produce chorioretinitis and/or uveitis. Such infections are a particularly common problem in immunocompromised patients.

Other causes of inflammation of the external or internal eye can involve autoimmune or allergic mechanisms, which may be provoked by infectious agents or diseases such as rheumatoid arthritis.

Common Clinical Features

Sites of infections and definitions

Blepharitis is an acute or chronic inflammatory disease of the eyelid margin. It can take the form of a localized inflammation in the external margin (hordeolum or sty) or a granulomatous reaction to infection and plugging of a sebaceous gland of the eyelid (chalazion).

Dacryocystitis is an inflammation of the lacrimal sac. It usually results from partial or complete obstruction within the sac or nasolacrimal duct, where bacteria may be trapped and initiate either an acute or a chronic infection.

Conjunctivitis is a term used to describe inflammation of the conjunctiva; it may extend to involve the eyelids, the cornea (keratitis), or the sclera (episcleritis). Extensive disease involving the conjunctiva and cornea is often called *keratoconjunctivitis.* Progressive keratitis can lead to ulceration, scarring, and blindness.

Ophthalmia neonatorum is an acute, sometimes severe, conjunctivitis or keratoconjunctivitis of newborn infants.

Endophthalmitis is rare, but often leads to blindness even when treated aggressively. The term refers to infection of the aqueous or vitreous humor, usually by bacteria or fungi.

Uveitis consists of inflammation of the uveal tract—iris, ciliary body, and choroid. Although most inflammations of the iris and ciliary body (iridocyclitis) are not of infectious origin, some agents have been implicated. The acute disease may be associated with severe eye pain, redness, and photophobia; other cases may progress quite silently, with decreased visual acuity as the only symptom in the late stages. The most common infective involvement of the uveal tract is chorioretinitis, in which inflammatory infiltrates are seen in the retina; this infection can lead to destruction of the choroid and inflammation of the optic nerve (optic neuritis) and may extend into the vitreous humor to cause endophthalmitis. If the disease is not treated adequately, the end result can be blindness.

Common Etiologic Agents

Blepharitis and keratitis

Acute conjunctivitis

The major infectious causes of various inflammatory diseases of the eye are listed in Table 55.1. *Staphylococcus aureus* is the principal offender in bacterial infections of the eyelid and cornea. *Haemophilus influenzae* and *Streptococcus pneumoniae* are common causes of acute bacterial conjunctivitis. In young infants, *Neisseria gonorrhoeae* and *Chlamydia trachomatis* are significant causes of external eye disease, contracted from the mother's birth canal, that must

Table 55.1 Major Infectious Causes of Eye Disease

Disease	Bacteria and *Chlamydia*	Viruses	Fungi	Parasites
Blepharitis	*Staphylococcus aureus*			
Dacryocystitis	*Streptococcus pneumoniae; Staphylococcus aureus*			
Conjunctivitis; keratitis; keratoconjunctivitis	*Streptococcus pneumoniae; Haemophilus influenzae; Haemophilus aegyptius; Streptococcus pyogenes; Staphylococcus aureus; Chlamydia trachomatis; Neisseria gonorrhoeae; Neisseria meningitidis*	Adenoviruses; herpes simplex; measles; varicella-zoster	*Fusarium* species *Aspergillus* species	
Ophthalmia neonatorum	*Neisseria gonorrhoeae; Chlamydia trachomatis*	Herpes simplex		
Endophthalmitis	*Staphylococcus aureus; Pseudomonas aeruginosa;* other Gram-negative organisms		*Candida* species *Aspergillus* species	
Iridocyclitis	*Treponema pallidum*	Herpes simplex; varicella-zoster		
Chorioretinitis	*Mycobacterium tuberculosis*	Cytomegalovirus; herpes simplex	*Histoplasma capsulatum; Coccidioides immitus; Candida* species	*Toxoplasma gondii; Toxocara canis*

Chronic conjunctivitis

be diagnosed and treated promptly. Chronic conjunctivitis, keratoconjunctivitis, or episcleritis at any age must also prompt consideration of *C. trachomatis* infection. Herpes simplex is also a major cause of chronic conjunctivitis, especially in infections of the external structures, and specific therapy is available. Epidemic conjunctivitis or keratoconjunctivitis is most commonly associated with a variety of adenovirus serotypes. Outbreaks have been associated with inadequately chlorinated swimming pools, contaminated equipment or eyedrops in physicians' offices, and communal sharing of towels, which facilitates direct transmission. Chorioretinitis is frequently a manifestation of systemic disease (for example, histoplasmosis, tuberculosis); it is particularly common in immunocompromised patients, who are liable to develop disseminated *Candida,* cytomegalovirus, or *Toxoplasma gondii* infections.

Epidemic adenovirus conjunctivitis

Chorioretinitis

Periorbital cellulitis

Infection of the soft tissues surrounding the eye (periorbital or orbital cellulitis) is potentially severe and can spread to involve the functions of the eye itself. Major causes are *S. aureus, H. influenzae,* and *Streptococcus pyogenes.*

General Diagnostic Approaches

In external bacterial infections of the eye, etiologic diagnoses can usually be established by Gram stain and culture of surface material or, in the case of viral infections, by tissue culture. Conjunctival scrapings for *C. trachomatis* can be prepared for immunofluorescent or cytologic examination and for appropriate tissue culture. Infections of internal sites pose a more difficult problem. Some, such as acute endophthalmitis, may require removal of infected aqueous humor for microbiologic studies. Infections involving the uveal tract may require indirect methods of diagnosis, such as serologic tests for toxoplasmosis and deep mycoses, blood cultures to demonstrate evidence of disseminated disease (for example, *Candida* sepsis), and efforts to demonstrate infection in other sites (for example, chest radiography and sputum culture to diagnose tuberculosis). Careful ophthalmologic examination using slit lamps and retinoscopy often helps to suggest specific etiologic agents based on the morphology of the lesions observed.

General Principles of Management

Topical agents for superficial bacterial infections

Various topical antimicrobial agents have been used effectively in external eye infections of presumed or proved bacterial origin. In addition, topical antiviral treatment is available for herpes simplex infections, but has not been proved efficacious for other viral diseases of the eye.

need for ophthalmologic consultation with severe or deep infection

Severe infections, whether external or internal, require specialized treatment that nearly always includes ophthalmologic consultation because they may threaten vision. Systemic infection associated with eye disease (for example, fungemia, tuberculosis) must be treated vigorously with appropriate antimicrobial agents.

Ear Infections

Most infections of the ear involve the external otic canal (otitis externa) or the middle ear cavity, which contains the ossicles and is bound by bony structures and the tympanic membrane (otitis media).

Otitis externa

Factors of importance in the pathogenesis of otitis externa include local trauma, furunculosis, foreign bodies, or excessive moisture, which can lead to maceration of the external ear epithelium (swimmer's ear). Occasionally, external otitis occurs as an extension of infection from the middle ear, with purulent drainage through a perforated tympanic membrane.

pathogenesis of otitis media and predisposing factors

The eustachian tube, which vents the middle ear to the nasopharynx, appears to play a major role in predisposing patients to otitis media. The tube performs three functions: ventilation, protection, and clearance via mucociliary transport. Viral upper respiratory infections or allergic conditions can cause inflammation and edema in the eustachian tube or at its orifice. These developments disturb its functions, of which ventilation may be the most important. As ventilation is lost, oxygen is absorbed from the air in the middle ear cavity, producing negative pressure. This pressure in turn allows entry of potentially pathogenic bacteria from the nasopharynx into the middle ear, and failure to clear these normally can result in colonization and infection. Other factors that can lead to compromise of eustachian tube function include anatomic abnormalities, such as tissue hypertrophy or scarring around the orifice, muscular dysfunction associated with cleft palate, and lack of stiffness of the tube wall. The latter is common in infancy and early childhood and improves with age. It may explain in part why otitis media occurs most often in infants 6–18 months old, then decreases in frequency as patency of the eustachian tube becomes established.

Common Clinical Features

P. aeruginosa in swimming pool and malignant otitis externa

Otitis externa is characterized by inflammation of the ear canal, with purulent ear drainage. It can be quite painful, and cellulitis can extend into adjacent soft tissues. A common form is associated with swimming in water that may be contaminated with aerobic, Gram-negative organisms such as *Pseudomonas* species. "Malignant" otitis externa is a considerably more severe form of external ear canal infection that can progress to invasion of cartilage and adjacent bone, sometimes leading to cranial nerve palsy and death. It is seen most frequently in elderly patients with diabetes mellitus and in immunocompromised hosts of any age. *Pseudomonas aeruginosa* is the most common causative pathogen.

Acute bacterial otitis media

Otitis media is arbitrarily classified as acute, chronic, or serous (secretory). Acute otitis media, nearly always caused by bacteria, is usually a complication of acute viral upper respiratory illness. Fever, irritability, and acute pain are common, and otoscopic examination will reveal bulging of the tympanic membrane and poor mobility and obscuration of normal anatomic landmarks by fluid and inflammatory cells under pressure. In some cases, the tympanic membrane will also be acutely inflamed, with blisters (bullae) on its external surface (myringitis). If treated inadequately, the infection can progress to involve adjacent structures such as the mastoid air cells (mastoiditis) or lead to perforation with spontaneous drainage through the tympanic membrane. Potential acute, suppurative sequelae include extension into the central nervous system and sepsis.

myringitis

mastoiditis

perforation of tympanic membrane

Chronic otitis media

risk of hearing loss

Chronic otitis media is usually a result of acute infection that has not resolved adequately, either because of inadequate treatment in the acute phase or because of host factors that perpetuate the inflammatory process (for example, continued eustachian tube dysfunction, caused by allergic or anatomic factors, or immunodeficiency). Sequelae include progressive destruction of middle ear structures and a significant risk of permanent hearing loss.

Serous otitis media

Serous otitis media may represent either a form of chronic otitis media or allergy-related inflammation. It tends to be chronic, causing hearing deficits, and is associated with thick, usually nonpurulent secretions in the middle ear.

Common Etiologic Agents

The usual causes of ear infections are listed in Table 55.2. *Streptococcus pneumoniae* is the single most common cause of acute otitis media after the first 3 months of life, accounting for 35–40% of all cases. *Haemophilus influenzae* is also common, particularly in patients less than 5 years of age. Viruses and *Mycoplasma* are rare primary causes of acute or chronic otitis media; however, they predispose patients to superinfection by the bacterial agents.

General Diagnostic Approaches

direct Gram stain and culture of infected sites in special cases

The diagnosis is established on the basis of clinical examination. Tympanometry can be performed in suspected cases of otitis media to detect the presence of fluid in the middle ear and to assess tympanic membrane function. The specific etiology of otitis externa can be determined by culture of the affected ear canal; one must keep in mind, however, that surface contamination and normal skin flora may lead to mixed cultures, which may be confusing. In otitis media, the most precise diagnostic method is careful aspiration with a sterile needle through the tympanic membrane after decontamination of the external canal. Gram stain and culture of such aspirates is highly reliable; however, this procedure is generally reserved for cases in which etiologic possibilities are extremely varied, as in young infants, or when clinical response to the usual antimicrobial therapy has been inadequate.

respiratory tract cultures unhelpful

Respiratory tract cultures, such as those from the nasopharynx, cannot be relied upon to provide an etiologic diagnosis.

General Principles of Management

Topical treatment of otitis externa

Except in severe cases, otitis externa can usually be managed by gentle cleansing with topical solutions. The Gram-negative bacteria most commonly involved are often susceptible to an acidic environment, and otic solutions buffered to a low pH (3.0 or less), as with 0.25% acetic acid, will often be effective. Various preparations are available, many of which also contain antibiotics.

Table 55.2 Common Causes of Ear Infection

Otitis externa	*Pseudomonas aeruginosa* is common; occasionally *Proteus* species, *Escherichia coli,* and *Staphylococcus aureus.* Bacteria found in otitis media may also be recovered if the process is secondary to middle ear infection with perforation and drainage through the tympanic membrane. Fungi, such as *Aspergillus* species, are occasionally implicated.
Acute otitis media	
Infants < 3 mo old	*Streptococcus pneumoniae,* group B streptococci, *Haemophilus influenzae, Staphylococcus aureus, Pseudomonas aeruginosa,* and Gram-negative enteric bacteria.
Infants > 3 mo old	*Streptococcus pneumoniae* and *Haemophilus influenzae* are most common; others include *Streptococcus pyogenes, Branhamella catarrhalis,* and *Staphylococcus aureus.*
Chronic otitis media	Mixed flora in 40% of cases cultured. Common organisms include *Pseudomonas aeruginosa, Haemophilus influenzae, Staphylococcus aureus, Proteus* species, *Klebsiella pneumoniae, Branhamella catarrhalis,* and Gram-positive as well as Gram-negative anaerobic bacteria.
Serous otitis media	Same as chronic otitis media; however, many more of these effusions are sterile, with relatively few acute inflammatory cells.

Antimicrobic therapy for otitis media

Acute otitis media requires prompt antimicrobial therapy and careful follow-up to ensure that the disease has resolved. The choice of antibiotic is usually empirical, designed specifically to cover the most likely bacterial pathogens because direct aspiration for diagnostic purposes is usually unnecessary. In the usual case these pathogens would be *S. pneumoniae* and *H. influenzae.*

If there is extreme pressure with severe pain, drainage of middle ear exudates by careful incision of the tympanic membrane may be necessary.

In patients with chronic or serous otitis media, management can be more complex, and it is often advisable to seek otolaryngologic consultation to determine further diagnostic procedures as well as to plan medical and possible surgical measures.

Sinus Infections

The paranasal sinuses (ethmoid, frontal, and maxillary) all communicate with the nasal cavity. In health, these sinuses are ciliated, epithelium-lined, air-filled cavities that are normally sterile. They are poorly developed in early life and, in contrast to otitis media, sinus infections are a rare problem in infancy.

Factors causing predisposition to sinusitis

The pathogenesis of sinus infection can involve several factors, most of which act by producing obstruction or edema of the sinus antrum, which impedes normal drainage. Consequently, bacterial infection and inflammation of the mucosal lining tissues develop. Predisposing factors may be 1) local, such as upper respiratory infections producing edema of antral tissues, mucosal polyps, deviation of the nasal septum, enlarged adenoids, or a tumor or foreign body in the nasal cavity; or 2) systemic, such as allergy, cystic fibrosis, or immunodeficiency. Occasionally, maxillary sinusitis can result from extension of a maxillary dental infection.

Common Clinical Features

Signs and symptoms vary according to which sinuses are affected and whether the illness is acute or chronic. Fever is sometimes present; cough, nasal discharge, fetid breath, pain over the affected sinus, headache, and tenderness to percussion over the frontal or maxillary sinuses are all features that may appear in different combinations and that suggest the diagnosis.

Complications

Complications of sinusitis can include local involvement of infection in nearby soft tissues, such as the orbit, and occasionally extension, either directly or via vascular pathways, into the central nervous system.

Common Etiologic Agents

Table 55.3 summarizes the usual etiologies of sinus infections. Respiratory viruses are also occasional causes, but appear most important in predisposing patients to bacterial superinfection of inflamed sinuses and their antral open-

Table 55.3 Common Causes of Sinus Infection

Acute sinusitis	*Streptococcus pneumoniae* and *Haemophilus influenzae* are most common; also *Streptococcus pyogenes, Staphylococcus aureus,* and *Branhamella catarrhalis.*
Chronic sinusitis	Same as for acute sinusitis; also Gram-negative enteric bacteria and anaerobic Gram-negative and Gram-positive bacteria. Mixed aerobic and anaerobic infections are relatively common. *Mucor* species may be found in compromised patients, e.g., those with diabetes mellitus.

ings. Together, *S. pneumoniae* and *H. influenzae* account for more than 60% of cases of acute sinusitis. Mucormycosis (zygomycosis), an unusual fungal infection, is a specific sinus infection that may be seen in compromised hosts, such as those with severe diabetes mellitus. It has a particular tendency to spread progressively to adjacent tissues and to the central nervous system and is very difficult to treat.

General Diagnostic Approaches

Gram stain and cultures of sinus aspirates

Radiographic studies of the sinuses will confirm the diagnosis. If it becomes necessary to determine the specific infectious agent, fluid should be obtained directly from the affected sinus by needle puncture of the sinus wall or by catheterization of the sinus antrum after careful decontamination of the entry site. Gram smears and cultures are then made. Cultures of drainage from the antral orifices or nasal secretions are unreliable because of contaminating aerobic and anaerobic normal flora.

General Principles of Management

In uncomplicated acute sinusitis, prompt antimicrobial therapy is initiated. The choice of antibiotics is usually empirical, based on the most likely bacterial causes and their usual susceptibility. For example, ampicillin is effective against nearly all strains of *S. pneumoniae* and most strains of *H. influenzae.* Additional therapy consists of topical vasoconstricting agents, which may reduce edema of the antral orifices and facilitate drainage.

Severe, complicated acute infections and chronic sinusitis often require otolaryngologic consultation. In such cases, it is often necessary to obtain cultures directly from the sinuses to select specific antimicrobial therapy, consider the need for surgical procedures to adequately remove the pus and inflammatory tissues, and correct any anatomic obstruction that may exist.

Murray R. Robinovitch

Dental and Periodontal Infections

56

Dental caries, chronic marginal periodontal disease, and the sequelae of these two diseases constitute the majority of oral and dental infections. In both, the source of the causative bacteria is the microbial plaque that forms on the teeth. Thus, although dental caries and chronic marginal periodontal disease are distinctly different, the prevention and/or halting of the progression of these diseases relies upon the elimination of dental plaque from the tooth surfaces. In addition to causing caries and chronic marginal periodontitis, the bacteria of dental plaque play a role in acute necrotizing ulcerative gingivitis (Vincent's infection), another important oral infection.

role of
dental plaque

Dental plaque is a soft, adherent dental deposit that forms as a result of bacterial colonization of the tooth surface. It is rather insoluble, as well as adherent, and thus resists removal by water spray or mouth rinsing. Only more vigorous means such as tooth brushing and flossing between the teeth will remove it.

caries from
acid production
by plaque bacteria

progressive
demineralization

periodontal infection

Dental caries is the progressive destruction of the mineralized tissues of the tooth, primarily caused by the production of organic acids resulting from the glycolytic metabolic activity of plaque bacteria. The basic characteristic of the carious lesion is that it progresses inward from the tooth surface, be that the enamel-coated crown or the cementum of the exposed root surface, involving the dentin and finally the pulp of the tooth. From here, infection can extend out into the periodontal tissues at the root apex or apices.

Chronic marginal periodontal disease encompasses two separate disease entities: gingivitis and periodontitis. These diseases are believed to be related in that gingivitis is thought to be an early stage leading ultimately to periodontitis. The term *gingivitis* is used when the inflammatory condition is limited to the marginal gingiva and bone resorption around the necks of teeth has not yet appeared. *Periodontitis* is used to connote the stage of chronic marginal periodontal disease in which there is progressive loss of tooth support. Periodontitis can also lead to periodontal abscess when the chronic inflammatory state around the necks of the teeth becomes acute at a specific location.

loss of tooth
support

Chronic marginal periodontitis is responsible for most tooth loss in people more than 35–40 years of age. The adjectives *chronic* and *marginal* indicate that the disease progresses slowly and results in the progressive destruction of the supporting tissues of the tooth (peridontal ligament and alveolar bone) from the margins of the gingiva toward the apices of the roots of the teeth.

Acute periodontitis

There is also an acute form of periodontitis that affects young children (prepubertal periodontitis), a form with an age of onset of around puberty that affects adolescents and results in more rapid loss of tooth support (juvenile periodontitis), and an adult form of the disease that progresses quite rapidly (rapidly progressive periodontitis). These diseases are thought to be caused by plaque organisms different from those responsible for chronic marginal periodontitis and/or an altered host resistance to the disease.

Dental Plaque

attachment of bacteria to dental pellicle

The formation of dental plaque is the result of a very specific colonization of tooth surfaces by oral bacteria. The mineralized tooth surface is always coated with a thin organic film called the *dental cuticle* or *pellicle.* This coating results from adsorption and binding of specific salivary macromolecules, mainly proteins and glycoproteins, to the tooth surface. As this cuticle or pellicle can form in a matter of minutes after the tooth surface is exposed to the oral fluid, bacteria never interact directly with the mineralized tooth surface. Instead, bacterial adherence to the tooth, which begins the colonization of the tooth surface, is mediated by this organic film.

dental plaque comprises many species of bacteria, including anaerobes

A number of oral bacteria adhere readily to the cuticle-coated tooth. Primary among them are Gram-positive cocci, such as *Streptococcus sanguis,* and short Gram-positive rods, which are the initial colonizers. After 2–4 days, fusiform and filamentous organisms appear. Anaerobic vibrios, spirochetes, and Gram-negative, motile, anaerobic organisms appear at about 6–10 days. Thus, as the dental plaque increases in thickness, Gram-negative anaerobic organisms appear and multiply. The extent and complexity of involved bacteria is shown in Figure 56.1. Dental plaque would coat the tooth surfaces uniformly but for its physical removal during chewing and other oral activities. Characteristically, plaque remains in the non-self-clean-

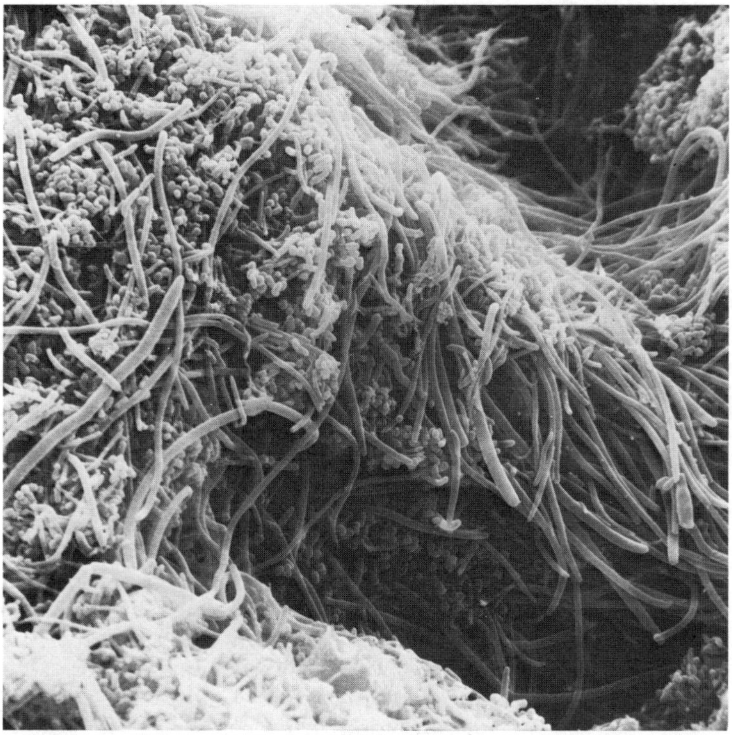

56.1 Scanning electronmicrograph of supragingival plaque. (*Kindly provided by Dr. W. Fischlsweiger and Dr. Dale Birdsell*).

plaque accumulates in non-self-cleansing areas of teeth and gingiva

subgingival plaque

sing areas of the teeth such as pits and fissures, along the margins of the gingiva, and between the teeth. In addition to this supragingival plaque, the sulcus around the tooth and periodontal pockets, which are pathologic extensions of this space, contain subgingival plaque. Subgingival plaque differs from supragingival plaque in that the former has an adherent zone next to the tooth surface and a nonadherent zone containing large numbers of Gram-negative, free-swimming, anaerobic microorganisms. Supragingival plaque lacks this nonadherent zone.

removal of plaque in oral hygiene

As the causative organisms of both dental caries and chronic marginal periodontal disease are believed to be in the dental plaque, a prime method for maintaining oral health is regular home care practices for plaque removal. Dental plaque cannot be effectively dispersed by chemical or enzymatic means, and the use of antibiotics for prophylactic inhibition of plaque formation cannot be clinically justified, although patients undergoing long-term antibiotic treatment for other medical reasons demonstrate a lower incidence of caries and periodontal disease. Antiseptic substances that bind to tooth surfaces and inhibit plaque formation, such as certain *bis*-biquanides (chlorhexidine, alexidine), have failed to gain approval by the U.S. Food and Drug Administration because of their side effects or lack of long-term effectiveness. Thus, tooth brushing and flossing, along with some other special means of physical plaque removal, remain virtually the only approach for eliminating the causative organisms and thus preventing caries and periodontal disease.

Dental Caries

greatest cause of tooth loss in child and young adult

factors in caries development

Dental caries is the single greatest cause of tooth loss in the child and young adult. Its onset can be very soon after the eruption of the teeth. The first carious lesions usually develop in pits or fissures on the chewing surfaces of the deciduous molars and result from the metabolic activity of the dental plaque that forms in these sites. Later in childhood, the incidence of carious lesions on smooth surfaces increases; these lesions are usually found between the teeth. The factors involved in the formation of a carious lesion are 1) a susceptible host or tooth; 2) the proper microflora on the tooth; and 3) a substrate from which the plaque bacteria can produce the organic acids that result in tooth demineralization.

The newly erupted tooth is most susceptible to the carious process. It gains protection against this disease during the first year or so by a process of posteruptive maturation believed to be attributable to improvement in the quality of surface mineral on the tooth.

role of saliva

Saliva provides protection against caries, and patients with dry mouth (xerostomia) suffer from high caries attack rates unless suitable measures are taken. In addition to the mechanical flushing and diluting action of saliva and its buffering capacity, the salivary glands also secrete several antibacterial products. Thus, saliva is known to contain lysozyme, a thiocyanate-dependent sialoperoxidase, and immunoglobulins, principally those of the secretory immunoglobulin A class. The individual importance of these antibacterial factors is unknown, but they clearly play some role in determining the ecology of the oral microflora.

protective effect of fluoride

Proper levels of fluoride, either systemically or topically, administered result in dramatic decreases in the incidence of caries (50–60% reduction by water fluoridation, 35–40% reduction by topical application). In the case of systemic fluoridation, the protective effect is thought to result from the incorporation of fluoride ions in place of hydroxyl ions of the hydroxyapatite during tooth formation, producing a more perfect and acid-resistant mineral phase of tooth structure. Topical application of fluoride is believed to achieve the same result on the surface of the tooth by initial dissolution of some of the hydroxyapatite, followed by recrystallization of apatite that incorporates fluoride ions into its lattice structure. Thus, the tooth can be made less susceptible to the cariogenic activity of dental plaque.

Role of microflora

The microbial basis of dental caries is well established, and Koch's postulates have been fulfilled for a number of microorganisms that cause the disease. This confirmation was achieved by using gnotobiotic (sterile) animals whose oral cavities could be colonized with a single organism. At times during the past half-century, a single microorganism was considered responsible for all caries; *Lactobacillus acidophilus* was regarded in this manner in the 1920s, and *Streptococcus mutans* enjoyed this reputation beginning in the 1960s. Currently, it is safe to say that any oral microorganism with a mechanism for colonizing the tooth surface or preexisting plaque and the ability to produce acid (acidogenic) and survive its action (aciduric) can be cariogenic. Organisms isolated from human carious lesions and shown to be cariogenic in gnotobiotic animals include some strains of *S. mutans, Streptococcus salivarius, Streptococcus sanguis, L. acidophilus, Lactobacillus casei, Actinomyces viscosus,* and *Actinomyces naeslundii.* Not all strains of these species are cariogenic.

several species may be cariogenic

substrate factors

Cariogenic organisms must be provided with an appropriate substrate for glycolysis to cause tooth demineralization, and dietary monosaccharides and disaccharides such as glucose, fructose, sucrose, lactose, and maltose are readily utilized by most oral bacteria. These carbohydrates permeate the dental plaque, are absorbed by the bacteria, and are metabolized sufficiently rapidly that organic acid products accumulate and cause the pH of the plaque to drop to levels sufficient to demineralize the tooth structure. Production of acid and the decreased pH are maintained until the substrate supply is exhausted. Obviously, high-sugar-content foods that adhere and have long oral clearance times are more cariogenic than less retentive foodstuffs such as sugar-containing liquids. Once the substrate is exhausted, the plaque pH returns slowly to its resting level. Frequency of application of substrate is extremely important, as the plaque pH may never reach its resting level.

significance of degree and duration of acid production

significance of synthesis of extracellular polyglycans from sucrose; adherence and carbohydrate storage

Dietary sucrose is also used in the synthesis of extracellular polyglycans such as dextrans and levans by some microorganisms that possess glucose transferase or fructose transferase enzymes on their cell surfaces. Synthesis of polyglycans is considered an additional virulence factor for two reasons: 1) The polyglycan-producing microorganisms are usually aggregated in its presence, which is believed to aid in the colonization of the tooth surface. *Streptococcus mutans* is a major cariogenic microorganism that acts in this way. 2) Extracellular polyglycan production may increase cariogenicity by serving as an extracellular storage form of substrate. Certain microorganisms synthesize extracellular polyglycan when sucrose is available, but then break it down into monosaccharide units to be used for glycolysis when dietary carbohydrate is exhausted. Thus, these microorganisms can prolong acidogenesis beyond the oral clearance time of the substrate.

significance of intracellular glycogen

Some oral bacteria also use dietary monosaccharides and disaccharides internally to form glycogen, which is stored intracellularly and used for glycolysis after the dietary substrate has been exhausted; thus, the period of acidogenesis is again prolonged and the cariogenicity of the microorganism increased. It is therefore clear that the ability to synthesize extracellular or intracellular storage polysaccharides, to colonize tooth surfaces, and to produce and survive in acid contributes to the microorganism's cariogenicity.

complications

The most common complications of dental caries are extension of the infection into the pulp chamber of the tooth (pulpitis), necrosis of the pulp, and extension of the infection through the root canals into the periapical area of the periodontal ligament. Periapical involvement may take the form of an acute inflammation (periapical abscess), a chronic nonsuppurating inflammation (periapical granuloma), or a chronic suppurating lesion that may drain into the mouth or onto the face via a sinus tract. A cyst may form within the chronic nonsuppurating lesion as a result of inflammatory stimulation of the epithelial rests normally found in the periodontal ligament. If the infectious agent is sufficiently virulent or host resistance is low, the infection may spread into the alveolar bone (osteomyelitis) or the fascial planes of the head and neck (cellulitis) or ascend along the venous channels to cause septic thrombophlebitis. As most carious lesions represent a mixed infection by the time cavities have developed, it is not surprising that most oral infections resulting from the extension of carious lesions are mixed and frequently caused by anaerobic organisms.

Chronic Marginal Periodontal Disease

Both chronic marginal gingivitis and periodontitis are now believed to be caused by certain bacteria in the dental plaque lying next to the gingival tissues. Thus, subgingival plaque found within the gingival crevice or the sulcus around the necks of the teeth is thought to house the etiologic agent(s). The characteristic histopathologic picture of gingivitis is of a marked inflammatory infiltrate of polymorphonuclear leukocytes, lymphocytes, and plasma cells in the connective tissue that lies immediately adjacent to the epithelium lining the gingival crevice and attached to the tooth. Collagen is lost from the inflamed connective tissue. There does not seem to be any direct invasion of the gingival tissues by intact bacteria.

role of subgingival plaque

mechanisms of tissue destruction

It has been proposed that tissue destruction is mediated by bacterial substances that pass through the epithelial barrier and cause either direct (for example, by bacterial enzymes or toxins) or indirect injury. Several mechanisms for indirect injury of the periodontal tissues have been proposed. These hypotheses include initiation of an unresolvable inflammatory response with excessive release of the lysosomal contents of polymorphonuclear leukocytes; activation of complement, which further magnifies the inflammatory response; and development of a host of humoral and cell-mediated immune responses, which can also magnify the inflammatory response as well as lead to tissue destruction through lymphokine release. Recently, because many oral bacteria have been found to contain potent polyclonal activators, it has been suggested that bacterial substances may lead to polyclonal activation of lymphocytes in the gingival tissues. Regardless of the mechanism of tissue destruction, the true source of the disease, namely, the causative bacteria, remains outside the gingival tissues and is therefore not susceptible to the body's defense mechanisms. For this reason, the disease continues to progress unless the dental plaque is removed and the involved tooth is kept plaque-free. If these measures are taken, chronic marginal gingivitis can resolve completely and the tissues return to normal.

bacterial source of disease is outside the affected tissues

bone resorption

As the disease progresses, a point may be reached at which the alveolar bone around the necks of the teeth is resorbed; the condition is then no longer termed gingivitis, but *periodontitis*. With resorption of the bone the attachment of the periodontal ligament is lost and the gingival sulcus deepens into a periodontal pocket. If unchecked, bone resorption progresses to loosening of the tooth, which may ultimately fall out. Occasionally, the neck of a periodontal pocket becomes constricted, the bacteria proliferate, causing an acute inflammatory response in the occluded pocket, and a periodontal abscess results. This acute exacerbation requires drainage in the same way as abscesses elsewhere for the patient to obtain relief from the symptoms.

periodontal abscess

Chronic marginal gingivitis will develop within 2 weeks in those who

Associated microflora

fail to practice effective tooth cleansing. It is not known whether particular species of plaque bacteria are responsible for gingival inflammation, but among those suspected of pathogenicity in the case of chronic marginal periodontitis are anaerobic Gram-negative rods (*Bacteroides gingivalis, Bacteroides melaninogenicus,* subspecies *intermedius, Fusobacterium nucleatum*), *Eikenella corrodens*, and some large spirochetes. Many of these organisms produce periodontal disease in monoinfected animals.

There is some evidence that the causative agents in rapidly progressing periodontal disease may differ from those associated with chronic marginal disease. In the condition known as juvenile periodontitis, a small anaerobic Gram-negative rod (*Actinobacillus actinomycetemcomitans*) and several species of another genus (*Capnocytophaga*) have been indicted based on studies of the flora of disease sites. In addition, it has been found that a significant proportion of patients with this condition demonstrate high serum antibody titers to *A. actinomycetemcomitans.*

Acute Necrotizing Ulcerative Gingivitis

Acute necrotizing ulcerative gingivitis is also known as *Vincent's infection* or *trench mouth.* This disease is distinctly different from chronic marginal periodontal disease. It has an acute onset, frequently associated with periods of stress and poor oral hygiene. There is rapid ulceration of the interdental areas of the gingiva, resulting in destruction of the interdental papillae. The inflammatory condition can quickly lead to pathologic bone resorption. Unlike chronic marginal periodontal disease, acute necrotizing ulcerative gingivitis is painful. As the oral epithelium is destroyed, the causative bacteria come into direct contact with the underlying tissues and may invade them. Spirochetes and fusiform bacteria have been implicated; thus, the term *fusospirochetal disease* has been used to describe this infection, which can also be manifested as ulceration in other areas of the pharynx or oral cavity. The disease may be treated with systemic antibiotics for immediate relief of symptoms, but resolution is dependent on thorough professional cleaning of the teeth and institution of good home care. Further details of fusospirochetal disease are provided in Chapter 24.

painful ulcerative lesions

fusospirochetal disease

Dental Plaque and Oral Flora in the Compromised Patient

As it can be the source of transient bacteremia, dental plaque must be viewed as a hazard in the compromised patient. The best example is the patient with heart valve damage as a result of a congenital anomaly, rheumatic fever, or a heart prosthesis. If transient bacteremia develops, the blood-borne bacteria may form vegetative growths in the heart and cause subacute bacterial endocarditis (Chapter 62). Such patients should always be placed on a course of prophylactic antibiotic therapy before any dental procedure is performed, including routine dental prophylaxis.

It has also been established that dental plaque organisms and other oral bacteria may give rise to serious systemic infections in patients whose host defense mechanisms are compromised. Patients who have undergone extensive radiation treatment of the jaw area, for example, are prone to develop osteomyelitis. Furthermore, one of the most frequent sources of fatal infections in leukemic patients is the oral cavity. Therefore, for these patients scrupulous home care and professional dental treatment are required.

Additional Reading and References

Genco, R.J., and Mergenhagen, S.E., Eds. 1982. *Host–Parasite Interactions in Periodontal Diseases.* Washington, D.C.: American Society for Microbiology.

Newbrun, E. 1983. *Cariology.* 2nd ed. Baltimore: Williams & Wilkins. These are authoritative reviews of caries and periodontal disease and new advances in understanding these conditions.

C. George Ray

Upper Respiratory Tract Infections and Stomatitis

57

Upper respiratory infections usually involve the nasal cavity and pharynx, and most (more than 80%) are caused by viruses. Like middle and lower respiratory illnesses, the diseases of the upper respiratory tract are named according to the anatomic sites primarily involved. *Rhinitis* (or coryza) implies inflammation of the nasal mucosa, *pharyngitis* denotes pharyngeal infection, and *tonsillitis* indicates an inflammatory involvement of the tonsils. Because of the close proximity of these structures to one another, infections may simultaneously involve two or more sites (for example, rhinopharyngitis or tonsillopharyngitis). All such infections are grouped under the general term *upper respiratory infections. Stomatitis* is a term used to describe infections primarily localized to the mucous membranes of the oral cavity. These infections can sometimes also involve the tongue (glossitis) or the gingival and periodontal tissues (gingivostomatitis or acute necrotizing ulcerative gingivitis (Chapter 56)).

Two other infections considered herein are peritonsillar abscess (quinsy), or retrotonsillar abscess, and retropharyngeal abscess. These infections are the result of direct invasion from mucosal sites and localization in deeper tissues to produce inflammation and abscess formation.

Common Clinical Features

Rhinitis and the common cold

Rhinitis is the most common manifestation of the common cold. It is characterized by variable fever, inflammatory edema of the nasal mucosa, and an increase in mucous secretions. The net result is varying degrees of nasal obstruction; the nasal discharge may be clear and watery at the onset of illness, becoming thick and sometimes purulent as the infection progresses over several days.

Pharyngitis and tonsillitis

Ulcerated lesions

Pharyngitis and tonsillitis are associated with pharyngeal pain (sore throat) and the clinical appearance of erythema and swelling of the affected tissues. There may be exudates, consisting of inflammatory cells overlying the mucous membrane, and petechial hemorrhages; the latter may be seen in viral infections, but tend to be more prominent in bacterial infections. Viral infections, particularly herpes simplex, may also lead to the formation of vesicles in the mucosa, which quickly rupture to leave ulcers. Pharyngeal candidiasis can also erode the mucosa under the plaques of "thrush." On rare occasions, the local inflammation may be sufficiently severe to produce *pseudomembranes,* which consist of necrotic tissue, inflammatory cells, and

Pharyngeal pseudomembranes

bacteria. This finding is particularly common in pharyngeal diphtheria, but may be mimicked by fusospirochetal infection (Vincent's angina) and sometimes by infectious mononucleosis. In acute tonsillitis or pharyngitis of any etiology, regional spread of the infecting agents with inflammation and tender swelling of the anterior cervical lymph nodes is also common.

Lymphadenitis

Stomatitis

Multiple ulcerative lesions of the oral mucosa, seen most frequently with severe primary herpes simplex infections, may extend to the tongue, lips, and face. In extreme cases, the pain may be so severe that the patient requires relief with topical anesthetics during the usual 9- to 12-day period of acute symptoms. *Candida* species can also invade oral surfaces to produce plaques identical to those of pharyngeal thrush. This infection is particularly common in young infants.

aphthous stomatitis (canker sores)

Aphthous stomatitis is a recurrent disease of the oral mucosa characterized by single or multiple painful ulcers with irregular margins, usually 2–10 mm in diameter. Healing usually occurs in a few days. The term commonly used to describe this condition is *canker sore.* The cause is unknown. It can easily be confused with recurrent herpes simplex lesions and, like herpes, tends to recur in relation to stress, menses, and other nonspecific stimuli.

noma

A severe, gangrenous stomatitis that progresses beyond the mucous membranes to involve soft tissues, skin, and sometimes bone can complicate a variety of acute illnesses in patients who are severely debilitated and whose oral hygiene is poor. This infection, called *noma* or *cancrum oris,* is rarely seen in the United States. Typical cases occur in underdeveloped countries among children with severe protein-calorie malnutrition. Measles will sometimes precipitate noma. Etiologic agents thought to be involved include *Fusobacterium* and *Bacteroides* species, as well as *Pseudomonas aeruginosa.*

Milder forms of stomatitis are seen in a variety of other common viral infections. Examples include Koplik's spots in measles, buccal or palatal ulcers in chickenpox, and similar phenomena in some enteroviral infections such as hand-foot-and-mouth disease.

Peritonsillar abscess

Abscesses in the peritonsillar area are usually a complication of tonsillitis. They are manifested by local pain, and examination of the pharynx reveals tonsillar asymmetry with one tonsil usually displaced medially by the abscess. This infection is most common in children more than 5 years of age and in young adults. If not properly treated, the abscess may spread to adjacent structures. It can involve the jugular venous system, erode into branches of the carotid artery to cause acute hemorrhage, or rupture into the pharynx to produce severe aspiration pneumonia.

Retropharyngeal abscess

Retropharyngeal abscesses occur most frequently in infants and children less than 5 years of age. They can result from pharyngitis or from accidental perforation of the pharyngeal wall by a foreign body. The infection is characterized by pain, inability or unwillingness to swallow, and, if the pharyngeal wall is displaced anteriorly near the palate, a change in phonation (nasal speech). The neck may be held in an extended position to relieve pain and maintain an open upper airway. Examination of the pharynx will usually reveal anterior bulging of the pharyngeal wall; if this finding is not apparent, lateral X-rays of the neck may demonstrate a widening of the space between the cervical spine and the posterior pharyngeal wall. The complications of retropharyngeal abscesses are basically the same as those described for peritonsillar abscesses; in addition, the suppurative process can extend posteriorly to the cervical spine to produce osteomyelitis or inferiorly to cause acute mediastinitis.

oral and pharyngeal lesions in immunocompromised hosts

In the immunocompromised patient, all of the various forms of stomatitis and pharyngitis described previously can be accentuated. Leukemia, agranulocytosis, chronic ulcerative colitis, congenital or acquired immunodeficiency, and treatment with cytotoxic or immunosuppressive drugs are commonly associated with such lesions. The marked damage to mucosal tissues that sometimes occurs can provide a portal of entry into deeper structures and then to the systemic circulation, creating a risk of bacterial or fungal sepsis. Conversely, oral lesions may also result from dissemination of infection from other remote sites. Examples include disseminated histoplasmosis and sepsis caused by *Pseudomonas* species.

Common Etiologic Agents

predominance of viral infections

S. pyogenes and *C. diphtheriae* infections

Gonococcal pharyngitis

Table 57.1 lists the more common causes of upper respiratory infections and stomatitis. Viral infections predominate. The most frequent bacterial cause to be considered is *Streptococcus pyogenes. Corynebacterium diphtheriae,* although rare in the United States, is a major pathogen that continues to cause infection in many other countries and must not be overlooked, particularly if clinical and epidemiologic findings suggest this possibility. *Neisseria gonorrhoeae,* isolated from adults with symptomatic pharyngitis in whom no other etiologic agent can be demonstrated, must now be considered a pharyngeal pathogen that is usually transmitted by oral–genital contact. Other bacteria occasionally implicated in acute pharyngitis and tonsillitis include *Corynebacterium pyogenes, Corynebacterium ulcerans, Francisella tularensis,* and β-hemolytic streptococci other than those of Lancefield group A; these are rare causes that are not specifically sought except in very unusual situations.

In patients with purulent rhinitis, sinusitis should also be considered in the differential diagnosis (Chapter 55). Unilateral and foul-smelling purulent discharge suggests the presence of a foreign body in the nose.

General Diagnostic Approaches

Viral infections

Although viruses cause the vast majority of upper respiratory infections, they are generally not amenable to specific therapy, and laboratory tests for viral infections are usually reserved for investigating outbreaks or in cases in which the illness seems unusually severe or atypical.

laboratory diagnosis of *S. pyogenes* infections

The primary diagnostic approach in pharyngitis and tonsillitis is to attempt to determine whether there is a bacterial cause requiring specific treatment. The only reliable method is to collect a throat swab for culture, taking care to thoroughly swab the tonsillar fauces as well as the posterior pharynx, and to include any purulent material from inflamed areas. Cultures are usually made only to detect the presence or absence of *S. pyogenes.*

For the laboratory diagnosis of diphtheria or pharyngeal gonorrhea, the clinical suspicion should be indicated to the laboratory so that specific cultures for *C. diphtheriae* or *N. gonorrhoeae* may be made.

evidence for pathogenic role of opportunists

Candida albicans species, fusospirochetal bacteria, *Pseudomonas* species, and other Gram-negative organisms are often found in pharyngeal or oral cultures from healthy individuals as well as in certain infections. Their probable pathogenic significance in association with disease in these sites, largely based on the appearance of the lesions and the presence of the organisms in large numbers, can be supported by histologic demonstration of tissue invasion by the organisms. It is important to remember that other bacterial pathogens such as *Streptococcus pneumoniae, Staphylococcus aureus, Haemophilus influenzae,* and even *Neisseria meningitidis* may be present in the pharynx. These organisms are *not* primary etiologic agents in rhinitis, pharyngitis, and tonsillitis, and their presence in the throat does *not* implicate them as causes of the illnesses described herein; they should instead be regarded as colonizers.

pathogens that may be present in normal flora but do not cause pharyngitis

The laboratory diagnosis of causes of peritonsillar and retropharyngeal abscesses is based on Gram staining and culture of purulent material obtained directly from the lesion, including anaerobic cultures.

Table 57.1 Major Infectious Causes of Upper Respiratory Disease

Disease	Viruses	Bacteria and Fungi
Rhinitis	Rhinoviruses; adenoviruses; coronaviruses; parainfluenza viruses; influenza viruses; respiratory syncytial virus; some Coxsackie A viruses	Rare
Pharyngitis or tonsillitis	Adenoviruses; parainfluenza viruses; influenza viruses; rhinoviruses; Coxsackie A or B viruses; herpes simplex virus; Epstein–Barr virus	*Streptococcus pyogenes*; *Corynebacterium diphtheriae*; *Neisseria gonorrhoeae*
Stomatitis	Herpes simplex virus; some Coxsackie A viruses	*Candida* species; *Fusobacterium* species and spirochetes
Peritonsillar or retropharyngeal abscess	None	*Streptococcus pyogenes* (most common); oral anaerobes such as *Fusobacterium* species; *Staphylococcus aureus* (rare); *Haemophilus influenzae* (usually in infants)

General Principles of Management

ten days of therapeutic levels of penicillin needed for *S. pyogenes* infections

Viral infections of the upper respiratory tract can only be treated symptomatically. If *S. pyogenes* is the bacteriologically proved cause, penicillin therapy is required unless specifically contraindicated, and therapeutic levels of the antibiotic should be maintained for at least 10 days. Such treatment prevents suppurative or toxigenic complications (for example, pharyngeal abscess, cervical adenitis, and scarlet fever) and the development of acute rheumatic fever. The latter, a serious complication, may occur in 1–3% of patients in certain population groups if they are not adequately treated. In addition, treatment of acute streptococcal infections can aid in reducing spread of the organisms to other persons. When the duration of therapy is less than 10 days, the risk of relapse and failure to eradicate the organisms is significantly increased.

Corynebacterium diphtheriae infections involve more complex management, which includes antitoxin as well as antibiotic treatment (detailed in Chapter 13). Infections caused by *N. gonorrhoeae* are treated with appropriate antibiotics (Chapter 16).

The management of stomatitis includes maintenance of adequate oral hygiene. If invasive *Candida* infection is present, topical and/or systemic antifungal therapy is sometimes necessary. Vincent's angina and other fusospirochetal infections are usually treated with systemic penicillin therapy as well as with appropriate dental and periodontal care. There is no specific, widely accepted treatment for aphthous stomatitis. Peritonsillar and retropharyngeal abscesses are treated aggressively with antibiotics and surgical drainage, taking care to prevent accidental aspiration of the abscess contents into the lower respiratory tract.

C. George Ray and Kenneth J. Ryan

Middle and Lower Respiratory Tract Infections

58

Middle Respiratory Tract Infection

most severe infections in childhood

For the purpose of this discussion, the middle respiratory tract will be considered to comprise the epiglottis, surrounding aryepiglottic tissues, larynx, trachea, and bronchi. Inflammatory disease involving these sites may be localized (for example, laryngitis) or more widespread (for example, laryngotracheobronchitis). The majority of severe infections occur in infancy and childhood. Disease expression varies somewhat with age, partly because the diameters of the airways enlarge with maturation and because immunity to common infectious agents increases with age. For example, an adult with a viral infection of the larynx (laryngitis) who was exposed to the same virus in childhood will have a relatively better immune response; in addition, the larger diameter of the larynx in the adult permits greater air flow in the presence of inflammation. An infant or child with the same infection in the same site can develop a much more severe illness, known as *croup,* which can lead to significant obstruction of air flow.

Common Clinical Features

Epiglottitis: swelling, edema, and inflammation of epiglottis

risk of acute airway obstruction

Epiglottitis is often characterized by the abrupt onset of throat and neck pain, fever, and inspiratory stridor (difficulty in moving adequate amounts of air through the larynx). Because of the inflammation and edema in the epiglottis and other soft tissues above the vocal cords (supraglottic area), phonation becomes difficult (muffled phonation or aphonia), and the associated pain leads to difficulty in swallowing. If this disease is not treated promptly, death may result from acute airway obstruction.

Laryngitis and Croup

subglottic infection

Laryngitis or its more severe form, croup, may have an abrupt onset (spasmodic croup) or develop more slowly over hours or a few days as a result of spread of infection from the upper respiratory tract. The illness is characterized by variable fever, inspiratory stridor, hoarse phonation, and a harsh, barking cough. In contrast to epiglottitis, the inflammation is localized to the subglottic, laryngeal structures, including the vocal cords. It sometimes extends to the trachea (laryngotracheitis) and bronchi (laryngotracheobronchitis), where it is associated with a deeper, more severe cough that may provoke chest pain and variable degrees of sputum production. When vocal cord inflammation is severe, transient aphonia may result.

Bronchitis

Bronchitis or tracheobronchitis may be a primary manifestation of infection or a result of spread from upper respiratory tissues. It is characterized by cough, variable fever, and sputum production, which is often clear at the onset but may become purulent as the illness persists. Auscultation of the chest with the stethoscope often reveals coarse bubbling rhonchi, which are a result of inflammation and increased fluid production in the larger airways.

association of chronic bronchitis with smoking, air pollution, and other diseases

acute exacerbations often associated with nontypable *H. influenzae* and with *S. pneumoniae*

Chronic bronchitis is a result of long-standing damage to the bronchial epithelium. A common cause is cigarette smoking, but a variety of environmental pollutants, chronic infections (for example, tuberculosis), and defects that hinder normal clearance of tracheobronchial secretions and bacteria (for example, cystic fibrosis) can be responsible. Because of the lack of functional integrity of their large airways, such patients are susceptible to chronic infection with members of the oropharyngeal flora and to recurrent, acute flare-ups of symptoms when they become colonized and infected by viruses and bacteria, particularly nontypable *Haemophilus influenzae* and *Streptococcus pneumoniae.* A vicious cycle of recurrent infection may evolve, leading to further damage and increasing susceptibility to pneumonia.

Common Etiologic Agents

With the exception of epiglottitis, acute diseases of the middle airway are usually caused by viral agents (Table 58.1). When acute airway obstruction is present, noninfectious possibilities must also be considered, such as aspirated foreign bodies and acute laryngospasm or bronchospasm caused by anaphylaxis.

Table 58.1 Major Causes of Acute Middle Respiratory Tract Disease

Syndrome	Viruses	Bacteria	Percentage Caused by Viruses
Epiglottitis	Rare	*Haemophilus influenzae* type b most common; also *Streptococcus pyogenes, Streptococcus pneumoniae, Corynebacterium diphtheriae, Neisseria meningitidis*	10
Laryngitis and croup	Parainfluenza virus, influenza virus, adenoviruses; occasionally respiratory syncytial virus, rhinoviruses, coronaviruses, echoviruses	Rare	90
Laryngotracheitis and laryngotracheobronchitis	Same as for laryngitis and croup	*Haemophilus influenzae* type b; *Staphylococcus aureus*	90
Bronchitis	Parainfluenza virus; influenza virus; respiratory syncytial virus; adenoviruses; measles	*Bordetella pertussis; Bordetella parapertussis; Haemophilus influenzae; Mycoplasma pneumoniae*	80

General Diagnostic Approaches

When a viral etiology is sought, the usual method of obtaining a specific diagnosis is by inoculation of tissue culture with material from the nasopharynx and throat. Acute and convalescent sera can also be collected to determine antibody responses to the common respiratory viruses and *Mycoplasma pneumoniae.* In bacterial infections, the following approaches are valuable.

high incidence of bacteremia in *H. influenzae* epiglottitis

local culture collection contraindicated in epiglottitis

Epiglottitis. Haemophilus influenzae type b, the most common cause of epiglottitis, produces an associated bacteremia in 85% of cases or more. Attempts to obtain local cultures from the epiglottis or throat are contraindicated because they may provoke acute reflex airway obstruction in patients who have not undergone intubation to ensure proper ventilation; furthermore, the yield is lower than that of blood culture. In addition, other bacterial agents that cause epiglottitis less frequently can often be isolated from the blood. The exception is *Corynebacterium diphtheriae* infection, in which local cultures of the nasopharynx or pharynx are required.

Laryngotracheitis and laryngotracheobronchitis. Although most cases of laryngotracheitis and laryngotracheobronchitis have a viral etiology, a severe purulent process is seen occasionally. Gram staining and culture of sputum or, better yet, purulent secretions obtained by direct laryngoscopy help to establish the causative agent. Blood cultures are again useful in such cases when bacteria are suspected.

nasopharyngeal specimens for diagnosis of pertussis

sputum examination for other bacteria

serodiagnosis of *Mycoplasma* infection

Acute bronchitis. A major bacteriologic consideration in acute bronchitis, especially in infants and preschool children, is *Bordetella pertussis.* Deep nasopharyngeal cultures plated on the appropriate media constitute the best specimens. Gram staining and examination of nasopharyngeal smears by direct fluorescent antibody methods are also useful adjuncts to establishing the diagnosis. When purulent sputum is produced, Gram staining and culture may be useful in suggesting other bacterial causes (Table 58.1). An exception is *M. pneumoniae* infection, which is most readily diagnosed by serologic testing of acute and convalescent sera.

General Principles of Management

maintenance of airway

chemotherapy for bacterial infections

The primary initial concern is ensuring an adequate airway. It is particularly crucial in epiglottitis, but can become a major issue in laryngitis or laryngotracheobronchitis as well. Thus, some patients will require placement of a rigid tube that provides communication between the tracheobronchial tree and the outside air (a nasotracheal tube or a surgically placed tracheostomy). Other adjunctive measures, such as highly humidified air and oxygen, may also provide relief in acute diseases involving the structures in and around the larynx. In proved or suspected bacterial infections, specific antibiotic therapy is required; other treatment, such as antitoxin administration in diphtheria, may also be necessary.

Lower Respiratory Tract Infection

Lower respiratory tract infection develops with invasion and disease of the lung, including the alveolar spaces and their supporting structure, the interstitium, and the terminal bronchioles. Infection may occur by extension of a middle respiratory tract infection, aspiration of pathogens past the upper airway defenses, or, less commonly, by hematogenous spread from a distant infection by inhalation, aspiration, extension from middle tract, or blood-borne route

infection through air passages associated with compromised local defenses

site such as an abscess or an infected heart valve. When infection develops through the respiratory tract, there is usually some compromise of the upper airway mechanisms for filtering or clearing inhaled infectious agents. The most common are those that impair the epiglottic and cough reflexes; such as drugs, anesthesia, stroke, and alcohol abuse. Toxic inhalations and cigarette smoking may also interfere with the normal mucociliary action of the tracheobronchial tree. In healthy persons, the most common antecedent to lower respiratory infection is infection of the middle respiratory structures (usually viral), allowing an otherwise innocuous aspiration of oropharyngeal flora to reach the lower tract and progress to disease rather than undergo rapid clearance. Some small infectious particles can accomplish airborne passage through the middle airway and bypass mucociliary defenses; if they can survive or multiply in alveolar macrophages, they may produce a primary infection. Examples include arthroconidia of *Coccidioides immitis* and cells of *Mycobacterium tuberculosis.*

Clinical Features

origin and characteristics of sputum

clinical signs

Acute pneumonia is an infection of the lung parenchyma that develops over hours to days and, if untreated, runs a natural course lasting days to weeks. The onset may be gradual, with malaise and slowly increasing fever, or sudden, as with the bed-shaking chill associated with the onset of pneumococcal pneumonia. The only early symptom referable to the lung may be cough, which is caused by bronchial irritation. In adults the cough becomes productive of sputum, which is purulent material generated in the alveoli and small air passages. In some cases the sputum may be blood streaked, rusty in color, or foul smelling. Shortness of breath (dyspnea), rapid respiratory rate, and sometimes cyanosis are signs of increasing loss of alveolar air-exchange surface through spread of exudate. Chest pain from involvement of the pleura is common. Physical signs on auscultation reflect the filling and eventual consolidation of alveoli by fluid and inflammatory cells. Consolidation of an entire area adjacent to the chest wall results in dullness to percussion over the site.

radiologic changes

The radiologic pattern of inflammatory changes in the lung is very useful in the diagnosis of pneumonia and for clinical differentiation into likely etiologic categories. The most common pattern is patchy infiltrates related to multiple foci centering on small bronchi (bronchopneumonia), which may progress to a more uniform consolidation of one or more lobes (lobar pneumonia). A more delicate, diffuse, or "interstitial" pattern, which is also common, is particularly associated with viral pneumonia.

Symptoms and signs

abscesses and cavities may develop

noninfectious causes

Chronic pneumonia has a slow insidious onset that develops over weeks to months and may last for weeks or even years. The initial symptoms are the same as those of acute pneumonia (fever, chills, and malaise), but they develop more slowly. Cough can develop early or late in the illness. As the disease progresses, appetite and weight loss, insomnia, and night sweat are common. Cough and sputum production may be the first indication of a vague constitutional illness referable to the lung. Bloody sputum (hemoptysis), dyspnea, and chest pain appear as the disease progresses. The physical findings and radiologic features can be similar to those of acute pneumonia, except that the diffuse interstitial infiltrates of viral pneumonia are uncommon. There may be parenchymal destruction and the formation of abscesses or cavities communicating with the bronchial tree. The clinical features of chronic pneumonia may also be caused by a number of infectious diseases or by noninfectious syndromes such as neoplasms, vasculitis, allergic conditions, infarction, radiation or toxic injury, and diseases of unknown etiology (for example, sarcoidosis).

infectious or noninfectious effusions

Pleural effusion is the transudation of fluid into the pleural space in response to an inflammatory process in adjacent lung parenchyma. It may result from a wide variety of causes, both infectious and noninfectious. *Empyema* is a purulent infection of the pleural space that develops when the infectious agent gains access by contiguous spread from an infected lung through a bronchopleural fistula or, less often, by extension of an abdominal infection through the diaphragm. Symptoms are usually insidious and related to the primary infection until enough exudate is formed to produce symptoms referable to the chest wall or to compromise the function of the lung. The physical and radiologic findings are characteristic, with dullness to percussion and localized opacities on X-ray that can be demonstrated by appropriate manipulation of the patient. In contrast to noninfectious effusions, empyema is frequently loculated.

purulent infection

Lung abscess is usually a complication of acute or chronic pneumonia caused by organisms that can cause localized destruction of lung parenchyma. It may occur as part of a chronic process or as an extension of an acute, destructive pneumonia, often after aspiration of oral or gastric contents. The symptoms of lung abscess, which are usually not specific, resemble those of chronic pneumonia or an acute pneumonia that has failed to resolve. Persistent fever, cough, and the production of foul-smelling sputum are typical. Lung abscess can be diagnosed and localized with certainty only radiologically; it appears as a localized area of inflammation with single or multiple excavations or as a cavity with an air–fluid level. Multiple abscesses may develop as a result of blood-borne infection.

freuquently follows aspiration pneumonia

blood-borne infection

Common Etiologic Agents

The infectious agents that cause lower respiratory infection most frequently are listed in Table 58.2. The etiology of acute pneumonia is strongly dependent on age. More than 90% of pneumonias in infants and children are caused by viruses, whereas less than 10–20% of pneumonias in adults are viral. The reasons are probably the same as those indicated previously for middle respiratory tract infections. Influenza and other viruses, however, may provide the initial predisposition toward bacterial infection. Viruses are extremely rare as a cause of chronic as opposed to acute lower respiratory tract infections, although some symptoms of the acute infection, such as cough, may persist for weeks until the bronchial damage has healed. Influenza virus is noteworthy as a cause of acute life-threatening pneumonia, even in previously healthy young adults. Pneumonia caused by bacteria such as enteric Gram-negative rods, *Pseudomonas,* and *Legionella* is primarily limited to adult patients with serious debilitating underlying disease or as a complication of hospitalization and its procedures (nosocomial infection). *Klebsiella pneumoniae* has been known to produce community-acquired pneumonia under conditions similar to those for *S. pneumoniae* infection. At any age the pneumococcus is the most common bacterial cause of acute pneumonia, and Gram-negative infections other than *Haemophilus* are rare in children unless they have cystic fibrosis.

most pneumonias viral in infants and children

viral infections cause predisposition to acute bacterial pneumonia

Gram-negative pneumonias in debilitated hosts

pneumococcus most common cause of acute bacterial pneumonia

Causes of lung abscess

Lung abscess and empyema follow infections with the more destructive organisms or massive aspiration of mixed anaerobic flora from the oropharynx. Several clinical clues can suggest some of the etiologic agents, given a typical clinical syndrome. For example, *Nocardia* and mycobacteria, which are strict aerobes, tend to produce upper lobe infiltrates, whereas aspiration pneumonia caused by anaerobes tends to develop in the most dependent parts of the lung. Textbooks on infectious disease should be consulted for further details regarding these features.

Table 58.2 Major Causes of Lower Respiratory Tract Infection

Syndrome	Viruses	Bacteria	Fungi	Other Agents
Acute pneumonia	Influenza Parainfluenza Adenovirus Respiratory syncytial (infants)	*Streptococcus pneumoniae* *Staphylococcus aureus* *Haemophilus influenzae* Enterobacteriaceae *Legionella* Mixed anaerobes (aspiration) *Pseudomonas aeruginosa*[b]	*Candida albicans*[b] *Aspergillus* species	*Mycoplasma pneumoniae* *Pneumocystis carinii*[b]
Chronic pneumonia	Rare	*Mycobacterium tuberculosis,* Other Mycobacteria; *Nocardia*	*Coccidioides immitis*[c] *Blastomyces dermatitidis*[c] *Histoplasma capsulatum*[c] *Cryptococcus neoformans*	*Paragonimus westermani*[c]
Lung abscess	None	Mixed anaerobes *Actinomyces* *Nocardia* *Staphylococcus aureus*[d] Enterobacteriaceae[d] *Pseudomonas aeruginosa*[b,d]	*Aspergillus* species	*Entamoeba histolytica*
Empyema	None	Mixed anaerobes *Staphylococcus aureus*[d] *Streptococcus pneumoniae*[d] Enterobacteriaceae *Pseudomonas aeruginosa*[b,d]	Rare	

[a]Occurrence limited to seasonal epidemics.
[b]Primarily infects the immunologically compromised host.
[c]Geographically limited.
[d]Infection develops during or after acute pneumonia.

Diagnosis

The degree of difficulty in establishing an etiologic diagnosis for a lower respiratory tract infection depends on the number of organisms produced in respiratory secretions and on whether the causative species is normally found in the oropharyngeal flora. In the presence of typical clinical findings, the isolation of influenza virus from the throat or of *M. tuberculosis* from sputum is sufficient for diagnosis of influenza or tuberculosis, because these organisms are not normally found in such sites. The same cannot be said for *S. pneumoniae* and most bacterial pathogens, as they may be found in the throat in a significant number of healthy persons (Chapter 12).

Sputum collection and evaluation: Problems of contamination

The examination of expectorated sputum has been the primary means of diagnosing the causes of bacterial pneumonia, but this approach has several advantages and disadvantages. The advantages are ease of collection and absence of risk to the patient. The primary disadvantages are confusing results from contamination of the sputum with oropharyngeal flora in the process of expectoration and excessive contamination with saliva. Efforts to remove saliva from sputum by washing or to accomplish interpretive differentiation of infective from normal flora by quantitative culture (as with urine specimens) (Chapter 60) have been unsuccessful. The quality of a sputum sample can be enhanced by collection early in the morning (just after the patient arises), careful instruction of the patient, and occasionally

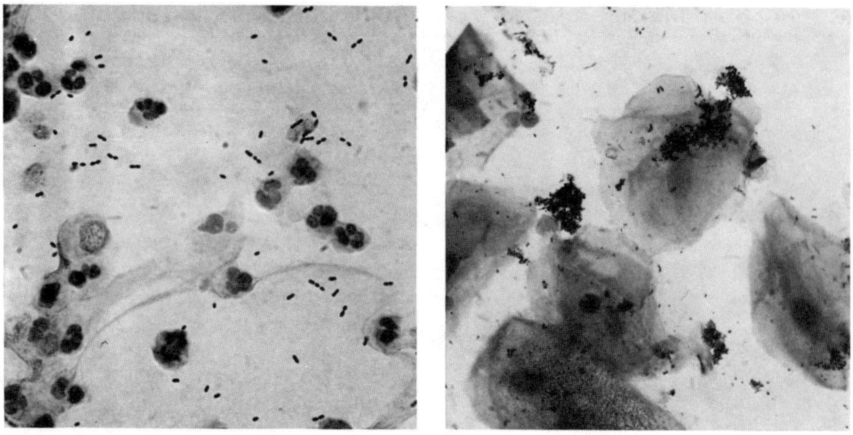

A B

58.1 Comparison of findings in sputum and saliva. True sputum (**A**) should show an abundance of inflammatory cells and no squamous epithelial cells. In acute bacterial pneumonia, large numbers of a single organism are usually present. This Gram smear shows large numbers of polymorphonuclear leukocytes and *Streptococcus pneumoniae.* Saliva (**B**) typically contains squamous epithelial cells and a mixed bacterial population.

by the use of saline aerosols or mists under the supervision of an inhalation therapy specialist. The worst results can be expected when the physician's only involvement is writing an order, which is then passed down the ward chain of command to an orderly, who directs the patient to put his "sputum" in a cup placed at the bedside.

Microscopic characteristics of sputum and saliva

Microscopic examination before culture of direct Gram smears of specimens alleged to be sputum has proved useful. Polymorphonuclear leukocytes and large numbers of a single morphologic type of organism are typical findings in sputum from a patient with bacterial pneumonia. Squamous epithelial cells from the oropharynx and a mixed bacterial population are characteristic of saliva (Figure 58.1). Unfortunately, most specimens are a mixture of both, which makes interpretation more difficult. Studies of such specimens have shown that more than 10–25 squamous epithelial cells per low-power ($\times 10$) microscopic field are evidence of excessive salivary contamination, and such specimens should not be cultured because the results may be misleading. Thus, the direct Gram smear is crucial to the use of expectorated sputum for diagnosis of acute bacterial pneumonia. The smear may be useful in the absence of cultural results, but cultures are useless without a Gram smear to assess specimen quality.

Salivary specimens should not be cultured

Another approach is to attempt a more direct collection from the lung using methods that bypass the oropharyngeal flora. This approach may be used in patients who are not producing sputum (children rarely do) or in cases where analysis of expectorated sputum has been inconclusive. The major techniques are shown in Figure 58.2. In transtracheal aspiration, an incision is made in the cricothyroid membrane and a catheter advanced deep into the tracheobronchial tree to aspirate sputum directly. This method is useful in diagnosis of both pneumonia and lung abscess, but is not considered safe in children. Any aspiration method that involves initial passage through the upper airway (including bronchoscopy) is less reliable than transtracheal aspiration, because the collection instruments become contaminated with oropharyngeal secretions. Aspirates from tracheostomies are also of limited value, because these sites become colonized with Gram-negative bacteria within hours of their implantation. Direct aspiration through the chest wall can be used for diagnosis of pneumonia or empyema if the involved area can be well localized and is at the lung periphery. In some cases an open lung biopsy is the only way to obtain diagnostic material. Bacteremia may occur in acute pneumonia, particularly in its early stages, and a positive

Transtracheal aspiration

Direct transpleural aspiration and open biopsy

Value of blood culture in acute pneumonia

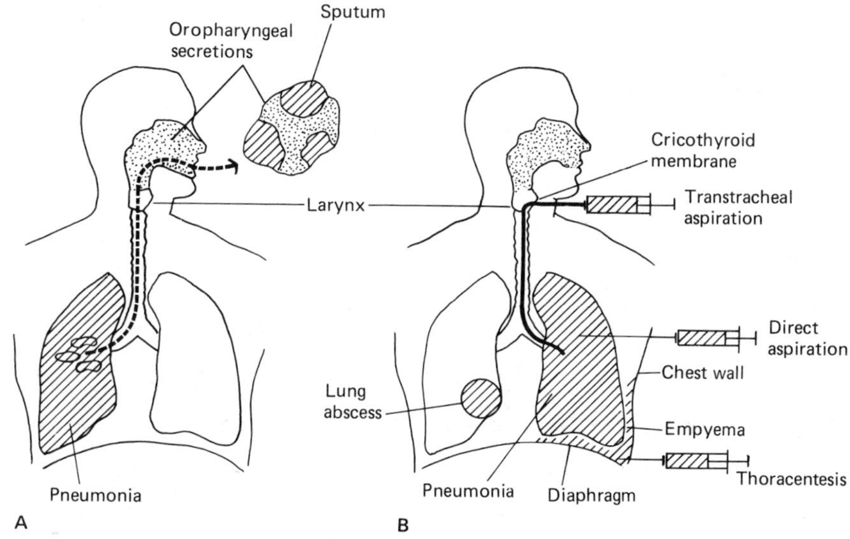

58.2. Techniques of specimen collection for diagnosis of lower respiratory tract infection. (**A**) Expectorated sputum must pass through the area above the larynx, which contains the normal oropharyngeal flora. The "sputum" may then be a mixture of both true sputum and other secretions. (**B**) Invasive collection techniques bypass the oropharyngeal flora to collect the purulent material directly. Some infections, such as empyema or lung abscess, may only be reached by direct aspiration or surgical procedures. Transtracheal aspiration collects material from below the larynx via a catheter inserted through the cricothyroid membrane.

blood culture will serve to confirm a diagnosis based on clinical findings or those of expectorated sputum culture. For this reason blood cultures are considered an essential part of the diagnostic workup of pneumonia.

anaerobic infections cannot be diagnosed from sputum

Once an appropriate specimen is obtained, diagnosis is usually readily made by culture using the methods described in Chapter 9 and in the sections on the individual etiologic agents. Only specimens collected by one of the invasive techniques should be used for anaerobic culture, because expectorated sputum is invariably contaminated with oropharyngeal anaerobes and results are meaningless. With some agents (*S. pneumoniae, H. influenzae*), detection of circulating antigen in the blood or urine by counterimmunoelectrophoresis may establish the diagnosis.

Management

The general principles of management of lower respiratory tract infections are similar to those of middle tract infections. Drainage and surgical measures are needed more often as an adjunct to antimicrobial therapy in the case of chronic pneumonia, lung abscess, and empyema. When bacterial infection is considered, empirical therapy is usually given until the results of cultures and antimicrobial susceptibility tests are available. Treatment may vary from penicillin alone for a child, in whom the most reasonable nonviral possibility is *S. pneumoniae,* to multiple drugs for a debilitated or immunosuppressed patient, in whom the possibilities are much broader. A direct Gram stain on a properly collected specimen may indicate the probable diagnosis and be helpful in selecting therapy.

Kenneth J. Ryan

Enteric Infections and Food Poisoning

59

High mortality from diarrheal diseases in developing countries

Acute infections of the gastrointestinal tract are among the most frequent of all illneses, exceeded only by respiratory tract infections such as the common cold. Diarrhea is the most common manifestation of these infections; however, because it is usually self-limiting within hours or days, most of those afflicted do not seek medical care. Nonetheless, in the United States gastrointestinal infection remains one of the three most common syndromes seen by physicians who practice general medicine. Worldwide, diarrheal disease remains one of the most important causes of morbidity and mortality among infants and children. It has been estimated that in Asia, Africa, and Latin America, depending on socioeconomic and nutritional factors, a child's chance of dying of a diarrheal illness before the age of 7 years can be as high as 50%. In developed countries mortality is lower, but still significant. This chapter will summarize the known etiologies and epidemiologic circumstances of these infections, as well as diagnostic methods and some aspects of management. Chapters on the individual etiologic agents should be consulted for details.

Clinical Features

The most prominent clinical features of gastrointestinal infections are fever, vomiting, abdominal pain, and diarrhea. Their presence varies with different diseases and different stages of infection. The occurrence of diarrhea is a central feature, and its presence and nature form the basis for classification of gastrointestinal infections into three major syndromes: watery diarrhea, dysentery, and enteric fever.

Watery Diarrhea

loss of fluid from proximal small intestine

The most common form of gastrointestinal infection is the rapid development of frequent intestinal evacuations of a more or less fluid character known as diarrhea (*dia-* + the Greek *rhein,* to flow through, as a stream). Nausea, vomiting, fever, and abdominal pain may also be present, but the dominant feature is intestinal fluid loss. Diarrhea is produced by pathogenic mechanisms that attack the proximal small intestine, the portion of the bowel in which more than 90% of physiologic net fluid absorption occurs. The purest form of watery diarrhea is that produced by enterotoxin-secreting bacteria such as *Vibrio cholerae* and *Escherichia coli,* which cause fluid loss without fever. Other common pathogens that damage the epithelium, such as rotaviruses, also cause fluid loss, but are more likely to cause fever and vomiting as well. Most cases of watery diarrhea run an acute but brief (1–3 days) self-limiting course. Exceptions are those caused by *V. cholerae,* which usually produces a more severe illness, and those caused by *Giardia lamblia,* which produces a watery diarrhea that may last for weeks.

Dysentery

colonic infection with inflammation

pus and blood in stools

Dysentery begins with the rapid onset of frequent intestinal evacuations, but the stools are of smaller volume than in watery diarrhea and contain blood and pus. If watery diarrhea is the "runs," dysentery is the "squirts." Fever, abdominal pain, cramps, and tenesmus are frequent complaints. Vomiting occurs less often. In dysentery the focus of pathology is the colon. Organisms causing dysentery can produce inflammatory and/or destructive changes in the colonic mucosa either by direct invasion or by production of cytotoxins. This damage produces the pus and blood seen in the stools, but does not result in substantial fluid loss because the absorptive and secretory capacity of the colon is much less than that of the small bowel. Dysenteric infections generally last longer than the common watery diarrheas, but most cases still resolve spontaneously in 2–7 days.

Enteric Fever

serious systemic disease with lymphoid and reticuloendothelial invasion

Enteric fever is a systemic infection, the origin and focus of which are the gastrointestinal tract. The most prominent features are fever and abdominal pain, which develop gradually over a few days in contrast to the abrupt onset of the other syndromes. Diarrhea is usually present, but may be mild and not appear until later in the course of the illness. The classic enteric fever is typhoid fever, which is produced by *Salmonella typhi* and described in detail in Chapter 20. The pathogenesis of enteric fever is more complex than that of watery diarrhea or dysentery. It generally involves penetration of the mucosa of the distal small bowel with subsequent spread outside the bowel to the biliary tract, liver, mesentery, or reticuloendothelial organs. Bacteremia is common, occasionally causing metastatic infection in other organs. Typhoid fever is the only infection for which these events have been well studied. Although it is usually self-limiting, enteric fever carries a significant risk of serious disease and even death. The duration of illness is not well established except for typhoid fever, which lasts 3–4 weeks when untreated.

Etiology

In the past 15 years, great advances have been made in our understanding of gastrointestinal infections. Before the late 1960s, fewer than 20% of the infectious syndromes described previously could be linked to a specific etiologic agent by any diagnostic method. The organisms listed in Table 59.1 now account for 60–80% of cases, although diagnostic methods for all of them are not yet available in all laboratories. The primary clinical syndrome caused by each agent is also listed in Table 59.1, but should not be regarded as absolute because symptoms and signs vary significantly from patient to patient and even at different times in the course of the same illness. For example, *Shigella* infections frequently go through a brief watery diarrhea stage before localizing in the colon, and *Campylobacter* enteritis usually begins with fever, malaise, and abdominal pain, followed by dysentery. In any single case the clinical findings may suggest a range of etiologic

Table 59.1 Features of Infectious Gastrointestinal Syndromes

Organism	Common Distribution	Clinical Syndrome
1. *Salmonella enteritidis*	Worldwide	Dysentery
2. *Salmonella typhi*	Tropical, underdeveloped countries	Enteric fever
3. *Shigella* sp.	Worldwide	Dysentery
4. *Shigella dysenteriae* (Shiga)	Tropical, underdeveloped countries	Dysentery
5. *Campylobacter fetus*	Worldwide	Dysentery
6. *Escherichia coli* (invasive)	Worldwide	Dysentery
7. *Escherichia coli* (enterotoxigenic)	Worldwide	Watery diarrhea
8. *Vibrio cholerae*	Asia, Africa, Middle East, Louisiana	Watery diarrhea
9. *Vibrio parahemolyticus*	Seacoast	Watery diarrhea
10. *Yersinia enterocolitica*	Worldwide	Enteric fever[d]
11. *Clostridium difficile*	Worldwide	Dysentery
12. *Clostridium perfringens*	Worldwide	Watery diarrhea
13. *Bacillus cereus*	Worldwide	Watery diarrhea
14. Rotavirus	Worldwide	Watery diarrhea
15. Parvo/picornavirus	Worldwide	Watery diarrhea
16. *Giardia lamblia*	Worldwide	Watery diarrhea
17. *Entamoeba histolytica*	Worldwide	Dysentery

Abbreviations: WBCs = white blood cells; PMNs = polymorphonuclear leukocytes.

agents, but are not sufficiently specific to be diagnostic of any single organism.

Importance of epidemiologic setting in preliminary diagnosis

The epidemiologic setting of the infection is of great importance in assessing the relative probability of each of the agents listed in Table 59.1. When combined with clinical findings, the differential diagnosis can usually be limited to two or three organisms. The major epidemiologic settings are 1) endemic infection; 2) epidemic infection; 3) traveler's diarrhea; 4) food poisoning; and 5) hospital-associated diarrhea.

Endemic Infections

By definition, endemic diarrheas are those that occur sporadically in the usual living circumstances of the patient (from the Greek *endemos,* dwelling in a place). Some organisms are endemic worldwide, whereas others are geographically limited. There are also seasonal variations and age-related attack rates within the endemic foci. In developed countries the most common causes of endemic gastrointestinal infections are rotaviruses, parvo/picornaviruses, *Campylobacter, Salmonella,* and *Shigella.* All are more common in infants and children because they are more prone to fecal–oral spread and because development of immunity is related to age. Rotaviruses account for 40–60% of diarrheal infections occurring during the cooler months in

higher frequency in infants and children

Table 59.1 *(continued)*

	Laboratory Diagnosis[a]					
		Culture			Serology	
Pathogenic Mechanism	Stool Microscopy	Stool[b]	Blood	Toxin in Stools	Antibody Detection	Antigen Detection
1. Mucosal invasion	WBCs (PMNs)	+	–	–	–	–
2. Penetration, spread	WBCs (monocytes)	+	+	–	+	–
3. Mucosal invasion	WBCs (PMNs)	+	–	–	–	–
4. Mucosal invasion, cytotoxin	WBCs (PMNs)	+	+	–	–	–
5. Unknown	WBCs (PMNs)	+	–	–	–	–
6. Mucosal invasion	WBCs (PMNs)	+[c]	–	–	–	–
7. Enterotoxin(s)	–	+[c]	–	–	–	–
8. Enterotoxin	–	+	–	–	–	–
9. Unknown	–	+	–	–	–	–
10. Penetration, spread	–	+	+	–	–	–
11. Cytotoxin, enterotoxin	–	+	–	+	–	–
12. Enterotoxin	–	+	–	–	–	–
13. Enterotoxin	–	+	–	–	–	–
14. Mucosal destruction	Electron microscopy[c]	–	–	–	–	+[c]
15. Mucosal destruction	Electron microscopy	–	–	–	–	–
16. Mucosal irritation	Flagellates, cysts	–	–	–	–	–
17. Mucosal invasion	Amebas, WBCs (PMNs)	–	–	–	+	–

[a]Plus sign indicates procedure is useful and usually available in clinical laboratories.
[b]Which cultures are done routinely depends on the laboratory and/or the physician's request.
[c]Appropriate methods may be available only in a limited number of laboratories.
[d]Infection may also manifest watery diarrhea or dysentery.

infants and children less than 2 years of age, but are uncommon in older persons.

Geographic limitations of some agents

The geographically limited agents (Table 59.1) are common only in the endemic areas listed. These distributions are not fixed, making it necessary to keep abreast of geographic changes in the distribution of established agents as well as the recognition of new ones. For example, cholera has long been limited to warm-climate river deltas in Asia, Africa, and the Middle East, but recently an endemic focus of *V. cholerae* in the United States was discovered off the coast of Louisiana.

Epidemic Infections

spread of typhoid, cholera, and shigellosis where hygiene is poor or after major disasters

Under certain epidemiologic conditions some of the organisms responsible for endemic infections can spread beyond the family unit to cause epidemics involving regional, national, and even international populations. The diarrheal diseases most frequently associated with epidemics are typhoid fever, cholera, and shigellosis. For all three, epidemics are related to the failure of basic public health sanitary measures. For example, *S. typhi* and *V. cholerae* may be spread for some distance through the community water supply, a route blocked by modern sewage and water treatment practices. When these procedures are not employed or are interrupted by equipment failure or natural disasters (floods, earthquakes), these diseases can and do recur in epidemic form. Epidemics of shigellosis may be water-borne under the same conditions, but *Shigella* dysentery is more typically a disease "of wars and armies, and of crowds and movement."* The very low infecting dose of *Shigella* can make spread through direct contact reach epidemic proportions when crowding and poor sanitary facilities are combined.

Although such epidemics are usually associated with the 19th century, it is clear that the potential remains. In the late 1970s large epidemics of both typhoid fever and shigellosis spread through Central and South America. In 1973 more than 200 cases of typhoid fever in Florida were associated with a defective chlorinator in the local water system.

Traveler's Diarrhea

Travelers from developed to less developed countries all too frequently experience a diarrheal illness in the first week that is usually brief but can be serious. The common names applied to this syndrome, such as "Delhi belly" and "Montezuma's revenge," reflect geographic associations and the cumulative frustration of those forced to spend part of their vacation next to the toilet rather than the swimming pool.

Predominant role of enterotoxigenic *E. coli*

The most extensive studies of traveler's diarrhea have involved travelers from the United States to Latin American countries, particularly Mexico. In nearly one-half of these cases the diarrhea is caused by enterotoxigenic strains of *E. coli* acquired during travel. *Shigella* infections account for another 10–20%, and the remaining cases are attributable to various pathogens or unknown causes. Ingestion of uncooked or incompletely cooked foods is the most likely source of infection, but most epidemiologic studies have not shown specific food associations. An exception is the strong relationship between toxigenic *E. coli* diarrhea and the consumption of salads containing raw vegetables. "Don't drink the water" still seems like sound advice for travelers to countries where hygiene remains poor, but the adage is not well supported by studies relating infection to water or ice consumption.

Food Poisoning

Single-source outbreaks

Many gastrointestinal infections involve food as a vehicle of transmission. The term *food poisoning,* however, is usually reserved for instances in which a single meal can be incriminated as the source. This situation typically arises when multiple cases of the same gastrointestinal syndrome develop at the same time among persons whose only common experience is a meal shared at a social event or restaurant. The probable etiologic agent can usually be assessed from knowledge of the incubation period, the food vehicle, and the clinical findings.

Disease from ingestion of preformed toxin

Infective disease

The most common causes of food poisoning are shown in Table 59.2. Some are not infections but intoxications, caused by ingestion of a toxin produced by bacteria in the food before it was eaten. Intoxications generally have shorter incubation periods than infections and may involve extraintestinal symptoms (for example, botulism). Food poisoning does not differ from endemic diarrheal infections caused by the same species. The length of the incubation period and the severity of the symptoms are generally related to the number of organisms in the infecting dose.

*Christie, A. B. 1974. *Infectious Disease, Epidemiology and Clinical Practice.* 2nd ed. New York: Churchill Livingstone, p. 137.

Table 59.2 Clinical and Epidemiologic Features of Food Poisoning

Etiology	Percentage of Cases[a]	Typical Incubation Period	Primary Clinical Findings	Characteristic Foods
INTOXICATION[b]				
Bacillus cereus (vomiting toxin)	1–2	1–6 hr	Vomiting	Rice
Clostridium botulinum	5–15	12–72 hr	Neuromuscular paralysis	Improperly preserved vegetables, meat, fish
Staphylococcus aureus	15–25	2–4 hr	Vomiting	Meats, custards, salads
Chemical[c]	20–25	0.1–48 hr	Variable	Variable
INFECTIONS[d]				
Bacillus cereus (diarrheal toxin)	1–2	6–24 hr	Watery diarrhea	Meat, poultry, vegetables
Clostridium perfringens	5–15	9–15 hr	Watery diarrhea	Meat, poultry
Salmonella	10–30	6–48 hr	Dysentery	Poultry, eggs, meat
Shigella	2–5	12–48 hr	Dysentery	Variable
Vibrio parahemolyticus	1–2	10–24 hr	Watery diarrhea	Shellfish
Trichinella spiralis	5–10	3–30 days	Fever, myalgia	Meat, especially pork
Hepatitis A	1–3	10–45 days	Hepatitis	Shellfish

[a]Based on documented outbreaks reported to the Centers for Disease Control, Atlanta (variable from year to year).
[b]Disease caused by toxin in food at time of ingestion.
[c]Includes heavy metals, monosodium glutamate, mushrooms, and various toxins of nonmicrobial origin.
[d]Disease caused by infection after ingestion.

association with deficiencies in food preparation and storage temperature

The epidemiologic circumstances of food poisoning vary with the etiologic agent, but virtually always involve a breach in the recommended procedures for handling food. The organisms may be present as contaminants in raw food before cooking or introduced by a carrier or contaminated utensil involved in preparation. Causes of bacterial food poisoning include failure to kill the organisms by adequate cooking, almost always followed by a period of warming (incubation) long enough for the organisms to multiply to infectious numbers or, in the case of toxigenic disease, to produce sufficient toxin to cause disease. In 80–90% of investigated outbreaks of bacterial food poisoning, the most important contributing factor is the use of improper storage temperatures for the food. This factor may obtain in home-cooked meals as well as those prepared in restaurants, in schools, or at large social events such as church picnics. An example of typical circumstances for a *Salmonella* outbreak is provided in Chapter 20.

Frequency of reported outbreaks

The relative frequency of each etiologic agent and the foods most frequently involved are also shown in Table 59.2. This information is based on outbreaks investigated by public health agencies but because of differences in reporting rules and practices, may not reflect the actual incidence of each. Large outbreaks, restaurant-associated outbreaks, and outbreaks involving serious illness with hospitalization or death are all more likely to be reported to health authorities than are mild diarrheas after a dinner party. In recent years, of the 400–500 outbreaks (10,000–15,000 cases) reported each year in the United States, fewer than 200 are "solved." Food poisoning characterized by a short incubation period (for example, *Staphylococcus aureus*) is more likely to be recognized because it can easily be associated with a specific meal and because the food itself may still be available for examination. There are also large geographic differences in reporting. For example, in 1979, New York City, in which 50% of the state population resides, reported 98% of New York State's food-borne outbreaks, and Connecticut reported more outbreaks than all of the southeastern states combined.

Determination of causes

Sampling problems aside, the food poisoning syndromes listed in Table 59.2 are well recognized, with *Salmonella, Clostridium perfringens,* and *S. aureus* accounting for more than 70% of those for which a microbial etiology can be found. For bacterial infections such as *Salmonella* and *Shigella,* which are not normal members of the stool flora, establishing the diagnosis by isolating the causative organism is relatively easy. If the circumstances indicate *C. perfringens* or *S. aureus* food poisoning, investigation will involve cultures of vomitus, stool from several cases, and the suspect food. In some cases, toxin detection will be required to establish the etiology and source. Such investigations are best coordinated by public health authorities, who can also address the legal and community implications of the outbreak. For example, one investigation of *Salmonella* food poisoning led to the discovery that the owner of a restaurant was keeping and slaughtering chickens at the restaurant. Although this practice may have provided very fresh chicken, it guaranteed *Salmonella* contamination of the entire kitchen.

Hospital-Associated Diarrhea

Enteropathogenic *E. coli* and *C. difficile*

The hospital environment should not allow spread of the usual causes of endemic intestinal infection. When such infection occurs, it can usually be traced to an employee who continues working while ill or to contaminated food prepared outside the hospital that is "smuggled" in by the patient's friends. Two special causes of hospital-associated diarrhea are *E. coli* in infants and *C. difficile* in patients treated with antimicrobial agents. The relative role of enterotoxigenic and the so-called enteropathogenic strains of *E. coli* in nursery outbreaks of diarrhea is controversial and is discussed in Chapter 20. The disease is highly infectious among newborns. Fortunately, such outbreaks have become rare. *Clostridium difficile* accounts for more than 90% of cases of a syndrome that ranges from mild diarrhea to fulminant pseudomembranous colitis during or after treatment with antibiotics. The disease is mediated by a cytotoxin and/or an enterotoxin produced in vivo by *C. difficile.* Rotaviruses can also cause hospital outbreaks in infants.

Diagnosis

Laboratory diagnostic procedures, summarized in Table 59.1, include microscopic examination, culture, toxin detection, and serologic procedures. The relative value of each is different for the various etiologies. The diagnostic approach therefore requires that the physician assess the clinical and epidemiologic features of the case, decide which organisms are potential causes, and provide this assessment to the laboratory so that appropriate procedures will be used.

Microscopic Examination

Stool cytology

Microscopic examination is of limited value in the assessment of bacterial infections. The presence of polymorphonuclear leukocytes in the stool correlates with organisms that produce disease by invasion, particularly colonic invasion. The leukocytes may be seen in unstained or methylene-blue-stained wet mount preparations; the absence of fecal leukocytes, however, does not exclude invasive diarrhea. The observation and morphologic characterization

Direct detection of intestinal parasites

of amebas and flagellates on wet or stained preparations are the primary means by which amebic (*Entamoeba histolytica*) and flagellar (*G. lamblia*) infections are diagnosed. Direct electron microscopy can be used to diagnose viral diarrhea, as the rotaviruses and parvo/picornaviruses have a characteristic morphology but cannot be grown in cell culture.

Electron microscopic detection of rotaviruses and parvo/picornaviruses

Culture

blood cultures negative in diarrheal and dysenteric infections

Stool culture on selective media

Isolation of the etiologic agent is the primary means by which bacterial enteric infection is diagnosed. In enteric fever the organism is typically present in the blood in the early stages of disease. Blood cultures are, however, usually negative in watery diarrhea and dysenteric infections, and stool culture must be relied upon for diagnosis. Fortunately, several good selective media have been developed for both direct plating and enrichment culture, which allow isolation of the infecting organism in the presence of a predominant normal flora. Selective media are then used for the various enteric pathogens. Some of these are listed in Table 9.1. Media routinely employed may vary between clinical laboratories, but should include those appropriate for *Salmonella, Shigella,* and *Campylobacter fetus.* Three or four primary plates and one or two enrichment broths are required. After incubation the enrichment broths are subcultured to new sets of selective plates, and suspect colonies on all plates are screened with multiple biochemical tests. Diarrhea caused by *E. coli* is a special problem, because none of the methods that define the enterotoxigenic and invasive strains is practical for clinical laboratories.

Toxin Assay

Cytopathic effect of *C. difficile*

Colony DNA hybridization probe

The cytotoxin of *C. difficile* can be detected by its cytopathic effect in a cell culture system. In most clinical cases, enough toxin is present for direct detection in a stool specimen. This assay is currently available only in reference laboratories. *Escherichia coli* enterotoxin can be assayed from cultures in specialized laboratories, but not directly from stool specimens. A DNA probe for the toxin gene developed by recombinant DNA techniques can be applied directly to colonies to detect enterotoxigenicity.

Serologic Diagnosis

At present, antibody detection is useful in the diagnosis of amebic dysentery caused by *E. histolytica* and of typhoid fever. Both are considered ancillary to the primary diagnostic tests, which involve specific detection of the organism by microscopic and cultural methods. Reagents are commercially available for the detection of rotavirus antigen in stool by enzyme-linked immunosorbent assay or radioimmunoassay. These methods have a sensitivity roughly comparable to that of electron microscopy. Serologic methods have been described for many other causes of gastrointestinal infection, but are not generally used because of lack of sensitivity, specificity, or availability of reagents.

Other Causes of Intestinal Infection

Despite recent advances in defining the etiologies of enteric infections, there are surely more to be discovered. Organisms not listed in Table 59.1, such as *Aeromonas, Citrobacter, Plesiomonas,* and others, have occasionally been associated with intestinal infections, but the evidence for their enteropathogenicity is not yet strong enough to interpret their isolation from individual cases. At our present state of knowledge it is not useful to attempt isolation of these organisms unless strong epidemiologic evidence supports interpretation of the results.

Treatment

Maintenance of fluid and electrolyte balance

Factors influencing decisions on antibiotic therapy

In most gastrointestinal infections the primary goal of treatment is relief of symptoms, with particular attention to maintaining fluid and electrolyte balance. The effect of common antidiarrheal medications such as bismuth compounds (Pepto-bismol) or antispasmotics (Lomotil) is variable depending on the etiology. In general, they may be helpful for the watery diarrhea caused by enterotoxins, but not for dysentery caused by mucosal invasion, and antispasmotics may be harmful or dangerous in the latter instance. Antimicrobial agents are usually not indicated for self-limited watery diarrhea, but are required for more severe dysenteric infections. Some enteric infections, such as typhoid fever, are always treated with antimicrobics. One set of recommendations concerning traveler's diarrhea suggests that the traveler make his own diagnosis of watery diarrhea versus dysentery by gross examination of the initial stools. If blood and pus are present (shigellosis), antibiotics should be taken; if not (toxigenic *E. coli*), Pepto-bismol is recommended, because it appears to absorb the enterotoxin and reduce its activity.

For specific therapeutic measures, the chapters on the individual etiologic agents or books on infectious disease should be consulted.

James J. Plorde

Urinary Tract Infections

60

A physycyen, truely, can lyttel descerne Ony maner sekeness wythout syght of uryne.

Hawes, S. 1509. *The Pastime of Pleasure* (The Oxford English Dictionary)

The examination of urine has been used to assist medical practitioners in the diagnosis and management of human illness for centuries. So great an emphasis did medieval physicians place on the color, sediment, smell, and even taste of this effluent that a urine-filled flask became the symbol of their profession. This fluid, which so faithfully reflects the maladies of the urinary tract, is produced by the kidney, collected by the renal pelvis, and transported through the ureters to the bladder for storage. Here it remains until the discomfort of bladder distention stimulates its evacuation via the urethra.

Definitions

Bacterial contamination of the urine within this tract (*bacteriuria*) is common and can, at times, result in microbial invasion of the tissues responsible for the manufacture, transport, and storage of urine. Infection of the upper urinary tract, consisting of the kidney and its pelvis, is known as *pyelonephritis*. Infection of the lower tract may involve the bladder (*cystitis*), urethra (*urethritis*), or prostate (*prostatitis*), the genital organ that surrounds and communicates with the first segment of the male urethra. Because all portions of the urinary tract are joined by a fluid medium, infection at any site may spread to involve other areas of the system.

prevalence of bacteriuria

It has been estimated that approximately 10% of humans are afflicted with a urinary tract infection at some time during their lives. The exact prevalence is age and sex dependent. Approximately 1% of male infants acquire infection but, unexpectedly, few show evidence of congenital urinary tract abnormalities. Thereafter, infection in the male is uncommon until the sixth decade of life, when enlargement of the prostate interferes with emptying of the bladder. In contrast, the prevalence of bacteriuria in schoolage girls is 1–2% and as many as 5% eventually are involved at some time during their childhood years. Although most recover uneventfully, this population group is at substantially increased risk of recurrent urinary tract infection during adult life. Accordingly, the prevalence of bacteriuria in the female population increases gradually with time, reaching 5% in women of childbearing age and 10–20% in postmenopausal women. These infections may be morbid or asymptomatic, acute or chronic, singular or recurrent. At times they can produce permanent damage to the kidney.

Pathogenesis

Host Factors

Ascending infections in women of child bearing age

Infections are seen most frequently in women of childbearing age. They are caused by gut flora, which reach the bladder via the urethra, after colonization of the external periurethral area and distal urethra. The circumstances that lead to this colonization are not fully understood, but it is known that certain types of bacteria adhere more readily to the vaginal introitus of infection-prone women than controls. Bacteria can reach the bladder more easily in the female host than in the male because the urethra is shorter, lies in close proximity to the moist perirectal area, and is subjected to the massaging effect of sexual intercourse. Once in the bladder, organisms that cause cystitis can multiply in the contained urine.

Factors contributing to colonization and infection

Catheter-associated infections

Bacteria can also be carried easily to the bladder in both men and women by passage of a catheter or other instrument, such as a cystoscope. This mode of transmission constitutes the most common single cause of hospital-acquired bacteriuria in either sex. A single transient catheterization of the bladder induces bacteriuria in approximately 1% of ambulatory and 10% of bed-ridden patients. An indwelling catheter, by providing a fluid-filled conduit for the migration of organisms from the external environment to the bladder, is more frequently associated with urinary tract infection. Even with meticulous attention to aseptic technique, most patients harboring a catheter for more than 2 weeks develop infection.

The factors that determine whether the bacteriuria persists after the removal of the initiating event include the number and type of bacteria introduced and the adequacy of the host's response to these organisms. In the overwhelming majority of cases, the number of bacteria is small and the host's defense mechanisms prove adequate. The urine itself is inhibitory to anaerobes and other fastidious organisms that are part of the normal flora of the urethral mucosa, and these bacteria seldom cause persistent infections.

Inhibitory properties of concentrated urine

Even organisms known for their ability to multiply in urine may be inhibited when exposed to the very high osmolality and concentration of urea and hydrogen ions that characterize the urine of many normal individuals. It is likely that the moderation of these urinary parameters during pregnancy accounts, at least in part, for the increased incidence of bacteriuria in this population. The antibacterial properties of the bladder mucosa and the few neutrophils that reach the surface contribute to the clearance of introduced organisms.

Flushing effects of micturation

Perhaps the most important of the host defenses, however, is the act of voiding. The constant flushing of contaminated urine from the body and its dilution with newly formed, uncontaminated urine eliminates bacteria or maintains their numbers at low levels.

Causes and effects of interference with urine flow

Any interference with this clearing mechanism results in bacterial multiplication and a greatly increased probability of developing or sustaining an infection. The interference may be by mechanical obstruction to urine flow (stone, stricture, or hypertrophied prostate), neurogenic impairment of bladder control (spinal cord injury, multiple sclerosis), or functional impairment, such as the vesicoureteral reflux seen in many children with urinary tract infections. The latter appears to result from the effect of the inflammatory reaction, which interferes with the integrity of the vesicoureteral junction and allows regurgitation of urine from the bladder into the ureters. Such reflux, not only returns a pool of infected urine to the bladder after voiding is completed, but also can carry bacteria to the renal pelvis and thus initiate infection in a previously uninvolved kidney.

Infections in pregnancy

A similar functional abnormality has been described in pregnant women. The hormonal changes in pregnancy lead to a decrease in bladder tone, diminished ureteral peristalsis, and dilatation of the renal pelvis and ureters. All enhance the likelihood of reflux and explain, at least in part, the frequency with which pregnant women with bacteriuria develop upper urinary tract disease. Congenital or acquired anatomic derangements of the vesicoureteral junction produce similar results.

Blood-borne infections

Occasionally, urinary tract infection occurs when bacteria seed the renal parenchyma directly from the blood. It is possible to infect the kidneys of experimental animals by intravenous injection of a variety of bacterial species other than Gram-negative bacilli. Hematogenous pyelonephritis in humans is uncommon, however, except during periods of sustained *Staphylococcus aureus* bacteremia.

Microbial Factors

fecal origin of infecting organisms

determinants of uropathogenicity of *E. coli*

infections associated with few serotypes

Human feces contain a rich diversity of bacterial species. Surprisingly, only a few regularly produce urinary tract infection. In fact, *Escherichia coli* accounts for more than 90% of acute infections in patients with structurally normal urinary tracts. The factors responsible for this extraordinary monopoly are incompletely understood, but the relative resistance of *E. coli* to the inhibitory effects of vaginal fluid, its possession of pili that aid its attachment to the epithelial cells of the urinary tract, and its motility appear to contribute to its effectiveness as a uropathogen. Some or all of these features, however, are found in other, less successful, enteric species. It has been shown that the relationship of *E. coli* to acute symptomatic urinary tract infection is limited to relatively few of the more than 150 O serotypes of this organism found in the stool. Interestingly, these serotypes, 01, 02, 04, 06, 07, and 075, are more resistant to the bactericidal effects of serum, suggesting that seroresistance also contributes to virulence. Finally, strains of *E. coli* isolated from patients with upper urinary tract disease possess K surface antigens absent from organisms isolated from the lower urinary tract.

Chronic and recurrent infections

Nosocomial infections with opportunists

effects of urease activity of *Proteus*

Patients with urinary tract abnormalities that interfere with the free flow of urine are particularly apt to experience chronic or recurrent infection. This exposes them to multiple courses of antimicrobial therapy, which eventually leads to the replacement of antibiotic-susceptible strains of *E. coli* with more resistant pathogens. Hospitalized patients are particularly susceptible to cross-infection with nosocomial strains of *Proteus, Providencia, Pseudomonas, Klebsiella, Enterobacter, Serratia*, coagulase-negative staphylococci, and enterococci, many of which are passed directly from catheterized patient to catheterized patient on the hands of medical personnel. Once established in the urinary tract, *Proteus* strains appear to be particularly virulent. Experimental evidence suggests that *Proteus mirabilis* possesses pili that facilitate its adherence to the mucosa of the renal pelvis. In addition, urease production by all species of *Proteus* leads to hydrolysis of urea, formation of ammonium hydroxide, and alkalinization of the urine. The elevated pH in the urine is directly toxic to renal cells and stimulates the formation of magnesium and ammonium phosphate struvite urinary calculi (stones), which can contribute to the chronicity of the infection by producing ureteral obstruction and sheltering the bacteria from the patient's defensive mechanisms and the physician's antimicrobial agents. Species of *Klebsiella*, because of their more limited urease production or through production of an extracellular polysaccharide slime layer, are also associated with the presence of urinary calculi.

S. saprophyticus infections

Staphylococcus saprophyticus, a coagulase-negative, urease-positive staphylococcus, is now recognized as the cause of as much as 20% of symptomatic urinary tract infections in young, sexually active women. *Staphylococcus aureus* infections usually result from the bacteremic seeding of the urinary tract, as described previously.

Yeasts, particularly species of *Candida*, may be isolated from catheterized

Candida infections

Chlamydia infections

patients receiving antibacterial therapy and from diabetics, but they seldom produce symptomatic disease. *Chlamydia trachomatis*, in contrast, can produce the acute urethral syndrome described subsequently.

Common Clinical Features

The clinical manifestations of urinary tract infection are variable. Approximately one-half of infections do not produce recognizable illness and are discovered incidentally during a general medical examination. Infections in infants produce symptoms of a nonspecific nature, including fever, vomiting, and failure to thrive. Manifestations in older children and adults, when present, often suggest the diagnosis and sometimes the localization of the infection within the urinary tract.

Urethritis

Dysuria and discharge

Infections confined to the urethra are characterized by painful urination (dysuria) and discharge of mucoid or purulent material from the urethral orifice. They are most commonly produced by sexually transmitted agents. This syndrome is discussed more fully in Chapter 64.

Cystitis

urgency, frequency, and dysuria

Causative bacteria multiply in urine

suprapubic tenderness and turbid urine

Acute urethral syndrome

The symptoms of cystitis—dysuria, frequent voiding (frequency), and an imperative "call to toilet" (urgency)—are similar to those of urethritis. This symptom complex is, in fact, produced by irritation of the mucosal surface of the urethra as well as the bladder. Unlike urethritis associated with sexually transmitted agents, cystitis is produced by the multiplication of enteric organisms in the bladder urine. It is clinically distinguished from urethritis by a more acute onset, the presence of bacteriuria, and the absence of a urethral discharge. The urine is often cloudy and malodorous and occasionally bloody; unlike patients with urethritis, those with cystitis often experience pain and tenderness in the suprapubic area. Fever and systemic manifestations of illness are usually absent unless the infection spreads to involve the kidney. Approximately one-third of women presenting with dysuria and frequency lack cultural evidence of either bacteriuria or sexually transmitted disease. Use of more sensitive culturing techniques in such patients has defined an acute urethral syndrome associated with the presence in the urethra of small numbers of enteric bacteria or agents of sexually transmitted infections, such as *C. trachomatis.*

Pyelonephritis

fever, flank pain, and systemic signs

association with premature birth

The typical presentation of upper urinary infection consists of flank pain and fever that exceeds 38.3°C. These findings may be preceded or accompanied by manifestations of cystitis. Rigors, vomiting, diarrhea, and tachycardia are present in the more severely ill. Physical examination reveals tenderness over the costovertebral areas of the back and, occasionally, evidence of septic shock. In the absence of obstruction, the clinical manifestations usually abate within a few days, leaving the kidneys functionally intact. It has been estimated, however, that 20–50% of pregnant women with acute pyelonephritis give birth to premature infants, one of the most serious consequences of urinary tract infection. In the presence of obstruction, a neurogenic bladder, or vesicoureteral reflux, clinical manifestations are more persistent, occasionally leading to necrosis of the renal papillae

Chronic pyelonephritis

and progressive impairment of kidney function with chronic bacteriuria. If a renal calculus or necrotic renal papilla impacts in the ureter, severe flank pain with radiation to the groin occurs.

Prostatitis

Symptoms and signs

Infection of the prostate is typically manifested as pain in the lower back, perirectal area, and testicles. In acute infection, the pain may be severe and accompanied by high fever, chills, and the signs and symptoms of cystitis. Inflammatory swelling can lead to obstruction of the neighboring urethra and urinary retention. On rectal palpation, the prostate is boggy and exquisitely tender. Response to antibiotic therapy is good, but occasionally abscess formation, epididymitis, and seminal vesiculitis develop. Typically, acute prostatitis develops in young adults; however, it can also follow placement of an indwelling catheter in an older man. Patients with chronic prostatitis seldom give a history of an acute episode. Many are totally without symptoms; others experience low-grade pain and dysuria. Periodic spread of prostatic organisms to the urine in the bladder produces recurrent bouts of cystitis. In fact, chronic prostatitis is probably the major cause of recurrent bacteriuria in men.

acute prostatitis in young men

Chronic prostatitis

General Diagnostic Approaches

Specimen Collection

The diagnosis of urinary tract infection is based on examination of the normally sterile urine or prostatic secretions for evidence of bacteria or an accompanying inflammatory reaction. Critical to this examination is the use of appropriate techniques for specimen collection. Urine is most easily obtained by spontaneous micturation. Unfortunately, voided urine is invariably contaminated with urethral flora and, in the case of the female, vaginal secretions, which can confound the results of laboratory testing. Although the contaminants can never be completely eliminated, their quantity may be diminished by carefully cleansing the periurethrum before voiding and allowing the initial part of the stream to flush the urethra before collecting a specimen for examination. This clean-voided midstream urine collection procedure is preferred to catheterization for routine purposes because it avoids the risk of introducing organisms into the bladder. When the laboratory examination of such a specimen produces equivocal results or the patient cannot comply with the requirements of the clean-voided technique, catheterization may be needed. Alternatively, urine may be aspirated from the bladder with a needle and syringe. In this procedure, the patient refrains from voiding until the bladder is distended. The suprapubic skin is then disinfected and a small needle passed through the skin into the bladder. The procedure has proved to be safe and well tolerated.

contamination of voided urine

Clean-voided urine collection

Suprapubic aspiration

Microscopic Examination

Pyuria

Approximately three-quarters of patients with urinary tract infection have pyuria (that is, more than 100 white cells per milliliter of urine). This finding is also common, however, in a number of noninfectious diseases. More specific is the presence of white cell casts, which occur almost exclusively, although not uniformly, in patients with acute pyelonephritis. The most sensitive and specific microscopic procedure is a Gram-stained smear of uncentrifuged urine (Plate P). The presence of at least one organism per oil-immersion field is almost always indicative of bacterial infection. The absence of bacteria in several fields makes the diagnosis unlikely.

Direct Gram staining

Urine Culture

significance of bacterial counts with clean-voided urine

significance in catheterized patients or suprapubic specimens

prevention of growth in urine after collection

Urine specimens collected even by the clean-void midstream procedure contain small numbers of bacterial contaminants. This finding can be distinguished from true bacteriuria only with quantitative cultures, which allow colony counts. Contaminated specimens usually yield less than 1000 colonies of mixed bacterial flora per milliliter of urine. In urinary tract infections, in contrast, more than 100,000 colonies of a single bacterial species are generally seen. Occasionally colony counts fall between these two values. If the patient is asymptomatic, the culture should be repeated. In symptomatic patients, counts in this range are considered significant if a single bacterial species is isolated. Intermediate counts on urine specimens collected by catheterization or suprapubic aspiration are always considered significant because contamination is minimal in such specimens. Colony counts must be performed on freshly collected or refrigerated specimens to prevent bacterial growth from occurring before processing.

Localization Studies

detection of antibody-coated bacteria

Urine specimens from ureters and bladder

Infections involving the kidney and prostate are more likely to relapse than those confined to the bladder and urethra; consequently they require more prolonged antimicrobial therapy. Accordingly, various laboratory tests have been designed to locate infection within the urinary tract and assist the physician in the selection of appropriate therapy. Perhaps the test most widely used is detection of antibody coating of urinary bacteria by means of fluorescein-labeled antibodies against human immunoglobulin. Antibody coating is characteristic of upper urinary tract infections. Unfortunately, the procedure yields both false-positive and false-negative results, which somewhat limits its usefulness. Bacterial counts on urine obtained simultaneously from the bladder and from each ureter may help to locate upper urinary tract infection. Similarly, simultaneous quantitative cultures of midstream urine and expressed prostatic secretions have been used to distinguish prostatic disease from bladder and renal infections.

Miscellaneous Studies

Blood cultures

If acute pyelonephritis or prostatitis is suspected, blood cultures should be obtained to exclude bacteremia. Infected children, men, and those who experience a relapse of urinary tract infection should be investigated with intravenous pyelography to allow detection and correction of any factor causing predisposition to infection.

General Principles of Management

Single-dose treatment of uncomplicated cystitis

Need to establish microbial diagnosis in other cases

The principal goal in the treatment of urinary tract infection is eradication of the offending organism from the urine and tissues. In simple isolated instances of cystitis in a young woman, the diagnosis may be confirmed by a simple Gram smear of urine and treatment for an assumed *E. coli* infection given empirically. Many antimicrobics are successful in controlling such infections, and knowledge of the susceptibility of community-acquired *E. coli* in a particular area serves as the best guide. In many cases, single-dose therapy has been shown to be as effective as a course covering several days. Sulfonamides and trimethoprim alone or in combination, ampicillin, and amoxicillin are the agents most commonly used.

In all other instances it is imperative to establish the presence of bacteriuria with one or, in asymptomatic bacteriuria, two quantitative urine cultures. Except in cases of clinical emergency, treatment should be delayed until the

Test of cure

diagnosis is established. As bacteriuria may persist despite the spontaneous abatement of symptoms, the success of treatment should be checked with follow-up urine cultures. The first should be obtained 48–72 hr after initiation of therapy. If the offending microorganism is still present at that time, the chemotherapeutic agent should be withdrawn and a substitute selected on the basis of susceptibility tests. If bacterial clearance has been achieved, the therapeutic course should be completed and repeat cultures obtained 2 weeks after termination of therapy. Sterile cultures at this time suggest eradication of the bacteriuria. A recurrence is classified as either *relapse* or *reinfection*. Relapses are recurrent infections produced by the organism responsible for the initial infection. They usually indicate an upper urinary tract infection or, in a male case, prostatitis, and require the initiation of a urologic evaluation. If an abnormality causing predisposition to urinary tract infection is discovered, it should be corrected whenever possible. If none is found, prolonged antibiotic therapy should be administered in hopes of eradicating the residual focus of infection.

Investigation and treatment of recurrences

Reinfections recurrences caused by a new species or serotype are usually indicative of a bladder infection. They respond readily to standard courses of treatment. Some patients, usually women of childbearing age, suffer repeated bladder reinfections. Those with several symptomatic episodes annually may be helped with long-term, low-dose chemoprophylaxis. In women whose recurrences are related to sexual activity, administration of the chemoprophylactic agent may be limited to immediately after intercourse.

Prophylaxis in patients prone to reinfection

Patients experiencing an episode of acute pyelonephritis should be hospitalized and treated, at least initially, with appropriate parenteral antibiotics. This treatment is particularly important if Gram-negative bacteremia is suspected. Asymptomatic bacteriuria developing in a patient with an indwelling catheter often remits spontaneously after the removal of the catheter. It need not be treated unless the patient is at high risk of sepsis because of an underlying problem. Symptomatic infections in catheterized patients require treatment.

Treatment of pyelonephritis and catheter-associated infections

Additional Reading and References

Farrar, W.E. Jr. 1983. Infections of the urinary tract. *Med. Clin. North Am.* 67:187. An up-to-date review of the topic and of the management of urinary tract infections in office practice.

Platt, R. 1983. Diagnosis and empiric therapy or urinary tract infections in the seriously ill patient. *Rev. Infect. Dis.* (*suppl. 1*) 5:S65–73. An excellent review of the factors determining immediate therapy in severe urinary tract infection.

Souney, P., and Polk, B.F. 1982. Single-dose antimicrobial therapy for urinary tract infections in women. *Rev. Infect. Dis.* 4:29–34. A review of studies on the effectiveness of single-dose therapy of uncomplicated infections in nonpregnant women.

C. George Ray

Central Nervous System Infections

61

Anatomy and pathophysiology

The cerebrum, cerebellum, brain stem, spinal cord, and their covering membranes (meninges) constitute the central nervous system (CNS). Because of the unique anatomic and physiologic features of the CNS, infections in this site can represent unique challenges to the microbiologist and clinician.

The CNS is encased in a rigid, bony vault, and it is highly vulnerable to the effects of inflammation and edema. The critical life-regulatory functions of the CNS and the metabolic requirements to sustain these functions can also be easily disrupted by infection, with resultant local acidosis, hypoxia, and neuronal destruction. Thus, the effects of increased pressure, biochemical abnormalities, and tissue necrosis can be profound and sometimes irreversible.

One specialized defense mechanism of the CNS is the so-called *blood–brain barrier,* which serves to minimize passage of infectious agents and potentially toxic metabolites into the cerebrospinal fluid (CSF) and tissues, as well as to regulate the rate of transport of plasma proteins, glucose, and electrolytes. When CNS infection develops, however, this barrier also poses difficulties in treatment: some antimicrobial agents are not transported as readily from the blood to the site of infection as they are to other tissues.

Within the brain are the ventricles, where CSF is actively produced, primarily by a specialized structure called the *choroid plexus.* The CSF fills the lateral ventricles in each half of the brain, circulates into a central third ventricle, and then passes through the cerebral aqueduct to emerge through foramina at the brain stem. From cisterns at the base of the brain, the CSF circulates in the subarachnoid space over the entire CNS, including the spinal cord, to supply nutrients and serve as a hydraulic cushion for these tissues. It is reabsorbed primarily by the major venous system in the meninges. Obstruction of the normal flow of CSF in either the internal (ventricular) or external (subarachnoid) systems can result in increased intracranial pressure, as production of CSF by the choroid plexus will continue within the ventricles. Such impairment of flow or normal reabsorption can occur during certain infections as a result of inflammation or subsequent fibrosis, leading to dilatation of the ventricles, compression of brain tissue, and a condition known as *hydrocephalus.*

Routes of Infection

Blood-borne spread

Most CNS infections appear to result from blood-borne spread; for example, bacteremia or viremia resulting from infection of tissue at a site remote from the CNS may result in penetration of the blood–brain barrier. Examples of infectious agents that commonly infect the CNS by this route are *Haemophilus influenzae, Neisseria meningitidis, Streptococcus pneumoniae, Mycobacterium tuberculosis,* and viruses such as enteroviruses and mumps. The initial source of infection leading to bloodstream invasion may be occult (for example, infection of reticuloendothelial tissues) or overt (for example, pneumonia, pharyngitis, skin abscess or cellulitis, or bacterial endocarditis).

Direct spread from infected focus

Occasionally, the route of infection is from a focus close to or contiguous with the CNS. These possible sources include otitis media, mastoiditis, sinusitis, or pyogenic infections of the skin or bone. Infection may extend directly into the CNS, indirectly via venous pathways, or in the sheaths of cranial and spinal nerves.

Traumatic, surgical, or congenital lesions

In some cases, a contiguous or distant infectious focus may not be necessary to produce CNS infection. If an anatomic defect exists in the structures encasing the CNS, infectious agents may readily gain access to the vulnerable site and establish themselves. Such defects may be traumatically or surgically induced or result from congenital malformatioms. For example, basilar skull fractures may produce an opening between the CNS and the sinuses, nasal passages (defects in the cribriform plate), mastoid, or middle ear. All of these sites are contiguous with the upper respiratory tract, which enables a number of potentially pathogenic respiratory flora to gain ready access to the CNS. Neurosurgical procedures also create transient communications between the external environment and the CNS that can be readily contaminated. This risk can be compounded when foreign bodies, such as shunts or external drainage tubes, must be left in place for the treatment of hydrocephalus. These foreign bodies, when colonized, can serve as chronic foci of infection. Congenital defects, such as meningomyeloceles or sinus tracts through the cranium or spine, may also be sources. The latter may be overlooked; the orifice of the sinus may be a small cleft on the skin surface, or occasionally it may open internally into the intestinal tract. Recurrent purulent meningitis or unusual pathogens in an otherwise healthy host should prompt a careful search for such defects.

Implanted foreign bodies

Intraneural pathways

Perhaps the least common route of CNS infection is via intraneural pathways. Agents capable of direct intraneural spread to the CNS include rabies virus (presumably along peripheral sensory nerves), herpes simplex virus (often, but not exclusively, via the trigeminal nerve root or sacral nerves), and perhaps some togaviruses.

Abscesses

Abscesses of the CNS deserve special mention. Although relatively uncommon compared with other CNS infections, they represent a special microbiologic and clinical problem. Such abscesses may be within the tissues of the CNS (for example, brain abscess see Figure 61.1) or localized in the subdural or epidural spaces. They sometimes develop as a complication of pyogenic meningitis. More commonly, abscesses of the CNS result from embolization of bacteria or fungi from a distant focus, such as endocarditis or pyogenic lung abscess; extension from a contiguous focus of infection (for example, sinusitis or mastoiditis); or a complication of surgery or nonsurgical trauma.

Common Clinical Features

Several terms commonly applied to CNS infections need to be understood. Purulent meningitis refers to infections of the meninges associated with a marked, acute inflammatory exudate and is usually caused by a bacterial infection. Such infections frequently involve the underlying CNS tissue to

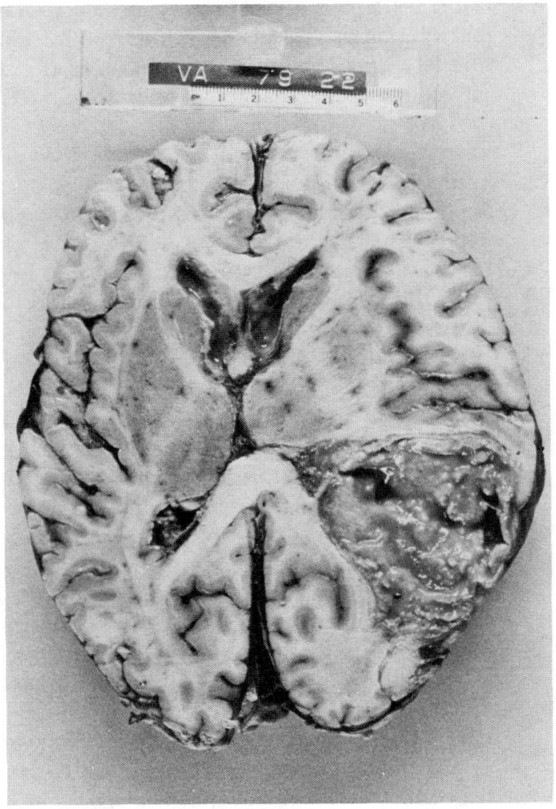

61.1 Coronal section of a brain, demonstrating a poorly encapsulated abscess.

Purulent meningitis

Ventriculitis

a variable degree, and it is now appreciated that often the ventricular system is also involved (ventriculitis). Most cases of purulent meningitis are acute in onset and progression and are characterized by fever, stiff neck, irritability, and varying degrees of neurologic dysfunction that, if untreated, usually progress to a fatal outcome.

Chronic meningitis

Chronic meningitis has a more insidious onset, with progression of signs and symptoms over a period of weeks. This infection is usually caused by mycobacteria and fungi that produce granulomatous inflammatory changes, but occasionally protozoal agents are responsible (see Table 61.3).

Aseptic meningitis

Aseptic meningitis implies the absence of the previously mentioned agents from the etiology and suggests viruses, nonspecific inflammatory reactions to chemical agents injected into the CSF, tumor cell responses, and bleeding as potential causes. Most aseptic meningitis syndromes are viral; the term implies that the primary site of inflammation is in the meninges, without clinical evidence of involvement of the neural tissue. Such patients may have fever, headache, a stiff neck or back, nausea and vomiting, and inflammatory cells in the CSF (CSF pleocytosis).

Encephalitis

Encephalitis also implies a primary viral etiology; however, acute or chronic demyelinating diseases with or without inflammation are included. This latter group includes the so-called *postinfectious* or *allergic* encephalomyelitis syndromes, in which the etiology and pathogenesis are not always clearly defined. Clinically, this term is reserved for patients who may show signs and CSF findings compatible with aseptic meningitis, but who also show objective evidence of CNS dysfunction (for example, seizures, paralysis, disordered mentation, and the like). Many clinicians use the term

Meningoencephalitis

meningoencephalitis to describe patients with both meningeal and encephalitic manifestations.

Poliomyelitis

Poliomyelitis refers to the selective destruction of anterior motor horn cells in the spinal cord and/or brain stem, which leads to weakness or paralysis of muscle groups and occasionally respiratory insufficiency. It is usually associated with aseptic meningitis, sometimes with encephalitis. The polioviruses are the major causes of this syndrome, although Coxsackie viruses (primarily type A_7) and other enteroviruses, such as enterovirus 71, have been implicated. The hallmark of poliomyelitis is asymmetric flaccid paralysis.

Acute polyneuritis

Two other nervous system syndromes presumably associated with infection deserve brief mention. Acute polyneuritis, an inflammatory disease of the peripheral nervous system, is characterized by symmetric flaccid paralysis of muscles. In most cases, no specific etiology is found; some, however, have been associated with *Corynebacterium diphtheriae* toxin, administration of inactivated influenza A virus vaccine (the swine flu vaccination campaign of 1976–1977 was incriminated as a factor in a number of adult cases), and infections by cytomegalovirus or Epstein–Barr virus. Reye's syndrome (encephalopathy with fatty infiltration of the viscera) is an unusual, acute, complex, noninflammatory process, usually observed in childhood, in which cerebral edema, hepatic dysfunction, and hyperammonemia develop within 2–12 days after onset of a systemic viral infection. Although the influenza A and B and varicella-zoster viruses have been most frequently implicated as contributors to this syndrome, the precise pathogenesis is not yet known.

Reye's syndrome

Common Etiologic Agents

The causes of CNS infections are numerous, as illustrated in Tables 61.1, 61.2, and 61.3. Acute purulent meningitis is usually caused by one of three organisms: *Haemophilus influenzae* type b, *Neisseria meningitidis,* or *Streptococcus pneumoniae.* The major exception is neonatal infection, in which *Escherichia coli* or group B streptococci are most frequently implicated. However, many other bacteria can occasionally cause the disease if they gain access to the meninges.

Acute viral disease

Of the viral causes of acute CNS disease, the categories most commonly encountered are the enteroviruses, mumps, herpes simplex, Epstein–Barr virus, and arthropod-borne viruses. In the United States, enteroviruses account for the greatest proportion of infections. Viral CNS infections can be manifested clinically as aseptic meningitis, encephalitis, or, with poliovirus and some other enterovirus infections, poliomyelitis. The age of the patient and the season of occurrence help somewhat in predicting some of the agents that may be involved, as illustrated in Table 61.2; other epidemiologic, ecologic, and clinical factors associated with these infections are discussed in the individual chapters on specific virus groups.

Slow viral infections

Slow viral infections of the CNS, such as Creutzfeldt–Jakob disease and subacute sclerosing panencephalitis, are discussed in detail in Chapter 43.

Chronic meningitis

Other important causes of CNS infections (Table 61.3) that must not be overlooked include *Mycobacterium tuberculosis* and the deep mycoses (especially *Cryptococcus neoformans* and *Coccidioides immitis*). These chronic infections can be insidious in onset and can mimic other processes in the clinical findings and CSF examination, thus delaying consideration of the proper diagnosis.

Noninfectious diseases mimicking infections

Finally, there are noninfectious causes of CNS disease to be considered in the differential diagnosis. These include 1) metabolic disturbances, such as hypoglycemia, diabetic coma, and hepatic failure; 2) toxic conditions,

Table 61.1 Common Causes of Purulent Central Nervous System Infections

Age Group	Agent
Newborns (<1 mo old)	Group B streptococci and *Escherichia coli* (most common); *Listeria monocytogenes; Klebsiella* species; other enteric Gram-negative bacteria
Infants and children	*Haemophilus influenzae* type b; *Neisseria meningitidis; Streptococcus pneumoniae*
Adults	*Streptococcus pneumoniae; Neisseria meningitidis*
Special circumstances	
Meningitis or intracranial abscesses associated with trauma, neurosurgery, or intracranial foreign bodies	*Staphylococcus aureus; Staphylococcus epidermidis; Streptococcus pneumoniae;* anaerobic Gram-negative and Gram-positive bacteria; *Pseudomonas* species
Intracranial abscesses not associated with trauma or surgery	Microaerophilic or anaerobic streptococci, anaerobic Gram-negative bacteria (often mixed aerobic and anaerobic flora of upper respiratory tract origin)

Table 61.2 Primary Acute Viral Infections of the Central Nervous System

Agent	Major Age Group Affected	Seasonal Predominance
Enteroviruses (Coxsackie A, Coxsackie B, echoviruses, polioviruses)	Infants, children	Summer–fall
Mumps	Children	Winter–spring
Herpes simplex		
Type 1	Adults	None
Type 2	Neonates, young adults	None
Arboviruses		
Western equine encephalitis	Infants, children	Summer–fall
St. Louis encephalitis	Adults over 40 yr old	Summer–fall
California encephalitis	School-aged children	Summer–fall
Eastern equine encephalitis	Infants, children	Summer–fall
Rabies	All ages	Summer–fall
Measles	Infants, children	Spring
Varicella-zoster	Infants, children	Spring
Lymphocytic choriomeningitis	Adults	None
Epstein–Barr virus	Children, young adults	None
Other (myxoviruses, paramyxoviruses, cytomegaloviruses, adenoviruses, etc.)	Infants, children	Variable

Table 61.3 Other Causes of Central Nervous System Infections

Disease	Agent
Chronic granulomatous infection	*Mycobacterium tuberculosis*[a]
	Coccidioides immitis
	Cryptococcus neoformans
	Histoplasma capsulatum
Parasitic infection	
Protozoa	*Toxoplasma gondii*[b]
	Trypanosoma
	Naegleria (ameba) species
Nematodes	*Toxocara* species
	Trichinella spiralis
	Angiostrongylus cantonensis
Cestodes	*Taenia solium* (cysticercosis)
Other	*Leptospira species*
	Treponema pallidum

[a] Tuberculous meningitis can appear as acute or chronically progressive disease.
[b] Toxoplasmosis of the central nervous system is usually seen in congenital infections or immunocompromised hosts.

such as those caused by bacterial toxins (diphtheria, tetanus, botulism), insect toxins (tick paralysis), poisons (lead), and drug abuse; 3) mass lesions, such as acute trauma, hematoma, and tumor; 4) vascular lesions, such as intracranial embolus, aneurysm, and subarachnoid hemorrhage; and 5) acute psychiatric episodes.

General Diagnostic Approaches

lumbar puncture

cells, protein, and glucose in CSF

Except in unusual circumstances, in which severe increases in intracranial pressure make the procedure dangerous, a lumbar puncture is the first step in the workup of a patient with suspected CNS infection. The CSF pressure is determined at the time of the procedure, and CSF is removed for analysis of cells, protein, and glucose. Ideally, the glucose content of the peripheral blood is determined simultaneously for comparison with that in the CSF. Table 61.4 presents guidelines for interpretation of results of CSF analysis;

Table 61.4 Findings of Cerebrospinal Fluid Analysis: Normal versus Infection

Age Group	Cells/mm^3	Polymorphonuclear Cells (%)	Glucose (% of Blood)	Protein (mg/dl)
Adults				
Normal	0–5	0	≥60	≤30
Viral infection	2–2000 (80)[a]	≤50	≥60	30–80
Bacterial infection	5–5000 (800)	≥60	≤45[b]	>60
Tuberculosis and mycoses	5–2000 (100)	≤50	≤45	>60
Neonates (normal)				
Term	0–32 (8)	≤60	≥60	20–170 (90)
Preterm	0–29 (9)	≤60	≥60	65–150 (115)

[a] Numbers in parentheses represent mean values.
[b] Usually very low or absent.

these guidelines represent generalizations, however, and must not be considered as absolute findings in all cases. For example, although a patient with bacterial, mycobacterial, or fungal meningitis will usually have a glucose level in the CSF of less than 40 mg/dl, or less than half the blood glucose level (hypoglycorrhachia), this finding may not be present in the early stages of infection. Although uncommon, viral infections of the CNS occasionally produce low glucose values in the CSF; in addition, the early stages of viral infection may be associated with a preponderance of polymorphonuclear leukocytes.

Interpretation of findings

Realizing the limitations, it is possible to make some general interpretations that are helpful in the diagnosis: Viral CNS infections are usually associated with a preponderance of lymphocytes, a normal glucose value, and a normal or moderately elevated protein level in the CSF. In contrast, acute bacterial meningitis usually causes a CSF pleocytosis consisting primarily of polymorphonuclear cells, a low glucose value, and a high protein level. Mycobacterial and fungal infections are more commonly associated with lymphocytosis (and sometimes moderate eosinophilia) in the CSF; like the acute bacterial infections, however, they tend to lower glucose and increase protein levels markedly.

Normal values for CSF are also shown in Table 61.4. Although no polymorphonuclear cells should appear in normal CSF, as many as four lymphocytes per cubic millimeter may be found occasionally in health. Neonatal CSF is considerably more difficult to interpret, as cell counts are often elevated in the absence of infection; glucose values, however, should be within the normal range.

Direct staining and culture

The other major procedures that must be performed on all CSF samples in which any infection is suspected include bacterial cultures and Gram staining. If the CSF is grossly purulent, a Gram stain of the uncentrifuged sample is often done; otherwise, the centrifuged sediment is used. According to the clinical indication, other microbiologic tests may be used, including viral cultures, special stains and cultures for fungi and mycobacteria, and immunologic methods to detect fungal or bacterial antigens (for example, latex agglutination for *Cryptococcus*, counterimmunoelectrophoresis for selected bacteria).

Tests for free antigens

Other laboratory tests

Tests on specimens other than CSF are selected on the basis of the clinical diagnostic possibilities. If acute bacterial meningitis is suspected, blood cultures may be used to ensure the diagnosis. Viral cultures of the pharynx, stool, or rectal swabs may provide indirect evidence of CNS infection. Herpes simplex encephalitis poses a unique situation: to establish the diagnosis, a biopsy specimen of the brain is sometimes required to demonstrate viral antigen by immunofluorescence and/or growth of virus. Other studies may include acute and convalescent sera for viral serology and serologic tests to detect antibodies to certain fungi, such as *Coccidioides immitis*.

Intracranial abscesses can often be detected with radiologic techniques, such as brain scanning. A definitive etiologic diagnosis is established by careful aerobic and anaerobic culture of the contents of the abscess.

General Principles of Management

chemotherapy

In bacterial, mycobacterial, and fungal infections of the CNS, prompt and aggressive antimicrobial therapy is required. The duration of treatment varies from as little as 10 days for uncomplicated bacterial meningitis to 12 months or longer for tuberculous meningitis and several years for some cases of fungal meningitis.

correction of metabolic defects and of raised intracranial pressure

In addition to antimicrobial therapy, correction of associated metabolic defects (acidosis, hypoxia, saline depletion, inappropriate antidiuretic hormone secretion) is necessary. Increased intracranial pressure as a result of vasogenic edema or hydrocephalus must be monitored and controlled accordingly; osmotic agents such as intravenous mannitol are often used to control acute cerebral edema, and neurosurgical shunting procedures may be needed to treat progressive hydrocephalus. Abscesses require drainage or, whenever possible, total surgical excision.

abscess drainage

treatment of viral infection

Except for those with herpes simplex encephalitis, which may respond to early treatment with antiviral agents, patients with viral infections of the CNS receive supportive care only. This therapy includes specific attention to the metabolic and ventilatory problems that may develop in severe cases.

C. George Ray and Kenneth J. Ryan

Intravascular Infections, Bacteremia, and Endotoxemia

62

In many cases the presence of circulating microorganisms in the blood is either a part of the natural history of the infectious disease or a reflection of serious, uncontrolled infection. Depending on the class of agent involved, this process is described as *viremia, bacteremia, fungemia,* or *parasitemia.* Viremia is usually a very early, even prodromal, event accompanied by fever, malaise, and other constitutional symptoms such as muscle aches. With the exception of a few specific infections, the detection of viremia does not play a role in the diagnosis or management of viral infections. The presence of bacteremia defines some of the most serious and life-threatening situations in medical practice, and it has a marked impact on the management and outcome of bacterial infections. This chapter will focus on the causes and implications of bacteremia and, to a lesser extent, fungemia. Diseases in which parasitemia is a feature are covered in Chapters 44–48.

Sepsis

The terms *sepsis* and *septicemia* are used somewhat loosely, but generally refer to the clinical symptom complexes associated with bacteremia. They include fever, chills, hypotension, shock, and evidence of spread to multiple body systems. The clinical findings may develop acutely, as in Gram-negative septic shock, or slowly, as in most forms of infective endocarditis. Because the bloodstream is sterile in health, bacteremia is considered serious regardless of the symptoms present; however, transient bacteremia may occur when there is manipulation or trauma to a body site that has a normal flora. After such events, species indigenous to the site may appear briefly in the blood, but are eventually cleared. Such transient bacteremias usually have no clinical significance, but they are important in the pathogenesis of infective endocarditis.

Transient bacteremia

Intravascular Infection

Intracardiac infections (endocarditis) and those primarily involving veins (thrombophlebitis) or arteries (endarteritis) are usually caused by bacterial agents, although fungi, rickettsiae, chlamydiae, and even viruses have been occasionally implicated. This discussion will focus primarily on the bacterial causes, because they are the most numerous and important. Infections of the cardiovascular system are usually extremely serious and, if not promptly and adequately treated, can be fatal. They commonly produce a constant shedding of organisms into the bloodstream that is often characterized by continuous, low-grade bacteremia (1–20 colony-forming units per milliliter of blood) in untreated patients.

Infective Endocarditis

Sites of endocardial infection

The term *infective endocarditis* is preferable to the commonly used term *bacterial endocarditis*, simply because not all infections of the endocardial surface of the heart are caused by bacteria. Most infections occur on cardiac valves, but can also develop on septal defects, shunts (for example, patent ductus arteriosus), or the mural endocardium. Infections involving coarctation of the aorta are also classified as infective endocarditis because the clinical manifestations and complications are similar.

The pathogenesis of infective endocarditis involves several factors that, if concurrent, result in infection:

cardiac abnormalities and hemodynamic effects

1. The endothelium is altered to facilitate colonization by bacteria and deposition of platelets and fibrin. Most infections involve the mitral or aortic valves, which are most vulnerable when abnormalities such as valvular insufficiency, stenosis, intracardiac shunts (for example, ventricular septal defect) or direct trauma (for example, catheters) exist. The turbulence of intracardiac blood flow that results from such abnormalities can lead to further damage to endothelial surfaces and facilitates platelet and fibrin deposition. These factors produce a potential nidus for colonization and infection.

bacteremia with normal flora as infection source

2. Transient bacteremia is common, but usually of no clinical importance. Often seen for a few minutes after a variety of dental procedures, it has also been shown to develop after manipulations such as bronchoscopy, sigmoidoscopy, cytoscopy, normal childbirth, and some surgical procedures. Even simple activities such as tooth brushing or chewing candy can cause such bacteremia. The organisms responsible for transient bacteremia are usually common surface flora of low pathogenicity, such as viridans streptococci. Other, more virulent strains may also be involved, however; for example, intravenous drug abuse may lead to bacteremia with *Staphylococcus aureus* or a variety of Gram-negative aerobic and anaerobic bacteria. Whether the organisms causing bacteremia (or fungemia) are of high virulence or not, they can colonize and multiply in the heart if local endothelial changes are suitable.

adherence and development of vegetation

3. Other factors that contribute to the pathogenesis of infective endocarditis include adherence of organisms to the damaged surface, complement activation, inflammation, tissue destruction, and fibrin and platelet deposition at the site of colonization. The resultant entrapment of organisms in this thrombotic "mesh" of platelets, fibrin, and inflammatory cells leads to a mature vegetation, which provides relative protection to the organisms from host humoral and phagocytic immune defenses as well as antimicrobial agents. As a result, the infection can be exceedingly difficult to treat. In addition, the vegetation can create greater hemodynamic alterations in terms of both obstruction to flow and increased turbulence, or parts of it may break off and be deposited in smaller blood vessels (embolization) with resultant obstruction and secondary sites of infection. Emboli may be transported to the brain or coronary arteries, for example, with disastrous results.

embolization

circulating immune complexes

Another phenomenon shown to contribute to infective endocarditis syndrome is the development of circulating immune complexes of microbial antigen and antibody. These complexes can activate complement and contribute to many of the peripheral vascular manifestations of the disease, including nephritis, arthritis, and cutaneous vascular lesions.

host immune and hyperimmune responses

Frequently, there is a widespread stimulus to host cellular and humoral immunity, particularly if the infection continues for more than a couple of weeks. This condition is characterized by hyperglobulinemia, splenomegaly, and the occasional appearance of macrophages in the peripheral blood. Some patients will develop circulating rheumatoid factor (IgM anti-IgG antibody), which may play a deleterious role in blocking IgG opsonic antibodies and causing microvascular damage. Antinuclear antibodies, which also appear occasionally may contribute to the pathogenesis of the fever, arthralgia, and myalgia that is often seen.

In summary, infective endocarditis involves an initial complex of endothelial damage or abnormality, which facilitates colonization by organisms that may be circulating through the heart. This colonization, in turn, leads to the propagation of a vegetation, with its attendant local and systemic inflammatory, embolic, and immunologic complications.

Acute, subacute, and chronic infective endocarditis

Common clinical features. Infective endocarditis has often been classified by the progression of the untreated disease. The acute course is generally fulminant with high fever and toxicity, and death may occur in a few days or weeks. Subacute endocarditis progresses to death over 6 weeks to 3 months, and chronic cases continue for longer than 3 months. These latter two forms of the disease are characterized by low-grade fever, night sweats, weight loss, and vague constitutional complaints. The clinical course is substantially related to the virulence of the infecting organism; *S. aureus,* for example, usually produces acute disease, whereas infections by the otherwise avirulent viridans streptococci are more likely to be subacute or chronic. Before the advent of antimicrobial therapy, death was considered inevitable in all cases. Physical findings often include a new or changing heart murmur, splenomegaly, various skin lesions (petechiae, splinter hemorrhages, Osler's nodes, Janeway's lesions), and retinal lesions.

Complications

Complications include the risk of congestive heart failure as a result of hemodynamic alterations, rupture of the chordae tendinae of the valves, or perforation of a valve. Abscesses of the myocardium or valve ring can also develop. Other common complications relate to the immunologic and embolic phenomena that can occur. The kidney is commonly affected, and hematuria is a typical finding. Renal failure, presumably on the basis of immune-complex glomerulonephritis, is possible. Left-sided endocarditis can readily lead to coronary artery embolization and "mycotic" aneurysms; the latter will be discussed later in this chapter. In addition, more distant emboli to the central nervous system can lead to cerebral infarction and infection. Right-sided endocarditis often causes embolization and infarction or infection in the lung.

streptococci most common cause

culture-negative endocarditis

Common etiologic agents. Table 62.1 summarizes the most common causes of infective endocarditis. Streptococci are involved in most cases. In the so-called culture-negative group, infective endocarditis is diagnosed on clinical grounds, but cultures do not confirm the etiologic agent. This group of patients is difficult to treat, and the overall prognosis is considered poorer than when a specific etiology has been determined. Negative cultures may result from 1) prior antibiotic treatment; 2) fungal endocarditis with entrapment of these relatively large organisms in capillary beds; 3) fastidious, nutritionally deficient, or cell-wall-deficient organisms that are difficult to isolate; 4) infection caused by obligate intracellular parasites, such as chlamydiae (*Chlamydia psittaci*), rickettsiae (*Coxiella burnetii*), or viruses; 5) immunologic factors (for example, antibody acting on circulating organisms); or 6) subacute endocarditis involving the right side of the heart, in which the organisms are filtered out in the pulmonary capillaries.

predisposing factors of unusual etiologies

Some special circumstances alter the relative etiologic possibilities, for example, intravenous drug addiction, prosthetic valves, and immunocom-

Table 62.1 Common Etiologic Agents in Infective Endocarditis

Agent	Approximate Percentage of Cases
Viridans streptococci (several species)	30–40
Group D streptococci (enterococci)	5–18
Other streptococci	15–25
Staphylococcus aureus	10–27
Staphylococcus epidermidis	1–3
Enterobacteriaceae and *Pseudomonas*	2–13
Fungi (*Candida* sp., *Aspergillus* sp., etc.)	2–4

promise. The major associations in these cases are summarized in Table 62.2.

Blood cultures

General diagnostic approaches. The diagnosis of infective endocarditis is usually suspected on clinical grounds; however, the most important diagnostic test for confirmation in the laboratory is the blood culture. In untreated cases, the organisms are generally present continuously in low numbers (1–20/ml) in the blood. If an adequate volume of blood is obtained, the first culture will be positive in over 95% of culturally confirmed cases. Most authorities recommend three cultures over 24 hr to ensure detection, and an additional three if the first set is negative. Multiple cultures yielding the same organism support the probability of an intravascular or intracardiac infection. In acute endocarditis, the urgency of early treatment may require collection of only two or three cultures within a few minutes of beginning antimicrobial therapy.

Other specific cardiologic procedures can delineate the nature of the lesion, size of vegetations, and progression of disease. Of these techniques, one of the most useful is two-dimensional echocardiography.

need for bactericidal agents

use of antimicrobic combinations

General principles of management. Because of the nature of the lesions and their pathogenesis, response to therapy may be slow and cure is sometimes difficult. Therefore, specific antimicrobial therapy must be aggressive, using agents that are bactericidal (rather than bacteriostatic) and can be given in amounts that will achieve high continuous blood levels without causing toxicity to the patient. Treatment may involve a single antimicrobial if the organism is highly susceptible in vitro, or antimicrobial combinations if

Table 62.2 Etiologic Agents More Commonly Observed in Special Circumstances

Situation	Agent
Intravenous drug abuse	*Staphylococcus aureus*; group D streptococci; Enterobacteriaceae and *Pseudomonas*; fungi
Prosthetic valve infection	*Staphylococcus epidermidis*; *Staphylococcus aureus*; Enterobacteriaceae and *Pseudomonas*; diphtheroids; *Candida* and *Aspergillus* sp.
Immunocompromise, chronic illness	Any of the above organisms

parenteral therapy and blood level monitoring

synergistic effects are possible (for example, a penicillin and an aminoglycoside for enterococcal endocarditis). Therapy is begun by the parenteral route to produce adequate blood levels, and the patient is monitored frequently to ensure antimicrobial activity in the serum sufficient to kill the organisms without causing unnecessary toxicity. Therapy is usually prolonged, lasting longer than 4 weeks in most cases. In some cases, surgery may be required to excise the diseased valve and replace it with a valvular prosthesis. The decision for surgery is sometimes difficult, requiring consultation with both a cardiologist and a surgeon.

candidates for antimicrobial prophylaxis

Prophylaxis can sometimes prevent the development of endocarditis. Candidates for prophylaxis include persons with known congenital or acquired intracardiac (or intravascular) shunts (for example, ventricular septal defect), deformities of the cardiac valves (for example, rheumatic heart disease), or prosthetic valves. These patients are at a particularly high risk of developing endocarditis when undergoing procedures known to cause transient bacteremia (for example, dental manipulations or surgical procedures involving the upper respiratory, gastrointestinal, or genitourinary tracts). Administration of high doses of antibiotics is begun just before the procedure and continued for 12–48 hr thereafter. An example of prophylaxis is the case of a patient with rheumatic valvular disease who is planning to undergo dental work. The organisms most likely to produce transient bacteremia would be a penicillin-sensitive member of the oral flora, especially viridans streptococci. Thus, an intramuscular dose of penicillin within 30 min before the procedure, followed by oral penicillin for 2 days afterward, would be expected to afford protection. Several regimens similar to this approach are recommended, depending upon the patient, the nature of the procedure, and the organisms that might be expected to be involved.

Mycotic Aneurysm

The term *mycotic aneurysm* is somewhat misleading, as it suggests infection by fungi. Originally used by William Osler to describe the mushroom-shaped arterial aneurysm that can develop in patients with infective endocarditis, the term now applies to infection with any organism that causes inflammatory damage and weakening of an arterial wall with subsequent aneurysmal dilatation. This sequence can progress to rupture, with a fatal outcome.

Pathogenesis of intraarterial infection

Arterial infection can result from direct extension of an intracardiac infection or from septic microemboli from a cardiac focus, with seeding of vasa vasorum within the arterial wall. As such, these infections frequently complicate infective endocarditis. Other pathogenetic factors include 1) seeding of a previously damaged arterial intima by bacteria from a distant infection (the intima may have been altered by atherosclerotic plaques, vascular thrombi, congenital malformations such as coarctation of the aorta, or trauma from needle puncture, surgery, and the like); 2) trauma to the arterial wall with direct contamination; and 3) spread from a contiguous focus of infection directly into the artery.

The clinical features vary according to the site of involvement. Common findings may include pain at the site of primary arterial supply (for example, back or abdominal pain in abdominal aortic infections) and fever. In many cases, a pulsatile mass may be palpated.

Etiologic agents

The etiologic agents are similar to those listed in Tables 62.1 and 62.2 for infective endocarditis, and diagnostic measures (for example, blood culture) are also the same. *Salmonella* species and *S. aureus* are particularly common offenders in this disease. Management requires vigorous, prolonged antimicrobial therapy. Surgical excision and vascular grafting are often necessary.

Suppurative Thrombophlebitis

Categories

Suppurative (or septic) thrombophlebitis is an inflammation of the vein wall frequently associated with thrombosis and bacteremia. There are four basic forms: superficial, pelvic, intracranial venous sinus, and portal vein infection (pylephlebitis). With the steadily increasing use of intravenous catheters, the incidence of superficial thrombophlebitis has risen and represents a major complication in hospitalized patients.

Pathogenesis

The pathogenesis of suppurative thrombophlebitis appears to first involve thrombus formation, which may result from trauma to the vein, extrinsic inflammation, hypercoagulable states, stasis of blood flow, or combinations of these factors. The thrombotic site is then seeded with organisms, and a focus of infection is established. In superficial thrombophlebitis, an intravenous cannula or catheter may cause local venous wall trauma, as well as serve as a foreign body nidus for thrombus formation. If bacteria are introduced into this site of thrombus formation, via intravenous fluid or local wound contamination or by bacteremic seeding from a remote site of infection, the infection will evolve.

I.V. catheter associated thrombophlebitis

Thrombophlebitis of pelvic, portal, or intracranial venous systems most often occurs as a result of direct extension of an infectious process from adjacent structures, or via venous and lymphatic pathways near sites of infection. For example, infections of intracranial venous sinuses usually result from orbital or sinus infections (causing cavernous sinus thrombophlebitis) or from infections of the mastoid and middle ear (causing lateral and sagittal sinus thrombophlebitis). Pelvic thrombophlebitis is a potential sequela of intrauterine infection (endometritis), particularly after pelvic surgery or 2–3 weeks after childbirth. Pelvic or intraabdominal infections may also spread to the portal venous system to produce pylephlebitis.

Common clinical features. Clinical manifestations vary according to the site of involvement. Common features often include fever and, in superficial thrombophlebitis, warmth, erythema, tenderness, and swelling over the infected vein. Signs of septicemia may also be present. Pelvic or portal vein thrombophlebitis is usually associated with high fever, chills, nausea, vomiting, and abdominal pain. Jaundice may develop in portal vein infections.

Intracranial thrombophlebitis varies in its presentation. Headache, facial or orbital edema, and neurologic deficits are variably present: for example, cavernous sinus thrombophlebitis often causes palsies of the third, fourth, fifth, and sixth cranial nerves. A major clue to the diagnosis is the presence of recent or current infection in adjacent structures (for example, mastoids, sinuses).

Complications

Complications of thrombophlebitis include extension of suppurative infection into adjacent structures, further propagation of thrombi, bacteremia with sepsis, and septic embolization. Embolization, particularly from pelvic or leg veins, is to the lungs, and pulmonary embolism with infarction may be the primary manifestation of the remote infection.

Common etiologic agents. The major infectious causes of suppurative thrombophlebitis are outlined in Table 62.3. In superficial thrombophlebitis, which often follows intravenous therapy, organisms that are common nosocomial offenders predominate (*S. aureus*, Gram-negative aerobes). Deeper infec-

Table 62.3 Common Etiologic Agents in Suppurative Thrombophlebitis

Site	Agent
Superficial veins (saphenous, femoral, antecubital, etc.)	*Staphylococcus aureus*; Gram-negative aerobic bacilli
Pelvic veins, portal veins	*Bacteroides* sp.; microaerophilic or anaerobic streptococci; *Escherichia coli*; β-hemolytic streptococci (group A or B)
Intracranial venous sinuses (cavernous, sagittal, lateral)	*Haemophilus influenzae*; *Streptococcus pneumoniae*; β-hemolytic streptococcus (group A); anaerobic or microaerophilic streptococci; *Staphylococcus aureus*

tions are more frequently caused by organisms that reside on adjacent mucous membranes (for example, *Bacteroides* species in intestinal and vaginal sites) or commonly infect adjacent sites (for example, *Haemophilus influenzae* and *Streptococcus pneumoniae* in acute otitis media and sinusitis).

Direct culture and blood culture

General diagnostic approaches. The diagnosis is often suspected on clinical grounds and from associated events known to create predisposition to such infections (for example, surgery, presence of indwelling venous cannulas). Direct cultures of the infected site or blood cultures will usually yield the infecting organism, because bacteremia is often present. Cultures of purulent material from adjacent infected sites may also suggest the etiologic agent.

Radiologic procedures, including scanning methods, may be necessary to localize the process and support the diagnosis. In some cases, surgical exploration is required, both for definitive treatment and obtaining specimens for culture.

Chemotherapy

General principles of management. Antimicrobial agents are an important aspect of treatment, with the choice of antibiotics based upon culture results. In the absence of microbiologic data, therapy is chosen to cover the most likely possibilities listed in Table 62.3. Other important aspects of management include prompt removal of possible offending sources, such as intravenous catheters, vigorous treatment of adjacent infections, and sometimes surgical excision and drainage. Severe cases may also benefit from systemic anticoagulant therapy to prevent further propagation of thrombi and embolization.

removal of source of infection

Many cases are preventable. Long-term intravenous cannulation should be avoided. Whenever possible, it is better to use short needles such as "scalp vein" cannulas than venous catheters or plastic cannulas. Careful asepsis is essential with all intravenous procedures to prevent contamination of intravenous fluids, tubing, and the site of venous entry.

Intravenous Catheter Bacteremia

Source of endocarditis and metastatic infection

A variant of intravascular infection develops when a medical device such as an intravenous catheter or any of several types of monitoring devices placed in the bloodstream becomes colonized with microorganisms. The event itself does not have immediate clinical significance but, unlike transient bacteremia from manipulation of normal floral sites, the bacteremia is continuous rather than transient. This persistence greatly increases the chances of secondary

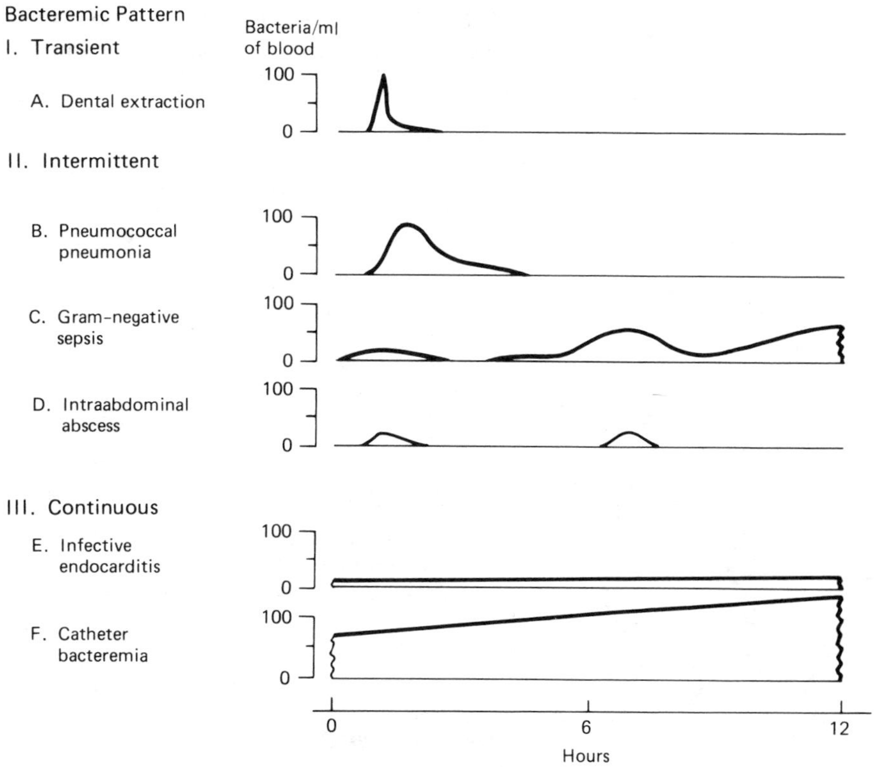

62.1 Patterns of bacteremia. The magnitude and timing of bacteremia for six typical patients (A–F) are depicted. These findings have implications for blood culture sampling plans. Cases such as **A** and **B** will only be detected by cultures taken early in their course. Cases such as **C** and particularly **D** are more variable and more likely to be detected by cultures spaced over the time period shown. Continuous bacteremia (**E** and **F**) should be detected by any sampling plan. It could be confused with transient bacteremia on single blood cultures, as both are caused by organisms of low virulence (viridans streptococci, *Staphylococcus epidermidis*); in cases such as E and F, however, bacteremia is sustained, whereas cases of transient bacteremia will yield multiple positive results only if they are collected at or near the same time.

complications such as infective endocarditis and metastatic infection, depending on any underlying disease and the virulence of the organism involved.

The organisms involved are usually those found in the skin flora, such as *Staphylococcus epidermidis* or *S. aureus.* In debilitated patients already on antimicrobial therapy, *Candida* species may be involved. Occasionally the sources of contamination are the intravenous solutions themselves rather than the skin. In these cases, members of the Enterobacteriaceae, *Pseudomonas,* or other Gram-negative rods are more likely.

discrepancy between degree of bacteremia and clinical manifestations

The clinical findings in catheter bacteremia are usually mild despite the large numbers of organisms in the bloodstream (Figure 62.1). Signs of inflammation may or may not be present, in addition to low-grade fever. Management is by removal of the contaminated catheter. Antimicrobial therapy will not eradicate the organisms in the presence of a foreign body (the catheter).

Extravascular Infection

Although bacteremia is a more constant feature of intravascular infection, most cases of clinically significant bacteremia are the result of extravascular infection. In these cases, the organisms drained or escaping from the infected focus reach the capillary and venous circulation through the lymphatic vessels. Depending on the magnitude of the infection and the degree of local control, these organisms may be filtered in the reticuloendothelial system or circulate more widely, producing bacteremia or fungemia. The process is dependent on the timing and interaction of multiple events and is thus much less predictable than the bacteremia of intravascular infection. If the infection is extensive and uncontrolled, such as an overwhelming staphy-

bacteremia more variable than with intravascular infection

Table 62.4 Frequency of Detection of Bloodstream Invasion by Bacteria and Some Fungi During Significant Infection at Extravascular Sites

Large (>90%) Proportion of Cases	
Haemophilus influenzae type b	*Brucella*[a]
Neisseria meningitidis	*Salmonella typhi*
Streptococcus pneumoniae (meningitis)	*Listeria*
Variable (10–90%) Depending on Stage and Severity of Infection	
β-hemolytic streptococci	Enterobacteriaceae
Streptococcus pneumoniae	*Pseudomonas*
Staphylococcus aureus	*Bacteroides*
Neisseria gonorrhoeae	*Clostridium*
Leptospira[a]	Anaerobic cocci
Borrelia[a]	*Candida*
Acinetobacter	*Cryptococcus neoformans*[a]
Small (<10%) Proportion of Cases	
Shigella (except *S. dysenteriae*)	*Pasteurella multocida*
Salmonella enteritidis	*Haemophilus*, noncapsulated
Campylobacter fetus, subspecies *jejuni*[a]	
Isolation Too Rare to Justify Attempt	
Vibrio	*Clostridium tetani*
Corynebacterium diphtheriae	*Clostridium botulinum*
Bordetella pertussis	*Clostridium difficile*
Mycobacterium	*Legionella*[b]

[a]Isolation and/or demonstration requires special methods or prolonged incubation.
[b]Infrequent isolation may be due to inadequate cultural methods.

lococcal pneumonia, there may be hundreds or even thousands of organisms per milliliter of blood, a poor prognostic sign. An intraabdominal abscess may only seed a few organisms intermittently until it is discovered and drained. Most infections that produce bacteremia fall between these extremes, with bloodstream invasion more common in the acute phases and intermittent at other times.

association with severe infections such as meningitis

The causative organisms and the frequencies with which they usually produce bacteremia (or fungemia) are listed in Table 62.4. There is considerable overlap, and the probability of bacteremia is dependent on the site as well as the organism. Any organism producing meningitis is likely to produce bacteremia at the same time. Infections with *H. influenzae* type b are usually bacteremic whether the site is the meninges, epiglottis, or periorbital tissues. Meningitis caused by *S. pneumoniae* can be expected to be bacteremic, but only 20–30% of pneumococcal pneumonias yield positive blood cultures.

bacteremia from respiratory, urinary, wound, and other primary sites of infection

The most common sources of bacteremia are urinary tract infections, respiratory tract infections, and infections of skin or soft tissues, such as wound infections or cellulitis. The organisms most frequently isolated from cases of bacteremia in a recent 6-month period at the Arizona Health Sciences Center are shown in Table 62.5. The frequency with which any organism causes bacteremia is related to both its propensity to invade the bloodstream (Table 62.4) and the frequency with which it produces infections. For example, the numerous cases of *Escherichia coli* bacteremia are mostly attributable to the fact that *E. coli* is the most common cause of urinary tract

Table 62.5 Cases of Bacteremia Reported in a 6-Month Period at the Arizona Health Sciences Center

Organism	Number of Cases	Percentage of All Cases
Staphylococci		
S. aureus (coagulase positive)	23	11
S. epidermidis (coagulase negative)[a]	5	2
Streptococci		
β-hemolytic	8	4
S. pneumoniae	10	5
Other	21	10
Listeria	2	1
Enterobacteriaceae		
Escherichia coli	46	22
Klebsiella	25	12
Enterobacter	10	5
Salmonella	3	1
Other	7	3
Pseudomonas	13	6
Haemophilus influenzae	4	2
Anaerobes	9	4
Miscellaneous bacteria	10	5
Fungi	12	6

[a]Probable contaminants such as *S. epidermidis*, diphtheroids, and propionibacteria excluded unless multiple isolates were obtained from same patient.

infection, a disease with a high prevalence but low incidence of associated bacteremia.

Gram-Negative Septic Shock

Clinical manifestations of endotoxic shock

Gram-negative shock may develop in patients with bacteremia caused by a Gram-negative organism. It is manifested by fever and chills, followed by hypotension, hypothermia, thrombocytopenia, intractable shock, and organ failure. It occurs most commonly in infections caused by Gram-negative rods such as the Enterobacteriaceae and *Pseudomonas aeruginosa,* but Gram-negative cocci such as *Neisseria meningitidis* may also be the cause. Once fully developed, the shock and organ failure may be irreversible and are responsible for the high mortality (25–60%) associated with Gram-negative sepsis.

Pathophysiology

The initial events in shock appear to be vasodilatation with resultant decreased peripheral resistance and increased cardiac output. The patient is flushed and febrile. Capillary leakage and reduced blood volume follow, which may lead to a whole series of events identical to those seen in shock resulting from blood loss. These manifestations include vasoconstriction, reflex capillary dilatation, and local anoxic damage. Once this stage is reached, the patient may develop both hypotension and hypothermia, and acidosis, hypoglycemia, and coagulation defects ensue with failure of highly perfused organs such as the lungs, kidneys, heart, brain, and liver.

Direct effects of endotoxin

The mechanisms involved in Gram-negative septic shock have been studied extensively in experimental animals. Most of the features seen in humans can be produced with the lipopolysaccharide endotoxin of the Gram-negative cell wall, although there is some variation between animal species and with different endotoxin preparations. The central events associated with the effect of endotoxin are 1) release of vasoactive substances such as histamine, serotonin, noradrenaline, and plasma kinins, which may cause arterial hypotension directly and trigger coagulation abnormalities; 2) disturbances in temperature regulation, which may be direct central nervous system effects or mediated by an endogenous protein pyrogen released from monocytes; 3) plasma complement depletion; and 4) direct metabolic effects in which endotoxin disturbs the mechanisms for controlling glucose metabolism. Oxidative phosphorylation by liver mitochondria is also impaired, and the action of corticosteroid hormones may be affected.

Immunologically mediated effects

Immune mechanisms may also be involved, as there are similarities between some features of endotoxin shock and allergic reactions. If so, previous sensitization by enterobacterial antigens in the gastrointestinal flora would be required. The acute events could then be triggered by the endotoxin released during the bacteremic phase of an infection. It is of interest in this regard that sterile (gnotobiotic) animals are resistant to the effects of endotoxin.

Management

Although the clinical and physiologic features described previously are typical of Gram-negative bacteremia with endotoxemia, they are not invariably present and are not reliable for distinguishing these cases from other overwhelming causes of bacteremia without endotoxic effects. The sudden appearance of one or more of these features, however, should alert the physician to the possibility of Gram-negative septic shock, because management requires more than antimicrobial therapy. Other therapeutic measures include maintenance of adequate tissue perfusion through careful fluid and electrolyte management and the use of vasoactive amines. Corticosteroids and anticoagulants may also be used, but their value is controversial.

Blood Culture

The primary means for establishing a diagnosis of sepsis is by blood culture. The microbiologic principles involved are the same as with any culture. A sample of the patient's blood is obtained by aseptic venipuncture and placed into an enriched broth. Growth is detected in the broth, and the organisms are isolated, identified, and tested for antimicrobial susceptibility. Because of the importance of blood cultures in the diagnosis and therapy of most bacterial and fungal infections, considerable attention must be paid to details of sampling if the prospects of obtaining a positive culture are to be maximized. In recent years older dogma has been replaced by a more scientific approach based on clinical studies of blood culture procedures. The approach to blood culture must be tailored to the individual patient, as no single procedure is best for all. The important features are as follows.

Skin decontamination

Venipuncture. Before venipuncture, the skin over the vein must be carefully disinfected to reduce the probability of contamination of the blood sample with skin bacteria. Although it is not possible to "sterilize" the skin, quantitative counts can be markedly reduced with a combination of 70% alcohol and a disinfectant containing iodine. Mechanical cleansing is as important as use of the disinfectant. Blood may be drawn with a needle and syringe or into a sterile blood collection tube containing an anticoagulant free of antimicrobial properties.

Anticoagulants

Sodium polyanethol sulfonate is currently preferred, as other anticoagulants such as citrate and ethylenediaminetetraacetic acid have antibacterial activity. Blood should not be drawn through indwelling venous or arterial catheters unless it cannot be obtained by venipuncture.

number of organisms in blood often < 1/ml

Volume. The number of organisms present in blood is often low (less than 1 organism/ml) and cannot be predicted in advance. Thus, small samples yield fewer positive cultures than larger ones. For example, as the volume sampled increases from 2 to 20 ml, the diagnostic yield increases by 30–50%. Samples of at least 10 ml should be collected from adult patients. The same principles apply with infants and young children, but the sample size is reduced to take account of the smaller total blood volume of a child. Although it should be possible to obtain at least 1 ml, smaller volumes should still be cultured because bacteremia at levels of more than 1000 bacteria/ml is found in some infants.

Number. If the volume is adequate, it is rarely necessary to collect more than two or three blood cultures to achieve a positive result. In intravascular infections (for example, infective endocarditis), a single blood culture will be positive in more than 95% of cases. Studies of sequential blood cultures from bacteremic patients without endocarditis have yielded 80% positive results on the first culture, more than 90% with two cultures, and 99% in at least one of a series of three cultures.

timing of intermittent bacteremia not predictable

interference of antimicrobic therapy with blood culture results

Timing. The best timing schedule for a series of two or three blood cultures is dependent on the bacteremic pattern of the underlying infection and the clinical urgency of initiating antimicrobial therapy. Figure 62.1 illustrates some typical bacteremic patterns that can be related to the probability of obtaining positive blood cultures. Transient bacteremia is usually not detected, because organisms are cleared before the appearance of any clinical findings suggesting sepsis. The continuous bacteremia of infective endocarditis is usually readily detected, as timing is not critical. Intermittent bacteremia presents the greatest problem for detection: there is no consistent way to predict when the organisms will be in the bloodstream, and fever spikes generally occur after, rather than during, the bacteremia. Little is known about the periodicity of bloodstream invasion, except that the bacteremia is more likely to be present and sustained in the early acute stages of infection. Closely spaced samples are less likely to isolate the organism than those spaced an hour or more apart. In urgent situations, when antimicrobial therapy must be initiated, two or three samples should be collected at brief intervals and therapy begun as soon as possible. It is generally not useful to collect blood cultures while the patient is receiving antimicrobics unless none were collected before therapy or there is a change in the clinical course suggesting superinfection. The laboratory should be advised when such cultures are submitted, because it is sometimes possible to inactivate the antibiotic prior to culture.

In summary, two or three collections of 10–20 ml of blood spaced over a 24-hr period one or more hours apart provide the optimal sampling conditions for detection of bacteremia or fungemia. Decreasing the number, volume, or sampling interval may be appropriate under certain conditions, such as those discussed previously. Likewise, it is appropriate to repeat and modify the blood culture procedure if the initial cultures are negative despite strong suspicion of bacteremia. The clinician should consult directly with the laboratory in such cases.

Laboratory processing. The basic blood culture procedure of incubating blood in an enriched broth is quite simple, but considerable effort must be expended to ensure detection of the broadest range of organisms in the least possible time. Daily examination of cultures for a week or more and a routine schedule of stains and/or subcultures of apparently negative cultures to detect organisms such as *H. influenzae* or *N. meningitidis,* which usually do not produce visual changes in the broth, are required. An automated blood culture system that measures ^{14}C-labeled carbon dioxide released from labeled substrates in the broth may be used in place of the conventional visual and cultural examinations. Some laboratories employ procedures that allow direct isolation of colonies, which is useful for quantitation and rapid identification.

Cultural conditions for aerobes and anaerobes

Modifications of laboratory blood culture procedures have been shown to favor certain classes of microorganisms, such as fungi and anaerobic bacteria. Isolation of fungi is facilitated by venting the bottles to achieve maximum aeration and by prolonged incubation. Anaerobes are favored by a highly reduced environment in unvented bottles. Because the latter conditions may inhibit strict aerobes and fungi, unvented bottles are usually paired with a vented counterpart to give optimal conditions for both aerobes and anaerobes.

Some bacteria, such as *Leptospira,* will not be isolated by routine blood culture procedures. The laboratory must be notified in advance so special media can be employed.

Interpretation. As the blood is normally sterile, the interpretation of blood cultures growing a pathogenic organism is seldom a problem. The major decision is the differentiation of agents causing transient bacteremia and skin contaminants from those opportunists associated with an intravascular or extravascular infection. Transient bacteremia is of short duration (Figure 62.1), is associated with manipulation of or trauma to a normal site possessing a normal flora, and involves species indigenous to that site. Despite skin disinfection, 2–4% of venipunctures result in contamination of the culture with small numbers of cutaneous flora such as *S. epidermidis,* corynebacteria (diphtheroids), and propionibacteria. The presence of these organisms in blood cultures can be considered a result of skin contamination unless quantitative procedures indicate large numbers (more than five organisms/ml) or repeated cultures are positive for the same organism. These findings should suggest diseases such as infective endocarditis or catheter bacteremia, which may be caused by these same organisms.

Normal floral contamination

C. George Ray

Infections of the Fetus and Newborn

63

The usual 10-month period from conception through birth and the first 4 weeks of extrauterine life is a unique period for host determinants of susceptibility and resistance to infection. It includes some paradoxes in which special mechanisms for defense are operating in the face of unusual susceptibility:

1. During normal development, the fetus is in a protected intrauterine environment, with fetal membranes serving as a physical barrier to external infection and the placenta contributing, with maternal immunity, to protection against many blood-borne infections. Transplacental transmission of specific immunoglobulins, particularly of the immunoglobulin G class (IgM does not normally cross the placental barrier), continues to provide some immunologic protection to the infant for weeks to months after birth, while lymphokines from the mother can provide transient cell-mediated immune support. If the infant is breast-fed, specific immunoglobulins (predominantly of the IgA class) in maternal colostrum afford some protection against pathogens that involve or invade through the infant's gastrointestinal tract.

immaturity of fetal immune system and suppression of maternal cell-mediated immunity

2. On the other hand, the fetal immune system is immature and there is relative suppression of maternal cell-mediated immunity as pregnancy progresses. These immune deficiencies serve an important biologic purpose, as they protect fetus and mother from activation of specific immunologic recognition and response mechanisms to differences in their histocompatibility locus antigens. If these processes did not occur normally, the fetus could be immunologically rejected by the mother or the fetal immune mechanisms activated to respond against maternal antigens in a form of "graft versus host" disease.

specific deficiencies of neonate

3. Specific and nonspecific immune responses begin to develop in early fetal life, perhaps as early as 8 weeks of gestation; however, a nearly normal immunocompetent state is usually not achieved until the infant is more than 2 years of age. Deficiencies commonly seen in the early period include decreased phagocytic capability and variability in intracellular killing of certain infectious agents, lower levels of complement components, and decreased opsonic capacity.

teratogenic effects of infection

4. Cell growth and organ differentiation are at their highest rates in the fetal–neonatal period, making the host especially susceptible to permanent damage when an infectious process intervenes.

Factors influencing risk of infection

The actual risk of infection and the types of pathogens encountered are influenced by a variety of interacting factors, including state of maternal health and susceptibility to specific agents, adequacy of fetal and neonatal nutrition, integrity of fetal membranes, and degree of maturity at birth. This chapter will outline the major types of infection of concern to those caring for the fetus and neonate and the general approaches to their diagnosis. Specific biologic characteristics and aspects of prevention and treatment for each of the agents have been addressed in previous chapters.

Definitions

Times and sources of infection

A number of terms are commonly used to describe the infections that can affect the fetus and newborn. *Prenatal infections* include those acquired by the mother and/or fetus at any time before birth. When fetal infection develops, it is usually either blood-borne to the placenta, with subsequent spread to the fetus (transplacental), or by the ascending route from the vagina through torn or ruptured fetal membranes. *Natal infections* are those acquired during delivery. They are often caused by agents in the maternal genital tract, but occasionally by organisms introduced from exogenous sources through attendants, fetal monitors, or other instruments. *Postnatal infections*, which constitute the remainder of the group, include all infections acquired after delivery throughout the newborn (or neonatal) period, defined as the first 4 weeks of life.

Another commonly used term is *congenital infection,* which describes infection occurring at any time before or at birth (prenatal or natal). Consequently, the infection is usually still active in the newborn period and sometimes persists for months or years.

The term *perinatal infection* is often used to include a period extending from 20–28 weeks of gestation to 7–28 days after birth. Because this definition is loose, it will not be used in this chapter.

Chorioamnionitis is an inflammatory response to infectious agents involving the chorionic and amnionic fetal membranes. It usually results from entry of pathogens from the vagina through tears or ruptures in the membranes, and it places the fetus at risk of direct exposure just before or at delivery. The risk of chorioamnionitis increases rapidly when membranes have been ruptured for longer than 12 hr before birth. When infection is by the blood-borne maternal route, there may be evidence of infection of the placenta, termed *placentitis.* Endometritis may be observed occasionally if the infection is an extension from a maternal pelvic focus along venous or lymphatic pathways.

Sepsis is a term employed to indicate a severe systemic bacterial infection associated with bacteremia.

Common Etiologic Agents

rarity of some childhood infections in infancy

postnatal *S. aureus* infections

Table 63.1 lists the major pathogens affecting the fetus and newborn, according to the usual modes of acquisition. Some, such as *Mycobacterium tuberculosis* and *Plasmodium* species, are exceedingly rare, but require consideration in certain clinical and epidemiologic circumstances. It should also be noted that some pathogens that commonly affect older infants and children are quite rarely observed in newborns. This phenomenon is partially attributable to the protective effect of maternally derived immunity to organisms such as *Haemophilus influenzae* type b, *Streptococcus pneumoniae, Neisseria meningitidis,* and mumps and measles viruses, but also reflects less opportunity for exposure to some agents early in life. Some organisms, such as *Staphylococcus aureus,* very rarely cause prenatal or natal infections, but commonly colonize in the postnatal period and most often cause disease after the first week of life.

Table 63.1 Modes of Infection and Major Agents

Mode	Agents: Bacteria	Agents: Viruses	Agents: Other
Prenatal			
Transplacental	*Listeria monocytogenes; Mycobacterium tuberculosis* (rare); *Treponema pallidum*	Rubella; cytomegalovirus; enteroviruses; Epstein–Barr virus	*Toxoplasma gondii; Plasmodium* sp.
Ascending	Group B streptococci; *Escherichia coli; Listeria monocytogenes*	Cytomegalovirus; herpes simplex	*Chlamydia trachomatis*
Natal	Group B streptococci; *Escherichia coli; Listeria monocytogenes; Neisseria gonorrhoeae*	Herpes simplex; cytomegalovirus; enteroviruses; hepatitis B; varicella-zoster	*Chlamydia trachomatis*
Postnatal	*Escherichia coli;* group B streptococci; *Listeria monocytogenes;* miscellaneous Gram-negative bacteria; *Staphylococcus aureus; Staphylococcus epidermidis; Clostridium tetani*	Cytomegalovirus; herpes simplex; enteroviruses; varicella-zoster; respiratory syncytial virus; influenza viruses	

Sources of colonization with pathogens

If one views the fetus as existing normally in a protected, "germ-free" intrauterine environment before emerging into a milieu of potential pathogens, it is easy to see how the newborn can be colonized with the first organisms encountered, which can then cause disease. The initial external pathogenic flora often acquired can include organisms frequently present in the maternal genital tract, such as group B streptococci and *Escherichia coli, Neisseria gonorrhoeae, Listeria monocytogenes, Chlamydia trachomatis,* and herpes simplex, which are important causes of natal infection.

Factors determining common neonatal infections

Postnatal infections may be late manifestations resulting from prenatal or natal colonization by pathogens such as those mentioned previously, but additional organisms may be acquired after birth. Particular risks include contamination of the nursery environment by a variety of Gram-negative bacteria, staphylococci, and some common viruses (Table 63.1) and attendants who are infected with or carrying such organisms. The risks are increased if the infant is born prematurely or otherwise physically compromised, and they are amplified by prolonged hospitalization and invasive procedures such as respiratory intubation, mechanical ventilation, and intravenous treatment.

risks of prematurity, prolonged hospitalization, and invasive procedures

Common Clinical Features, Diagnosis, and Management

Acute Bacterial Sepsis

When a physician first encounters a sick newborn, the primary concern is whether the illness represents sepsis and/or meningitis caused by bacteria. This determination is important, because treatment is both feasible and extremely urgent. Clinical disease apparent at birth or developing within the first 3 days of life (early onset) has usually been acquired prenatally. Mortality can exceed 70%, even with prompt treatment. Later onset of symptoms is commonly associated with natal or postnatal acquisition of pathogens; however, these infections can also be exceedingly severe. If meningitis develops, the overall mortality, even with treatment, ranges from

Severity of neonatal infections

group B streptococci and *E. coli*

Diagnostic clues

25 to 40%, and permanent neurologic damage may occur in 30–50% of survivors. The two pathogens most commonly associated with neonatal sepsis and meningitis are group B streptococci and *E. coli.*

The diagnosis of neonatal infections is based first on clinical suspicion. There is sometimes a history of recent maternal febrile illness immediately before or at birth. Other suggestive features include fetal distress, prolonged rupture of membranes, foul-smelling amnionic fluid, and premature delivery. The first signs and symptoms of illness in the infant may be subtle and extremely variable, including respiratory distress, apneic episodes, cyanosis, irritability, unexplained jaundice, poor feeding, abdominal distention, and fever. Initial laboratory findings often include either leukocytosis, with an increased proportion of immature neutrophils, or leukopenia. The development of seizures, hypotension, or disseminated intravascular coagulation indicates a particularly grave prognosis.

Cultures of blood and cerebrospinal fluid

Initial therapy

Diagnostic tests for suspected infections must be initiated as quickly as possible, followed by empirical antimicrobial therapy while waiting for culture results. The major tests include examination and culture of cerebrospinal fluid and a blood culture. The antibiotics initially chosen are those known to be effective against the pathogens most commonly encountered. They often include penicillin or ampicillin for the streptococci (also useful for *L. monocytogenes*) and an aminoglycoside such as gentamicin for *E. coli.*

Other Bacterial and Chlamydial Infections

Chlamydial and gonococcal conjunctivitis

Although *N. gonorrhoeae* and *C. trachomatis* are common natally acquired infections, they are usually not associated with sepsis. Both can produce a severe conjunctivitis in the newborn that requires prompt diagnosis and treatment. Gonococcal ophthalmia is usually apparent in the first 5 days after birth, whereas the onset of chlamydial conjunctivitis is frequently delayed until after the first week of life.

Chlamydial infant pneumonia syndrome

Another significant illness associated with natally acquired *C. trachomatis* infection is infant pneumonia syndrome. The onset of respiratory symptoms is often delayed, with most cases occurring between 2 weeks and 6 months of age. This illness is also considered in Chapter 28.

Postnatal infections by *S. aureus*

Scalded skin syndrome

Localized infections, such as cutaneous or subcutaneous abscesses, show a particular association with postnatally acquired infections with *S. aureus* and occasionally with various Gram-negative bacteria. If the newborn is affected by a staphylococcal strain that produces exfoliative toxin, the local lesion may be relatively trivial in contrast to the more widespread effect of circulating toxin on the skin, which is termed the *staphylococcal scalded-skin syndrome.* Prompt treatment with an antistaphylococcal antimicrobial agent results in resolution of the disease within 2 weeks, usually with complete healing.

Syphilis

Congenital syphilis

Prenatal infection by *Treponema pallidum* (congenital syphilis) is now unusual in the United States, but if left untreated, the organism can produce long-term damage, often without apparent signs or symptoms in the newborn period. To minimize these risks, serologic screening is recommended for all pregnant women when first seen in early gestation and at delivery. An alternative to testing the mother at delivery is to screen sera from newborn infants. In addition, serologic testing is recommended whenever clinical or epidemiologic circumstances suggest the possibility of exposure at any time during pregnancy. Prompt treatment of infected mothers during pregnancy, preferably with penicillin, will markedly reduce the risk of fetal infection. Similar treatment is also effective for the infected infant.

TORCH Complex

Toxoplasmosis, rubella, cytomegalovirus, herpes simplex, and other infections

Common clinical manifestations

Delayed manifestations

When bacterial, spirochetal, and chlamydial infections have been reasonably excluded from consideration, other possibilities can best be remembered by the convenient acronym TORCH (*T*oxoplasmosis, *O*ther, *R*ubella, *C*ytomegalovirus, *H*erpes simplex). This term comprises major infections that can be particularly severe if acquired prenatally. There is often significant overlap of clinical manifestations associated with the various agents in the TORCH complex. Common features may include low birth weight, rash, jaundice, and hepatosplenomegaly. On the other hand, many infants with TORCH infections can go undiagnosed, because the clinical signs may be inapparent at birth, only to appear weeks, months, or even years later. For example, congenital cytomegalovirus infection may be manifested only as mild mental retardation and/or hearing loss that may not become apparent until after the first year of life. Toxoplasmosis also presents a dilemma. It is estimated that as many as 1 in 200 pregnancies in the United States is complicated by primary infection with *Toxoplasma gondii,* which is usually subclinical. Of these cases, approximately 45% result in fetal infection, but only 8–11% of the infected offspring demonstrate clinical symptoms in the newborn period. The remainder are at risk, however, and can ultimately develop neurologic deterioration and/or chorioretinitis, which may not be recognized until 5 or more years later. These observations only partially illustrate the importance of TORCH complex infections and our relative impotence in controlling many of them.

Sources, risks, and prevention of hepatitis B infection

Neonatal varicella from infected mother

Of the array of miscellaneous agents grouped in the "other" category, two viruses deserve specific mention. If the mother has active infection with hepatitis B virus during pregnancy, the risk of natal or postnatal transmission to the infant is high (range, 20–80%, depending on the status of virus activity). Although it is unlikely that clinical disease will be apparent in the newborn period, it is important to undertake specific measures to prevent infection in the infant when the mother is infected. They include immediate administration of hepatitis B immune globulin after birth and consideration of subsequent immunization of the infant with hepatitis B vaccine. Primary varicella is infrequent in pregnancy. If the mother develops varicella less than 5 days before or 2 days after delivery, however, the risk is great of severe neonatal varicella, with a mortality of approximately 20%. It is recommended that the infant be given varicella-zoster immune globulin (or zoster immune globulin) immediately in an attempt to prevent or modify subsequent disease. Maternal zoster infections are not associated with a significant risk to the offspring, presumably because of adequate transplacental transmission of specific antibody.

The approach to a suspected TORCH complex infection requires some thought in selection of appropriate tests. Appendix 63.1 summarizes the major clinical and historic features of specific agents and the diagnostic procedures that can be used. The following general comments should also be kept in mind:

1. Clinical and epidemiologic data are used as much as possible in ascertaining likely specific agents.
2. Probabilities must be weighed; for example, congenital cytomegalovirus

infection is by far the most frequent TORCH complex agent encountered in the United States (more than 90% of all proved cases).

3. Potentially treatable infections must be considered most urgent. If toxoplasmosis or herpes simplex is suggested by the historic and clinical findings, it may be controlled by prompt and aggressive therapy. Other infections, which are potentially preventable by early specific immunoglobulin therapy of the infant, include maternal varicella and hepatitis B infections. The remaining agents involved in the TORCH array are not amenable to specific therapy at present. Their importance lies more in long-term prognosis, planning of continuing care, and epidemiologic management.

focus on treatable conditions

4. Serologic testing, when indicated, should be done on both infant and maternal sera collected at the same time to facilitate interpretation of specific antibody titer levels in the infant. This approach is based upon the following principles: Passive transplacental transmission of IgG antibodies occurs, but these maternal antibodies normally wane and disappear in the infant over 3–6 months. If the infant is actively infected, it usually produces its own specific antibodies to the agent, which then persist for much longer periods. Thus, a specific antibody titer in the infant's serum during the first month of life equal to or less than that of the mother may merely reflect passive transfer, and does not support a diagnosis of active infection. On the other hand, if the infant's titer is significantly higher than the mother's (fourfold or greater) or rises progressively in serial samples obtained in later months, active infection by the agent in question is suggested.

value of comparisons of maternal and infant antibody titers

Determination of infant IgM antibodies

In active congenital and neonatal infections, the infant's early responses often include IgM antibodies. As maternal IgM antibodies rarely cross the placental barrier, specific IgM antibody determinations early in life may be useful for the diagnosis of congenital toxoplasma, rubella, and cytomegalovirus infections. These tests are not readily available in many areas, however, and both false-positive and false-negative results have been noted. The presence of rheumatoid factor has been a major cause of false-positive results. Newer tests that show promise of high specificity include solid-phase IgM assays with antihuman IgM as a "capture" antibody and enzyme-linked antibody markers.

Lack of value of nonspecific tests

Nonspecific tests, such as quantitation of total IgM or IgA or detection of rheumatoid factor, have limited or no usefulness. Negative results do not rule out infection, and positive results must be regarded cautiously. Other tests, such as lymphocyte stimulation with specific antigens, show some promise, but are not yet available in enough centers to recommend them routinely.

Conclusion

Fetal and neonatal infections remain a highly significant and often frustrating challenge. They can be severe, and permanent sequelae are common. At the onset of infection, clinical signs and symptoms are often exceedingly subtle; thus, the physician must be quickly alerted to the infectious possibilities, particularly when specific treatment is available.

Of all of these infections, that most preventable currently is rubella, and assurance of immunity before conception is a mandatory goal. Better control of the remainder may become possible in the future with newer bacterial and viral vaccines, better early diagnostic methods, and improved treatment methods.

Appendix 63.1 TORCH Complex: Salient Features and Diagnostic Tests

Toxoplasmosis

Suggestive Clinical Findings. Chorioretinitis (found in more than 90% of symptomatic neonatal cases); lymphadenopathy.

Maternal History. Usually negative; occasional cervical lymphadenopathy during pregnancy.

Tests of Choice. Specific maternal and infant antibody titers; follow-up titers may be helpful.

Other Infections

The list of causes includes enteroviruses, hepatitis B, varicella-zoster, Epstein–Barr virus, arthropod-borne viruses, malaria, and tuberculosis. As the agents in this category most commonly encountered are the enteroviruses, the features summarized here pertain primarily to them.

Suggestive Clinical Findings. Sepsislike syndromes; meningitis; myocarditis (findings are variable).

Maternal History. Fever common at or near parturition.

Tests of Choice. Viral cultures of throat, rectum, and cerebrospinal fluid.

Rubella

Suggestive Clinical Findings. Congenital malformations, often multiple. In severe cases, "celery stalking" of metaphyses of long bones may be seen in early radiographs (see also cytomegalovirus).

Maternal History. Rubellalike illness or epidemiologic history of exposure in early pregnancy is common. If available, maternal serologic and immunization history can aid in supporting or refuting this diagnostic possibility.

Tests of Choice. Specific maternal and infant antibody titers. Serial determinations over 6 months may be of additional help. Culture is not a readily available routine test in most hospitals; special arrangements must be made.

Cytomegalovirus

Suggestive Clinical Findings. None very specific in differentiating infection from most others in the group. Statistically, cytomegalovirus is the most common congenital infection encountered. In florid cases, early radiographs of the long bones may resemble those of congenital rubella (celery stalking).

Maternal History. Usually none; occasionally, an account of a mononucleosislike syndrome may be elicited.

Tests of Choice. Urine culture is the most sensitive test. If results are negative, this diagnosis is highly unlikely; if positive, the diagnosis is supported (especially if cultures are done in the first 3 weeks of life). With advancing age of the infant, however, positive cultures may require careful interpretation before an unequivocal diagnosis is made.

Herpes Simplex

Suggestive Clinical Findings. Cutaneous vesicles and/or ocular or mucous membrane ulcerations; however, these lesions may not become apparent until other signs of illness have developed.

Maternal History. Up to 70% have no history of genital lesions or symptoms. Others may have a history of recent primary symptomatic infection. It is also important to ascertain whether genital lesions were known to exist in recent sexual partners.

Tests of Choice. Culture of lesions; immunofluorescent and cytologic studies may be available for rapid diagnosis. If no lesions are present, throat culture is also a valuable source. Brain biopsy, urine, and cerebrospinal cultures may also be necessary in some cases. Maternal cultures, if positive, may give indirect support regarding etiology.

Additional Reading and References

Feigin, R.D., and Callanan, D.L. 1983. Postnatally acquired infections. In *Behrman's Neonatal–Perinatal Medicine. 3rd ed.* Fanaroff, A.A., and Martin, R.J., Eds. St. Louis: Mosby, pp. 650–691.

Glasgow, L.A., and Overall, J.C., Jr. 1983. Viral and protozoal perinatal infections. In *Behrman's Neonatal–Perinatal Medicine. 3rd ed.* Fanaroff, A.A., and Martin, R.J., Eds. St. Louis: Mosby, pp. 692–707. This and the previous citation are up-to-date, well-referenced contributions that can add appropriate detail to the specific infections discussed in this chapter.

Lawrence Corey

Sexually Transmitted Diseases

64

Sexually transmitted infections are an important public health problem in all population groups and social strata. Over the past two decades, agents such as *Chlamydia trachomatis* and hepatitis B have been newly recognized as important sexually transmitted pathogens, whereas others such as the genital herpesvirus and *Neisseria gonorrhoeae* have increased in prevalence. Table 64.1 lists the prominent sexually transmitted pathogens and the disease syndromes associated with them. The most important are discussed as follows.

Gonorrhea

Gonorrhea is an acute pyogenic infection of columnar and transitional epithelium caused by *N. gonorrhoeae.* The urethra, endocervix, anal canal, pharynx, and conjunctivae can be infected directly. Spread of the organism along contiguous mucosal surfaces results in endometritis, salpingitis, peritonitis, and bartholinitis in the female host and epididymitis in the male. Systemic complications of bacteremic spread (gonococcemia) include inflammation of tendon sheaths (tenosynovitis), arthritis, dermatitis, myopericarditis, hepatitis, endocarditis, and meningitis. The microbiology of this organism is discussed in Chapter 16.

range of diseases

Epidemiology

The prevalence and clinical manifestations of gonorrhea differ according to the patient population surveyed. Gonorrhea was detected in cultures taken by private physicians in 2% of women in a 1977 survey conducted by the Centers for Disease Control; however, a much higher prevalence of infection (approaching 20%) has been found in women reporting to venereal disease clinics who are under 30 years of age, unmarried, and of low socioeconomic status. The risk of transmission of gonorrhea from an infected woman to a man during one sexual exposure is estimated to be about 30%, whereas the risk of transmission from an infected man to a woman may be as high as 90%.

Genital manifestations

urethritis

Gonococcal infection of the genital tract may be symptomatic or asymptomatic in men or women. Persons with symptomatic disease generally have sexual contacts with ignored or absent symptoms. The most common manifestation of gonococcal infection in men is urethritis with purulent discharge, dysuria, frequency, and meatal erythema. The usual incubation period is 2–7 days after exposure. In the absence of treatment, symptoms persist for an average of 8 weeks, with unilateral epididymitis in 5–10% of cases. In

Table 64.1 Sexually Transmitted Agents and Diseases Caused

Agent	Disease or Syndrome
Bacterial	
Neisseria gonorrhoea	Urethritis; cervicitis; proctitis; pharyngitis; conjunctivitis; endometritis; pelvic inflammatory disease; perihepatitis; bartholinitis; disseminated gonococcal infection
Chlamydia trachomatis	Nongonococcal urethritis; epididymitis; cervicitis; salpingitis; inclusion conjunctivitis; infant pneumonia; trachoma; lymphogranuloma venereum
Ureaplasma urealyticum	Nongonococcal urethritis
Treponema pallidum	Syphilis
Gardnerella vaginalis	Nonspecific vaginitis[a]
Haemophilus ducreyi	Chancroid
Calymmatobacterium granulomatis	Granuloma inguinale
Viral	
Herpes simplex virus	Primary and recurrent genital herpes; aseptic meningitis; neonatal herpes
Hepatitis B virus	Hepatitis B, acute and chronic infections
Cytomegalovirus	Heterophil-negative infectious mononucleosis; congenital birth defects
Genital wart virus	Condylomata accuminata; laryngeal papilloma of newborn
Molluscum contagiosum virus	Genital molluscum contagiosum
Protozoan	
Trichomonas vaginalis	Trichomonal vaginitis
Fungal	
Candida albicans	Vulvovaginitis; penile candidiasis
Ectoparasitic	
Phthirus pubis	Pubic louse infestation
Sarcoptes scabiei	Scabies

[a] Association remains unproved.

cervicitis

women, gonorrhea is manifested by discharge and pain associated with infection of the cervix. Characteristically, the endocervix is dusky red and friable with mucopurulent yellow exudate emanating from the endocervical os. Urethral infection causes urinary frequency and dysuria.

spread to upper genital tract

PID

association of PID with intrauterine devices

risk of infertility and ectopic pregnancy

Upward spread of the gonococcus to the endometrium causes endometritis associated with abnormal menstrual bleeding and midline abdominal pain. Further extension into the fallopian tubes results in pelvic inflammatory disease (PID) or acute salpingitis. The symptoms of gonococcal PID include bilateral lower abdominal pain, tenderness localized to the fallopian tubes and ovaries, fever, chills, and leukocytosis. The onset is generally during or shortly after menses, and the risk is increased in women using an intrauterine contraceptive device. The inflammatory response to gonococcal infection of the upper genital tract can result in scarring or dysfunction of the fallopian tubes and a decrease in fertility. The average risk of infertility is 13% after one episode of salpingitis, 35% after two episodes, and 75% after three or more episodes. In addition, salpingitis appears to increase the risk of subsequent ectopic pregnancies. Occasionally, spread of gonococci into the upper abdomen may lead to gonococcal perihepatitis with abdominal pain bilaterally or in the right upper quadrant, tenderness, and a hepatic friction rub. This diagnosis is often confused with acute cholecystitis.

Disseminated gonococcal infection

skin manifestations

arthritis

Spread beyond the pelvic area can produce disseminated gonococcal infection, which may proceed through two phases. The first is an early bacteremic phase characterized by fever, asymmetric tenosynovitis, and petechial, papular, or hemorrhagic skin lesions on the distal extremities. Without treatment, the systemic manifestations of bacteremia may subside only to be followed by infection at another site, most often an isolated joint. Septic arthritis may develop without a prior history to suggest bacteremia. The infection occasionally leads to endocarditis or meningitis. In contrast to strains causing urethritis, those causing disseminated gonococcal infection are usually resistant to killing by serum, often produce asymptomatic infections, have more fastidious growth requirements, and are almost always highly sensitive to penicillin.

Diagnosis

A presumptive diagnosis of gonococcal infection may be made when Gram staining of the infected material reveals typical Gram-negative intracellular diplococci (Plate **M**). In experienced hands, the sensitivity of the Gram stain exceeds 95% for urethral exudate from men and 60% for endocervical exudate from women. Cultures of exposed sites, such as the pharynx, urethra, cervix, and anal canal, should be obtained from all patients in whom the disease is suspected, except for men with smear-positive urethritis.

Treatment

penicillins

agents for β-lactamase-producing strains

Currently, recommended treatment of gonorrhea has undergone change because of the emergence of penicillin-resistant *N. gonorrhoeae* and the frequent association between *N. gonorrhoeae* and *C. trachomatis* infection. Detailed recommendations from the Centers for Disease Control are provided by the Sexually Transmitted Disease Treatment Guidelines in the supplement to *Morbidity and Mortality Weekly Report* (Vol. 31, No. 2-S, August 22, 1982). In areas where penicillinase-producing gonococci are rare and concurrent chlamydial infection is not expected, high single-dose oral therapy with ampicillin or amoxicillin is used with probenecid to block renal excretion and raise and prolong blood levels. High-dose intramuscular injection of procaine penicillin G with probenecid can also be used. A course of oral tetracycline is effective for tetracycline-susceptible strains and will treat simultaneous chlamydial infection; however, because of difficulty in ensuring patient compliance, antibiotics curative with single high doses are usually preferable. It should be remembered the treatment plan must also include the sexual partner. The recent emergence of β-lactamase-producing gonococci (Chapter 16) has made it important to follow treatment with cultural tests for cure. At present, spectinomycin is the drug of choice for penicillinase-producing strains or when their presence is likely because of epidemiologic associations (disease contracted in Southeast Asia) or treatment failure with penicillin G. Some of the newer third-generation cephalosporins, such as cefotaxime, are also effective in treating infections caused by gonococci resistant to penicillin and/or spectinomycin.

Syphilis

Syphilis is a chronic systemic infection caused by *Treponema pallidum,* which is usually sexually transmitted. The primary lesion is an ulcer with regional lymphadenopathy. Secondary syphilis is a bacteremic stage associated with generalized mucocutaneous lesions. This stage is followed by a latent period of subclinical infection that lasts for many years and eventually leads to tertiary syphilis in 30–50% of untreated cases. Tertiary syphilis may present as aortitis, central nervous system disease, or destructive mucocutaneous, musculoskeletal, and parenchymal lesions. *Treponema pallidum* and the pathogenesis of the different syphilitic stages are discussed in Chapter 24.

Epidemiology

Nearly all cases of noncongenital syphilis are acquired by sexual contact with infectious lesions. Fomite spread and transmission via blood transfusion

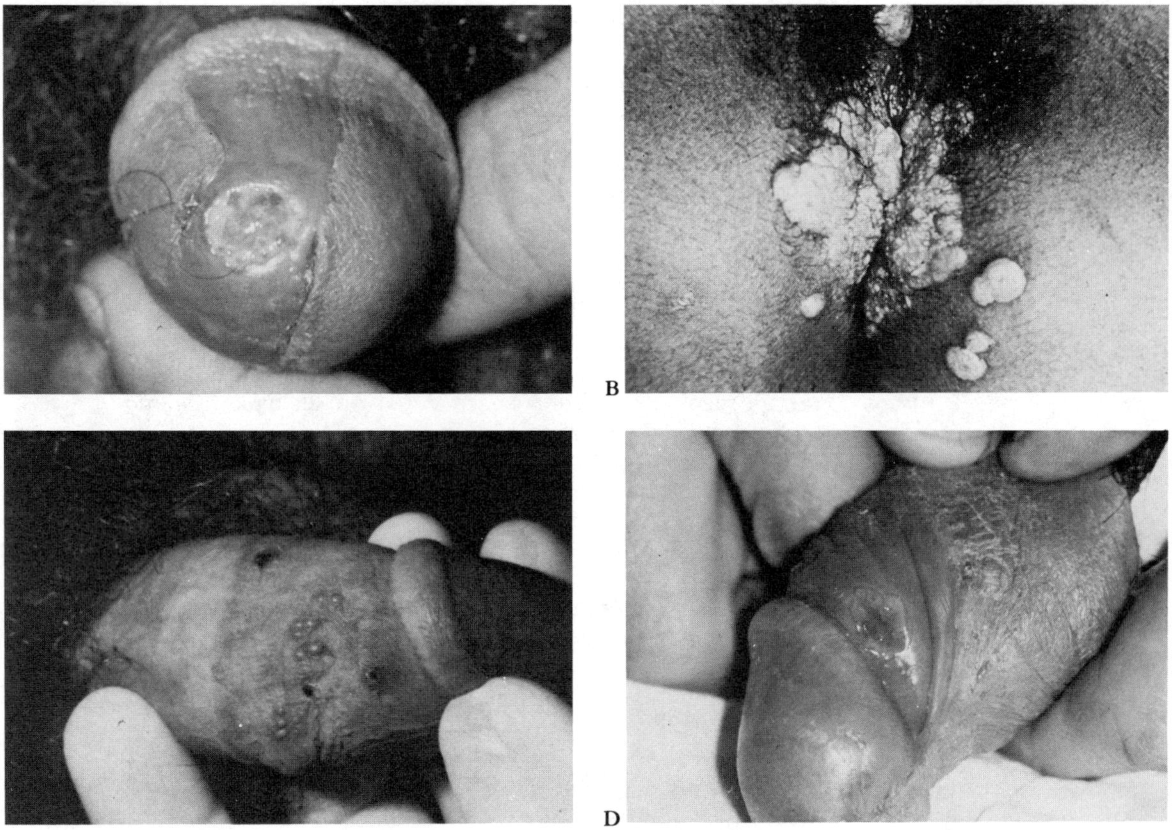

64.1 Some manifestations of sexually transmitted diseases. (**A**) Syphilitic chancre, showing rolled borders and indurated margin. Lesion is nontender when touched. (**B**) Condylomata lata in secondary syphilis. (**C**) Multiple grouped vesicles of genital herpes. (**D**) Chancroid infection. Lesion is tender and ulcerated. Patient also had a large, fluctant inguinal lymph node.

are both extremely rare. Most cases of syphilis occur in individuals 18-24 years of age. In the United States, the incidence is highest in nonwhite urban residents and about one-half of all men with primary, secondary, or early latent syphilis are homosexual or bisexual. About one-third of sexual contacts of those with infected primary or secondary lesions will develop the disease. New cases of syphilis must be reported to health departments to permit identification and treatment of contacts.

Primary syphilis

chancre

Syphilis must always be considered in the differential diagnosis of a genital ulcer. The median incubation period from contact until the appearance of the primary syphilitic chancre is about 21 days, but inversely proportional to the size of the infecting inoculum. The chancre (Figure 64.1A) develops at the site of infection. Typically, it begins as an indurated, painless papule, usually of the penis, external genitalia, anal area, or lips, that becomes ulcerated. Bilateral, firm, nonsuppurative, painless enlargement of the inguinal lymph nodes usually develops within 1 week of the primary lesion and may persist for months. Primary lesions teeming with *T. pallidum* can be found by dark-field or direct fluorescent antibody microscopy. They heal spontaneously after 4–6 weeks.

Secondary syphilis

Secondary syphilis may develop 2–10 weeks after the primary lesion has healed. It is characterized by a symmetric mucocutaneous maculopapular rashes and systemic manifestations

condylomata lata

dark-field examination positive

rash and generalized nontender lymph node enlargement with manifestations of systemic infection. Skin lesions are distributed on the trunk and extremities, often including the palms, soles, and face, and can mimic a variety of infectious and noninfectious skin eruptions. About one-third of cases develop painless mucosal warty erosions called *condylomata lata* (Figure 64.1B). These erosions usually develop in warm, moist sites such as the genitals and perineum. They are often elevated and pale or pink, and must be differentiated from infectious genital warts (condylomata accuminata). The VDRL and FTA test are invariably positive in secondary syphilis. Large numbers of *T. pallidum* are present in all lesions, and dark-field or direct fluorescent antibody examination of exudate from secondary lesions readily establishes the diagnosis. In one-third of untreated cases, host immune responses appear to resolve the infection. In the remainder the illness enters a dormant or latent state.

Latent syphilis

Latent syphilis is characterized by positive results of serologic tests in the absence of clinical signs or symptoms or of abnormal findings in cerebrospinal fluid. It is divided into two stages. Early latent syphilis, which occurs within 2 years of infection, is potentially transmissible because relapses associated with spirochetemia are possible. Late latent syphilis, which occurs more than 2 years after infection, is associated with immunity to relapse and resistance to reinfection. About one-third of cases do not progress beyond this stage.

Tertiary syphilis

neurosyphilitic manifestations

general paresis

tabes dorsalis

asymptomatic neurosyphilis

About one-third of patients with untreated syphilis will develop clinically evident tertiary manifestations (that is, cardiovascular syphilis, neurosyphilis, or gumma formation). Tertiary syphilis may appear as early as 5 years after infection, but characteristically occurs after 15–20 years. Neurosyphilis may be manifested as meningovascular syphilis, general paresis, or tabes dorsalis. Meningovascular syphilis involves diffuse gummatous and obliterative vascular changes of the meninges associated with increased cells and protein in the cerebrospinal fluid and focal neurologic changes. In general paresis, there is extensive cortical degeneration of the brain, and, unlike other tertiary syphilitic diseases, large numbers of *T. pallidum* are found in the affected areas. Some changes develop in the cerebrospinal fluid, but the major disease manifestations are personality changes ranging from decreased memory to hallucinations or frank psychosis. Delusions of grandeur are characteristic but not diagnostic, as they may also occur in healthy politicians, medical administrators, or senior house staff! Tabes dorsalis involves demyelination of the posterior columns and dorsal roots and damage to dorsal root ganglia. The latter produces ataxia, wide-based gait, foot slap, and loss of the sensations of position, pain, and temperature. Not all patients with central nervous system involvement have symptomatic disease. The diagnosis of asymptomatic neurosyphilis is made in those who have a reactive serum treponemal antibody test (for example, FTA-ABS) with increased cells and protein and a reactive VDRL in the cerebrospinal fluid.

Cardiovascular syphilis

aortic aneurysm

The most characteristic lesion of late cardiovascular syphilis is the development of an aneurysm of the ascending and transverse segments of the aortic arch as a result of gummatous changes in the middle coat of the aorta and loss of elasticity. This aneurysm can lead to aortic valve incompetence, pressure necrosis of structures adjacent to the aorta, or rupture of the aorta.

Gumma

The isolated gumma is a granulomatous reaction to *T. pallidum* infection. It occurs most often in skin, bones, or joints, but may involve any organ. Clinical manifestations of gumma are similar to those of other mass-producing lesions in the tissues, such as tumors. The diagnosis of a gumma involves serologic evidence of the disease and characteristic histologic features. Because of its protean sites of attack, syphilis, like tuberculosis, is a great mimic of other diseases.

Table 64.2 Frequency, in percent, of Positive Serologic Tests in Untreated Syphilis

Stage of Syphilis	VDRL[a]	FTA[b]-ABS	MHA[c]-TP
Primary	70	80	15
Secondary	100	100	100
Latent or late	70	98	98

[a]Nontreponemal antigen test.
[b]Fluorescence treponemal antibody test.
[c]Treponemal microhemagglutination test.

Congenital syphilis

routine serologic testing of pregnant women

The fetus is susceptible to syphilis only after the fourth month of gestation, and adequate treatment of an infected mother before that time will prevent fetal damage. Thereafter, treatment of the mother involves treatment of an already infected fetus. Because active syphilitic infection is devastating to the infant, routine serologic testing is performed in early pregnancy and should be repeated in the last trimester in women at high risk of acquiring syphilis. Untreated maternal infection may result in fetal loss or congenital syphilis, which is analogous to secondary syphilis in the adult, with involvement of the eyes, meninges, bones, and skin. Anemia, jaundice, and thrombocytopenia may also occur, and the disease in the infant must be differentiated from other congenital infections such as toxoplasmosis, rubella, and cytomegalovirus.

Diagnostic tests

dark-field examination and direct fluorescent antibody staining

All primary and secondary lesions should be evaluated by dark-field examination by an expert or by direct fluorescent antibody staining. The surface of a lesion is gently abraded and squeezed to express a drop of serous transudate, which is then examined directly for characteristic motile treponemes by dark-field microscopy or for the presence of *T. pallidum* by direct fluorescent antibody staining of a smear. A positive test is diagnostic of syphilis.

Serodiagnosis

specificity of treponemal antigen tests

VDRL as a test for cure

false-negative VDRL results

false-positive VDRL results

The basis of treponemal and nontreponemal serologic tests for *T. pallidum* infection is discussed in Chapter 24. Table 64.2 illustrates the frequency of positive test results in untreated syphilis by stage of disease for the VDRL, FTA, and microhemagglutination tests. Treponemal tests are highly specific, but remain positive after cure. Nontreponemal tests such as the VDRL are less specific, but the titers reflect the activity of disease and can be used as a test of cure. The VDRL titers should decrease at least fourfold after successful treatment of primary, secondary, or early latent syphilis, and 75% of primary and 40% of secondary cases revert to completely negative within 3–12 months. Failure of titers to decrease suggests inadequate therapy. An initial decrease followed by an increase during the first year suggests reinfection or relapse. The VDRL test results are falsely negative in 25% of patients with early primary syphilis and 25–30% of those with late or late latent syphilis. Many acute conditions that cause cell damage result in transient false-positive VDRL results. Chronic (more than 6 months) false-positive results are associated with drug addiction, autoimmune diseases, and aging.

Treatment

penicillin therapy

Treponema pallidum is killed by low concentrations of penicillin G; long exposure to the drug is required in established disease, however, probably because of the slow generation time of the organism. There is no evidence of resistance *T. pallidum* to penicillin, which remains the antimicrobic of choice. Erythromycin, tetracyclines, chloramphenicol, and cephalosporins are alternative antibiotics in penicillin-hypersensitive patients.

Jarisch–Herxheimer reaction

Fever, chills, myalgia, headache, tachycardia, leukocytosis, and vasodilatation, known as the *Jarisch–Herxheimer reaction,* may develop 2–24 hr after penicillin treatment of syphilis is begun. This reaction occurs in about one-half of patients with primary syphilis, 90% of those with secondary syphilis, and 25% of those with latent disease. In secondary syphilis, erythema and edema of the mucocutaneous lesions may occur. The pathogenesis of the reaction is not completely understood, but appears to result from an immune response to release of antigen by large numbers of lysed spirochetes.

prevention

At present, no vaccine against syphilis is available. Prevention and control depends upon detection and treatment of infectious cases. Because about one-third of those exposed to syphilis will develop disease, prophylactic therapy of all sexual contacts with penicillin G is recommended.

Genital Herpes Simplex

Genital herpes simplex virus (HSV) infection has emerged as a disease of increasing public health importance. It differs from other sexually transmitted diseases in the chronicity of the infection and the frequency of recurrences. The biology of this organism is described in Chapter 39. Genital HSV infections can be caused by viral types 1 or 2. The symptoms and signs of infection are similar for both HSV-1 and HSV-2.

Epidemiology

As genital herpes is not a reportable disease in the United States, the annual incidence is unknown; however, approximately half a million new cases have been estimated to occur yearly. It is the most common cause of genital ulceration in industrialized nations. Antibody prevalence data indicate that the incidence of genital herpes depends on the past sexual activity of the population studied. In some, such as prostitutes, HSV-2 antibody is detected in up to 80% of individuals. It is estimated that in middle-class American populations, the prevalence of antibody to HSV-2 is approximately 15–30%. Genital herpes infection is contracted by direct spread. It may be transmitted by asymptomatic shedding of virus from the cervix, from the urethra, in the semen, or from seemingly trivial infected lesions.

Clinical manifestations

painful vesicles

multiple primary lesions

The mean incubation period from sexual contact to onset of lesions is 5 days. Lesions begin as small erythematous papules that soon form vesicles and then pustules. Within 3–5 days the vesiculopustular lesions break to form painful coalesced ulcers that subsequently dry; some form crusts and heal without scarring (Figure 64.2). With primary disease the genital lesions are usually multiple (mean, 20), bilateral, and extensive (Figure 64.1C). The urethra and cervix are also infected frequently, with discrete or coalesced ulcers on the exocervix. Bilateral tenderness of the inguinal lymph nodes

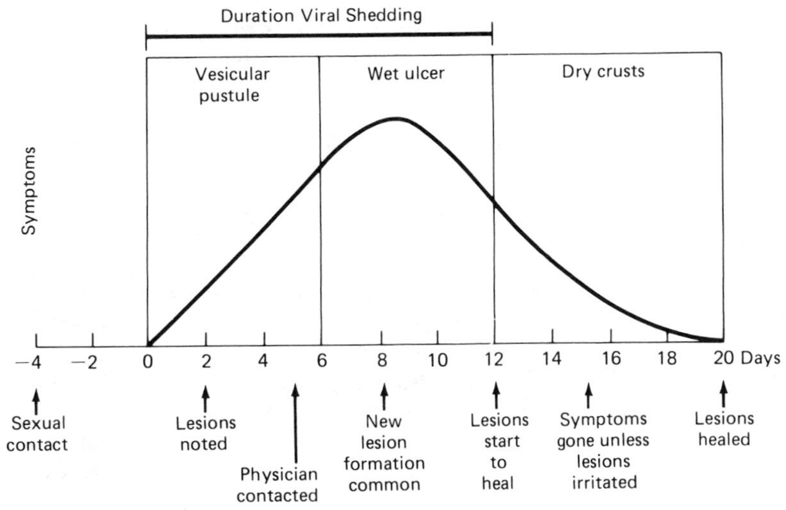

64.2 Typical course of first episode of herpetic infection.

cervical ulcers

inguinal adenopathy

systemic manifestations

other complications

and slight enlargement are usually present, are most apparent during the second week of the disease, and may persist as long as 1–2 months after infection. Lymph nodes do not become suppurative as in *Haemophilus ducreyei* infection. About one-third of patients show systemic symptoms such as fever, malaise, and myalgia, and 10% develop aseptic meningitis with neck ridigity and severe headache. Other complications include herpetic pharyngitis and autoinoculation of virus to other body sites, including fingers, lips, buttocks, and thighs. Bacterial superinfection is very uncommon. First episodes of disease usually abate after 20–30 days of illness.

recurrent infection

In contrast to primary infection, recurrent genital herpes is a disease of shorter duration, usually localized in the genital region, without systemic symptoms. One of the characteristic symptoms is prodromal paresthesia in the perineum, genitalia, or buttocks 12–24 hr before the appearance of lesions. Recurrent genital herpes usually presents with grouped vesicular lesions in the external genital region. Local symptoms such as pain and itching are mild and last for 4–5 days. The mean duration of viral shedding is 4 days, and lesions usually last for 10–14 days.

At least 60% of patients with primary genital HSV-2 infection develop recurrent episodes of genital herpes within 6 months. Genital HSV-1 infection appears to recur less frequently. In cases that recur, the median number of recurrences is four or five per year. They are not evenly spaced, and some patients experience a succession of monthly attacks followed by a period of quiescence. Most recurrences result from reactivation of virus from S_3–S_4 dorsal root ganglia. Recently, occasional episodes of reinfections with different strains of HSV have been documented.

Diagnosis

viral culture

Tzanck test

Although some genital HSV infections can be diagnosed clinically, the etiologic diagnosis of any genital ulceration should be determined; confirmation is best made by viral culture of the fluid from a fresh lesion. A smear prepared from the base of the lesions and treated with either Giemsa or Papanicolaou stain may show intranuclear inclusions or multinucleated giant cells typical of herpes (Tzanck test). This test is less sensitive than viral culture.

Treatment with acyclovir

The antiviral agent acyclovir has been used to shorten the course of primary and recurrent episodes, but it does not affect the latent state of the virus in the dorsal nerve root ganglia. Patients with genital herpes should not have sexual activity until lesions are completely healed.

relationship of herpes to cervical neoplasia

Women with genital herpes should undergo annual cervical cytologic (Papanicolaou) smear examinations, because their risk of cervical neoplasia is increased four to five times. Women with recurrent genital herpes should be monitored during pregnancy. If lesions are active, cesarean section is indicated to avoid transmission of infection to the neonate (Chapter 39).

Chancroid

painful nonindurated ulcer

inguinal bubo

Chancroid, a disease caused by *H. ducreyi,* is characterized by painful genital ulcerations and suppurative inguinal adenopathy. It is common in tropical areas, although outbreaks have recently occurred in Canada and the United States. The classic chancroid ulcer is a superficial, exudative, ragged ulcer measuring 1–2 cm (Figure 64.1D). It is painful and tender, but nonindurated. Involvement of the inguinal lymph nodes appears rapidly and may develop into an abscess within a node (bubo), which can rupture. The differential diagnosis includes genital herpes and syphilis; some distinguishing features are listed in Table 64.3. Genital HSV lesions may be difficult to differentiate from chancroid, although inguinal adenopathy in genital herpes is usually discrete and nonsuppurative. Microbiologic diagnosis of chancroid by culture on a special selective medium should be attempted in

Table 64.3 Causes of Genital Ulcerations

Disease	Type of Lesion	Type of Inguinal Adenopathy[a]
Genital herpes	Multiple grouped lesions; vesicles to coalesced ulcers	Tender on palpation
Chancroid	Tender, shallow, painful, ulcerated lesion	Suppurative
Syphilis	Nontender, indurated	Rubbery consistency
Lymphogranuloma venereum	Painless, small ulceration, usually healed at time of presentation	Suppurative
Granuloma inguinale	Chronic indolent, papular lesions	"Pseudobubo" caused by induration of subcutaneous tissue in inguinal area

[a]Involvement of inguinal lymph nodes.

sulfonamide therapy

all cases. The recommended treatment is sulfisoxazole or sulfonamide-trimethoprim combination. Fluctuant lymph nodes should be aspirated.

Lymphogranuloma Venereum

painless ulcer

Multiple inguinal bubos and fistulas

Complications

Isolation of organism and serodiagnosis

Tetracycline therapy

Lymphogranuloma venereum (LGV) is a chlamydial infection characterized by transient genital lesions followed by multilocular suppurative involvement of the inguinal lymph nodes. The primary genital lesion is usually a painless ulcer or papule, which heals in a few days and may go unnoticed. The most common presenting complaint is inguinal adenopathy. Nodes are initially discrete, but as the disease progresses they become matted and suppurative (bubos). The skin over the node may become thin and multiple draining fistulas develop. Systemic symptoms such as fever, chills, headaches, arthralgia, and myalgia are common. Late complications include urethral or rectal strictures and perirectal abscesses and fistulas. In homosexual men, LGV strains can cause a hemorrhagic ulcerative proctitis. The most satisfactory method for diagnosis is isolation of an LGV strain of *C. trachomatis* from aspirated bubos. In 80–90% of patients, the LGV complement fixation test is positive (titer of more than 1:64) shortly after the appearance of the bubo. The treatment of choice for acute LGV is tetracycline. Lymph nodes should also be aspirated to prevent rupture.

Granuloma Inguinale

persistent papules or ulcers

C. granulomatis

Donovan bodies

Tetracycline therapy

Granuloma inguinale is a very uncommon disease characterized by chronic, persistent genital papules or ulcers. It is caused by *Calymmatobacterium granulomatis,* a Gram-negative bacillus morphologically and antigenically similar to *Klebsiella.* The genital ulcerations persist for months and may extend into the inguinal region. The diagnosis of granuloma inguinale is usually made by examination of impression smears from biopsy specimens of the lesion. Wright- or Giemsa-stained smears demonstrate clusters of encapsulated coccobacilli in the cytoplasm of mononuclear cells. These aggregates, called *Donovan bodies,* are considered diagnostic. *Calymmatobacterium granulomatis* has been isolated in culture using specialized media containing egg yolk. Tetracycline is the treatment of choice.

Acquired Immunodeficiency Syndrome

A serious and apparently new immunodeficiency syndrome has been described recently in which previously healthy persons become predisposed to unusual neoplasms such as Kaposi's sarcoma or to the range of opportunistic infections described in Chapter 65, including *Pneumocystis carinii* pneumonia (Chapter 48). Clinical and laboratory findings indicate a severe and apparently irreversible cellular immunodeficiency, which particularly involves a reduced number of helper T lymphocytes relative to suppressor cells. The disease appears to be spreading, and in many reported cases death has resulted from persistent or recurrent opportunistic infections.

Epidemiologic evidence suggests that the disease is infectious and usually sexually transmitted. Through the first half of 1983, over 70% of the 1641 documented cases developed in homosexual or bisexual men. Most of the remainder were in intravenous drug users (17%) and persons born in Haiti now living in the United States (5%). Cases have also occurred in hemophiliacs (1% of all cases), indicating that a causative agent may be transmitted by some blood product concentrates. Only 7% of all cases have been in women, often in sexual partners of bisexual individuals or intravenous drug users. A few cases of AIDS appear to have occurred in children, again usually following the therapeutic use of blood or blood products.

Recently, evidence has accumulated that a retrovirus, tentatively called human T-cell lymphotrophic type 3 (HTLV-III), may be the cause of AIDS. The virus has been isolated from about 50 cases of AIDS in homosexual men, and about 95% of those with the disease have antibody to HTLV-III. The agent appears to affect T-cells, although B-cell infections also occur in vitro. While definite proof is still lacking that HTLV-III is the cause of AIDS, it appears at the time of writing to be the best candidate (see Chapter 43 for further consideration and references).

Other Specific Diseases

Several specific skin diseases may be acquired by sexual contact, including scabies, pubic louse infestation, and genital warts. Details should be sought in textbooks of dermatology or venereology.

Clinical Syndromes of Multiple Etiology

As indicated previously, nongonococcal urethritis, cervicitis, epididymitis, vaginitis, and PID may have multiple etiologies. The range of known infecting organisms is shown in Table 64.1, and the clinical manifestations are discussed as follows.

Nongonococcal Urethritis

The terms *nongonococcal urethritis* (NGU) and *postgonococcal urethritis* are used to describe cases not attributable to infection by *N. gonorrhoeae.* Patients present with dysuria and/or urethral discharge. In men, urethritis is established when purulent exudate is produced by milking the urethra from the base of the penis to the meatus. In the absence of expressible discharge, the presence of polymorphonuclear leukocytes in a urine sediment or on a urethral swab suggests urethritis.

C. trachomatis

U. urealyticum and HSV

The major cause of NGU is *C. trachomatis,* which accounts for 30–50% of cases. *Ureaplasma urealyticum* appears to be responsible for an additional 30% of cases. Herpes simplex virus has been implicated as the etiologic agent in about 2% of cases. About one-fourth of all cases have no established etiology; response to tetracycline therapy in some of these cases, however, indicates that an infectious etiology is likely.

Epidemiology

The age distribution of patients with NGU is similar to that of patients with gonococcal urethritis, but the ratio of NGU to gonorrhea is highest for individuals of high socioeconomic status. In most Western industrialized nations, NGU is now three times as common in men as gonococcal urethritis, possibly because treatment of sexual contacts of patients with NGU is not generally emphasized. This finding may also explain why cervical infection with *C. trachomatis* has been found to be several times more common than gonococcal infection in most population studies.

Clinical manifestations

Diagnosis

Clinical signs and symptoms of NGU are similar to those of *N. gonorrhoeae* infection. Patients present with urethral discharge, dysuria, and meatal swelling. There tends to be less urethral discharge with NGU than with gonococcal urethritis, but the diseases cannot be differentiated clinically in the individual patient. Gram stain of urethral exudate in the untreated patient with NGU demonstrates the presence of neutrophils, but not the Gram-negative intracellular gonococci seen in gonorrhea. Where available, specific cultural diagnosis of *C. trachomatis, U. urealyticum,* or HSV can be attempted. In practice, most patients in whom smear and cultured results are negative for gonococci are treated empirically without a specific etiologic diagnosis.

Tetracycline therapy

Tetracycline is usually effective, but approximately one-third of patients with nonchlamydial NGU fail to respond or have recurrences after treatment. Some are caused by tetracycline-resistant strains of *U. urealyticum,* but others may be related to HSV or unknown pathogens. Alternative drugs include erythromycin or a combination of spectinomycin and a sulfonamide.

Postgonococcal urethritis

Postgonococcal urethritis appears in men 2–3 weeks after curative penicillin treatment of gonorrhea. It is usually due to *C. trachomatis* infection that was acquired simultaneously with gonorrhea, but which has a much longer incubation period. Penicillin therapy cures only the *N. gonorrhoeae* component of this mixed infection.

Epididymitis

Unilateral swelling of the epididymis is a common clinical illness seen in sexually active men. It is usually quite painful, with fever and acute unilateral swelling of the testicle that is sometimes confused with testicular torsion. In the preantibiotic era, approximately 10–15% of untreated gonococcal infections resulted in epididymitis. In developed countries, the two most common causes of epididymitis are *N. gonorrhoeae* and *C. trachomatis.* In men over 35 years of age and in homosexual men, *Enterobacteriaceae* and *S. epidermidis* may also cause the disease, probably from reflux of infected urine into the epididymis. This condition is often associated with obstruction by the prostate gland. Treatment depends on demonstration of the etiologic agent in urethral specimens of epididymal aspirates.

gonococcal and chlamydial infection in young men

Enterobacterial and *S. epidermidis infection* in older men

Cervicitis

The microbial etiology of cervical infections is varied; *N. gonorrhoeae* and *C. trachomatis* cause endocervicitis, and HSV can infect the stratified squamous epithelium of the ectocervix. The major clinical manifestation of cervicitis is a mucopurulent vaginal discharge. The cervix is friable and inflamed, and polymorphonuclear leukocytes are present in the exudate. Viral, chlamydial, and gonococcal cultures are needed to demonstrate the etiologic agent. Occasionally, other pathogens such as cytomegalovirus and *Trichomonas vaginalis* are associated with symptomatic cervicitis. Therapy depends on the etiologic agent involved.

gonococcal, chlamydial, and HSV infections most common

Vaginitis and Vaginal Discharge

Symptomatic vaginal discharge may accompany salpingitis, endometritis, cervicitis, or a simple vaginitis. Evaluation includes pelvic examination, cervical cultures for *N. gonorrhoeae,* and microscopic examination of the discharge. Measurement of the pH of the discharge may also be helpful. Pelvic examination is valuable in determining whether uterine, adnexal, or cervical tenderness is present and whether the source of the discharge is the cervix or the vagina.

Candida vaginitis

The clinical and laboratory findings vary with the etiologic agent. *Candida albicans* generally produces a vulvovaginitis associated with pruritis and erythema of the vulvar area and a discharge with the consistency of cottage cheese. Microscopic demonstration of yeast and pseudomycelia in a potassium hydroxide preparation of the exudate confirms the diagnosis. *Candida* vaginitis can be treated with local nystatin or with miconazole.

Trichomonas infection

Trichomonas vaginalis typically produces a foamy, purulent vaginal discharge. The pH is variable (usually greater than 5.0), and numerous polymorphonuclear cells and motile trichomonads will be seen on a wet mount examination. Metronidazole is effective therapy for *T. vaginalis* vaginitis. Sexual partners should also be treated.

association of *Gardnerella* with nonspecific vaginitis

Clue cells

uncertain role of *G. Vaginalis*

The "nonspecific vaginitis" or bacterial vaginosis associated with *Gardnerella vaginalis* characteristically produces a discharge that is yellowish, homogeneous, and adherent to the vaginal wall. The pH is greater than 5.0. Addition of KOH to the vaginal secretions produces a fishy smell as a result of volatilization of amines. The Gram stain shows a shift from the usual *Lactobacillus* flora to one with many Gram-negative coccobacilli. Clue cells, which are vaginal epithelial cells heavily coated with tiny *G. vaginalis,* may also be seen. It remains uncertain whether *Gardnerella* is the primary cause of the disease or whether anaerobic bacteria are involved. Treatment may be difficult, but metronidazole is most effective, suggesting that anaerobic organisms are contributory. Relapses are common. It is uncertain whether treatment of sexual partners has any effect on the remission rate.

Pelvic Inflammatory Disease

multiple etiologies; *N. gonorrhoeae* predominant

Higher incidence with use of intrauterine devices

Clinical manifestations of PID vary, but generally include lower abdominal pain elicited by movement of the cervix or palpation of the adnexal or endometrial areas. In most clinical studies, about one-half of all cases of PID are caused by *N. gonorrhoeae.* Nongonococcal PID has a complex and sometimes polymicrobial etiology, including *C. trachomatis, Bacteroides,* anaerobic streptococci, and *Mycoplasma hominis* alone or in various combinations. In general, nongonococcal PID is milder than that associated with *N. gonorrhoeae* infection. The incidence of PID is 5–10 times higher in women with intrauterine devices than in those not using this form of contraception. The diagnosis is established most reliably by culture of peritoneal aspirates from the vaginal cul-de-sac.

Additional Reading and References

Holmes, K.K., and Mardh, P-A. 1983. *International Perspectives on Neglected Sexually Transmitted Diseases.* New York: McGraw–Hill. A monograph on sexually transmitted diseases and their effect on maternal complications.

Holmes, K.K., Mardh, P.A., Sparling, F., and Wiesner, P. 1984. *Sexually Transmitted Diseases.* New York: McGraw–Hill. This treatise on sexually transmitted diseases is the definitive textbook on the subject.

Sexually Transmitted Disease Treatment Guidelines. 1982. *Morbid. Mortal. Weekly Rep. Suppl.* 31 (2-S). Up-to-date details of recommended therapy are provided.

Lawrence Corey

Infections in the Immunocompromised Patient

65

Immunocompromised patients are those with some disorder or deficit in host defense mechanisms that predisposes them to increased frequency and morbidity or infections. Many such infections are caused by organisms that are members of the normal flora in health; they gain the ability to infect because of disruptions or disorders of the skin or mucosal barriers, neutropenia (shortage of neutrophils), impairment of phagocyte chemotaxis or intraphagocytic killing, and defects in antibody production or cell-mediated immunity. An immunocompromised state may result from trauma, the use of cytotoxic or immunosuppressive therapeutic agents, or genetic abnormalities, or it may be acquired as, for example, in acquired immunodeficiency syndrome (Chapter 64).

causes of immunocompromise and associated infecting organisms

In evaluating nontraumatic defects in host defenses, it is useful to categorize them as 1) defects to nonspecific immune responses (for example, the phagocytic response); 2) defects in the complement system; 3) defects in antibody-mediated immunity; and 4) defects in cell-mediated immunity. Each of these tends to be associated with infections caused by specific groups of organisms (Table 65.1 and Appendix 65.1). For example, neutropenia and disorders of phagocytosis are often associated with infections by Gram-positive cocci, Enterobacteriaceae and *Pseudomonas*, and sometimes fungi. In contrast, patients with defects in cell-mediated immunity tend to have severe viral, parasitic, and fungal infections or disease caused by bacteria that can multiply intracellularly (for example, mycobacteria). Those with defects in antibody production, such as agammaglobulinemia, are prone to infection with encapsulated organisms such as *Streptococcus pneumoniae* and *Haemophilus influenzae*.

Combined defects

In many immunosuppressed patients, several specific deficits in host defense mechanisms may be present concurrently. For example, cytotoxic drugs and glucocorticoids may impair phagocytosis, cell-mediated immunity, and humoral immunity and cause ulcerations of mucosal barriers, particularly of the oropharynx and gastrointestinal tract. Such patients are susceptible to the range of organisms associated with each of the individual deficits.

Defects in Mucosal Barriers

Defects in mucosal barriers allow access to the tissue by organisms that normally colonize the skin, gastrointestinal tract, or upper airway. Burns, extensive trauma, or decubitus ulcers remove the epithelial defense of the skin; however, less obvious factors, such as inhalation of toxic materials and

Table 65.1 Infections in the Compromised Host

Type of Compromise	Examples	Pathogens
↓ Leukocyte number or functions	Myelocytic leukemias Chronic granulomatous disease Granulocytopenia Acidosis Burns	*Staphylococcus* *Serratia* *Pseudomonas* *Candida* *Aspergillus* *Nocardia* *Legionella*
↓ Humoral immune response and complement deficits	Lymphocytic leukemias Multiple myeloma Nephrosis Antimetabolites Hypogammaglobulinemia	*Pneumococci* *H. influenzae* *Streptococci* *Pseudomonas* *Pneumocystis* *Enteroviruses*
↓ Cellular immune response	Hodgkin's disease Steroids Uremia Antimetabolites Malnutrition	*Mycobacteria* *Candida* *Coccidioides, Histoplasma, Blastomyces, Cryptococcus* Herpes group viruses Adenoviruses *Toxoplasma* *Pneumocystis* *Legionella* *Listeria*
↓ Reticuloendothelial system function	Splenectomy Chronic hemolysis	*Pneumococci* *Salmonella* *Listeria*

immunosuppressive therapy, may cause the damage to mucosal surfaces that predisposes to attachment and replication of potentially pathogenic organisms and can cause loss of host clearing mechanisms (for example, ciliary function). Defects in intestinal mucosal barriers are often associated with infections caused by Gram-negative aerobic and anaerobic enteric bacteria from the gut flora. Staphylococcal, streptococcal, or pneumococcal infections of the lung are particularly likely when the respiratory epithelium is damaged, whereas *Pseudomonas aeruginosa* infections are a common feature of severe burns. Bacteremia is a common complication of severe infections of these types.

Defects in Numbers or Functions of Phagocytes

When the natural barriers of the skin and mucosal surfaces are breached, the next major line of defense is the circulating phagocyte. To defend against infection, there must be an adequate number of these cells, which must be able to move to the site of infection and ingest and kill invading organisms. Numerous defects in these processes have been described.

Neutropenia

causes and significance of neutropenia

Although normal neutrophil granulocyte counts vary greatly according to the age, sex, and race of the patient, the usual value is 2500–7500 cells/mm^3 of blood in adults. Neutropenia may result from inherited or acquired diseases, use of cytotoxic drugs, or adverse reactions to therapeutic agents such as chloramphenicol. If the neutrophil count decreases to less than 500 cells/mm^3, especially less than 100 cells/mm^3, the incidence of infections increases markedly. Severe neutropenia is accompanied most frequently by bacterial infections caused by the pyogenic Gram-positive cocci, Enterobacteriaceae, *P. aeruginosa*, and *H. influenzae*. Fungal infections with *Candida, Aspergillus*, or the Phycomycetes are also common.

associated infections

Defects in Chemotaxis and Leukocytic Function

failure to produce chemoattractants

Occasionally, defects in phagocytic defenses are caused by inadequate leukocyte chemotaxis or function (Table 65.2). Deficiencies of complement or immunoglobulins can decrease chemoattractants at the site of an infection, and certain metabolic diseases such as diabetes and uremia can alter the microenvironment of leukocytes to reduce their mobility and responsiveness to tactic stimuli. This phenomenon has also been shown to occur in immune complex diseases such as lupus erythematosus. In each case, removal of the leukocyte to a normal environment restores its mobility and ability to respond chemotactically.

reversible inhibition of chemotaxis in metabolic diseases

Chronic granulomatous disease

Several genetic diseases produce specific defects in granulocyte bactericidal mechanisms that result in an immunocompromised host. Because they frequently diminish life span, these illnesses are usually seen in children. That most studied is chronic granulomatous disease, an X-linked disease of childhood associated with frequent pyogenic infections, usually caused by *Staphylococcus aureus*. The basic deficit is an inability to generate superoxide in phagocytes. In another disease, the Chédiak–Higashi syndrome, neutrophil lysosomes fail to fuse with the phagosome and the cells fail to destroy ingested organisms. These children also suffer recurrent infections with pyogenic organisms.

Chédiak–Higashi disease

sites and causes of infection

The spectrum of infections in patients with phagocytic dysfunction is wide and includes repeated bouts of cellulitis, pharyngitis, perirectal and other abscesses, pneumonia, osteomyelitis, and bacteremia. Many pyogenic organisms other than staphylococci can be involved. Antimicrobic treatment given either therapeutically or prophylactically has helped greatly in the care of these patients, but they still suffer repeated bouts of infection that

Table 65.2 Disorders of Phagocytosis and Intracellular Phagocytic Killing

Chemotactic Defects	*Ingestion*
Complement component deficiency	Actin–myosin dysfunction
Immunoglobulin deficiency	Drugs (colchicine, tetracycline, cyclophosphamide)
Intrinsic defects	Hyperosmolar states
"Lazy leukocytes"	Acute infections
Burns	
Hyperimmunoglobulin syndrome (Job's syndrome)	*Degranulation*
Collagen vascular disease	Chédiak–Higashi syndrome
Opsonization	*Killing*
Immunoglobulin deficiency	Lysosomal enzyme deficency
Complement component deficiency	Chronic granulomatous disease
Interference by immune complexes (systemic lupus erythematosus)	Glucose 6-phosphate dehydrogenase deficiency
Inhibition by drugs	Drugs (phenylbutazone, chloramphenicol)
Sickle cell anemia	Glutathione reductase deficiency

may ultimately prove fatal. Recently, new techniques have been developed to allow rapid collection and transfusion of functioning leukocytes in sufficient numbers to benefit some patients.

Defects in Immune System

Antibody Deficiency

IgA deficiency and giardiasis

IgG and IgM deficiency and susceptibility to encapsulated organisms

immunodeficiency in multiple myeloma and lymphocytic leukemia

Several congenital and acquired disorders can lead to inadequate synthesis of immunoglobulins as a result of deficiency or dysfunction of B lymphocytes. The most common and least serious is immunoglobulin A deficiency, which is associated with increased risk of gastrointestinal tract infection, especially with the parasite *Giardia lamblia*. Individuals with severe defects in IgG and IgM production (hypogammaglobulinemia or agammaglobulinemia) are prone to recurrent infections with encapsulated organisms such as *S. pneumoniae* or *H. influenzae*, which require opsonizing antibody for adequate phagocytosis (Chapter 7). Sinusitis, otitis media, bacterial pneumonia, and bacteremia are the most common types of infection. Selective deficiency in immunoglobulin production may also occur in multiple myeloma and certain types of chronic lymphocytic leukemia that involve monoclonal proliferation of one immunoglobulin-producing cell line and relative deficiencies of cells producing other antibodies. These patients are also prone to infections by systemically invasive organisms.

Treatment of antibody deficiency

use of pneumococcal vaccine

Repeated injections of immunoglobulins (immune serum globulin) may decrease the incidence and morbidity of infections in patients with agammaglobulinemia. In those capable of some immune responses, the use of pneumococcal vaccine may provide a degree of protection against overwhelming infection with this organism.

Complement Deficiency

systemic *Neisseria* infections

most serious defects involve both classic and alternate pathways

Defects of the complement system also predispose the patient to infection with encapsulated organisms that require opsonization. Individuals with deficiencies in C3 or later components of complement usually present with infections similar to those seen in patients with hypogammaglobulinemia, but they may also develop recurrent bacteremia caused by *Neisseria meningitidis* or *Neisseria gonorrhoeae* if they are infected with these species. Patients with defects in the early complement components, C1, C2, or C4, have less of a problem than those with later complement deficiencies, because they retain the ability to utilize the alternate complement pathway to activate C3 and hence C5–C9.

Disorders in Cell-Mediated Immunity

rare congenital abnormalities

effects of immunosuppressive cytotoxic drugs

multiple effects of glucocorticoids

Cell-mediated immunity is the part of the immune system that involves previously sensitized thymus-derived lymphocytes and is independent of circulating antibody. Both congenital and acquired abnormalities of the cell-mediated immune system are possible. Congenital abnormalities, which are uncommon, include thymic dysplasia syndrome, ataxia telangiectasia, and severe combined immunodeficiency (both T- and B-cell deficiency). A much more common defect develops in patients on treatment with immunosuppressive or cytotoxic agents that damage both macrophage precursors and T lymphocytes. Cytotoxic chemotherapy for cancer with cyclophosphamide and other antimetabolites has these effects and also inhibits humoral immune responses. Glucocorticoids can have multiple effects, causing neutropenia, lymphopenia, and monocytopenia through suppression of cell production, inhibition of mobilization of neutrophils to the site of inflammation, and interference with cell-mediated immune responses by altering the responsiveness of monocytes and macrophages to lymphokines. In addition, glucocorticoids impair the function of cells lining the mucosal surfaces, thus increasing the chance of microbial invasion by this route. Combinations of glucocorticosteroids and immunosuppressive drugs are essential in the treatment of certain diseases, but are particularly likely to interfere with the ability of a patient to combat new or established infections.

A detailed analysis of the infections associated with the different causes of cell-mediated and combined immune deficits is beyond the scope of this chapter. In general, defects in cell-mediated immunity are associated with increased susceptibility to infection with some opportunistic pathogens, particularly facultative or obligate intracellular pathogens (Appendix 65.1). Because of the wide range of potential infecting organisms, the sites of infection associated with defects in cell-mediated immunity are varied. They include superficial skin infections, lung infections, pharyngitis, otitis, sinusitis, bacteremia, and abscesses. Infections with multiple organisms are common. Clinical recognition and treatment of these infections is often difficult, because they may be relatively silent. Laboratory diagnosis can also be difficult, because many of the organisms listed in Appendix 65.1 require special culture media and grow slowly; others cannot be grown at all. It must be remembered that colonization of a peripheral site by an opportunistic organism does not necessarily mean that it is the cause of invasive disease. Thus, isolation of *Candida albicans* from the urine or the pharynx does not indicate that it is the cause of a concurrent renal abscess pneumonitis. Diagnostic procedures such as biopsy of involved organs are often needed to identify the causative agent.

susceptibility to intracellular pathogens

difficulties in clinical and laboratory diagnosis of infections

Attempts to enhance cell-mediated immune responses specifically or nonspecifically with agents that have shown some activity in animals generally have had little if any effect in reducing the frequency and severity of opportunistic infections in humans. Transfer factor has been used with limited success. It is a substance of low molecular weight secreted by circulating lymphocytes that can passively transfer delayed hypersensitivity to nonreactive individuals. Clinical trials are under way with thymosin, a product of the thymus gland that enhances the production and function of T lymphocytes in animals. Interferon also shows some promise and is under study.

Treatment of deficiency

Treatment of Infections in Immunocompromised Patients

need for early diagnosis and treatment

Successful treatment of infections in the compromised host depends on recognition of the deficit, early diagnosis, and prompt intervention. In neutropenia, the clinical signs of infection and even of abscess formation may not be apparent when the patient is first seen because of lack of reaction to the disease. It is thus usually necessary to initiate antibiotic treatment before results of culture and antibiotic susceptibility tests are available. Broad-spectrum antimicrobic coverage is used initially and replaced with narrower-spectrum agents, when the etiologic agent and its susceptibility are known, to reduce the risk of superinfection. In general, bactericidal antimicrobics are needed to control infections when host defenses are inadequate, and with severe infections a combination of synergistic agents may be necessary to provide increased bactericidal action.

Use of bactericidal agents

Patients with neutropenia have high rates of infection, and mortality is 20–30% if bacteremia develops. Therefore, short-term prophylactic antibiotic treatment has been advocated for these cases and can be effective in preventing infection until the neutrophil count improves. Selection of resistant organisms and "breakthrough" bacteremia as a result of overwhelming infection are major risks in these susceptible patients, and the physician must be alert to the possibility of superinfection with other pathogens during treatment.

Antimicrobic prophylaxis in neutropenia

Problems of resistance, breakthrough bacteremia, and superinfection

Appendix 65.1 Agents Commonly Infecting Immunocompromised Patients

Agent	Decreased Phagocytosis	Complement Deficiency	Agamma-globulinemia	Defects in Cell-Mediated Immunity
Bacteria				
Staphylococcus aureus and β-hemolytic streptococci	+++	++	++	
Streptococcus pneumoniae	+++		+++	
Enterobacteriaceae	+++	+	+	
Pseudomonas aeruginosa	+++	++	+	
Haemophilus influenzae	+	+	+++	
Salmonella species	+	+		+++
Listeria monocytogenes				+++
Mycobacterium species				+++
Legionella				+++
Nocardia asteroides				+++
Neisseria species		++	+	
Fungi				
Candida species				
Systemic	++			
Chronic mucocutaneous				+++
Aspergillus species	+++			
Phycomyces species	+++			
Cryptococcus neoformans				+++
Coccidioides immitis				+++
Histoplasma capsulatum				+++
Viruses				
Herpes simplex			+	+++
Varicella-zoster			++	+++
Cytomegalovirus				+++
Epstein–Barr				+++
Papovaviruses				++
Enteroviruses			+++	
Hepatitis B				+++
Influenza			+	+
Adenoviruses			+	+++
Parasites				
Pneumocystis carinii			++	+++
Giardia lamblia			++	+
Toxoplasma gondii				+++
Strongyloides sterocoralis				+++

Note: Number of pluses indicates relative susceptibility to the organisms listed according to the immune deficits.

Additional Reading and References

Grieco, M.H., Ed. 1980. *Infections in the Abnormal Host.* Yorke Medical Books. This multiauthored volume, which provides encyclopedic coverage of the subject, is recommended as a reference source.

Kenneth J. Ryan

Nosocomial Infections and Infection Control

66

Nosocomial is a medical term for hospital associated. Nosocomial infections are those that arise during hospitalization as a complication of another illness. Infection control is a hospital-based discipline, the purpose of which is prevention of nosocomial infections by application of epidemiologic concepts and methods.

The shining example of the fundamental importance of epidemiology in detection and control of nosocomial infections is the work of Ignaz Semmelweis, which preceded the microbiologic discoveries of Pasteur and Koch. His recognition, definition, and solution of the problem of childbed (puerperal) fever will be outlined as much as an example of still-valid epidemiology as for its historic importance.

Semmelweis and control of childbed fever

Semmelweis was Assistant Obstetrician at the Vienna General Hospital, where more than 7000 infants were delivered each year. Childbed fever (puerperal endometritis), which we now know was caused primarily by *Streptococcus pyogenes* (group A), was a major problem accounting for 600–800 maternal deaths per year. By careful review of hospital statistics, Semmelweis clearly showed that the death rate in one of the two divisions of the hospital was 10 times that in the other. Division I, which had the high mortality, was the teaching unit in which all deliveries were by obstetricians and students. In Division II, all deliveries were by midwives. No similar epidemic existed elsewhere in the city of Vienna. Mortality was very low in mothers delivering at home.

Semmelweis postulated that the key difference between Divisions I and II was participation of the physicians and students in autopsies. One or more cadavers were dissected daily, some from cases of childbed fever and other infections. Hand washing was perfunctory, which Semmelweis believed to allow the transmission of "invisible cadaver particles" by direct contact between the mother and the physician's hands during examinations and delivery. In 1847, as a countermeasure, he required hand washing with a chlorine solution until the hands were slippery and the odor of the cadaver was gone. The results were dramatic. The full effect of the chlorine hand washing can be seen by comparing mortality in the two divisions for 1846 and 1848 (Table 66.1). The mortality in Division I was reduced to that of Division II, and both were below 2%.

critical importance of hand washing in infection control

Unfortunately, because of his personality and failure to publish his work until 1860, Semmelweis' contribution was not generally appreciated in his

Table 66.1 Childbed Fever at the Vienna General Hospital

	Division I (Teaching Unit)			Division II (Midwife Unit)		
Year	Births	Maternal Deaths	Percentage	Births	Maternal Deaths	Percentage
1846[a]	4010	459	11.4	3754	105	2.7
1848[b]	3556	45	1.3	3219	43	1.3

[a]No hand washing.
[b]First full year of chlorine hand washing.

lifetime. As his frustration mounted over lack of acceptance of his ideas, he became abusive and irrational, eventually alienating even his early supporters. Some believe that he also suffered from presenile dementia (Alzheimer's disease). He died in an insane asylum in 1865, unaware that his concept of spread via direct contact would later be recognized as the most important mechanism of nosocomial infection and that hand washing would remain the most important means of infection control in hospitals.

Nosocomial Infections

Definitions

Infections associated with any hospitalization may be divided into two categories, community acquired and nosocomial. The Centers for Disease Control (CDC) in Atlanta defines community infections as those present or incubating at the time of hospital admission. All others are considered nosocomial, including those that appear within 14 days of hospital discharge. For example, a case of chickenpox erupting on the fifth hospital day would be classified as community acquired (incubating), but the same infection would be nosocomial if the patient had been in the hospital beyond the limits of the known incubation period (20 days). A staphylococcal skin infection appearing 12 days after discharge would be called nosocomial despite the distinct possibility that it was acquired at home. The purpose is to identify all infections that are truly a complication of hospitalization, at the risk of including a few others that were acquired elsewhere. It is important to recognize the peculiar infection hazards posed by the hospital: it is there that the most seriously infected and most susceptible patients are housed and often cared for by the same staff. Antibiotic therapy, by reducing competing flora, may create a predisposition to hospital-acquired infection often with resistant organisms.

Special hazards to hospitalized patients

Sources

Endogenous infections

The infectious agents responsible for nosocomial infections arise from various sources. Many are endogenous, originating from the patient's own normal flora. The factors involved in the pathogenesis of such infections are essentially the same in or out of the hospital. They include any debilitating disease plus the additional risks imposed by treatments that breach the normal defense barriers. Surgery, urinary or intravenous catheters, and invasive diagnostic procedures all may provide normal flora with access routes to usually sterile sites. The risk of infection is generally related to the extent of the trauma and the severity of the underlying illness. Minimizing or controlling both is the primary preventive measure. Of particular concern in infection control are nosocomial infections in which the source of organisms is the hospital rather than the patient. These sources include hospital personnel, the environment, and medical equipment.

Exogenous infections

Hospital personnel. Physicians, nurses, students, therapists, and any others who come in contact with the patient may transmit infection. Transmission of an organism causing infection in one patient to another patient is called *cross-infection.* The mechanism is usually direct contact via the hands of the medical attendant. Another source is the infected medical attendant. Many hospital outbreaks have been traced to hospital personnel, particularly physicians, who continue to care for patients despite an overt infection. Transmission is usually by direct contact, although airborne transmission is also possible. A third source is the person who is not ill but is carrying a virulent strain. *Staphylococcus aureus* and group A streptococcal infections are those in which carriers are most frequently involved. Nasal carriage is most important, but sites such as the perineum and anus have also been involved in outbreaks. An occult carrier is less often the source of nosocomial infection than a physician covering up a boil or a nurse minimizing "the flu." The carrier is difficult to detect unless the epidemic strain has distinctive characteristics or the epidemiologic circumstances indicate a single person.

cross-infection

infected medical attendants

carriers

Environmental sources. The hospital air, walls, floors, linens, and the like are not sterile, and thus could serve as a source of organisms causing nosocomial infections. Since Joseph Lister sprayed carbolic acid into the air of operating theaters in Glasgow, the importance of this route of infection has generally been exaggerated. With the exception of the immediate vicinity of a case or carrier, transmission through the air or on fomites is much less important than that caused by personnel or equipment. Exceptions are instances in which organisms are numerous and patients particularly susceptible or when a particular site is unusually vulnerable (valvular heart surgery).

environmental contamination least important source

Medical devices. Much of the success of modern medicine is related to medical devices that support or monitor basic body functions. By their very nature, devices such as catheters and respirators carry a risk of nosocomial infection, because they bypass normal defense barriers, providing microorganisms access to normally sterile fluids and tissues. Most of the recognized causes are bacterial or fungal. The risk of infection is related to the degree of debilitation of the patient and various factors concerning the design and management of the device.

infection from equipment that crosses epithelial or other defenses

Any device that crosses the skin or a mucosal barrier will allow flora in the patient or environment to gain access to deeper sites around the outside surface. Possible access inside the device (for example, in the lumen) adds another and sometimes greater risk. In some devices, such as urinary catheters, contamination is avoidable; in others, such as respirators, complete sterility is either impossible or impractical to achieve.

The risk of contamination leading to infection is increased if the organisms can multiply within the system. This process requires moisture, because no bacteria or fungi will grow in a totally dry system. The nutrient content and temperature of the available fluid largely determine which organism will survive and multiply. In general, Gram-positive bacteria such as staphylococci require near-physiologic fluid, whereas many of the Gram-negative rods are much less demanding. Once organisms such as *Pseudomonas, Acinetobacter,* and members of the Enterobacteriaceae gain access, they can frequently multiply in an environment containing water and little else.

Importance of moist environment

Even with proper growth conditions, many hours are required before contaminating organisms become numerous. In devices studied in detail, the risk of infection begins to increase after 24–48 hr and is cumulative even if the device is changed or disinfected at intervals. It is thus important to discontinue transcutaneous procedures as soon as medically indicated.

need to remove transcutaneous and urethral devices as soon as possible

The medical devices most frequently associated with nosocomial infections are listed below. The infectious risk of others can be estimated from the principles discussed previously. New devices are constantly being introduced into medical care, occasionally without adequate consideration of their potential to cause nosocomial infection.

Closed systems

Urinary catheters. The infectious risk of a single urinary catheterization has been estimated at 1–5%. Indwelling catheters carry a risk that may be as high as 10% for each day the catheter is in place. The major preventive measure is maintenance of a completely closed system through the use of valves and aspiration ports designed to prevent bacterial access to the inside of the catheter or collecting bag. The urine itself serves as an excellent culture medium once contamination occurs.

Sources of intravenous contamination

Vascular catheters. Needles and plastic catheters placed in veins (or, less often, in arteries) for fluid administration, monitoring vital functions, or diagnostic procedures are a leading cause of nosocomial bacteremia. These sites should always be suspected as a source of organisms whenever blood cultures are positive with no apparent primary site for the bacteremia. Contamination may originate from the skin flora with growth in the catheter tip or somewhere in the lines, valves, bags, or bottles of intravenous solutions proximal to the insertion site. The latter circumstance usually involves Gram-negative rods, whereas infections originating from the catheter tip are predominantly staphylococcal. Preventive measures include aseptic insertion technique and appropriate care of the lines, including changes at regular intervals.

Nebulizer contamination

Respirators. Machines that assist or control respiration by pumping air directly into the trachea have a great potential for infection if the aerosol they deliver becomes contaminated. Bacterial growth is significant only in the parts of the system that contain water; in systems using nebulizers, bacteria can be suspended in water droplets small enough to reach the alveoli. This combination of circumstances has been documented as a cause of lung infection when large numbers of Gram-negative rods contaminate the respirator aerosol. These organisms include *Pseudomonas,* Enterobacteriaceae, and a wide variety of environmental bacteria such as *Acinetobacter, Flavobacter,* and *Alcaligenes.* The primary control measure is periodic disinfection of the tubing, reservoirs, and nebulizer jets. Studies of contamination indicate that equipment should be changed every 24–48 hr.

Risk of hepatitis B infection to patients and staff

Hemodialysis. Bacterial infections of shunts and cannulas, a possible complication of chronic hemodialysis, are generally similar in origin to other infections arising from catheterization. Contamination of the dialysis fluid or artificial kidney is now an uncommon problem, but remains possible because the fluid contains bacterial nutrients and is maintained at body temperature. A far greater problem in hemodialysis units is the risk of hepatitis B infection as a result of the many procedural manipulations involving blood. If a patient carrying hepatitis B virus is treated in a hemodialysis unit, the most immediate risk is to the dialysis staff, but transmission to other patients also occurs. In a 1970 CDC report, 80% of hemodialysis units surveyed had experienced hepatitis in patients, staff, or both. Some units have had substantial epidemics. Control requires meticulous attention to procedures that prevent direct contact with blood, such as the use of gloves and gowns. Identification of hepatitis B carriers so that they can be treated separately is very important. Most units have established serologic surveillance procedures to detect both carriers and evidence of transmission among patients and staff.

Table 66.2 Nosocomial Infection Rates, Frequencies, and Most Common Pathogens

Infection	Infections/10,000 Hospital Discharges[a,b]	Percentage of All Nosocomial Infections[b]	Most Common Pathogens
Primary bacteremia[c]	7–30	3–7	*Staphylococcus aureus*; *Escherichia coli*; *Klebsiella*
Surgical wound	52–98	18–27	*Staphylococcus aureus*; *Escherichia coli*
Lower respiratory tract	35–72	14–18	*Klebsiella*; *Staphylococcus aureus*; *Pseudomonas aeruginosa*
Urinary tract	112–151	34–46	*Escherichia coli*; group D streptococci; *Pseudomonas aeruginosa*
Cutaneous	15–33	4–8	*Staphylococcus aureus*
All others	23–70	8–16	*Staphylococcus aureus*; *Escherichia coli*

[a] Data from 1979 National Nosocomial Infection Study, published by Centers for Disease Control in March 1982.
[b] Ranges reflect differences among community, community–teaching, federal, municipal, and university hospitals.
[c] No documented site of origin.

Etiologic Agents and Infection Rates

The rates and relative frequencies of the most common forms of nosocomial infection are shown in Table 66.2, together with the most common etiologic agents for each. These data are taken from the 1979 National Nosocomial Infections Study, a voluntary surveillance program directed by the CDC. Using the CDC definition of nosocomial infection, the rates in U.S. hospitals range between 0.8 and 8.9%. Most have nosocomial infection rates of 3–5%. If extrapolated to the more than 40 million persons hospitalized in the United States each year, this percentage translates to well over 1 million cases annually.

Differences between hospitals

The ranges shown in Table 66.2 reflect differences among community, community–teaching, federal, municipal, and university hospitals. In general, the rates are lowest in community hospitals and highest in municipal and university hospitals. This finding probably reflects differences in the types of patients treated in these institutions. For example, municipal hospitals usually have a higher proportion of elderly and debilitated patients and university hospitals a higher proportion of immunosuppressed patients. Both groups are more susceptible to infection and tend to have prolonged hospital stays. Table 66.2 also shows that urinary tract infections are the most common nosocomial infections, constituting one-third to one-half of all cases. Most of these infections are associated with the use of urinary catheters.

Urinary tract infections most common

The most common pathogens isolated are *Escherichia coli* and *S. aureus,* which together account for 25–30% of nosocomial infections. Other members of the Enterobacteriaceae, group D streptococci, *Pseudomonas aeruginosa,* and *Candida* species are also common causes. In general, the organisms most resistant to antimicrobics, such as *Klebsiella, Serratia,* and *Pseudomonas,* are

Antimicrobic resistant organisms more common in hospitals

much more common as causes of hospital-acquired than of community-acquired infections. For example, Table 66.2 shows *E. coli* to be the most common cause of urinary infection in the hospital; its proportion (32%), however, is much smaller than its share of community-acquired urinary infections, which exceeds 90%. Other organisms such as the group A streptococcus are currently uncommon, but occasionally cause outbreaks of serious infections, including puerperal fever.

Viral infections

Viruses tend to be underestimated in or excluded from surveys of nosocomial infections, because most hospitals still lack adequate viral diagnostic laboratories. Respiratory viruses such as influenza virus and respiratory syncytial virus have been shown to spread in hospitals by respiratory droplet inhalation or direct contact. Some of the highly infectious viruses, such as varicella (chickenpox, herpes zoster) and rubella (German measles), have caused outbreaks among susceptible patients and medical staff. Hepatitis B virus is responsible for hospital-associated infections in which transmission is from patient to medical staff, rather than the reverse.

Infection Control

Infection control is the sum of all the means used to prevent nosocomial infections. Historically such methods have been developed as an integral part of the study of infectious diseases, often serving as key elements in the proof of infectious etiology. Semmelweis' hand washing is the first example. Later in the 19th century, Joseph Lister achieved a dramatic reduction in surgical wound infections by infusion of a phenolic antiseptic into wounds.

Change from antisepsis to asepsis

This local destruction of organisms was known as *antisepsis* and sometimes included liberal applications of disinfectants, including sprays. As it became recognized that contamination of wounds was not inevitable, the emphasis gradually shifted to preventing contact between microorganisms and susceptible sites, a concept called *asepsis*. Asepsis, which utilizes the methods of sterilization and disinfection discussed in Chapter 4, is the central concept of infection control. The measures taken to achieve asepsis vary, depending on whether the circumstances and environment are most similar to the operating room, hospital ward, or outpatient clinic.

Asepsis

Surgical aseptic procedures and attitudes

Operating room. The surgical suite and operating room represent the most controlled and rigid application of aseptic principles. The procedure begins with the use of a disinfectant scrub of the skin over the operative site and the hands and forearms of all who will have contact with the patient. The use of sterile drapes, gowns, and instruments serves to prevent spread through direct contact, and caps and face masks reduce airborne spread from personnel to the wound. As all students learn the first time they scrub, even the manner of dressing and moving in the operating room are rigidly specified, and those involved assume a strict aseptic attitude as well as their masks and gowns. In some hospitals the air entering the operating room is filter sterilized, but this practice is expensive and its value unproved. The level of bacteria in the air is generally more related to the number of persons and amount of movement in the operating room than to incoming air. The net effect of these procedures is to draw a sterile curtain around the operative site, thus blocking any contact with microorganisms. Surgical aspesis is also employed in other areas where invasive special procedures such as cardiac catheterization are performed.

Hospital ward. Although theoretically desirable, strict aseptic procedures as used in the operating room are impractical in the ward setting. Asepsis is

Critical importance of hand washing

Isolation procedures

practiced by the use of sterile needles, medications, dressings, and other items that could serve as transmission vehicles if contaminated. A "no touch" technique for examining wounds and changing dressings eliminates direct contact with any nonsterile item. Invasive procedures such as catheter insertion and lumbar punctures are done under aseptic precautions similar to those used in the operating room. In all circumstances hand washing between patient contacts is the single most important aseptic precaution.

Patients with infections pose special problems, because they may transmit their infections to other patients either directly or by contact with a staff member. This additional risk is managed by the techniques of isolation, which separate the infected patient from others on the ward. The appropriate isolation techniques vary with the communicability of the infectious agent and the route(s) of transmission. These criteria have been formalized into specific isolation categories recommended by the CDC for use in hospitals. The isolation categories most commonly used are listed in Table 66.3 with the general techniques used for each. Details, including a list of recommendations for all communicable diseases, can be found in the CDC manual *Isolation Techniques for Use in Hospitals.* It is the physician's responsibility not only to recognize the presence of the infection, but to institute the appropriate isolation restrictions.

Outpatient clinic. The general aseptic practices used on the hospital ward are also appropriate to the outpatient situation as preventive measures. The potential for cross-infection in the clinic or waiting room is obvious, but has been little studied regarding preventive measures. Patients who may be infected should be segregated whenever possible using techniques similar to those of hospital ward isolation. The examining room may be used in a manner analogous to the private rooms on a hospital ward. This approach is difficult because of patient turnover, but should be attempted for infections that would require strict or respiratory isolation in the hospital.

Table 66.3 Isolation Techniques Used in Hospitals

Isolation Category	Route of Transmission Blockage	Isolation Techniques	Typical Infections
Strict	All	Private room[a]; gowns; gloves; masks; all articles[b]	Congenital rubella; chickenpox; plague (pneumonic); generalized staphylococcal skin infections
Respiratory	Respiratory route	Private room[a]; masks; contaminated articles[c]	Measles; tuberculosis; pertussis
Enteric	Contact spread from stools	Private room (children)[a]; gowns[e]; gloves[e]; contaminated articles[c]	*Salmonella*; *Shigella*; hepatitis
Wound and skin	Contact spread from lesions	Private room (desirable); gowns[e]; gloves[e]; masks[f]; contaminated articles[c]	Infected burns[d] Draining wounds[d]
Protective	Staff to patient	Private room[a]; gowns; masks; gloves[e]	Agranulocytosis; extensive burns; immunosuppression

[a] Door must be kept closed.
[b] All articles leaving room must be either discarded or wrapped for future sterilization or disinfection.
[c] Articles contaminated with pus or potentially infected secretions must be discarded or wrapped for future sterilization or disinfection.
[d] Wound or burn infections with *Staphylococcus aureus* or group A streptococci, which cannot be easily contained by dressings, require strict isolation.
[e] For those touching patient.
[f] For those changing dressings.

Organization

Modern hospitals are required by regulatory agencies to have formal infection control programs. Although the exact arrangements vary among hospitals, all have an Infection Control Committee and some kind of epidemiology service.

The infection control committee. The Infection Control Committee is composed of representatives of various medical and surgical services, as well as of pathology, hospital administration, nursing, housekeeping, food services, central supply, and other hospital departments. The chairman is usually a microbiologist, infectious disease specialist, pathologist, or some other person with a special interest in and knowledge of infection control. The committee is a policy-making and review body. The institution's infection control procedures and information on the status of nosocomial infections in the hospital are periodically reviewed by the committee. When epidemiologic circumstances warrant it, the committee may have to take drastic action such as closing a hospital unit or suspending a physician's privileges.

The epidemiology service. The epidemiology service is the working arm of the Infection Control Committee. Its functions are performed by one or more epidemiologists who usually have a nursing background. This work requires familiarity with clinical microbiology, epidemiology, infectious disease, and hospital procedures. The main activities are as follows.

1. *Patient surveillance.* It is necessary to collect ongoing information about the frequency and nature of nosocomial infections in the hospital to detect deviations from the institutional or national norm. Such reviews are conducted by the epidemiologist and reported to the Infection Control Committee.
2. *Environmental surveillance.* Routine sampling of the microbial flora of the hospital (air, floors, and the like) is of no value, but programs to sample some of the medical devices known to be nosocomial hazards can be useful. The epidemiology service usually oversees such programs, although the sampling itself may be done by others.
3. *Outbreak investigation.* On-the-spot investigation of true or potential outbreaks allows early implementation of preventive measures. This activity is probably the single most important function of the epidemiology service. Suspicion of an increased number of infections may be communicated to the epidemiologist by a physician, nurse, or microbiologist or be indicated by surveillance data. An investigation must then be conducted to verify the facts and establish basic epidemiologic associations. The primary concern is cross-infection, in which a virulent organism is being transmitted from patient to patient. Solution of the problem may require additional microbiologic investigations, such as bacteriophage typing of *S. aureus.* Other circumstances may indicate the failure of ward personnel to follow an established procedure, such as aseptic care of a closed-drainage urinary catheter.
4. *Education.* The epidemiology service should take the initiative in education of the hospital staff regarding infection control. This information may be imparted informally as rounds are made on hospital wards or in the course of surveillance or outbreak investigation. Formal in-service teaching sessions on subjects such as urinary catheter care, isolation procedures, and the like are also important. All hospital personnel, from housekeeping to medical staff, must be involved in continual review of infection control procedures, because the most common problem is be-

havioral. It cannot be stressed sufficiently that the most important procedure for preventing cross-infection is adequate hand washing between contacts with patients.

Summary

The prevention of nosocomial infections is contingent on basic and applied knowledge drawn from all parts of this book. Applied with common sense, these principles can both prevent disease and reduce the costs of medical care.

Additional Reading and References

Bennett, J.V., and Brachman, P.S., Eds. 1979. *Hospital Infections.* Boston: Little, Brown & Co. All aspects of nosocomial infections and infection control are covered in detail.

Isolation Techniques for Use in Hospitals. 2nd ed. DHEW Publication No. (CDC) 76-8314. Washington, D.C.: U.S. Government Printing Office, 1975. This 104-page manual gives specific recommendations on the management of infected patients on hospital wards. Model isolation signs for use on doors to patient rooms are included.

ADDENDUM

New Developments in Medical Microbiology

Any textbook in a dynamic field of science and medicine will, inevitably, be somewhat out-of-date before it is reprinted and sometimes between writing and publication. We believe, however, that the thrust of emerging fronts in our field is reasonably clear and projections can be made from present progress to probable future advances.

New Developments in Laboratory Diagnosis

In principle, it appears likely that the major new developments in laboratory diagnosis of infection will involve improvement and exploitation of techniques already available and discussed throughout this text. Molecular cloning now allows the large-scale production of DNA probes, which can then be used to detect small amounts of homologous microbial nucleic acid in preparations taken directly from patients. Until now, the practicality of this approach has been limited by the need to use radio-labeled DNA (usually with ^{32}P), which requires special handling precautions and a day or two for detection on photographic film. Recently, biotin linked to a nucleotide base has been employed as a DNA label. It can be detected by its extraordinary avidity for egg-white protein (avidin) to which an enzyme is linked. The presence of the labeled material can then be detected by addition of a substrate that is altered in color when acted on by the enzyme. A similar procedure can be used employing fluorescein as the label. This has opened up procedures for rapid and simple identification of specific genetic sequences by in situ hybridization, allowing detection of some microorganisms without the need for culture in material taken directly from the patient. The procedure can also be employed to detect gene coding for production of specific products, such as some microbial exotoxins. Kits and automated procedures to exploit these approaches can be expected to become available increasingly and to provide greater rapidity and specificity to the diagnosis of many infections.

A second major development involves the exploitation of procedures for selecting and producing monoclonal (hybridoma) antibodies against single, unique microbial antigens. This provides a degree of specificity attainable with antisera produced by simple immunization of animals. When used in conjunction with highly sensitive enzyme-linked immunoassay (ELISA) or similar procedures, these approaches have already been shown to detect microorganisms or microbial antigens rapidly in amounts that could previously only be recognized after amplification in culture. Both hybridoma and DNA homology-based procedures can also be combined with short periods of growth in culture to increase their sensitivity, and they have been shown to be effective in the early diagnosis of a range of bacterial, viral, protozoal, and fungal infections.

These approaches can be expected to be extended to cover most diseases for which a limited number of etiologic agents are usually responsible. They will thus supplement and often replace the immunofluorescent, immunoelectrophoretic, and coagglutination procedures that are already widely used.

Serodiagnostic procedures for infections due to organisms with complex antigenic structures (e.g., bacteria, protozoa, and fungi) can be expected to improve with the development of new knowledge of antigenic structures gained from two dimensional electrophoretic analyses and the application of immunoblotting techniques that combine SDS-page peptide separation with immunodetection techniques. Purification of specific antigens will reduce cross-reactions and may provide useful tests for diseases for which serodiagnostic procedures have previously been unhelpful. Molecular cloning will permit production of antigens, including antigens for organisms that are difficult to cultivate. This has already been accomplished, for example, with *Treponema pallidum*.

Automation is being applied increasingly in clinical microbiology laboratories. This trend can be expected to continue, thus providing advantages in speed, precision, and accuracy to a wide range of clinical microbiologic procedures.

Molecular Epidemiology

Just as molecular biologic procedures have now become of immediate value in diagnostic microbiology, their power and precision are opening new understanding of the epidemiology of microorganisms and of extrachromosomal and transposable genetic elements. Hybridization techniques and gel electrophoretic analyses of extrachromosomal DNA and viral genomes have provided more sensitive measures of similarity between strains than have been achieved by traditional serologic tests. Comparisons of restriction endonuclease fragments of DNA from different isolates have provided still more sensitivity and have also made it possible to trace the spread of plasmids and transposable elements within and between microbial species and from zoonotic reservoirs to humans. In the future, these approaches can be expected to become as much a routine in the typing and tracing of microbial strains and genetic determinants as has bacteriophage typing been in the past.

Antimicrobics

The development of many new antibacterial antimicrobics, particularly among the β lactams and aminoglycoside group, can be confidently predicted to continue, and the spectra of activity will extend to include many organisms that are currently naturally resistant or resistant through plasmid-coded antimicrobic modifying enzymes. Agents with little antimicrobic action but that are able to block β-lactamase activity have already been developed and found to extend the activity of some β-lactam antibiotics: this approach may be expected to become increasingly important. Past experience, however, offers little expectation that the development of new antimicrobics will finally overcome the problems of bacterial resistance because of the genetic plasticity and diversity of prokaryotes and their ability to acquire properties that ensure their survival under adverse conditions. Conservative and selective use of antimicrobics and avoidance of nosocomial cross-infection still appear to be the most promising approaches to the control of resistance.

Adhesion and Infectivity

The need for microbial attachment to surfaces as a means of colonization and as a prelude to invasion is being found to apply to increasing numbers of organisms, diseases, and even to the microbial growth that often occurs on and around prosthetic devices. Understanding of this process offers an opportunity of interrupting the earliest stage of infection by blocking adherence with free adhesins or receptors, by stimulating local sIgA production against adhesins, and by selecting materials for prosthetic devices, which are resistant to the mechanisms of microbial adherance. There is evidence that some microbial mediators of adherance may reduce the access of antimicrobics and inhibit the effectiveness of immunologic and phagocytic defense mechanisms, and we can anticipate increasing attention to efforts to abrogate these effects.

Vaccine Development

Until very recently, the most successful vaccines have been rather pure preparations of protective antigens (such as tetanus toxoid or pneumococcal polysaccharide) or attenuated live organisms that establish low-grade infections when conferring immunity (such as small pox, live poliomyelitis, and B.C.G. vaccines). With few exceptions, vaccines have been delivered parenterally by subcutaneous or intradermal routes. Improved ability to purify antigens, to produce them by cloning procedures, and to analyze the responses that occur to them during infection are now offering the opportunity of developing simpler and more specific vaccines for a wider range of bacterial and viral diseases, and to reduce the level of antigenic stimulation and undesirable effects produced by components that are irrelevant to protection. For example, component vaccines from *Bordetella pertussis* are under development and that should help avoid the reactions and systemic manifestations associated with vaccines now in use. In the case of some immunizing viral polypeptide molecules, complete amino acid sequences have been determined and the immunogens have been produced synthetically. These approaches can lead to the development of vaccines that will immunize against several diseases simultaneously and which will avoid unnecessary antigenic stimuli.

Immunization procedures in the past have been unsuccessful with many respiratory and intestinal infections, even though the course of the disease indicates that immunity develops. As we have indicated elsewhere in the book, there is much evidence to indicate the importance of local immunity by sIgA in these diseases. There is thus increasing interest in stimulating such immunity by the use of live vaccines of attenuated organisms or of genetically engineered chimeras that synthesize the protective antigens of one or more pathogen in situ, but are themselves avirulent. Success in immunizing against *Shigella dysenteriae* has already been achieved using a live streptomycin-dependent strain in the absence of the antibiotic, and thus under conditions in which it cannot multiply.This has clearly shown the potentiality of such approaches for vaccines that stimulate local immunity, and we can anticipate the development of new oral vaccines against enteric infections and of locally applied vaccines against some respiratory viral infections.

New and Disappearing Diseases

The past decade or so has been a time in which several important infectious diseases have been recognized or have developed. Examples include Legionnaires disease, detection of the cause of Lyme disease, the recognition of *Campylobacter jejuni* as a major cause of endemic and epidemic intestinal infection, and the discovery of Delta virus, which is associated with hepatitis B infection and can itself cause severe episodes of hepatitis. Acquired immune deficiency syndrome (AIDS) has also arisen or become a major problem during the past five years, and has now been shown to be due to a retrovirus (HTLV-III) related to the human T cell leukemia virus. Cryptosporidiosis, a protozoal disease of animals, was first recognized in humans as a serious intestinal infection in AIDS and other immunocompromised patients, and has been shown to be a significant cause of self-limiting diarrheal disease in otherwise healthy children. Various factors have contributed to these changes. Campylobacter and cryptosporidial infections are almost certainly not new, but their extent has only recently been recognized. The increase in legionellosis appears to have reflected changes in building construction, ventilation, cooling, and water distribution systems, while the current epidemic of AIDS partially reflects social and behavioral changes. It is very probable that future changes in human ecology, behavior, demography, and medicine will lead to the development or recognition of other "new" diseases, and will increase the proportions of opportunistic infections among those whose normal defenses are compromised through age, disease, or therapy.

Conversely, the eradication of smallpox has shown that eradication of some other extant diseases in developed countries, if not worldwide, is possible and in some cases probable; success will depend first on absence of a significant healthy carrier state or of a zoonotic reservoir in wildlife. Other factors of great importance will be effective vaccines or therapeutics, ease of recognition of the disease, specific laboratory diagnostic tests, and the appropriation of the necessary resources in money and personnel. Measles is already largely under control in developed countries, and national eradication is clearly feasible. Rubella, mumps, syphilis, and tuberculosis are all potentially eradicable within a community if the will, resources, and political support are available, but significant reductions in these diseases will continue or may be expected to occur, even with present approaches to their control.

Glossary

A

Prefixes
Arthro- Pertaining to joints
Auto- Self, or arising from within
Auxo- Pertaining to growth

Suffix
-algia Pain

Acanthosis Hypertrophy of prickle cell layer of skin
Accessory sinuses Blind-ended cavities in bone draining into nasal cavity
Achlorhydria Absence of hydrochloric acid in stomach
Acidosis Increased acidity of body fluid
Adnexal (uterine) Fallopian tubes and ovaries
Agammaglobulinemia Absence of immunoglobulins in blood
Agranulocytosis Failure of white blood cell production in bone marrow
Alveoli (lung) Microscopic air sac in lung
Amniotic fluid Fluid in amnion surrounding fetus
Analog Structurally or functionally similar
Anamnestic Immunological: enhanced memory response on exposure to antigen
Anaphylaxis Immediate antibody-mediated hypersensitivity
Anergic Absence of ability to respond to antigen
Aneurysm Localized abnormal dilatation of blood vessel
Anicteric Absence of clinical jaundice
Anorexia Loss of appetite
Anoxia Lack of adequate oxygenation of blood/ or tissues
Antibiogram Pattern of in vitro susceptibilities to different antibiotics
Antisera Sera containing specific antibodies
Antispasmodic Drug that relieves spasm
Antitussive Substance that helps control coughing
Antrum Cavity or chamber within the body
Aplastic anemia Failure of red cell production in bone marrow
Apnea Temporary absence of breathing
Aqueduct of Sylvius Canal connecting the third and fourth ventricles of brain
Arrythmia Irregularity of heart beat
Arteriole Smallest artery leading to capillary
Arthralgia Pain in a joint
Ascites Fluid in peritoneal cavity
Asepsis Exclusion of pathogenic organisms
Asphyxia Suffocation
Astrocyte Connective tissue cell of nervous system
Ataxia Disturbance of muscular coordination
Atelectasis Collapse of part of the lung
Atherosclerosis Hardening of the arteries
Atrophy Wasting
Attenuation Lessening (of virulence)
Autochthonous flora Organisms with intimate and permanent association with an epithelial surface
Autolysis Destruction by enzymes of the cell itself

B

Prefixes
Bio- Pertaining to life
Brady- Slowing
Broncho- Pertaining to bronchial tree

Suffix
-blast Precursor cell

Bacteremia Bacteria in the blood
Bacteriocins Proteins produced by one bacterium that kill another of the same or other species

Bacteriuria Bactèria in the urine
Bartholin's glands Lubricating glands on either side of the vaginal opening
Basophilic Affinity for staining with a basic dye
Biliary Pertaining to the bile and bile ducts
Bilirubin Bile pigment
Biotype Subtype within a species characterized by physiologic properties
Blepheral Pertaining to the eyelids
Bolus Rounded mass that may obstruct (e.g., fecal bolus) or a concentrated mass (e.g., an antibiotic) given rapidly intravenously
Bradycardia Unusually slow heart beat
Bronchiectasis Pathologic dilatation of terminal bronchi
Bronchiole Smallest subdivision of bronchial tree
Bronchoscopy Examination of interior of bronchi through an optical instrument

C

Prefixes
Cardio- Pertaining to the heart
Cysto- Pertaining to the bladder
Cyto- Pertaining to the cell

Suffix
-cidal Killing

Cardiomyopathy Disease of heart muscle
Caseous Cheesy in consistency
Cementum Layer of modified bone on tooth root
Chelators Compounds that bind metallic ions
Chemoprophylaxis Use of antimicrobics to prevent infection
Chemotaxis Attraction of a motile cell
Chitin Polysaccharide exoskeletons of some insects or walls of some fungi
Cholecystitis Inflammation of gallbladder
Cholinergic nerves Nerve fibers that release acetylcholine at their terminals
Chorioamnionitis Inflammation of fetal membrane
Chorioretinitis Inflammation of choroid and retina of the eye
Clone Identical progeny of a single cell, gene, or genes
Coartation Stricture or narrowing (e.g., of aorta)
Cocultivation Process that can be used for unmasking latent virus by growing susceptible cells with those from the affected tissue
Coloboma Defect of the eye
Colostrum Initial secretion of the breast after delivery (contains antibodies and lymphocytes)
Comedo Blocked sebaceous duct with retention of sebum (blackhead)
Commensal Organism of the normal flora that has a symbiotic relationship with the host
Coprolith Stony hard stool
Cornea Clear anterior portion of the eyeball
Corticosteroid Steroid hormone from adrenal gland—some are antiinflammatory
Cribriform plate Area of bone above the nasal cavity through which pass the olfactory nerves
Cuticle Skin or surface layer
Cyanosis Blue color of skin caused by lack of oxygen
Cystic fibrosis Congenital disease of secreting glands affecting pancreas, respiratory tract, and sweat glands—associated with viscid respiratory mucus
Cystoscope Optical instrument for examining inside of urinary bladder

D

Prefixes
Dermo- Pertaining to the skin
Dys- Difficult or painful

Debridement Removing foreign matter and dead tissue
Decubitus ulcer Pressure sore (bed sore)
Demyelination Loss of nerve sheaths
Desquamation Loss of skin epithelial cells
Dextran A polymer of D-glucose
Dimorphism Occurring in two morphologic forms under different conditions
Diverticulum Blind-ended extrusion from a hollow organ
Dyspareunia Difficult or painful intercourse
Dyspnea Shortness of breath
Dysuria Difficulty or pain on urinating

E

Prefixes
Ecto-, Exo- Outside or outer
Endo- Within
Entero- Pertaining to intestines
Epi- Upon or additional to

Suffixes
-ectomy Surgical removal of
-emia Of the blood

Ecchymosis Bruise
Ecthyma Eroded, scabbed lesion of the skin
Ectopic pregnancy Fetal development outside the uterus (usually in the fallopian tubes)
Edema Excessive fluid in tissues

Elastosis Disorder of fibrous elastic proteins
Embolism Sudden blocking of an artery
Emphysema (pulmonary) Irreversible enlargement of alveolar sacs of lung
Empyema Pus in a body (e.g., pleural) cavity
Encephalitis Inflammation of brain tissue
Endocardium Inner lining of the heart
Endocervix Columnar-celled lining of the interior passage of the uterine cervix
Endogenous Originating within an organism
Endometrium Interior epithelial lining of uterus
Endophthalmitis Inflammation of interior tissues of the eye epithelial
Enteric Pertaining to the intestinal tract
Enzootic Disease present at low levels at all times in an animal community
Eosinophils Subpopulation of granulocytic white cells
Epicardium Outer lining of the heart
Epididymis Tubular structure attached to the testes in which spermatozoa mature
Epiphysis Growing end of a bone
Episome Plasmid or viral DNA that can replicate extrachromosomally or can integrate into chromosomes
Epitope Structural part of an antigen that determines specificity of an antigen–antibody reaction (also called antigenic determinant)
Epitrochlear node Lymph node above inner side of elbow
Erythema Red color of skin caused by dilatation of blood vessels
Erythema nodosum Red raised skin nodules usually on the legs—manifestation of hypersensitivity

F

Fallopian tubes Tubes extending from ovaries to uterus
Fascia Sheets of specialized connective tissue
Felinophobe Cat hater
Fibrin Insoluble protein of blood clots
Fibroblast Specialized cell producing collagen and elastic connective tissue
Fibrosis Formation of collagenous connective tissue
Fistula An abnormal passage from a hollow organ (e.g., intenstine)
Fluorochrome A fluorescent dye
Follicle A small sac or cavity
Fomites Inanimate objects transmitting infectious agents
Foramina Outlets to cavities
Fungemia Fungi in the bloodstream

G

Prefix

Gastro- Pertaining to the stomach

Suffix

-genic Arising from, origin

Ganglion Group of nerve cells outside the spinal cord
Gangrene Death of tissue
Geophagia Eating soil or other inedible substances
Gingival crevice Area between tooth and gum
Glaucoma Excessive pressure in eyeball, which can lead to blindness
Glial Connective tissue of the central nervous system (neuroglia)
Glomerulus Microscopic organ of specialized capillaries in the kidney, which filter waste products from the blood
Glucans Polymers of glucose
Gnotobiotic animals Animals reared under aseptic conditions which may either be sterile ("germ free") or in which defined microflora are introduced
Gonads Ovaries or testes
Granuloma Chronic inflammation lesion infiltrated with macrophages and lymphocytes and accompanied by fibroblast activity
Gravid Pregnant

H

Prefixes

Hemo, Hema- Pertaining to blood
Hepato- Pertaining to the liver
Hetero- Of different origin
Hyper- Greater than, above normal
Hypo- Less than, below normal

Haploid Half the number of chromosomes of eukaryotic tissue cells (see meiosis), or number of chromosomes in asexual organisms
Hematocrit Volume of erythrocytes in blood as a percentage of the total volume of blood (adult normal = 45%)
Hematoma Extravasation of blood in the tissues' cells causing a swelling
Hematopietic system Precursor cells that produce blood cells
Hemianopsia Loss of vision in half the visual field
Hemoglobinemia Free hemoglobin in the blood
Hemolysis Liberation of hemoglobin from red cells
Hemoptysis Coughing up of blood
Hemothorax Blood in the pleural cavity of the chest

Hepatocytes Liver cells
Hepatoma Malignant tumor of liver cells
Hepatomegaly Enlargement of the liver
Heterologous Derived from a different clone, strain, species, or tissue
Heterophil antibody Antibody reacting with an antigen other than that which elicited its production
Heteroploid Cell with abnormal number of chromosomes
Hilar lymph nodes Nodes at the root of the lung
Histocompatibility antigens Antigens on tissue cells that are recognized by the host as self or foreign
Homeostasis Tendency to stability of conditions within a complex biologic system
Hybridoma A clone derived from fused cells of different origin, e.g., from an antibody producing lymphocyte and a tumor cell
Hydrocele Fluid accumulation within the scrotum
Hyperalimentation Intravenous administration of nutrients for treatment or avoidance of malnutrition
Hyperammonemia Excessive amounts of ammonia in the blood
Hyperbaric oxygen Oxygen under increased pressure relative to the atmosphere
Hyperemia Increased blood flow to a tissue
Hypernatremia Increased serum sodium
Hyperplasia Increase in number of cells in a tissue
Hypertension Increased blood pressure
Hypochlorhydria Reduced hydrochloric acid in the stomach
Hypoglycemia Blood sugar below normal levels

I

Prefixes
Inter- Between
Intra- Within

Suffix
-itis Inflammation of

Ideopathic Of unknown origin
Ileitis Inflammation of the lower ileum
Infarct Interference with blood supply producing local death of tissue
Integument Skin
Interstitial Spaces between the cells of a tissue
Intertriginous Pertaining to area between folds of skin
Intima Endothelial inner lining of a blood vessel
Intrathecal Within the membranes of the spinal cord
Introitus Opening
Isoantigen Normal substance present in one individual that may elicit an antibody response in another

J

Jejunum Portion of intestinal tract between duodenum and ileum

K

Karyotype Size, structure, and organization of chromosomes within a cell
Keratin Major protein of the skin, hair, and nails
Keratitis Inflammation of the cornea of the eye
Kinetoplast Structure at the base of a protozoal flagellum
Kwashiorkor Condition caused by severe protein malnutrition in a child

L

Lamina propria Connective tissue supporting the epithelial cells of a mucous membrane
Leukemia Malignant tumor of white blood cells
Leukocytosis Increased blood leukocyte count
Leukopenia Abnormally low leukocyte count
Lupus erythematosis (systemic) Autoimmune inflammatory disease of skin, joints, and other tissues
Lymphadenitis Enlarged inflamed lymph nodes
Lymphocytosis Increased blood lymphocyte count
Lymphoma Tumor of lymphatic tissues
Lymphopenia Abnormally low lymphocyte count
Lymphoreticular Relating to the reticuloendothelial cells of the lymphatic system
Lysis Dissolution of cells

M

Prefixes
Macro- large
Mega- Large
Micro- Small
Myo- Pertaining to muscle

Suffix
-metry Measure

Mastitis Inflammation of breast tissue
Mastoid Process of temporal bone behind the ear that contains air cells
Meatus Orifice
Meckel's diverticulum Congenital diverticulum of the lower part of the ileum

Mediastinum Mid-portion of the chest, including heart, bronchial bifurcation, and esophagus
Medulla oblongata Portion of central nervous system between brain and spinal cord
Megacolon Dilatation of the colon
Meiosis Cellular division process yielding haploid gametes
Meningomyelocele Malformation of vertebral column with protrusion of meninges
Mentation Mental activity—thinking
Mesenchymal Derived from the embryonic mesoderm layer
Mesentery Fold of the peritoneum surrounding the intestinal tract and attaching it to the posterior abdominal wall
Metastases Satellite tumors or infections spread through lymphatics or blood stream from a primary site
Microcephaly Small head with failure of development of the brain
Microphthalmia Failure to develop normal sized eyes
Monoclonal Derived from a single cell
Mordant Substance that enhances the effect of a stain
Mucolytic Substance that dissolves mucus
Multiple sclerosis Chronic disorder involving disseminated focal damage to nerve cells
Myalgia Pain in the muscles
Myelin Component of the insulated covering (myelin sheath) around the axon of a neuron, which increases the conduction velocity of the nerve impulse

N

Prefixes
Neo- New
Nephrito- Pertaining to the kidney
Neuro- Pertaining to nerves or nervous system

Nares Interior of the nostrils
Nasolacrimal duct Duct draining the conjunctiva into the nasal cavity
Necrosis Death of tissue
Neoplasm Tumor
Nephritogenic Producing inflammation of the kidneys
Neurone Nerve and its nerve cell
Neutropenia Reduced number of circulating neutrophil leukocytes
Neutrophils Major class of polymorphonuclear phagocytic leukocytes
Nosocomial Acquired within a hospital

O

Prefixes
Oligo- Small, few
Onco- Pertaining to tumors
Osteo- Pertaining to bone

Oligodendroglia Specialized connective tissue cells of the central nervous system
Oncogenic Causing tumors
Ontogeny Origin and course of development of an individual organism
Operculum A lid or cover
Opisthotonus Several spasm of back muscles leading to hyperextension of the spine
Opthalmia Severe inflammation of the eye
Orchitis Inflammation of a testis
Organogenesis Formation of the organs of the body
Ossicles Small bones (e.g., of hearing)
Osteomyelitis Inflammation of bone marrow and adjacent bone

P

Prefixes
Pan- All, throughout
Para- Beside, abnormal
Peri- Around, covering
Pleo- More
Poly- Many, repeated

Pandemic Worldwide severe epidemic
Panencephalitis Inflammation of all tissues of the brain
Papilla Small nipplelike swelling
Papilledema Edema of the optic nerve and adjacent retina
Papilloma Warty or projecting tumor of the epithelium
Parenchymal Substance of body organs in contrast to their coverings
Paresis Paralysis
Paresthesia Disorders of sensation, or tingling
Paronychia Infection of nail fold
Parotid glands Salivary glands beneath the cheek
Periapical Beside the root of a tooth
Pericardium Membranous lining around the heart
Perinephric Around the kidneys
Perineum Area between vulva or scrotum and the anus
Periodontal Area around the tooth, including supporting tissues
Periosteum Membrane around the bone
Peristalsis Normal contractile waves of a hollow organ

Petechiae Small hemorrhages in the skin
Peyer's patches Lymphoid follicles in the ileum
Photophobia Intolerance of light
Phylogeny Pertaining to the evolution history of a species
Pilo-sebaceous Unit of hair follicle and sebaceous gland
Plasma Liquid part of whole blood
Plasmin Derived from plasminogen—dissolves fibrin
Plasminogen Normal constituent of blood—precursor of plasmin
Platelet Small anucleate cell involved in filling small holes in blood vessels and in clotting mechanisms
Pleocytosis Increased number of cells in a particular area
Pleomorphism Variation in shape and size
Pleurodynia Pain caused by inflammation or irritation of the pleura
Pneumonitis Inflammation of the lung
Pneumothorax Air in the pleural cavity
Polyarthralgia Pain in several joints
Polyclonal activation Simultaneous activation of different antibody producing clones or lymphocytes
Polymorphonuclear Two or more lobes to the nucleus
Polymyositis Inflammation of many muscles
Polyneuritis Inflammation of many nerves
Polyp A sessile benign or malignant tumor of a mucous membrane (usually of colon)
Polyposis Presence of many polyps
Portal venous system Veins carrying blood from the intestinal tract to the liver
Premenarchal Prepubertal years in the female (before onset of menses)
Prepuce Foreskin
Proctoscopy Use of an instrument to examine interior of rectum
Prodromal Initial symptoms before characteristic manifestations of disease
Prophylaxis Measures or treatment designed to prevent disease
Prostate gland Gland surrounding male urethra, which produces part of the seminal fluid
Prosthesis Artificial replacement of a missing part of the body
Proteinurea Protein in the urine indicating abnormality
Prothrombin Precursor of thrombin; thrombin activates the terminal blood clotting mechanism
Pruritis Itching
Puerperal Following childbirth
Purpura Multiple hemorrhages in the skin, mucous membranes, or other organs
Pyelonephritis Infection of the pelvis and tissue of the kidney
Pyuria Pus in urine

R

Prefix
Rhino- Pertaining to the nose

Receptor Component of the cell surface to which another substance or organism attaches specifically
Renal Pertaining to the kidney
Reservoir of infection Natural habitat or source of an infecting organism
Reticuloendothelial system System of phagocytic monocytes, particularly those fixed in the spleen, bone marrow, and lymph nodes
Retinoblastoma Malignant tumor of the retina
Rhinitis Inflammation of the nasal mucosa

S

Prefixes
Sub- Below
Supra- Above

Salpingitis Inflammation of the fallopian tubes
Saprophyte Organism living on dead organic material in environment
Sarcolemma Membrane surrounding muscle fiber
Sclera White part of the eyeball
Sebum Waxy secretion of sebaceous glands
Sequestrum Necrotic fragment within a bone
Serotype Subtype of species detectable with specific antisera
Serpiginous Moving irregularly from one place to another
Serum Liquid part of blood separable after clotting
Shunt Deviation of blood or other body fluid, e.g., from artery to vein
Siderophore Compound that binds ion
Sigmoid colon Lower portion of the colon between descending colon and rectum
Sinusoid A wide thin-walled venous passage
Sphincter Circular muscle controlling a natural orifice
Splanchnic Pertaining to the viscera
Squamous epithelium Composed of layers of flattened cells
Stasis Stagnation or cessation of flow of body fluids

Stenosis Reduction in diameter of a blood vessel or tubular organ
Steroids Derivatives of cholestrol, including hormones, some of which have antiinflammatory effects
Strabismus Squint
Stratum corneum Outer keratinized part of the skin
Submandibular Below the jaw
Subphrenic Below the diaphragm
Sulcus Groove
Syndrome Group of clinical manifestations characterizing a particular disease or condition
Synovium Lining membrane of a joint, tendon, or bursa

T

Prefixes
Tachy- Increased rate, swift
Thrombo- Pertaining to thrombosis
Tracheo- Pertaining to the trachea

Tachycardia Abnormally high heart rate
Tachypnea Abnormally rapid rate of breathing
Tamponade (cardiac) Increased fluid around the heart leading to interference of cardiac function
Tenesmus Ineffective and painful straining at stool or in urination
Tenosynovitis Inflammation of tendon sheaths
Teratogenic Causing abnormalities of fetal development
Thrombocyte (See platelet)
Thrombosis Blood clot within a blood vessel
Titer Highest dilution of an active substance (e.g., antibody in serum) that still causes a discernable reaction (e.g., with another substance)
Tracheostomy Surgically produced artificial air passage into trachea
Tropism Having an infinity for a particular organ, or moving towards or away from a particular stimulus
Tumorigenesis The property of causing tumors
Turbinates Baffles in the nasal cavity designed to warm and humidify the air
Tympanic membrane Ear drum

U

Suffix
-uria Pertaining to urine

Ureter Tube carrying urine from the kidney to bladder
Urticaria Local edema and itching of the skin
Uvea Inner vascular coat of the eyeball, including the iris
Uvula Small extension hanging from the back of the soft palate

V

Prefix
Vaso- Pertaining to blood vessels

Vacuole Microscopic hole or cavity
Vagotomy Surgical division of the vagus nerve
Vasa vasorum Small blood vessels in walls of veins and arteries
Vasculitis Inflammation of blood vessels
Vector An animate transmitter of disease, e.g., an insect
Venipuncture Insertion of a hypodermic needle into a vein—usually to draw blood
Ventricle Fluid filled cavity, e.g., a chamber of the heart
Venule Smallest component of venous system
Vesicle Small fluid filled cavity, e.g., a blisterlike lesion of the skin
Vesicoureteral Junction of ureter with urinary bladder
Villus Small epithelial projections of the mucous membrane

Z

Zymodemes Subtypes differentiated according to their isoenzyme profiles

Index

The page ranges given for citations of organisms, which are covered in detail, include considerations of habitat, morphology, antigenic structure, cultural characteristics, virulence determinants, pathogenesis of disease, antimicrobic susceptibility, and life cycles when appropriate. Only unusual properties, those of special interest, or those discussed elsewhere in the text, are included as subcitations.

A similar approach has been adopted for specific diseases, in which the major citation includes clinical manifestations, epidemiology, laboratory diagnosis, prevention, and treatment, when these are covered in the text. Pages cited for individual antimicrobics include consideration of structure, mode of action, spectrum, and resistance mechanisms when appropriate. As with the citations for organisms, subcitations for diseases and antimicrobics relate to unusual characteristics or those considered elsewhere in the text.

The marginal headings in the cited pages should be used to find the specific information needed.

A

Abscesses
- anaerobic Gram-negative rods, anaerobic cocci, 202
- brain, 155, 308, 609
- hepatic, amebiasis, 487
- *Peptostreptococcus*, microaerophilic streptococci, 203
- peritonsillar and retropharyngeal, 581, 582
- *Pseudomonas pseudomallei*, 268
- pulmonary, 588
- *Staphylococcus aureus*, 155, 158

Acanthamoeba, 489

Acetylglucosamine (N-acetylglucosamine in cell wall structure), 12

Acetylmuramic acid (N-acetylmuramic acid in cell wall structure), 12

Acid-fast stain, 291, 309

Acne vulgaris, 556

Acquired immune deficiency syndrome, 459, 646

Actinobacillus actinomycetemcomitans, 579

Actinomyces, 305–307, 577
- *A. israelii*, 305
- *A. naeslundii*, 577
- *A. propionicus*, 305
- *A. viscosus*, 577

Actinomycosis, 305–307

Acyclovir (acycloguanosine), 144, 420
- Epstein–Barr virus, 426
- genital herpes simplex, 144, 416, 420, 644
- varicella-zoster infection, 422

Adenine arabinoside (vidarabine), 144
- herpes simplex, 416, 419

Adenosine triphosphate
- in bacterial metabolism, 16
- *Chlamydia* requirement, 318
- *Rickettsia* requirement, 311

Adenoviruses, 372–375, 456, 568, 569, 585, 589

Adenyl cyclase
- cholera toxin effect, 259
- enterotoxigenic *E. coli* toxin effect, 242

Adherence, 66
- *Bordetella pertussis*, 223
- in dental and periodontal infections, 575, 577
- *Escherichia coli*, 241, 242
- *Neisseria gonorrhoeae*, 211
- normal flora, 51
- pili, 15
- *Streptococcus pyogenes*, 168
- *Vibrio cholerae*, 259

Adsorption, viral, 28

Aeromonas, 269

African trypanosomiasis (sleeping sickness), 503–505

Agammaglobulinemia (hypogammaglobulinemia), 650

Agar diffusion and dilution susceptibility tests, 140, 141

Agar media. *See* Culture media

Age
- and infectious diseases, 77, 78
- influenza A viral attack rates, 365
- and paralytic poliomyelitis, 398

Agglutination
- in bacterial identification, 101–102
- in viral identification, 118

Aging
- reactivation tuberculosis, 296
- varicella-zoster infection, 420

AIDS. *See* Acquired immune deficiency syndrome

Airway obstruction
- diphtheria, 184
- *Haemophilus influenzae* epiglottitis, 219
- middle respiratory tract infections, 584

Alastrim (variola minor), 390

Alcaligenes fecalis, 270

Alcohol disinfection, 38

Algae, association with *Legionella pneumophila*, 235

Alimentary tract infections, 592–600

Allergic encephalitis, 610

Amantadine treatment of influenza, 144, 368, 369

Amebas, 484–489

Amebiasis, 486–488

Amebic dysentery, 461, 487

Amebomas, 486, 487

Amikacin, 132, 133

para-Aminobenzoic acid, competetive inhibition of sulfonamides, 137

Aminoglycoside-aminocyclitol antimicrobics, 131–133
- anaerobic organism resistance, 132, 193–194
- spectra, 148
- synergism with β lactams, 133

p-Aminosalicylic acid, 139
Amphotericin B, 142–143
systemic fungal infections, 343, 346, 349, 352, 354, 357, 360
toxicity, 143, 333
Ampicillin, 127, 128
for enteric fever, 253
enterococcal infections, 175
Haemophilus influenza resistance, 221
resistance mechanisms, 128, 129
for sinus infections, 573
spectrum, 148
Anabolic pathways, 16
Anaerobes, 193–204
clostridia, Gram negative, and cocci, 193–204
cultural techniques, 193
facultative and strict, 16
normal microbial flora, 53
oxygen toxicity, 193
Anaerobic cellulitis, 196, 557
Anaerobic myositis. *See* Gas gangrene
Anaerobic respiration, 17
Anal cellophane tape test, 517, 538
Ancylostoma duodenale, 516, 521–522
Anemia
aplastic, 135
hemolytic, *Mycoplasma pneumoniae,* 229
hookworm infections, 522
macrocytic, fish tapeworm infection, 542
malaria, 474
sickle cell, osteomyelitis, *Salmonella* infections, 252
Anesthesia and lower respiratory tract infections, 587
Animal inoculation, viral isolation, 110–111
Anthrax infections, 188–192
Antibiotics. *See* Antimicrobics and chemotherapy
Antibodies
coating, in urinary tract infections, 606
complement fixing, 118, 119
heterophile, Epstein–Barr virus, 424–426
passive immunization, 84–86
serologic diagnosis of infection, 116–120
to toxins and toxoids, 70
see also Serology
Antifungal antimicrobics, 142–143
Antigenic shifts and drifts, influenza A virus, 363–365
Antigens
analysis, bacterial identification, 103–105
bacterial cell wall, 13
Borrelia recurrentis variation, 287
Duffy, in plasmodial infections, 472
Enterobacteriaceae, cell wall, capsule slime layer, flagella, 239
sandwich method of detection, 115
variation in malarial parasites, 475
viral, 27, 112
Antimicrobic susceptibility
spectra, 130, 139, 148
tests for, 140–141
Antimicrobics and chemotherapy, 123–149
aminoglycoside-aminocyclitol antibiotics, 131–133
antifungal agents, 142–143
antituberculous agents, 139, 298
antiviral agents, 143–145
beta-lactam antibiotics
cephalosporins, 129–131
penicillins, 126–131
chloramphenicol, 135–136
clinical pharmacology, 124
epidemiology of resistance to, 145–149
erythromycin and lincosamide antibiotics, 136
laboratory tests, 140–142
polypeptide antibiotics, 138
resistance, innate and acquired, 125–126
selective toxicity, 123
sources and terminology, 124
sulfonamides, 136–138
superinfections, 57–58, 146
tetracyclines, 133–135
therapeutic index, 123
trimethoprim, 138
vancomycin, 139
Antiphagocytic mechanisms, 67
Antisepsis and antiseptics, 33, 38–40
Antispasmotics in gastrointestinal infections, 600
Antistreptolysin O, 173
Antitoxin, 72
Aortic aneurysm, syphilis, 641
Appendix, enterobiasis, 517
Arachnia propionicus, 305
Arboviruses, 434–442
Arenaviruses, 443
Arizona, 254
Arthritis
Haemophilus influenzae, 220
hepatitis B, 408
Mycoplasma pneumoniae, 229
Neisseria gonorrhoeae, 212–213
Neisseria meningitis, 208
septic, 564–566
Staphylococcus aureus, 155
Streptococcus pneumoniae, 178
Arthroconidia, *Coccidioides immitis,* 354
Arthroderma benhamiae, 330
Arthropod-borne viruses, 434–442
Ascaris lumbricoides (round worm), 515, 519–521
Ascomycetes, 330
Aspergillosis, 345–346
allergic and pulmonary, 345
in immunocompromised patients, 345
Aspergillus, 344–346
Assay of antimicrobics, 142
Astroviruses, 433
Ataxia telangiectasia, 652
Athlete's foot, 334, 336
ATP. *See* Adenosine triphosphate
Attenuation, 83
Australia antigen, 407
Autoclave, 35–36
Axoneme, flagellate protozoa, 491

B

Bacillus, 188–189
B. anthracis
anthrax infection, 189–191
capsule polypeptide, 10
B. cereus, 191
B. subtilis, 191
B. thuringiensis, 16
Bacitracin test, *Streptococcus pyogenes,* 173
Bacteremia, 616–628
catheter infections, 622–623, 658
causative organisms, 624
extravascular infection, 623–625
gonococcal, 212–213, 638–639
Gram negative, 240, 616
Haemophilus influenzae, 221
infective endocarditis, 617–620
meningococcal, 208
pneumococcal, 178, 180
staphylococcal, 155
and trematode infections, 552
see also Blood culture
Bacteria
classification, 20–21
determinants of virulence, 67–70
fetal and newborn infections, 630, 631
Gram reaction, 11–12, 92–93
growth kinetics, 18–20
metabolism, 16
of normal flora, 50–58
pathogens, 21
structures, 9–16
appendages, 15–16
basic shapes, 9
capsule, 9–10
cell surface, 9–16
cell wall, 11–13
cytoplasm, 14–15
variation and genetics, 41–48
gene (DNA) transfer, 43–46
gene expression, 42
mutation, 42–43
plasmid phenotypes, 46–47
recombinant DNA techniques, 47–48
see also specific bacteria and laboratory diagnosis of infectious diseases
Bacterial endocarditis, 617–620
Bacterial superinfection
with chemotherapy, 57–58, 146
influenza complication, 366–367, 369
measles complication, 381
vaccinia infection, 393
Bactericidal activity, 123
Bactericidal tests, 141
Bacteriocins, 46
Bacteriophages, 30–32
lysogenic conversion, 32, 168, 183, 200
replication, 30
Salmonella typhi typing, 251
Staphylococcus aureus typing, 152
T phage morphology, 31

temperate, 31–32
transduction, 45
virulence, 31
Bacteriostatic activity, 123
Bacteroides, 202
B. fragilis, 202, 560
B. melaninogenicus-asaccharolyticus, 202
normal microbial flora in feces, 54
B.C.G. vaccine, 296
Bear meat trichinosis, 529
Beef tapeworm *(Taenia saginata),* 537–539
Bejel (endemic syphilis), 285
β-hemolysis, 163
β-lactam antimicrobics, 126–131
β-lactam ring, 126
β-lactamases, 126, 129
Bicarbonate loss in cholera, 259, 260
Bifidobacteria, breast-fed infants, 54, 57
Bile solubility of pneumococci, 176
Biliary tract
cholecystitis, 196
Salmonella carriage, 252–253
strongyloidiasis, 523
trematode infections, 548
Binary fission, 3
Bismuth compounds, gastrointestinal infections, 600
Black Death (plague), 275
Blackwater fever in malaria, 474
Bladder
cystitis, urinary infection, 241, 604
trematode infections, 552
Blastoconidia, 328
Blastomyces dermatitidis and blastomycosis, 352–354
Blepharitis, 567
Blepharoplast, 491
Blind-loop syndrome, role of normal microbial flora, 56
Blood
loss in hookworm infections, 521–522
normal microbial flora, 51
transmission of infection, 78–80
Blood agar, 94, 120
Blood brain barrier, CNS infections, 608
Blood culture, 626
CNS infections, 614
gastrointestinal infections, 599
Gram-negative septic shock, 626, 628
infective endocarditis, 619
lower respiratory tract infections, 590
middle respiratory tract infections, 586
suppurative thrombophlebitis, 622
urinary tract infections, 606
yeast infections, 343
see also Bacteremia
Blood fluke, *Schistosoma,* 550–554
Boil. *See* Furuncle
Bone and joint infections, 562–566
Blastomyces dermatitidis, 353
cryptococcal, 349
pyogenic osteomyelitis, 562–564
septic arthritis, 564–566
sequestrum formation, 562, 564
Sporothrix schenckii, 359
Staphylococcus aureus, 155
Bone marrow
chloramphenicol inhibition of blood formation, 135
depression with sulfonamides, 137
dysfunction, arbovirus infection, 437
in inflammatory response, 63
phagocytic cells, 65
transplants
cytomegalovirus infection, 423
varicella-zoster infections, 421
Bordet–Gengou medium, *Bordetella pertussis,* 223, 225
Bordetella pertussis (whooping cough), 223–226
ciliary inhibition, 66
culture media, 97, 223, 225
toxins and pathogenesis, 223–224
Bornholm disease, 402
Borrelia recurrentis, relapsing fever, 287–289
Bothria, 535
Botulism, 70, 81, 200–201
Branhamella, 206, 215
Breast feeding, infant's normal flora, 54, 57
Brill's disease, 315
Bronchi, middle respiratory tract infections, 584–586
Bronchiolitis, respiratory syncytial virus, 370–372
Bronchitis, 220
Brucella, 271–274
erythritol stimulation of growth, 273
multiplication in macrophages, 273
species and antigenic structure, 271–272
see also Brucellosis
Brucellosis, 271–274
clinical course, 274
epidemiology, 273
reticuloendothelial infection, 271
transmission in unpasteurized milk, 273, 274
treatment and prevention, 274
Brugia malayi, 527
Bubo, 276
Bubonic plague, 276
Bullous impetigo, *Staphylococcus aureus,* 155, 158
Bullous myringitis, 229, 230
Bunyaviridae, 27, 436
Burkitt's lymphoma, Epstein–Barr virus involvement, 426, 457
Burn infections
group A streptococcal, 169
immunization and prophylaxis, 7–8
Pseudomonas aeruginosa, 266, 560

C

Calabar swellings, 534
Calciviruses, 433
California virus, 441
Calymmatobacterium granulomatis, 645
Campylobacter fetus, 262
bacteremia, 262
cultural conditions, 96, 97
Campylobacter jejuni, C. fetus ss. *jejuni,* 262–263
arthritis, 565
infectious diarrhea, 262–263
Cancer and viruses, 455–459
Candida albicans, 339–343
esophagitis, 342
infection with hyperalimentation, 340
respiratory infections, 342
septic arthritis, 564
skin infections, 339, 341, 556
stomatitis, 581
thrush, 341
vaginitis, 341, 648
see also Candidiasis
Candida glabrata (Torulopsis glabrata), 343
Candida tropicalis, 343
Candidiasis, 339–343
chronic mucocutaneous, 341
disseminated, 340, 342
secondary to antibiotic therapy, 57, 134
Cannibalism and kuru, 454–455
Canning and botulism, 200
Capillaria and capillariasis, 514
Capsids, viral, 23–26 , 31
virus structure, 23–26, 31
Capsomer, 24
Capsule
antiphagocytic effects, 67, 68, 72
Bacillus anthracis, 189
bacterial, visualization and composition, 9–10
Brucella, 271
Cryptococcus neoformans, 347
Enterobacteriaceae, 238, 239
Haemophilus influenzae, 216, 218
Klebsiella, 247
Neisseria, 205
Staphylococcus aureus, 154
Streptococcus pneumoniae, 175–176
antigenic specificity, 164, 176
DNA transformation, 43–44
free polysaccharide, 178
opsonization, 178
swelling reaction, 10, 180
virulence, 176, 180
Carbenicillin, 127
anti-*Pseudomonas* activity, 127, 128
spectrum, 148
Carbohydrate fermentation and oxidation in bacterial classification, 99
Carbol-fuchsin stain, 91
Carbon, bacterial growth requirement, 17–18
Carbon dioxide
in bacterial cultures, 96–98
bacterial growth, 17–18
Carbuncles, *Staphylococcus aureus,* 155
Carcinoma
cervical, and herpes simplex, type 2, 417
hepatocellular, and hepatitis B, 410
nasopharyngeal, Epstein–Barr virus involvement, 426, 457
Cardiolipin, *Treponema pallidum,* 282, 283
Caries, 574, 576–578

Carriage
amebiasis, 487
Corynebacterium diphtheriae, 184
definition, 77
group A streptococcus, 172
Haemophilus influenzae, 217
hepatitis B, 409–410
meningococcus, 206
normal microbial flora, 50
Rickettsiae, 312
Salmonella, 252–253
Shigella, 245
Staphylococcus aureus, 54, 150
Vibrio cholerae, 260
Cat, host of *Toxoplasma,* 478–480
Catalase in bacterial classification, 99
Catheters, intravenous and bacteremia, 622–623, 658
Catheters, urinary and infection, 602, 657–658
Cavity, pulmonary, 296, 351, 356
Cefamycins, 129
Cell culture, 106–110
C. difficile toxin detection, 201
Chlamydia growth, 319
Rickettsia growth, 310–311
virus growth and isolation, 106–112
see also individual viruses
Cell division, 18
Cell-mediated hypersensitivity, 71, 73
Cell-mediated immunity, 73–74
Cell wall, bacterial, 11–13
Cellulitis, 557
anaerobic, 196
Haemophilus influenzae, 220
Central nervous system infections, 608–615
Cephalosporin antimicrobics, 129–131
β lactam structure, 129
generations of cephalosporins, 130–131
spectra, 130, 148
Cercariae, trematodes, 545–550
Cerebrospinal fluid
analysis, normal vs. infection, 613
Haemophilus influenzae morphology, 216
measles antibodies, in subacute sclerosing panencephalitis, 452
see also CNS infections and meningitis
Cervicitis in sexually transmitted diseases, 647
Cervix, uterine
dysplasia, and papilloma viruses, 456–457
neoplasia, and genital herpes simplex, 644
strawberry, trichomoniasis, 494
Cestode infections, 535–544
attachment mechanisms, 535
beef tapeworm *(Taenia saginata),* 537–539
fish tapeworm *(Diphyllobothrium latum),* 541–542
hermaphrodite units, 535
hydatid disease *(Echinococcus granulosus, E. multilocularis),* 542–544
pork tapeworm *(Taenia solium),* 539–540
Chagas' disease, 461, 505–507
Chancre, syphilitic, 282, 640
Chancroid, 644–645
Chediak–Higashi syndrome, 651
Chemoprophylaxis
clostridial infections, 196, 199
Haemophilus meningitis, 219
meningococcal meningitis, 209
rheumatic fever, 170
surgical infections, 147, 160, 559
tuberculosis, 298–299
Chemotaxis of phagocytes, 64
in immunocompromised patients, 651
Chemotherapy. *See* Antimicrobics and chemotherapy
Chickenpox (varicella) virus, 77, 422
Children. *See* Infants and children
Chinese liver fluke, *Clonorchis sinensis,* 548, 549
Chitin, fungal cell wall, 326
Chlamydia, 318–325
antigenic structure, 319
antimicrobic susceptibility, 132, 135, 137, 320, 321
cell culture, 319
C. psittaci, 321
C. trachomatis, 322–325
eye infections, 322, 568–569
genital tract infections, 80, 323–324
glycogen synthesis, 319
infant pneumonia syndrome, 324
lymphogranuloma venereum, 324
reproductive cycle, 318, 319
species differentiation, 321
Chlamydoconidia
Candida albicans, 339
tuberculate, *Histoplasma capsulatum,* 349
Chloramphenicol, 135–136
in enteric fever, 253
in rickettsial infections, 314
spectrum, 148
toxicity, 135
Chloramphenicol acetyl transferase, 135
Chlorhexidine, 40
Chloride hypersecretion, in cholera, 259, 260
Chlorine disinfection, 39
Chloroquine, malaria treatment, resistant strains, 476–477
Chocolate agar, 121
fungal culture, 332
Haemophilus influenzae, 217
Cholera. *See Vibrio cholerae* and gastrointestinal infections
Chorioamnionitis
fetal and newborn infections, 630
Ureaplasma urealyticus, 232
Chorioretinitis, 481, 568
Chromatoid bodies, *Entamoeba histolytica,* 484
Chromoblastocosis, 360
Chromosomes
structure in bacteria, 14
temperate bacteriophages, 31
see also Bacteria, variation and genetics
Cigarette smoking, middle respiratory tract infections, 585
Ciliates, 462–463
Citrate in bacterial classification, 99
Citrobacter, 254
Classification
bacteria, 20, 21
fungi, 330–331
genetic and molecular approaches, 20
numerical taxonomy, 20
parasites, 462–464
viruses, 26–27
Clindamycin, 136
pseudomembranous enterocolitis, 57, 136, 201
spectrum, 148
susceptibility of anaerobes, 136
Clonorchis sinensis (liver fluke), 548–549
Clostridum
C. botulinum, 200–201
C. difficile, 201
culture medium, 97
enterotoxin, clindamycin resistance, 136
hospital-associated diarrhea, 598
pseudomembranous enterocolitis, 57
C. perfringens, 194–197
anaerobic cellulitis, 196
endometritis, 196
exotoxins, 195
food poisoning, 195, 197, 597–598
gas gangrene, 194–196, 560
heat-resistant spores, 195
lecithinase activity, 70, 195
wound infections, 560
C. tetani, 197–200
toxin, 198
see also Tetanus
Clotrimazole, antifungal activity, 333, 337
Coagglutination, 102, 151
Coagulase, staphylococcal, 99, 150–153, 159–160
Cocci, 9
Coccidioides immitis, 354–355
arthrospores, 354–355
spherules, 354, 356
Coccidioidomycosis, 78, 355–357
erythema nodosum, 356
meningitis, 356
pulmonary lesions, 356
valley fever, 356
Cold, common, viruses, 375–376
Cold hemagglutinins, *Myoplasma pneumoniae,* 230–231
Cold sores, herpes simplex, 415
Collagenase, bacterial infection, 70
Colon
dilatation, American trypanosomiasis (Chagas' disease), 507
normal flora, 53–54
Colonies, bacterial, 94
Colorado tick fever, 435, 436, 442
Commensalism, 50
Common cold virus (rhinovirus), 375–376
Complement
deficiency, immunocompromised patients, 652
in inflammatory response, 63–65, 72
Complement fixation, 118, 119
Computer, bacterial classification, 20, 101

Concentration methods for cysts and ova, 467
Conidia, 329, 334
Conjugation, DNA transfer, 45
Conjunctiva, defenses against microbial invasion, 60
Conjunctival sac, normal microbial flora, 52
Conjunctivitis, 568–569
  adenoviruses, 373
  chlamydial, 322
  description, 567
  enterovirus, 402
  gonococcal, 212
  Haemophilus, 222
  tularemia, 278
Coracidium of *Diphyllobothrium latum*, 536
Cord factor, *Mycobacterium tuberculosis*, 292, 293
Corneal transplantation
  Creutzfeldt–Jakob infection, 455
  rabies, 448
Coronaviruses, 27
Corticosteroid therapy
  for Gram-negative spectic shock, 626
  Pneumocystic carinii infection, 511
  risks with hepatitis B, 411
  tissue nematode infections, 528, 530, 533
Corynebacteria, diphtheroids, 186
Corynebacterium diphtheriae, 182–186
  lysogenic conversion, 32, 183
  metachromatic granules, 182
  Schick test, 186
  selective media, 182
  toxin production, 183
  see also Diphtheria
Corynebacterium hemolyticum, 186
Corynebacterium sp., group JK, 186
Corynebacterium ulcerans, 186
Cough reflex, lower respiratory tract defense, 587
Counterimmunoelectrophoresis, in antigen detection, 101, 102, 105
Cowpox, 393
Coxiella burnettii, 316–317
  intraphagocytic multiplication, 67
  Q fever, 316–317
Coxsackie viruses, 401–402
Cresol disinfection, 40
Creutzfeldt–Jakob disease, 455, 611
Croup, middle respiratory tract infection, 369–370, 584
Cryptococcosis, 347–349
  in immunocompromised hosts, 348
  meningitis, 348
  pulmonary infection, 348
Cryptococcus neoformans, 347–349
  capsule, 347
  India ink preparation, 348, 349
Cryptosporidiosis, 668
Crystal violet stain, 91
C-type particle, 458
Cultivation of bacteria, 93–98
Culture media
  agar, 94, 120–121
  anaerobic, 121
  blood agar, 94, 120
  Bordet–Gengou, 223, 225
  broth, 94, 120
  chocolate agar, 121, 217, 227
  cysteine-glucose, 277
  defined and undefined, 93
  differential, 96
  enrichment, 96
  general purpose, 97
  Hektoen enteric agar, 121
  indicator, 96
  MacConkey agar, 121
  routine isolation systems, 98
  selective, 96, 97, 121
  special purpose, 97
  Thayer–Martin, 121
Cyclic adenosine-monophosphate (cAMP) and enterotoxins, 259
Cycloguanil pamoate treatment, *Leishmania* infections, 501
Cystic fibrosis, *Pseudomonas aeruginosa* infections, 267
Cysticercosis, 540
Cystitis, 241, 604
  acute hemorrhagic, adenoviruses, 373
Cysts, parasitic
  Entamoeba histolytica, 484
  Giardia lamblia, 495
  Toxoplasma gondii, 478–480
Cytomegalovirus, 422–424
  fetal and newborn infections, 422, 633–635
Cytopathic effects of virus in cell culture, 107–110
Cytoplasmic membrane, bacterial, 13–14
Cytotoxicity, antibody-dependent cell-mediated, 74

D

Dacryocystitis, 567
Dane particles (hepatitis B), 406, 408
Dark repair of DNA, 33
Dark-field microscopy, 91
Death, microbial, 33–40
Defective interfering (DI) particles, 29, 30
Delta agent, hepatitis B, 411
Dengue, 441
Dental infections, 574–579
Deoxyribonucleases, bacterial, 167, 195, 248
Deoxyribonucleic acid. *See* DNA
Dermatophytoses, 334–338
Deuteromycetes, fungi imperfecti, 330
Diabetes
  Candida albicans infection, 340, 342
  and Coxsackie virus infection, 402
  reactivation tuberculosis, 296
  zygomycete infections, 346
Diaper rash, *Candida albicans* infection, 341
Diarrhea
  amebiasis, 486–488
  Campylobacter infection, 262–263
  cholera, 259–261
  giardiasis, 496
  salmonellosis, 251
  shigellosis, 246
  traveler's, *Escherichia coli*, 242–243, 594
  Vibrio parahemolyticus, 262
  viral, 427–433
Dick test, 168
Dicloxacillin, 127
Dientamoeba fragilis, 494
Diethylcarbamazine, filarial infections, 533, 534
Diffusion susceptibility tests, 140–141
Dihydrofolate reductase, competetive inhibition by trimethoprim, 138
Dihydropterate synthetase, 137
Diiodohydroxyquin treament, amebiasis, 488
Dimorphism, 329
Diphtheria, 182–186
  cutaneous, 184
  exotoxin production, 69, 70, 183
  treatment and prevention, 185–186
Diphyllobothrium latum (fish tapeworm), 541–542
Dipicolinic acid, 15
Disease
  communicable and noncommunicable, epidemiology, 76–77
  and infection, distinction between, 77
Disinfection, 33, 38–40
Disseminated gonococcal infection, 211–213
Disseminated intravascular coagulation syndrome, 208
DNA
  bacteriophage, 31, 41
  base ratios and homology tests, 104
  chromosomal, 41–47
    bacterial classification, 20–21
  homology tests, bacterial identification, 104
  plasmid, 14, 41
  recombinant techniques, 47–48
  recombination, 43–46
  repair, 33
  synthesis: inhibition by antimicrobics, 139
  synthesis, T phages, 31
  thymine dimer formation by UV light, 33
  viral, 23–31
DNA viruses
  classification, 26–27
  transformation, 30
  tumor viruses, 456–457
Dog
  hydatid disease, 542, 544
  Leishmania reservoir, 500–503
  toxocariasis, 526–528
  rabies, 448
Dog or cat, transmission of *Pasteurella multocida*, 279
Donovan bodies, granuloma inguinale, 645
Down's syndrome, hepatitis B, 410
Downey cells, 424
Doxycycline, 134
Drug abuse
  endocarditis, 618–619
  hepatitis B, 410
  and lower respiratory infections, 587

Drug abuse *(cont.)*
staphylococcal infections, 156
Duodenal secretions in *Giardia* diagnosis, 497
Dust spread of infection
coccidioidomycosis, 355
intestinal nematodes, 516
Dysentery, 593
Escherichia coli, 243
fulminating amebic, 487
Shigella, 244
see also Enteric infections and food poisoning

E

Ear infections
causes of infection, 571
otitis externa, 267, 569–571
otitis media, 570–571
Eastern equine encephalitis, 434, 441
Ebola virus, 443–444
Echinococciasis, 542–544
Echinococcus granulosus and *Echinococcus multilocularis,* 542–544
Echoviruses, 401–402
Ecthyma contagiosum (orf), 393
Ecthyma gangrenosum, *Pseudomonas aeruginosa,* 267
Eggs
cestode, 535–544
embryonated in viral isolation, 110, 111
nematode, 513–525
trematode, 545–554
Eikenella corrodens, 270, 579
Elephantiasis, 530–533
ELISA. *See* Enzyme-linked immunosorbent assay
Embden–Meyerhof pathway, 16
Encephalitis, 610
arbovirus infections, 437
herpes simplex, 416
rabies, 446
slow viruses, 451–453
Encephalopathies, subacute spongiform, 453–455
Endocarditis, 616–623
culture negative, 618
enterococcal, 175, 619
pneumococcal, 178
role of normal flora, 55
staphylococcal, 155, 160, 617, 619
viridans streptococcal, 55, 180, 619
Endocervicitis, gonococcal, chlamydial, 212
Endolimax, 484
Endometritis, clostridial, 196
Endophthalmitis, 568
Endospores, *Coccidioides,* 354–355
Endothrix, 335
Endotoxemia (Gram-negative septic shock), 625–628
Endotoxin
Gram-negative bacteria, determinant of disease, 13, 68, 69
meningococcus, 207
Energy synthesis, bacterial, 16
Entamoeba coli, 484, 485
Entamoeba histolytica, 461, 484–486
Enteric fever, *Salmonella typhi,* 249–253
Enterobacter, 248
Enterobacteriaceae, 238–253
antimicrobic susceptibility, 240–241
capsules and slime layer, 238–239
classification, 239–240
endotoxins, 250
flagella, 15
general characteristics, 257
habitat, 238
Enterobius vermicularis (pinworm, threadworm), 513–518
Enterochelin, iron chelation, 67
Enterococci. *See* Streptococcus, group D
Enterocolitis
Salmonella, 249–251, 253
Staphylococcus aureus, 156
Yersinia enterocolitica, 256
Enterotoxins
Bacillus cereus, 191
Clostridium perfringens, 195
Entamoeba histolytica, 486
Escherichia coli, 242–243
Staphylococcus aureus, 153, 157
Vibrio cholerae, 258–260
Enteroviruses, 394–402
Enveloped viruses, 23
Enzyme-linked immunosorbent assay, 114, 120
Enzymes
bacterial, role in virulence, 70
extracellular
bacterial metabolism, 16
Clostridium perfringens, 195
Pseudomonas aeruginosa, 265–266
Staphylococcus aureus, 153–154
Streptococcus pneumoniae, 176–177
Streptococcus pyogenes, 166–167
restriction, recombinant DNA techniques, 47–48
viral, 24–25, 30, 31
Eosinophilia
in helminthic infections, 467, 528, 530, 532, 540, 549
tropical eosinophilia syndrome, 532
Epidemiology of infectious diseases, 76–87
epidemics, 81–83
immunization principles, 83–86
incubation period and communicability, 80–81
infection and disease, 77–78
nosocomial (hospital) infections, 662
Epidermodysplasia verruciformis, 456
Epidermophyton, 334, 335
Epididymitis, 211–212, 647
Epiglottitis, 584, 585, 586
acute, *Haemophilus influenzae,* 219, 586
Epithelium
barrier to microbial invasion, 60–62
microbial adherence, 66
Epstein–Barr virus, 424–426
and Burkitt's lymphoma, 426, 457
infectious mononucleosis, 78, 424–426
and nasopharyngeal carcinoma, 426, 457
Equine encephalitides. *See* Eastern equine encephalitis and Western equine encephalitis
Ergosterol, fungal cell membranes, 142
Erysipelas, skin infection, 169, 557
Erysipeloid, 187
Erysipelothrix rhusiopathiae, 187
Erythema infectiosum, 388
Erythema multiforme, *Mycoplasma pneumoniae,* 229
Erythema nodosum, *Coccidioides immitis,* 356
Erythrocyte, in plasmodia infection, 469–472
Erythrogenic toxin of *Streptococcus pyogenes,* 168, 170
Erythromycin, 136
in diphtheria, 185
in Legionnaires' disease, 236–237
spectrum, 148
Escherichia coli, 241, 244
antigens, 241
bacteremia, 624
in diarrheal diseases, 594, 596
enteroinvasive, 242
enterotoxigenic, 242–243
meningitis in the newborn, 243–244
normal fecal flora, 54
nosocomial (hospital) infections, 659
surface antigen K 88, 66
toxins LT and ST, 242–243
urinary tract infections, 241–242, 603
Esophagus
Candida albicans infections, 341
dilatation, American trypanosomiasis (Chagas' disease), 507
Espundia, leishmaniasis, 462
Ethambutol, 139
tuberbulosis treatment, 294
Ethylene oxide sterilization, 36–37
Eukaryote and prokaryote distinction, 2, 3
Exfoliatin, 153, 156
Exosporium, 15
Exotoxins, disease determinants, 68–70
Eye infections, 567–569
defense mechanisms, 567
herpes simplex, 416
Pseudomonas aeruginosa, 267
Sporothrix schenkii, 359
syphilis, 642
toxocariasis, 527–528
toxoplasmosis, 481
see also Conjunctivitis

F

Facultative anaerobes, 16
Fallopian tubes
gonorrhea, 211–212
salpingitis, gonococcal, chlamydial, 212, 323
Farmer's lung, 345
Fasciola, 547, 548
Fat malabsorption, role of normal flora, 56
Fatty acids of skin, defense against microbial invasion, 60
Feces, normal microbial flora, 54

Fermentation, 16
Fetus and newborn, infections, 629–635
acute bacterial sepsis, 631–632
bacterial and chlamydial infections, 632
blood and CSF cultures, 632, 635
chlamydial and gonococcal conjunctivitis, 632
chorioamnionitis, 630
common etiologic agents, 630, 631
congenital toxoplasmosis, 481
cytomegalovirus, 633–635
definitions, 630
diagnosis, 632–635
hepatitis B infection, 633
herpes simplex, 633–635
immune system immaturity, 629
immunoglobulin M antibodies, 634
infant pneumonia syndrome, 632
neonatal deficiencies, 629
neonatal varicella, 633
prematurity risks, 631
rubella, 383–387, 633–635
scalded skin syndrome, 632
serologic testing, 634
syphilis, 632–633, 642
TORCH complex, 633–634
toxoplasmosis, 633–635
Fever
endotoxin release, 68
in inflammatory response, 64
malarial, 474
Filaments, axial, 15, 280
Filariasis, 462, 530–533
Filter, sterilization, 37
Fimbriae (pili), 15
Fish tapeworm, *Diphyllobothrium latum*, 541–542
Flagella, 15
Flagellar antigens, 15, 239
Flagellate infections, 491–507
giardiasis, 494–497
leishmaniasis, 498–503
trichomoniasis, 492–494
trypanosomiasis, 503–507
Flavobacterium, 270
Fleas, transmission of *Yersinia pestis*, 274–275
Flora, normal, 50–58
Flucytosine, antifungal agent, 143, 333
Candida albicans, 343
Cryptococcus neoformans, 349
Flukes. *See* Trematodes
Fluorescent antibody microscopy, 91, 113–114
Fluorescent treponemal antibody absorption test, FTA-ABS, 284, 614–642
Fluorescin produced by *P. aeruginosa*, 265
Fluoride, and dental caries, 576–577
Fluorochrome stain, 93
Folate deficiency, trimethoprim side effect, 138
Folic acid
deficiency, role of normal flora, 56
synthesis, sulfonamide effect, 137
Food poisoning
Bacillus cereus, 191
botulism, 200–201
characteristic foods, 597
clinical findings, 597
Clostridium botulinum, 200
Clostridium perfringens, 195, 197
common causes and epidemiology, 596–597
Salmonella, 251
Staphylococcus aureus, 153, 157
Formaldehyde disinfection, 40
F plasmid of *E. coli*, 45
Francisella tularensis, 277–279
culture medium, 97
upper respiratory tract infection, 582
Freshwater swimming, *Naegleria* infections, 489
Fungi and fungal diseases
antifungal antimicrobics, 142–143, 333
cell structure, 326
classification, 330–331
conidia and spores, 329
culture media, 332
dermatophytes, 334–338
dimorphism, 329, 332
fungi imperfecti (deuteromycetes), 330
growth and morphology, 327–330
hyphae and mycelium, 328–329
infections in immunocompromised patients, 654
KOH preparation, 331
lactophenol cotton blue preparations, 332
opportunistic mycoses, 339–346
subcutaneous mycoses, 358–360
superficial mycoses, 334–337
systemic mycoses, 347–357
yeast and mold forms, 327–330
Fungus ball, *Aspergillus*, 345
Furuncle *Staphylococcus aureus*, 155, 158, 556
Fusobacterium, 194, 202
fusospirochetal disease (Vincent's infection), 56, 202, 289, 579, 581
normal fecal flora, 54

G

Gallbladder infections. *See* Biliary tract
Ganglioside receptor, cholera toxin, 259
Garnerella (Haemophilus) vaginalis, 226–227, 648
Gas gangrene, 195–196, 560
Gastrointestinal tract infections
adenoviruses, 373
amebiasis, 486
endemic infections, 594–595
epidemic infections, 595–596
epithelium, defense against microbial invasion, 61
exotoxin effects, 70
hospital-associated diarrhea, 598
mortality, 592
normal microbial flora, 53–54, 305
transmission routes, 78–79
traveler's diarrhea, 596
treatment, 600
viral, acute gastroenteritis, 427–433
see also Diarrhea and Food poisoning
Gene transfer by transformation, transduction, and conjugation, 43–46
Genetic factors
bacterial variation, 41–48
in infectious disease, 77–78, 82
in malaria, 472
in rheumatic fever, 171
Genital herpes simplex, 643–644
and cervical neoplasia, 644
Ureaplasma urealyticum, 231–232
Genotype, definition, 41
Gentamicin, 132, 133
spectrum, 148
see also Aminoglycoside antimicrobics
Germ tube tests, *Candida albicans*, 339, 343
German measles. *See* Rubella
Ghon complex, tuberculosis, 296
Giardia lamblia and giardiasis, 494–497
Giemsa stain. *See* Staining
Gingivitis, 574, 578–579
Glanders, 268
Glandular fever. *See* Infectious mononucleosis
Glomerulonephritis
acute, immune complex disease, 71
group A streptococcal, 171–172
immune complex, kala azar, 502
in malaria, 475
Glucose 6-phosphate dehydrogenase deficiency, protection against malaria, 472
Glutaraldehyde disinfection, 40
Glycogen in vaginal epithelium, 55
Glycogen synthesis, *Chlamydia trachomatis*, 319
Gnotobiotic animals, 57
Gonococcus. *See Heisseric gonorrhoeae*
Gonorrhea, 637–639
Gram stain mechanisms and procedure, 11, 92–93
Gram-negative bacteria
cell wall composition, 12–13
endotoxin, 13
septic shock (endotoxemia), 625–628
Gram-positive bacteria
cell wall composition, 11–12
Granuloma inguinale, 645
Granulomatosis infantisepticum, 187
Granulomatous uveitis, 481
Gray syndrome, with chloramphenicol treatment, 135
Griseofulvin, 143, 333
Ground itch, hookworm infection, 522
Growth factors
bacterial requirements, 18
Haemophilus influenzae, 216–217, 222
Gumma, syphilis, 641

H

Haemophilus
H. aegyptius, 222
H. ducreyi, 222
H. influenzae, 216–221
arthritis, 220, 564

Haemophilus {cont.}
cellulitis, 220
epiglottitis, 219
eye infections, 568, 569
IgA protease, 66
immunity, 218
meningitis, 219, 609–612
respiratory infections, 220, 582, 583
satellite phenomenon, 217
H. parainfluenzae, 222
Hair
follicle infections, 555–556
superficial fungal infection, 334–337
Hakuri, 429
Halogen disinfection, 38–39
Halophilic bacteria, 261
Hand-foot-and-mouth disease, 402
H antigen, 15, 239
Hearing
aminoglycoside toxicity, 133
see also Ear infections
Heart
African trypanosomiasis (sleeping sickness), 504
American trypanosomiasis (Chagas' disease), 506
Aspergillus infections, 345
Candida albicans infections, 342
diphtheria toxin effects, 184
hookworm infections, 522
infective endocarditis, 617–620
inflammation, Coxsackie B virus, 402
tissue nematode infections, 527
Heat sterilization, 35–36
Hektoen agar. *See* Culture media
Helminths
parasitic pathogens, 463–464
see also Cestodes, Nematodes, and Trematodes
Helper T-cells, 73
Hemadsorption, viral, 107, 110
Hemagglutination
inhibition, 112–113
passive, 102
viral, 107, 110, 113, 118, 362–365, 380
Hematin, *Haemophilus influenzae* growth factor, 216
Hemoflagellates, 503–507
Hemolysins, 153, 166–167, 195
Hemolysis, α and β, 163
Hemorrhagic fever
arbovirus infections, 437
arenaviruses, 443
Hemozoin, malarial pigment, 470, 472
Hepatic encephalopathy, role of normal flora, 56
Hepatitis
amebic, 486
infectious mononucleosis, 424–425
leptospirosis, 286
sepsis in newborn, 632
in TORCH syndrome, 633
yellow fever, 441
see also individual hepatitis viruses
Hepatitis A virus and disease, 403–406
immune electron microscopy, 403
passive protection, 86, 406
serodiagnosis, 406
Hepatitis B virus and disease, 406–411
antigenemia and immune response, 408–409
antigens HBcAg, HBeAg, HBsAg, 407–411
Dane particle, 406, 408
liver carcinoma association, 410
passive protection, 86, 410
vaccine, 84, 411
Hepatitis non-A non-B, 411
Hermaphrodite unit
cestodes, 535
trematodes, 545
Herpangina, 402
Herpes simplex, 414–420, 634–644
fetal and newborn infections, 633–635
fusospirochetal disease complication, 289
intercellular bridges, 68, 73, 418
latency and disease, 418–419
reactivation, 419
type 1 infections, 415–416
type 2 infections, 416–417, 643–644
Herpesviruses, 413–426
Herpetic whitlow, 416, 557
Heterophil antibodies, 425–426
see also Epstein–Barr virus
Hexachlorophene, 40
High pressure liquid chromatography, antimicrobic assays, 142
Histamine in inflammatory response, 63
Histiocytes, phagocytosis, 63
Histoplasma capsulatum and histoplasmosis, 349–352
dimorphism, 349
disseminated, 351
histoplasmin skin test, 350–352
tuberculate macroconidia, 349
Hodgkin's disease, varicella–zoster infections, 421
Homofermentation, 16
Hookworm infections, 521–523
Hosts of parasites, definitive and intermediate, 466
Hyaluronic acid, streptococcal capsules, 162
Hyaluronidase, in bacterial infection, 70, 154, 167
Hybridoma antibodies, 665–666
Hydatid disease, 542–544
Hydrochloric acid, gastric, defense against microbial invasion, 61
Hydrophobia, rabies, 447
Hymenolepsis nana, 537
Hyperalimentation procedures, *Candida* infections, 340
Hypersensitivity reactions
delayed type, pathologic changes, 71, 73
to fungi, 350, 352, 355
in leprosy, 302
to mycobacteria, 292, 293, 295
tissue nematode infections, 533
trematode infections, 551, 553
Hyphae, fungal, 328–329, 334
Hypoalbuminemia, hookworm infections, 522
Hypothalamus, in inflammatory response, 64

I

Icosahedral symmetry, 24
Idoxuridine (5-iodo-2'-deoxyuridine), 144, 416
Imidazoles, antifungal agent, 143, 333, 343
Immune complex, and tissue damage, 70–71
Immune response
adaptive, of host to systemic infection, 72–74
to infection, overview, 5
priming by normal flora, 57
Immune serum globulin and passive immunization, 83–85, 86, 406, 422
Immunity
antibody-mediated, 72–73
cell-mediated, 73–74
immunocompromised host infections, 649–654
see also Immunocompromised patients
population factors in epidemics, 82
racial, species, 59, 77–78, 82, 296, 356
Immunization, 83–85
active and passive, 83–86
Immunocompromised patients, defects, and etiologic agents, 649–654
Acanthamoeba infections, 489
Bacillus infections, 191
Candida albicans infections, 342
Coccidioides immitis infections, 356
Cryptococcus neoformans infections, 348
cytomegalovirus infection, 423
ear infections, 570
Epstein–Barr virus, 425
eye manifestations, 569
fusospirochetal diseases, 289
giardiasis, 496
intestinal nematode infections, 524–525
lower respiratory tract infections, 588
measles infection, 381
opportunistic infections, 56, 649–654, 657–659
oral and dental infections, 579
osteomyelitis, *Salmonella* infections, 252
Pneumocystis carinii infections, 509–512
Pseudomonas aeruginosa infections, 266
skin infections, 558
toxoplasmosis, 481–483
upper respiratory tract infections, 581
vaccinia infection, 393
varicella–zoster virus, 420, 422
zygomycosis, 346
Immunofluorescence
bacterial detection, 91, 102
in serodiagnosis, 119
viral detection, 110, 113–114
see also individual organisms
Immunoglobulin A (IgA), 62, 260
deficiency, giardiasis, 496

proteases, 66
in saliva, 576
Immunoglobulin G (IgG), 72
course and duration of immune response, 117
Immunoglobulin M (IgM), 72
course and duration of immune response, 117–118
fetal and newborn infections, 634
rubella, 386–387
Immunoglobulins, general
antibody-mediated immunity, 72–73
deficiencies in immunocompromised patients, 652
passive immunization, 84–86
Impetigo, pyoderma, 169, 172, 556–557
Inclusion bodies, 114–116
Inclusion (storage) granules, 15, 233
Incubation period, infectious disease, 80–81
India ink preparations, *Cryptococcus neoformans,* 348, 349
Indole, bacterial classification, 99
Infants and children
American trypanosomiasis (Chagas' disease), 506
blood culture, septic shock, 627
bone and joint infections, 562–566
botulism, 201
central nervous system infections, 612
Chlamydia trachomatis infection, 322–325
cytomegalovirus infections, 423
enteroviruses, 396–402
eye and ear infections, 567–572
gastrointestinal infections, 243, 594–595
giardiasis, 496, 497
group B streptococcal infections, 174
hepatitis B, 410
herpes simplex, type 1, 415
inclusion conjunctivitis, 322
lower respiratory tract infections, 588
middle respiratory tract infections, 586
mumps, measles, rubella, 378–388
neonatal herpes, 417
neonatal meningitis, *Escherichia coli,* 243–244
normal microbial flora, 51
opthalmia neonatorum, 212
parainfluenza infection (croup), 369–370
Pneumocystis carinii infection, 511
respiratory syncytial virus, 370–372
Reye's syndrome, 366
roseola infantum (exanthem subitum), 387–388
rubella, 383–387
subacute sclerosing panencephalitis, 451–452
upper respiratory tract infections, 581
urinary tract infections, 601
viruses of diarrhea, 427–433
Infection, general characteristics
definition, 77
endogenous and exogenous, 4–5
epidemiology, 76–86
epithelial barrier, 60–62
immune response of host, 72–74
infectivity requirements, 66
inflammatory response, 63–64, 68
initial environment, 63
laboratory diagnosis, 88–122
normal microbial flora, 55–56
pathogenesis, 59–75
persistent and latent, 29–30
phagocytic defenses, 64–68
species differences in host susceptibility, 59
virulence mechanisms, 67–71
zoonotic, epidemiology, 76, 80
Infectious mononucleosis (Epstein–Barr virus), 424–426
epidemiology, 78, 425
similarities of toxoplasmosis, 481
Infectivity, 77
Inflammatory response
to microbial invasion, 63–64, 68
to superficial fungal infections, 334
Influenza, 361–365
age-specific attack rates, 365
bacterial superinfection, 366–367, 369
doctrine of original antigenic sin, 365
mortality, 361, 367
pandemic, 82, 361
Reye's syndrome, 366
Influenza viruses, 361–364
antigenic drifts and shifts, 363–364
hemagglutinin antigens, 363–365
history and habitat, 361–362
influenza A, 363–365
neuraminidase antigens, 363–365
Insect vectors, 78, 80
arthropod-borne viruses, 435
enteroviruses, 396
lymphatic filariasis, 531
malaria, 469–470, 473, 477
of rickettsia, 310–317
Insertion sequences, 41
Interference, viral detection in cell culture, 110
Interferons, 74, 144, 145
influenza recovery, 367
varicella–zoster treatment, 422
Interleukins, cell-mediated immunity, 73
Intravascular infections, 616–623
infective endocarditis, 617–620
intravenous catheter bacteremia, 622–623
mycotic aneurysm, 620–621
suppurative thrombophlebitis, 621–622
Invasiveness, 66
Inverted repeat DNA base sequences, 42
Iodide, *Sporothrix schenckii* treatment, 360
Iodine disinfection, 38
Iron
and bacterial growth, 63, 67
complexes with siderophores, 18
deficiency, hookworm infections, 522
and humoral immunity, 72
Legionella pneumophila growth, 233
Isolation procedures for patients, 660–661
Isoniazid, 139
tuberculosis treatment, 294, 298, 299
IUDR, idoxuridine, 144, 416

J

Japanese B encephalitis, 434, 435, 442
Jarisch–Herxheimer reaction, 642
J.C. virus, 453, 457
Jenner, Edward, 390
Jock itch, 334
Junin virus (Argentinian hemorrhagic fever), 443

K

Kala azar (disseminated visceral leishmaniasis), 462, 502–503
K antigen, 239
Kanamycin, 131–133
see also Aminoglycoside antimicrobics
Kaposi's sarcoma, *Pneumocystis carinii* association, 510
Katayama syndrome, 552, 553
Keratoconjunctivitis, acute hemorrhagic, enterovirus infection, 402
Ketaconazole, antifungal antimicrobic, 143, 333
Kidney
cestode infections, 544
in infective endocarditis, 618
renal disease in malaria, 475, 476
see also Glomerulonephritis and Urinary tract infections
Killer T-cells, 73
Kinetics of bacterial growth, 18–20
Kinetics of microbial killing, 34
Kinetoplast, flagellate protozoa, 491, 498
Kirby–Bauer diffusion test, 141
Klebsiella, 247–248
capsule, resistance to macrophage killing, 66
cross-reactions with *Streptococcus pneumoniae* and *Haemophilus influenzae,* 247
see also Enterobacteriaceae
Koplik's spots (measles), 381
Korean hemorrhagic fever, 444–445
Kuru, 454–455
Kwashiorkor in hookworm infections, 522

L

Laboratory diagnosis of infectious diseases
bacteria
agglutination, 101–102
antigenic analysis, 103–105
biochemical characteristics, 99–100
culture, media and conditions, 93–98, 120–121
DNA probes, 104
Gram stain, direct, 92
identification, 98–106
immunofluorescence methods, 102–103
microscopy, 90–91
serologic methods in identification, 101–105
stains, 91–93
serodiagnosis
agglutination, 118
complement fixation, 118, 119

Laboratory diagnosis of infectious diseases
bacteria *(cont.)*
hemagglutination inhibition, 118
immunoassays, 120
immunofluorescence, 119
neutralization, 118
principles, 116–117
specimen types and transport, 88–90
virus
antigen detection, 114
cytology and histology, 114–116
electron microscopy, 113–114
identification, 112–116
isolation methods, 106–112
animal inoculation, 110–111
cell culture, 106–110
embryonated egg, 110
serologic detection, 112–113
specimen selection and transport, 105–106
β-Lactamases, 126, 129
Haemophilus influenzae, 221
Legionella pneumophila, 234
Neisseria gonorrhoeae, 214
Staphylococcus aureus, 154
Lactic acid formation
bacterial metabolism (homofermentation), 16, 17
skin, defense against microbial invasion, 60
Lactobacillus, morphology and normal distribution, 56, 187
Lactoferrin, antimicrobial properties, 62, 63
Lactophenol cotton blue, fungal morphology, 332
Lactose
fermentation, Enterobacteriaceae, 240
intolerance, giardiasis, 496, 497
Lag phase of bacterial growth, 19
Lancefield serologic classification of streptococci, 104, 163
Langhans giant cells, 295
Larva, rhabditiform and filariform. *See* Nematodes, intestinal
Laryngitis, middle respiratory tract infections, 584, 586
Lassa fever virus, 443
Latent infections
adenoviruses, 374
herpesviruses, 413–415, 418
syphilis, 283, 641
typhus, 315
viral diseases, 30
Lecithinase, *Clostridium perfringens,* 195
Legionella pneumophila, 233–237
epidemiology, 76, 77, 234–235
erythromycin in therapy, 136, 236–237
Legionnaires' disease. *See Legionella pneumophila*
Leishman–Donovan bodies, 499–502
Leishmania species, 498–503
Leishmaniasis
diffuse cutaneous, 501–502
disseminated visceral (kala azar), 502–503
distribution of infection, 462
localized cutaneous, 500–501
mucocutaneous, 501
tapir nose, 501
Leishmanin skin test, 499–502
Lepromin skin test, 302
Leprosy. *See Mycobacterium leprae*
Leptospira
culture medium, 97
leptospirosis. *See* Spirochetes
Leukemia viruses, 458–459
Leukocidins, 67, 153
Leukocytes, polymorphonuclear, in inflammatory response, 63–64
Leukoencephalopathy, progressive multifocal, 452–453
L forms, 11
Lincomycins, 136
Lincosamide antibiotics, 136
Lipid, *Mycobacterium tuberculosis* cell wall, 291, 293
Lipopolysaccharide, bacterial cell wall, 13, 239, 264, 310
Lipoprotein
bacterial cell wall, 13
viral external coat, 23–25
Lipoteichoic acid, 166, 168
Listeria monocytogenes, 186–187
Liver infections. *See* Hepatitis
Liver fluke, *Clonorchis sinensis,* 545, 548–549
Loa loa and Loiasis, 534
Lockjaw, tetanus, 199
Loeffler's medium, *Corynebacterium diphtheriae,* 182, 185
Log (exponential) phase of bacterial growth, 19
Loiasis, 534
Lowenstein–Jensen medium, *Mycobacterium tuberculosis* culture, 292
Lumbar puncture, central nervous system infections, 613
Lung
alveolar macrophages, defense against microbial infections, 62
ascariasis, 519, 521
Aspergillus infections, 345
Blastomyces dermatitidis infection, 353
cestode infection, 544
Coccidioides immitis infection, 356
Cryptococcus neoformans infections, 347, 348
Histoplasma capsulatum infections, 350
hookworm infections, 522
Legionnaires' disease, 235
lower respiratory tract infections, 586–591
malaria effects, 476
nocardiosis, 308
paragonimiasis, 546–548
Pneumocystis carinii infections, 510–511
Sporothrix schenkii infections, 359
tissue nematode infections, 527, 530
trematode infections, 552
see also Pneumonia
Lung fluke. *See* Trematode infections
Lupus erythematosus, immunocompromised patients, 651
Lyme disease, 289
Lymph, and microbial invasion, 63
Lymph nodes, phagocytic cells, 65
Lymphadenitis, acute mesenteric, *Yersinia pseudotuberculosis,* 255–256
Lymphatic filariasis, 530–533
Lymphocytes, T and B, 72
Lymphocytic choriomeningitis virus, 442–443
Lymphogranuloma venereum, 324, 645
Lymphokines
fetal and newborn infections, 629
interferon, 74
in phagocytosis, 65
Lymphoma, Burkitts, 424, 426, 457
Lysogenization and lysogenic conversion, 32, 168, 183, 200
Lysozyme
antimicrobial properties, 62, 63
in saliva, 576
viral enzymes, 24, 25

M

MacConkey agar, Enterobacteriaceae, 121, 239, 240, 246
Machupo virus (Bolivian hemorrhagic fever), 443
Macroconidia, fungal, 328–329
Macrolide antimicrobics, 136
Macrophage migration inhibition factor, 73
Macrophages, 62, 64–65, 73, 295
Malabsorption
ascariasis, 520
blind-loop syndrome, 56
giardiasis, 496
sprue, tropical, 56
Malaria, 469–478
blackwater fever, 474
circulatory and renal diseases, 474–476
endemic disease, 474
fetal and newborn infections, 635
frequency of infection, 460–461
hosts, definitive and intermediate, 466
immunity, 475
mortality, 461, 473
Plasmodium species, differential characteristics, 471
protection by red cell abnormalities, 472
resistant strains, 461, 476, 477
vector transmission, 78, 80, 470, 477
Malignant pustule,anthrax, 190, 191
Malignant transformation, 30, 456
Malnutrition, reactivation tuberculosis, 296
Malta fever. *See* Brucellosis
Mammary carcinoma virus (mouse), 456
Mannitol fermentation by *Staphylococcus aureus,* 151
Marburg virus, 443–444, 446
Maurer's dots, 471
Measles, 380–383
central nervous system effects, 381
depression of cell-mediated immunity, 381
epidemiology, 77–78, 382
immune response, 382

immunization, 83–85, 383
Koplik's spots, 381
Measles, German. *See* Rubella
Meat, uncooked
cestode infections, 537, 538, 540
trichinosis, 529
Mebendazole treatment
cestode infections, 539
intestinal nematodes, 517, 519, 521, 522
Meckel's diverticulum, 56
Media. *See* Culture media
Melarsoprol for African trypanosomiasis (sleeping sickness), 505
Meleney's ulcer, 203
Melioidosis, 268
Membrane, cytoplasmic, 13, 14
Meningitis, 608–615
aseptic, 610
enterovirus infection, 402
herpetic, 416
leptospirosis, 286
mumps, 379
poliomyelitis, 399
central nervous system infections, 610–612
coccidioidal, 356
cryptococcal, 348
Haemophilus influenzae, 219
Listeria monocytogenes, 186
meningococcal, 208–209
neonatal, 611
bacterial sepsis, 631
Escherichia coli, 243–244
group B Streptococcal infections, 174
pneumococcal, 178
tuberculous, 296, 609, 611, 613
Meningoencephalitis, 610–611
African trypanosomiasis (sleeping sickness), 504
Mycoplasma pneumoniae, 229
primary amebic, 488–489
see also Encephalitis
Merozoites, protozoa, 469–471
Merthiolate, microbial death, 33
Mesosomes, 14
Metabolism, bacterial, 16, 17
Methenamine silver stain for fungi, 331, 351
Histoplasma capsulatum stain, 351
Pneumocystis carinii, 509
Methicillin, 127
Staphylococcus aureus resistance, 154
Methylene blue stain, 91
Metronidazole, 139
amebiasis, 488
anaerobic infections, 204
giardiasis, 497
trichomoniasis, 494
Miconazole, antifungal activity, 143, 333, 337
Microaerophilic streptococci, 203
Microbial death, 33–40
definitions, 33–34
disinfection, antisepsis, and sanitization, 38–40
kinetics of killing, 34
pasteurization and tyndallization, 37–38
sterilization, 34–37
Micrococcus, 161
Microhemagglutination test for *T. pallidum,* 284
Microscopy
bright-field, 91
dark-field, 91
immune electron, 403
fluorescence, 91, 93, 113, 114
Microsporum, 334, 335
Milk
immunoglobulins, antimicrobial effects, 62
and normal fecal flora in infants, 54
Milker's nodules, 393
Minimum bactericidal concentration, 124
Minimum inhibitory concentration, 124
Minimum lethal concentration, 124
Minocycline, 134
Miracidia, 545
Molds. *See* Fungi
Molluscum contagiosum, 393
Monocytes, phagocytosis, 64
Mononucleosis, infectious, 424–425
Moraxella, 269
Morganella, 254
Motility, bacterial, 15
Mouth infections. *See* Stomatitis
M protein of S. pyogenes, 166, 168, 173
Mucociliary blanket, 54, 60
Mucopeptide, cell wall, 11–12
Mumps, 378–380
Muscles
masseter, tetanus, 199
tissue nematode infections, 527–529
Mutation and mutagenesis, 42–43, 294
Myalgia, epidemic, Coxsackie B virus, 402
Mycelium, fungal, 328–329
Mycetoma, 360
Mycobacteria, 291–304
acid fastness, 291
cell wall structure, 291
growth rates, 291, 304
hypersensitivity to proteins, 292
M. africanum, 292
M. avium-intracellulare complex, 301
M. bovis, 292
M. fortuitum complex, 303
M. kansasii, 301
M. leprae and leprosy, 302–303
M. marinum, 303, 558
M. scrofulaceum, 301
M. smegmatis, 300
M. tuberculosis
central nervous system infections, 609–612
cord factor, 292
culture media, 292
generation time, 18, 292
intraphagocytic survival, 67, 294
resistance to chemicals, 293
resistant mutants, 294
tuberculin (PPD), 297
virulence mechanisms, 71, 293–294
see also Tuberculosis
M. ulcerans, 303
N-glycolylmuramic acid content, 291
pathogenicity, 292, 304
pigment production, 291, 300, 304
Mycology. *See* Fungi and fungal infections
Mycoplasma, 228–232
cell wall absence, 228
growth in artificial media, 228
membrane sterols, 228
M. hominis, 232
M. pneumoniae, 229–231, 585–586
erythromycin and tetracycline susceptibility, 136, 148
septic arthritis, 564
species differentiation, 228, 229
Mycotic aneurysm, 620–621
Myringitis, 570

N

Naegleria infections, 489
Nails, superficial fungal infections, 334–337
Nalidixic acid, 139
Nasopharyngeal cultures, middle respiratory tract infections, 225, 586
Necator americanus, hookworm, 514, 516, 521–522
Negri body, rabies pathology, 447
Neisseria, 205–215
N. gonorrhoeae, 210–214
conjunctivitis and ophthalmia neonatorum, 212
culture media, 96, 97, 213
eye infections, 212, 568
gonorrheal infections, 212–213, 638–639
pharyngitis, 212, 582, 583
pili, 15, 210
see also Sexually transmitted diseases
N. lactamica, 214
N. meningitidis, 206–210
carrier state, 50, 206
central nervous system infections, 208, 609–612
meningococcemia, 208
vaccine, 209
Nematodes, intestinal, 513–525
Nematodes, tissue, 526–534
Neomycin, 132
Netilmicin, 132, 133
Neuralgia, postherpetic, 420
Neuraminidase
influenza virus, 362–365
Streptococcus pneumoniae, 176
Neurotoxins, *Clostridium botulinum,* 200
Neutralization, serodiagnosis of viral infection, 118
Neutropenia, immunocompromised patients, 650–653
Neutrophils, in phagocytosis, 64
Niclosamide treatment, cestode infections, 539
Nicotinamide adenine dinucleotide
bacterial metabolism, 16
Haemophilus influenzae growth factor, 216–217

Nitrofuramox treatment, American trypanosomiasis (Chagas' disease), 507
Nitrofurantoin, 139
Nitrogen, bacterial growth requirement, 17–18
O-Nitrophenyl-beta-galactoside, in bacterial classification, 100
Nocardia, 307–309
in immunocompromised hosts, 650, 654
infections, sulfonamide therapy, 137, 309
Normal flora, 50–58
beneficial effects, 57–58
of different sites, 51–55
physiologic and ecologic determinants, 51
role in disease, 55–56
Norwalk agent, 431
Nosocomial (hospital) infections, 655–663
catheters, 658
diarrhea outbreaks, 598
environmental sources, 657
epidemiology, 83
epidemiology service, 662
hemodialysis, 658
hospital ward, 661
infection control, 660–663
isolation procedures, 661
medical devices, 657–658
operating room, 660
outpatient clinic, 661
pathogenic agents, 659–660
respirators, 658
Semmelweis' discoveries, 655–656
sources, 656–658
suppurative thrombophlebitis, 621–622
urinary tract infections, 602–603, 659–660
see also individual organisms
Novobiocin, *Staphylococcus saprophyticus* resistance, 151
Nuclear body, nucleoid, 14
Nucleic acids. *See* DNA and RNA
Nucleocapsid, 24
Nucleotide cofactors, rickettsiae, 311
Null cells, 74
Nystatin antifungal agent, 142–143
Candida albicans, 343
toxicity, 333

O

O antigen, 13, 239
Oleic acid-albumin agar, *Mycobacterium tuberculosis* culture, 292
Onchocerca volvulus, 531, 533
Onchocerciasis (river blindness), 461, 462
Oncogenes, RNA tumor viruses, 458
Oocyst, *Toxoplasma gondii,* 478–480
Operons, 42
Ophthalmia neonatorum (gonococcal), 212, 568, 632
Opisthotonus, 199
Opportunistic pathogen, 59
Opsonization
phagocytic defenses, 65
pneumococcus, 176, 178
Staphylococcus aureus, 151
Oral and dental infections, 574–579
bacterial species, 575, 577, 579
bone resorption, 578
caries, 574, 576–578
in children and young adults, 576
cuticle (pellicle), 575
extracellular polyglycans, 577
fluoride effects, 576–577
gingivitis and periodontitis, chronic marginal, 574, 578–579
glycogen role, 577
in immunocompromised patients, 579
plaque, 574–576
saliva role, 576
tooth support, 575
ulcerative gingivitis, acute necrotizing, 579
Vincent's infection (trench mouth), 289, 579
xerostomia, 576
Orbivirus, 26, 435, 442
Orchitis, mumps, 379
Orf, 393
Organ culture, virus isolation, 106
Oriental sore, leishmaniasis, 462, 499, 500
Ornithosis, 321–322
Orthomyxoviruses, 28
Osteomyelitis, 562–564
common causes, 563
in sickle cell anemia and immunocompromised patients, *Salmonella* infections, 252
Staphylococcus aureus, 155, 158
Otitis externa, 267, 569–571
Otitis media, 570–572
Haemophilus influenzae, 220
pneumococcus, 178
tetanus, 198
Oxidase test, 100, 205, 213, 265
Oxygen
hyperbaric in treatment of gas gangrene, 196
sensitivity of anaerobes, 193, 204
spirochete requirements, 280
therapy, *Pneumocystis carinii* infection, 512
Ozena, *Klebsiella,* 248

P

PABA. *See* p-Aminobenzoic acid
Pancreatic duct strongyloidiasis, 523
Pandemic influenza, 82, 361
Panencephalitis, subacute sclerosing, 381, 451–452, 611
from chronic measles virus infection, 381, 451, 452
Papovaviruses, 456–457
Parabasal body, flagellate protozoa, 491
Paracoccidioides brasiliensis, 357
Paragonimus westermani (lung fluke), 546–548
Parainfluenza viruses, 369–370
Paralysis
poliomyelitis, 399
respiratory, rabies, 447
Paramyxoviruses, 27
Parasites (eukaryotic), introduction, 460–468
control and treatment, 468
definition, 50, 460
diagnosis, 467
helminths, morphology, classification, and physiology, 463–464
human infections, significance, 460–462
infections in immunocompromised patients, 654
life cycles, transmission and distribution, 465–466
pathogenesis, 466
protozoa, biology, morphology, and classification, 462–463
toxicity of antiparasitic drugs, 468
Paronychia, *Staphylococcus aureus,* 155
Parotid glands, mumps infection, 379
Parvoviruses, 26
Pasteur
anthrax vaccination, 189
rabies vaccine, 448
Pasteurella multocida, 279
Pasteurella pestis. See Yersinia pestis
Pasteurization, 37
Pathogenesis of infection, 59–75
see also individual organisms and disease syndromes
Pathogens, primary and opportunistic, 59
Pelvic inflammatory disease
Chlamydia trachomatis, 323
gonorrhea, 212, 638
intrauterine devices, 638, 648
Mycoplasma hominis, 232
Penicillins, 126–129
and aminoglycosides, synergism, 125
benzyl-penicillin G, 126, 127
broad spectrum, 127, 128
classification, 126–128
inhibition of cell wall synthesis, 128
narrow spectrum, 127, 128
penicillinase resistant, 127, 128
pneumococcal resistance, 177
spectrum, 148
structure, 126, 127
toxicity, 129
Penicillinase, plasmid-coded, 129
H. influenzae, 129, 221
N. gonorrhoeae, 129, 214
S. aureus, 129, 154
Pentamidine treatment
African trypanosomiasis (sleeping sickness), 505
Leishmania infections, 502
Pentons, toxic, adenoviruses, 374
Peptide kinins, in inflammatory response, 63
Peptidoglycan
Gram-negative cell wall, 12
Gram-positive cell wall, 11–12
rickettsial cell wall, 310
Peptococcus, 194, 203

Peptostreptococcus, 194, 202–203
Periodic acid-Schiff stain for fungi, 331
Periodontitis. *See* Oral and dental infections
Periplasmic space, 14
Peritonitis, *Streptococcus pneumoniae,* 178
Permeases, 14
Pertussis, 223–226
Petriellidium boydii, 360
pH indicator, culture media for bacteria, 96
Phagocyte defects, immunocompromised patients, 650–651
Phagocytosis, microbicidal mechanisms, 64–66
Pharyngitis
  diphtheritic, 184
  epidemiology, 172
  gonococcal, 212, 582
  herpes simplex, type 1, 415–416
  Mycoplasma pneumoniae, 229, 230
  nonstreptococcal exudative, adenoviruses, 373
  streptococcal, 169, 170
  upper respiratory infections, 580–583
Pharyngoconjunctival fever, adenoviruses, 373
Phenol disinfection, 39–40
Phenotype
  definition, 41
  plasmid, 46–47
Phialophora, 360
Phospholipids, bacterial cell wall, 13
Picornaviruses, 26, 394–402, 403
Piedra, 338
Piedraia hortai, 338
Pili (fimbriae), 15
  Enterobacteriaceae, 238
  Neisseria, 205, 210, 211
  Pseudomonas aeruginosa, 264
  sex, bacterial conjugation, 45
  Streptococcus pyogenes, 166
Pilosebaceous units, 52
Pinta, 284
Pinworm. *See Enterobius vermicularis*
Plague. *See Yersinia pestis*
Plasmids, 14
  and antimicrobic resistance, 125, 145–147
  bacterial conjugation, 45–46
  and beta-lactamase production, 129
  phenotypes, 46–47
  and resistance to antimicrobics, 133, 244
  virulence determinants, 47, 71, 242
Plasminogen activators, 154, 167
Plasmodium falciparum, malariae, ovale, vivax, Malarial parasites, 469–478
Platyhelminthes, 545–554
Plerocercoid, 536
Plesiomonas, 366
Pleurodynia, 37
Pneumococcus. *See Streptococcus pneumoniae*
Pneumocystis carinii, 509–512
  cyst and trophozoite forms, 509
  infections in immunocompromised patients, 509–512
  stains, 509
  taxonomy and tissue culture, 509
Pneumolysin, 176
Pneumonia
  chlamydial infant syndrome, 632
  cryptococcal, 348
  Haemophilus, 220
  influenzal, 366
  Klebsiella, 247
  lower respiratory tract infections, 587–589
  neonatal, group B streptococcal infection, 174
  pneumococcal, 177–178
  Pseudomonas aeruginosa, 267
  respiratory syncytial virus, 370–371
  staphylococcal, 156
  walking, *Mycoplasma pneumoniae,* 229–231
Poliomyelitis
  central nervous system infections, 611
  clinical syndrome, 399
  epidemiology, 78, 395–396
  vaccine, 399–401
  virus serotypes, 398
Polioviruses, 398–401
  replication, 29
Polyene, antifungals, 142–143
Polymorphonuclear leukocytes in host defense, 63–64
Polymyxin B, polypeptide antimicrobic, 138
Polyoma viruses, 457
Polysaccharide
  bacterial capsules, 10
  Haemophilus influenzae capsule, 216
  meningococcal capsule, 206
  pneumococcal capsule, 176, 178
Pontiac fever, 234
Pork tapeworm, *Taenia saginata,* 539–540
Postpartum fever
  group A streptococci, 170, 655
  Ureaplasma, 232
Powassan virus, 442
Poxviruses, 390–393
P.P.D. (tuberculin) skin test, 293–297
Praziquantel treatment
  cestode infections, 540
  trematode infections, 549, 554
Precipitin tests, bacterial identification, 101
Pregnancy
  ectopic, and gonorrhea, 638
  genital herpes simplex, 644
  transplacental spread of infection, 78, 480, 631
  trichomoniasis, 493–494
  urinary tract infections, 602, 604
Primaquine, malaria treatment, 477
Proglottids, 464
Prokaryotes, 2, 3
Prontosil rubrum, 136
Prophylaxis
  hepatitis A, 86, 406
  hepatitis B, 86, 410–411
  meningococcal infections, 137
  newborns, conjunctivitis, 325
  see also Chemoprophylaxis
Propionibacterium, 52, 187
Prostate infection
  Blastomyces dermatitidis infection, 353
  gonorrhea, 211–212
  trichomoniasis, 494
  trimethoprim treatment, 138
  see also Urinary tract infections
Protein, outer membrane, 13
Protein A, *Staphylococcus aureus,* 102, 151, 154
Protein synthesis
  aminoglycoside inhibition, 132
  chloramphenicol inhibition, 135
  erythromycin and lincomycin inhibition, 136
  genetic control, 42
  tetracycline inhibition, 134
Proteus species, 254, 255, 603
Protoplast, 11
Protozoa, 462–463
Providencia, 254
Pruritis ani, intestinal nematodes, 517, 522
Pseudohyphae, fungal, 332
Pseudomembranous enterocolitis and clindamycin, 136
Pseudomonas aeruginosa, 39, 264–268
  antimicrobic susceptibility, 133, 138, 267
  burn and wound infections, 266–267, 560
  cystic fibrosis infection, 267
  ear and eye infections, 267
  ecthyma gangrenosum, 267
  pigment production, 264, 265
  toxins and extracellular products, 265–266
Pseudomonas cepacia, 268
Pseudomonas mallei, 268
Pseudomonas pseudomallei, 268
Psittacosis (ornithosis), 321–322
Puerperal fever, 170, 655
Pustular dermatitis (orf), 393
Pyelonephritis, 604–605
Pyoderma, streptococcal, 556
Pyrantel pamoate treatment, intestinal nematodes, 517, 521, 522
Pyridoxal kinase deficiency, protection against malaria, 472
Pyrimethamine
  and sulfadoxine, malaria pervention, 477
  and sulfonamides, toxoplasmosis treatment, 483
Pyrogen, endogenous, in inflammatory response, 64

Q

Q fever, *Coxiella* infection, 316–317
Quaternary ammonium compounds, 38–39
Queensland tick fever, 311
Quellung reaction
  Haemophilus influenzae, 216
  Klebsiella, 247
  Streptococcus pneumoniae, 10, 180
Quinacrine hydrochloride treatment, giardiasis, 497

R

Rabies, 80, 85, 446–449
Race and infectious disease, 77–78, 82, 296, 356
Radiation, ionizing
bacterial mutagen, 43
microbial death, 37
Radioimmunoassay
antimicrobic levels, 142
bacterial antigen detection, 103, 105
viral antigen detection, 114, 120
Receptors
cholera toxin GM1 ganglioside, 259
glycoprotein, viral infections, 66
surface, phagocytic cells, 65
Recombinant DNA techniques, 47–48
Rectal gonorrhea, 212
Relapsing fever, *Borrelia recurrentis,* 287–289
Reoviruses, 376
Replication of viruses
animal viruses, 28–29
bacteriophages, 30
persistent and latent infection, 29–30
transformation and endogenous genes, 30
Resistance to antimicrobics, 46, 125, 145–149
see also individual antimicrobics and organisms
Respirator humidifier infections, 266, 658
Respiratory syncytial virus, 370–372
Respiratory tract
epithelial defense against microbial invasion, 60–61
normal microbial flora, 54
transmission of infection, 78, 79
Respiratory tract infections
lower, 586–591
middle, 584–586
upper, 580–583
see also Bronchitis, Bronchiolitis, Epiglottitis, Pharyngitis, and Pneumonia
Restriction endonucleases, 47–48
Reticuloendothelial system
Brucella infections, 271, 273
Histoplasma capsulatum infection, 350
and phagocytosis, 64, 65
Salmonella typhi infection, 250
Retroviruses, 457–459
Reverse transcriptase, 25, 30, 458
Reye's syndrome, influenza and varicella-zoster association, 366, 611
R factor, 125
see also Plasmids
Rhabditiform larvae, 516
Rhabdoviruses, 27, 434
Rheumatic fever, 170–171
penicillin prophylaxis, 173
tissue damage from immune reactions, 171
Rhinitis, upper respiratory infections, 580
Rhinoscleroma, *Klebsiella,* 247
Rhinoviruses, 375–376
Rhizopod (amebic) infections, 484–489
RIA. *See* Radioimmunoassay
Ribavirin, 144, 372
Ribonuclease H and RNA tumor viruses, 30
Ribosomes, bacterial, 14
effect of antimicrobics, 132, 134, 135, 136, 139
Rice-water stools (cholera), 260, 261
Rickettsia, 310–317
Brill's disease, 315
Coxiella burnettii (Q fever), 316
insect vectors, 310
R. akari (rickettsialpox), 314
R. rickettsii (Rocky Mountain spotted fever), 312–314
R. prowazekii (louse-borne typhus fever), 314–315
R. tsutsugamushi (scrub typhus), 316
R. typhi (murine typhus), 315–316
tissue culture, 310
Weil–Felix serodiagnostic test, 311
Rifampin, 139
Haemophilus influenzae prophylaxis, 219
meningococcal prophylaxis, 209
tuberculosis treatment, 294
Rimantidine, 144
Ringworm, 334–338
Risus sardonicus, 199
Ritter's disease. *See* Scalded skin syndrome
River blindness, 533–534
RNA and gene expression, 42
RNA viruses, 28–30
classification, 26–27
RNA tumor viruses (retroviruses), 30, 457–459
Rocky Mountain spotted fever, 312–314
Romana's sign, 506
Roseola infantum (exanthem subitum), 387–388
Rotaviruses, 428–431
Roundworms. *See* Nematodes
Rous sarcoma virus, 456
Rubella, 383–387
fetal and newborn infections, 78, 384–386, 633–635
Rubeola. *See* Measles
Russian spring summer encephalitis, 435

S

Sabin vaccine for poliomyelitis, 400
Sabin–Feldman dye test for toxoplasmosis, 482
Sabouraud's agar, 332
fungal culture, 332
Safranin stain, 91
Saliva
in dental and oral infections, 575, 576
in diagnosis of lower respiratory tract infections, 590
herpes simplex, type 1, 415
immunoglobulins, antimicrobial effects, 62
normal microbial flora, 53
transmission of infection, 78, 79
Salk vaccine for poliomyelitis, 399
Salmonella, 248–253
biochemical reaction patterns, 100
classification and serotypes, 248–249
isolation media, 97
S. choleraesuis, extraintestinal infections, 252
S. enteritidis
common-source epidemic, 81
enterocolitis, 251
extraintestinal infections, 252
serologic classification, 104, 248–249
S. typhi
carrier state, 77, 252–253
enteric fever, 249–250, 251–252, 593
see also Enteric infections and food poisoning
Sanitization
definition, 33
methods, 38–40
Sarcomas, cell transformation by RNA tumor viruses, 457
Scabby mouth (orf), 393
Scalded skin syndrome (Ritter's disease), 153, 155, 156, 632
Scarlet fever
erythrogenic toxin of group A streptococci, 69, 168, 170
"Staphylococcal scarlet fever," 156
Schick test, 186
Schistosoma haematobium, 550, 554
Schistosoma japonicum, 550–554
Schistosoma mansoni, 550–554
Schizogony in sporozoa, 463, 469–470, 478
Schuffner's dots, 471
Scolex, 535
Scotch (cellophane) tape test for *Enterobius* eggs, 517
Scrapie, 453
Scrub typhus *(R. tsutsugamushi),* 316
Sebaceous gland infection, 555–556
Selective toxicity, 123
Semmelweis, nosocomial infections, 655–656
Sepsis, fetal and neonatal, 174, 243, 631–632
Escherichia coli, 243
Listeria monocytogenes, 186
Streptococcus, group B, 174
Serology
bacterial identification, 101–104
basic principles, 116–117
methods of serodiagnosis, 118–120
parasitic infections, 467
viral identification, 112–113
Serotonin, in inflammatory response, 63
Serratia, 248
Sexually transmitted diseases, 637–648
acquired immunodeficiency syndrome, 646
chancroid, *Haemophilus ducreyi,* 644–645
Chlamydia trachomatis, 323–325
genital herpes simplex, 416–417, 643–644
gonorrhea, 211–213, 637–639
granuloma inguinale, 645
lymphogranuloma venereum, 645
nongonococcal urethritis, 646–647

pelvic inflammatory disease, 638, 648
skin diseases, 646
syphilis, 282–283, 639–643
trichomoniasis, 465, 493–494
Shigella, 244–247
classification, 244
Shigellosis, 245–249, 593, 595
Shingles, 420
Shock, Gram-negative, 68–69, 625–628
Shope papilloma, 456
Sialic acid, capsules, group B streptococci, 174
Sickle cell trait, protection against malaria, 472
Siderophores, iron complexes, 18
Sinus infections, 220, 572–573
Skin
coccidioidin test, 356
decontamination, blood culture sampling, 626
defenses against microbial invasion, 60
histoplasmin skin test, 350, 352
intestinal nematode penetration, 522, 523
normal microbial flora, 51
transmission of infections, 79–80
tuberculin test, 293, 297
Skin lesions and infections, 555–558
acne vulgaris, 556
bacteremia, 624
Blastomyces dermatitidis, 353
Candida albicans, 341, 556
bullous impetigo, *Staphylococcus aureus,* 155, 158, 557
cryptococcal, 349
dermatophyte fungi, 556
erysipelas, 557
folliculitis, staphylococcal and *Pseudomonas,* 555
furuncles, 155, 556
hair follicles, sebaceous glands, sweat glands, 555–556
herpes simplex, type 1, 415
infective endocarditis, 618
Leishmania, 449–502
lesions from bacterial toxins, 555
minor lesions, 556–557
nocardiosis, 308
scalded skin syndrome, 153, 155, 156, 632
Sporothrix schenckii, 359
Staphylococcus aureus, 155–156, 556–557
streptococcal pyoderma (impetigo), 556
superficial fungal, 334–337
ulcers and granulomatous lesions, 557–558
Sleeping sickness, trypanosomiasis, 461, 503–505
Slime layer
capsular, 9
Enterobacteriaceae, 238, 239
Pseudomonas aeruginosa, 264
Slow virus diseases, 451–455
Smallpox, 390–392
Snail. *See* Trematode infections
Spargana and sparganosis, 541
Species differences, host susceptibility for infection, 59
Specimen collection, 88–90, 105–106
Actinomyces, 307
anaerobic culture, 203–204
blood and tissue parasites, 467
intestinal parasites, 467
Mycobacterium tuberculosis, 300
urinary tract infections, 605–606
Spectinomycin, 139
treatment of penicillinase producing gonococci, 214
for *Ureaplasma urealyticus,* 232
Spectrum of antibiotics, 148
see also individual antimicrobics
Spheroplast, 11
Spherule of *Coccidioides immitis,* 354, 355
Spirilla, 9
Spirochetes, 280–289
axial filaments, 280
Borrelia recurrentis, 287–289
flagella, 15
fusospirochetal diseases, 289
Leptospira interrogans, 285–287
Lyme disease, 289
microscopy, 280
normal oral flora, 289
relapsing fever, 287, 289
shape, 9
staining methods, 280
Treponema pallidum, 280–284
Treponematoses, other, 284, 285
Spores
Bacillus, 188–191
Clostridium, 193–201
fungal, 329
killing by autoclave, 35–36
resistance, structure, and development, 15–16
Sporogony, sexual reproduction in *Sporozoa,* 463, 469–470
Sporothrix schenkii and sporotrichosis, 358–360
Sporozoan infections, 469–483
plasmodia, 469–478
differential characteristics, 471
see also Malaria
Toxoplasma gondii, 478–483
description of organism, 479
see also Toxoplasmosis
Spotted fevers (rickettsial), 311–314
Sputum
collection, 589–590
eggs, trematode infections, 548
eosinophilia, ascariasis, 519
in lower respiratory tract infections, 587–589
in middle respiratory tract infections, 586
St. Louis encephalitis, 435, 441
Stains
acid-fast, procedure, 93
modified stain for *Nocardia,* 309
Dieterle, *Legionella,* 233
fluorochrome, 93
Giemsa and Wrights
Borrelia recurrentis, 287
herpes simplex virus inclusions, 644
for malarial parasites, 476
microfilariae, 532
Pneumocystis carinii, 509
rickettsiae, 310
Gram, 11, 92–93
half-Gram for *Legionella,* 233
Gram and acid-fast, bacterial classification, 91–93
Gram–Weigert, *Pneumocystis carinii,* 509
hematoxylin-eosin, *Pneumocystis carinii,* 509
methenamine silver, *Pneumocystis carinii,* 509
Ponder–Kinyoun, 93
safranin, 91
toluidine blue O, *Pneumocystis carinii,* 509
Ziehl–Neelsen. *See* Acid-fast stain
Staphylococcus aureus and staphylococcal infections, 151–160
bacteriophage typing, 152
cell wall structure, 151
coagglutination, 102, 151
coagulase, 152, 153
endocarditis, 155, 618, 619
eye infections, conjunctivitis, 156, 568, 569
food poisoning, 77, 153, 157, 598
furuncles, 155, 556
infections, other, 155–156
leukocidins, 67
nosocomial infections, 659
osteomyelitis, 155, 562–564
pneumonia, 156, 589
slide clumping test, 152
surface protein A, 68, 151
teichoic acid of cell wall, 151
toxic shock syndrome, 153, 156–157
toxin-caused diseases, 156–157
wound infections, 156, 559
Staphylococcus enterocolitis, secondary to antibiotic therapy, 57, 156
Staphylococcus epidermidis, 52, 150, 160
Staphylococcus saprophyticus, 150–151, 160–161
Stationary phase of bacterial growth, 19
Sterilization
autoclave, 35–36
filtration, 37
gas, 36–37
heat, 35–36
ultraviolet light and ionizing radiation, 37
Sterols
fungal cell membrane, 326
Mycoplasma cell membrane, 228
Stevens–Johnson syndrome, 229
Stomatitis, 581, 582, 583
Stool culture, gastrointestinal infections, 599
Streptococci, 162–180
classification, 163–165
hemolytic, α and β, 163
infective endocarditis, 618, 619
group A. *See S. pyogenes*
group B, *S. agalactiae,* 173–174

Streptococci *(cont.)*
group D and enterococci, 174–175
S. mutans
capsule synthesis, 10
and caries, 577
normal microbial flora, 53
S. pneumoniae
capsule, 67, 176
capsule swelling reaction, 10
differentiation from viridans streptococci, 180
diseases, 177–179
ear infections, 571
eye infections, 568
meningitis, 178, 609–612
normal flora and pathogenesis, 582
pneumococcal pneumonia, 177–179
transient normal flora, 50
S. pyogenes (group A)
delayed noninfectious diseases
acute glomerulonephritis, 171–172
rheumatic fever, 170–171
diseases due to infection, 168–170
streptolysin O and S, 166–167
structure, 166
toxin-caused diseases, scarlet fever, 170
S. sanguis, dental infections, 575
viridans streptococci, 164, 180
Streptokinase, 167
Streptolysins, S and O, 165–167
Streptomyces, source of antibiotics, 124
Streptomycin, 131–133
in plague, 277
in tuberculosis, 294
in tularemia, 279
Strobila, 535
Strongyloides stercoralis, 516, 523–525
Subacute sclerosing panencephalitis and measles, 381, 451–452
Sudden infant death syndrome, and infant botulism, 201
Sulfonamides, 136–138
for *Haemophilus influenzae,* 221
mode of action, 137
Nocardia, 309
synergism with trimethoprim, 137, 138
trachoma, 322
urinary tract infections, 606
Sulfones, 139
leprosy therapy, 302–303
Sulfur granules in actinomycosis, 305–307
Superinfection, bacterial. *See* Bacterial superinfection
Suppressor T-cells, 73
Suramin treatment
African trypanosomiasis (sleeping sickness), 505
onchocerciasis, 534
Surfactant disinfection, 39
Surgical wound infections, 558, 559
SV 40 virus, 457
Swarming, of *Proteus,* 254
Sweat gland infection, 555–556
Sweating sickness, 82
Swimming pools
Myobacterium marinum infections, 303
Pseudomonas infections, 267
sanitation, 39
Symbiosis, overview, 2
Synergy, antimicrobic combinations, 125, 133, 142, 160
Synovial fluid, in septic arthritis, 565
Syphilis, 282–284, 639–643
aortic aneurysm, 641
central nervous system involvement, 283, 641
chancre, 282, 640
clinical stages, 282–283, 640–641
fetal and newborn infections, 283, 632–633, 642
gumma, 283, 641
Jarisch–Herxheimer reaction, 642
meningovascular, 641
transplacental infection, 78, 631, 642
see also Treponema pallidum
Systemic mycoses, 347–357

T

T-cell function, 73
brucellosis, 273
dengue, 438
enterovirus infections, 397
Epstein–Barr virus, 425
Immuno-compromised host, 652–653
Influenza, 366–367
Malaria, 475
T phage morphology, 31, 32
Tabes dorsalis, syphilis, 641
Taenia saginata, 537–539
Taenia solium, 539–541
Tapeworm (cestode) infections, 535–544
Tapir nose, *Leishmania* infections, 501
Taxonomy
Adansonian or numeric, 20
DNA base ratios and homology criteria, 20–21
fungi, 330
weighted, 20
Teeth
normal microbial flora, 53
tetracycline affinity, 134
Teichoic acid, Gram-positive cell wall, 12, 151, 166
Tellurite medium, *Corynebacterium diphtheriae,* 182, 185
Temperate bacteriophage, 31–32
Temperature
pasteurization, 33, 37
requirement for microbial infectivity, 66
virulence alterations, 71
Tetanospasmin, 198, 199
Tetanus, 198–200
immune globulin, 85, 199
predisposing conditions, 198
prevention and treatment, 84, 86, 87, 199
Tetracyclines, 134–135
amebiasis, 488
effect on teeth, 134
Haemophilus influenzae, 221
nongonococcal urethritis, 647
Rocky Mountain spotted fever, 314
spectrum, 148
trachoma, 322
Ureaplasma urealyticus, 232
Thalassemia, protection against malaria, 472
Thayer–Martin medium, *Neisseria gonorrhoeae,* 213
Therapeutic index, 123
Thiabedazole treatment, intestinal nematode infections, 525
Threadworm. *See Enterobius vermicularis*
Thrombocytopenia
malaria, 474
measles infection, 381
Thrombophlebitis
microaerophilic streptococci, 203
suppurative, 621–622
Thrush, 341
Thymic dysplasia syndrome, 652
Thymine dimers, 33
Tissue culture. *See* Cell culture
Tissue flagellates, 497–503
Titer, measure of antibody concentration, 117
Tobramycin, 131, 132, 133
Togaviridae. *See* Viruses, zoonotic
Tolerance to antimicrobics, definition, 128
Tonsillitis, upper respiratory infections, 580–583
TORCH complex, fetal and newborn infections, 633–635
Torula histolytica. See Cryptococcus neoformans
Torulopsis glabrata (Candida glabrata), 343
Toxic shock syndrome, 153, 156–157
Toxins. *See* Exotoxins and Endotoxin
Toxocara canis and toxocariasis, 526–528
Toxoids, antigenicity
diphtheria toxoid, 183, 185–186
immunization procedures, 84–86
tetanus toxoid, 199
Toxoplasmosis, *T. gondii,* 478–483
chorioretinitis, 481
fetal and newborn infections, 480–483, 633–635
in immunocompromised host, 481–483
prevalence and distribution, 462, 479
Sabin–Feldman dye test, 482
similarity to infectious mononucleosis, 481
transmission of infection, 479–480
transplacental infection, 78, 480
Trachea, middle respiratory tract infections, 584, 586
Trachoma, 322
Transaminase, in hepatitis A, 404
Transduction of DNA, 45
Transferrin, iron binding, 63
Transformation
of bacteria (DNA-mediated), 43–45
of eukaryotic cells, 30, 456
Transmission of infection, 78–80
See individual organisms and diseases
Transpeptidation reaction in cell wall synthesis, 128
Transposons, 42, 46
Transtracheal aspiration, 590
Trematode infections, 545–554

Clonorchis sinensis (liver fluke), 548–549
Paragonimus westermani (lung fluke), 546–548
Schistosoma species (blood fluke), 550–554
Trench mouth, 579
Treponema pallidum, 280–284
antigenic structure, 282
cardiolipin antigen, 282, 283
in endemic syphilis (Bejel), 284, 285
fluorescent treponemal antibody test, 284
microhemagglutination test for antibody, 284
see also Syphilis
Trichinella spiralis, 528–530
Trichomonas vaginalis, 463, 491–492, 494–495, 648
Trichomoniasis, 463, 493–495
Trichophyton, 330, 334, 335
Trichuris trichiura (whipworm), 515, 518–519
Trifluorothymadine treatment, herpes simplex, type 1, 144, 416
Trimethoprim, 138
for enteric fever, 253
Pneumocystis carinii infections, 512
Shigella infections, 247
spectrum (with sulfonamide), 148
synergy with sulfonamides, 138
Trophozoites
Entamoeba histolytica, 484–486
Giardia lamblia, 494–497
Plasmodium species, 471
Pneumocystis carinii, 509
Toxoplasma gondii, 479
Tropical sprue, role of normal flora, 56
Trypanosoma brucei, 503–505
Trypanosoma cruzi, 461, 505–507
Trypanosomiasis, 503–507
Tsetse fly, *Trypanosoma brucei* development cycle, 503–505
Tsutsugamushi fever, 312, 316
Tuberculin skin test (purified protein derivative), 293, 297
Tubercule bacillus. *See Mycobacterium tuberculosis*
Tuberculosis, 294–300
BCG vaccine, 299
caseation, 296
delayed-type hypersensitivity, 71, 295–297
Ghon complex, 296
history and prevalence, 294
miliary, 296
primary infection, 295–296
reactivation, 296
transmission routes, 295
see also Tuberculin skin test
Tularemia. *See Francisella tularensis*
Tumors, viral, 455–459
Tyndallization, 37–38
Typhoid fever, 251–252, 593
treatment, 136, 138
endotoxin role, 69
mortality, 593
pathogenesis, 593
trimethoprim treatment, 138
see also Salmonella
Typhus fever. *See Rickettsia*

U

Ultraviolet light
bacterial mutagen, 43
sterilization, 33, 37
Undulant fever. *See Brucellosis*
Ureaplasma urealyticum, 231–232
Urease
Cryptococcus neoformans, 347
Proteus, 255
Urethritis
gonorrhea, 212, 637
nongonococcal infections, 323, 646–647
trichomoniasis, 494
Ureaplasma urealyticum, 232
see also Urinary tract infections
Urinary tract infections, 241–242, 601–607
bacteremia, 624
cystitis, 604, 641
diagnosis
microscopy, 605
specimen collection, 605
cultures, 606
epithelial defense against microbial invasion, 61
Escherichia coli, 241–242, 603–608
incidence and prevalence, 601
localization studies, 606
nosocomial (hospital) infections, 659
prostatitis, 605
Pseudomonas aeruginosa, 266, 267
pyelonephritis, 604–605
role of normal flora, 55
Staphylococcus saprophyticus, 160
transmission of, 79, 80
urethritis, 604
Urine
eggs in *Schistosoma* infection, 553
growth of bacteria, 61
Uveitis, 568

V

Vaccines, 83–86
adenoviruses, 375
BCG, for tuberculosis, 299
diphtheria, pertussis, tetanus, 226
equine encephalitis, 440
Haemophilus influenzae, 218–221
hepatitis B, 411
influenza virus, 368
Leptospira interrogans, 287
live and inactivated, 83, 84–85
measles, 383
meningococcal, 209–210
mumps virus, 380
poliovirus, 398–401
Pseudomonas aeruginosa, 267–268
rabies, 448–449
rubella, 387
Salmonella typhi, 253
Schistosoma bovis, 554
Shigella, 247
smallpox, 390–393
Streptococcus pneumoniae, 179
varicella–zoster virus, 422
Vibrio cholerae, 261
yellow fever, 440
Yersinia pestis, 277
Vaccinia virus, 392–393
Vagina and vaginitis
Candida albicans infections, 341, 648
epithelial defenses against microbial invasion, 60
Gardnerella vaginalis, 226–227, 648
normal microbial flora, 55, 57
sexually transmitted diseases, 648
Trichomonas vaginalis, 493–494, 648
Valley fever, *Coccidioides immitis,* 356
Vancomycin, 139
Clostridium difficile, 201
Staphylococcus aureus, 160
Varicella–zoster virus, 420–422
Variola (smallpox), 390–392
VDRL tests, syphilis, 641–642
Veillonella, 203
Venereal disease. *See* Sexually transmitted diseases
Venezuelan equine encephalitis, 435
Vesicular stomatitis virus, 444
Vi antigen of *Salmonella typhi,* 250
Vibrio cholerae, 258–261
carriage, 260
eltor biotype, 258, 260
rice-water stools, 260, 261
thiosulfate-citrate-bile salt-sucrose agar, 261
toxin, 259
Vibrio parahemolyticus, 262
Vincent's infection (trench mouth), fusospirochetal disease, 56, 202, 279, 289, 581
Viridans streptococci, and bacterial endocarditis, 55, 180, 618, 619
Virion, 23
Viroid, 23
Virulence, 59, 77
determinants, 5, 68–71
iron requirements, 18
see also Bacteria, variation and genetics, and individual organisms
Viruses, general consideration, 23–32
adenoviruses, 372–375
antiviral agents, 143–145
arboviruses, 434–442
arenaviruses, 442–443
bacteriophage, 30–32
capsid protein, 23–24
cell transformation, 30, 456, 457
classification, 26–27
coronaviruses, 376
defective, 29–30
of diarrhea, 427–433
adenoviruses, 433
astroviruses, 433
caliciviruses, 433
coronaviruslike agents, 433
parvo/picornaviruses, 431–432
rotaviruses, 428–431
Ebola virus, 443–444

Viruses, general consideration *(cont.)*
enteroviruses, 394–402
Coxsackie viruses, 401–402
echoviruses, 401–402
polioviruses, 398–401
erythema infectiosum, 388
hepatitis viruses, 403–412
hepatitis A, 403–406
hepatitis B, 406–411
hepatitis, non-A non-B, 411
herpesviruses, 413–426
cytomegalovirus, 422–424
Epstein–Barr virus, 424–426
herpes simplex viruses, types 1 and 2, 414–417
varicella–zoster, 420–422
host specificity, 23
infections in immunocompromised patients, 654
influenza viruses, 361–369
J.C. virus, 453, 457
latency, 30
see also Latent infections
Marburg virus, 443–444, 446
measles virus, 380–383
mumps virus, 378–380
papilloma viruses, 456–457
papovaviruses, 453
parainfluenza viruses, 369–370
poxviruses, 390–393
molluscum contagiosum, 393
orf, 393
vaccinia, 392–393
variola, 390–392
primate polyoma SV40, 457
rabies virus, 446–450
reoviruses, 376
replication, 28–30
respiratory syncytial virus, 370–372
rhinoviruses, 375–376
roseola infantum (exanthem subitum), 387–388
rubella virus, 383–387
slow viruses, 451–455
conventional agents
progressive multifocal leukoencephalopathy, 452–453
subacute sclerosing panencephalitis, 451–452
unconventional agents
biologic and physical properties, 454
Creutzfeldt–Jakob disease, 455
kuru, 454–455
structure, 23–26
symmetry, helical or icosahedral, 24
transformation and endogenous genes, 30
tumor viruses
DNA tumor viruses, 456–457
RNA tumor viruses (retroviruses), 457–459
vesicular stomatitis virus, 444
Vitamin B_{12}
deficiency, fish tapeworm infection, 542
malabsorption, giardiasis, 496
Vitamins, bacterial production, 58
Vocal cord inflammation, 584
Voges–Proskauer test, 100
Vulvovaginitis, gonococcal, 212
see also Vagina and vaginitis
VW antigens of *Yersinia*, 255

W

Warthin–Finkeldey cells (measles), 382
Warts, viral, 456–457
Water, hypersecretion in cholera, 259, 260
Waterhouse–Friderichsen syndrome, 208
Wax, skin, defense against microbial invasion, 60
Weil Felix serologic test, 311, 312
Weil's disease, leptospirosis, 286
West Nile fever, 435
Western equine encephalitis, 434–440
Whipworm. *See Trichuris trichiura*
Whitlow, herpetic, 416, 557
Whooping cough. *See Bordetella pertussis*
Widal test, 253
Winter vomiting disease, 432
Woolsorter's disease, 191
World Health Organization
BCG immunization for tuberculosis, 299
smallpox eradication, 390-391
Wound infections, 558–561
anaerobic, 193–204, 560
bacteremia, 624
etiologic agents, other, 559–560
group A streptococcal, 169, 172
immunocompromised patients, 559
nutritional and immunologic status, 559
prevention and treatment, 160, 560–561
Pseudomonas aeruginosa, 267, 560
sources and classification, 558–559
Staphylococcus aureus, 156, 160
vascular integrity, 559
Wuchereria bancrofti, lymphatic filariasis, 527, 530–533

X

Xenodiagnosis, 507
Xerostomia, 576

Y

Yaws, 284
Yeasts and yeast infections
Candida albicans, 339–343
Candida, other species, 343
Cryptococcus neoformans, 347–349
treatment, 143, 343, 349
Yellow fever, 434, 441
Yersina enterocolitica, 256
cultural conditions, 96
enterocolitis, 256
Yersinia pestis, 255
plague, 272, 274–277
transmission by fleas, 272, 274–277
urban and sylvatic, 275
Yersinia pseudotuberculosis, 255–256
mesenteric lymphadenitis, 255
Yogurt, lactobacilli, 56, 187

Z

Ziehl–Neelsen stain, 93
see also Stains, acid-fast
Zoonotic diseases, 80
bacterial, 250–251, 255–256, 271–279, 285–289
rickettsial, 310–314, 315–317
viral, 434–445, 446–450
Zoster, varicella–zoster, 420–421